Department of Family Medicine

Williams
OBSTETRICS
Fourteenth Edition

LOUIS M. HELLMAN

Deputy Assistant Secretary for Population Affairs, Department of Health, Education, and Welfare, Washington, D.C.; Emeritus Professor, Department of Obstetrics and Gynecology, State University of New York, Downstate Medical Center, Brooklyn, New York

JACK A. PRITCHARD

Gillette Professor, Department of Obstetrics and Gynecology, University of Texas (Southwestern) Medical School at Dallas; Director of Obstetrics, Parkland Memorial Hospital, Dallas, Texas

with the collaboration of
RALPH M. WYNN

Professor and Head, Department of Obstetrics and Gynecology, Abraham Lincoln School of Medicine, University of Illinois at the Medical Center, Chicago, Illinois

APPLETON-CENTURY-CROFTS
EDUCATIONAL DIVISION/MEREDITH CORPORATION
New York

To the men of high purpose
who have sometimes jeopardized their careers
in defense of the right of all children to be well born,
this text is respectfully dedicated.

This volume represents the Fourteenth Edition of *Williams Obstetrics*, the first six of which were written by the late J. Whitridge Williams, Professor of Obstetrics in Johns Hopkins University, and Obstetrician-in-Chief to the Johns Hopkins Hospital from 1896 to 1931; the seventh, eighth, and ninth editions were prepared by the late Henricus J. Stander, Professor of Obstetrics and Gynecology in Cornell University and Obstetrician and Gynecologist-in-Chief to the New York Hospital from 1931 to 1948; the tenth and eleventh were prepared by Nicholson J. Eastman; the twelfth and thirteenth by Nicholson J. Eastman and Louis M. Hellman.

PREFACE

The five years since publication of the thirteenth edition of this textbook have witnessed a growing concern for the social aspects of maternity care. During this period continued interest in the physiology and pathology of reproduction has generated a vast body of knowledge of basic biologic importance and direct applicability. The base of obstetrics has thus broadened to include fetal medicine and human ecology as integral to the specialty in the 1970s.

We have endeavored to strike a balance in introducing new concepts and restating established principles, with the aim of maintaining clinical excellence. Chapters dealing primarily with management of obstetric problems incorporate new scientific information, while reflecting the effects of the social and economic status of women on their reproductive efficiency. To emphasize the importance of the patient's emotions on her reproductive behavior, we have replaced the single chapter on psychiatric aspects of pregnancy and childbirth with relevant comments in appropriate sections throughout the book.

The material on therapeutic abortion, sterilization, and contraception has been entirely rewritten in order to present significant technical information within the context of current social trends that influence practice in these areas. Here, where science and philosophy meet, a particular effort to minimize bias was exerted. The chapters dealing with coincidental diseases of pregnancy and with the fetus and newborn have incorporated current concepts in the clinical and basic scientific areas related to modern obstetrics.

Revision of the chapters on reproductive anatomy, physiology, and endocrinology summarizes the significant biochemical and ultrastructural findings of the last five years. An entirely rewritten chapter on the hypertensive disorders in pregnancy incorporates significant laboratory data as well as important new clinical findings that stress the influence of social and familial factors. The relation of preeclampsia to the ultimate development of persistent hypertension has received detailed attention.

Despite these extensive revisions and additions, we have by continued judicious deletion and economy of phrase not added substantially to the number of pages in the last edition.

In keeping with the concept of J. Whitridge Williams, the author of the first six editions of this textbook, we have eschewed undue emphasis of our special areas of interest and points of view. We have instead attempted to present the current consensus in obstetric diagnosis and therapy. Where opinion remains divided, we have presented the rationale of each suggested form of management. Where our combined experience has been extensive and consistent, we have outlined our currently employed plans of treatment, with no implication that alternate methods are inapplicable.

Maintaining another tradition of this textbook, we have selected all references with great care in the belief that accurate documentation of scientific data is a prerequisite to scholarship. Each reference list has therefore been checked by a professional bibliographer.

The modern format for this text was established by Doctor Nicholson J. Eastman, Professor of Obstetrics at Johns Hopkins, with the publication of the tenth edition. Although each subsequent edition has been extensively revised the standards of scholarship and readability set by Dr. Eastman during the 20 years of his authorship have been scrupulously respected.

With the exception of Chapter 26, all the material has been written by the authors, each of whom edited and approved the entire text. We express deep appreciation to Dr. Leon C. Chesley, Professor of Obstetrics and Gynecology, State University of New York, Downstate Medical Center, for his scholarly monographic revision of the chapter on hypertensive disorders in pregnancy.

We are particularly grateful to Dr. Arthur Lesser, Director, Maternal and Child Health, HSMHA, Department of Health, Education, and Welfare for compilation of the data for the charts and tables in Chapter 1, and to Dr. Paul C. MacDonald, Professor of Obstetrics and Gynecology at the University of Texas (Southwestern) Medical School at Dallas, for valuable help with the sections on endocrinology. We are also grateful to Dr. Rita Harper, Assistant Professor of Pediatrics, State University of New York, Downstate Medical Center, for her help with the chapters on the Newborn and Diseases of the Newborn. In addition, we owe gratitude to Doctors Hall, Jones, Kobayashi, Kohl, Nelson, Solish, Tricomi, and Valenti of Dr. Hellman's staff, Dr. Peggy Whalley of Dr. Pritchard's staff, and Doctors Kernis and Savage of Dr. Wynn's staff for their help and advice in their special areas of competence.

Special mention must be made of our debt to Doctors Hall and MacDonald who assumed our administrative chores during the writing of this text.

We are indebted to our secretaries for typing the manuscript and to Mrs. Edith Gelfand who supervised the preparation of figures. We owe a special debt of gratitude to Mrs. Florence Gubitz for supervision and direction of flow of the manuscript. Miss Madeleine Steele has checked each reference for accuracy. For this arduous task we are grateful.

Finally, it is our pleasure to thank Appleton-Century-Crofts for the meticulous attention they have devoted to the preparation of this volume.

Louis M. Hellman

Jack A. Pritchard

CONTENTS

Preface

Section One: ORIENTATION

1. OBSTETRICS IN BROAD PERSPECTIVE   1

Section Two: ANATOMY AND PHYSIOLOGY OF REPRODUCTION

2. THE ANATOMY OF THE FEMALE REPRODUCTIVE ORGANS   19
3. THE OVARIAN CYCLE AND ITS HORMONES   58
4. THE ENDOMETRIAL CYCLE AND MENSTRUATION   90
5. GAMETOGENESIS AND EARLY DEVELOPMENT OF THE OVUM   108
6. THE PLACENTA AND ITS HORMONES   143
7. THE MORPHOLOGIC AND FUNCTIONAL DEVELOPMENT OF THE FETUS   199
8. MATERNAL PHYSIOLOGY IN PREGNANCY   236

Section Three: MANAGEMENT OF NORMAL PREGNANCY

9. DIAGNOSIS OF PREGNANCY   277
10. THE NORMAL PELVIS   290
11. PRESENTATION, POSITION, ATTITUDE, AND LIE OF THE FETUS   320
12. PRENATAL CARE   332

Section Four: PHYSIOLOGY AND CONDUCT OF LABOR

13. THE FORCES CONCERNED IN LABOR   349
14. THE MECHANISM OF LABOR IN VERTEX PRESENTATIONS   374
15. THE CLINICAL COURSE OF LABOR   387
16. THE CONDUCT OF NORMAL LABOR AND DELIVERY   400
17. ANALGESIA AND ANESTHESIA   430

Section Five: THE PUERPERIUM AND THE NEWBORN

18. THE PUERPERIUM   465
19. THE NEWBORN   477

Section Six: ABNORMALITIES OF PREGNANCY

20. ABORTION AND PREMATURE LABOR   493
21. ECTOPIC PREGNANCY   535
22. DISEASES AND ABNORMALITIES OF THE PLACENTA AND FETAL MEMBRANES   564
23. PLACENTA PREVIA AND ABRUPTIO PLACENTAE   609
24. COMPLICATIONS CAUSED BY DISEASES AND ABNORMALITIES OF THE
     GENERATIVE TRACT   639
25. MULTIPLE PREGNANCY   656
26. HYPERTENSIVE DISORDERS IN PREGNANCY—LEON C. CHESLEY   685
27. MEDICAL AND SURGICAL ILLNESSES DURING PREGNANCY
     AND THE PUERPERIUM   748

Section Seven: ABNORMALITIES OF LABOR

28. DYSTOCIA CAUSED BY ANOMALIES OF THE EXPULSIVE FORCES   835
29. DYSTOCIA CAUSED BY ABNORMALITIES IN POSITION, PRESENTATION, OR
     DEVELOPMENT OF THE FETUS   853
30. DYSTOCIA CAUSED BY PELVIC CONTRACTION   894
31. DYSTOCIA CAUSED BY ABNORMALITIES OF THE GENERATIVE TRACT   921
32. INJURIES TO THE BIRTH CANAL   932
33. ABNORMALITIES OF THE THIRD STAGE OF LABOR   956

Section Eight: ABNORMALITIES OF THE PUERPERIUM

34. PUERPERAL INFECTION   971
35. DISORDERS OF THE PUERPERIUM OTHER THAN PUERPERAL INFECTION   993

Section Nine: ABNORMALITIES OF THE NEWBORN

36. INJURIES SUSTAINED BY THE FETUS IN PREGNANCY AND LABOR   1007
37. DISEASES OF THE NEWBORN   1026
38. MALFORMATIONS OF THE FETUS   1063

Section Ten: OPERATIVE OBSTETRICS

39. THERAPEUTIC ABORTION, INDUCTION OF LABOR, STERILIZATION, AND
     CONTRACEPTION   1085
40. FORCEPS   1115
41. BREECH EXTRACTION AND VERSION   1145
42. CESAREAN SECTION   1163

Index   1191

Williams
OBSTETRICS
Fourteenth Edition

1

OBSTETRICS IN BROAD PERSPECTIVE

Definition. *Obstetrics* is the branch of medicine that deals with parturition, its antecedents, and its sequels. It is concerned principally, therefore, with the phenomena and management of pregnancy, labor, and the puerperium, in both normal and abnormal circumstances.

In a broader sense obstetrics is concerned with reproduction of a society. Maternity care aims to promote health and well-being, both physical and mental, among young people and to help them develop healthy attitudes toward sex, family life, and the place of the family in society. Obstetrics is concerned with all of the social factors that greatly influence both the quantity and the quality of human reproduction. The problems of population growth are obstetrics' natural heritage. The vital statistics of the nation, published monthly by the National Center for Health Statistics, attest society's concern with the charge of this specialty.

The word *obstetrics* is derived from the Latin term *obstetrix*, meaning *midwife*. The etymology of obstetrix, however, is obscure. Most dictionaries connect it with the verb *obstare*, which means *to stand by* or *in front of*. The rationale of this derivation is that the midwife stands by or in front of the parturient. This etymology has long been attacked by Seligmann, who believed that the word was originally *adstetrix* and that the *ad* had been changed to *ob*. In that case, obstetrix would mean *the woman assisting the parturient*. The fact that on certain inscriptions *obstetrix* is also spelled *opstetrix* has led to the conjecture that it was derived from *ops* (*aid*) and *stare*, meaning *the woman rendering aid*. According to Temkin, the most likely interpretation is that obstetrix meant *the woman who stood by the* parturient. Whether it alluded merely to the midwife's standing in front of or near the parturient or whether it carried the additional connotation of rendering aid is not clear.

The term *obstetrics* is of relatively recent usage. The Oxford English Dictionary gives the earliest example from a book published in 1819, indicating that in 1828 it was necessary to apologize for the use of the word *obstetrician*. Kindred terms, however, are much older. For example, *obstetricate* occurs in English works published as early as 1623; *obstetricatory*, in 1640; *obstetricious*, in 1645; and *obstetrical*, in 1775. These terms were often used figuratively. As an example of such usage the adjective *obstetric* appears in Pope's *Dunciad* (1742) in the famous couplet:

> There all the Learn'd shall at the labour stand,
> and Douglas lend his soft, obstetric hand.

The much older term *midwifery* was used instead of *obstetrics* until the latter part of the nineteenth century in both the United States and Great Britain. It is derived from the Middle English *mid*, meaning *with*, and *wif*, meaning wife in the sense of a *woman*. The term *midwife* was used as early as 1303, and *midwifery*, in 1483. In England today the term midwifery carries the same connotation as obstetrics, and the two words are used synonymously.

Aims of Obstetrics. The transcendent objective of obstetrics is that every pregnancy culminate in a healthy mother and a healthy baby. Obstetrics strives to minimize the number of women and infants who die as a result of the reproductive process or who are left injured therefrom. It aims further to minimize the discomforts and hazards of pregnancy, labor, and puerperium, so that both mother and child will conclude the experience in physical and mental health. Obstetrics is concerned further with the number and spacing of children so that both mother and offspring may enjoy optimal physical and emotional well-being. Finally, obstetrics strives to analyze and influence the social factors that impinge on reproductive efficiency.

Vital Statistics: Definitions. To aid in the reduction of the number of mothers and infants that die as the result of pregnancy and labor, it is important to know how many such deaths occur in this country each year and in what circumstances. To evaluate these data intelligently, it is essential to know the following standard definitions:

Birth rate. The number of births per 1,000 population.

Fertility rate. The number of live births per 1,000 female population aged 15–44 years.

Marriage rate. The number of marriages per 1,000 population.

Neonatal death. Death of a newborn infant within the first four weeks of life. This definition is used chiefly in the United States; the World Health Organization defines the neonatal period as the first seven days of life.

Neonatal death rate. The number of neonatal deaths per 1,000 live births.

Infant mortality rate. Infant deaths (under 1 year of age) per 1,000 live births.

Stillbirth. An infant with no heartbeat who neither breathes nor cries nor shows any other sign of movement.

Fetal death. Death in utero of a fetus weighing 500 g or more. This weight corresponds roughly with a fetus of 20 weeks or more gestational age, that is, with a "viable" fetus. (Note: this term is often used loosely and *incorrectly* to designate the sum of fetal and neonatal loss. The term is also used by the National Center for Health Statistics to include fetal deaths irrespective of the duration of pregnancy. These divergent practices lead to lack of statistical precision. Death is defined in the following context: after expulsion the fetus does not breathe or show any other evidence of life, such as the beating of the heart, pulsation of the umbilical cord, or definite movement of voluntary muscles.)

Fetal death rate. The number of fetal deaths per 1,000 births (live births and stillbirths).

Perinatal death rate. The sum of fetal and neonatal death rates (theoretically, the denominator for both these rates should be the total number of births).

Maternal death rate or mortality. The number of maternal deaths that occur as the direct result of the reproductive process per 100,000 live births. (Note: this rate is calculated per *one hundred* thousand live births and not per *one* thousand.)

The Birth Rate and Fertility Rate. One index of the need for obstetric personnel is the number of births each year. Additional indices are the crude birth rate and the general fertility rate. From these data, particularly the fertility rate, the expected number of births in future years can be estimated. In 1968 there were 3,470,000 live births registered in the United States, a decline of 6 per cent from the number in 1966. It was also the tenth year in which the number of births continued to decline since the peak of approximately 4,300,000 in 1957. This decline is about 20 per cent from the peak value (Fig. 1).

There were approximately 2,965,000 births in the United States when the birth registration area was established in 1915. The number rose steadily except for a slight decline during World War I. It declined again during the depression,

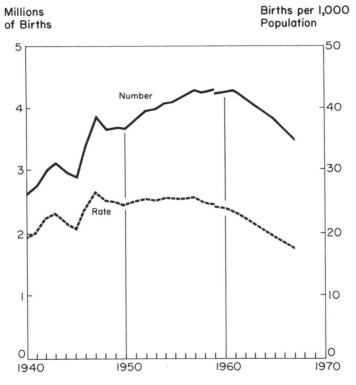

Fig. 1. Live births and birth rates, 1940-1968. (Monthly Vital Statistics Report, Provisional Statistics Annual Summary for the United States, 1968, National Center for Health Statistics, HSMHA, U.S. Department of Health, Education, and Welfare.)

reaching a low of 2,307,000 per year in 1933. Although there was another decline related to movements of military personnel overseas in the Second World War, it was followed by the "baby boom," which continued almost uninterrupted until 1957. Since then, the declining trend in births has been reflected in almost all measures of fertility. The crude birth rate declined from 25.3 per 1,000 population in 1957 to 17.4 in 1968. The general fertility rate, which is a much more sensitive indicator of births and trends because it takes into account the population at risk (women between the ages of 15 and 44), dropped about 30 per cent during this period. The declines have been somewhat faster for white women, but the difference in trends at most ages is not great. At higher birth orders, however, the rates for nonwhites have been falling faster than those for whites.

Projections of Live Births.   Nothing could be of greater concern to obstetricians and to obstetric practice than the future number of live births. The course of fertility in the United States depends on a number of factors, including future migration, mortality, marriage, and patterns of childbearing, as well as the composition by age and sex of the future population. Although the number of children born to any population at a projected date in the future cannot be calculated with precision, reasonable projections can be based upon explicit assumptions regarding the future effect of these factors. The precision of these predictions depends on how closely the projected economic and demographic factors apply to the population concerned.

The number of women of childbearing age through 1985 can be projected with reasonable certainty, as shown in Table 1.

Table 1. **Projection of Number of Women of Childbearing Age in the United States, 1965–1985**

Year	Women 15–44 Years (in thousands)
1965	38,939
1970	42,336
1975	46,881
1980	51,887
1985	56,000

From Department of Commerce, Bureau of Census Current Population Reports, Series P-25, Nos. 381 and 388, 1968.

The Bureau of the Census has recently taken these figures as a basis for projecting the number of births. In any case, it is evident that the number of women capable of childbearing will increase in the United States, and the number of anticipated births will be greater than today. This trend has already begun with an increase of about 2 per cent in the number of births in 1969 over 1968. This increase in the number of births, which is of tremendous economic importance for the country in general, bears specifically on the need for more maternity beds and for more medical manpower in this specialty.

Maternal Mortality.   The number of women who died in 1967 as the direct result of childbearing was 987 in the course of 3,512,000 live births, a mortality rate of 28 per 100,000 live births. Figure 2 shows the dramatic reduction in the maternal mortality rate during the past three decades, from a plateau above 600 in white women before 1930 to a level of less than one twentieth that rate in 1967, in which year the rate in white women was 19.5. The corresponding figures for the nonwhite were 1,170 in 1930 and 69.5 in 1967. Whereas the overall decline has been spectacular, there is a persistent differential between the white and nonwhite maternal mortality rates. This differential appears to be increasing as the rates fall. In 1930 the rate for nonwhites was about twice that for white women, and by 1967, about three and a half times.

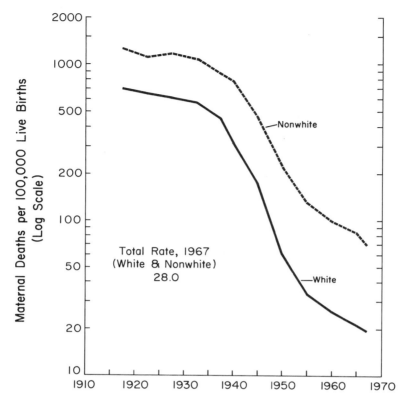

Fig. 2. Maternal mortality, 1915–1967, United States Birth Registration Area. (Vital Statistics of the United States, 1967, Vol. II—Mortality, Part A, Table 1-16, National Center for Health Statistics HSMHA, U.S. Department of Health, Education,and Welfare.)

These differences in maternal mortality rates result primarily from social and economic factors, such as lack of a medical attendant at delivery, lack of ante-partum care, dietary deficiencies, poor hygiene, lack of contraceptive services, and faulty health education. As these unfavorable social and economic conditions are improved, the racial difference in the maternal death rates will doubtless decrease.

The maternal mortality rate varies also with the age of the mother, as plainly shown in Figure 3. In all races the tremendous increase in mortality with advancing age can be explained only on the basis of an intrinsic maternal factor. The increasing frequency of hypertension with advancing years and the greater tendency to uterine hemorrhage contribute significantly to the elevation of mortality. Advanced age and high parity act independently to increase the risk of childbearing, but their effects are usually additive. In the actual analysis of cases, it is difficult to dissociate these two factors. Figure 3 must therefore be interpreted as showing, for the most part, the additive effects of age and parity. It shows in addition that the lowest maternal mortality rates occur in mothers between 20 and 30 years of age, the reproductive period when the outlook for the baby also is best.

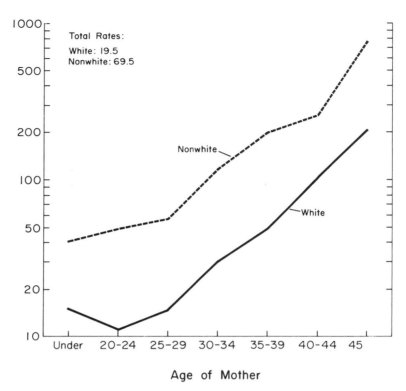

Fig. 3. Maternal mortality rate by age of mother, 1967. (Vital Statistics of the United States, 1967, Vol. II—Mortality, Part A, Table 1-16, National Center for Health Statistics, HSMHA, U.S. Department of Health, Education and Welfare.)

Geographic Distribution.   Maternal mortality shows a large geographic variability, reflecting the social and economic status of the population as well as the distribution of medical care and facilities. In general, the mortality rates are lower in metropolitan areas. Deaths from hemorrhage and toxemia predominate in rural areas. This generalization may no longer be valid when the central metropolitan areas become filled with a nonwhite population.

As a result of improvements in obstetric care, ready access to blood for transfusion, and antibiotics, the death rates from toxemia, hemorrhage, and sepsis have fallen to the point that this classic triad no longer accounts for the overwhelming majority of maternal deaths. Figure 4 presents the national picture rather than that of well-equipped and properly manned metropolitan centers, where hemorrhagic death is a rarity, and deaths from illegal abortion rather than from the classic triad are likely to predominate.

Abortion has assumed a prominent place among causes of maternal mortality. These cases may well be underreported, for although sepsis in general causes deaths among the white and nonwhite populations with equal frequency, abortion with sepsis accounts for twice as many deaths among nonwhite as it does among white women. It is possible that white women can buy safer abortions; if so, it remains to be explained why the importance of sepsis in general among the causes of death is equal for white and nonwhite women.

Fig. 4. The relative frequency of the most common causes of maternal death, based on 987 deaths in the United States in 1967, as tabulated by the National Center for Health Statistics. Hemorrhage includes deaths from ectopic pregnancy and abortion without sepsis or toxemia as well as deaths from other types of obstetric hemorrhage. As explained in the text, deaths associated with maternal heart disease and other coincidental conditions are not included. (Vital Statistics of the United States, 1967, Vol. II—Mortality, Part A, Table 1-15, National Center for Health Statistics, HSMHA, U.S. Department of Health, Education, and Welfare.)

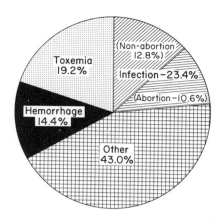

Common Causes of Maternal Mortality. Hemorrhage, toxemias of pregnancy, and infection still account for nearly 60 per cent of reported maternal deaths for the United States. The official reports differ from those of individual hospitals, which include deaths not strictly related to pregnancy, such as those from cardiac disease. The individual institutional reports, based on findings at autopsy rather than the death certificate alone, often provide a more accurate diagnosis. The causes of obstetric hemorrhage are multiple: uterine bleeding immediately after birth (postpartum hemorrhage); shock and bleeding in association with abortion; bleeding from rupture of the fallopian tube (extrauterine or ectopic pregnancy); bleeding as the result of abnormal placental location or separation (placenta previa and abruptio placentae); and bleeding from rupture of the uterus. The toxemias of pregnancy, occurring in about 6 or 7 per cent of gravid women, are characterized by various combinations of hypertension, edema, and proteinuria, and in some severe cases by convulsions and coma. Puerperal infection of the genital tract usually originates in endometritis, which sometimes undergoes extension to cause peritonitis, thrombophlebitis, bacteremia, and other distant foci of infection. Details of the origin, prevention, and treatment of these conditions form a large portion of the subject matter of obstetrics.

Hemorrhage is probably a relatively more important cause of maternal death than is apparent from Figure 4 and from the national vital statistics. In official classifications of causes of death, it is customary to list only the *direct* cause; predisposing factors are necessarily ignored. For example, if the final and direct cause of death is puerperal infection, it is so classified. A common sequence of events in fatalities from puerperal infection, however, is as follows: the patient suffers a serious hemorrhage and her resistance to infection is thereby weakened; operative attempts to correct the cause of the hemorrhage may traumatize tissues and introduce infection; death occurs days or weeks later from puerperal infection. Hemorrhage thus acts as a most important predisposing factor, but it does not appear as the cause of death in the official statistics. Only if a woman actually bleeds to death is the fatality classified as hemorrhagic.

As the number of maternal deaths declines, the data from the death certificates become less informative. For example, in Figure 4 deaths classified as "other" (no specified complication mentioned) account for over 40 per cent of the deaths.

Furthermore, the death of a gravid or puerperal woman with a complication such as heart disease or diabetes is not classified by the National Center for Health Statistics as a "maternal death," but appears under the direct medical cause of the death. Many coincidental diseases are therefore excluded from "maternal mortality" despite the overriding influence of the pregnancy on the fetal outcome.

For these reasons studies based on hospital experience often provide a more accurate estimate of the overall toll of pregnancy. Currently these studies mention heart disease, vascular accidents, anesthesia, and a host of other medical conditions as factors that assume an increasingly important role in total maternal mortality. These conditions will be discussed in detail in Chapter 27.

Reasons for Recent Decline in Maternal Mortality.   Many factors and agencies are responsible for the dramatic fall in the maternal death rate in this country over the past 20 years. Obviously there has been a general improvement in medical practice. The widespread use of blood transfusion and antibiotics and the maintenance of fluid, electrolyte, and acid-base balance in the serious complications of pregnancy and labor have materially changed obstetric practice. Equally important is the development of widespread obstetric training and educational programs, which have provided more and better qualified specialists and, at the same time, more competent general practitioners. The American Board of Obstetrics and Gynecology has been especially instrumental in this advance. Although lacking legal authority, it is the generally endorsed body that certifies specialists in this field. Approximately 8,000 specialists whom the board has certified have established high levels of obstetric care in their own practices and, by example and precept, have provided tutelage of high caliber for thousands of medical students, interns, and residents.

Obstetrics is unique in that no other branch of medicine is subject to such careful public scrutiny. Not only are births a matter of public record, but maternal and perinatal deaths are examined by municipal and state health authorities. In many areas, local medical or obstetric and gynecologic societies also examine such deaths, and mortality conferences are frequently conducted as part of the continuing medical education of the obstetrician.

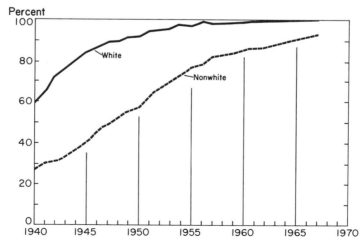

Fig. 5. Percentage of live births occurring in hospitals, by color, 1940–1967. (Vital Statistics of the United States, 1967, Vol. I—Natality, Table 1-23, National Center for Health Statistics, HSMHA, U.S. Department of Health, Education, and Welfare.)

Postgraduate courses in obstetrics designed especially for general practitioners have been held in such large numbers throughout the country that there is scarcely a practitioner who has not had the opportunity of receiving instruction in his own vicinity. The records, furthermore, show that tens of thousands of physicians have attended. In this connection, the American College of Obstetricians and Gynecologists is entitled to great credit for its annual and district meetings, which have afforded instruction and stimulation to its huge roster of over 9,000 obstetricians and gynecologists.

The *sine qua non* of good work in any field is well-trained personnel, but they could not have achieved the excellent results shown in Figure 2 had there not been a great expansion in facilities for good obstetric care. Almost every state has experienced widespread expansion of facilities for prenatal care. Under the guidance of state health departments with federal financial aid distributed through the Children's Bureau, many additional prenatal clinics have been established. Where such clinics are adequately staffed, there is excellent screening of pregnant women needing specialized care as well as supervision of routine problems. Despite increased facilities, there are many areas in the United States where prenatal services are woefully inadequate, particularly in the Deep South and in many of our large inner cities. Even where facilities are adequate, there is a nationwide decrease in the percentage of women receiving adequate prenatal care. Understanding of these factors led Congress to appropriate approximately $36,000,000 for the fiscal year 1969 for maternity care and further expansion of maternity and infant care centers and $12,000,000 for family planning projects. Bricks and mortar, however, even with adequate manpower, will not by themselves achieve the final solution. There are other deterrents to adequate prenatal care that are but poorly understood.

From the viewpoint of safer care during labor, the outstanding advance of the past 25 years has been the great increase in the proportion of hospital deliveries. As shown in Figure 5, as recently as 1940 only three out of five white births took place in hospitals; this figure is now close to 100 per cent. In recent years the nonwhite population has come to accept hospital services but not to the same degree as have white women (Fig. 5); 7 per cent of nonwhite women do not receive hospital care. In Mississippi, Alabama, and Arkansas nearly one quarter of the births take place outside the hospital. Hospital births not only mean better facilities but imply care by physicians.

The United States and Other Nations.   The United States ranks eleventh in maternal mortality compared with a group of other developed nations (Table 2).

Table 2. **Maternal Mortality, 1963–1965**

Sweden	20.0
Denmark	20.6
Norway	21.7
England and Wales	26.6
Belgium	30.3
Australia	31.0
New Zealand	31.3
Netherlands	31.5
Israel	31.8
Canada	32.6
U.S.A.	33.6 (22.4*)

* ( ) *Nonwhite population eliminated.*
From Statistical Bulletin, Metropolitan Life Insurance Co. Vol. 49, December 1968.

If only the white population is considered, this country ranks fourth. That a significant proportion of our mothers do not receive optimal obstetric care is obvious from the data relating to maternal mortality.

Perinatal Mortality.   The sum of stillbirths and neonatal deaths accounts for the perinatal mortality. With the current very low incidence of maternal deaths, perinatal loss rates not only are a better index of the level of obstetric care, but also give a valid indication of an equally important datum, the infant morbidity. To some extent, the total perinatal loss is correlated with the age and parity of the mother. The rate is highest for infants born to mothers under 20 and over 40 years of age, and lowest for infants born to women 20 to 29. Similarly, the rates tend to be highest for first births and births of the order of six and over.

The total number of stillbirths in the United States during 1967 was approximately 55,000, and the number of neonatal deaths was approximately 58,000. Of the total perinatal loss (approximately 113,000), the vast majority resulted directly from antepartum and intrapartum causes. Expressed differently, the number of infants lost in close association with the reproductive process accounts for

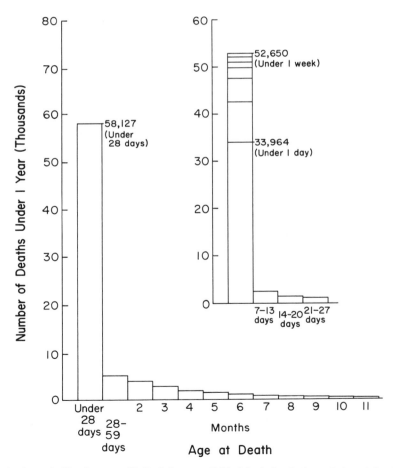

Fig. 6. Infant mortality, by age, United States, 1967. (Vital Statistics of the United States, 1967, Vol. II—Mortality, Part A, Table 2-8, National Center for Health Statistics, HSMHA, U.S. Department of Health, Education, and Welfare).

almost 6 per cent of all of the deaths in the United States at all ages and from all causes. The same results are observed year after year, indicating the magnitude of the infant loss associated with pregnancy, labor, and the early weeks of life.

Factors Affecting the Stillbirth Rate. Stillbirths tend to decline as the quality of care before and during birth improves. Many of these deaths stem from maternal disease, such as diabetes, hemorrhagic disorders of pregnancy, and toxemia, and accidents of labor, such as prolapse of the cord. Fetal death may also be the result of injudicious conduct of labor or traumatic delivery. With improvement in prenatal care and proper hospitalization, some of these accidents need not cause perinatal deaths. In a large proportion of deaths in utero, however, there is no obvious explanation.

Neonatal Deaths. Nearly half of the neonatal deaths occur in the first day of life (Fig. 6). The number of deaths during those 24 hours exceeds that from the second month to the completion of the first year. The causes of this huge wastage during the neonatal period are numerous, but by far the most important is premature birth (Fig. 7). For example, of the 58,127 neonatal deaths occurring in 1967, nearly one half involved premature infants (less than 2,500 g in weight) who, for the most part, were born a month or more before term. The proportion of premature births (based on weight) differs among ethnic groups, ranging from 70 to 75 per 1,000 in white mothers to approximately 150 per 1,000 births in nonwhites in 1967. The interracial difference in the rates of prematurity accounts for nearly three quarters of the difference in neonatal mortality between these two groups. Social and environmental factors probably weigh more heavily than race,

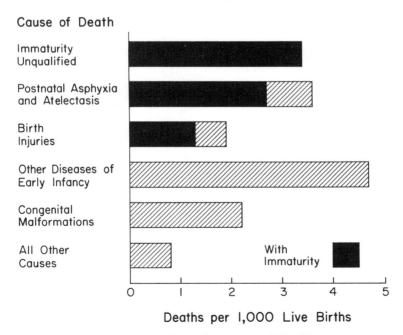

Fig. 7. Main causes of neonatal mortality, United States, 1967. (The terms prematurity and immaturity are used interchangeably. A better term is "low birth weight," recommended by WHO.) (Vital Statistics of the United States, 1967, Vol. II—Mortality, Part A, Table 2-12, National Center for Health Statistics, HSMHA, U.S. Department of Health, Education and Welfare.)

however, in the cause of this difference. Prematurity accounts for a high proportion of infant morbidity and for a large fraction of the neurologic deficits that are tragic individually and costly to society. Why many women go into labor prematurely and give birth to infants that are often unable to survive is one of the greatest unsolved problems of obstetrics.

The second most common cause of neonatal death is injury to the central nervous system. Here the word "injury" is used in its broad sense to indicate both cerebral injury resulting from hypoxia in utero and traumatic injury to the brain during labor and delivery. Many of these deaths could be prevented by more judicious management of labor. Another important but less frequent cause of neonatal death is congenital malformation.

Neonatal mortality rates have gradually fallen from 34.0 in 1933 to 24.0 in 1946 to approximately 16.5 in 1967. This decrease, though significant, is not comparable to the fall in maternal mortality (Fig. 8). From 1950 to 1965 there was a marked slowing in the rate of decline in neonatal mortality; even a reversal of the trend was noted for a short period of time. This static situation was reflected also in infant mortality. In only 3 of our 21 largest cities was there a significant annual reduction during the period 1960–1965. The infant mortality rate for the nation as a whole fell only 5 per cent during the decade 1956–1965. An increased social awareness and a willingness of our federal government to expend significant funds on maternity and infant care have accelerated the rate of decline in infant mortality. In the two years 1967–1968 the rate fell twice as fast as in the preceding decade. The 1969 provisional rate of 20.7 per 1,000 live births shows

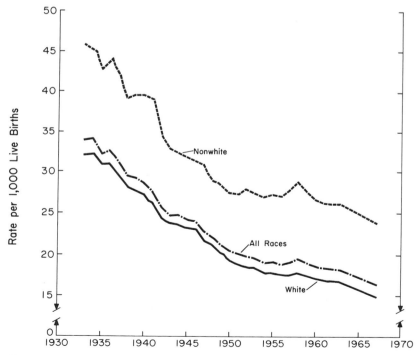

Fig. 8. Neonatal mortality rates by color, United States, 1933–1967. (Statistical Abstract of the United States, 1969, Table 70.)

a continuation of this decline in infant mortality. This rate represents a decrease of 4.6 per cent from the rate of 21.7 in 1968. The United States ranks seventh, however, among countries of the Western world in neonatal mortality rates (Table 3).

Table 3. **Neonatal Death Rates in the United States and Six West European Countries**

Country	Deaths under 28 Days per 1,000 Live Births
Sweden (1966)	10.2
Netherlands (1966)	11.2
Norway (1965)	12.0
England and Wales (1966 provisional)	12.8
Denmark (1965)	14.8
Scotland (1966)	15.2
United States (1966)	17.1 (approx. 15.5*)

* *White only.*
From United Nations Demographic Year Book, 1967, Table 16.

Removal of the data for nonwhites, moreover, does not improve our standing. Despite recent efforts, our improvement has not been so rapid as that of several other developed countries. Our relative standing in prenatal mortality has been carefully reviewed by Chase. She believes that although comparative data are not available, it is likely that the United States has a higher proportion of babies weighing less than 2,500 g than do countries with prenatal loss rates lower than ours.

Abortion. Far exceeding stillbirths and neonatal mortality as a cause of wastage in pregnancy is abortion. In medical parlance, abortion connotes both spontaneous and artificial termination of pregnancy before the period of viability. Since about 15 per cent of all pregnancies terminate spontaneously in abortion, the number of these accidents occurring annually in the United States may be estimated to be of the order of 600,000. Defective germ plasm is the causative factor in a large proportion of spontaneous abortions; others may be the result of unsatisfactory environmental conditions, including hormonal factors; many, perhaps most, are of unknown cause. To ascertain the total number of potential human lives lost each year in this country from abortion, it is necessary to add to the spontaneous accidents a huge but unknown number of criminal abortions. The total may be over one million.

The Birth Certificate. Statutes in all 50 states and the District of Columbia require that a birth certificate be completed for every birth and submitted promptly to the local registrar. After the birth has been duly registered, notification is sent to the parents of the child and a complete report is forwarded to the National Center for Health Statistics in Washington. Most states now require registration of all births, including stillbirths, in which the pregnancy has exceeded 20 weeks in duration.

There are many reasons why the complete and accurate registration of births is essential. Certification of the facts of birth is needed as evidence of age, citizenship, and family relationships. In connection with military service and passports they are indispensable; moreover, the data they provide are of immeasurable importance to all agencies (social, public health, demographic, or obstetric) dealing with human reproduction. For instance, the data presented in the foregoing paragraphs were culled almost entirely from information published by the National Center for Health on the basis of birth certificates; they represent, furthermore, only a small fraction of the information obtainable from that source. A birth certificate, such as that shown in Figure 9, provides even more data of direct obstetric importance. Hence, the prompt and accurate completion of this certificate after each birth is not only a legal duty but a contribution to the broad field of obstetric knowledge.

Obstetrics and Other Branches of Medicine.   Obstetrics is a multifaceted subject, with close 'and numerous relations to other branches of medicine. It is so intimately related to the kindred subject of gynecology that obstetrics and gynecology are generally regarded as one specialty. Gynecology deals with the physiology and the pathology of the female reproductive organs in the nonpregnant state, whereas obstetrics deals with the pregnant state and its sequels. Correct differential diagnosis in either obstetrics or gynecology entails an intimate acquaintance with the clinical syndromes met in both; in addition, the methods of examination and many operative technics are common to both disciplines. It is therefore obligatory that every obstetrician have extensive experience in gynecology, and vice versa.

The concern of obstetrics with the newborn infant brings the subject into close relation with pediatrics also. Although in many of our larger medical centers the newborn is turned over immediately to the pediatrician, such a practice is not always feasible. Even in metropolitan centers, inconvenient hours of birth often impose on the obstetrician the management of the newborn for the first few, most critical hours of life. He must be expert, therefore, in the management of the infant at this time. Current concern with fetal well-being has opened the new field of fetal medicine. By examination of the cells in the amniotic fluid it is now possible to diagnose about 28 fetal diseases and to treat at least one. In the near future the scope of intrauterine diagnosis and treatment will undoubtedly broaden. In this area the boundaries between obstetrics and pediatrics are blurred.

Since pregnant and nonpregnant women are subject to the same diseases, the obstetrician constantly encounters the more common diseases in his patients. The clinical picture presented by some of these disorders is altered greatly during pregnancy and the immediate puerperium; conversely, these diseases affect the course of gestation. For example, in rheumatic heart disease, diabetes, tuberculosis, and pyelonephritis, the prognosis and management may be altered by pregnancy. Psychiatric problems manifest themselves more frequently in the care of pregnant patients than even the obstetrician himself may recognize. For example, in most cases of so-called morning sickness there is an important emotional element.

Among the preclinical sciences, obstetrics is most intimately related perhaps to embryology. The study of spontaneous abortion, for example, depends on knowledge of anomalies in the development of the early embryo and trophoblast. Abortion may result also from hormonal defects, which link the subjects of obstetrics and endocrinology, and from chromosomal defects, which forge a link to cytogenetics. The concept of Rh isoimmunization has shown how immunologic factors may interfere with the successful outcome of pregnancy. Obstetrics and general pathology meet most closely in the rapidly developing field of perinatal pathology. Other important relations of obstetrics to preclinical sciences include the study of bacteriology in connection with puerperal infection, biochemistry in relation to the toxemias of pregnancy and placental transfer, physiology as it ap-

U.S. STANDARD

CERTIFICATE OF LIVE BIRTH

FORM APPROVED
BUDGET BUREAU NO. 68—R1900

TYPE, OR PRINT IN PERMANENT INK
SEE HANDBOOK FOR INSTRUCTIONS

CHILD

1. CHILD—NAME — FIRST / MIDDLE / LAST
2a. DATE OF BIRTH (MONTH, DAY, YEAR) — BIRTH NUMBER
2b. HOUR — M.
3. SEX
4a. THIS BIRTH—SINGLE, TWIN, TRIPLET, ETC. (SPECIFY)
4b. IF NOT SINGLE BIRTH—BORN FIRST, SECOND, THIRD, ETC. (SPECIFY)
5a. COUNTY OF BIRTH
5b. CITY, TOWN, OR LOCATION OF BIRTH
5c. INSIDE CITY LIMITS (SPECIFY YES OR NO)
5d. HOSPITAL—NAME (IF NOT IN HOSPITAL, GIVE STREET AND NUMBER)

MOTHER

6a. MOTHER—MAIDEN NAME — FIRST / MIDDLE / LAST
6b. AGE (AT TIME OF THIS BIRTH)
6c. STATE OF BIRTH (IF NOT IN U.S.A., NAME COUNTRY)
7a. RESIDENCE—STATE
7b. COUNTY
7c. CITY, TOWN, OR LOCATION
7d. INSIDE CITY LIMITS (SPECIFY YES OR NO)
7e. STREET AND NUMBER

FATHER

8a. FATHER—NAME — FIRST / MIDDLE / LAST
8b. AGE (AT TIME OF THIS BIRTH)
8c. STATE OF BIRTH (IF NOT IN U.S.A., NAME COUNTRY)

CERTIFIER

9a. INFORMANT — RELATION TO CHILD
9b. ATTENDANT—M.D., D.O., MIDWIFE, OTHER (SPECIFY)
10a. I CERTIFY THAT THE ABOVE NAMED CHILD WAS BORN ALIVE AT THE PLACE AND TIME AND ON THE DATE STATED ABOVE.
10b. DATE SIGNED (MONTH, DAY, YEAR)
10c. SIGNATURE
10d. CERTIFIER—NAME (TYPE OR PRINT)
10e. MAILING ADDRESS (STREET OR R.F.D. NO., CITY OR TOWN, STATE, ZIP)
11a. REGISTRAR—SIGNATURE
11b. DATE RECEIVED BY LOCAL REGISTRAR (MONTH, DAY, YEAR)

CONFIDENTIAL INFORMATION FOR MEDICAL AND HEALTH USE ONLY

FATHER

12. RACE—FATHER — WHITE, NEGRO, AMERICAN INDIAN, ETC. (SPECIFY)
13. EDUCATION—SPECIFY HIGHEST GRADE COMPLETED — ELEMENTARY (0, 1, 2, 3, 4, . . . OR 8) / HIGH SCHOOL (1, 2, 3, OR 4) / COLLEGE (1, 2, 3, 4, OR 5+)
14a. PREVIOUS DELIVERIES—HOW MANY OTHER CHILDREN — ARE NOW LIVING
14b. WERE BORN ALIVE BUT ARE NOW DEAD
14c. WERE BORN DEAD (FETAL DEATH AT ANY TIME AFTER CONCEPTION)

MOTHER

15. RACE—MOTHER — WHITE, NEGRO, AMERICAN INDIAN, ETC. (SPECIFY)
16. EDUCATION—SPECIFY HIGHEST GRADE COMPLETED — ELEMENTARY (0, 1, 2, 3, 4, . . . OR 8) / HIGH SCHOOL (1, 2, 3, OR 4) / COLLEGE (1, 2, 3, 4, OR 5+)
17a. DATE OF LAST LIVE BIRTH — MONTH / DAY / YEAR
17b. DATE OF LAST FETAL DEATH — MONTH / DAY / YEAR
18. DATE LAST NORMAL MENSES BEGAN — MONTH / DAY / YEAR
19a. MONTH OF PREGNANCY PRENATAL CARE BEGAN — FIRST, SECOND, THIRD, ETC. (SPECIFY)
19b. PRENATAL VISITS—TOTAL NUMBER (IF NONE, SO STATE)
20. LEGITIMATE (SPECIFY YES OR NO)
21. BIRTH WEIGHT

DEATH UNDER ONE YEAR OF AGE
ENTER STATE FILE NUMBER OF DEATH CERTIFICATE FOR THIS CHILD.

22. COMPLICATIONS RELATED TO PREGNANCY (DESCRIBE OR WRITE "NONE")
23. BIRTH INJURIES TO CHILD (DESCRIBE OR WRITE "NONE")
24. COMPLICATIONS NOT RELATED TO PREGNANCY (DESCRIBE OR WRITE "NONE")
25. CONGENITAL MALFORMATIONS OR ANOMALIES OF CHILD (DESCRIBE OR WRITE "NONE")
26. COMPLICATIONS OF LABOR (DESCRIBE OR WRITE "NONE")

MULTIPLE BIRTHS
ENTER STATE FILE NUMBER FOR MATE(S)
LIVE BIRTH(S)
FETAL DEATH(S)

LOCAL FILE NUMBER

1968 REVISION

DEPARTMENT OF HEALTH, EDUCATION, AND WELFARE—PUBLIC HEALTH SERVICE—NATIONAL CENTER FOR HEALTH STATISTICS

PHS—796—REV. 1-68

U.S. GOVERNMENT PRINTING OFFICE : 1967 OF—241-658

Fig. 9. United States standard birth certificate contains data for statistical information and confidential data to be used only for medical statistical purposes.

plies to labor, and pharmacology of oxytocic and anesthetic agents. The numerous applications of the preclinical sciences to problems of human reproduction are evidenced by the expansion of the National Institute of Child Health and Human Development.

In the international field of public health the World Health Organization has manifested its interest in the broader aspects of obstetrics by sponsoring the activities of two committees: its Expert Committee on Maternity Care and its Expert Committee on Midwifery Training. The objectives of maternity care, as set forth by these committees, reflect their broad goals.

Obstetrics is related also to certain fields that are not strictly medical. Since a dietary origin is suspected in many disturbances of pregnancy, obstetrics requires knowledge of the science of nutrition. In studies of fetal malformations, genetics is obviously of prime importance. Since the mother-child relationship is the basis of the family unit, the obstetrician is continually dealing with psychologic and sociologic problems, among the more important of which is the enormous number of illegitimate births in the United States each year. In addition, obstetrics has important legal aspects, especially in regard to the changing abortion laws, alleged traumatic abortion (taxicab accidents, for example), and legitimacy of the offspring.

The Future.   Although the recent decline in maternal mortality has been enormous, the millennium is neither here nor close by. If the nonwhite mortality were reduced to the level of the white by providing equal care, if the maternal deaths from criminal abortion were eliminated, and if the half of white deaths considered preventable by many mortality studies were prevented, approximately two thirds of these mothers' lives could be saved each year. Maternal mortality affects most seriously the socially and economically deprived. Many of these deaths result from sheer lack of adequate facilities including lack of properly distributed antepartum clinics, of suitable hospital arrangements, and of readily available blood. Others are caused by gross errors of management by the obstetric personnel. Errors of omission include failure to provide antepartum care, to follow the patient carefully throughout labor and the early puerperium, and to obtain appropriate consultation. Among errors of commission, unnecessary operative interference looms large. The great decline in maternal mortality over the past third of a century is the result of changes in obstetric principles. Modern obstetrics stresses conservatism in obstetric surgery and, above all, the avoidance of trauma. The obstetrician who operates unnecessarily, and by the same token often traumatically, practices the obstetrics of the 1930's and encounters a corresponding mortality.

These several deficiencies in maternity care must obviously be corrected first if maternal mortality is to be brought to the irreducible minimum. It can and doubtless will be lowered to that level by the same methods that have proved efficacious in the past: more, superior, and more equitably distributed personnel and facilities.

Many of the tasks required by the broadened implications of maternity care can be performed by allied health professionals. Obstetrics has already made a good beginning in the use of these personnel for a wide variety of maternity services. Whether they are called nurse midwife, nurse clinician, or maternity assistant, they will fill a void created by unavailability of obstetric manpower now and in the future.

In the present state of our knowledge, despite the promising new science of fetal medicine, the outlook for a dramatic reduction in perinatal mortality is less than assured. Nor are we likely to reduce the infant morbidity or the incidence of physical and neurologic handicaps, let alone the more obscure defects of personality and learning, until we can control prematurity. As maternal mortality was the paramount obstetric problem of the first half of this century, so will prematurity loom transcendent in the latter half. Its abolition depends upon the discovery of the physiologic factors that determine the onset of labor. In this area of research, we have made a modest beginning. Complete solution of the problem, however, requires not only physiologic discoveries but the union of obstetrics with those social sciences that bear on the epidemiology of prematurity and detailed knowledge of the etiologic significance of social and environmental factors.

By acknowledging the prime importance of the problem of prematurity, we recognize the corollary of the right of every child to be physically, mentally, and emotionally "well-born." This concept is fundamental to human dignity. If obstetrics is to play a role in its realization, the specialty must broaden its base to include the dynamics and control of population. The right to be "well-born" in its broadest sense is simply incompatible with unrestricted fertility. Yet our knowledge of the forces operative in the fluctuation and control of population growth is still rudimentary. This concept of obstetrics as a social as well as a biologic science impels us to accept a responsibility unprecedented in American medicine.

REFERENCES[*]

Bureau of the Census, U.S. Department of Commerce. Projections of the population of the United States by age and sex to 1985. Current Population Reports, Series P-25, No. 279, 1964.

Chase, H. C. Perinatal and infant mortality in the United States and six west European countries. Amer J Public Health 57:1735, 1967.

Day, R. L. Factors influencing offspring: number of children, interval between pregnancies, and age of parents. Amer J Dis Child 113:179, 1967.

Eastman, N. J. Mt. Everest in utero. Amer J Obstet Gynec 67:701, 1954.

——— Problems in the evolution of obstetrics. JAMA 171:1292, 1959.

——— Current trends in population control. Fertil Steril 15:477, 1964.

——— The contribution of John Whitridge Williams to obstetrics. Amer J Obstet Gynec 90:561, 1964.

Grabill, W. H., Kiser, C. V., and Whelpton, P. K. The Fertility of American Women. New York, John Wiley & Sons, 1958.

Hellman, L. M. Nurse-midwifery in the United States. Obstet Gynec 30:883, 1967.

Hunt, E. P. Lags in reducing infant mortality. Welfare in Review 2:1, 1964.

——— Infant mortality and poverty areas. Welfare in Review 5:1, 1967.

——— and Goldstein, S. M. Trends in Infant and Childhood Mortality—1961, U.S. Department of Health, Education and Welfare, Children's Bureau, Statistical Series No. 76, 1964.

Kohl, S. G. Perinatal Mortality in New York City, Responsible Factors. A study of 955 deaths by the Subcommittee on Neonatal Mortality, Committee on Public Health Relations, and the New York Academy of Medicine. Published for The Commonwealth Fund by the Harvard University Press, Cambridge, Mass., 1955.

Lesser, A. J. The federal government in child health care. Pediat Clin N Amer 16:891, 1969.

[*] In this chapter only, the general references listed are not necessarily mentioned specifically in the text.

Mendelson, C. L.   Cardiac Disease in Pregnancy. Philadelphia, F. A. Davis, 1960.

Monahan, H. B., and Spencer, E. C.   Deterrents to prenatal care. Children 9:114, 1962.

National Center for Health Statistics, U.S. Department of Health, Education, and Welfare, Public Health Service, Natality Statistics Analysis, United States, 1962, Publication No. 1000, Series 21, No. 1, U.S. Government Printing Office, 1964.

——— U.S. Department of Health, Education and Welfare, Public Health Service, Monthly Vital Statistics Report; Advance Report, Final Natality Statistics, 1963, 13 (No. 6): Supplement, September 11, 1964.

Oxford English Dictionary.   Oxford at the Clarendon Press, 1933. The statements about the history of the term *obstetrics*, as well as the definition of obstetrics as stated in the first senence of this chapter, were obtained chiefly from this source.

Report of the Program Area Committee on Child Health, APHA requirements for data on infant and perinatal mortality. Amer J Public Health 57:1848, 1967.

Russell, J. K.   Pregnancy in the young teenager. Lancet 1:365, 1969.

Shapiro, S.   Development of birth registration and birth statistics in the United States. Population Studies, 4(1):86, 1950.

——— Schlesinger, E. R., and Nesbitt, R. E. L.   Infant, Perinatal, Maternal and Childhood Mortality in the United States. Cambridge, Harvard University Press, 1968.

Social Aspects in Teaching of Obstetrics and Gynaecology.   Fourth Report of the Expert Committee on Maternal and Child Health, WHO Technical Report Series No. 266, Geneva, 1963.

Temkin, O.   Personal communication. Dr. Owsei Temkin, Associate Professor of the History of Medicine, Johns Hopkins University School of Medicine, has graciously devoted time to a study of the etymology of the word *obstetrics,* and the comments cited are entirely his.

The Midwife in Maternity Care.   Report of a WHO Expert Committee, WHO Technical Report Series No. 331, Geneva, 1966.

World Health Organization, Expert Committee on Midwifery Training (First Report), Technical Report Series No. 93. New York, Columbia University Press, 1955.

ANATOMY AND PHYSIOLOGY OF REPRODUCTION

2

THE ANATOMY OF THE FEMALE REPRODUCTIVE ORGANS

The female organs of reproduction are classified as external and internal. The external organs and the vagina serve for copulation; the internal organs provide for development and birth of the fetus.

EXTERNAL GENERATIVE ORGANS

The *pudenda,* or the external organs of generation, are commonly designated the *vulva,* which includes all structures visible externally from the lower margin of the pubis to the perineum—namely, the mons veneris, the labia majora and minora, the clitoris, vestibule, hymen, urethral opening, and various glandular and vascular structures (Fig. 1).

Mons Veneris. The mons veneris is the fatty cushion over the anterior surface of the symphysis pubis. After puberty its skin is covered by curly hair, forming the *escutcheon.* The distribution of pubic hair generally differs in the two sexes. In the female it occupies a triangular area, the base of which is formed by the upper margin of the symphysis, and a few hairs extend downward over the outer surface of the labia majora. In the male the escutcheon is not so well circumscribed, the hairs extending upward toward the umbilicus and downward over the inner surface of the thighs. Although considered a secondary sexual characteristic, the female escutcheon occasionally resembles the male type. The mons veneris is known also as the mons pubis.

Labia Majora. Extending downward and backward from the mons veneris are two rounded folds of adipose tissue covered with skin, the labia majora. They vary in appearance, according to the amount of fat within them. The labia majora are homologous with the scrotum in the male. The round ligaments terminate at their upper borders. They are less prominent after childbearing, and in old age they usually shrivel. Ordinarily they measure 7 to 8 cm in length, 2 to 3 cm in width, and 1 to 1.5 cm in thickness. They are somewhat tapered at their lower extremities. In children and virginal adults they usually lie in close apposition, completely concealing the underlying parts, whereas in multiparous women they

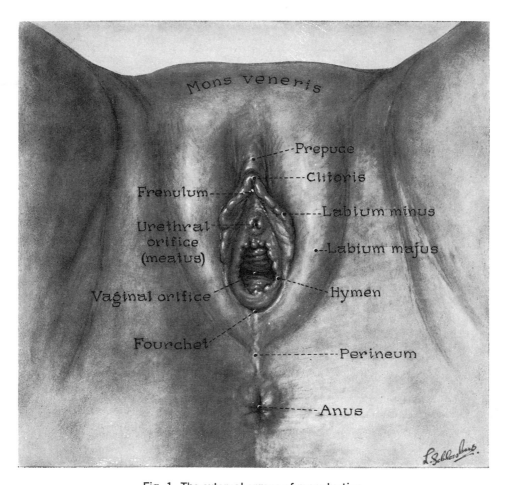

Fig. 1. The external organs of reproduction.

often gape widely. They are directly continuous with the mons veneris above and merge into the perineum posteriorly, medially joining to form the *posterior commissure.* The outer surface of the labium majus resembles the adjacent skin, and after puberty is covered with hair. In nulliparas the inner surface is moist, resembling a mucous membrane, whereas in multiparas it becomes more skinlike, but is not covered with hair. It is richly supplied with sebaceous glands. Beneath the skin there is a layer of dense connective tissue, which is rich in elastic fibers and adipose tissue but is essentially free of muscular elements. Unlike the squamous epithelium of normal vagina and cervix, parts of the vulvar skin contain many epithelial appendages (Fig. 2). Beneath this layer is a mass of fat, forming the bulk of the labium and supplied with a plexus of veins, which as the result of external injury may rupture to create a hematoma.

Labia Minora.   Separation of the labia majora reveals two flat reddish folds, the labia minora, or nymphae, which meet at the upper extremity of the vulva. They vary greatly in size and shape. In nulliparous women they are usually hidden by the labia majora; in multiparas they project beyond them.

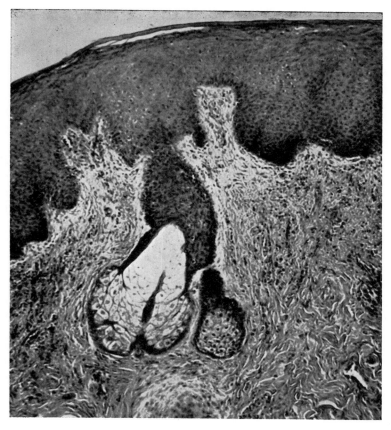

Fig. 2. Section through adult vulva, showing stratified squamous epithelium and epithelial appendages.

Each labium minus consists of a thin fold of tissue, which when protected presents a moist, reddish appearance, similar to that of a mucous membrane. It is, however, covered by stratified squamous epithelium, into which numerous papillae project. It contains no hair but many sebaceous follicles and occasionally a few sweat glands. The interior of the labial folds is made up of connective tissue, in which are many vessels and a few smooth muscular fibers, as in typical erectile structures. They are extremely sensitive and abundantly supplied with the several varieties of nerve endings.

The labia minora converge anteriorly, each dividing toward its upper extremity into two lamellae, of which the two lower fuse to form the *frenulum of the clitoris*, with the upper pair merging into the *prepuce*. Posteriorly they either pass almost imperceptibly into the labia majora or approach the midline as low ridges that fuse to form the *fourchet*.

Clitoris. The clitoris is a small, cylindric, erectile body situated at the anterior extremity of the vulva and projecting between the branched extremities of the labia minora, which form its prepuce and frenulum. It consists of a glans, a corpus, and two crura. It is the homologue of the penis, from which it differs in the lack of a corpus spongiosum and in the absence of the urethra. The glans is made up of spindle-shaped cells, and the corpus contains two corpora cavernosa, in the walls of which are smooth muscle fibers. The long narrow crura arise from the inferior surface of the ischiopubic rami and fuse just below the middle of the pubic arch to form the body of the clitoris. The clitoris rarely exceeds 2 cm in length, even in a state of erection. It is sharply bent by traction exerted by the labia minora. As a result, its free end points downward and inward toward the vaginal opening. The glans, which rarely exceeds 0.5 cm in diameter, is covered by stratified epithelium richly supplied with nerve endings and is extremely sensitive. The vessels of the highly erectile clitoris are connected with the vestibular bulbs (Fig. 3). The clitoris is a major female erogenous organ.

Krantz has studied the abundant nerve supply of the external genitalia. The labia majora, as well as the labia minora and clitoris, contain a delicate network of free nerve endings, with the fibers terminating in small knoblike thickenings in or adjacent to the cells. These endings are more frequently encountered in papillae than elsewhere. Tactile discs are also found in abundance in these areas. The genital corpuscles, which are considered the main mediators of erotic sensation, vary considerably. They are sparsely and randomly distributed in the labia majora deep in the corium, but the labia minora contain a great number of the corpuscles, particularly in the prepuce and skin overlying the glans clitoridis.

Vestibule.   The vestibule is the almond-shaped area enclosed by the labia minora and extending from the clitoris to the fourchet. It is the remnant of the urogenital sinus of the embryo and is perforated by four openings: the urethra, the vagina, and the ducts of Bartholin's glands. The posterior portion of the vestibule between the fourchet and the vaginal opening is called the *fossa navicularis*. It is rarely observed except in nulliparous women, since it is usually obliterated as the result of childbirth.

Related to the vestibule are the *major vestibular glands*, or *Bartholin's glands* (Fig. 3). They are a pair of small compound glands, about 0.5 to 1 cm in diameter; one is situated beneath the vestibule on either side of the vaginal opening. They lie under the constrictor muscle of the vagina and are sometimes found partially covered by the vestibular bulbs. Their ducts, from 1.5 to 2 cm long, open on the sides of the vestibule just outside the lateral margin of the vaginal orifice. Their small lumina ordinarily admit only the finest probe. During sexual excitement mucoid material is secreted by the glands. The ducts sometimes harbor gonococci, which may gain access to the gland, causing suppuration of the entire labium. The *glandulae vestibulares minores* are small mucous glands opening on the upper portion of the vestibule.

Urethral Opening.   The urinary meatus is in the midline of the vestibule, 1 to 1.5 cm below the pubic arch and a short distance above the vaginal opening. It is usually puckered. Its orifice appears as a vertical slit, which can be distended to 4 or 5 mm in diameter. The *paraurethral ducts* open usually on the vestibule on either side of the urethra, but occasionally on its posterior wall just inside its orifice. They are of small caliber, 0.5 mm in diameter, and of varying length. In this country, they are generally known as *Skene's ducts* (Fig. 3).

The urethra in its lower two thirds traverses the anterior vaginal wall, from which it is relatively inseparable. The circular muscle of the lower third of the vagina encircles the urethra superiorly and inferiorly.

Vestibular Bulbs.   Lying beneath the mucous membrane of the vestibule on either side are the vestibular bulbs, which are almond-shaped aggregations of

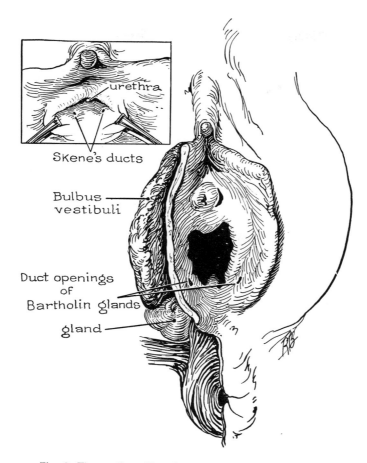

Fig. 3. The urethra, Skene's ducts, and Bartholin's glands.

veins, 3 to 4 cm long, 1 to 2 cm wide, and 0.5 to 1 cm thick. They lie in close apposition to the ischiopubic rami, partially covered by the ischiocavernosus and constrictor vaginae muscles. Their lower terminations are usually about the middle of the vaginal opening, and their anterior extremities extend upward toward the clitoris.

Embryologically, the vestibular bulbs correspond to the corpus spongiosum of the penis. During parturition they are usually pushed up beneath the pubic arch; but since their posterior ends partially encircle the vagina, they are subject to injury and rupture, which may give rise to a hematoma of the vulva or to profuse external hemorrhage.

Vaginal Opening and Hymen.   The vaginal opening occupies the lower portion of the vestibule and varies considerably in size and shape. In virgins it is entirely hidden by the overlapping labia minora; and when exposed, it appears almost completely closed by the membranous hymen.

The hymen presents marked differences in shape and consistency. It comprises mainly connective tissue, both elastic and collagenous. Both surfaces are covered by noncornified stratified squamous epithelium. Connective tissue papillae are more numerous on the vaginal surface and at the free edge. According to Mahran and Saleh, there are no glandular or muscular elements. It is not richly supplied with nerve fibers. In the newborn child it is very vascular and redundant; during pregnancy the epithelium is thick and rich in glycogen; after the menopause the epithelium thins, and slight focal cornification may appear. In adult virgins it is a membrane of varying thickness that surrounds the vaginal opening more or less completely and presents an aperture varying in size from that of a pinpoint to a caliber that admits the tip of one or even two fingers. The hymenal opening is usually crescentic or circular, but may occasionally be cribriform, septate, or fimbriated. Since the fimbriated variety may be mistaken for a ruptured hymen, it is necessary for medicolegal reasons to exercise caution in making definite statements regarding rupture of the hymen.

As a rule the hymen ruptures during the first coitus, tearing at several points, usually in its posterior portion. The edges of the tears soon cicatrize, and the hymen becomes permanently divided into two or three portions, separated by narrow slits extending down to its base. The extent to which rupture occurs varies with the structure of the hymen and the degree to which it is distended. Although it is commonly believed that rupture of the hymen is associated with slight bleeding, hemorrhage does not occur in all cases. There may, however, occasionally be profuse bleeding. Infrequently the membrane may be very resistant, requiring surgical incision before coitus can be accomplished.

The changes in the hymen after coitus are often of medicolegal importance, especially in cases of alleged rape, in which the physician is occasionally called upon to examine the victim and testify concerning his findings. The essence of the criminal act is penetration of the hymen, however slight. In virgins examined a few hours after the alleged attack, fresh tears, abrasions, or bleeding points on the hymen constitute corroborative evidence of the crime. Negative findings are of no significance, however, since the hymen may not be torn despite repeated coitus. In fact, many cases of pregnancy have been reported in women with unruptured hymens. It is not necessary to prove that ejaculation has occurred to justify a conviction of rape; the essence of the crime is the physical and emotional injury to the woman, consummated by penetration. Conversely, ejaculation without penetration is not sufficient to constitute the crime of rape (Wharton).

The changes produced by childbirth, as a rule, are readily recognized. After the puerperium the remnants of the hymen form several cicatrized nodules of varying size, the *myrtiform caruncles*. By and large they constitute incontrovertible evidence of previous childbearing. An imperforate hymen, a rare lesion, occludes the vaginal orifice completely, causing retention of the menstrual discharge.

The Vagina.   The vagina is a musculomembranous tube extending from the vulva to the uterus and interposed between the bladder and the rectum (Fig. 4). It represents the excretory duct of the uterus, through which its secretion and the menstrual flow escape; it is the female organ of copulation; and, finally, it forms part of the birth canal at labor. Anteriorly, the vagina is in contact with the bladder and urethra, from which it is separated by connective tissue often referred to as the vesicovaginal septum. Posteriorly, between its lower portion and the rectum, is similar tissue forming the rectovaginal septum. Approximately one fourth of the vagina is separated from the rectum by the rectouterine pouch, or cul-de-sac of Douglas.

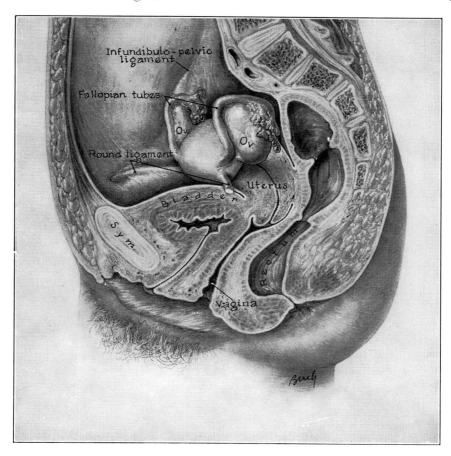

Fig. 4. Cross section of pelvis showing relations of pelvic viscera.

The significance of the rectovaginal septum has been lengthily debated. The definitive structure is probably homologous with the rectovesical septum in the male. Although well formed by the fourteenth week of fetal development, according to Milley and Nichols, the rectovaginal septum may be difficult to identify because it is closely adherent to the posterior aspect of the vaginal connective tissue.

The origin of the human vagina remains a subject of debate among embryologists. The vaginal epithelium is variously said to arise from (1) the müllerian system, (2) wolffian duct epithelium, and (3) the epithelium of the urogenital sinus. The most widely accepted view is that the vagina arises in part from the müllerian ducts and in part from the urogenital sinus.

Davies and Kusama, among others, however, have summarized evidence that the entire vagina may arise from the urogenital sinus. According to this concept, the fused müllerian ducts impinge on the posterior wall of the urogenital sinus. The vagina thus arises as a proliferation of the epithelium in the pars pelvina of the urogenital sinus and is therefore endodermal in origin. Canalization of the solid proliferation of the sinus occurs between the eighteenth and twenty-second weeks of development. The junction between the epithelium of the proliferation from the sinus and that of the fused müllerian ducts lies approximately in the region of the cervix.

Forsberg favors the view that the human vaginal epithelium is a wolffian derivative. According to him, the differentiated wolffian epithelium may induce a cranial growth of the sinus epithelium, thereby changing its character. Despite extensive work in rodents, the anatomic and developmental variations among species limit the value of the comparative approach to the question of origin of the human vagina.

Normally, the anterior and posterior walls of the vagina lie in contact, a slight space intervening between their lateral margins. When not distended, the canal is H-shaped on transverse section (Fig. 5). The vagina is capable of marked

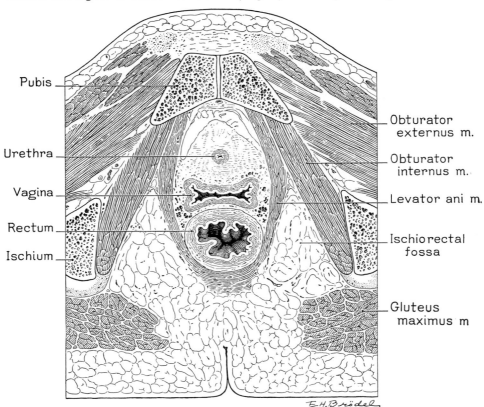

Fig. 5. Cross section through pelvis showing H-shaped lumen of vagina. (Adapted from Canton Atlas.)

distention, as manifested at childbirth. The upper end of the vagina is a blind vault into which the lower portion of the uterine cervix projects. The vaginal vault is subdivided into the anterior, posterior, and lateral fornices. Since the vagina is attached higher up upon the posterior than upon the anterior wall of the cervix, the posterior fornix is considerably longer than the anterior. The fornices are of great clinical importance because through their thin walls the internal pelvic organs can usually be palpated. The posterior fornix, moreover, provides ready surgical access to the peritoneal cavity. The vagina varies considerably in length. Since it is united to the uterus at an acute angle, its anterior wall is always shorter than its posterior. Anterior and posterior walls measure 6 to 8 and 7 to 10 cm, respectively.

Projecting into the lumen from the midlines of both the anterior and posterior walls are prominent longitudinal ridges, the anterior and posterior vaginal columns. In nulliparas numerous transverse ridges, or *rugae*, extend outward from, and almost at right angles to, the vaginal columns, gradually fading away as they approach the lateral walls. They form a corrugated surface, which is not present before menarche and which gradually becomes obliterated after repeated childbirth and after the menopause. In elderly multiparas the vaginal walls are often smooth. The mucosa of the vagina (Fig. 6) is composed of typical noncornified

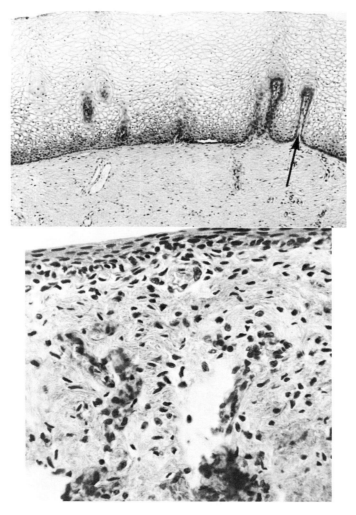

Fig. 6. Top, adult vagina, showing noncornified, thick, stratified squamous epithelium. Epithelial appendages are absent. Arrow indicates a papilla. Bottom, thin vaginal epithelium of a prepuberal girl.

stratified squamous epithelium. Beneath the epithelium is a thin layer of connective tissue, rich in blood vessels, with occasional small lymphoid nodules. The mucosa, very loosely attached to the underlying connective tissue, is easily dissected off at operations. Argument remains, however, as to whether this tissue is a definite fascial plane in the strict anatomic sense.

The significance and the very existence of the *endopelvic fascia* have been frequently questioned. In a careful study Roberts and associates concluded that the uterovaginal (endopelvic) fascia is a well-defined structure. They confirmed, furthermore, the division of the perineal fascia into superficial and deep portions, with the deep perineal fascia forming the inferior boundary of the superficial perineal space.

From early infancy until after the menopause, the cells of the superficial layer of the mucosa contain considerable glycogen. Examination of exfoliated cells from the vagina permits identification of the various stages of the sexual cycle in women as well as in many lower animals.

Typical glands are normally absent from the vagina. In parous women, fragments of stratified epithelium that sometimes give rise to cysts are occasionally embedded in the vaginal connective tissue. These vaginal inclusion cysts are not glands but remnants of mucosal tags that were buried during the repair of vaginal tears at delivery. Other cysts lined by columnar or cuboidal epithelium are derived from remnants of the wolffian or müllerian ducts.

The muscular coat is not sharply defined, although two layers of smooth muscle, an outer longitudinal and an inner circular, may usually be distinguished. At the lower extremity of the vagina there is a thin band of striated muscle, the *constrictor* or *sphincter vaginae;* the *levator ani,* however, is the principal muscle that closes the vagina. Outside of the muscular layer is connective tissue that joins the vagina to the surrounding parts. It contains many elastic fibers and an abundance of veins.

In the nonpregnant woman the vagina is kept moist by a small amount of secretion from the uterus; but in pregnancy there is extensive vaginal secretion, which normally consists of a curdlike product of exfoliated epithelium and bacteria, with a markedly acidic reaction. Bacilli are the predominant bacteria during pregnancy, although cocci are not infrequent. The acidic reaction has been attributed to lactic acid, which is thought to result from the breakdown of glycogen in the mucosa by the bacilli of Döderlein.

The pH of the vaginal secretion varies with ovarian activity. Before puberty it ranges between 6.8 and 7.2, whereas in the adult it is well below this range. According to Rakoff, Feo, and Goldstein the pH of the vagina in the adult woman ranges between 4.0 and 5.0. The pH was lowest at midcycle and highest premenstrually.

The vagina has an abundant vascular supply. Its upper third is supplied by the cervicovaginal branches of the uterine arteries, its middle third by the inferior vesical arteries, and its lower third by the middle hemorrhoidal and internal pudendal arteries. Immediately surrounding the vagina is an extensive venous plexus, the vessels from which follow the course of the arteries and eventually empty into the hypogastric veins. For the most part, the lymphatics from the lower third of the vagina along with those of the vulva empty into the inguinal lymph nodes, those from its middle third into the hypogastrics, and those from its upper third into the iliacs. The human vagina, according to Krantz, is devoid of any

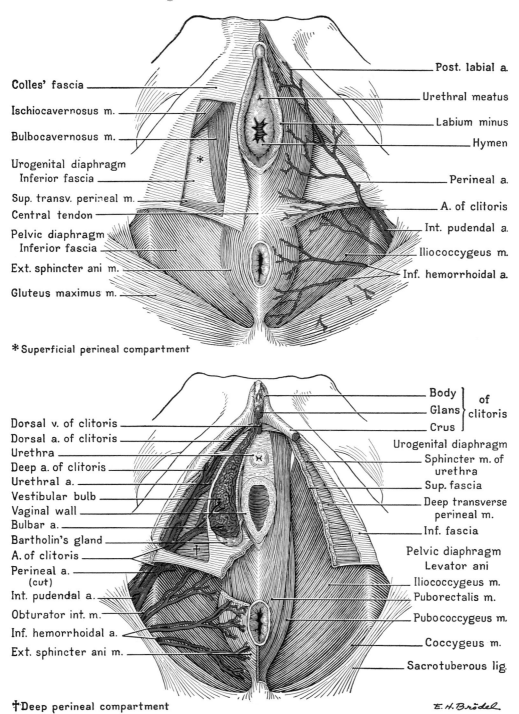

Post. labial a.

Colles' fascia

Urethral meatus

Ischiocavernosus m.

Labium minus

Bulbocavernosus m.

Hymen

Urogenital diaphragm
Inferior fascia

Perineal a.

Sup. transv. perineal m.

A. of clitoris

Central tendon

Int. pudendal a.

Pelvic diaphragm
Inferior fascia

Iliococcygeus m.

Ext. sphincter ani m.

Inf. hemorrhoidal a.

Gluteus maximus m.

*Superficial perineal compartment

Body ⎱
Glans ⎰ of clitoris
Crus ⎱

Dorsal v. of clitoris

Urogenital diaphragm

Dorsal a. of clitoris

Sphincter m. of
urethra

Urethra

Deep a. of clitoris

Sup. fascia

Urethral a.

Deep transverse
perineal m.

Vestibular bulb

Inf. fascia

Vaginal wall

Bulbar a.

Pelvic diaphragm
Levator ani

Bartholin's gland

A. of clitoris

Iliococcygeus m.

Perineal a.
(cut)

Puborectalis m.

Int. pudendal a.

Pubococcygeus m.

Obturator int. m.

Inf. hemorrhoidal a.

Coccygeus m.

Ext. sphincter ani m.

Sacrotuberous lig.

†Deep perineal compartment

E. H. Brödel

Fig. 7. Diagrams of the perineum.

special nerve endings (genital corpuscles), but occasionally free nerve endings are found in the papillae.

The Perineum.   The perineum consists of the muscles and fascia of the urogenital and pelvic diaphragms. The urogenital diaphragm, lying across the pubic arch above the superficial perineal (Colles') fascia, consists of the deep transverse perineal muscles and the constrictor of the urethra. The pelvic diaphragm is made up of two muscles, the coccygeus and levator ani, the latter consisting of three portions—iliococcygeus, pubococcygeus, and puborectalis. These muscles form a sling for the pelvic structures; between them pass the urethra, vagina, and rectum. The puborectalis and pubococcygeus constrict the vagina and rectum and form an efficient functional rectal sphincter (Fig. 7). The median raphe of the levator ani between the anus and the vagina is reinforced by the central tendon of the perineum, on which the bulbocavernosi, the superficial transverse perineal muscles, and the external sphincter ani converge. These structures contribute to the *perineal body* and form the main support of the perineal floor. They are often lacerated during delivery (see Ch. 16, Figs. 19 through 22). The ischiocavernosi enclose the crura of the clitoris and facilitate erection of that organ (see Ch. 13, Figs. 15 through 21).

INTERNAL GENERATIVE ORGANS

The Uterus.   The uterus is a muscular organ partially covered by peritoneum. Its cavity is lined by the endometrium. During pregnancy the uterus serves for reception, retention, and nutrition of the conceptus, which it expels during labor.

The nonpregnant uterus is situated in the pelvic cavity between the bladder and rectum, its inferior extremity projecting into the vagina. Almost its entire posterior wall is covered by peritoneum, the lower portion of which forms the anterior boundary of the pouch of Douglas. Only the upper portion of the anterior wall is so covered, since its lower portion is united to the posterior wall of the bladder by a well-defined layer of connective tissue.

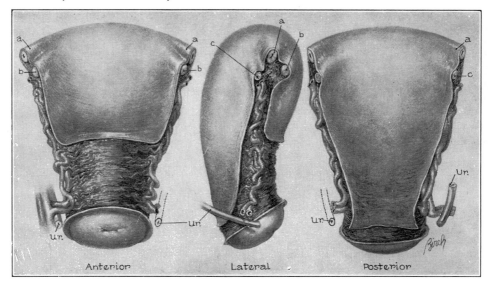

Fig. 8. Anterior, lateral, and posterior aspects of uterus. a, fallopian tube; b, round ligament; c, ovarian ligament; ur., ureter.

The uterus resembles a flattened pear in shape (Fig. 8) and consists of two unequal parts: an upper triangular portion, the *corpus,* and a lower, cylindric or fusiform portion, the *cervix.* The anterior surface of the corpus is almost flat, whereas its posterior surface is distinctly convex. The fallopian tubes arise from the *cornua* of the uterus, at the junction of the superior and lateral margins. The convex upper segment between the points of insertion of the fallopian tubes is called the *fundus uteri.* The lateral margins extend from the cornua on either side to the pelvic floor. Laterally the uterus below the insertion of the fallopian tubes is not directly covered by peritoneum but receives the attachments of the broad ligaments.

There are marked variations in size and shape of the uterus, depending on

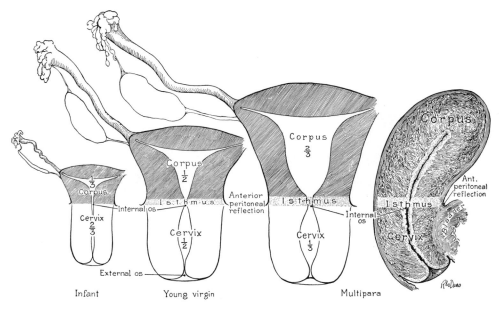

Fig. 9. Frontal and sagittal sections of normal uterus and appendages. The comparative size of infantile, adult nonparous, and multiparous uteri.

age and parity. The infantile organ varies from 2.5 to 3 cm in length; that of adult nulliparas measures from 5.5 to 8, 3.5 to 4, and 2 to 2.5 cm in its greatest vertical, transverse, and anteroposterior diameters, respectively, as compared with 9 to 9.5, 5.5 to 6, and 3 to 3.5 cm, respectively, in multiparous women. Nonparous and parous uteri differ considerably also in weight, the former normally ranging from 45 to 70 g, and the latter 80 g or more (Langlois). The relation between the length of the corpus and that of the cervix likewise varies widely (Fig. 9). In the young child the corpus is only half as long as the cervix. In young nulliparas the two are of about equal length. In multiparous women, the relation is reversed, the cervix representing only a little more than one third of the total length of the organ.

The great bulk of the organ consists of muscle, and the anterior and posterior walls of its body lie almost in contact, the cavity between them a mere slit (Fig. 10). The cervix is fusiform with a small opening at each end, the *internal os* and the *external os.* On frontal section, the cavity of the body of the uterus is triangular, whereas that of the cervix retains its fusiform shape. After childbearing, the triangular appearance becomes less pronounced as its margins become concave instead of convex. At the menopause the organ decreases in size, with atrophy of myometrium and endometrium.

The *isthmus* is of great obstetric significance because in pregnancy it contributes to the lower uterine segment.

Cervix Uteri. The cervix is the portion of the uterus below the isthmus and the internal os. On the anterior surface of the uterus its upper boundary is indicated roughly by the point at which the peritoneum is reflected upon the bladder.

It is divided by the attachment of the vagina into supravaginal and vaginal portions. The supravaginal segment is covered on its posterior surface by peri-

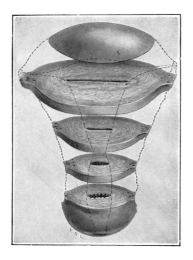

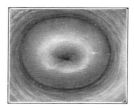

Fig. 11. Nonparous external os.

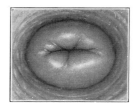

Fig. 10. Reconstruction of uterus showing shape of its cavity.

Fig. 12. Parous external os.

toneum, whereas its lateral and anterior surfaces are in contact with the connective tissue of the broad ligaments and bladder. The vaginal portion of the cervix, which is usually designated the *portio vaginalis*, projects into the vagina; at its lower extremity is the external os.

The external os may vary greatly in appearance. Before childbirth it is a small, regular oval opening. The nulliparous cervix has the consistency of the nasal cartilage. After childbirth the orifice is converted into a transverse slit that divides the cervix into so-called anterior and posterior lips. When the cervix has been deeply torn during labor it may become irregular, nodular, or stellate. These changes are sufficiently characteristic to permit the examiner to ascertain, in most instances, whether the woman has borne children (Figs. 11 and 12).

The cervix is composed basically of connective tissue, as Danforth has shown, with occasional smooth muscle fibers, many vessels, and elastic tissue. The transition from the collagenous tissue of the cervix to the muscular tissue of the corpus, although generally abrupt, may be gradual, extending over 10 mm. Studies by Danforth, Buckingham, and Roddick suggest that the physical properties of the cervix are determined by the state of the connective tissue, and that during pregnancy and labor the remarkable dilatability of the cervix results from dissociation of collagen. They were able to quantitate the proportion of collagen to muscle in the human cervix. In the normal cervix, muscle formed an average of about 10 per cent; in "incompetent cervices" (Ch. 20), however, the proportion of muscle was much greater (Buckingham and co-workers).

The mucosa of the cervical canal, although embryologically a direct continuation of endometrium, has differentiated characteristically in such a way that sections through the canal resemble a honeycomb. The mucosa is composed of a single layer of very high columnar epithelium, which rests upon a thin basement membrane. The oval nuclei are situated near the base of the columnar cells, the upper portions of which look rather clear because of their mucoid content. These cells are abundantly supplied with cilia.

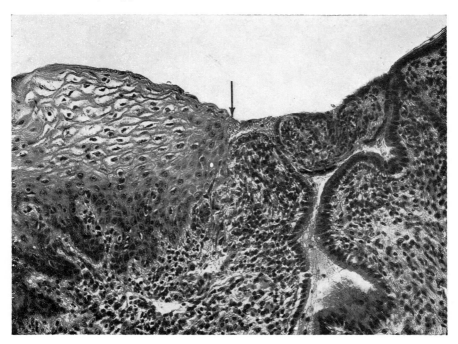

Fig. 13. Squamocolumnar junction of the pregnant cervix is shown at arrow. In this section tubular glands of the exposed portion of the endocervix lie outside the external os. (From Davies and Woolf. Clin Obstet Gynec 6:265, 1963.)

The cervical glands extend from the surface of the mucosa directly into the subjacent connective tissue, since there is no submucosa as such. Fluhmann has argued that the apparently racemose structure of the glands is actually the result of a complicated system of compound clefts. The mucous cells of this epithelium furnish the thick, tenacious secretion of the cervical canal.

The mucosa of the vaginal portion of the cervix is directly continuous with that of the vagina, both consisting of stratified squamous epithelium. Normally there are no glands beneath it, but frequently endocervical glands extend down almost to its surface. If their ducts are occluded, the glands may form retention cysts a few millimeters in diameter, the so-called *nabothian follicles*.

Normally the squamous epithelium of the vaginal portion and the columnar

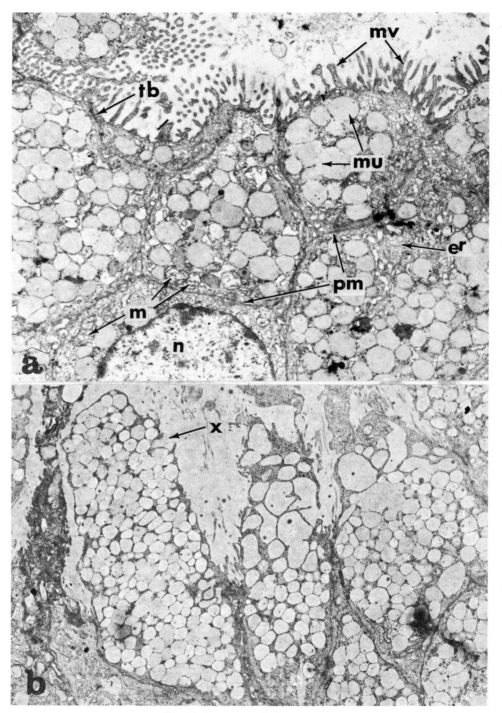

Fig. 14. Legend on facing page.

epithelium of the cervical canal form a sharp line of division near the external os (Fig. 13). In response to inflammation and trauma associated with aging, however, the stratified epithelium gradually extends up the cervical canal to line its lower third or occasionally lower half. This change is more marked in multiparas, in whom the lips of the cervix are often everted. Uncommonly the junction of the two varieties of epithelium occurs on the vaginal portion outside the external os, as in *congenital ectropion*.

The cyclic changes in the cervical mucosa are dependent upon the varying hormonal patterns of the menstrual cycle, as discussed on page 99.

During the past few years several technically satisfactory ultrastructural studies of the human cervix have been published. In an earlier study of the human cervical epithelium, Davies and Woolf reported that the basal cells, which were rich in ribonucleoprotein (RNP) granules, contained numerous mitochondria but few tonofilaments. In the parabasal and intermediate layers they found accumulations of tonofibrils and glycogen, paranuclear vacuoles, a great increase in complexity of intercellular spaces and of desmosomes, and a decrease in mitochondria and RNP particles. In the superficial layers, cytoplasmic detail was obscured by massive accumulations of tonofibrils. Small electron-dense bodies, possibly keratohyalin, were found, but there was no stratum granulosum corresponding to what is seen in the epidermis.

The endocervical epithelium, according to Davies and Woolf, contained highly convoluted basal plasma membranes. There were many RNP particles, but no glycogen or tonofilaments in the cytoplasm (Fig. 14). The supranuclear cytoplasm was filled with mucoid droplets, especially in pregnancy.

Several questions of clinical interest have recently been answered by histologic and electron microscopic studies. For example, Schueller showed that the endocervix contained ciliated cells, occurring singly or in patches. Growth of the cilia appeared to be stimulated by estrogen and depressed by progesterone.

The identity and significance of the basal lamina ("basement membrane") are still controversial. Younes and associates (1965) found half-desmosomes on the epithelial cell membranes of the ectocervix. Warren and his co-workers, on the contrary, could not find an ultrastructurally distinct basement membrane.

The derivation of the cervical epithelial cells has been elucidated by ultrastructural studies. Younes and colleagues described clear cells identical in fine structure with the Langerhans cells of the human epidermis. These elements, which were found in the intercellular spaces of squamous epithelium, appear to be more frequent in carcinoma in situ. Laguens and his co-workers described three cellular types in the human endocervix: mucous columnar, ciliated, and reserve. The highly differentiated mucus-producing cells are largely filled by secretion. Several forms of reserve cells were identified. Stegner and

Fig. 14. Top, luminal aspect of the epithelium of the endocervix of a nonpregnant woman. The plasma membrane adjoining the lumen is thrown up into slender branching microvilli (mv). There are terminal bars (tb) attaching the cells to one another close to the lumen. The cytoplasm is densely packed with mucous droplets (mu), which are limited externally by membranes studded with RNP granules. Between the droplets is a feltwork of membranous and vesicular elements of the endoplasmic reticulum (er), many scattered RNP granules, and mitochondria (m). Some of the mucous droplets are confluent. Nucleus (n). Bottom, apical aspect of the mucified epithelium of the endocervix of a pregnant woman. The cytoplasm is ballooned out into the lumen and distended with many mucous droplets, which reduce the intervening cytoplasm to narrow septa. Many of the droplets are confluent because of breakdown of the septa. A similar breakdown of septa close to the cervical lumen causes the release of the mucus into the lumen, as at x. (From Davies and Woolf. Clin Obstet Gynec 6:265, 1963.)

Beltermann described a random arrangement of ciliated and mucus-producing cells. They saw no transitions from ciliated to mucous columnar types, although poorly differentiated round cells with large nuclei (reserve cells) were considered capable of differentiating into either squamous or mucus-producing elements. The morphologically transitional stages are consistent with this concept.

Corpus Uteri. The wall of the uterine body is made up of three layers: serosal, muscular, and mucosal. The serosal layer is formed by the peritoneum covering the uterus, to which it is firmly adherent except just above the bladder and at the margins where it is deflected to the broad ligaments.

The innermost, or mucosal, layer, which lines the uterine cavity, is the endometrium. It is a thin, pinkish, velvety membrane, which on close examination is seen to be perforated by a large number of minute openings, the mouths of the uterine glands. Because of the constant cyclic changes during the reproductive period of life, the endometrium normally varies greatly in thickness, measuring from 0.5 up to 3 to 5 mm. It consists of surface epithelium, glands, and interglandular tissue in which are numerous blood vessels and tissue spaces.

The histologic appearance of the normal endometrium is shown in Figures 1 to 4 of Chapter 4; the ultrastructural features are illustrated in Figures 5 to 6 of that chapter. Since the uterus has no submucosa, the endometrium is attached directly to the underlying myometrium along an irregular boundary.

The epithelium of the endometrial surface is composed of a single layer of closely packed, high columnar ciliated cells. The oval nuclei during most of the endometrial cycle are situated in the lower portions of the cells but not so near the base as in the endocervix.

Cilia have been demonstrated in the endometria of many mammals. The ciliated cells occur in discrete patches, whereas secretory activity appears to be limited to nonciliated cells. The cilia persist throughout the entire period of sexual activity and disappear 8 to 10 years after the menopause. The ciliary current in both the tubes and the uterus is in the same direction, extending downward from the fimbriated end of the tubes toward the external os.

The tubular *uterine glands* are invaginations of the epithelium of the surface, which, in the resting state, resemble the fingers of a glove. They extend through the entire thickness of the endometrium to the myometrium, which they occasionally penetrate for a short distance. Histologically they resemble the epithelium of the surface and are lined by a single layer of columnar, partially ciliated epithelium that rests upon a thin basement membrane. They secrete a thin alkaline fluid that serves to keep the uterine cavity moist (Figs. 1 through 4 in Ch. 4).

The classic monograph of Hitschmann and Adler in 1908 clearly demonstrated that the endometrium undergoes constant hormonally controlled changes during each menstrual cycle. These three fundamental phases—*menstrual, proliferative* (follicular), and *secretory* (luteal)—will be considered in detail in Chapter 4 in the section on menstruation. In brief, immediately after menstruation the normal endometrium is quite thin, with the tubular glands well separated. It increases rapidly in thickness and, before the next menstrual period, usually contains many convoluted or sacculated glands. At the menopause the entire endometrium undergoes atrophy: its epithelium flattens; its glands gradually disappear; and its interglandular tissue becomes more fibrous.

The connective tissue of the endometrium between the surface epithelium and the myometrium is a mesenchymal stroma. Immediately after menstruation it consists of closely packed oval and spindle-shaped nuclei, around which there is very little cytoplasm. When separated by edema the cells appear stellate, with branching cytoplasmic processes that form anastomoses. The cells are more closely packed around the glands and blood vessels than elsewhere. Several days before menstruation they usually become larger and more vesicular, resembling decidual cells. At the same time there is a diffuse leukocytic infiltration.

The vascular architecture of the endometrium is of great importance in explaining certain phenomena of menstruation and pregnancy. Arterial blood is carried to the uterus by the uterine and ovarian arteries. As the arterial branches penetrating the uterine wall obliquely inward reach its middle third, they ramify in a plane parallel to the surface and are named the *arcuate arteries*. Radial branches extend at right angles toward the endometrium, as shown in Figure 15.

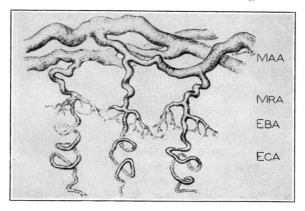

Fig. 15. Stereographic representation of myometrial and endometrial arteries in the macaque. Above are shown parts of myometrial arcuate arteries (MAA) from which myometrial radial arteries (MRA) course toward the endometrium. There are found larger endometrial coiled arteries (ECA) and smaller endometrial basal arteries (EBA). (From Okkels and Engle. Acta Path Microbiol Scand 15:150, 1938.)

The endometrial arteries consist of *coiled arteries*, essentially a continuation of the radial arteries, and *basal arteries*, which branch from the radial arteries at a sharp angle, as shown in Figure 15. The coiled arteries supply most of the middle and all of the superficial third of the endometrium. Their walls have been shown by Okkels and Engle to react sensitively to hormonal influences, especially by vasoconstriction, and thus they probably play a part in the mechanism of menstrual bleeding, as explained on page 93. The straight basal endometrial arteries are smaller in both caliber and length than the coiled vessels. They extend only into the basal layer of the endometrium, or at most a short distance into the middle layer, and are not affected by hormonal influences. Transitions between these two types are not uncommon.

The major portion of the uterus consists of bundles of smooth muscle, united by connective tissue containing many elastic fibers. According to Schwalm and Dubrauszky, muscle fibers progressively diminish caudally to the extent that the cervix contains only 10 per cent muscle. In the corpus the inner uterine wall contains relatively more muscle than do the outer layers, and the anterior and posterior walls contain more than do the lateral walls. In pregnancy, muscle in the upper portion of the uterus increases greatly, but there is no significant change in the muscle content of the cervix. Schwalm and Dubrauszky report that these differences in the various walls of the corpus disappear in pregnancy. On the basis of these findings, they reason that active participation of the cervix in dilatation during labor is unlikely. Anatomic changes in the myometrium during pregnancy are detailed in Chapter 8.

Ultrastructural studies of smooth muscle have lagged behind those of skeletal muscle, and fine structural knowledge of the myometrium is particularly meager. Electron microscopic investigations of uterine muscle, furthermore, have been confined largely to rodents, with the result that the correlation of human myometrial fine structure and function is still rudimentary (Nemetschek-Gansler).

Hashimoto and co-workers attempted to compare the ultrastructure of the nonpregnant human uterus with that of the pregnant organ at term. In the muscle cells of the pregnant uterus they noted a great increase in large mitochondria, a moderate development of Golgi complexes, and a considerable increase in endoplasmic reticulum. More recently, Yokoyama noted a tenfold increase in length and a threefold increase in width of human myometrial cells during pregnancy. He found no significant increase in nuclear size and no neogenesis of smooth muscle cells, however. According to Yokoyama, there were no direct intercellular cytoplasmic communications.

Several correlative ultrastructural and biochemical studies of the rat's uterus have recently been published. Bergman found that in the absence of estrogen the uterus is electrically and mechanically quiescent, showing no evidence of well-defined cellular junctions such as those found in physiologically active tissue. Bo, Odor, and Rothrock studied the ultrastructural effects of progesterone, alone or in combination with estrogen, on the smooth muscle cells of the rat's uterus. Progesterone alone alters the ultrastructure of smooth muscle cells, but not to the extent observed after preliminary stimulation by estrogen. The most prominent changes were accumulation of granular endoplasmic reticulum, free ribosomes, glycogen particles, and extensive Golgi complexes.

Needham and Shoenberg describe the relatively low content of actomyosin in uterine muscle. The explanation lies in the greater proportion of stromal protein intimately connected with smooth muscle cells than with skeletal muscle. The nonpregnant human uterus contains 22 mg of collagen per gram wet weight, whereas the comparable figure for striated muscle is 4.8 mg.

Ligaments of the Uterus.   Extending from either side of the uterus are the broad, round, and uterosacral ligaments.

The *broad ligaments* are two winglike structures extending from the lateral margins of the uterus to the pelvic walls and dividing the pelvic cavity into anterior and posterior compartments. Each broad ligament consists of a fold of peritoneum enclosing various structures and presents superior, lateral, inferior, and median margins. The inner two thirds of the superior margin form the mesosalpinx, to which is attached the fallopian tube. The outer third, extending from the fimbriated end of the tube to the pelvic wall, forms the *infundibulopelvic ligament* (suspensory ligament of the ovary), through which traverse the ovarian vessels. The portion of the broad ligament beneath the fallopian tube is the *mesosalpinx*. It consists of two layers of peritoneum between which is scant, loose connective tissue in which the *parovarium* may sometimes be found.

The parovarium consists of a number of narrow vertical tubules lined by ciliated epithelium. They connect at their upper ends with a longitudinal duct that extends just below the fallopian tube to the lateral margin of the uterus, where it ends blindly near the internal os. This canal, the remnant of the wolffian (mesonephric) duct in the female, is designated *Gartner's duct*. The parovarium, a remnant of the wolffian body, is homologous with the caput epididymidis in the male. Its cranial portion is the *epoophoron,* or organ of Rosenmüller. Its caudal portion, or *paroophoron,* is a vestigial group of mesonephric tubules in or around the broad ligament. It is homologous with the male paradidymis, or organ of Giraldès. The paroophoron usually disappears in the adult but occasionally forms macroscopic cysts.

At the lateral margin of the broad ligament the peritoneum is reflected on the side of the pelvis. The base of the broad ligament, which is quite thick, is continuous with the connective tissue of the pelvic floor; through it pass the uterine vessels. Its most dense portion—usually referred to as the cardinal ligament, the transverse cervical ligament, or Mackenrodt's ligament—is composed of connective tissue that is firmly united to the supravaginal portion of the cervix and the lateral margin of the uterus. It encloses the uterine vessels and ureter.

A vertical section through the uterine end of the broad ligament is triangular, with the uterine vessels in its broad base (Fig. 16). It is widely attached to the connective tissues adjacent to the cervix, the *parametrium*. A vertical section through the broad ligament shows that its upper part is made up mainly of three branches, in which the tube, ovary, and round ligaments are situated. Its lower portion is not ordinarily so thick as in the section shown in Figure 16.

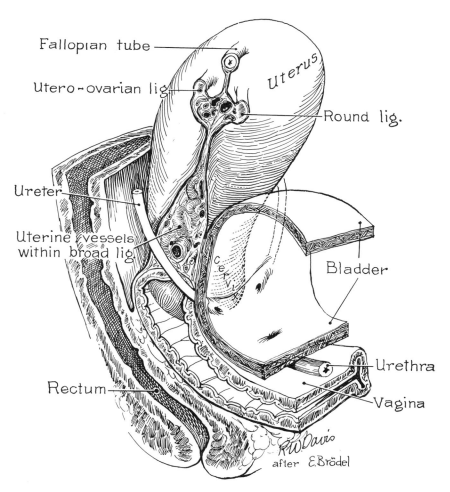

Fig. 16. Section through uterine end of broad ligament.

The *round ligaments* extend on either side from the anterior and lateral portion of the uterus just below the insertion of the tubes. Each lies in a fold of peritoneum continuous with the broad ligament and runs upward and outward to the inguinal canal, through which it passes, to terminate in the upper portion of the labium majus. The round ligament, in the absence of pregnancy, varies from 3 to 5 mm in diameter; it is composed of smooth muscle, which is directly continuous with that of the uterine wall, and a certain amount of connective tissue. Peripherally, in the inguinal canal, it may contain a few fibers of striated muscle. It corresponds to the gubernaculum testis of the male. In the nonpregnant condition it is a lax cord, but in pregnancy it undergoes considerable hypertrophy.

The *uterosacral ligaments* extend from the posterior and upper portion of the cervix, encircle the rectum, and are inserted into the fascia over the second and third sacral vertebrae. They are composed of connective tissue and muscle and are covered by peritoneum. They form the lateral boundaries of the cul-de-sac, or pouch of Douglas, and aid in retaining the uterus in its normal position by exerting traction upon the cervix.

Position of the Uterus.   The usual position of the uterus is slight anteflexion. When the woman is standing upright the uterus is almost horizontal and is somewhat flexed anteriorly, the fundus resting upon the bladder, whereas the cervix is directed backward toward the tip of the sacrum with the external os approximately at the level of the ischial spines. The position of the organ varies from that described according to the degree of distention of the bladder and rectum.

The normal uterus is a partially mobile organ. The cervix is anchored, but the body of the uterus is free to move in the anteroposterior plane. Posture and gravity therefore determine somewhat the position of the uterus. The forward tilt of the pelvis in the erect position probably results in the usually anterior position of the uterus.

The base of the broad ligament contains dense connective tissue, which is reflected laterally on the side of the pelvis and medially is firmly united to the supravaginal portion of the cervix. This parametrial connective tissue, usually called the *cardinal ligament,* is of importance in supporting the uterus. The upper portion of the broad ligament, which contains only scant loose connective tissue, does not influence the position of the uterus. The paravaginal connective tissue shares with the parametrial tissue the function of uterine support.

Blood Vessels of the Uterus.   The vascular supply of the uterus is derived principally from the uterine and ovarian arteries. The uterine artery, a main branch of the hypogastric (Fig. 17), after descending for a short distance, enters the base of the broad ligament, crosses over the ureter, and makes its way to the side of the uterus. Just before reaching the supravaginal portion of the cervix the uterine artery divides into two branches. The smaller cervicovaginal artery supplies the lower portion of the cervix and the upper portion of the vagina. The main branch turns abruptly upward and extends as a highly convoluted vessel along the margin of the uterus, giving off a branch of considerable size to the upper portion of the cervix and numerous smaller branches that penetrate the body of the uterus. Just before reaching the tube it divides into three terminal branches: the fundal, tubal, and ovarian. The ovarian branch anastomoses with the terminal branch of the ovarian artery; the tubal, making its way through the mesosalpinx, supplies the tube; and the fundal branch is distributed to the upper portion of the uterus.

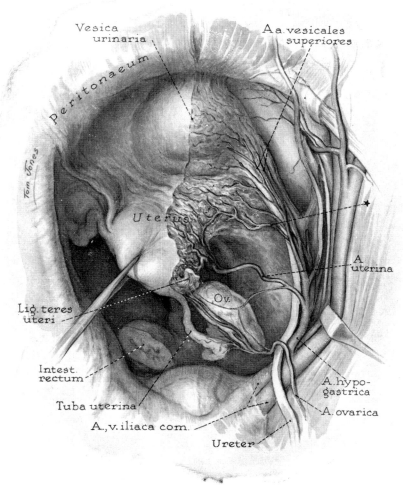

Fig. 17. Blood vessels of the uterus and pelvis. Star indicates vaginal artery. (From Curtis, Anson, Ashley, and Jones. Surg Gynec Obstet 75:421, 1942.)

After traversing the broad ligament, the uterine artery reaches the uterus approximately at the level of the internal os. About 2 cm to the side of the uterus it crosses over the ureter, as shown in Figures 8 and 18. The proximity of the uterine artery to the ureter at this point is of great surgical significance, because during hysterectomy the ureter may be injured or ligated in the process of clamping and tying the uterine vessels.

The ovarian artery, a direct branch of the aorta, enters the broad ligament through the infundibulopelvic ligament. On reaching the ovarian hilum it divides into a number of smaller branches that enter the ovary, whereas its main stem traverses the entire length of the broad ligament and makes its way to the upper portion of the margin of the uterus, where it anastomoses with the ovarian branch of the uterine artery. There are numerous additional communications between the vessels of the two sides of the uterus.

When the uterus is contracted the lumens of the abundant veins are collapsed,

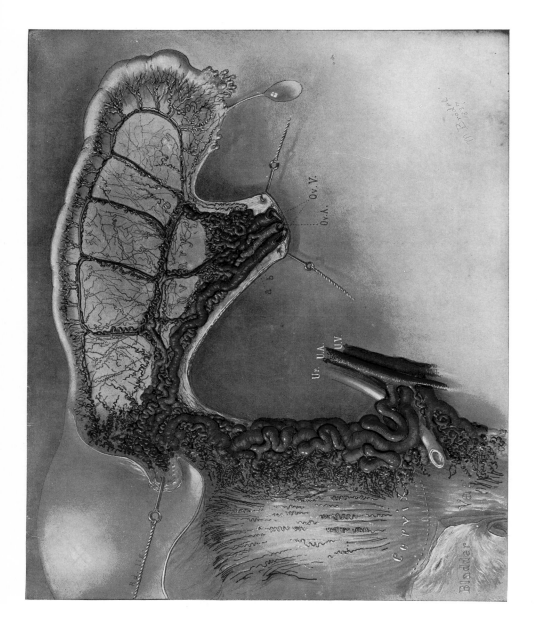

Fig. 18. Blood supply of uterus, tubes, and ovaries.

but in injected specimens the greater part of the uterine wall appears to be composed of dilated venous sinuses. On either side, the arcuate veins unite to form the uterine vein, which empties into the hypogastric vein and thence into the common iliac vein. The blood from the ovary and upper part of the broad ligament is collected by several veins that, within the broad ligament, form the large *pampiniform plexus,* the vessels from which terminate in the ovarian vein. The right ovarian vein empties into the vena cava, whereas the left empties into the left renal vein.

Lymphatics. The endometrium is abundantly supplied with lymphatics, but true lymphatic vessels are confined largely to the base. The lymphatics of the underlying myometrium increase toward the serosal surface and form an abundant lymphatic plexus just beneath it, especially on the posterior wall of the uterus and, to a lesser extent, anteriorly.

The lymphatics from the various portions of the uterus drain into several sets of nodes. Those from the cervix terminate mainly in the hypogastric nodes, which are situated at the bifurcation of the common iliac vessels between the external iliac and hypogastric arteries. The lymphatics from the body of the uterus are distributed to two groups of nodes. One set of vessels drains into the hypogastric nodes. The other set, after joining certain lymphatics from the ovarian region, terminates in the lumbar nodes, which are situated in front of the aorta at about the level of the lower pole of the kidneys.

Innervation. The abundant nerve supply of the uterus appears to be regulatory rather than primary. In experimental animals labor may progress satisfactorily after all nerves to the uterus have been severed; furthermore, human patients who become pregnant after transection of the spinal cord often have normal uterine activity during labor.

The nerve supply is derived principally from the sympathetic nervous system, but partly also from the cerebrospinal and parasympathetic systems (Fig. 19). The parasympathetic system is represented on either side by the pelvic nerve, which consists of a few fibers derived from the second, third, and fourth sacral nerves; it loses its identity in the cervical ganglion of Frankenhäuser. The sympathetic system enters the pelvis through the hypogastric plexus, which arises from the aortic plexus just below the promontory of the sacrum. After descending on either side, it also enters the uterovaginal plexus of Frankenhäuser, which consists of ganglia of varying size, but particularly of a large ganglionic plate situated on either side of the cervix just above the posterior fornix and in front of the rectum. Latarjet and Rochet state that Frankenhäuser's ganglion actually lies posterior to the cervix in the base of the uterosacral ligament.

Branches from these plexuses supply the uterus, bladder, and upper part of the vagina and comprise both myelinated and nonmyelinated fibers. Some of them terminate freely between the muscular fibers, whereas others accompany the arteries into the endometrium.

Both the sympathetic and parasympathetic nerves contain motor and a few sensory fibers. The sympathetic fibers cause muscular contraction and vasoconstriction, whereas the parasympathetics inhibit contraction and lead to vasodilatation. Since the Frankenhäuser plexus is derived from both sources, it has certain functions of both components of the autonomic nervous system. Mahon concluded that the sympathetic nerves maintain the tonus, and the parasympathetics affect the intermittent contractions of the uterus.

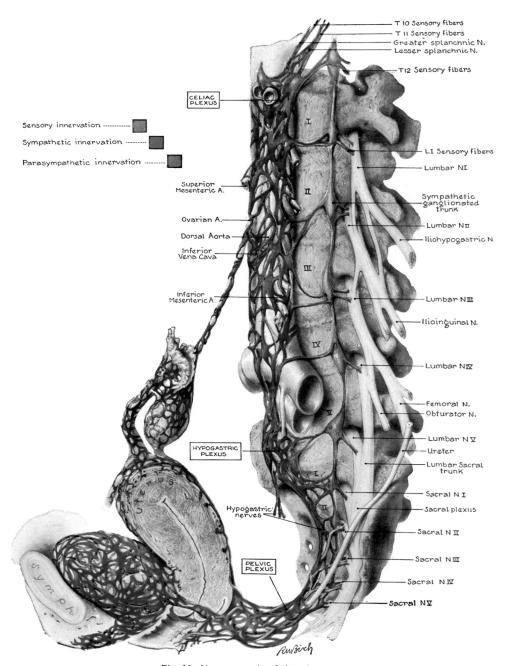

Fig. 19. Nerve supply of the uterus.

The nerve supply of the pelvic viscera is of clinical interest in that many types of pelvic pain may be permanently relieved by severing the hypogastric plexus. The eleventh and twelfth thoracic nerve roots carry sensory fibers from the uterus, transmitting pain of uterine contractions to the central nervous system. The sensory nerves from the cervix and upper part of the birth canal pass through the pelvic nerves to the second, third, and fourth sacral, whereas those from the lower portion of the canal pass through the ilioinguinal and pudendal nerves. The motor fibers to the uterus leave the spinal cord at the level of the seventh and eighth thoracic vertebrae. This separation of motor and sensory levels permits the use of caudal and spinal anesthesia in labor.

Development of the Uterus. The uterus and tubes arise from the müllerian ducts, which first appear near the upper pole of the urogenital ridge in the fifth week of development in embryos 10 to 11 mm long. This ridge consists of the mesonephros, the gonad, and their ducts. The first indication of the müllerian duct is a thickening of the celomic epithelium at the level of the fourth thoracic segment. The thickening becomes the fimbriated extremity (infundibulum) of the fallopian tube, invaginating and growing caudally to form a slender tube at the lateral edge of the urogenital ridge. In the sixth week the growing tips of the two müllerian ducts approach each other in the midline, reaching the sinus a week later (embryos of 30 mm). At that time the two müllerian ducts have begun to fuse at the level of the inguinal crest, or gubernaculum (primordium of the round ligament), to form a single canal. The upper ends of the ducts thus produce the fallopian tubes, the fused part giving rise to the uterus. The uterine lumen is completed from the fundus to the vagina during the third month. According to Koff, the vaginal canal is not patent throughout its length until the sixth month.

The Fallopian Tubes. The fallopian tubes, or oviducts, extending from the uterine cornua to the ovaries, are the ducts through which ova gain access to the uterine cavity. The oviducts vary from 8 to 14 cm in length, are covered by peritoneum, and have a lumen lined by mucous membrane. Each tube is divided into an interstitial portion, isthmus, ampulla, and infundibulum. The *interstitial* portion is included within the muscular wall of the uterus. Its course is roughly obliquely upward and outward from the uterine cavity. Blanchard has described variations in its course and length from 0.8 to 2 cm with a diameter of the lumen from 0.5 to 1 mm. The isthmus, or the narrow portion of the tube adjoining the uterus, gradually passes into the wider lateral portion, or *ampulla.* The *infundibulum,* or fimbriated extremity, is the funnel-shaped opening of the distal end of the tube (Figs. 20 and 21). The tube varies considerably in thickness, the narrowest portion of the isthmus measuring from 2 to 3 mm and the widest portion of the ampulla from 5 to 8 mm in diameter.

With the exception of its uterine portion the tube throughout its entire length is covered with peritoneum, which is continuous with the upper margin of the broad ligament. It is completely surrounded by peritoneum except at its lower portion, to which the mesosalpinx is attached. The fimbriated extremity opens into the abdominal cavity. One projection, the *fimbria ovarica,* which is considerably longer than the others, forms a shallow gutter, which approaches or reaches the ovary. The musculature of the tube is in general arranged in two layers, an inner circular and an outer longitudinal layer. In the distal portion of the tube the two layers become less distinct and, near the fimbriated extremity,

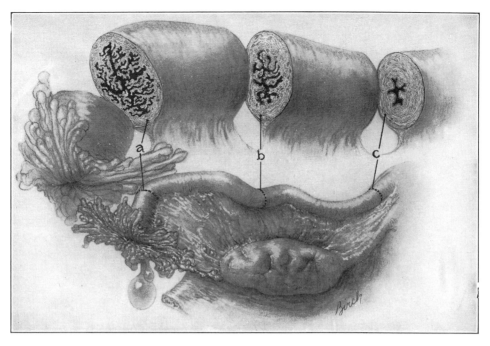

Fig. 20. The fallopian tube in cross section showing the gross structure of the epithelium in several portions: a, infundibulum; b, ampulla; and c, isthmus.

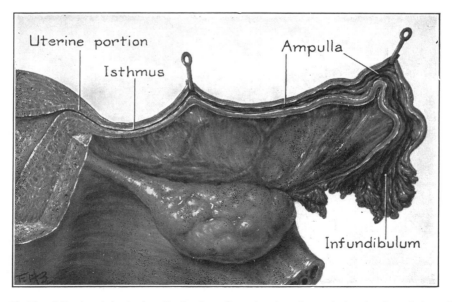

Fig. 21. The fallopian tube in longitudinal section, showing the variation in size of the tubal lumen, the longitudinal folds, and the relations of the tube to the mesosalpinx, the uterine cornu, and ovary.

are replaced by an interlacing network of muscular fibers. The tubal musculature is constantly undergoing rhythmic contractions, the rate of which varies with phases of the menstrual cycle. The contractions occur with greatest frequency and intensity during transport of ova, and are slowest and weakest during pregnancy. The contractions are influenced by hormones. The propagation of the waves of contraction is apparently facilitated by the nerves. The tube is lined by a mucous membrane, the epithelium of which is composed of a single layer of columnar cells, some ciliated and some secretory, which rest upon a thin basement membrane. The ciliated cells are most abundant at the fimbriated extremity; elsewhere they form discrete patches. There are differences in the proportions of these two types of cells in different phases of the cycle. Since there is no submucosa, the epithelium is in intimate contact with the underlying muscle. Only occasionally does it adjoin intermuscular strands of connective tissue.

The mucosa is arranged in longitudinal folds, which become more complicated toward the fimbriated end. Consequently, the appearance of the lumen varies from one portion of the tube to another. Cross sections through the uterine portion reveal four simple folds, forming a figure that resembles a Maltese cross. The isthmus is more complicated. In the ampulla the lumen is almost completely occupied by the arborescent mucosa, which consists of very complicated folds (Fig. 22).

The current produced by the tubal cilia is directed toward the uterus. Indeed, minute foreign bodies introduced into the abdominal cavities of animals eventually appear in the vagina after making their way down through the tubes and the cavity of the uterus. Tubal peristalsis is another important factor in transport of the ovum.

The tubes are richly supplied with elastic tissue, blood vessels, and lymphatics. Occasionally dilated lymphatics may occupy the entire substance of a tubal fold.

Diverticula may occasionally extend from the lumen of the tube for a variable distance into its muscular wall and reach almost to its serosa. They may play a role in the development of ectopic pregnancy (Ch. 21).

The tubal mucosa undergoes cyclic histologic changes similar to, but much less striking than, those in the endometrium. The postmenstrual phase is characterized by a low epithelium that rapidly increases in height. During the follicular phase the cells are taller; the ciliated elements are broad with nuclei near the margin, and the nonciliated cells are narrow with nuclei nearer the base. In the luteal phase the secretory cells enlarge, project beyond the ciliated cells, and extrude their nuclei. In the menstrual phase these changes become even more marked. Both Hellman and Andrews have shown characteristic changes in the fallopian tubes during late pregnancy and the puerperium, including a low mucosa, plugging of the capillaries with leukocytes, and a decidual reaction. If estrogen is given in the puerperium the mucosal cells increase in height. The secretory cells decrease in height and lose much of their cytoplasm, and some appear peglike. These cyclic changes in the tubal mucosa and the associated alteration in contractility of the tubal musculature may both be the result of changing proportions of estrogen and progesterone.

The pertinent gross anatomic, histologic, and ultrastructural information about the human fallopian tube is well summarized in the recent book by Woodruff and

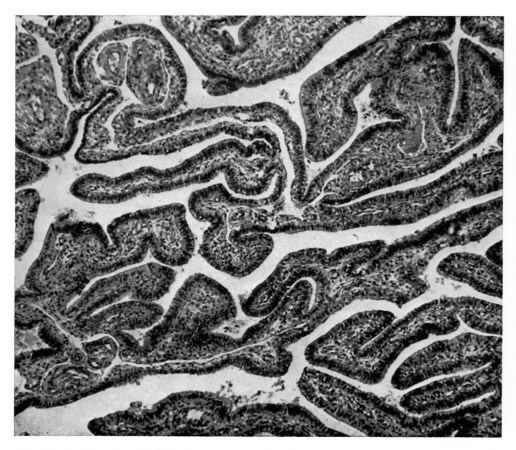

Fig. 22. Section through fallopian tube near fimbriated extremity, showing complexity of rugae.

Pauerstein. The ciliated and secretory cells described by Hashimoto and co-workers have now been studied by electron microscopy in several laboratories. These two cell types, as well as intercalary elements, have been identified (Fig. 23). Ultrastructural changes in the fallopian tube during the menstrual cycle have not been so consistent as those described in the human endometrium. Cyclic changes in tubal cilia, as well as differences among the various portions of the oviduct, of the rhesus monkey have recently been studied by Brenner.

The Ovaries.   *Gross Anatomy.*   The ovaries are more or less almond-shaped organs, the chief functions of which are the development and extrusion of ova and the elaboration of steroidal hormones. They vary considerably in size. During the childbearing period they measure from 2.5 to 5 cm in length, 1.5 to 3 cm in breadth, and 0.6 to 1.5 cm in thickness. After the menopause they diminish mark-edly in size, and in old women they often measure scarcely more than 0.5 cm in each diameter.

Normally the ovaries are situated in the upper part of the pelvic cavity, resting in a slight depression on the lateral wall of the pelvis between the divergent external iliac and hypogastric vessels—the ovarian fossa of Waldeyer. When the

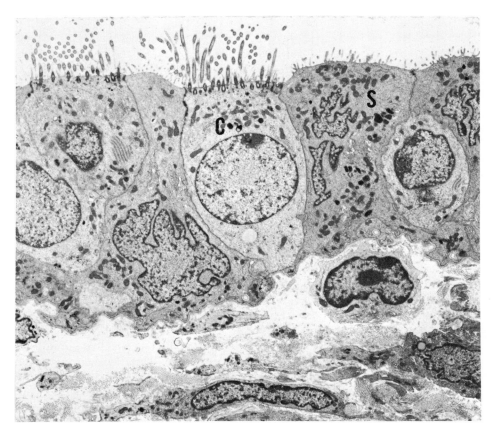

Fig. 23. Electron micrograph of human fallopian tube 48 hours postpartum. Ciliated (C) and secretory (S) cells are easily distinguished. × 4,500. (Courtesy of Dr. Ralph M. Wynn.)

woman is standing, the long axes of the ovaries are almost vertical, but they become horizontal when she is on her back. Their situation, however, is subject to marked variations, and it is rare to find both ovaries at exactly the same level.

The surface of the ovary in contact with the ovarian fossa is called the lateral, and that directed toward the uterus is known as the medial surface. The margin attached to the mesovarium is more or less straight and is designated the hilum, whereas the free margin is convex and is directed backward and inward toward the rectum.

The ovary is attached to the broad ligament by the *mesovarium*. The *ovarian ligament* extends from the lateral and posterior portion of the uterus, just beneath the tubal insertion, to the uterine, or lower pole, of the ovary. It is usually several centimeters long and 3 to 4 mm in diameter. It is covered by peritoneum and is made up of muscle and connective tissue fibers continuous with those of the uterus. The *infundibulopelvic* or *suspensory ligament of the ovary* extends from the upper, or tubal, pole to the pelvic wall. Through it course the ovarian vessels and nerves.

For the most part the ovary projects into the abdominal cavity and is free of a peritoneal covering except near its hilum, where a narrow band may be found continuous with the peritoneum covering the mesosalpinx. The greater part of its surface is dull white and moist.

The exterior of the ovary varies in appearance with age. In young women the organ presents a smooth, dull white surface through which glisten several small, clear follicles. As the woman grows older it becomes more corrugated, and in elderly women its exterior may be markedly convoluted.

The general structure of the ovary can best be studied in cross sections, in which two portions may be distinguished, the *cortex* and the *medulla*. The cortex, or outer layer, varies in thickness with age, thinning with advancing years. In this layer the ova and graafian follicles are located. It is composed of spindle-shaped connective tissue cells and fibers, among which are scattered primordial and graafian follicles in various stages of development. The follicles become less numerous as the woman grows older. The outermost portion of the cortex, which is dull and whitish, is designated the *tunica albuginea*. On its surface is a single layer of cuboidal epithelium, the germinal epithelium of Waldeyer.

The medulla, or central portion, of the ovary is composed of loose connective tissue, which is continuous with that of the mesovarium. It contains a large number of arteries and veins and a small number of smooth muscle fibers continuous with those in the suspensory ligament. The muscle may function in movements of the ovary.

Both sympathetic and parasympathetic nerves supply the ovaries. The sympathetic nerves are derived in great part from the ovarian plexus, which accompanies the ovarian vessels; a few are derived from the plexus surrounding the ovarian branch of the uterine artery. The ovary is richly supplied with nonmyelinated nerve fibers, which for the most part accompany the blood vessels. They are merely vascular nerves, whereas others form wreaths around normal and atretic follicles, giving off many minute branches that have been traced up to, but not through, the membrana granulosa.

Accessory Ovaries. Accessory bodies are occasionally found near the main ovary. These structures are usually small, although rarely they may attain considerable size. Frequently they result from peritoneal bands that cut off small portions of the ovary from the main body of the organ during fetal life.

Major has described ureteral obstruction caused by a retroperitoneal corpus luteum that arose from an ovarian remnant.

Development of the Ovary. The developmental changes in the human urogenital system have been followed from the third week after conception to maturity. At first the changes are the same in both sexes. The earliest sign of a gonad appears on the ventral surface of the embryonic kidney between the eighth thoracic and fourth lumbar segments at about four weeks. As Figure 24A shows, the peritoneal epithelium has thickened, and clumps of cells bud off into the underlying mesenchyme. This circumscribed area of the peritoneum is often called the *germinal epithelium*. At the fourth week, however, the region contains many large ameboid cells that have migrated into the body of the embryo from the yolk sac, where they have been recognized as early as the third week. These *primordial germ cells* are distinguished by their size and certain morphologic and cytochemical features. They react strongly in tests for alkaline phosphatase (McKay, Robinson, and Hertig) and are recognizable even after repeated divisions. Primordial germ cells have been studied in many animals. If these cells are destroyed before they have begun to migrate or if they are prevented from reaching the genital area, a "gonad" lacking germ cells will develop.

When the primordial germ cells reach the genital area, some enter the germinal epithelium and others mingle with the groups of cells proliferated from it or lie in the mesenchyme. Rapid division of all these types of cells results in development of a prominent *genital ridge* by the end of the fifth week. It projects into the body cavity medial to a fold that contains the mesonephric (wolffian) and the müllerian ducts (Fig. 24B). Since the growth of the gonad is most rapid at the surface, it enlarges centrifugally. By the seventh week (Fig. 24C) it has separated from the mesonephros except at the narrow central zone, the future hilum, where the blood vessels enter. At that time the sexes can be distinguished, since the testis can be recognized by well-defined radiating strands of cells (sex cords). They are separated from the germinal epithelium by mesenchyme that becomes the tunica albuginea. The sex cords, consisting of large germ cells and smaller epithelioid cells derived from the germinal epithelium, develop into the seminiferous tubules and tubuli recti. The rete, probably derived from mesonephric elements, establishes connection with the mesonephric tubules that develop into the epididymis. The mesonephric duct becomes the vas deferens.

In the female the germinal epithelium continues to proliferate for a much longer period. The groups of cells thus formed lie at first in the region of the hilum. As connective tissue develops between them, they appear as sex cords. They give rise to the medullary cords and persist for variable periods (Forbes). By the third month, medulla and cortex are defined as in Figure 24D. The bulk of the organ consists of cortex, a mass of crowded germ and epithelioid cells that show some signs of grouping, but there are no distinct cords as in the testis. Strands of cells extend from the germinal epithelium into the cortical mass, and mitoses are numerous. The rapid succession of mitoses soon reduces the size of the germ cells to the extent that they are no longer clearly differentiated from their neighbors. They are then called *oogonia*. Some of them in the medullary region are soon distinguished by a series of peculiar nuclear changes. Large masses of nuclear chromatin appear, very different from the chromosomes of the oogonial divisions. This change marks the beginning of *synapsis*, which involves interactions between pairs of chromosomes derived originally from father and mother. Various stages of synapsis can soon be seen throughout the cortex. Since similar changes occur in adjacent cells, groups (or "nests") appear. During one stage of synapsis the chromatin is massed at one side of the nucleus, and the cytoplasm becomes highly fluid. Unless the preservation is prompt and perfect, these cells appear to be degenerating. Such artifacts have frequently been misinterpreted as evidence of widespread degeneration among oogonia.

By the fourth month some germ cells, again in the medullary region, having passed through synapsis, have begun to enlarge. They are called *primary oocytes* (Fig. 25) at the beginning of the phase of growth that continues until they reach maturity. During this period of growth many oocytes undergo degeneration, both before and after birth. The primary oocytes soon become surrounded by a single layer of flattened *follicle* cells (Ch. 3, Fig. 1) derived originally from the germinal epithelium. They are then called *primordial follicles* and are seen first in the medulla and later in the cortex. Some begin to grow even before birth, and some are believed to persist in the cortex almost unchanged until the menopause.

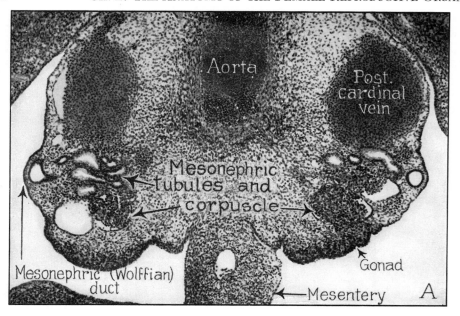

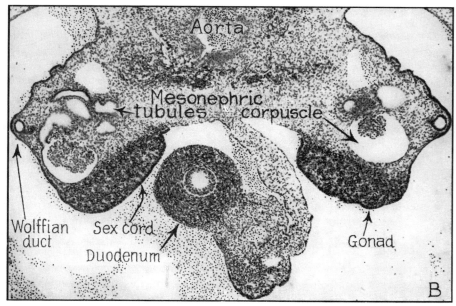

Fig. 24. Photomicrographs of sections of human embryos showing relations of gonads and metanephros. A, 11 mm embryo from fifth week after ovulation taken at level of arm bud. (Carnegie Collection No. 8773.) B, 14.2 mm embryo of five weeks from same level as A. Active proliferation has thickened gonad, which is still spread out on surface of mesonephros. On left, renal corpuscle opens into tubule. (Carnegie Collection No. 6520.)

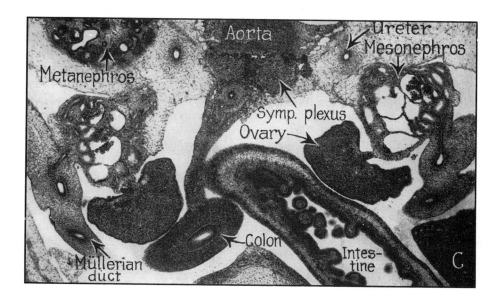

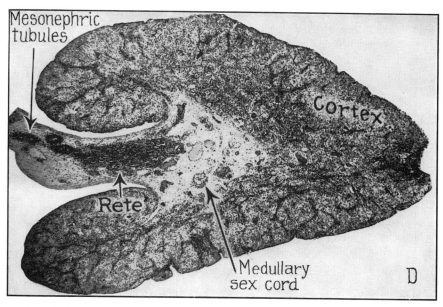

Fig. 24. (cont.). C, 31.5 mm embryo of seven weeks taken at level of duodenum. Ovary has separated from mesonephros and appears homogeneous in structure. At right a collecting tubule enters wolffian duct. (Carnegie Collection No. 6573.) D, five and a half month fetus, median section of ovary. Mesonephric tubules now included in mesovarium. Large mass of rete ovarii tubules, sex cords, and blood vessels in medulla. Cortex with nests of oocytes in stages of synapsis. Forbes 12-11A.)

By eight months the ovary has become a long, narrow, lobulated structure attached to the body wall along the line of the hilum by the *mesovarium*, in which lies the *epoophoron*. The germinal epithelium at that stage has been separated for the most part from the cortex by a band of connective tissue (tunica albuginea), which is absent in many small areas where strands of cells, usually referred to as cords of Pflüger, are in contact with the germinal epithelium. Among them are cells believed by many to be oogonia that have come to resemble the other epithelial cells as a result of repeated mitoses. The underlying cortex has two distinct zones. Superficially there are nests of germ cells in synapsis, interspersed with Pflüger cords and strands of connective tissue. In the deeper zone there are many groups of germ cells in synapsis, as well as primary oocytes, prospective follicle cells, and a few primordial follicles. There are in addition numerous scattered degenerating cells, although this zone is well vascularized. Such cellular degeneration is regularly present at certain stages in various rapidly growing regions of normal embryos.

At term the various types of ovarian cells may still be found. In some cases there are vesicular follicles in the medulla, which are all doomed to early degeneration. In some mammals oogonia have been recognized even during sexual maturity, and the cyclic production of crops of primary oocytes has been described (Allen in mouse; Evans and Swezy in rat, dog, cat, and guinea pig).

Microscopic Structure of Ovary. From the first stages of its development until after the menopause the ovary undergoes constant change. The number of oocytes at birth has been variously estimated at 100,000 to 600,000 (see Ch.

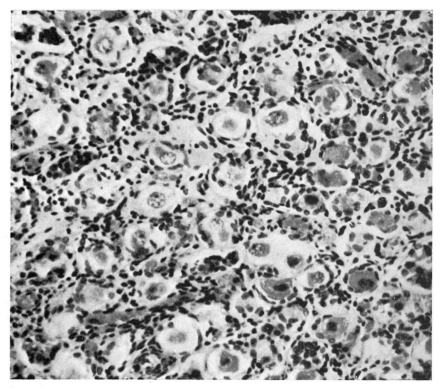

Fig. 25. Ovary of newborn child. Numerous primordial follicles are seen.

5, p. 113). The duration of the period of atresia for a given follicle is unknown, although such data are essential to resolution of the question of neogenesis of ova in the adult. Since only one ovum is ordinarily cast off during a menstrual cycle, it is evident that a few hundred ova suffice for reproduction. The mode by which the others disappear is discussed in the section dealing with the corpus luteum and follicular atresia (Ch. 3, p. 72).

Mossman and co-workers, in an attempt to clarify the terminology of glandular elements in adult human ovaries, distinguish interstitial, thecal, and luteal cells. The interstitial glandular elements are formed from cells of the theca interna of degenerating or atretic follicles; the thecal glandular cells are formed from the theca interna of ripening follicles; and the true luteal cells are derived from granulosal cells of ovulated follicles and from undifferentiated stroma surrounding them.

The huge store of primordial follicles at birth is gradually exhausted during the period of sexual maturity. Block has demonstrated a gradual decline from a mean of 439,000 oocytes in girls under 15 years to a mean of 34,000 in women over the age of 36. Allen, as well as Evans and Swezy, however, adduced evidence that in certain mammals oogenesis is a rhythmic process beginning before puberty and extending throughout sexual maturity and that all ova reaching maturity are of recent origin. Öhler and others, on the contrary, have refuted the concept of continued oogenesis in higher mammals including man. (For further discussion, see page 113)

In the young child the greater portion of the ovary is composed of the cortex, which is filled with large numbers of closely packed primordial follicles. Those nearest the central portion of the ovary are at the most advanced stages of development. In young women the cortex is relatively thinner but still contains a large number of primordial follicles separated by bands of connective tissue cells with spindle-shaped or oval nuclei. Each primordial follicle consists of an oocyte and its surrounding single layer of epithelial cells, which are small and flattened, spindle-shaped, and somewhat sharply differentiated from the still smaller spindly cells of the surrounding stroma (Fig. 25).

The oocyte is a single large roundish cell with a clear cytoplasm and a relatively large nucleus near the center. There are one large and several smaller nucleoli, and numerous masses of chromatin. The diameter of the smallest oocytes in the adult average 0.033 mm, and that of the nuclei, 0.020 mm (see Ch. 3, Fig. 1).

REFERENCES

Allen, E.   Ovogenesis during sexual maturity. Amer J Anat 31:439, 1923.

Andrews, M. C.   Epithelial changes in the puerperal fallopian tube. Amer J Obstet Gynec 62:28, 1951.

Bergman, R. A.   Uterine smooth muscle fibers in castrate and estrogen-treated rats. J Cell Biol 36:639, 1968.

Blanchard, O.   Histopathologic study of interstitial segment of Fallopian tube, Buenos Aires Universidad Nacional Fac. des Cien. Med Rev 2:1, 1955.

Block, E.   Quantitative morphological investigation of the follicular system in women. Acta Anat 14:108, 1952.

Bo, W. J., Odor, D. L., and Rothrock, M. L.   Ultrastructure of uterine smooth muscle following progesterone or progesterone-estrogen treatment. Anat Rec 163:121, 1969.

Brenner, R. M.   Renewal of oviduct cilia during the menstrual cycle of the rhesus monkey. Fertil Steril 20:599, 1969.

Buckingham, J. C., Buethe, R. A., Jr., and Danforth, D. N.   Collagen-muscle ratio in clinically normal and clinically incompetent cervices. Amer J Obstet Gynec 91:232, 1965.

Curtis, A. H., Anson, B. J., Ashley, F. L., and Jones, T.   Blood vessels of the female pelvis in relation to gynecological surgery. Surg Gynec Obstet 75:421, 1942.

Danforth, D. N.   The fibrous nature of the human cervix and its relation to the isthmic segment in gravid and nongravid uteri. Amer J Obstet Gynec 53:541, 1947.

———— Buckingham, J. C., and Roddick, J. W., Jr.   Connective tissue changes incident to cervical effacement. Amer J Obstet Gynec 80:939, 1960.

Davies, J., and Kusama, H.   Developmental aspects of the human cervix. Ann NY Acad Sci 97:534, 1962-1963.

———— and Woolf, R. B.   Histology and fine structure of the adult human cervix uteri. Clin Obstet Gynec 6:265, 1963.

Evans, H. M., and Swezy, O.   Ovogenesis and normal follicular cycle in adult mammalia. Mem Univ Calif 9:119, 1931.

Fluhmann, C. F.   The nature and development of the so-called glands of the cervix uteri. Amer J Obstet Gynec 74:753, 1957.

Forbes, T. R.   On the fate of the medullary cords of the human ovary. Contrib Embryol 30:9, 1942.

Forsberg, J. G.   Origin of vaginal epithelium. Obstet Gynec 25:787, 1965.

Hashimoto, M., Komori, A., Kosaka, M., Mori, Y., Shimoyama, T., and Akashi, K.   Electron microscopic studies on the smooth muscle of the human uterus. J Jap Obstet Gynec Soc 7:115, 1960.

———— Shimoyama, T., Kosaka, M., Komori, A., Hirasawa, T., Yokoyama, Y., and Akashi, K. Electron microscopic studies on the epithelial cells of the human fallopian tube. (Report I.) J Jap Obstet Gynec Soc 9:200, 1962.

———— Shimoyama, T., Kosaka, M., Komori, A., Hirasawa, T., Yokoyama, Y., Kawase, N., and Nakamura, T.   Electron microscopic studies on the epithelial cells of the human fallopian tube. (Report II.) J Jap Obstet Gynec Soc 11:92, 1964.

Hellman, L. M.   The morphology of the human fallopian tube in the early puerperium. Amer J Obstet Gynec 57:154, 1949.

Hitschmann, F., and Adler, L.   (The structure of the endometrium of the sexually mature woman). Mschr Geburtsh Gynaek 27:1, 1908.

Koff, A. K.   Development of the vagina in the human fetus. Contrib Embryol 24:59, 1933.

Krantz, K. E.   Innervation of the human vulva and vagina. Obstet Gynec 12:382, 1958.

Laguens, R. P., Lagrutta, J., Koch, O. R., and Quijano, F.   Fine structure of human endocervical epithelium. Amer J Obstet Gynec 98:773, 1967.

Langlois, P. L.   The size of the normal uterus. J Reprod Med 4:220, 1970.

Latarjet, A., and Rochet, P.   (The hypogastric plexus in women). Gynec Obstet 6:225, 1922.

Mahon, R.   (Extraperitoneal ruptures of the dome of the bladder of obstetric origin). Gynec Obstet 39:19, 1939.

Mahran, M., and Saleh, A. M.   The microscopic anatomy of the hymen. Anat Rec 149:313, 1964.

Major, F. J.   Retained ovarian remnant causing ureteral obstruction. Obstet Gynec 32:748, 1968.

McKay, D. G., Robinson, D., and Hertig, A. T.   Histochemical observations on granulosa-cell tumors, thecomas and fibromas of the ovary. Amer J Obstet Gynec 58:625, 1949.

Milley, P. S., and Nichols, D. H.   A correlative investigation of the human rectovaginal septum. Anat Rec 163:443, 1969.

Mossman, H. W., Koering, M. J., and Ferry, D., Jr.   Cyclic changes in interstitial gland tissue of the human ovary. Amer J Anat 115:235, 1964.

Needham, D. M., and Shoenberg, C. F.   Biochemistry of the myometrium, in Cellular Biology of the Uterus, R. M. Wynn (ed.). New York, Appleton-Century-Crofts, 1967, Ch. 9.

Nemetschek-Gansler, H.   Ultrastructure of the myometrium, in Cellular Biology of the Uterus, R. M. Wynn (ed.). New York, Appleton-Century-Crofts, 1967, Ch. 10.

Öhler, I.   (Contribution to the knowledge of the ovarian epithelium and its relationship to oogenesis). Acta Anat 12:1, 1951.

Okkels, H., and Engle, E. T.   Studies on finer structure of uterine blood vessels of Macacus monkey. Acta Path Microbiol Scand 15:150, 1938.

Rakoff, A. E., Feo, L. G., and Goldstein, L.   The biologic characteristics of the normal vagina. Amer J Obstet Gynec 47:467, 1944.

Roberts, W. H., Habenicht, J., and Krishingner, G.   The pelvic and perineal fasciae and their neural and vascular relationships. Anat Rec 149:707, 1964.

Schueller, E. F.   Ciliated epithelia of the human uterine mucosa. Obstet Gynec 31:215, 1968.

Schwalm, H., and Dubrauszky, V.   The structure of the musculature of the human uterus-muscles and connective tissue. Amer J Obstet Gynec 94:391, 1966.

Skene, A. J. C.   The anatomy and pathology of two important glands of the female urethra. Amer J Obstet 13:265, 1880.

Stegner, H. E., and Beltermann, R.   (The electron microscopy of the endocervical gland epithelium and the so-called reserve cells.) Arch Gynaek 207:480, 1969.

Warren, J. W., Dockerty, M. B., Wilson, R. B., and Welch, J. S.   Basement membrane in the uterine cervix. Amer J Obstet Gynec 95:23, 1966.

Wharton, F.   Criminal Law, 12th ed. Rochester, New York, Lawyer's Co-operative Publishing Company, 1932, Vol. I, pp. 698–700. Sect. 465: Neglect and Injury: Ch. 14: Homicide.

Woodruff, J. D., and Pauerstein, C. J.   The Fallopian Tube. Baltimore, The Williams & Wilkins Co., 1969.

Yokoyama, Y.   An electronmicroscope study of the human uterine smooth muscle cells. J Jap Obstet Gynec Soc 15:122, 1968.

Younes, M. S., Robertson, E. M., and Bencosme, S. A.   Electron microscope observations on Langerhans cells in the cervix. Amer J Obstet Gynec 102:397, 1968.

———— Steele, H. D., Robertson, E. M., and Bencosme, S. A.   Correlative light and electron microscope study of the basement membrane of the human ectocervix. Amer J Obstet Gynec 92:163, 1965.

3

THE OVARIAN CYCLE AND ITS HORMONES

This chapter and the next are devoted to the closely integrated and synchronized phenomena normally involving the ovary and endometrium of the non-pregnant woman each month during her reproductive years. Teleologically, the purpose of the ovarian cycle is to provide an ovum for fertilization, whereas that of the endometrial cycle is to furnish a suitable bed in which the fertilized ovum may implant and develop. Since, however, the endometrial changes are regulated by the ovarian hormones, the two cycles are very closely related.

Both the ovarian and menstrual cycles extend from the first day of one menstrual period to the first day of the next. The typical human female sexual cycle is 28 days, although variations are common and normal (Ch. 4, p. 99).

Development of the Follicle.   Throughout the reproductive years, and in childhood to a lesser degree, certain primordial follicles show evidence of growth and development (Fig. 1). As the oocyte increases in size the surrounding follic-

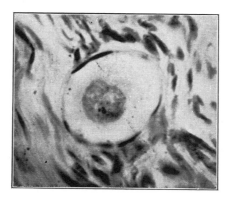

Fig. 1. Primordial follicle from adult ovary.

ular cells become cuboidal and their nuclei appear to be arranged in several layers (Figs. 2 and 3). The follicular growth soon becomes eccentric, causing the oocyte to lie at one side of the ball of follicular cells. Fluid accumulates be-

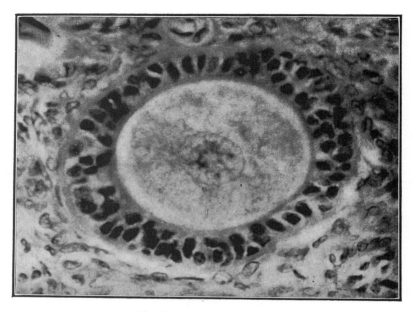

Fig. 2. Developing follicle.

tween the cells, forming a vesicle, with the ovum at one side (Fig. 4). While the follicle is still very small, a clear elastic membrane, the *zona pellucida,* appears about the ovum (Figs. 5 and 6). The zone pellucida envelops the ovum and probably persists until after it has reached the uterus. The mature follicle is known as a *graafian follicle,* after de Graaf, who discovered it in 1672. The follicular or granulosa cells that immediately surround the ovum constitute the *cumulus oophorus* or *discus proligerus,* which projects into the abundant follicular fluid of the antrum. As the graafian follicle grows, the surrounding stromal cells enlarge and the capillary net becomes closer, forming the theca interna, which is the site of formation of estrogens (Fig. 7). The cells of the theca interna develop lipid droplets and persist after ovulation immediately adjacent to the enlarged follicular cells or granulosa lutein cells. Measurements of ova in sections of a well-preserved ovary indicate that although the ovum grows slowly during the development of the graafian follicle, its volume increases about fortyfold before its maturity. The nucleus, however, increases only about threefold during this period. The large increase in cytoplasm includes the accumulation of nutrients such as yolk granules.

Mature Graafian Follicle.   There is no reliable evidence that human ova are normally formed after birth. Before puberty, mature graafian follicles are found only in the deeper portions of the cortex. Later, however, they develop in the superficial portions also. During each cycle, one makes its way to the surface, where it appears as a transparent vesicle varying from a few to 10 or 12 mm in diameter. As the follicle approaches the surface of the ovary, its walls become thinner and more abundantly supplied with vessels (Fig. 8), except in its most prominent projecting portion, which appears almost bloodless and is designated the *stigma,* the spot where rupture is to occur.

From without inward, the mature graafian follicle consists of (1) a layer

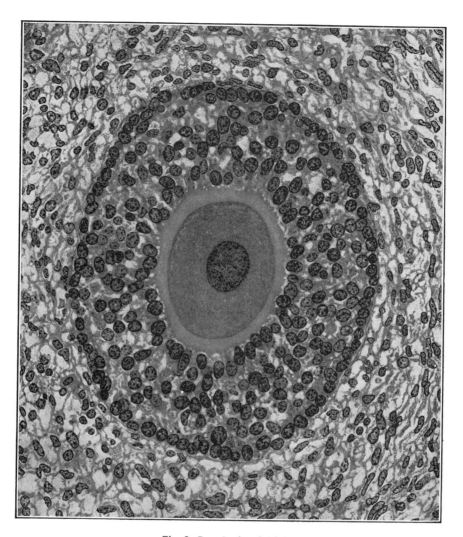

Fig. 3. Developing follicle.

of specialized connective tissue, the theca folliculi; (2) an epithelial lining, the membrana granulosa; (3) the ovum; and (4) the liquor folliculi. The theca folliculi comprises an outer theca externa and an inner theca interna. The theca externa consists of ordinary ovarian stroma arranged concentrically about the follicle, but the connective tissue cells of the theca interna are greatly modified.

Almost as soon as the primordial follicle begins to develop, mitotic figures appear in the immediately surrounding stroma followed by considerable multiplication of cells, which become distinctly larger than those of the surrounding connective tissue. As the follicle increases in size, these cells, the *theca lutein cells,* accumulate lipid and a yellowish pigment and appear granular. There is simultaneously a marked increase in the vascularity of the theca and in the number of lymphatic spaces.

The theca cells before ovulation are separated from the granulosa cells by

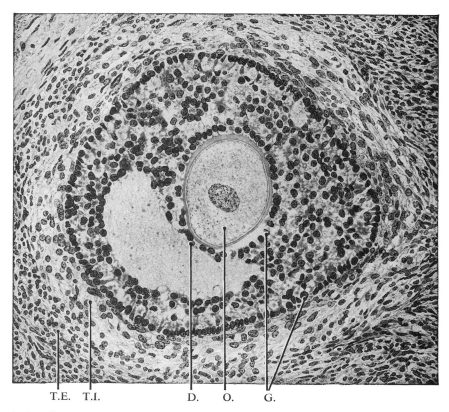

T.E.   T.I.   D.   O.   G.

Fig. 4. Graafian follicle approaching maturity. T.E., theca externa; T.I., theca interna; D., discus proligerus (cumulus oophorus); O., ovum; G., granulosa cell layer.

a highly polymerized membrane. It is possible that luteinizing hormone may depolymerize the membrane at about the time of ovulation and allow vascularization of the granulosa to take place.

The epithelial lining of the follicle, or membrana granulosa, consists of several layers of small polygonal or cuboidal cells with round, darkly staining nuclei; the larger the follicle, the fewer is the number of layers. At one point the membrana granulosa is much thicker than elsewhere, forming a mound in which the ovum is included, the cumulus oophorus (discus proligerus). While the follicle is developing, it is situated at the portion farthest from the surface of the ovary. The follicle is filled with a clear, proteinaceous fluid, the *liquor folliculi,* or follicular fluid. The granulosa cells do not take up the usual fat stains until the stage of preovulatory swelling, a period of rapid growth that occurs about 24 hours before ovulation and is apparently related to the onset of the secretion of progesterone.

As the human ovum approaches maturity, if it is brightly illuminated on a dark background, it' is barely visible to the naked eye. According to Allen and co-workers its average diameter in the fresh state is 0.133 mm. Hartman states that the average size of the human ovum varies from 0.133 mm to 0.140 mm in diameter.

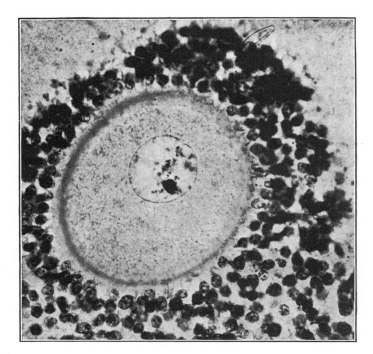

Fig. 5. Human oocyte from a large graafian follicle. (Carnegie Laboratory.)

If the nearly mature ovum is examined in the follicular fluid or in physiologic saline, the following structures may be distinguished in and about it: (1) a surrounding corona radiata; (2) a zona pellucida; (3) a perivitelline space; (4) a small clear zone of protoplasm; (5) a broad, finely granulated zone of protoplasm; (6) a central, deutoplasmic zone; (7) the nucleus, or germinal vesicle, with its germinal spot; and if appropriately stained (8) many small spheroidal mitochondria. The ovum can rotate freely within the zona pellucida although its outer vitelline membrane appears closely applied to it. The first polar body is extruded into the perivitelline space shortly before ovulation. At fertilization, shrinkage of the ovum results in its complete separation from the zona pellucida as it floats in the perivitelline fluid. During its growth the oocyte accumulates deutoplasm (yolk granules). According to Allen and others, before ovulation the ovum is transparent with a faint yellowish tinge in the living state. There are also larger lipoid granules, which in preserved material appear to surround the nucleus (germinal vesicle). Numerous mitochondria are distributed through the cytoplasm. The spherical nucleus is located near the center of the oocyte. It has a large nucleolus and sparsely distributed chromatin. Shortly before ovulation the nucleus migrates toward the periphery, and the formation of polar bodies begins.

Ovarian follicles develop throughout childhood and occasionally attain considerable size, but they do not normally rupture at this time, instead undergoing atresia in situ. The hypophysial hormones necessary for ovulation are not functionally coordinated until sexual maturity is attained (p. 82). Even in adults many follicles that reach a diameter of 5 mm or more undergo atresia. Usually

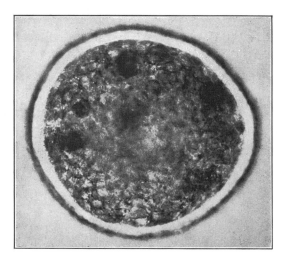

Fig. 6. Human ovum washed from tube. Fresh specimen, surrounded by semitransparent zona pellucida, consists largely of lipoid masses. Ovum measured 0.136 mm in the living state. (Carnegie Collection No. 6289, Dr. W. H. Lewis.)

Follicular fluid   Granulosa

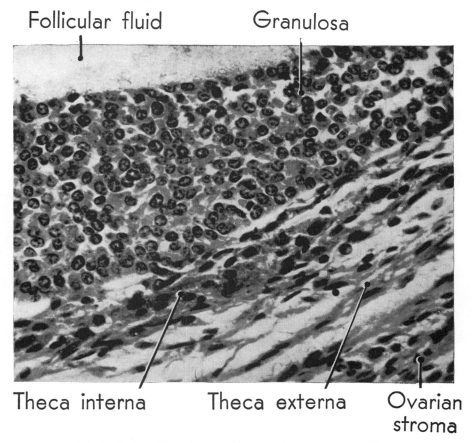

Theca interna   Theca externa   Ovarian stroma

Fig. 7. Section through the wall of a mature graafian follicle.

only one of a group of enlarging follicles continues to grow and to produce a normal mature egg that is extruded at ovulation. The mechanism that normally limits maturation and ovulation to only one of the enlarging follicles has not been elucidated.

Ovulation.   As the graafian follicle grows to a size of 10 to 12 mm in diameter, in response to the humoral mechanism described subsequently and schematically demonstrated on page 98, it gradually reaches the surface of the ovary and finally protrudes above it. Necrobiosis of the overlying tissues rather than the pressure within the follicle is the principal factor causing follicular rupture. The cells at the exposed tip of the follicle float away at the site of the pale stigma so that the region becomes transparent. The thinnest clear area then bursts, and the follicular liquid and the ovum surrounded by the zona pellucida and corona radiata are extruded, constituting ovulation. The actual rupture of the follicle is not explosive. The discharge of the ovum with its zona pellucida and attached follicular cells takes not more than two to three minutes, in the rabbit at least, and is expedited by the separation, just before rupture, of the ovum with the surrounding granulosa cells (corona radiata) from the follicular wall as the result of accumulation of fluid in the cumulus; hence, the ovum floats freely in the liquor.

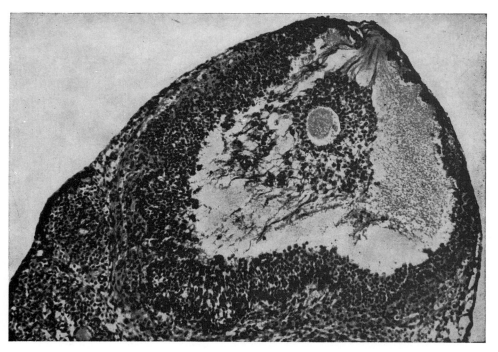

Fig. 8. Rat ovary just prior to ovulation. (Courtesy of Dr. Richard J. Blandau.)

Excellent motion pictures of the process of ovulation in the rat have been obtained by Blandau. In Figures 8 and 9, two frames show the follicle just before ovulation and the expulsion of the ovum. In the first, the stigma is clearly visible, whereas the second shows the actual expulsion of the ovum.

Time of Ovulation.   The exact time of ovulation within the cycle is of the utmost importance for several reasons. First, since the life-span of both the spermatozoon and the unfertilized ovum is limited, fertilization must take place within about 24 hours after ovulation if conception is to occur that month. In cases of female sterility, detection of the time of ovulation and appropriate adjustment of coitus are most important steps in therapy. Second, to avoid conception, coitus could be limited to that part of the cycle several days from the time of ovulation, or the "safe period." Finally, ovulation marks the midpoint of both the ovarian and menstrual cycles. The period from the first day of menstrual bleeding to ovulation is designated the *preovulatory* or follicular phase of the cycle. The follicular phase represents roughly the first half of the ovarian cycle; the second half is known as the luteal phase. Ovulation divides the ovarian cycle into these two main phases.

Various methods have been employed to ascertain the time of ovulation in women, the most dependable of which is the direct recovery of ova from the fallopian tube at operation. Allen and colleagues recovered mature unfertilized ova from the fallopian tube on the twelfth, fifteenth, and sixteenth days of the cycle, and concluded that ovulation occurs approximately on day 14 of a 28-day

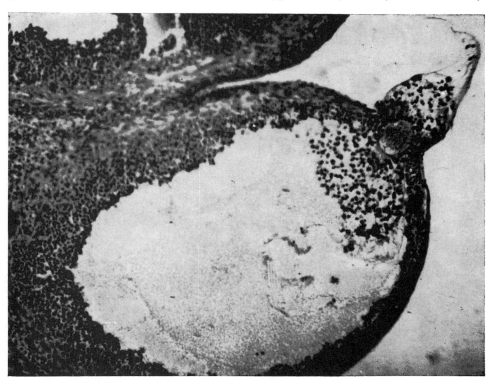

Fig. 9. Moment of ovulation in the rat. (Courtesy of Dr. Richard J. Blandau.)

cycle. Other dependable methods for ascertaining the time of ovulation are examination of fertilized ova and evaluation of the changes that have taken place at the site of the ruptured follicle. Investigation by these technics has demonstrated that although ovulation frequently occurs between the twelfth and sixteenth days of the cycle, there is considerable variation. It is not uncommon for

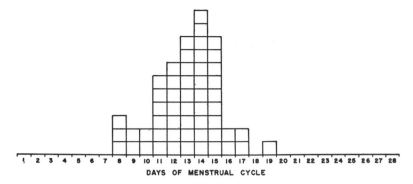

DAYS OF MENSTRUAL CYCLE

Fig. 10. Day of ovulation in 54 women calculated from the apparent age of the corpus luteum. Each block represents an observation of one woman. (After Brewer and Jones.)

ovulation to take place at any time between the eighth and twentieth days, as shown in Figure 10. Ovulation bears a closer temporal relation to the next menstrual period than to the previous menses, usually occurring approximately 14 days before the first day of the succeeding menstrual bleeding.

Signs and Symptoms of Ovulation. On or about the day of ovulation perhaps 25 per cent of women experience lower abdominal pain on the involved side. This so-called *Mittelschmerz* is thought to result from peritoneal irritation by follicular fluid or blood escaping from the ruptured follicle. The symptom rarely occurs during every cycle.

A useful means of detecting ovulation is the shift in basal body temperature from a lower relatively constant level during the follicular or preovulatory phase to a higher level early in the luteal or postovulatory phase, as shown in Figure 11. Ovulation occurs most likely just before or during the shift in temperature. The increase in the basal body temperature is the result of the thermogenic action of progesterone. A similar thermal response can be induced by injecting progesterone into a castrated subject. The rise in basal body temperature there-

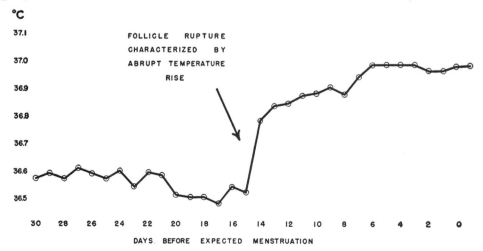

Fig. 11. Basal temperature shift characteristic of rupture of follicle. (From Palmer. Obstet Gynec Survey 4:1, 1949.)

fore may provide evidence of production of progesterone and the development of a corpus luteum. Extensive luteinization of the granulosa, however, may occur in a follicle that still contains an ovum.

Other Tests for Ovulation. During the follicular phase the cervical mucus increases in amount. Near the time of ovulation its appearance changes from opaque to clear. At this time its viscosity decreases considerably and the mucus can be drawn into long threads with considerable elastic recoil (*Spinnbarkeit*). Also at this time the cervical mucus, spread on a glass slide and allowed to dry, demonstrates marked arborization, or "ferning," because of its content of sodium chloride (Ch. 4, Fig. 10, and p. 101). All of these changes are maximal at about the time of ovulation. They offer no proof of ovulation, but in normal circumstances simply herald the imminent release of an ovum. Similar changes in cervical mucus may be induced in castrated women given appropriate doses of estrogen. After ovulation the changes in the mucus regress; the arborization of dried mucus is soon replaced by a beaded, or "cellular," pattern.

As discussed in Chapter 4, numerous characteristic morphologic changes take place in the endometrium after the formation of a corpus luteum and its production of progesterone. Since ovulation is nearly always associated with these changes, the demonstration of a secretory endometrium is very strong evidence that ovulation has previously occurred during the cycle.

Increased progesterone circulating in the blood of a nonpregnant woman is additional evidence that luteinization of a follicle and most likely ovulation have taken place. Although progesterone can be measured in the blood, in general such tests are not yet available for clinical use. Technics for measuring minute amounts of progesterone should, in the near future, become more readily available for clinical problems.

The detection in the urine of pregnanediol, a common metabolite of progesterone, does not prove that ovulation has occurred. Considerable amounts may be found, for instance, in the urine of women with sclerocystic ovaries and chronic anovulation.

Many other tests, ranging from detection of altered symptoms or physical findings to biochemical or biophysical changes, have been proposed for detecting ovulation. Most of these have been reviewed by Speck. There is still, however, no accurate test that can be readily carried out by women to warn them of impending ovulation.

Corpus Luteum   The corpus luteum normally forms in the ovary immediately after ovulation, at the site of the ruptured follicle. It is colored by a golden pigment, from which it derives its name, which means "yellow body." Microscopically the corpus luteum demonstrates four stages of development: proliferation, vascularization, maturity, and regression. White and co-workers have reviewed the life cycle of the corpus luteum using histochemical technics.

When the mature graafian follicle ruptures, the ovum, follicular liquid, and a considerable portion of the surrounding granulosa are discharged. The collapsed walls of the empty follicle form convolutions about the blood-filled cavity (Fig. 12). The remaining granulosa cells appear polyhedral with round, vesicular nuclei and frothy cytoplasm. There are many large lacunae containing extravasated blood but initially no blood vessels. The theca interna is invaginated, and its vascular channels are greatly dilated. Endothelial sprouts from these vessels penetrate the granulosa and the hemorrhagic cavity of the ruptured follicle. Hertig

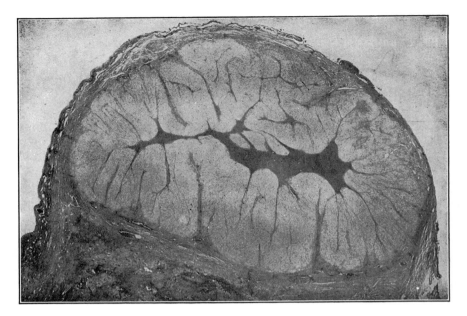

Fig. 12. Corpus luteum of pregnancy. Low power. See also Figure 14.

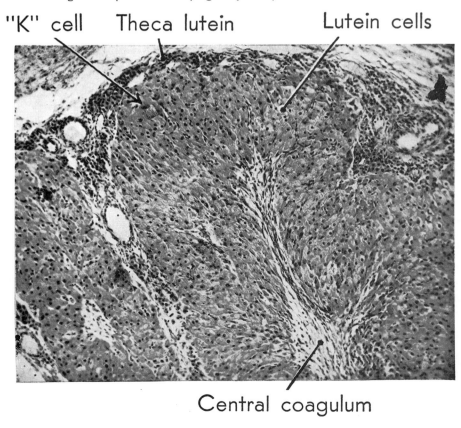

"K" cell   Theca lutein   Lutein cells

Central coagulum

Fig. 13. Section through the wall of a mature corpus luteum of menstruation.

has described the "K" cell (Fig. 13), which can be recognized in the mature graafian follicle as a stellate cell with deeply eosinophilic, homogeneous cytoplasm. During the proliferative stage, strands of K cells, having migrated from the theca, extend into the membrana granulosa as far as the central coagulum.

In the stage of vascularization that soon follows ovulation the blood-filled cavity of the ruptured follicle undergoes rapid organization. Grossly the central coagulum appears pale gray with only a few hemorrhagic foci. Microscopically there are fibroblasts but no capillaries within the coagulum. Elsewhere in the granulosa layer, dilated capillaries are conspicuous. As the stage of vascularization of the corpus luteum progresses to maturity, the luteinized cells originating from granulosa show peripheral vacuolation, suggesting physiologic activity. The theca interna cells are also vacuolated; when stained for lipid, they show much coarser droplets than do the granulosa lutein cells. The K cells continue to form a prominent portion of the corpus luteum at that stage and also contain lipid, as well as a high concentration of alkaline phosphatase.

The mature corpus luteum measures from 1 to 3 cm in diameter but occasionally occupies a third or more of the entire ovary. At this stage it is characteristically bright yellow.

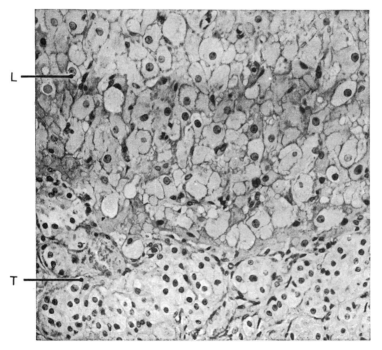

Fig. 14 Corpus luteum of pregnancy. High power. L, lutein cells; T, theca lutein cells.

Regressive changes occur in the corpus luteum occasionally as early as the twenty-third day of the cycle. These changes become progressively more marked up to the onset of menstruation until the central coagulum has been obliterated by connective tissue and blood pigment has been removed by leukocytes. There is no further capillary proliferation; the nuclei of the granulosa lutein cells lose their chromaticity, and peripheral vacuolization of the cytoplasm decreases as increasing accumulations of coarse lipid droplets appear. The theca cells can be seen only in widely separated clumps. The K cells develop hyperchromatic nuclei, and the cellular outlines almost disappear. There is progressive loss of lipid-staining material throughout the entire corpus luteum. With menstruation, complete regression of the corpus luteum takes place. If fertilization does not take place, the corpus luteum is designated the *corpus luteum of menstruation*. If fertilization occurs, a *corpus luteum of pregnancy* is initiated and the degenerative changes are postponed (Fig. 14).

Adams and Hertig have recently described the ultrastructure of human corpora lutea at approximately 2, 3, 5, 11, and 15 days after ovulation. The 5-day corpus luteum, compared with younger differentiating and older regressing specimens, has ultrastructural characteristics consistent with maximal production of progesterone. The 5-day luteal cell has a peripheral mass of agranular endoplasmic reticulum, which merges with a large paranuclear Golgi area. Parallel cisternae of granular endoplasmic reticulum are found peripherally. Lipid droplets and mitochondria with tubular cristae are numerous in the physiologically active cells, the complex plasma membranes of which suggest specialized activities.

Corpus Luteum of Pregnancy. The duration and the function of the corpus luteum of pregnancy have been subjected to much speculation and investigation. The scientific validity of hormonal therapy in the prevention of early abortion depends upon an understanding of the function of this structure.

Hertig has enumerated the morphologic criteria of a very early corpus luteum of pregnancy, including increased congestion; a surge of hyperplasia from the twenty-third to twenty-eighth days, after the last period, presumably resulting, at least in part, from the stimulus of chorionic gonadotropin; an increasing number of K cells; and the absence of any atrophic, ischemic, and regressive changes like those that appear when menstruation is imminent. The degenerative changes in the corpus luteum are delayed for a variable length of time but take place most frequently at about six months of gestation, although normal corpora lutea have been found at term.

Adams and Hertig recently compared the ultrastructure of human corpora lutea obtained during the sixth, tenth, sixteenth and thirty-fifth weeks of pregnancy with those of the menstrual cycle. In pregnancy, the luteal cell appears more highly compartmentalized, with a peripheral mass of endoplasmic reticulum and a central area where mitochondria and Golgi complexes are concentrated. The area rich in mitochondria and Golgi complexes extends to a cell surface with microvilli that face a vascular space. Certain luteal cells with irregular nuclear membranes contain vesicular aggregates within the peripheral nucleoplasm or the perinuclear cytoplasm. These nuclear vesicular aggregates and certain spherical bodies may reflect prolonged endocrine stimulation and secretory exhaustion, which ultimately produce electron-dense cells with pyknotic nuclei.

In a current ultrastructural study, Crisp and co-authors compared the granulosa and theca lutein cells of human corpora lutea. In early pregnancy, granulosa lutein cells are distinguished from theca lutein cells on the basis of their more homogeneous, electron-lucent matrix, enlarged pleomorphic mitochondria, abundant endoplasmic reticulum, and several other important ultrastructural features. They found, furthermore, that granulosa lutein cells of early pregnancy may be distinguished from those of the progestational phase of the menstrual cycle by their better developed endoplasmic reticulum, large spherical mitochondria, more numerous membrane-bound granules, and greater numbers of intercellular canaliculi. They suggested that these differences are related to the high titer of serum gonadotropin during early gestation. On the basis of morphologic specializations it seems likely that the corpus luteum may secrete, in addition to steroids, a proteinaceous product, perhaps relaxin.

The corpus luteum is necessary for maintenance of pregnancy for only a short period after implantation in the human being. Among animal species the need for the corpus luteum in order to prevent abortion is highly variable. Numerous human pregnancies have succeeded despite early ablation of the corpus luteum. Pratt has reported continuation of pregnancy after such an operation performed as early as the twentieth day after the last menstrual period, or about the time of implantation. In a review of cases in which the corpus luteum had been removed early in pregnancy, Hall reported a rate of abortion of a little over 20 per cent. He believes that rate is not higher than expected following any abdominal surgery in the first trimester. In a well-designed experiment Tulsky and Koff removed the corpora lutea from 14 women on whom they intended to perform sterilization and therapeutic abortion. Spontaneous abortion occurred in only 2. In the remainder the pregnancies were terminated by dilatation and curettage. Ten of the 14 patients, furthermore, continued to excrete normal quantities of pregnanediol until the conceptus was removed.

The degenerative changes in the corpus luteum are delayed by chorionic gonadotropin. The corpus luteum, of course, produces progesterone, but soon after implantation the human placenta secretes enough progesterone to maintain pregnancy. The corpus luteum, though necessary for implantation in the human being, is not required for pregnancy beyond the earliest stages.

Corpora Albicantia. In the absence of pregnancy, degenerated lutein cells are rapidly resorbed, and in a short time the corpus luteum is replaced by newly formed connective tissue closely resembling the surrounding ovarian stroma. These structures, the so-called corpora albicantia, appear on section dull and white, somewhat like scar tissue. They are, however, gradually invaded by the surrounding stroma and are broken up into increasingly small hyaline masses, which eventually are completely resorbed. Ultimately the site of the original

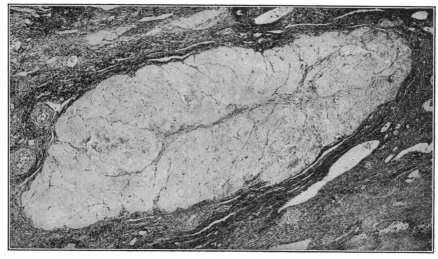

Fig. 15. Corpus albicans.

follicle is indicated only by an area of slightly thickened connective tissue. In older women this process may be slower and less complete. It is not uncommon to find the ovaries of women near the menopause almost filled by scars of varying size (Fig. 15).

Atretic Follicles.   Theca lutein cells are admixed somewhat with granulosa lutein cells, but for the most part the two types of cells are distinctive in their appearance. The granulosa lutein cells are larger, more highly vacuolated, and provided with a smaller nucleus; the theca lutein cells are somewhat smaller, more deeply stained, and have a relatively larger nucleus.

The theca lutein cells play a prominent part in the life history of follicles that degenerate without rupture. This process, *follicular atresia*, is particularly pronounced during pregnancy. In such circumstances, after the follicle has attained a certain size, the ovum undergoes cytolysis, while the membrana granulosa degenerates and is cast off into the liquor folliculi and eventually resorbed. While these changes are in progress, the theca lutein cells proliferate to form a tunic many layers thick about the follicle, which frequently becomes yellowish. Eventually, as the follicular fluid disappears, the walls of the follicle collapse and the thecal cells surrounding it undergo fatty and hyaline change. Finally there results an irregular hyaline body that cannot be distinguished from a similar structure derived from a corpus luteum.

Atresia is the fate of the vast majority of follicles that develop beyond the primordial stage; the process begins during intrauterine life and continues until after the menopause. Corpora lutea, however, nearly always develop only from the comparatively few follicles that rupture after reaching maturity. Possibly one of the functions of the corpus luteum is obliteration of the spaces left by the ruptured follicles without the formation of cicatricial tissue, thus preventing conversion of the entire organ to scar tissue.

The Ovarian Hormones

ESTROGEN

In 1900 Knauer in a classic experiment demonstrated that ovarian transplants would prevent atrophy of the uterus in ovariectomized rabbits. Twelve years later Adler extracted from ovaries a substance that caused estrus in the guinea pig, and in 1917 Stockard and Papanicolaou described cyclic variations in the vaginal smear of the guinea pig. This means of bioassay enabled Allen and Doisy in 1923 to isolate a potent estrogen from follicular fluid of the sow's ovary. In 1927 Aschheim and Zondek found that urine in pregnancy was rich in estrogenic substances. With a ready source of crude material and a satisfactory method of bioassay, the way was paved for final chemical identification. Within the next two years Doisy and Butenandt almost simultaneously announced the crystallization from urine of an estrogenic substance later designated as *estrone* (Fig. 16). In 1930 Browne, working in Collip's laboratory, isolated from placental tissue the much less potent estrogenic steroid *estriol* (Fig. 16). It was not until 1936, however, that MacCorquodale and his associates, working in Doisy's laboratory, crystallized *estradiol* (Fig. 16), the most potent of the three estrogenic substances.

Terminology.   In 1936 the Council on Pharmacy and Chemistry of the American Medical Association adopted *estrogen* as the collective term for all substances

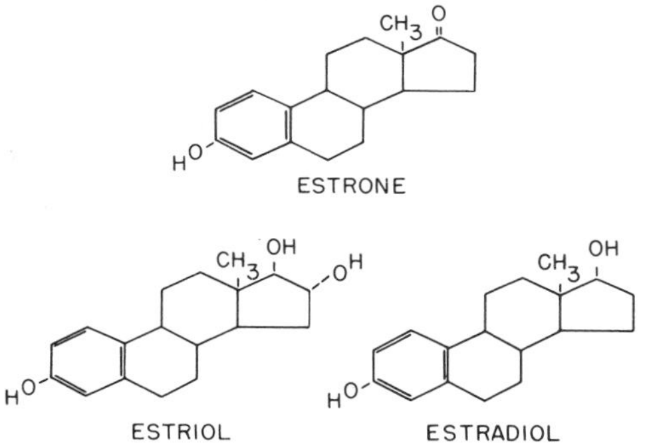

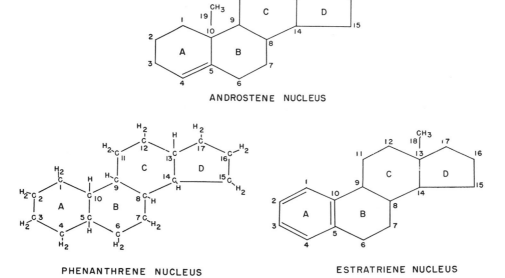

ESTRONE

ESTRIOL   ESTRADIOL

Fig. 16. Structural formulas of the three important estrogens.

capable of producing the typical changes of estrus: enlargement of the uterus, "cornification" of the vagina, and mating in immature or in oophorectomized adult animals. The chemical names of the common estrogens in the human being are estrone, estradiol, and estriol.

Chemistry of the Estrogens.   The parent hydrocarbon of the naturally occurring estrogens, estrane, possesses an 18-carbon skeleton and differs from the parent compound of the C_{19} series in that the angular methyl group at position 10 is absent. All of the estrogens that have been isolated from human sources possess this structure, and in addition, ring A is characteristically aromatic, as in estratriene (Fig. 17). The hydroxyl group at position 3 of the estrogens is therefore phenolic, that is, weakly acidic. The phenolic structure accounts for the solubility of these compounds in alkali and provides the basis for their separation from neutral steroids. This chemical property

ANDROSTENE NUCLEUS

PHENANTHRENE NUCLEUS   ESTRATRIENE NUCLEUS

Fig. 17. Theoretical structural nuclei from which the estrogens and androgens are derived.

also allows their estimation by extremely sensitive methods such as fluorescence and formation of radioactive derivatives. This fortuitous structure allows the detection of the extremely low levels of estrogen encountered in biologic fluids.

The biosynthesis and metabolism of the classical estrogens—estrone, estradiol, and estriol—have been well studied. In recent years, however, a large number of additional metabolites have been isolated and characterized from human urine and various other sources (Breuer). By the technic of isotope dilution in vivo it has been shown that most of these are metabolites derived from the classical estrogens, estrone, and estradiol. The biologic role, if any, of these compounds. however, is at present obscure.

The estrogens in both blood and urine occur mostly in conjugated forms, linked to either glucuronic or sulfuric acid.

Sources of Estrogens.   The histochemical investigations of Dempsey and Bassett and of McKay and Robinson indicate that the thecal cells elaborate estradiol. Additional experimental data involving implantation of granulosal or thecal cells into castrated animals showed endocrine activity associated only with the transplanted thecal cells. Furthermore, ovarian irradiation that resulted in destruction of the granulosa and proliferation of the theca allowed a persistence of estrogenic activity. Observations of experimentally produced ovarian tumors indicate that the thecal component of the granulosa cell tumor rather than the granulosa secretes estrogen. In pregnancy the placenta is the major source of estrogens (Ch. 6, p. 177).

Although the thecal cells are considered the site of formation of estrogen in the developing follicle, the luteinized granulosal cells of the corpus luteum become enzymatically competent to produce estrogen and may serve as a quantitatively significant source during the luteal phase of the menstrual cycle. This issue will not be settled until luteinized granulosa and theca cells can be adequately separated and tested. In addition, estrogen in the plasma and urine of nonpregnant women may also be derived from two other sources. First, the adrenal cortex has the enzymatic capability to synthesize estrogen, as evidenced by the in vitro conversion of radioactive precursors, such as progesterone, androstenedione, and testosterone, to estrone-estradiol. Whether this possible source of estrogen obtains in physiologic circumstances is unknown, but the existence of an extragonadal source of estrogen is established. This extragonadal estrogen, however, or a part thereof, may be derived from the extraglandular conversion of androstenedione to estrone. The importance of extragonadal sources of estrogen remains to be established.

Biosynthetic Pathways of the Formation of Estrogen in the Ovary.   Through the work of numerous investigators many of the steps involved in ovarian biosynthesis of estrogen have been elucidated. These steps are diagrammatically illustrated in Figure 18, which shows several noteworthy features of this biosynthetic system.

First, incubation of ovarian tissue with simple precursors such as acetate or cholesterol results in formation of estrogen (Ryan and Smith). Unlike the placenta, therefore (Ch. 6), the ovary does not require circulating steroidal precursors for biosynthesis of estrogen but has the capacity for de novo synthesis.

Second, in vitro studies have demonstrated that at least two separate pathways for synthesis of estrogen are operative in the human ovary. One proceeds via Δ^4-3-keto intermediates, progesterone, 17 α-hydroxyprogesterone, Δ^4-androstenedione, and testosterone to synthesis of estradiol; the other proceeds via Δ^5-3β-hydroxy intermediates, pregnenolone, 17 α-hydroxypregnenolone, and dehydroisoandrosterone. Ryan speculates

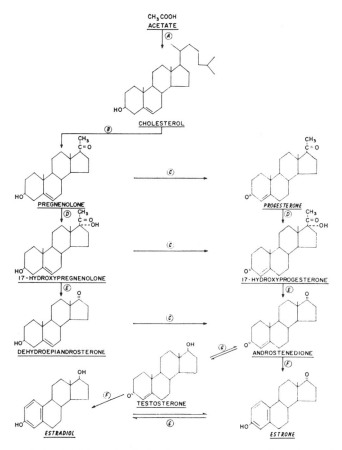

Fig. 18. Pathway of steroid biosynthesis in the ovary. A, formation of sterol from acetate; B, cleavage of cholesterol side chain—converts C_{27} to C_{21} compound; C, 3β-ol-dehydrogenase and Δ^4-Δ^5-isomerase reaction; D, 17α-hydroxylation; E, cleavage of side chain—converts C_{21} to C_{19} compounds; F, aromatizing reaction; G, 17β-ol-dehydrogenase (reversible). (From Smith and Ryan. Amer J Obstet & Gynec, 84:141, 1962.)

that the two pathways may have a histologic separation in the ovary. It is possible that the Δ^5-3β-hydroxy pathway is preferred in the theca cells, whereas the Δ^4-3 ketone pathway may be utilized principally in corpus luteum, which is known to be a rich source of 3β-ol-dehydrogenase, the enzyme required for the conversion of Δ^5-3-hydroxy steroids to the Δ^4-3-ketone moiety. Studies designed to ascertain the existence of this histologic difference in biosynthetic routes are currently under way in several laboratories. It is quite possible, of course, that the synthetic capacities of the two cellular types differ quantitatively rather than qualitatively, so that an absolute division of enzymatic capabilities is not demonstrable by in vitro technics.

Third, both proposed pathways of ovarian estrogen synthesis may proceed through "androgenic" intermediates, dehydroisoandrosterone, Δ^4-androstenedione, and testosterone. Not only is the enzymatic potential of the ovary to produce androgen established, but the secretion of androgen during the normal cycle has been amply demonstrated.

Nature of the Ovarian Secretion of Estrogen. Estimations of the daily "production rate" of estrogen in menstruating women have been made. This rate is a measure of the total daily production of estrogen—that is, the amount of estrogen produced from all sources, including ovarian secretion, adrenal secretion, peripheral or extraglandular formation from other substances such as androgen, and any as yet unidentified sources. Although it does not directly measure ovarian secretion, it is, of course, probable that the bulk of estrogen produced by menstruating women originates as an ovarian secretory product. The daily production rates of estradiol have been calculated from the amount of dilution by endogenously produced hormone of an intravenously administered tracer dose of isotope-labeled estradiol. The degree to which endogenous hormone dilutes the administered tracer is estimated by measuring the specific activity of the urinary metabolite estradiol. Utilizing this experimental design, Goering and Herrmann found that the production rate of estradiol in the immediate premenstrual and postmenstrual phases of the cycle was about 50 μg per 24 hours, rising to levels of 150–300 μg per 24 hours at the time of ovulation. These results are in excellent agreement with estimates made by many other indirect technics.

Isotope studies have also provided additional evidence that the principal ovarian secretory product is estradiol, which, in turn, is the parent precursor of the multiple urinary estrogenic metabolites. Fishman, Bradlow, and Gallagher showed that estradiol introduced into the circulation is quickly converted to estrone. Although intravenously administered estrone is also converted to estradiol, this transformation proceeds at a much slower rate. Furthermore, Gurpide and associates have found that the fraction of intravenously administered isotope-labeled estradiol converted to estrone is more than 90 per cent, whereas the fraction of intravenously administered radioactive estrone converted to estradiol is approximately 50 per cent. This relatively slow rate of interconversion (compared with the rate of irreversible metabolism) allowed Gurpide and co-workers to measure simultaneously the rate of production of estrone and estradiol in normal menstruating women. Their results indicate that the principal secretory product is estradiol, but in some instances the secretion of smaller amounts of estrone was also detected. Since these investigators based their calculations on the specific activities of the estrogenic metabolites contained in the glucuronide fraction of hydrolyzed urine (liberated by incubation with β-glucuronidase), the study cannot be considered as evidence against the possible secretion of estradiol by the ovary as a sulfate ester.

Estrogens in Biologic Fluids.   The estrogens circulating in blood are principally sulfuric acid conjugates, whereas those metabolites found in urine are principally glucuronic acid conjugates. Only a small fraction of the total amount of estrogens produced is excreted in the urine; substantial amounts have been identified in the feces.

Frank and associates first noted the tendency toward a biphasic curve of estrogen excretion in urine, with one peak at or near the time of ovulation and a second peak during the height of the luteal phase. During the four or five days before the next menstrual period the excretion of estrogens declines rapidly. Recently a similar pattern has been identified for estrogens in plasma, as shown schematically in Figure 19.

Actions of the Estrogens.   Estradiol may be regarded as essentially a growth hormone with selective affinity for tissues derived from the müllerian ducts: the fallopian tubes, the endometrium, the myometrium, and the cervix. Jensen and Jacobson, as well as others, have shown that while only a small amount of a physiologic dose of estradiol can be found in a growth-responsive tissue, the tissues derived from müllerian ducts have a much greater ability to "incorporate and retain estradiol (but not estrone) for a prolonged period of time" than do other tissues, such as liver, kidney, and skeletal muscle.

The developmental role, if any, of estrogens in sexual differentiation remains to be ascertained. Jost and others have reported that the male sex hormone testosterone is necessary for the development of the wolffian ducts into the male sexual apparatus as well as the differentiation of the genital tubercle into the male external genitalia. It has been assumed by inference that the female sex hormone is necessary in the embryo for the proper development of the müllerian ducts,

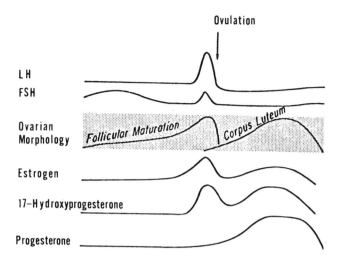

Fig. 19. A schematic drawing to demonstrate the changes in plasma of the various hormones involved in ovulation in women. LH, luteinizing hormone; FSH, follicle-stimulating hormone. (From Strott, Yoshimi, Ross, and Lipsett. J Clin Endocrin Metab 29:1166, 1969.)

although it has by no means been satisfactorily demonstrated. It is likely, however, that in the absence of the testis the müllerian ducts and the genital tubercle differentiate along female lines and that no positive stimulus is necessary.

At puberty the effects of estrogens are seen in the development of female habitus. Vaginal cornification occurs and the uterus attains the adult size and configuration. The fundus-to-cervix ratio changes from 1:1 to the adult ratio of 2:1. In addition to producing these end organ responses, estrogens also influence the actions of other endocrine glands and their hormones.

1. Effects on Uterus. Csapo has demonstrated that in the ovariectomized rabbit, estrogen determines the amount of actomyosin and adenosine triphosphate (ATP) present in the uterine musculature. In the intact immature and in the spayed adult monkey, estrogen causes hypertrophy of the uterine musculature, marked proliferation of the endometrium, and increased blood supply. The spiral arteries respond to the growth stimulus of estrogens even more actively than does the rest of the endometrium; as a result, their tips progressively approach the epithelial surface. In addition, estrogens affect the activity of the cervical epithelium in such a way that the cervical mucus increases in quantity and pH, attains a clear fluid state, and is more readily penetrated by spermatozoa. Microscopically the dried mucus is characterized by the formation of a "fern," as discussed on page 101.

2. Effects on Vagina. Estrogens produce thickening of the vaginal epithelium. In castrated monkeys and women, estrogens change the vaginal epithelium from a structure two or three cells deep to a thick membrane densely packed with compressed cells.

3. Effects on Fallopian Tubes. Estrogens stimulate growth of the fallopian tubes and appear to influence the activity of the tubal musculature. In experimental animals tubal contractions reach their height at estrus. Their dependence on estrogens is indicated by their disappearance after ovariectomy and their restoration by administration of estrogens.

4. Effects on Breasts. The administration of estrogens to the immature or ovariectomized animal in which the mammary glands are rudimentary or atrophic cause an extension of the ducts comparable to that seen in the sexually mature, nulliparous animal. The type of growth varies in different species. In the human being and monkey, partial lobule-alveolar growth is induced, as well as ductal development. In other animals the action is solely on the ducts, the simultaneous action of progesterone being necessary for the proliferation of the lobule-alveolar system.

5. Effects on Other Endocrine Organs. Estrogens suppress the pituitary follicle-stimulating hormone (FSH) function, as demonstrated long ago by Frank and Salmon, who showed the elevated urinary FSH titer found in menopausal or ovariectomized women could be lowered by the administration of estrogens. The actual pituitary content of FSH was lowered after estrogen administration, indicating that the effect was not just the result of secretory suppression and increased glandular storage. In women there is evidence that estrogens can trigger the release of luteinizing hormone, which, in turn, brings about ovulation in a mature ovarian follicle.

6. Effects on the Ovary. There is direct action of estrogenic hormones on ovarian tissue itself. Estradiol, by a local effect, stimulates the growth of the ovarian follicle even in the absence of follicle-stimulating hormone and potentiates the response to gonadotropins.

7. Effects on the Skeletal System. Estrogens favor epiphysial closure in immature animals, including human beings. Their role, if any, in osteoporosis is not clear.

PROGESTERONE

During the postovulatory phase of the ovarian cycle progesterone is secreted by the corpus luteum.

Prenant, in 1898, first suggested that the corpus luteum was an organ of internal secretion. Fraenkel, in 1910, demonstrated that the corpus luteum in the rabbit was necessary for the proper maintenance of pregnancy. In the same year Bouin and Ancel described histologically the progestational endometrium, providing the foundation upon which Corner and Allen established their classical method of bioassay, which enabled them in 1928 to isolate from sow's ovaries the hormone that they named "progestin" to indicate its specific role in gestation. Somewhat later, when Butenandt characterized it as a steroid he suggested the chemical nature be indicated in the nomenclature by the suffix "sterone." The term progesterone thus arose from the combination of the two words.

Butenandt described a urinary steroid excreted in large amounts during pregnancy and therefore named "pregnanediol." The significance of the compound, however, was not recognized until 1937, when Venning demonstrated a correlation between the excretion of pregnanediol in the urine and the presence of endogenous or exogenous progesterone. She showed that pregnanediol, excreted as sodium pregnanediol glucuronide, was a metabolite of progesterone and that its excretion usually reflected the amount of progesterone present. Previously only minute amounts of progesterone had been isolated from the corpus luteum itself and from the blood of the ovarian vein. No metabolites of progesterone had been identified, and therefore no means of monitoring the output of progesterone were available.

Definition.   Progesterone is defined as a specific, biologically active steroid producing progestational changes in the uterus of suitably prepared immature or ovariectomized rabbits.

Chemistry of Progesterone.   Progesterone, the principal hormone of the corpus luteum, is a derivative of the 21-carbon compound pregnane. In addition to the 2-carbon side chain at position 17, progesterone has a ketone group at carbon-20 and a Δ^4-3-keto grouping in ring A, a characteristic of several hormonally active steroids.

Sources of Progesterone.   Progesterone and two compounds closely related structurally, Δ^4-3-ketopregnen-20α-ol and Δ^4-3-ketopregnen-20β-ol, have been isolated from the corpus luteum, the ovarian vein blood, the placenta, and the adrenal. Progesterone may be found in peripheral venous blood, but none is found in the urine or feces. LeBlond and others were able to demonstrate progesterone in the endometrium and liver of the rat.

Metabolism of Progesterone.   In the human being the major known metabolite of progesterone is pregnanediol. Dorfman, Ross, and Shipley have demonstrated pregnanolone in the urine after administration of progesterone; the allo forms of both pregnanolone and pregnanediol are also recoverable in much smaller amounts. The liver has been identified as the major site of conversion of progesterone to these compounds.

Experiments of LeBlond indicated that there was some localization of progesterone in the rat's endometrium, where the hormone exerts its activity. Histologic studies by Jones, Wade, and Goldberg have shown that the glandular cells that are rich in glycogen are low in alkaline phosphatase, an enzyme that decreases greatly when large amounts of progesterone are given. Further experiments showed that progesterone blocks the formation of high-energy phosphate in hepatic mitochondria of the rat, favoring production of glycogen.

Progesterone and Metabolites in Blood and Urine.   Progestational activity in the blood of ovulating women reaches a maximum about one week after ovulation. Experiments with the injection of labeled progesterone now seem clearly to define its metabolic pathways. About 65 per cent of injected progesterone can be recovered in the excreta, with 20 per cent in the urine and 45 per cent in the bile or feces. In the urine, half is excreted as pregnanediol, 10 to 20 per cent as pregnanolone, and a small amount as other metabolites. The material in the bile is apparently from 50 to 60 per cent pregnanediol, 30 to 40 per cent pregnanolone, and about 10 per cent unidentifiable polar material. In women with normal cycles the peak excretion of pregnanediol occurs on the twentieth and twenty-first day, and the average value during the cycle amounts to 5 mg per 24 hours. Excretion of pregnanediol usually declines and may be absent for two days before menstruation.

These figures compare well with those of the progesterone assays of the corpus luteum of menstruation by Hoffman, who found the first measurable progesterone on the fourteenth day of the cycle. The values increased to a maximum by the sixteenth day and remained elevated until the twenty-fourth day of the cycle, after which there was a gradual decline until menstruation. The average total excretion of pregnanediol during the menstrual cycle is 30 mg. Reasoning therefrom, the corpus luteum of menstruation produces 600 mg of progesterone during the span of function. If, however, the amount of progesterone necessary for the production of progestational endometrium is used as the basis for calculation, the figure obtained is closer to 300 mg.

Effects of Progesterone.   The more profound effects of progesterone recognized thus far include the following: conversion of proliferative endometrium to secretory endometrium and then to decidua; inhibition of the contractility of smooth muscle, especially in the uterus; stimulation of natriuresis and, in turn, increased aldosterone production; stimulation of the respiratory center and an increased respiratory rate. More recently it has been shown by several investigators that small amounts of progesterone given to castrated or postmenopausal women who had been given estrogen leads to a sudden and transient rise in circulating luteinizing hormone. This action of progesterone appears to be of little physiologic significance.

   1. Effects on Endometrium.   A major function of progesterone is the preparation of the endometrium for implantation and maintenance of pregnancy. These progestational changes in the endometrium were classically described by Hitschmann and Adler and were later detailed by Noyes, Hertig, and Rock. In the properly estrogen-primed endometrium, progesterone produces manifold evidences of secretory activity. The tubular endometrial glands characteristic of the preovulatory phase are converted into tortuous structures. Subnuclear vacuoles in the epithelial cells are the first histologic evidence of glandular secretion. These vacuoles increase in size and migrate toward the luminal margin of the cell, which finally ruptures, allowing secretion to pour into the lumens of the glands. If these same glandular epithelial cells are suitably stained, glycogen can be demonstrated at about the time vacuolization first appears. Thereafter it steadily increases in amount until shortly before menstruation; the alkaline phosphatase activity, however, appears to reach its maximum around the time of ovulation. The stroma becomes edematous, and the constituent cells undergo hypertrophy with an increased amount of cytoplasm. If stimulation persists, the stromal cells form sheets of decidual cells. These characteristic histologic, cytochemical, and ultrastructural changes are discussed further in Chapter 4 (Figs. 1–6 and p. 94).

   The normal menstrual flow occurs from the progestational endometrium. The amount of progesterone necessary to produce these typical endometrial effects is influenced by the previous estrogenic stimulation as well as the duration of the stimulation by progesterone and the continuity of the dosage. Ten milligrams of progesterone given intramuscularly daily for seven days produce minimal secretory glandular changes. The level for vascular response, however, seems to be lower than that for the glandular reaction, since half this dose produces satisfactory withdrawal bleeding in the absence of any glandular progestational effect. To prevent menstruation in the presence of a regressing corpus luteum it is necessary to give large amounts of progesterone, 100 to 250 mg daily in divided doses. With these doses menstruation can be delayed from 10 to 14 days, but after this period women may bleed despite continued therapy.

   2. Effects on Maintenance of Pregnancy.   The progestational endometrium, with the deposition of glycogen that occurs under the influence of progesterone, furnishes proper nutritive conditions for the nidation and retention of the fertilized ovum. If, because of a deficiency of progesterone, the endometrial bed collapses, products of conception implanted therein are aborted. In many animals, such as the rat and mouse, the presence of the corpus luteum seems to be necessary throughout pregnancy, since its removal at any stage leads to abortion. As classically described by Corner and Allen, ovariectomy in the pregnant rabbit or destruction of all the corpora lutea before the last few days of its gestational period regularly causes abortion. By administering an extract of sow's corpora lutea they were able to maintain pregnancy to term (30 days, approximately) in rabbits ovariectomized shortly after mating. They found, furthermore, that if the corpora lutea of the pregnant rabbit are excised 14 to 18 hours after mating, the fertilized ova develop to the blastocystic stage and are then transported to the uterine cavity where they soon die. Pincus and Werthessen showed that if progesterone is administered to such animals, it promotes normal growth of the blastocyst in proportion to the degree of endometrial proliferation achieved. Since these workers could also promote growth of ova by keeping them in a suitable culture medium, they concluded that the arrest of ovular growth regularly after ovariectomy in the rabbit was a result of the unfavorable uterine condition. In other words, progesterone maintains pregnancy through its protective action on the endometrium.

The ability of women to carry pregnancy to completion in the absence of the corpus luteum in no way indicates that progesterone is unnecessary. The placenta, which normally produces progesterone and estrogen in large quantities throughout much of pregnancy, is able to manufacture these hormones even at a very early stage in gestation in sufficient quantities to maintain the gestation.

3. *Effect on Uterine Motility.* Knaus concluded that, in rabbits, progesterone acts on both endometrium and myometrium. He demonstrated decreased spontaneous uterine activity and complete inhibition of the response to the oxytocic hormone in the postovulatory phase of the cycle during the time of transportation, implantation, and early development of the fertilized ovum. He found that in the human uterus also progesterone inhibited spontaneous motility and the response to posterior pituitary extracts. Csapo found, using isolated muscle, that progesterone decreases the electrochemical gradient and, depending upon the extent of its domination, can inhibit myometrial function in the presence of a complete actomyosin and adenosine triphosphate system. The decrease of the electrochemical gradient makes the muscle insensitive to oxytocin, epinephrine, acetylcholine, and histamine.

4. *Effects on Fallopian Tubes.* Histologic studies show that to a degree the tubal mucosa undergoes cyclic changes. During the luteal phase, it undergoes changes that indicate secretory activity. This interpretation is substantiated by Joël's observation that the content of glycogen and ascorbic acid in the human tubal mucosa reaches its height during the luteal phase and that its lipid content is highest at the beginning of this phase. That the progestational hormone causes the tubal modification seen during the luteal phase has been demonstrated in the rabbit by Westman and by Caffier. Cyclic variations in the activity of the tubal musculature have also been ascribed to progesterone. There are rhythmic contractions, the amplitude of which is greatest at the height of the follicular phase and least during the luteal phase of the cycle; the relative quiescence in the latter phase, attributed to the action of progesterone, may play an important part in transport of the fertilized ovum to the uterine cavity.

5. *Effect on the Cervix.* The cervix produces different types of mucus during various phases of the cycle. Just before menstruation the secretions are scanty, viscid, full of leukocytes, impermeable to spermatozoa, and lacking in a ferning pattern. These characteristics are presumably the effect primarily of progesterone.

6. *Effect on Ovulation.* Hertz, Meyer, and Spielman showed that progesterone caused the copulatory response in the guinea pig. In women, most of the progesterone is produced after ovulation.

7. *Effect on Breasts.* Progesterone is largely responsible for the acinar and

lobular development during the luteal phase of the menstrual cycle, following the action of estrogen on the ductal epithelium. The two hormones, by dual action, are capable of bringing about complete mammary development, estrogen acting chiefly on the ductal system and progesterone on the lobular alveolar apparatus.

8. *Effect on Other Endocrine Systems.* Progesterone will not suppress the pituitary production of follicle-stimulating hormone, according to Greep and Jones, and thus perhaps is ineffective in the relief of menopausal symptoms. Salhanick and associates believe that progesterone may suppress the secretion of luteinizing hormone, but this point is still debated.

9. *Thermogenic Effects.* The induction by progesterone of an increase in the basal body temperature has been used to identify luteal function.

Synthetic Progestogens. Several synthetic steroid compounds with varying degrees of progesteronelike activities are being used in clinical medicine, especially combined with estrogens as oral contraceptives. The structures and the modes of action of a number of these compounds are discussed by Diczfalusy.

ANDROGENS

The human ovary is enzymatically capable of synthesizing dehydroisoandrosterone, Δ^4-androstenedione, and testosterone. Evidence that includes the results of in vitro isolations and incubations of ovarian tissue, analysis of ovarian venous blood, and measurements of secretory rate before and after adrenal suppression, indicates that the normal ovary actually secretes both dehydroisoandrosterone and Δ^4-androstenedione. Androstenedione levels in blood from the ovarian vein increase sharply in the late follicular phase, decrease slightly during the early luteal phase, and then rise again. Androstenedione and other plasma androgens in the general circulation, however, are derived to an important degree, either directly or indirectly, from adrenal secretion (Vande Wiele).

RELAXIN

Relaxin is a polypeptide that has been identified in many mammalian species. Its exact function is poorly understood; its effects vary from one species to another. The main source of the hormone is probably the ovary, but in many animals it may be produced by the placenta as well. Relaxin is said to cause softening of the cervix in several mammals. On that basis its use in slowly progressive human labors has been suggested. Even if relaxin produces cervical softening, however, it does not overcome the main problem of dysfunctional labor.

PITUITARY GONADOTROPIC HORMONES

With the work of Philip Smith in hypophysectomized animals the importance of the pituitary gland in the sexual cycle was first appreciated. Fluhmann in 1929 contributed early clinical information when he discovered large amounts of pituitary gonadotropin in the blood of menopausal women. In 1931 Fevold, Hisaw, and Leonard succeeded in demonstrating that this pituitary gonadotropic fraction actually contained two active components, the follicle-stimulating hormone (FSH) and the luteinizing hormone (LH), which has since been referred to as the interstitial cell-stimulating hormone (ICSH). In 1939 the Evans Laboratory in Berkeley, California, and the Squibb Biological Research Laboratory, directed by Van Dyke, almost simultaneously described the chemical separation and identification of these substances. These reports made possible experiments with relatively pure hormones and further elucidated the physiologic activity of the pituitary fractions.

The next major contribution in the control of the ovarian cycle by the pituitary hormones came from Harris, who demonstrated the presence of the hypophysial portal system, a series of blood vessels along the pituitary stalk communicating with the hypothalamic centers. Wislocki showed that the blood flow in this system was from the hypothalamus to the anterior pituitary gland rather than in the reverse direction. Markee demonstrated that the release of LH was dependent upon the excretion of certain adrenergic or cholinergic chemicals by the cells of this hypothalamic center. Further work indicated that changes in the hypothalamus are responsible for the onset of puberty, rather than maturation of the ovary or the pituitary, both of which are capable of adult function at birth if properly stimulated.

Follicle-Stimulating Hormone. The follicle-stimulating hormone (FSH) when administered to hypophysectomized immature female rats causes growth of the follicle, development of the antrum, and increased ovarian weight. Follicle-stimulating hormone is essential for the production of estrogen by the ovary. The metabolic fate of the follicle-stimulating hormone is unknown. It appears to be excreted in the urine in much the same form in which it is secreted by the pituitary.

Although FSH was one of the first gonadotropic hormones to be identified, it was the last to be isolated in a pure preparation in 1949. It is a readily water-soluble glycoprotein. The isoelectric point of the hormone isolated from pituitary

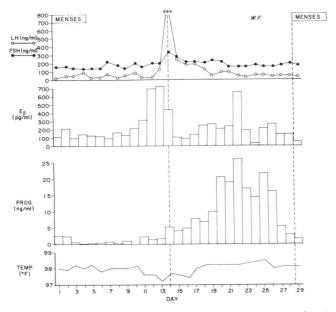

Fig. 20. Plasma levels throughout the menstrual cycle of the hormones involved in ovulation. LH, luteinizing hormone; FSH, follicle-stimulating hormone; E_2, estradiol; Prog., progesterone; Temp., basal body temperature; ng, nanogram; pg, picogram. (From Vande Wiele and co-workers. Recent Progr Hormone Res 126:63, 1970.)

of swine is pH 4.8. The carbohydrate fraction of the protein includes mannose and hexosamine.

Follicle-stimulating hormone usually is first detectable in the blood and urine of girls at about 11 years of age. During the normal menstrual cycle, before ovulation the FSH level remains relatively constant or changes only slightly until just prior to ovulation, when it probably rises somewhat. By the time of ovulation any previous increase in the FSH level has receded to nearly baseline levels. During the remainder of the menstrual cycle it either remains there or rises again very slightly (Figs. 19 and 20). The modest rise usually found in plasma FSH just before ovulation coincides with an increase in luteinizing hormone that is much greater in magnitude.

After the menopause, when production of estrogen by the ovary is negligible, the level of FSH in plasma and the amount excreted in the urine are very much increased. Administration of estrogen markedly lowers but does not completely abolish the secretion of FSH by the pituitary.

Luteinizing Hormone.   The luteinizing hormone (LH) is also referred to as interstitial cell-stimulating hormone. LH restores the interstitial cells in the ovary of a hypophysectomized mature female rat and stimulates testicular interstitial cells to secrete androgen in the hypophysectomized mature male rat.

An electrophoretically pure preparation was obtained from pituitary glands of sheep and swine in 1939; the fractions obtained from the two sources have slightly different chemical characteristics. LH, like FSH, is a highly water-soluble glycoprotein. The isoelectric point of LH from swine is pH 7.45. The molecular weight is approximately 90,000, and the carbohydrate fraction contains mannose and hexosamine. This hormone is produced also by a type of beta cell in the anterior pituitary.

According to Yussman and Taymor, the LH levels in plasma rise sharply 12 to 24 hours before the estimated time of ovulation and reach a peak about 8 hours later. These investigators also noted that FSH follows a similar but less marked pattern of response. Plasma progesterone levels were noted by them to increase after the rise in LH. Therefore, even though progesterone in small doses has been demonstrated to trigger LH release, the evidence is that in the normal menstrual cycle significant amounts of circulating progesterone are not present until after the LH surge.

Estradiol will trigger the release of LH and has been shown to reach a peak level at or probably just before the time of increased LH release. Vande Wiele and associates have treated the mature rat with antibody to estradiol and thereby not only successfully blocked the commonly recognized end-organ responses to estrogen but also prevented LH release and ovulation. Stilbestrol, however, the activity of which is not inhibited by antibodies to estradiol, restored ovulation. These results obtained by Vande Wiele with antiestradiol were in sharp contrast to those obtained with antibodies to progesterone. Although the antiprogesterone blocked the recognized end-organ response to progesterone, it did not prevent the discharge of LH or ovulation. Thus, a rise in circulating estrogen appears to be the important stimulus for the secretion of LH by the pituitary.

Luteotropic Hormones.   Even in the rat there does not appear to be a single luteotropic hormone. Instead, prolactin, luteinizing hormone, follicle-stimulating hormone, and estrogens all appear to be required for normal function of the corpus luteum.

Vande Wiele, Jewelewicz, and their associates have studied corpus luteum function in women who previously had undergone hypophysectomy. Ovulation and corpus luteum formation were induced by giving repeated injections of FSH and then LH (Fig. 21). In one experiment the dosage of LH, all given in one day, was such as to mimic the normal LH surge that occurs just before ovulation. There were increases initially in estrogens and progesterone in the plasma that were not sustained. Within five days the levels became very low; and on the sixth day after injecting the LH, the patient menstruated. These results were duplicated in other patients who received LH for only one day. The studies were then repeated, but the injection of LH was continued daily. Progesterone and estrogens were detectable in the plasma until the onset of menstruation 17 days after LH was started. Vande Wiele and co-workers were not able by giving LH to prolong the life of the corpus luteum and thereby delay the onset of menstruation much beyond the normal time of about 15 days. One patient conceived during the course of these studies. She subsequently gave birth to quintuplets that survived! These investigators conclude that luteinizing hormone is essential to maintain the normal life-span of the corpus luteum. The life-span of the corpus luteum, however, cannot be prolonged indefinitely by luteinizing hormone.

Luteolytic factors, the activities of which depend in some way on the presence of a uterus, have been suggested on the basis of experiments in several species, including sheep, sow, and guinea pig. No proof of a uterine luteolytic factor in women has yet been provided, however.

NEUROHUMORAL CONTROL

Anterior pituitary function is under neurohumoral control. Humoral agents, now called releasing factors, are liberated from nerve endings of the hypothalamic tracts into the capillaries of the portal vessels in the median eminence. The re-

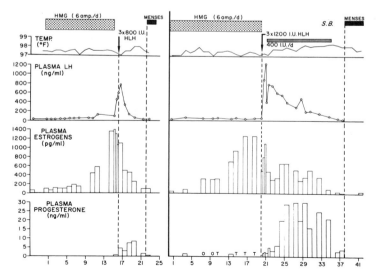

Fig. 21. Induction of ovulation in a woman without a pituitary by giving human menopausal gonadotropin (HMG) for 14 days followed by human luteinizing hormone (HLH). (From Vande Wiele and co-workers. Recent Progr Hormon Res 126:63, 1970.)

leasing factors are then carried through the hypophysial-portal circulation to the anterior pituitary (Harris).

During the past decade considerable evidence has accumulated for distinct releasing factors for each of the hormones secreted by the anterior pituitary. The releasing factors all appear to be peptides of quite low molecular weight. One of them, thyrotropin (TRF) releasing factor, has recently been synthesized.

Highly purified material with potent luteinizing releasing factor (LRF) activity has been prepared from pig, sheep, and cattle. Some of these preparations have been shown to evoke a rapid rise in circulating luteinizing hormone in men and children as well as in women.

Thus the hypothalamus is of fundamental importance in the control of the many mechanisms concerned with ovulation. Most likely a sudden surge in the secretion of LRF causes an outpouring of luteinizing hormone from the anterior pituitary. This hormone, in turn, causes ovulation if the follicle has achieved an appropriate state of maturity.

References

Adams, E. C., and Hertig, A. T.   Studies on the human corpus luteum. I. Observations on the ultrastructure of development and regression of the luteal cells during the menstrual cycle. J Cell Biol 41:696, 1969.

———— and Hertig, A. T.   Studies on the human corpus luteum. II. Observations on the ultrastructure of luteal cells during pregnancy. J Cell Biol 41:716, 1969.

Adler, L.   (Physiology and pathology of ovarian function). Arch Gynaek 95:349, 1912.

Allen, E., and Doisy, E. A.   An ovarian hormone: a preliminary report on its localization, extraction, and partial purification, and action in test animals. JAMA 81:819, 1923.

———— Pratt, J. P., Newell, Q. U., and Bland, L. J.   Human tubal ova; related early corpora lutea and uterine tubes. Contrib Embryol 22:45, 1930.

Aschheim, S., and Zondek, B.   (Anterior pituitary hormone and ovarian hormone in the urine of pregnant women). Klin Wschr 6:248, 1927.

Bouin, P., and Ancel, P.   (Research on the function of the corpus luteum). J Physiol et Path Gén 12:1, 1910.

Breuer, H.   The metabolism of the natural estrogens. Vitamins Hormones 20:285, 1962.

Browne, J. S. L.   Further observations on ovary stimulating hormone of placenta. Cited by Collip, J. B. Canad Med Ass J 22:761, 1930.

Butenandt, A.   (On "Progynon" a crystallized female sexual hormone). Naturwissenschaften 17:879, 1929.

———— (On pregnanediol, a new steroid derivative from pregnant urine). Ber chem Ges 63:659, 1930.

———— and Westphal, U.   (On the isolation and characterization of the corpus luteum hormone). Ber chem Ges 68:1850, 1934.

Caffier, P.   (On the hormonal influence of the human tubal mucosa and its therapeutic utilization). Zbl Gynaek 62:1024, 1938.

Corner, G. W.   On the origin of the corpus luteum of the sow from both granulosa and theca interna. Amer J Anat 26:117, 1919.

———— Physiology of the corpus luteum. I. The effect of very early ablation of the corpus luteum upon embryos and uterus. Amer J Physiol 86:74, 1928.

———— and Allen, W. M.   Physiology of the corpus luteum. II. Production of a special uterine reaction (progestational proliferation) by extracts of the corpus luteum. Amer J Physiol 88:326, 1929.

———— Alkaline phosphatase in the ovarian follicle and in the corpus luteum. Contrib Embryol 32:1, 1948.

Crisp, T. M., Dessouky, D. A., and Denys, F. R.   The fine structure of the human corpus luteum of early pregnancy and during the progestational phase of the menstrual cycle. Amer J Anat 127:37, 1970.

Csapo, A. I.   The molecular basis of myometrial function and its disorders, in La Prophylaxie en Gynécologie et Obstétrique, Congrès International de Gynécologie et Obstetrique. Geneva, Georg et Cie, 1954, p. 693.

de Graaf, R.   De mulierum organis generationi inservientibus. Lugd., Batav., 1677, p. 161.

Dempsey, E. W., and Bassett, D. L.   Observations on the fluorescence, birefringence and histochemistry of the rat ovary during the reproductive cycle. Endocrinology 33:384, 1943.

Diczfalusy, E.   Mode of action of contraceptive drugs. Amer J Obstet Gynec 100:136, 1968.

Doisy, E. A., Veler, C. D., and Thayer, S.   Folliculin from urine of pregnant women. Amer J Physiol 90:329, 1929.

Dorfman, R. I., Ross, E., and Shipley, R. A.   Metabolism of the steroid hormones. The metabolism of progesterone and ethynyl testosterone. Endocrinology 42:77, 1948.

Fevold, H. L., Hisaw, F. L., and Leonard, S. L.   The gonad-stimulating and the luteinizing hormones of the anterior lobe of the hypophysis. Amer J Physiol 97:291, 1931.

Fishman, J., Bradlow, H. L., and Gallagher, T. F.   Oxidative metabolism of estradiol. J Biol Chem 235:3104, 1960.

Fluhmann, C. F.   Anterior pituitary hormone in blood of women with ovarian deficiency. JAMA 93:672, 1929.

———   A new procedure for the demonstration of estrin in the blood of women. Endocrinology 18:705, 1934.

Frank, R. T., and Salmon, U. J.   Effect of administration of estrogenic factor upon hypophysical hyperactivity in the menopause. Proc Soc Exper Biol Med 33:311, 1935.

———and Goldberger, M. A.   The female sex hormone. JAMA 86:1686, 1926.

——— Goldberger, M. A., and Spielman, F.   Utilization and excretion of female sex hormone. Proc Soc Exper Biol Med 29:1229, 1932.

Fraenkel, L.   (New experiments on the function of the corpus luteum). Arch Gynaek 91:705, 1910.

Fraenkel-Conrat, H. L., Herring, V. V., Simpson, M. E., and Evans, H. M.   Mechanism of action of estrogen on insulin content of rat's pancreas. Proc Soc Exp Biol Med 48:333, 1941.

Goering, R. W., and Herrmann, W. L.   Estrogen secretion rate studies in normal women. Clin Res 12:115, 197, 1964.

Greep, R. O., and Jones, I. C.   Recent Progress in Hormone Research. New York, Academic Press, 1950, Vol. 5.

Gurpide, E., Hausknecht, R., Vande Wiele, R. L., and Lieberman, S.   Abs. 45 Meeting Endocrine Soc. (1963).

Hall, R. E.   Removal of the corpus luteum in early pregnancy. A review of the literature and report of 2 cases. Bull Sloane Hosp Wom 1:49, 1955.

Harris, G. W.   Hypothalamic control of the anterior pituitary gland. Ciba Foundation Colloquia on Endocrinology 4:106, 1952.

———   Ovulation. Amer J Obstet Gynec 105:659, 1969.

Hartman, C. G.   Uterine bleeding as early sign of pregnancy in the monkey (*Macacus rhesus*) together with observation on the fertile period of the menstrual cycle. Bull Hopkins Hosp 44:155, 1929.

———   How large is the mammalian egg? Quart Rev Biol 4:373, 1929.

——— and Corner, G. W.   Removal of the corpus luteum of the ovaries of the rhesus monkey during pregnancy: observations and cautions. Anat Rec 98:539, 1947.

Hertig, A. T.   The aging ovary: preliminary note. J Clin Endocr 4:581, 1944.

———   Gestational hyperplasia of endometrium: a morphologic correlation of ova, endometrium, and corpora lutea during early pregnancy. Lab Invest 13:1153, 1964.

Hertz, R., Meyer, R. K., and Spielman, M. A.   Specificity of progesterone in inducing sexual receptivity in the ovariectomized guinea pig. Endocrinology 21:533, 1937.

Hitschmann, F., and Adler, L.   (The structure of the endometrium of sexually mature women with special reference to menstruation). Mschr Geburtsh Gynaek 27:1, 1908.

Hoffman, F.   (On the content of progesterone in the ovary and blood during the cycle). Geburtsh Frauenh 8:723, 1948.

——— and von Lam, L.   (On the formation of progesterone during the cycle and in pregnancy). Zbl Gynaek 70:1177, 1948.

Jensen, E. V., and Jacobson, H. I.   Basic guides to the mechanism of estrogen action. Recent Progr Hormone Res 18:387, 1962.

Jewelewicz, R., Warren, M., Dyrenfurth, I., and Vande Wiele, R. L.   Human pituitary luteinizing hormone as an ovulation inducing agent. Presented before the Society for Gynecologic Investigation, New Orleans, April 1, 1970.

Joël, K.   The glycogen content of the fallopian tubes during the menstrual cycle and during pregnancy. J Obstet Gynaec Brit Emp 46:721, 1939.

Jones, H. W., Wade, R., and Goldberg, B.   Phosphate liberation by endometrium in the presence of adenosinetriphosphate. Amer J Obstet Gynec 64:1118, 1952.

———— and Weil, P. G.   The corpus luteum hormone in early pregnancy. Report of a case in which there was early removal of the corpus luteum. JAMA 111:519, 1938.

Jost, A.   Problems of fetal endocrinology. Recent Progr Hormone Res 8:379, 1953.

Knauer, E.   (Ovarian transplantation). Arch Gynaek 60:322, 1900.

Knaus, H.   The action of pituitary extract upon the pregnant uterus of the rabbit. J Physiol 61:383, 1926.

———— (A new method for estimation of the end of ovulation). Zbl Gynaek 53:2193, 1929.

LeBlond, C. P.   Isotopes in Biochemistry. The Ciba Foundation, London, Blakiston, 1951.

———— Simpson, M. E., and Evans, H. M.   Isolation of pituitary follicle-stimulating hormone

Li, C. H., Simpson, M. E., and Evans, H. M.   Isolation of pituitary follicle-stimulating hormone (FSH). Science 109:445, 1949.

MacCorquodale, D. W., Thayer, S. A., and Doisy, E. A.   The isolation of the principal estrogenic substance of liquor folliculi. J Biol Chem 115:435, 1936.

Markee, J. E., Sawyer, C. H., and Hollinshead, W. H.   Andrenergic control of release of luteinizing hormone from hypophysis of rabbit. Recent Progr Hormone Res 2:117, 1948.

Marrian, G. F.   The urinary estrogens and their quantitative determination. Cancer 10:704, 1957.

McKay, D. G., and Robinson, D.   Observations on fluorescence, birefringence and histochemistry of human ovary during menstrual cycle. Endocrinology 41:378, 1947.

———— Robinson, D., and Hertig, A. T.   Histochemical observations on granulosa-cell tumors, thecomas and fibromas of the ovary. Amer J Obstet Gynec 58:625, 1949.

Noyes, R. W., Hertig, A. T., and Rock, J.   Dating the endometrial biopsy. Fertil Steril 1:3, 1950.

Pincus, G., and Werthessen, N. T.   Quantitative method for bioassay of progestin. Amer J Physiol 120:100, 1937.

Pratt, J. P.   Corpus luteum in its relation to menstruation and pregnancy. Endocrinology 11:195, 1927.

———— Human corpus luteum. Arch Path 19:380, 1935.

Prenant, A.   (On the morphologic importance of the corpus luteum, and its physiologic and possible therapeutic action). Rev Médicale de Liest 30:385, 1898.

Ryan, K. J.   Biological aromatization of steroids. J Biol Chem 234:268, 1959.

———— The Ovary. Grady, H. G., and Smith, D. E. (eds.). Baltimore, Williams and Wilkins, 1963, p. 69.

———— and Smith, O. W.   Biogenesis of estrogens by the human ovary. I. Conversion of acetate-l-ΔC^{14} to estrone and estradiol. J Biol Chem 234:268, 1959.

Salhanick, H. A., Hisaw, F. L., and Zarrow, M. X.   The action of estrogen and progesterone on the gonadotrophin content of the pituitary of the monkey. J Clin Endocr 12:310, 1952.

Smith P. E.   The disabilities caused by hypophysectomy and their repair. JAMA 88:158, 1927.

Speck, G.   The determination of the time of ovulation. Obstet Gynec Survey 14:798, 1959.

Stockard, C. R., and Papanicolaou, G. N.   The existence of a typical oestrous cycle in the guinea pig, with a study of its histological and physiological changes. Amer J Anat 22:225, 1917.

Strott, C. A., Yoshima, T., Ross, G. T., and Lipsett, M. B.   Ovarian physiology: relationship between plasma LH and steroidogenesis by the follicle and corpus luteum; effect of HCG. J Clin Endocr 29:1157, 1969.

Tulsky, A. S., and Koff, A. K.   Some observations on the role of the corpus luteum in early human pregnancy. Fertil Steril 8:118, 1957.

Vande Wiele, R. L., Bogumil, J., Dyrenfurth, I., Ferin, M., Jewelewicz, R., Warren, M., Rizkallah, T., and Mikhail, G.   Mechanisms regulating the menstrual cycle in women. Recent Progr Hormone Res 126:63, 1970.

Venning, E. H.   Excretion of various hormone metabolites in normal pregnancy. Obstet Gynec Survey 3:661, 1948.

———— and Browne, J. S. L.   Isolation of a water soluble pregnanediol complex from human pregnancy urine. Proc Soc Exp Biol Med 34:792, 1936.

———— and Browne, J. S. L.   Urinary excretion of sodium pregnanediol glucuronidate in the menstrual cycle. (An excretion product of progesterone). Amer J Physiol 119:417, 1937.

———— and Browne, J. S. L.   Studies on corpus luteum function. I. The urinary excretion of sodium pregnanediol glucuronidate in the human menstrual cycle. Endocrinology 21:711, 1937.

Westman, A., Jorpes, E., and Widström, G.   (Investigation of the mucosal cycle in the uterine tube, its hormonal regulation and the significance of the tubal secretion for vitality of the fertilized eggs). Acta Obstet Gynec Scand 11:279, 1931.

White, R. F., Hertig, A. T., Rock, J., and Adams, E.   Histological and histochemical observations on the corpus luteum of human pregnancy with special reference to corpora lutea associated with early normal and abnormal ova. Contrib Embryol 34:55, 1951.

Wislocki, G. B.   The vascular supply of the hypophysis cerebri of the rhesus monkey and man. Proc A Res Nerv Ment Dis 17:48, 1938.

Yussman, M. A., and Taymor, M. L.   Serum levels of follicle stimulating hormone and luteinizing hormone and of plasma progesterone related to ovulation by corpus luteum biopsy. J Clin Endocr 30:396, 1970.

4

THE ENDOMETRIAL CYCLE AND MENSTRUATION

The endocrine changes during the ovarian cycle, as described in the preceding chapter, may be summarized as follows: (1) During the preovulatory, or follicular, phase of the cycle estradiol is produced in increasing quantity. (2) During the postovulatory, or luteal, phase of the cycle progesterone is produced in addition to estradiol. (3) During the premenstrual phase the corpus luteum regresses and both kinds of hormones are withdrawn. Consequent upon these phases of the ovarian cycle are the four main stages of the endometrial cycle, which comprise (1) phase of postmenstrual reorganization and *proliferation* in response to stimulation by estrogen; (2) phase of abundant glandular *secretion*, resulting from the combined action of progesterone and estrogen; (3) phase of *premenstrual ischemia* and involution; and (4) *menstruation* with collapse and desquamation of the superficial layers of the endometrium, resulting from the withdrawal of the ovarian hormones. The follicular, preovulatory, or proliferative phase and the postovulatory, luteal, or secretory phase are customarily divided into early and late stages. The normal secretory phase may be subdivided rather finely, according to histologic criteria, from shortly after ovulation until the onset of menstruation.

Early Proliferative Phase.   An early proliferative stage of the endometrial cycle is shown in Figure 1. The endometrium is thin, usually less than 2 mm in depth. The glands are narrow tubular structures pursuing almost a straight course from the surface toward the basal layer. The glandular epithelium is low columnar, and its lumens are narrow. The nuclei are round and basal. In the deeper part of the endometrium the stroma is rather dense, and the nuclei are deep-staining and small. In the superficial reorganizing layer the stroma is looser, and the nuclei are more nearly round, more vesicular, and larger than in the deeper layers; mitotic figures are numerous, especially in the glands. Although the blood vessels are numerous and prominent, there is no extravasated blood or lymphocytic infiltration at this stage.

Late Proliferative Phase.   Figure 2 shows that the endometrium has become thicker, as a result of both hyperplasia and increase in stromal ground substance. The loose stroma is especially prominent superficially, where the glands are

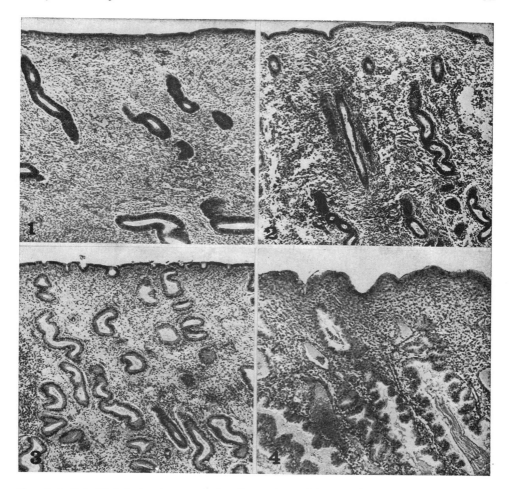

Figs. 1, 2, 3, 4. Histologic changes during the endometrial cycle. (Courtesy of Dr. Ralph M. Wynn.)

Fig. 1. Early proliferative endometrium. Shortly after menstruation. Glands are short and relatively straight and narrow. Stroma moderately dense.

Fig. 3. Early secretory endometrium. About three days after ovulation. Subnuclear secretory vacuoles are evident in epithelium. Total thickness of endometrium not significantly greater than in Figure 2.

Fig. 2. Late proliferative endometrium. Endometrium thicker than in Figure 1. Glands are more tortuous with higher epithelium. Stroma is more edematous.

Fig. 4. Late secretory endometrium. Several days before menstruation. Glands are tortuous, serrated, and exhausted of secretion. Early predecidual change of superficial stroma.

widely separated compared with those of the deeper zone, which are crowded and tortuous. Basally the stroma is denser. This zoning becomes more pronounced in the secretory phase. The glandular epithelium becomes gradually taller and pseudostratified toward the time of ovulation. After ovulation there is often a variable increase in the density of the stroma.

Early Secretory Phase. The total thickness of the endometrium may decrease slightly because of loss of fluid from the tissues. During this stage three zones become well defined: the basal layer, or zona basalis, adjacent to the myometrium;

the compact layer, or zona compacta, immediately beneath the endometrial surface; and the spongy layer, or zona spongiosa, between the compact and basal layers. The basal layer undergoes little if any histologic alteration during the menstrual cycle, but mitoses are found in the glands. The spongy middle layer comprises a lacy labyrinth with little stroma between the tortuous and serrated glands, which are the most characteristic feature of the luteal phase. In the compact superficial layer the glands are more nearly straight and narrower, but their lumens are often filled with secretion. Edema of the abundant stroma is an important factor in the thickening of the endometrium, but there is also a true increase in dry weight. The secretory endometrium may often attain a thickness of 4 to 5 mm (Fig. 3).

Late Secretory Phase.   This stage represents the culmination of the histologic changes of the endometrial cycle. The endometrium has become extremely vascular, succulent, rich in glycogen, and therefore ideal for the implantation and growth of the ovum. At the time of the cycle corresponding to implantation, or about a week after ovulation, the endometrium is 5 to 6 mm thick, and the secretory changes preparatory to nidation of the ovum are maximal (Fig. 4).

The stromal cells, particularly those around the blood vessels, undergo hypertrophic changes similar to, but less extensive than, those of the true decidua in pregnancy (p. 149).

Since the cyclic changes in the endometrium affect, by and large, only the compact and spongy layers, the zona compacta and zona spongiosa together are often designated the *zona functionalis,* or functional layer.

A further characteristic of the secretory phase is the striking development of the coiled arteries, which become more tortuous. They branch in the compact layer, and the arterioles break up into capillaries within this zone. During the first weeks of the menstrual cycle the arteries extend only about halfway through the endometrium. Since the arterioles lengthen more rapidly than the endometrium thickens, their distal ends reach progressively closer to the surface of the endometrium. Mitoses are common in their walls. This unequal growth results in a disproportion between the length of the arterioles and the thickness of the endometrium; in consequence the vessels become increasingly coiled.

Premenstrual Phase.   The premenstrual phase of the cycle occupies the two or three days before menstruation and corresponds to the regression of the corpus luteum. The chief histologic characteristic of this phase is infiltration of the stroma by polymorphonuclear or mononuclear leukocytes, producing a pseudoinflammatory appearance. At the same time, the reticular framework of the stroma in the superficial zone disintegrates. As a result of the loss of tissue fluid and secretion, the thickness of the endometrium often decreases significantly during the two days before menstruation (Fig. 4). In the process of reduction the glands and arteries collapse.

In a classic study, Markee described the vascular changes occurring before menstruation, as observed in intraocular transplants of endometrium in the rhesus monkey. He found that as the result of the compression of the endometrium, the coiling of the arterioles increases markedly. Although the coils are fairly regular earlier in the cycle, just before menstruation they become quite irregular.

Markee's work, furthermore, has shown two entirely different vascular phenomena in endometrial transplants for the few days preceding menstrual bleeding. Beginning one to five days before the onset of menstruation there is a period of slowed circulation, or relative stasis, during which vasodilatation may occur. There follows a period of vasoconstriction beginning 4 to 24 hours before the escape of any blood. The period of stasis is extremely variable, ranging from less than 24 hours to four days. In Markee's opinion, the slowing of the circulation leading to stasis is caused by the increased resistance to blood flow offered by the coiled arteries. As more coils are added, the blood flow becomes increasingly slower. Another explanation, however, must be invoked for the bleeding during anovulatory cycles and for bleeding following the withdrawal of estrogens, in which circumstances the arteries may be quite simple or relatively uncoiled. In such cases, there may be a more direct mechanism involving arteriolar vasoconstriction.

Vasoconstriction of the coiled arteries precedes the onset of menstrual bleeding by 4 to 24 hours, corresponding to the premenstrual ischemic phase. After the constriction has begun, the superficial half to two thirds of the endometrium receives an inadequate supply of blood during the remainder of that menstrual cycle; the anemic appearance of the functional zone may be striking. When, after a period of constriction, an individual coiled artery relaxes, hemorrhage occurs from that artery or its branches. Then, in sequence, these constricted arteries relax and bleed, the succession of small hemorrhages from individual arterioles or capillaries continuing for a variable period of time. Although this sequence of vasoconstriction, relaxation, and hemorrhage appears to be well established, the mechanism that actually brings about the escape of blood from the vessels remains an enigma. It is entirely possible that the damage to the walls of the vessels during the period of vasoconstriction results in their rupture when the constricted segment relaxes and the blood flow is resumed.

Menstrual Phase. Menstrual bleeding may be either arterial or venous, with the former predominating. It occurs at first as the result of rhexis of a coiled artery with consequent formation of a hematoma, but occasionally it takes place by leakage through the vessel. When a hematoma forms, the superficial endometrium becomes distended and ruptures. Fissures subsequently develop in the adjacent functional layers, and bloody fragments of tissue of various sizes become detached. Autolysis occurs to some extent, but as a rule fragments of tissue may be found in the vagina and in the menstrual discharge. Hemorrhage stops when the coiled artery returns to a state of constriction. The changes accompanying partial necrosis seal off the tip of the vessel; and in the superficial portion, often only the endothelium remains. The endometrial surface is restored, according to Markee, by growth of the flanges, or collars, forming the everted free ends of the uterine glands. These flanges increase in diameter very rapidly, and the continuity of the epithelium is effected by the fusion of the edges of these sheets of thin migrating cells. The spongy zone is not entirely lost, and even some of the compact layer may remain after menstruation. By the end of menstruation the reduction in cellular size and loss of both tissue fluid and secretion result in a histologic picture superficially resembling the basalis of the secretory phase. These findings have led to the widespread idea that the entire endometrium except the basal zone is lost during menstruation. There is no direct evidence for that assumption, however. In the days immediately after menstruation the compact and spongy zones are reorganized, and the cell division therein is extensive.

The histologic changes during the human endometrial cycle have recently been reevaluated. Among the more thorough studies of menstruation are those of McLennan and Rydell, who believe that loss of endometrial tissue is less extensive than previous investigators have suggested. In their opinion, regeneration of the uterine surface occurs from residual spongiosa rather than from the most basal elements. If parts of the compact and spongy layers remain, most of the superficial portion of the endometrium during the so-called early proliferative phase cannot be considered new growth, but rather reorganization of tissue under a new epithelial cover. McLennan and Rydell confined their comments to menstruation, properly defined as bleeding associated with an ovulatory cycle, but another endocrine basis must be sought for anovulatory bleeding. According to Ramsey's summary of anatomic changes in the uterus during the menstrual cycle, it becomes increasingly clear that the spiral arteries are responsible for many functions of the endometrium. They maintain it, through successive menstrual cycles, in a recurringly receptive state and, after implantation of a fertilized ovum, enable it to provide a suitable circulatory mechanism for embryonic and fetal development to term.

Ultrastructure.   According to Wynn's ultrastructural studies, the endometrium reveals cytoplasmic secretion into the glandular lumens throughout the cycle. The terms "secretory" and "proliferative" therefore less accurately reflect the histologic pattern than do "preovulatory" ("follicular") and "postovulatory" ("luteal").

Since varying degrees of differentiation may occur in the same endometrium at different sites and even from cell to cell, the dating is based on the most advanced consistent pattern in the specimen. The basal endometrium remains essentially unchanged throughout the proliferative phase, whereas cyclic changes affect the superficial epithelium and particularly the glands in the zona spongiosa. The pseudostratification noted with the light microscope is not seen in thin sections if tangential cuts are avoided. The epithelial cytoplasm is poorly differentiated, containing numerous ribosomes but relatively few extensive channels of endoplasmic reticulum or elaborate Golgi complexes.

The mitochondria are randomly scattered throughout the cytoplasm in the early proliferative phase. Near the time of ovulation, they are located primarily near the base of the cell. They then enlarge, forming prominent cristae and developing in relation to polyribosomes and perinuclear patches of glycogen. Shortly before ovulation the small accumulations of glycogen coalesce to form large deposits between the nucleus and the basal plasma membranes, resulting in a well-defined structure that may be detected with the electron microscope about two days before the appearance of the typical "subnuclear vacuole" noted with the light microscope.

The Golgi apparatus increases in size during the midproliferative period, with the addition of lamellae and vesicles. Microvilli project from all well-preserved epithelial cells, but extensive pinocytosis is not evident. Occasional endometrial cells with typical cilia are found throughout the cycle, but they are much more common in the lower uterine segment and endocervix.

The stromal changes in the preovulatory phase vary temporally and topically. The late proliferative stroma resembles that of the early secretory phase, which also is variable. The stromal nuclei are relatively large and usually more dense than those of the epithelial cells. The usually scant cytoplasm may be reduced to a mere rim, forming the "naked nuclei" seen with the light microscope. Large numbers of endometrial granulocytes are uncommon, and plasma cells are rare except around the time of the menses.

The changes in endometrial organelles during the proliferative phase thus reflect a pattern consistent with endogenous growth and metabolism rather than elaboration of complex proteins for export. The end of the proliferative phase is characterized by cessation of development of these organelles, possibly a "braking" effect of progesterone.

Ultrastructural characteristics confined to the secretory phase have been identified by Wynn and others. Confluent subnuclear patches of glycogen and large mitochondria can first be detected by electron microscopy on or about day 14, approximately 36 to 48 hours before subnuclear vacuolation can be recognized by light microscopy. The mitochondria that first appear about the time of ovulation are several times larger than the typical organelles of the proliferative phase. Not more than a few of the giant mitochondria are found in any individual cell (Fig. 5). By day 17, deposits of glycogen are diffusely scattered through the cyto-

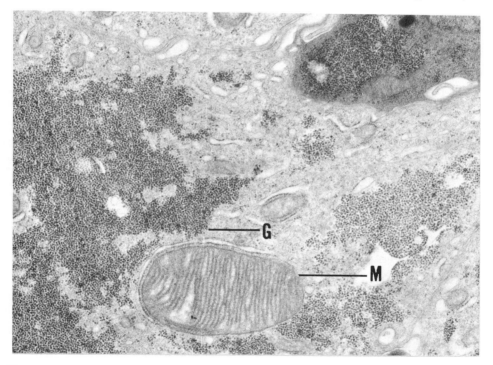

Fig. 5. Electron micrograph of postovulatory endometrium, showing association between giant mitochondrion (M) and deposit of glycogen (G) in epithelium. In this patient a Lippes loop had been in place for almost three years. (Courtesy of Dr. Ralph M. Wynn.)

plasm, and supranuclear Golgi complexes are dense and well developed. Smaller mitochondria are prominently distributed between convolutions of the plasma membranes.

Between days 17 and 20, a characteristic nucleolar channel system is maximally conspicuous (Fig. 6). Endoplasmic reticulum is not prominent, but mitochondria continue to enlarge and elongate, and convolutions of the plasma membranes continue to increase. By day 19 or 20, large projections from the surface of the glandular epithelial cells are found in association with extensive intraluminal secretion. At this time, the cytoplasm has ceased to differentiate further. The

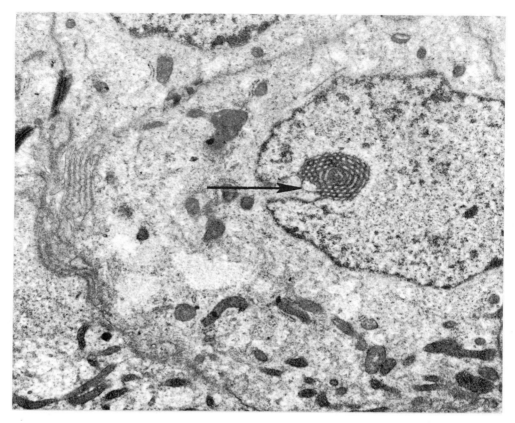

Fig. 6. Electron micrograph of early secretory (day 17) endometrium, showing characteristic nucleolar channel system (arrow). (Courtesy of Dr. Ralph M. Wynn.)

Golgi apparatus, however, remains fairly complex, and the nuclei have returned from luminal to basal positions.

By day 22, intraluminal secretion is prominent and the cells contain fewer intracytoplasmic secretory granules. There is little suggestion of pseudostratification. The microvilli are somewhat shorter and the epithelial cells themselves are lower. Basal laminas are thicker and plasma membranes are maximally folded.

By day 23 the granular endoplasmic reticulum has become less prominent, and the number of nucleolar channel systems has decreased greatly. Occasional Golgi complexes still appear well developed, and deposits of glycogen and lipids are scattered throughout the epithelial cells. The slender, elongated mitochondria resemble those of decidual cells, and the plasma membranes are highly convoluted. Mitochondria are distributed basally and peripherally, and small patches of glycogen are seen apically.

On day 24, isolated deposits of glycogen, large Golgi complexes, fragments of endoplasmic reticulum, and numerous small mitochondria are seen. The plasma membranes remain maximally convoluted, and complex intercellular spaces develop. Basal laminas of capillary and epithelium may be separated by only wisps of connective tissue.

In a cycle in which pregnancy does not occur, signs of cytoplasmic degeneration appear by day 25, including stromal hemorrhage, increased numbers of lysosomes and lipid granules, and clumping of nuclear chromatin. The decidual cell of pregnancy does not regress but maintains its numerous characteristic slender mitochondria and short fragments of endoplasmic reticulum. The fibrillar connective tissue is condensed to form a "capsule" around the cell, and the characteristic epithelioid pattern is established.

The first half of the postovulatory phase is concerned with elaboration and secretion of cytoplasmic products into the glandular lumens. The appearance of the giant mitochondria and nucleolar channel systems is probably related to a particular balance of estrogen and progesterone rather than to ovulation itself. The second postovulatory week is concerned with development of the stroma into predecidual tissue.

Ultracytochemical studies of the human endometrial cycle have suggested another means of correlating morphologic changes with metabolic functions. In the study by Sawaragi and Wynn, alkaline phosphatase, identified on epithelial plasma membranes, was found throughout the proliferative and into the midsecretory phase. Acid phosphatase was observed in lysosomes of glandular epithelium after day 21. Glucose-6-phosphatase was most evident around the time of ovulation and in the early secretory phase, localized most prominently in the endoplasmic reticulum. The timed localization of these enzymes suggests that they are biochemical determinants of the intracellular metabolic activity required to support implantation and early nutrition of the conceptus.

The Endometrial Cycle in Retrospect. The correlation of the ovarian cycle and its hormones with the endometrial cycle and the action of the pituitary gonadotropic hormones is summarized in Table 1 and in Figures 7 and 8. Although

Table 1. **Correlation of the Ovarian and Endometrial Cycles (Ideal 28-Day Cycle)**

Phase	Menstrual	Early Follicular	Advanved Follicular	Ovulation	Early Luteal	Advanced Luteal	Premenstrual
Days	1–3 to 5	4 to 6–8	9 to 12–16	12–16	15–19	20–25	26–32
Ovary	Involution of corpus luteum	Growth and maturation of graafian follicle		Ovulation	Active corpus luteum		Involution of corpus luteum
Estrogen	Diminution	Progressive increase		High concentration	Secondary rise		Decreasing
Progesterone	Absent			Appearing	Rising		Decreasing
Endometrium	Menstrual desquamation and involution	Reorganization and proliferation	Further growth and watery secretion	—	Active secretion and glandular dilatation	Accumulation of secretion and edema	Regressive
Pituitary secretion							
FSH	Fairly constant until just before ovulation			Moderate increase just before	Rapid decrease to previous levels		
LH	" "	"	"	"	Marked increase just before	" "	" "

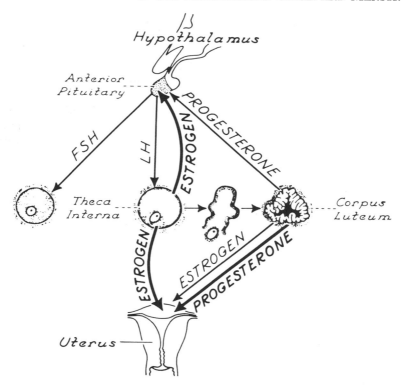

Fig. 7. Diagram illustrating hormonal relationships of the hypothalamus, pituitary, ovaries, and endometrium in the menstrual cycle.

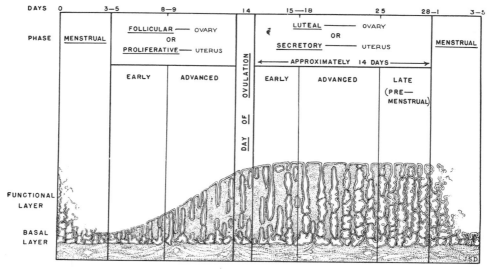

Fig. 8. Diagram illustrating cyclic changes in thickness and in form of glands and arteries of endometrium and their relation to ovarian cycle.

the cycle is divided into phases for descriptive purposes and convenience in diagnosis, the changes are continuous throughout an ovulatory cycle. There is, furthermore, considerable variation in both the activity of the endocrine glands and the response of the target organ, the uterus. Secretory changes closely resembling those of the luteal phase may occasionally appear before ovulation. Although the postovulatory phase of the cycle is generally very close to 14 days in length, the normal follicular phase may vary from 7 to 21 days. Finally, whereas the bleeding of a typical ovulatory menstrual cycle is preceded by endometrial ischemia, bleeding may appear at the expected time even without prior ovulation, formation of a corpus luteum, or secretion of progesterone. The histologic features of anovulatory cycles are reproduced in the bleeding endometria of patients after abrupt withdrawal of estrogens. Anovulatory cycles sometimes occur in otherwise apparently normal women, but the incidence is difficult to ascertain because adequate observations of the ovaries are rarely possible. It appears that in some such cycles a follicle enlarges but becomes cystic and degenerates. In others no follicles grow beyond a few millimeters throughout an entire cycle. Withdrawal of progesterone, therefore, is not essential for cyclic uterine bleeding. It is rare, however, for women with persistent anovulation to menstruate regularly.

At about 27 to 35 days after the last menstrual period there may be bleeding around the site of implantation of the ovum, resulting in slight vaginal bleeding that is sometimes mistaken for a menstrual period. According to Hartman, this "placental sign" bleeding always occurs during pregnancy in the rhesus monkey.

The histologic changes in the endometrium during the menstrual cycle are summarized in Figure 9, from Noyes, Hertig, and Rock. So characteristic are these alterations that an experienced pathologist can "date" an endometrium accurately from its microscopic appearance.

The Cervical, Vaginal, and Tubal Cycles.   As described and illustrated in the monograph of Papanicolaou, Traut, and Marchetti, cyclic changes occur in the endocervical glands, especially during the follicular phase of the cycle. During the early follicular phase, the glands are only slightly tortuous and the secretory cells are not very tall. Mucous secretion is meager. The late follicular phase is characterized by pronounced tortuosity of the glands, deep invagination, tumescence of the epithelium, high columnar cells, and abundant secretion. The connective tissue acquires a looser texture and shows better vascularization. Ovulation is followed by regression.

The increasing secretory activity of the endocervical glands reaches its height about the time of ovulation and is the result of estrogenic stimulation. Only at that time, in most women, is the cervical mucus of such a quality as to permit passage of the spermatozoa. The property of the cervical mucus that permits it to be drawn out in long strands is termed *Spinnbarkeit,* which is maximal at the time of ovulation. As pointed out by Papanicolaou, Traut, and Marchetti, the synchronization of the height of secretory activity in the cervical and endometrial cycles is precise and purposeful. In the cervix, where the mucus facilitates passage of the spermatozoa, it occurs when the ovum is just ready to be fertilized, a period of probably not more than about 15 hours. In the endometrium, where the purpose of the highly developed secretory activity seems to be to help provide a site favorable for nidation of the fertilized ovum, the changes are maximal about six days later, when the ovum is ready to implant.

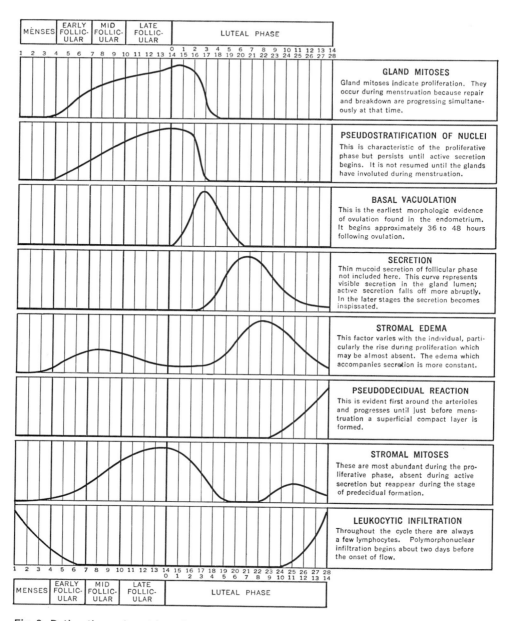

Fig. 9. Dating the endometrium. Correlation of important morphologic findings. (From Noyes, Hertig, and Rock. Fertil Steril 1:3, 1950.)

The "Fern Pattern."   If cervical mucus is aspirated, spread on a glass slide, allowed to dry for about ten minutes, and examined microscopically, characteristic patterns may be discerned, depending on the stage of the menstrual cycle and the presence or absence of pregnancy. From about the seventh day of the menstrual cycle to about the eighteenth day, a fernlike pattern is seen (Fig. 10); it is sometimes called "arborization" or the "palm leaf pattern." After the twenty-first

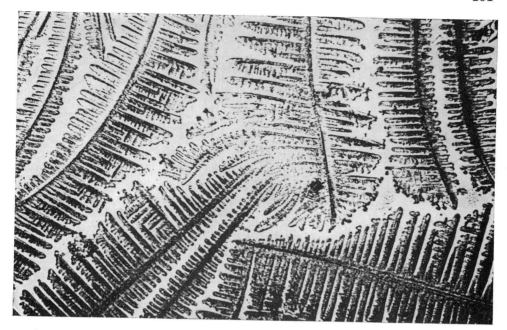

Fig. 10. Typical "fern arborization" pattern in cervical smears at midcycle in normal men-struating women. Note fullness and regular branching.

day, approximately, this fern pattern has disappeared and is replaced by a quite different, beaded or cellular picture (Fig. 11). This beaded pattern is usually encountered also in pregnancy.

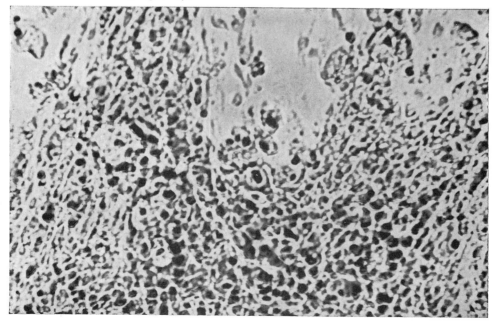

Fig. 11. A smear of cervical mucus from a pregnant patient at eight months. The beaded pattern is evident. (Courtesy of Dr. J. C. Ullery.)

The crystallization of the mucus, which is necessary for the production of the fern, or arborized, pattern, is dependent upon the concentration of electrolytes, mainly sodium chloride, in the secretion. In general a 1 per cent concentration of sodium chloride is required for the full development of a fern pattern; below that concentration either a beaded pattern or atypical, incomplete arborization is seen. The salt concentration in the cervical mucus, in turn, is under hormonal control, as demonstrated by the following facts: The typical fern pattern can be produced in postmenopausal women by injections of estrogen, and the days of the menstrual cycle during which the fern pattern is observed correspond with the days of estrogenic dominance, with the pattern most pronounced at the time of ovulation. Once progesterone is being produced in appreciable amounts, the fern pattern is rapidly replaced by a beaded, or "cellular," pattern, even though estrogen continues to be produced in relatively large amounts.

In summary, the presence or absence of the fern pattern is determined by hormonal action. Whereas the cervical mucus is relatively rich in sodium chloride when estrogen but not progesterone is being produced, the secretion of progesterone without a reduction in the secretion of estrogen promptly lowers the sodium chloride content of the mucus, either cervical or nasal, to a level at which ferning will not occur in the dried specimen. Progesterone during pregnancy usually exerts a similar effect, even though the amount of estrogen produced is tremendous compared with that of a normal menstrual cycle.

Because of the constant desquamation of the vaginal epithelium the cellular content of the vaginal fluid reflects to some degree the changes in the epithelium of the surface of the vagina. The human vaginal epithelium, under estrogenic stimulation, exhibits cyclic changes during which it reaches its greatest development at the end of the follicular phase. As shown in Figure 12, this stage is characterized by enlargement, flattening, and spreading of these cells and by relative leukopenia, whereas the smear in the luteal phase shows an increase in the number of basophilic cells and leukocytes, as well as irregular grouping.

As discussed on page 47, the fallopian tubes undergo characteristic cyclic changes with respect to both epithelium and muscular activity. The most characteristic morphologic variation in the epithelial cells of the tubal mucosa is a change in height. This difference has been carefully measured; in the follicular phase the height of the epithelium is over 30 microns, whereas in the luteal phase it averages not more than 20 microns.

CLINICAL ASPECTS OF MENSTRUATION

Menstruation is a periodic, physiologic discharge of blood, mucus, and cellular debris from the uterine mucosa, occurring at more or less regular intervals from puberty to the menopause except for pregnancy and lactation.

The Menarche and Puberty.   The age at which menstruation begins has declined steadily until recent years (Fig. 13). Treloar believes this decline has ceased in the United States and the age of menarche may possibly be on the rise. The average time at which menstruation begins is now between the twelfth and thirteenth year but in a small minority of apparently normal girls its onset may occur as early as the tenth or as late as the sixteenth year. The menarche refers specifically to the onset of the first menstruation, whereas puberty is a broader term, referring to the entire transitional stage between childhood and maturity. The menarche, hence, is just one sign of puberty.

The Menopause and Climacteric.   Menopause is the cessation of menstrual function, which occurs, on the average, at 47 years of age. There are wide varia-

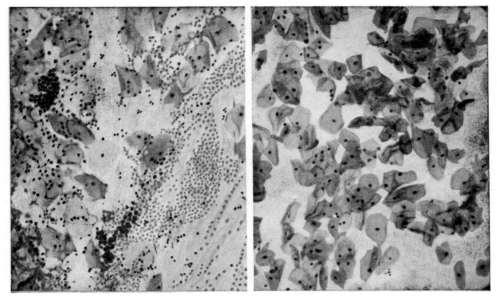

Menstrual phase.   Early follicular phase.

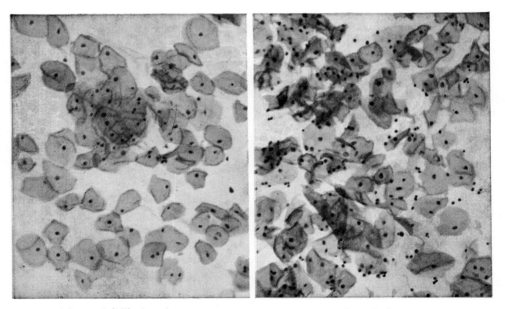

Advanced follicular phase.   Luteal phase.

Fig. 12. Vaginal smears in normal menstrual cycle stained with OG6-EA36. Acidophilic cells red; basophilic cells blue-green. Photomicrographs colored by H. Murayama. (From Papanicolaou, Traut, and Marchetti. The Epithelia of Woman's Reproductive Organs. New York, Commonwealth Fund, 1948.)

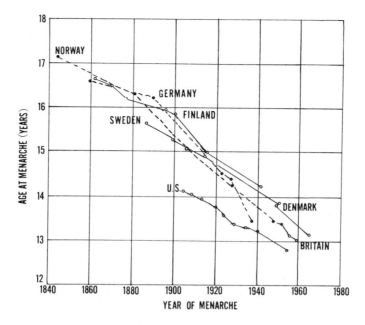

Fig. 13. Age of menarche has declined steadily in the United States and other countries. (From "Earlier Maturation in Man" by J. M. Tanner. Copyright 1968 by Scientic American, Inc. All rights reserved.)

tions in the age at which menopause occurs, however. About one half of all women cease menstruating between 45 and 50, about one quarter stop before 45, and another one quarter continue to menstruate until past 50. The term *climacteric* is derived from the Greek word meaning "rung of a ladder" and bears the same relation to the menopause as the term *puberty* bears to menarche. The climacteric refers to the critical period in a woman's life known to the laity as the "change of life."

Interval and Duration.   Although the *modal interval* at which menstruation occurs is 28 days, there is great variation among women in general as well as in the cycles of any individual woman. Marked irregularity in the length of the menstrual cycle is not incompatible with fertility in women. Arey, who analyzed 12 different studies comprising about 20,000 calendar records from 1,500 women and girls, reached the conclusion that there is no evidence of perfect regularity. In a study of 479 normal British women by Gunn, Jenkin, and Gunn, the typical difference between the shortest and longest cycle was 8 or 9 days; in 30 per cent it was over 13 days; in no case was it less than 2 or 3 days. Arey found that in an average adult woman one third of all her cycles depart more than 2 days from the mean length of her cycle. Arey's analysis of 5,322 cycles in 485 normal white women indicated an average interval of 28.4 days; his figure for the average cycle in puberal girls was longer, 33.9 days. More recently Chiazze and associates analyzed the length of 30,655 menstrual cycles of 2,316 women. The mean for all cycles was 29.1 days. For cycles ranging from 15 to 45 days the average length was 28.1 days. The degree of irregularity was such that only 13 per cent of the women had cycles that varied in length by less than 6 days. Haman surveyed 2,460 cycles in 150 housewives attending a clinic where special attention was directed to recording accurately the length of the menstrual cycles. Haman's data and Arey's figures for white women, superimposed in the distribution curves shown in Figure 14, indicate that the findings in the two series are almost identical.

The *duration* of menstrual flow is also variable; the usual duration is 4 to 6 days, but lengths between 2 and 8 days may be considered physiologic. In any individual woman, however, the duration of the flow is usually fairly constant.

Character and Amount.   The menstrual discharge consists of shed fragments of endometrium mixed with a variable quantity of blood. Usually the blood is liquid, but if the rate of flow is excessive, clots of varying size may appear. Considerable attention has been directed to the usual state of incoagulability of menstrual blood. The most logical explanation for its incoagulability is that the blood, having already undergone coagulation as it was shed, was promptly liquefied by fibrinolytic activity. Endometrium possesses not only potent thrombo-

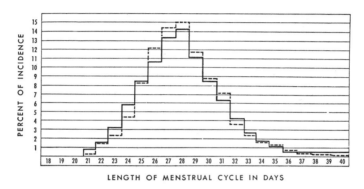

LENGTH OF MENSTRUAL CYCLE IN DAYS

Fig. 14. Duration of menstrual cycle based on distribution data of Arey (continuous line) and of Haman (broken line). (Courtesy of Eli Lilly and Co.)

plastic properties, which promptly initiate clotting, but also a potent activator of plasminogen, which effects prompt lysis of the clot.

The toxic properties of the menstrual discharge formerly attracted considerable interest. The discharge undoubtedly contains toxic proteins and peptides (Smith and Smith), resulting most likely both from proteolytic activity inherent in the mixture of blood and endometrium and also from bacterial contamination (Zondek).

The average amount of blood lost by normal women during a menstrual period has been found by several groups of investigators to range from about 25 to 60 ml (Hallberg and associates; Baldwin and co-workers; Hytten and associates; Millis; Barker and Fowler). With a normal hemoglobin concentration of 14 g per 100 ml and a hemoglobin iron content of 3.4 mg per gram, these volumes of blood contain from 12 to 29 mg of iron and represent a loss equivalent to 0.4 to 1.0 mg of iron every day of the cycle, or about 150 to 400 mg per year. Finch has measured the rate of decrease in the specific activity of the miscible ion of the body for a period of years after the injection of Fe^{55} to ascertain the rate of loss of iron from the body. Women who menstruated lost on the average 0.6 mg of iron per day more than did men and postmenopausal women. Since the amount of iron that is absorbed from the usual diet is quite limited, this "negligible" iron loss is important because it contributes to the low iron stores found in a majority of women (Scott and Pritchard; Hallberg and associates).

Changes in Body Weight.   It has been reported frequently that about 30 per cent of women shortly before the onset of menstruation gain one to three pounds, which they lose promptly as menstruation begins. Although only a minority of women manifest gains, there has been a tendency to regard the increase in weight as a normal characteristic of the cycle, reflecting the influence of steroid hormones. Actually, the average gain is insignificant, perhaps a quarter of a pound, as shown in a statistical study of this question by Chesley and Hellman, and more recently by Golub and associates. It would appear, therefore, that the concept of appreciable premenstrual weight gain as a physiologic phenomenon is not valid. Pronounced, regularly recurring weight gain before menstruation, or "premenstrual edema," is abnormal.

The many additional reported systemic changes during the menstrual cycle have been reviewed by Southam and Gonzaga. It is quite probable that many of these systemic changes, alleged to occur normally during the menstrual cycle, would fail to be substantiated by more critical studies.

REFERENCES

Arey, L. B.   The degree of normal menstrual irregularity. An analysis of 20,000 calendar records from 1,500 individuals. Amer J Obstet Gynec 37:12, 1939.

Baldwin, R. M., Whalley, P. J., and Pritchard, J. A.   Measurements of menstrual blood loss. Amer J Obstet Gynec 81:739, 1961.

Barker, A. P., and Fowler, W. M.   The blood loss during normal menstruation. Amer J Obstet Gynec 31:979, 1936.

Chesley, L. C., and Hellman, L. M.   Variations in body weight and salivary sodium in the menstrual cycle. Amer J Obstet Gynec 74:582, 1957.

Chiazze, L., Brayer, F. T., Macisco, J. J., Parker, M. P., and Duffy, B. J.   The length and variability of the human menstrual cycle. JAMA 203:377, 1968.

Finch, C. A.   Body iron exchange in man. J Clin Invest 38:392, 1959.

Golub, L. J., Menduke, H., and Conly, S. S., Jr.   Weight changes in college women during the menstrual cycle. Amer J Obstet Gynec 91:89, 1965.

Gunn, D. L., Jenkin, P. M., and Gunn, A. L.   Menstrual periodicity; statistical observations on a large sample of normal cases. J. Obstet Gynaec Brit Emp 44:839, 1937.

Hallberg, L., Hallgren, J., Hollender, A., Hogdahl, A.-M., and Tibblin, G.   Occurrence of iron deficiency anemia in Sweden. Symposia of Swedish Nutrition Foundation 6:19, 1968.

———— Hogdahl, A.-M., Nilsson, L., and Rybo, G. Menstrual blood loss, a population study: Variation at different ages and attempts to define normality. Acta Obstet Gynec Scand 45:320, 1966.

Haman, J. O.   The length of the menstrual cycle. A study of 150 normal women. Amer J Obstet Gynec 43:870, 1942.

Hartman, C. G.   Studies in the reproduction of the monkey *Macaca (Pithecus) rhesus* with special reference to menstruation and pregnancy. Contrib Embryol 23:1, 1932.

Hytten, F. E., Cheyne, G. A., and Klopper, A. I.   Iron loss at menstruation. J Obstet Gynaec Brit Comm 71:255, 1964.

Markee, J. E.   Menstruation in intraocular endometrial transplants in the rhesus monkey. Contrib Embryol 28:219, 1940.

McLennan, C. E., and Rydell, A. H.   Extent of endometrial shedding during normal menstruation. Obstet Gynec 26:605, 1965.

Millis, J.   The iron losses of healthy women during consecutive menstrual cycles. Med J Aust 2:874, 1951.

Noyes, R. W., Hertig, A. T., and Rock, J.   Dating the endometrial biopsy. Fertil Steril 1:3, 1950.

Papanicolaou, G. N., Traut, H. F., and Marchetti, A. A. The Epithelia of Woman's Reproductive Organs. New York, Commonwealth Fund, 1948.

Ramsey, E. M. Vascular anatomy of the uterus, in Wynn, R. M. (ed.), Cellular Biology of the Uterus. New York, Appleton-Century-Crofts, 1967, Ch. 3, p. 33.

Sawaragi, I., and Wynn, R. M. Ultrastructural localization of metabolic enzymes during the human endometrial cycle. Obstet Gynec 34:50, 1969.

Scott, D. E., and Pritchard, J. A. Iron deficiency in healthy young college women. JAMA 199:897, 1967.

Smith, O. W., and Smith, G. V. Menstrual discharge of women. I. Its toxicity in rats. Proc Soc Exp Biol Med 44:100, 1940.

Southam, A. L., and Gonzaga, F. P. Systemic changes during the menstrual cycle. Amer J Obstet Gynec 91:142, 1965.

Treloar, A. National Institutes of Health, Bethesda, personal communication, 1970.

Wynn, R. M., and Harris, J. A. Ultrastructural cyclic changes in the human endometrium. I. Normal preovulatory phase. Fertil Steril 18:632, 1967.

—— and Woolley, R. S. Ultrastructural cyclic changes in the human endometrium. II. Normal postovulatory phase. Fertil Steril 18:721, 1967.

Zondek, B. Does menstrual blood contain a specific toxin? Amer J Obstet Gynec 65:1065, 1953.

5

GAMETOGENESIS AND DEVELOPMENT OF THE OVUM

The process by which mature *germ cells,* or gametes, are formed from their respective primordial cells is called *gametogenesis,* a phenomenon associated with all forms of sexual reproduction. In the human being it entails the morphologic changes in the primitive germ cells, which are present in the embryo by the end of its third week of development. Both *oogenesis,* in the course of which mature ova are formed from primitive oogonia, and *spermatogenesis,* which results in the production of spermatids, share the basic biologic feature of maturation, or reduction, division.

Such special cellular division, known as *meiosis,* is characterized by a long and unusual prophase, and results in reduction of the *diploid* number of chromosomes, constant for each species, to the *haploid* number. In man the 46 chromosomes, comprising 44 autosomes and 2 sex chromosomes, are halved during a meiotic division, with the result that each mature gamete contains 23 chromosomes, or 22 autosomes and 1 sex chromosome. The diploid number is not restored until union of the egg and sperm during fertilization (Fig. 1). *Spermiogenesis,* comprising the final changes leading to production of mature male gametes, involves alterations in the shape of the spermatids and their transformation to spermatozoa. The fact that the mature germ cells are derived directly from primitive cells that may have migrated to the developing gonads from the yolk sac as early as the fifth week of embryonic life underlies the concept of *continuity of the germ plasm.* It explains, moreover, how some germ cells, reaching maturity at a very late date, as in the case of human ova, may have remained dormant for as long as 40 years.

Meiosis. The essential biologic feature of gametogenesis is meiotic cellular division. All primitive germ cells, *oogonia* and *spermatogonia,* contain the diploid number of 46 chromosomes. The former have the female complement of 44 autosomes and 2 X chromosomes; the latter, in common with ordinary male somatic cells, have 44 autosomes, one X and one Y chromosome. When these stem cells divide to produce primary oocytes and spermatocytes, each chromosome un-

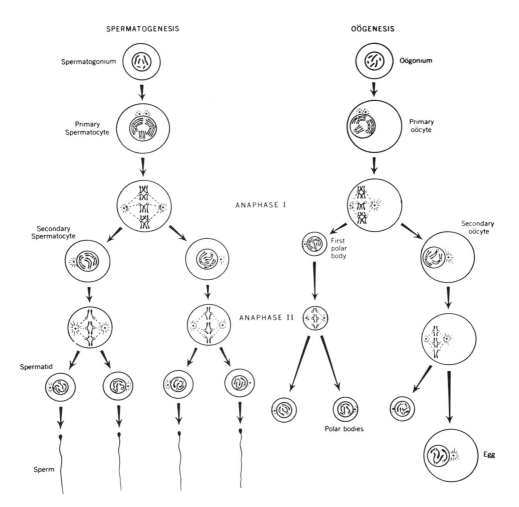

Fig. 1. Diagram representing the meiotic sequence in the male and female animal. Left, process of spermatogenesis resulting in the formation of four spermatozoa. Right, oogenesis resulting in the formation of one egg and three polar bodies. (From Gardner. Principles of Genetics. Courtesy of John Wiley & Sons, Inc.)

dergoes replication by splitting longitudinally, forming a double-stranded structure. During this typical *mitosis,* one strand of each chromosome enters each daughter cell, which thus obtains the identical chromosomal components of the parent cell (Fig. 2).

When, however, the primary oocytes and spermatocytes continue their maturation to form secondary oocytes and spermatocytes, respectively, the ensuing meiotic division is quite different, in that each of the newly formed cells receives only 23, or the haploid number of chromosomes. The basic difference between meiosis and ordinary mitosis is the prolonged meiotic prophase, in which there is preliminary pairing of homologous chromosomes before division. During the *leptotene* stage of meiotic prophase, the 46 chromosomes appear as single slender threads; in the next, or *zygotene,* stage, the homologous chromosomes are aligned

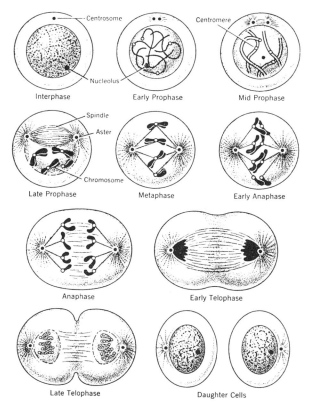

Fig. 2. Diagram of mitosis in an animal cell with four chromosomes. (From Gardner. Principles of Genetics. Courtesy of John Wiley & Sons, Inc.)

parallel to each other in *synapsis*, with the formation of 23 bivalent components. Each chromosome then splits longitudinally except at the *centromere*, as in ordinary mitosis, and the ensuing *pachytene* stage comprises *tetrads* of four chromatids, the shape of which depends on the position of the centromere, a thickened point of attachment of the spindle fibers to the chromatid pairs; at this point the chromatids may break and recombine with strands from the homologous chromosome. During the next, or *diplotene*, stage the homologous strands separate, but recombination in the form of *chiasmata* may occur, effecting interchange of genetic material. During the metaphase of the first meiotic division the bivalents (two chromatids making up each chromosome) become oriented on the spindle; when the cell divides, the members of each pair move toward opposite poles into the daughter cells, which then contain the haploid number of chromosomes, still double-stranded except at the centromere, and are no longer genetically identical with the parent cell. Each secondary oocyte will thus receive 22 autosomes and an X chromosome, and each secondary spermatocyte will receive 22 autosomes and either an X or a Y chromosome (Fig. 3).

At the second meiotic division the *diad* splits at the centromere to form two *monads,* one of which passes into each daughter cell, probably having already undergone a typical mitotic longitudinal replication. The mature ovum (22 + X),

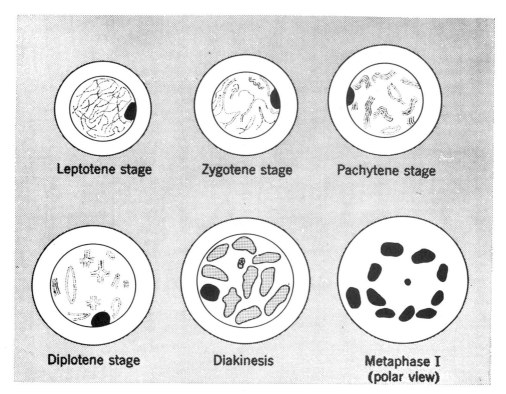

Fig. 3. Diagram of the meiotic prophase, illustrating pairing and duplication of chromosomes in the zygotene and pachytene stages, respectively. (From Gardner. Principles of Genetics. Courtesy of John Wiley & Sons, Inc.)

if fertilized by a spermatozoon containing 22 + Y chromosomes, will produce a male zygote (44 + XY) (Fig. 4); if fertilized by an X-containing spermatozoon, the result will be a female (44 + 2X).

Biochemistry of Cellular Division. The helical structure of DNA (deoxyribonucleic acid) is shown in Figure 5. During mitotic interphase, synthesis of DNA occurs simultaneously with the duplication of the chromosomes. Autoradiographic studies of the incorporation of tritiated thymidine into chromosomes indicate that duplication is accomplished by separation of the two original DNA subunits ,of each chromosome and by subsequent synthesis of two new subunits. At the following cellular division each chromatid receives one original and one new subunit. Alkylating agents, for example, may owe their effectiveness in the chemotherapy of cancer to their prevention of cellular division by bridging across the DNA helix, precluding separation of the subunits.

Oogenesis. In the sections of Chapters 2 and 3 dealing with the embryology of the ovary, the derivation of the primitive germ cells from the yolk sac and the histogenesis of the granulosal and thecal elements were described. Pinkerton and colleagues were able to trace the development of the human ovum by histochemical technics depending mainly upon the high content of alkaline phosphatase characteristic of the germ cells. In the first phase (migration), the germ cells

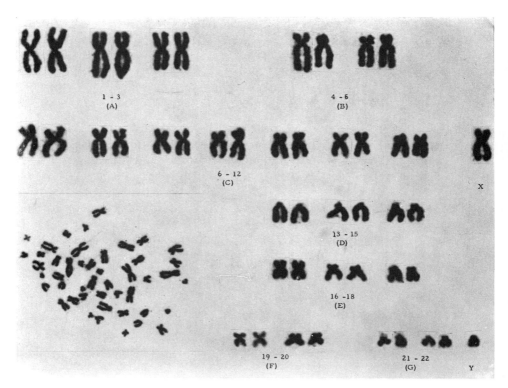

Fig. 4. Chromosomes from a normal male cell. The numbering and placement are based on the Denver Convention. The female karyotype has two X chromosomes instead of the XY. (Courtesy of Dr. Carlo Valenti.)

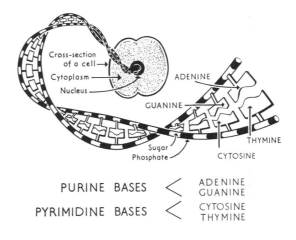

Fig. 5. Diagram of the double helix of the DNA molecule.

reach the medial slope of the mesonephric ridge, where the gonads arise, divide rapidly, and become oogonia; in the second phase (division), the germ cells divide mitotically at a rate that is maximal during the eighth to twentieth week, gradually slowing, and finally ceasing at birth; in the third phase (maturation), the cells enter the prophase of the first meiotic division, acquiring a ring of granulosa cells and becoming definitive oocytes within the primary follicles.

It is well to remember that all oocytes are derived from the primitive germ cells. The celomic mesoblast overlying the medial aspect of the mesonephric ridge supplies mesenchymal cells to the gonad until at least the fifteenth week and possibly until the last trimester, when it becomes a definite surface epithelium with a well-defined basement membrane. There is no evidence that this epithelium ever functions as a germinal layer, and hence no evidence of *neogenesis* of human ova. In Hartman and Leathem's review are reproduced several frames of a film by Blandau, which cinematographically records, in the mouse, the ameboid migration of primitive germ cells from the yolk sac to the germinal ridges. The primitive oogonia, furthermore, continue localized movements within the developing ovary even after reaching the pachytene stage of meiosis.

In man there is some indirect evidence that neogenesis of ova does not occur. Of the total number of primary oocytes at birth, variously estimated at 40,000 to 300,000, the majority degenerate. After puberty, several oocytes may begin to enlarge during each cycle, but ordinarily only one reaches full maturity. Winter, studying the ovaries of healthy nonpregnant women, found that at 30 years of age, for example, there were about 10,000 primary follicles, whereas at one month of age there were from 100,000 to 200,000. He interpreted the steady decrease in the number of primary follicles throughout life as indicative of a predetermined number of ova at birth.

Oogenesis, according to Raven, fundamentally involves the "storage of developmental information." Whereas in ordinary mitotic division there is exact reduplication of the genetic code at each cycle, in meiosis the genetic material undergoes only one reduplication before the two maturation divisions. By measuring DNA quantitatively, it can be shown that the reduplication occurs early in oogenesis, presumably in the premeiotic stages. Even early oocytes contain in their nuclei about twice the quantity of DNA found in diploid somatic cells and four times the amount in spermatids. Raven points out, furthermore, that essentially the same quantity of DNA is found in the germinal vesicle of the growing oocyte as in the equatorial plate of the first maturation division. From these data it appears that the reduplication of DNA in preparation for meiosis occurs in the earliest stages of oogenesis. By as early as the third fetal month, clusters of oogonia may be found in the ovarian cortex. Mitoses may be seen in some, whereas others have already differentiated into primary oocytes and entered the leptotene and zygotene stages of the first meiotic prophase. By the seventh fetal month almost all the oogonia have been transformed into primary oocytes, largely in the pachytene stage. By the time of birth, oogonia can no longer be detected, having differentiated into primary oocytes, which with their surrounding layer of follicular cells make up the primordial follicles. The oocytes have already entered the *dictyotene,* or resting, stage, in which they remain until maturation, only then to enter the metaphase of the first meiotic division.

The primary oocytes increase in size, while proliferating cuboidal follicular cells form increasingly thick coverings around them (Fig. 6). The follicular cells,

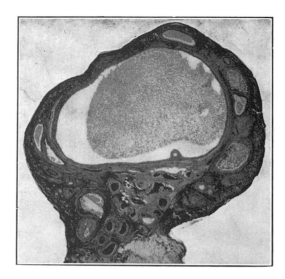

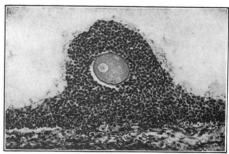

Fig. 6. Transverse section of macaque ovary showing ovum in almost fully grown 5 mm follicle. Top, × 10. Bottom, same ovum × 100. (Macaque No. 100, collection of Dr. G. W. Corner.)

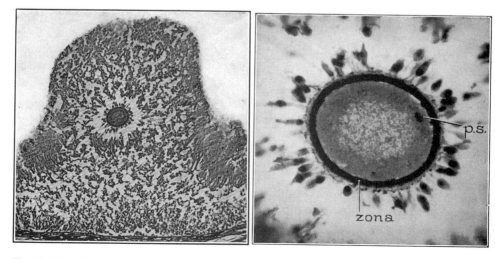

Fig. 7. Ovum in mature 7 mm follicle. Left, × 50. Note loosening of cells of cumulus oophorus. Right, same ovum × 358, containing first polar spindle, p.s., and surrounded by corona radiata. (Macaque No. 109, collection of Dr. G. W. Corner.)

furthermore, deposit on the surface of the oocyte an acellular glycoprotein mantle, which gradually thickens to form the *zona pellucida.* Irregular fluid-filled spaces between the follicular cells then coalesce to form an antrum. The radially elongated follicular cells surrounding the zona pellucida form the *corona radiata.* A solid mass of follicular cells surrounding the ovum in the side of a developing vesicular ovarian follicle is the *cumulus oophorus (discus proligerus)* (Fig. 7). As the follicle nears maturity, the cumulus projects farther into the antrum, with the result that the oocyte appears to be supported by a column of follicular cells. At this stage the follicle varies from 6 to 12 mm in diameter and lies immediately beneath the surface of the ovary.

During the final stage of transformation of the primordial into the mature graafian follicle, the primary oocyte completes its first meiotic division, which it began before birth (Fig. 8). The important result is the formation of two daughter cells, each with 23 chromosomes but of greatly unequal size. One receives almost all the cytoplasm of the mother cell to become a secondary oocyte; the other, the first polar body, receives hardly any. The polar body lies between the zona pellucida and the vitelline membrane of the secondary oocyte. The studies of tubal ova by Hertig and Rock indicate that the first polar body is cast off while still in the ovary. Before the nucleus of the secondary oocyte returns to a resting stage, following the first maturation division, the second division begins. The final result is the formation of a large mature oocyte and a second polar body. Just as a spindle begins to form in the secondary oocyte, ovulation occurs.

One of the most interesting unsolved problems in this field is elucidation of the mechanisms that prevent all ova but one from undergoing simultaneous maturation and ovulation during the first cycle. The factors responsible for allowing only one ovum normally to reach full maturity each month are still poorly understood.

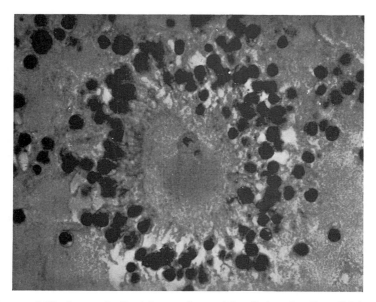

Fig. 8. A human follicular egg in the late anaphase of the first maturation division. Note the mitotic figure close to the center of the field. (From Hertig and Rock. Amer J Obstet Gynec 47:149, 1944.)

In man, the second maturation division is probably completed only if the ovum is fertilized. Failing to meet a spermatozoon within 24 hours of ovulation, the ovum begins to degenerate. Although it is not certain that the first polar body always undergoes subsequent division, fertilized ova have been found accompanied by three polar bodies. During maturation the diameter of the human ovum increases from 19 μ in the original oocyte to 135 μ in the fully mature ovum, a sevenfold increase.

Spermatogenesis.   In the male embryo, as previously described in the female, the primordial germ cells enter the developing gonad during the fifth week of development. There they are incorporated into irregularly shaped primitive sex cords composed of cells derived from the surface epithelium.

The sex cords at birth are solid, only later developing a lumen to become the seminiferous tubules. Two kinds of cells are found in the sex cords; the larger type, located along the basement membrane, has a pale-staining nucleus with one or more nucleoli and probably represents the primordial germ cell; the other type, also found along the basement membrane, is much smaller and has coarsely granulated nuclei; these cells cease to proliferate at birth and become sustentacular (Sertoli) cells.

The primitive germ cells in the testicular epithelium undergo division to form spermatogonia, some of which (Type A) divide to form new spermatogonia; others give rise to more highly differentiated spermatogonia (Type B), which develop into primary spermatocytes. These cells have large spherical nuclei with finely dispersed chromatin, either free in the nucleoplasm or attached to the nuclear membrane.

Clermont studied the mode of proliferation, differentiation, and renewal of spermatogonia in man. In his thorough investigations he described three main types of spermatogonia: dark (Ad) and pale (Ap) spermatogonia of Type A and spermatogonia of Type B. According to Clermont, Type A cells are present in all stages of the cycle. A pair of Type Ad spermatogonia act as stem cells. One member of the pair divides to form a pair of new Type Ad stem cells, while the other member divides to form a pair of more highly differentiated spermatogonia, the pale Type A. The Type Ap spermatogonia, in turn, give rise to spermatocytes. Clermont's model suggests that at each cycle of the seminiferous epithelium the spermatogonia renew themselves by producing new stem cells, while they simultaneously form spermatocytes, which later give rise to the mature germ cells, the spermatozoa.

The ensuing nuclear changes during spermatogenesis are entirely analogous to those in oogenesis. Each primary spermatocyte enters the long prophase of the first meiotic division. Upon completion of the first reduction division, two secondary spermatocytes are formed, with the haploid number of chromosomes; but unlike the products of the first meiotic division of the ovum, the secondary spermatocytes receive equal shares of cytoplasm from the parent cell. Almost immediately after formation, the secondary spermatocytes begin the second meiotic division, which results in the production of four spermatids. Theoretically, each primary spermatocyte after two meiotic divisions gives rise to four spermatids, which are chromosomally analogous to the mature ovum and second polar body, and which subsequently develop into spermatozoa (Figs. 1 and 9).

Spermiogenesis.   Immediately after they are formed, the spermatids undergo extensive changes in shape to become spermatozoa, by the process of spermio-

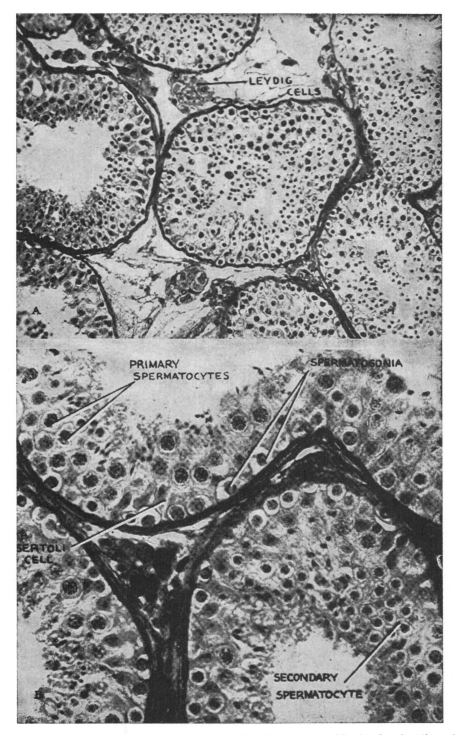

Fig. 9. Sections of normal human testes. A, testis of male aged 26, showing Leydig cells. B, testis of male aged 34 with sperm count 120 million per ml, showing stages of spermatogenesis. (From W. O. Nelson, in Greep. Histology. Courtesy of The Blakiston Company, Inc.)

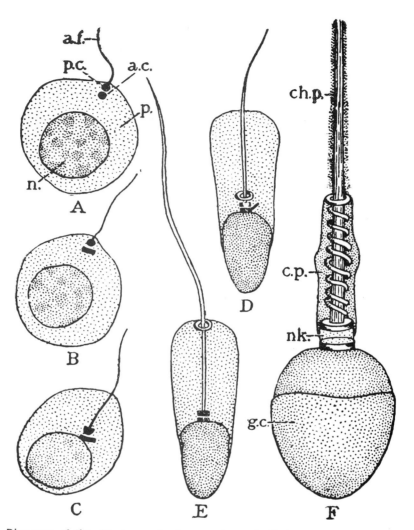

Fig. 10. Diagrams of the development of spermatozoa (A-F) (Meves): anterior centrosome, a.c.; axial filament, a.f.; connecting pieces, c.p.; chief piece, ch.p.; galea capitis, g.c.; nucleus, n.; neck, nk.; protoplasm, p.; posterior centrosome, p.c. (From Greep. Histology. Courtesy of The Blakiston Company, Inc.)

genesis. The newly formed spermatid has a spherical nucleus, a prominent Golgi zone, and numerous mitochondria. An initial change in the Golgi zone is the appearance of the dense *acrosomic granule,* which later forms a thin membrane over the surface of the nucleus, the head cap. The centrioles migrate to the pole of the nucleus opposite the head cap and form the flagellum, while the nucleus itself becomes condensed and slightly flattened and elongated. At the same time, mitochondria move toward the flagellum to form a collar around the axial filament. Distally the mitochondrial collar is limited by an annular structure, and together with the centriole, the collar and ring form the middle piece of the spermatozoon. At the completion of spermiogenesis the cytoplasm and the Golgi material not

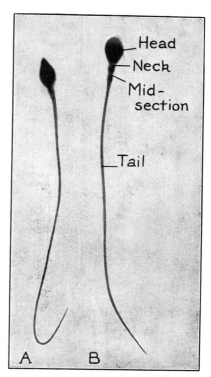

Fig. 11. Human spermatozoa. Re-touched photomicrographs. Head viewed in profile in A and from flat surface in B. The head contains the deeply staining nucleus, above which is the light cap. (From Hotchkiss. Fertility in Men. Courtesy of J. B. Lippincott Co.)

incorporated into the spermatozoa are cast off. Though only slightly motile when they first enter the seminiferous tubules, the spermatozoa become fully motile in the epididymis (Figs. 10 and 11).

TRANSPORT OF OVA AND SPERMATOZOA

Tubal Transport.   After ovulation the human ovum must normally gain access to the fallopian tube for fertilization. The mechanism by which ova are transported is more obvious in animals such as the rabbit, with ovaries completely enclosed in a peritoneal bursa into which the oviduct opens. In women, however, the ovaries lie free in the peritoneal cavity, and only the fimbria ovarica may actually touch their upper poles. Of the numerous factors implicated in the pickup and transport of ova, only ciliary current and muscular action of the tube and adnexal ligament have been subjected to direct observation. Westman, for example, showed that the infundibulum of the tube moves in the direction of the ovary and that the ovary itself rotates on its long axis. By injecting radiopaque contrast medium beneath the tunica albuginea of the ovary at laparotomy and performing subsequent hysterosalpingography, he was able to demonstrate the same muscular action in women as in rabbits and monkeys. Mastroianni, furthermore, has described a functional sphincter just beyond the tubal ostium. Since movements of the fimbriated extremity have been directly observed through the culdoscope, and since suction has not been demonstrated, adopting Clewe's analogy, he likened tubal action to that of a carpet sweeper rather than a vacuum cleaner. The role of even muscular activity as a prime factor in human tubal function may be questioned by the occurrence of successful pregnancies following the Pomeroy sterilization operation. In that procedure, in the event of recanalization of the tube, there is no regeneration of muscle and hence no true peristalsis or even successive muscular contractions in the direction of the uterus.

The role of hormones in tubal function is far from clear. In general, however, estrogens appear to increase and progesterone to decrease muscular activity. The endocrine effects, furthermore, are distinctly dose-related. Greenwald has shown, for example, that in the rabbit a low dose of estrogen accelerates the transport of eggs, whereas ten times the dose may lock the egg in the oviduct for five days or longer. The tubal anatomy and endocrinology of the rabbit are sufficiently unusual, however, that results based on studies of that species cannot be applied directly to man. Chang has shown, furthermore, that the tubal transport of rabbit ova may be modified by certain antifertility agents. Norethynodrel, a commonly used oral contraceptive, may cause retention of ova in the fallopian tube or acceleration of transtubal passage.

Kendle and Bennett showed that transport of ova through the oviduct of the mouse was inhibited or delayed by reserpine, which is said to cause major changes in the endocrine environment. Since restoration of the hormonal milieu had no effect on transport of ova, it seemed that endocrine control was not the principal regulatory factor. Chlorpromazine and tetrabenazine also cause a reduction in the rate of transport of ova, and all three drugs studied cause hypothermia. Kendle and Bennett found that maintaining the drug-treated mice in hyperthermic conditions led to a normal rate of transport of ova. They reasoned that hypothermia and the drugs causing it may result in altered muscular contraction, which may be of the greatest importance in tubal transport of ova.

The accurate synchronization of ova and endometrium as a prerequisite for normal subsequent development has been studied by Noyes and Dickmann, who showed that rats' ova of the same age as, or slightly older than, the endometrium to which they were transferred had a greater chance of survival than ova one day or more younger than the endometrium. Any factor that rushes the eggs prematurely through the tubes into the endometrium may thus upset the critical timing and exert thereby a contraceptive effect. It was formerly thought that intrauterine devices exerted their effect in this manner.

By recording intraluminal pressure changes in the oviduct of the rabbit in vivo, Greenwald observed differences in motility of the ampullary and isthmic portions. Since the changes in tubal motility were not necessarily related to the rate of migration of the ovum, he concluded that the timing of the relaxation of the ampullary-isthmic junction, where delay normally occurs, was a crucial factor in transport. Since fertilization in mammals usually occurs in the ampulla, whatever the roles of the tubal cilia and peristalsis may be, an adequate theory must explain how ova are moved down and spermatozoa up the fallopian tube.

Migration of the Ovum.   In most mammals the ovum requires three to three and one half days for transit through the oviduct, reaching the cavity of the human uterus about three to four days after fertilization. In animals with a bicornuate uterus and a single cervix, corpora lutea may be found in one ovary, and embryos in the contralateral horn, providing presumptive evidence of *migration of the ovum.* In women the ovum may wander across the pelvis to be picked up by the opposite tube (*external migration*) or, theoretically, may cross inside the uterus and migrate up the opposite tube (*internal migration*). Presumptive clinical evidence of migration of the ovum includes the finding of a corpus luteum on one side and an ectopic pregnancy in the contralateral tube, as well as successful intrauterine pregnancy in women who have only one tube and the contralateral ovary. It is likely that the entire subject of migration of the ovum in women has received more attention than it deserves. In their normal anatomic relations, as observed at laparotomy, both tubes usually hang freely, with their fimbriated extremities posterior to the uterus and rather closely approximated. In view of the known motility of the tubes and ovarian ligaments, it is entirely reasonable that the ovum may easily be picked up by the opposite tube, without recourse to complicated mechanisms of internal or external migration.

Transport of Spermatozoa. During human coitus an average ejaculate of 2 to 3 ml with an average sperm count of 120 million per milliliter is deposited in the vagina. According to Hotchkiss, of these 300-odd million spermatozoa, of which between 80 and 90 per cent are normal forms, only one must meet, in the upper portion of the fallopian tube, the single mature ovum released during each normal ovulatory cycle. MacLeod believes that a count of 20 million spermatozoa is compatible with fertility, provided the sperm are of normal motility and not more than 15 to 20 per cent are abnormal forms.

Whereas mammalian spermatozoa are normally highly motile, their rapid rate of movement requires the participation of contractions of the female genital tract. Although Hartman showed that rat semen is rapidly aspirated into the uterus, it is doubtful whether a similar event occurs in women, in whom the roles of peristalsis, tubal spasm, and myometrial contractions in the transport of sperm remain to be clarified. Freund, Saphier, and Wiederman demonstrated a contractile response in vitro of the uterus and vagina of the guinea pig to the deposition of semen, explaining thereby the rapidity of transport of sperm in that species. Bickers indicated that spermatozoa may pass through the cervical canal on their own power, but require uterine contractions to ascend beyond the internal os. Moghissi, studying the excised human genital tract, reported that in the absence of neural and hormonal regulation viable and motile sperm were incapable of passing the internal cervical os. Sperm could reach the internal os only in the presence of suitable mucus characteristic of the midcycle. He concludes that sperm penetrate as far as the internal os on the basis of their own motility, but that reaching the oviduct requires extrinsic forces.

Capacitation. In rats and rabbits, and possibly in human beings, spermatozoa must be conditioned before they can effect fertilization. In a comprehensive review of the subject, Noyes has indicated that, although there are still many questions regarding the changes in the spermatozoa before attainment of the capacity for fertilization, or capacitation, the alterations are related to time, incubation, and removal of seminal fluid. Adams and Chang demonstrated that acquisition of the capacity to penetrate ova took place gradually in the tube and uterus.

Within the past few years considerable attention has been devoted to the mechanisms of capacitation in a variety of animals. Marston and Kelly found that in the rhesus monkey penetration of the egg by the sperm occurs within six hours of introduction of spermatozoa into the uterus. They conclude, therefore, that if capacitation occurs in this animal, it does so within three to four hours.

Mattner noted that bovine sperm exposed to, cervical mucus are more refractory to the "dilution effect"—that is, they are longer-lived. He postulates that the protection afforded by mucus is related more to its structural and physical than to its chemical properties. Zaneveld and co-workers described a trypsinlike enzyme in the acrosomes of ejaculated and capacitated sperm in the rabbit. The enzyme is said to aid in removal of the zona pellucida from the ovum. According to Zaneveld and co-authors, the acrosomes contain also an inhibitor of the trypsinlike enzyme, as does seminal fluid. Capacitation may thus be regarded as the removal of an inhibitor.

Chang achieved in vitro fertilization of rabbit ova by capacitated sperm, as proved by transfer and subsequent development of fertilized donor's eggs in a recipient's uterus. Although experimental attempts of this kind date back to Spallanzani in 1776, human "genetic surgery" utilizing frozen human semen, as described in Sherman's review, has only recently become a possibility. The most highly publicized recent work has perhaps been that of Edwards and co-workers in England, who reported in vitro fertilization of human oocytes that were themselves matured in vitro. The human "test tube baby" is, of course, far from an accomplishment, or even a necessarily desirable possibility, but it is no longer entirely within the realm of science-fiction.

FERTILIZATION

Although only one of the many millions of spermatozoa deposited in the female genital tract actually effects fertilization, the others may aid the fertilizing sperm in penetration of the ovum. In the union of egg and sperm, the essence of fertilization, there are several significant biologic implications. First, the diploid number of chromosomes is restored and thereby variation of species is maintained; second, the sex of the offspring is determined and a primary sex ratio established and maintained; and third, fertilization initiates the sequence of mitotic divisions that result in cleavage and further development of the zygote.

The union of ovum and sperm in most mammals ordinarily occurs in the ampulla of the oviduct, and much more rarely on the surface of the ovary. In ferrets and certain insectivores, however, spermatozoa normally enter the ovarian follicles and penetrate the mature ova before ovulation. In the human being, such an event is a great rarity, possibly accounting for certain instances of primary ovarian pregnancy (p. 559). In mammals, except for unusual examples of parthenogenesis, the union of sperm and egg is requisite to the development of the normal adult. In insects such as the bee, however, the males or drones may develop from unfertilized eggs. In other insects there are male- and female-producing eggs that develop without fertilization into adults; as a result an alteration of sexually produced and parthenogenetic generations results. In certain vertebrates too, notably the frog, unfertilized eggs may, by various means, be artificially stimulated to divide.

The principal function of the spermatozoa is to contribute paternal genes to the offspring. Although only one spermatozoon actually penetrates the ovum, the others possibly help by detaching the corona radiata, presumably by enzymatic action. Tubal ova may be recovered surrounded by up to 60 spermatozoa, some of which may be embedded in the zona pellucida. How the spermatozoa traverse the zona pellucida and by what means the vitelline membrane becomes refractory to the penetration of other spermatozoa after fertilization remain to be discovered. The ultrastructural changes accompanying the fusion of gametes are well described in Austin's monograph.

Zona Pellucida. Blandau has provided informative electron micrographs, reproduced in Hartman and Leathem's review, that shed some light on the nature of the zona pellucida. In the rat, the ampullar ova are normally free of cumulus cells within 24 to 36 hours after ovulation. Ultrastructural examination of preovulatory eggs shows, however, that small protoplasmic processes of the oocytes and follicular cells extend into or across the zona pellucida. The cytoplasmic extension of the corona anchors the granulosa cells firmly to the zona in the follicular and early postovulatory egg. Microvilli on the surface of the egg extend into the zona pellucida and greatly increase the total surface area. They are no longer obvious at the time that the perivitelline space appears. The cytoplasmic extensions are of probable significance in the transport of metabolites from the follicular cells to the oocytes during the period of active growth.

Dickmann and Noyes have shown that the zona pellucida in the rat is shed from the blastocyst during the fifth day after fertilization. The shedding, moreover, appears unrelated to a specific uterine environment, but is rather an intrinsic manifestation of growth and maturation of the blastocyst. Since the blastocyst, free of the zona pellucida, may survive and develop normally to term when transferred to the uterine horns of recipient animals, the zona is clearly not necessary for implantation; on the contrary, its removal is a prerequisite for implantation, at least in the laboratory rodents thus far studied. The precise timing and mechanism of loss of the zona pellucida and its function are problems that remain to be solved.

Changes Preceding Implantation. In a study of the development of mouse eggs in diffusion chambers within the peritoneum, Bryson showed that the ova continue to develop normally up to the stage of implantation and to that apparently critical period when the zona pellucida is normally shed. Doyle, Gates, and Noyes had previously shown that with mouse as well as rat eggs development proceeds normally when the transferred eggs are the same age or slightly more advanced than the endometrium. The older eggs, however, sometimes developed into heavier fetuses than did the eggs of synchronous transplants. The younger ova, however, disintegrated at the time when the zona pellucida of synchronously transplanted ova were normally shed. Bryson's experiments in particular indicated that the early development of the ova was not correlated with the endocrine state of the host; although hormones have no apparent effect on free blastocysts of the mouse in other normal or extrauterine locations, they have indeed a critical effect on intrauterine development, especially at the time of and after implantation. During its free sojourn in the uterine cavity there is, in general, considerable freedom of the unattached blastocyst from extrinsic influences. In the stages of development immediately after implantation, however, the conceptus is remarkably sensitive. At such a time teratogenic agents, whether drugs, ionizing radiation, or viruses, may exert profound effects.

Abnormal Sexual Differentiation. Since there are two chromosomally different kinds of spermatozoa in mammals, the male gamete determines the sex of the offspring. In birds, on the contrary, the ovum or the female parent determines chromosomal sex. Although heredity is the principal determinant of sex in mammals, environmental factors must also be operative, as evidenced by the various inter-sexes and, in the opossum, for example, the phenomenon of sexual transformation. In general, in mammals a Y chromosome will lead to male sexual differentiation, even in the presence of more than one X chromosome. Miller has shown that nor-mally only one X is active; the others undergo late replication and form the planoconvex sex chromatin masses (Barr bodies) seen on the nuclear membranes. The number of *sex chromatin* masses in interphase nuclei is, therefore, one less than the number of X chromosomes in the cells at mitotic metaphase.

Although in *mosaicism* involving sex chromosomes the sex chromatin bodies and the sex chromosomes themselves may vary from tissue to tissue, the two are constant with respect to each other. In the study of human intersex and certain forms of sterility, analyses of sex chromatin and sex chromosomes provide impor-tant data. The latter, though more difficult to study, provide more accurate infor-mation, since the sex chromatin frequency may vary in certain types of cells, in newborns, and in disease. Platt and Karling, for example, have reported in the exfoliated vaginal cells of healthy women a sex chromatin frequency of about 56 per cent. Since during mitosis the sex chromatin migrates from its peripheral location, cells undergoing rapid replacement and malignant cells are more likely to have low chromatin body counts, in contrast to stable cells such as neurons. Similarly, reversible intranuclear edema or intranuclear migration of the chroma-tin body may explain the low counts in situations of stress. Since, furthermore, the chromatin masses may not be fully manifest during fetal life, a calculation of the primary sex ratio based on aborted tissue may be erroneously weighted in favor of the male (see p. 498). It may be reasonable to consider the normal human female as a mosaic of X chromosomes. One X in a normal female is genetically inert and morphologically condensed to form the Barr body; the active X can be contributed by either parent. Beutler and co-workers have supported the concept of X mosaicism with studies using the gene for glucose-6-phosphate dehydroge-nase deficiency as a marker.

Many abnormalities of sexual development may result from meiotic *nondis-junction* of the monads and diads of the sex chromosomes of either parent during diakinesis, the final stage of prophase. Thus, instead of producing two cells with one X each, a primary oocyte may give rise to one cell with two X chromosomes, and one with none. Similarly, a primary spermatocyte may give rise to two cells, with XY and O chromosomal complements, respectively. If then, a normal mature oocyte (X) is fertilized by a spermatozoon with no sex chromosome, an individual with 45 chromosomes and an XO karyotype results. Clinically such a patient represents the variety of *Turner's syndrome* that is *chromatin-negative* and sterile. By analogy, nondisjunction of the homologous X chromosomes may result in an XX mature oocyte, which, if fertilized by a normal Y-bearing spermatozoon, pro-duces an XXY individual. Such a person, representing a common type of *Kline-felter's syndrome*, will have 47 chromosomes and *chromatin-positive* cells. Cases of Klinefelter's syndrome with more than 47 chromosomes—for example, the XXXY karyotypes—may be explained either on the basis of nondisjunction of the gametes of both parents, or on the statistically much more likely basis of non-disjunction of the female gamete during both the first and second meiotic divi-sions.

Chromosomal mosaicism, however, requires a different explanation. An XXX/ XO mosaic, for example, might result from mitotic nondisjunction, with the shift of an X from one strain to another, but an XXX/XX chromosomal pattern is more difficult to explain. Nondisjunction or translocation of an *autosome* (a chromosome other than an X or a Y), furthermore, may result in other clinically significant genetic abnormalities, such as Down's syndrome (mongolism), which typically is characterized by 47 chromosomes, or an autosomal trisomy.

The most profound chromosomal disturbances may result not merely in genetic anomalies but in abortion. Thiede and Salm studied the chromosomes of tissues derived from human abortions. In the spontaneous abortions, there was a high proportion of chromosomal anomalies, particularly polyploidy and trisomy, whereas in the therapeutic abortions the chromosomal pictures, or *idiograms*, were essentially normal (Ch. 20, Fig. 6).

Aging of Gametes. Lanman discusses the deleterious effects of delays in reproduction, including aging of eggs and sperm and delays in parturition. The increased incidence of the trisomy 21 variety of Down's syndrome late in reproductive life is well recognized. It may be related to an increased tendency toward nondisjunction in eggs that may have remained dormant in the ovary for 40 years or more. Although the incidence of this syndrome in the population as a whole is only 3 per 2,000 live births, it rises to about 1 in 40 in women over the age of 45. The proper placement of chromosomes during cell division depends on their attachment to the spindle. This connection is normally established by about 20 to 30 threads attached to the centromere. According to Lanman, aging during the prolonged dictyotene stage might progressively impair the attachment.

Tesh and Glover noted that aging of the male gametes also exerted deleterious effects on the embryo and fetus. They reported that aging of rabbit sperm in the male reproductive tract led to loss of fertilizing capacity. If these sperm fertilized eggs, moreover, an increase in embryonic anomalies resulted.

Vickers noted that delayed fertilization also led to an increase in chromosomal anomalies of the embryo. In mice in which fertilization was delayed (7 to 13 hours), triploidy, for example, was increased ninefold. Vickers postulates that the chromosomal aberrations may result from errors in meiosis, fertilization, or cleavage.

DEVELOPMENT OF THE OVUM

Cleavage of the Ovum. After fertilization, the mature ovum becomes a zygote, which then undergoes segmentation, or cleavage, into blastomeres. With the accumulation of fluid between the blastomeres, the blastocyst is formed. Although it is not strictly correct to refer to segmenting zygotes as ova, the earliest stages of human development have traditionally been so designated. The blastocyst, or "ovum," then implants on or in the endometrium, while the fetal membranes and germ layers of the embryo are formed. Although the distinction between embryo and fetus is essentially arbitrary, it is customary to refer to the human conceptus from fertilization through the first eight weeks of development as an *embryo,* and from eight weeks until term as a *fetus.* During the embryonic period the major organ systems are formed, and during fetal life histogenesis, or differentiation of the tissues, proceeds. Sexual differentiation, however, is not completed until puberty.

The first typical mitotic division of the segmentation nucleus of the zygote results in the formation of two blastomeres. A photomicrograph of the living

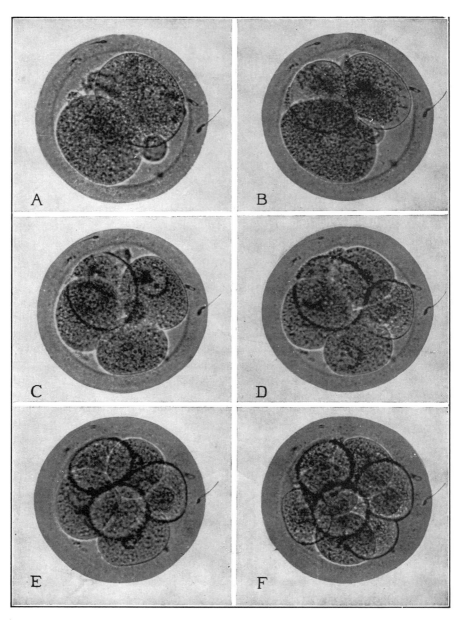

Fig. 12. Photomicrographs (× 300) of living monkey ovum showing its cleavage divisions. The fertilized ovum was washed out of the tube and cultivated in plasma; its growth changes were recorded cinematographically. The illustrations are enlargements from single frames of the film. A, two-cell stage, 29 hours and 30 minutes after ovulation. B, three-cell stage, 36 hours and 4 minutes after ovulation. C, four-cell stage, 37 hours and 35 minutes after ovulation. D, five-cell stage, 48 hours and 39 minutes after ovulation. E, six-cell stage, 49 hours exactly after ovulation. F, eight-cell stage, 49 hours and 48 minutes after ovulation. These cleavages normally occur as the ovum passes down the fallopian tube. Note the spermatozoon in the zona pellucida. (After Lewis and Hartman. Contrib Embryol 24:187, 1933.)

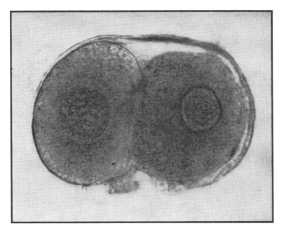

A

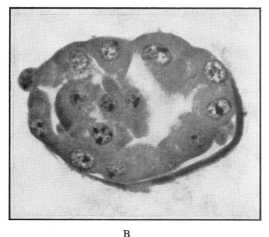

B

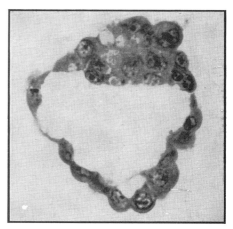

C

Fig. 13. Human preimplantation stages. A, two-celled stage. Intact ovum surrounded by zona pellucida, photographed after fixation. Washed from fallopian tube about one and a half days after conception. Nuclei shimmer through granular cytoplasm. Polar body in perivitelline space. (Carnegie Collection No. 8698. × 500.) B, 58-celled blastula with intact zona pellucida found in uterine cavity three to four days after conception. Thin section showing outer (probably trophoblastic) and inner (embryo-forming) cells and beginning segmentation cavity. (Carnegie Collection No. 8794. × 600.) C, 107-celled blastocyst found free in uterine cavity about five days after conception. A shell of trophoblastic cells enveloping fluid-filled blastocele, and inner mass consisting of embryo-forming cells. (Carnegie Collection No. 8663. × 600.) (From Hertig, Rock, Adams, and Mulligan. Contrib Embryol 35:199, 1954.)

segmenting monkey's ovum (Fig. 12) shows the blastomeres and polar bodies suspended in the perivitelline fluid and surrounded by the zona pellucida. The human ovum (Fig. 13) undergoes similar changes. In fact, mammalian eggs in general are remarkably similar in their earliest stages in that the entire egg divides, in contrast to the situation in the megalecithal eggs of birds and certain reptiles, in which cleavage is restricted to one pole.

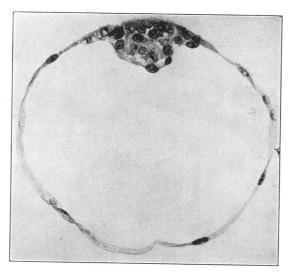

Fig. 14. Section through blastula of monkey. × 300. Ovulation age 9 days. The delicate trophoblast forms the outer wall of the segmentation cavity; the embryo develops from the inner cell mass at the pole uppermost in this figure. (C 522, Carnegie Collection.) (Retouched photomicrograph.)

During its three days within the fallopian tube, the egg undergoes slow cleavage, as indicated by the recovery from the uterine cavity of human ova with only 12 blastomeres. As the blastomeres continue to divide, a solid mulberrylike ball of cells, the *morula,* is produced. With time-lapse cinematography, Lewis and Gregory photographed all these stages in the development of the rabbit's egg before implantation. The gradual accumulation of fluid within the morula results in formation of the blastocyst, at one pole of which is a compact mass of cells destined to produce the embryo (Figs. 14 and 15); the outer layer of cells is the *trophoblast,* which nourishes the ovum until establishment of the placental circulation (p. 159). Krishnan and Daniel have isolated from the uterus of the rabbit early in pregnancy a protein fraction that is said to be capable of induction

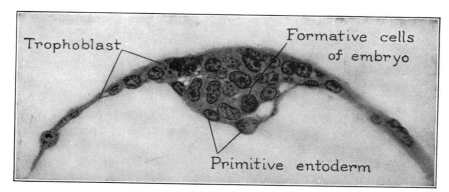

Fig. 15. Section through embryonic area of monkey. × 500. (Retouched photomicrograph.)

of blastulation in the morula. Partial purification of this fraction indicates that the activity is restricted to a single homogeneous protein component. This important work needs confirmation and extension to other species.

The Early Human Ovum. Most of our knowledge of the earliest stages of human development is derived from the material obtained by Hertig and Rock and prepared by Heuser with unsurpassed histologic skill. The earliest human ovum available for study is the pronuclear form discovered by Noyes and co-workers (Fig. 16). In the normal two-celled egg flushed from the fallopian tube (Fig. 13A), Hertig and Rock found the blastomeres and a polar body free in the perivitelline fluid and surrounded by a thick zona pellucida (compare with monkey's ovum, Fig. 12A). They provisionally considered as abnormal the four cleavage stages with 5, 8, 9, and 11 to 12 blastomeres that they found in the uterine cavity, but recovered morphologically normal stages comprising 12 and 58 cells. The normal ova, still surrounded by a zona pellucida, measured 0.150 and 0.154 mm, respectively, in the fresh state. In the 58-cell morula (Fig. 13B) can be distinguished the outer cells, presumably destined to produce the trophoblast, and the inner cells that form the embryo. The next stage that Hertig and Rock obtained is a 107-cell blastocyst (blastodermic vesicle), which is not larger than the earlier cleavage stages, despite the accumulated fluid (Fig. 13C). It measured 0.153 × 0.155 mm in diameter before fixation and after the disappearance of the

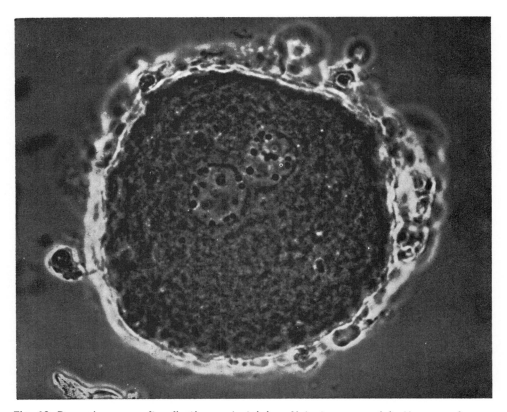

Fig. 16. Pronuclear egg after fixation and staining. Note two pronuclei. Absence of zona pellucida is an artifact of processing. Phase contrast. (Courtesy of Dr. Zeev Dickmann and Dr. Robert W. Noyes.)

zona pellucida. The 8 formative (embryo-producing) cells are surrounded by 99 trophoblastic cells. The "ovum," now a blastocyst, is ready to implant.

Implantation.   Before implantation, the zona pellucida disappears and the blastocyst adheres to the endometrial surface. After erosion of the epithelium, the blastocyst sinks into the endometrium. The Hertig-Rock ova indicate that in man, as in the majority of mammals, the pole of the blastocyst at which the inner cell mass is located enters first. The extent to which the blastocysts grow varies greatly among mammals, but eventually all implant on or in the endometrium.

One of the earliest implantation sites discovered by Hertig is shown in Figure 17. It measured only 0.36 × 0.31 mm, its discovery remaining a remarkable achievement. The blastocyst shown in Figure 17 was in the process of entering the endometrium, with its thin outer wall still within the uterine cavity. An ovum at a similar stage, with dimensions of 0.45 × 0.30 × 1.125 mm, is shown in Figure 18. It appears to have flattened out in penetrating the uterine epithelium, in the fashion of the blastocyst of the rhesus monkey. The enlargement and multiplication of the trophoblastic cells in contact with the endometrium are alone responsible for the increase in size of the implanted, as compared with the free, blastocyst. The hole in the uterine epithelium created by the ovum as it implants indicates the size of the egg at the onset of erosion of the surface. The defect is bounded by a zone of maternal epithelium that shriveled as the trophoblast spread out beneath it (Fig. 18). When correction is made for the additional shrinkage resulting from preparation of the histologic sections, the diameter of the ovum at the moment of implantation can be estimated as 0.23 mm. A monkey's blastocyst at a corresponding stage, estimated by Streeter and by Heuser as nine days after fertilization, measured 0.42 × 0.34 mm. In man, therefore, the ovum enters the endometrium earlier than in the monkey and soon becomes completely buried. According to Hertig and Rock, the smaller human ovum implants at about six days after fertilization.

Mechanism of Implantation.   Although practically nothing is known of the fundamental nature of implantation in man, some information based on studies of the rabbit and rodents is available. In the rat there is no destruction of uterine epithelium by the trophoblast until the embryo comes to lie deep within the decidual crypt and an extensive decidual response has been initiated. In the guinea pig and man, however, a full decidual response is not elicited until the trophoblast has eroded the superficial uterine epithelium. Shelesnyak and Tic concluded that the nonspecific stimulus to decidualization was either histamine or a histaminelike substance present at the site of injury at the time of blastocystic attachment. They postulated, furthermore, that a surge of estrogen releases the histamine from the endometrium.

The blastula, or blastocyst, of most placental mammals makes no firm contact with the endometrium for several (three to more than ten) days after reaching the uterus. Whereas in man the free blastocystic period is four to six days, in some species there is a "developmental diapause," or delayed implantation, in which the blastocysts may remain unattached for much longer intervals (six months or more in the pine marten, for example).

Böving's anatomic analysis of implantation in the rabbit, though probably applicable in detail only to that species, is virtually the only attempt, even partially successful,

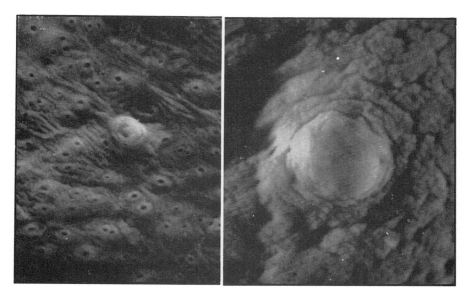

Fig. 17. Low and high power photographs of surface view of an early human implantation obtained on day 22 of cycle, less than 8 days after conception. Site was slightly elevated and measured 0.36 by 0.31 mm. Left, the actual size of the ovum is indicated by the white square at the lower right. Mouths of uterine glands appear as dark spots surrounded by halos. (Carnegie Collection No. 8225.)

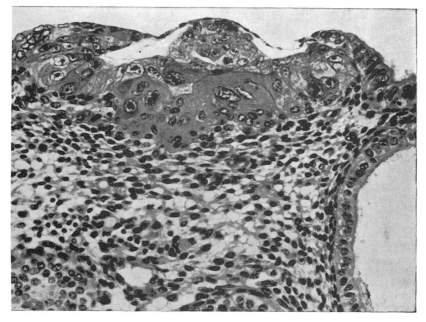

Fig. 18. Youngest human ovum (about seven and a half days). × 300. (Carnegie Collection No. Mu-8020.) Implantation is still shallow so that the characteristics of the collapsed blastocyst wall continue in evidence. Ovum is well anchored to the endometrium, however, by its trophoblast. The embryo is the small globular mass situated between the blastocyst wall above and the proliferating trophoblast underneath it. (From Hertig and Rock. Amer J Obstet Gynec 47:149, 1944.)

to formulate a unified concept of the basic biologic mechanisms. In the first, or muscular, stage of implantation, the blastocysts are scattered randomly along the uterine cornu. Progesterone stimulates blastocystic expansion, causing uterine distention and waves of contractions that progress in both directions from the blastocyst. The blastocysts are then pushed as far apart from one another as possible, becoming evenly spaced along the cornu. As the blastocysts eventually become too large to be moved along the uterus, the stimulus for the mechanism of spacing thus becomes its inhibitor.

In the second, or adhesive, stage, the mucopolysaccharide envelopes secreted around the conceptus by the oviduct and uterus are perforated by the trophoblast, which then becomes adherent. The adhesion is induced by a local rise in pH that accompanies discharge of bicarbonate from the abembryonic hemisphere of the blastocyst and removal of carbon dioxide where there is a capillary at the base of the uterine epithelium. The reaction is speeded by carbonic anhydrase, the activity of which is greatly augmented by progesterone at the time of implantation.

The third, or penetrative, stage of implantation is probably also a consequence of the preceding local rise in pH. Böving believes that alkalinity causes dissociation of the cellular uterine epithelium, but that the trophoblast, being syncytial, remains intact. Although progesterone plays a central role in the process of implantation, the specific order of events and their efficient coordination require local interplay of the various components of the mechanism.

The variations in blastocystic spacing and implantation among other mammals, however, are extensive. Böving has theorized that the fundamental difference between invasion by trophoblast and by cancer lies essentially in the cellular character of malignant tissue. An objection to the theory has been raised by Kirby and Malhotra, however, who examined the invading trophoblast of the mouse with the electron microscope. In that species, at least, the invasive trophoblast is cellular rather than syncytial.

In their recent ultrastructural analysis of the cellular relations of endometrium and trophoblast at the sites of implantation in a variety of mammals, Enders and Schlafke found that in all species studied the trophoblastic cells extend over several uterine epithelial cells at the "apposition stage." The trophoblast can adhere to the apical ends of uterine epithelial cells by means of primitive junctional complexes. In most species, desmosomal junctions are formed in addition between trophoblast and the lateral aspects of uterine epithelial cells. Enders and Schlafke suggest that the capacity of trophoblast to form junctions with epithelial cells is an important part of the process of implantation, facilitating penetration of the endometrium without dislodgment of the blastocyst.

Tachi and co-workers provide interesting ultrastructural documentation of the sequence of events surrounding implantation in the rat. After shedding its zona pellucida, the blastocyst of the rat makes contact with tips of microvilli and bleblike cytoplasmic protrusions of the epithelial cells during the afternoon of the fifth day postcoitum. Sperm tail inclusions were observed in both trophoblast and inner cell mass as late as the fifth day postcoitum. By the sixth day uterine epithelial microvilli were usually lost and trophoblastic plasma membranes were interlocked with those of endometrial epithelium, often forming tight junctions. Highly electron-dense cells were frequently wedged between trophoblast and uterine epithelium. The earliest morphologic responses of stromal cells to blastocystic attachment were changes in nuclear shape, distribution of chromatin, and nucleolar structure in the subepithelial layer. During the seventh day, basal laminas generally disappeared and the trophoblast was in close contact with stromal cells. The distance between the two unit membranes was around 100 to 200 angstroms. A periplacental "fibrinoid" barrier was not recognized at this stage, but Tachi and co-workers leave open the question that this postulated immunologic barrier may appear at a later stage (see Ch. 6, p. 169).

Development of Ovum After Implantation.   At seven and a half days, the stage shown in Figure 18, the wall of the blastocyst facing the uterine lumen consists of a single layer of flattened cells, whereas the thicker opposite wall comprises two zones, the trophoblast and the embryo-forming inner cell mass. The maternal tissues in contact with the trophoblast show definite signs of injury, and the decidua immediately adjacent appears condensed, perhaps as a result of withdrawal of water by the invading trophoblast. Within the trophoblast, two subdivisions are soon distinguishable, the *cytotrophoblast,* comprising individual cells with relatively pale-staining cytoplasm, and the *syncytiotrophoblast,* in which dark-staining nuclei are irregularly distributed within a common baso-philic cytoplasm. In the trophoblast, mitotic figures are confined to the cellular elements. Evidence for the derivation of the syncytium from the cytotrophoblast, based on autoradiographic and ultrastructural studies, is presented on page 154. By as early as seven and a half days, the inner cell mass, now the *embryonic disc,* has already differentiated into a thick plate of primitive ectoderm and an under-lying layer of endoderm. Between the embryonic disc and the trophoblast appear some small cells that soon enclose a space that will become the amniotic cavity.

In the next stage of the Hertig-Rock series, the nine and a half day ovum (Fig. 19), the increase in size is due mainly to development of the syncytium, which comprises a complex network of protoplasmic strands, enclosing irregular fluid-filled spaces, the *lacunae,* which later become confluent. The embryonic disc now consists of a "dorsal" ectoderm, made up of tall columnar cells, and a "ven-tral" endoderm, formed of somewhat irregular cells. The remainder of the blasto-cyst is occupied by a proteinaceous coagulum, limited externally by a layer of flattened cells (the *exocelomic,* or *Heuser's, membrane*) of uncertain origin. The amniotic cavity dorsal to the embryonic disc is now well defined. Its very early

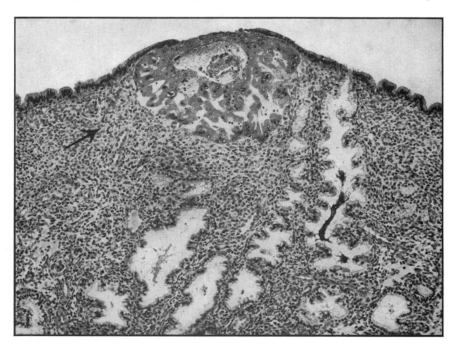

Fig. 19. A thin section of ovum obtained on twenty-fifth day of cycle, nine and a half days or less after conception. Area still exposed to uterine lumen, 0.38 × 0.26 mm bordered as in Figure 20. Syncytiotrophoblast, a complex network filling enlarged implantation site. Within cytotrophoblastic shell, two-layered embryo and amnion-forming cells. Arrow indicates zone of enlarged stromal cells. (Carnegie Collection No. 8004.) Photomicrograph × 100. (From Her-tig and Rock. Contrib Embryol 31:65, 1945.)

origin by cavitation is characteristic of the anthropoids and certain of the chiroptera (bats), whereas amniogenesis by folding of fetal membranes most intimately enveloping the fetus occurs in most mammalian orders. In reptiles, birds, and many mammals, the amnion morphologically appears to be an extension of the fetal ectoderm, continuous with the skin. Streeter, Hertig, and others previously associated with the Carnegie Institution, however, conclude that in man the embryonic and extraembryonic structures are sharply demarcated in the blastocystic stage. In other words, they believe that both epithelium and mesenchyme of all the fetal membranes are derived directly from the primitive trophoblast, leaving the inner cell mass to produce only the body of the embryo. With regard to the amnion, it seems reasonable that at least the epithelium is delaminated from the trophoblast. There is, furthermore, no convincing evidence that the inner cell mass produces any of the extraembryonic mesoderm. Details of the controversy are discussed by Wynn and others.

As the ovum enlarges, more maternal tissue is destroyed and the walls of its capillaries are eroded, with the result that maternal blood enters the lacunae. With deeper burrowing of the ovum into the endometrium, the trophoblastic

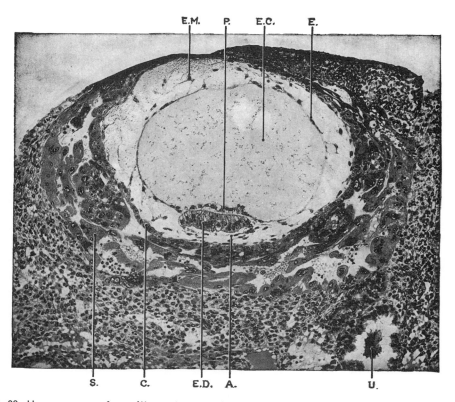

Fig. 20. Human ovum of previllous stage. × 120. (Carnegie Collection No. 7700.) Free cells are delaminating from inner surface of trophoblast around its entire circumference, forming amnion adjacent to germ disc. E.D., embryonic disc; P., primitive entoderm; A., amnion; E., exocelomic membrane; E.C., exocelomic cavity; C., cytotrophoblast; S., syncytium; E.M., extraembryonic mesoblast; U., uterine gland removed on the twenty-ninth day after the onset of the last menstrual period. Its age is estimated as about 12 days. (From Hertig and Rock. Contrib Embryol 31:65, 1945.)

strands branch to form the solid primitive villi traversing the lacunae. Located originally over the entire surface of the ovum, the villi later disappear except over the most deeply implanted portion, the future placental site. The mesenchyme first appears as isolated cells within the cavity of the ovum. When the cavity is completely lined with mesoderm, it is termed the *chorionic vesicle,* and its membrane, now called the *chorion,* is composed of trophoblast and mesenchyme.

The 12-day ovum shown in Figure 20 has reached a diameter of almost 1 mm. The mesenchymal cells within the cavity are most numerous about the embryo, where they eventually condense to form the *body stalk,* which serves to join the embryo to the nutrient chorion and later develops into the umbilical cord. The site of entry of the blastocyst into the endometrium is then covered by regenerated epithelium. The defect itself is plugged by an operculum (Teacher), consisting of fibrin and cellular debris. The syncytiotrophoblast of the chorionic shell is permeated by a system of intercommunicating channels or trophoblastic lacunae containing maternal blood. At the same time the surrounding endometrial stroma shows a decidual reaction, characterized by enlargement of the connective tissue cells and storage of glycogen therein. The amniotic cavity is then lined by ectoderm, apparently continuous with that of the embryonic disc. At this stage the endoderm probably delaminates from the inferior surface of the embryonic disc and soon spreads peripherally beyond the disc to line the blastocele. The process results in the formation of the endodermal primary yolk sac. The rest of the blastocyst is filled with primary mesoderm, consisting of sparse mesenchymal

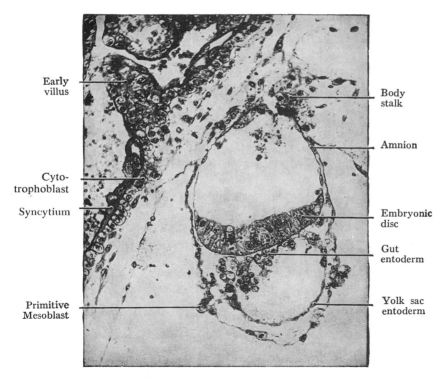

Fig. 21. Embryo. × 180. (After Brewer.)

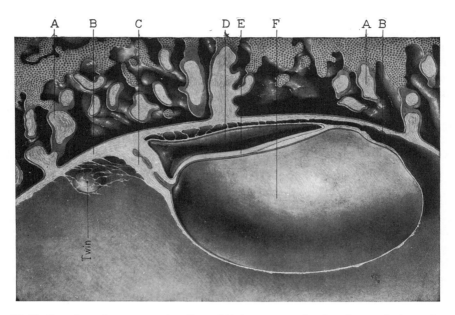

Fig. 22. Median view of wax reconstruction of Mateer ovum, showing the amniotic cavity and its relations to chorionic membrane and yolk sac. × 50. A, chorionic villi; B, chorionic membrane; C, body stalk with allantois; D, flattened amniotic cavity; E, embryonic area; F, yolk sac. (After Streeter.)

cells in a loose matrix. The mesoderm, according to one school of thought, arises from the trophoblast, but its precise mode of origin in man remains to be elucidated. It appears possible, however, to trace some of this early mesoderm into the embryonic disc, between ectoderm and endoderm.

The Germ Layers.   In Figures 21 and 22 the amnion and yolk sac with both epithelial and mesenchymal components can be seen. The body stalk, representing the future caudal end of the embryo, can also be recognized at this stage. Cellular proliferation in the embryonic disc marks the beginning of a thickening in the midline that clearly indicates the embryonic axis and is called the *primitive streak.* Cells spread out laterally from the primitive streak between ectoderm and endoderm to form the mesoderm. These three germ layers then give rise to the various organs of the body. From the *ectoderm* are derived the entire nervous system, central and peripheral, and the epidermis with such derivatives as the crystalline lens and the hair. The *endoderm* develops into the lining of the gastrointestinal tract, from pharynx to rectum, and such derivative organs as the liver, pancreas, and thyroid. The dermis, the skeleton, the connective tissues, the vascular and urogenital systems, and most skeletal and smooth muscle arise from the *mesoderm.* The cavity that later divides the somatic and visceral sheets of intraembryonic mesoderm is the *celom.*

Formation of the Somites.   During the third week of development the primitive streak becomes a prominent feature, leading to recognition of cephalic and caudal ends of the embryo. As cells proliferate rapidly and spread laterally from the primitive streak, a midline *primitive groove* develops. Simultaneously, the yolk

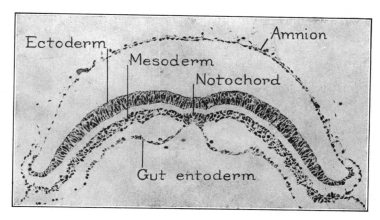

Fig. 23. Photomicrograph of transverse section through presomite human embryo. × 125. (No. 5960 Carnegie Collecton.) (From Heuser, Hertig, and Rock. Contrib Embryol 31:85, 1945.)

sac enlarges, with the result that the embryonic disc is spread out upon it, as in the megalecithal eggs of reptiles and birds. Figure 22 shows a well-defined body stalk, into which a narrow endodermal diverticulum, the allantois, has extended. In many mammals the allantois develops into a large sac that vascularizes the chorion. A forward extension of the primitive streak, the *notochord* (Fig. 23), constitutes the primordial supporting structure of vertebrates and remains as a continuous column of cells throughout embryonic life. Remnants of the notochord persist in the adult as the nucleus pulposus of the intervertebral discs.

Since differentiation of structure proceeds from cephalic to caudal ends, a sequence characteristic of all vertebrate embryos, most of the substance of the early embryo will enter into formation of the head, the subsequent development of the primitive streak providing material for the rest of the body. Figure 24 shows the thickened ectoderm that forms the *neural plate,* which soon develops a *neural groove* (Fig. 25), as neural folds arise on either side. Connecting the cavity of the future neural tube with the future lumen of the gut is the *neurenteric canal.* As the neural folds develop, the underlying lateral mesoderm is divided into discrete blocks, the *somites* (Figs. 24 through 26), which give rise to the skeletal and connective tissues, the muscles, and the dermis. The first three or four somites enter into formation of the occipital region of the head. The primordium of the heart has already appeared beneath the pharynx as it is separated from the yolk sac by a fold that also lifts the cephalic end of the embryo above the level of the yolk sac. Figure 27 (A to D) shows the elevation of the neural folds and their closure to form a tube, which is wider from the outset in the region of the fourth pair of somites. Although the head remains relatively enormous during the embryonic period, the rest of the body takes form after the fourth week, and the head becomes smaller in proportion. By the seventh week of embryonic life the neck can be recognized, the tail filament has disappeared, and the embryo can be identified as human. From the eighth week on, changes in the shape of the human fetus are less striking. Some of the principal features are outlined in Chapter 7.

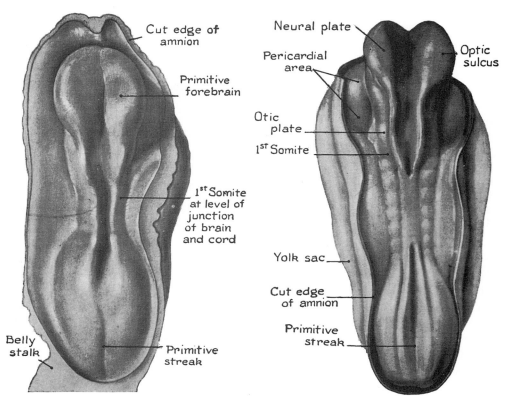

Fig. 24. Human embryo at beginning of segmentation. × 67. Dorsal view of model showing open neural groove. (Carnegie Collection No. 1878. Drawing by Didusch after Ingalls. Contrib Embryol 11:61, 1920. From Streeter. Scientific Monthly 32:495, 1931.)

Fig. 25. Seven-somite human embryo. × 45. Estimated (Streeter) ovulation after 21 days. Note closure of neural tube in middle region. (Carnegie Collection No. 4216. Drawing by Didusch after Payne. Contrib Embryol 16:115, 1925. From Streeter. Scientific Monthly 32: 495, 1931.)

Comparative Embryology. To summarize the features of early embryology described in this chapter and to simplify the explanation of human placental development to follow (Ch. 6), a brief consideration of homologies among mammalian fetal membranes is in order. The first attachment of the blastocyst to the uterus may be mesometrial or antimesometrial. Since the midsagittal plane of the simplex uterus of man is the homologue of the antisometrial surface of the bicornuate uterus, the site of first attachment in the human being, which is usually in the midline dorsally or ventrally, may be regarded as basically *antimesometrial*. Implantation of the blastocyst may be *interstitial*, or deep, as in man, or superficial, as in the macaque. The orientation of the embryonic disc to the uterus, furthermore, may be mesometrial or antimesometrial. Since in man both the first attachment of the blastocyst and the orientation of the embryonic disc are antimesometrial, the human "ovum" implants with the inner cell mass down. In many of the important laboratory rodents, however, the first attachment is antimesometrial but the inner cell is oriented mesometrially, with the result that in such animals as the guinea pig the inner cell mass is directed upward. An unusual situation is found in the tarsier, in which the embryonic area is directed upward, as a result of an antimesometrial orientation of disc to uterus and a mesometrial first attachment. In

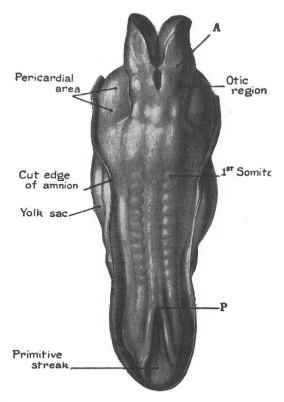

Pericardial area

Otic region

Cut edge of amnion

1st Somite

Yolk sac

A

P

Primitive streak

Fig. 26. Ten-somite human embryo. × 25. A and P mark superior and inferior limits of neural tube closure. (Carnegie Collection No. 5074. Drawing by Didusch after Corner. Contrib Embryol 20:81, 1929. From Streeter. Scientific Monthly 32:495, 1931.)

summary, human implantation is characterized by an antimesometrial first attachment, an antimesometrial, downwardly directed inner cell mass, and a location deep within the endometrium that accounts for the development of both basal and capsular deciduas. The decidua capsularis is, of course, absent in forms with superficial implantation.

The details of origin of the human amnion, allantois, and extraembryonic mesoderm in man require further investigation. It is believed, however, that the human amnion arises precociously by cavitation in the ectodermal portion of the embryonic disc, its epithelium, at least, derived more or less directly by delamination from the trophoblast. The human endoderm, at first comprising a scattered layer of cells ventral to the amnionic vesicle, resembles somewhat the earliest stages of the inverted yolk sac characteristic of the higher rodents, as described in detail by Mossman. The mesoderm then spreads rapidly around the inside of the blastocyst, soon differentiating into parietal and visceral layers. In the monkey, and very likely also in man, it does not arise directly from the inner cell mass of the morula. In the visceral portion vitelline vessels form, while in the parietal or somatic part the allantoic vessels develop. It is an important generalization that since no blood vessels develop in the true somatopleure, amnionic or chorionic, the chorion must be vascularized by neighboring mesoderm, either vitelline or allantoic. The human placenta, vascularized by homologues of allantoic vessels, is therefore a typically *chorioallantoic* mammalian organ.

By the time hematopoiesis is evident in the mesoderm, the rudimentary human endodermal allantois has grown into the preformed body stalk or mesodermal allantois. The endodermal portion indicates that the human body stalk is homologous with the

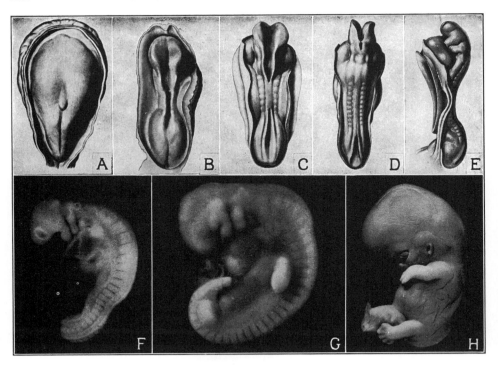

Fig. 27. Human embryogenesis. (Carnegie Collection.) A, Heuser, × 30, 19 days. B, Ingalls, × 28. C, Payne, × 23. D, Corner, × 23. E, Atwell, × 15.5, 21 to 22 days. F, × 12, fourth week. G, × 8.5, fifth week. H, × 2.5, eighth week. (Form Streeter. Scientific Monthly 32:495, 1931.)

large allantoic stalks of animals such as the rabbit. It is therefore just as reasonable to regard the vascular chorionic mesoderm as allantoic in man as in the rat and mouse, in which there is an even slighter trace of allantoic endoderm. Thus the human body stalk can be considered most simply as the precociously differentiated mesenchyme of the allantois.

In light of the interest in congenital anomalies engendered by the recent thalidomide disaster and the epidemic of rubella, as well as the increasing emphasis on protection of the pregnant woman from the teratogenic effects of ionizing radiation and other external influences such as drugs, the importance of basic embryologic information in obstetrics becomes evident. Furthermore, the earlier in embryogenesis the teratogen exerts its effect, the more profound are the changes likely to be. As a result of the liberal abortion laws in Japan, Nishimura and colleagues have had the opportunity of studying over 1,200 intact normal and abnormal human embryos. Their valuable data supplement the classic material of Streeter described in Chapter 7 and provide standards for subsequent studies of human embryogenesis and teratogenesis. An understanding of normal development makes the mode of origin of congenital anomalies largely self-explanatory to the obstetrician.

References

Adams, C. E., and Chang, M. C. Capacitation of rabbit spermatozoa in the fallopian tube and in the uterus. J Exp Zool 151:159, 1962.

Austin, C. R. Ultrastructure of Fertilization. New York, Holt, Rinehart & Winston, 1968.

Beutler, E., Yeh, M., and Fairbanks, V. F. The normal human female as a mosaic of X-chromosome activity: Studies using the gene for G-6-PD-deficiency as a marker. Proc Nat Acad Sci USA 48:9, 1962.

Bickers, W.   Sperm migration and uterine contractions. Fertil Steril 11:286, 1960.

Blandau, R. J., White, B. J., and Rumery, R. E.   Observations on the movements of the living primordial germ cells in the mouse. Fertil Steril 14:482, 1963.

Böving, B. G.   Implantation, in Wynn, R. M. (ed.). First Conference on Fetal Homeostasis. New York, New York Academy of Sciences, 1965, p. 138.

Brewer, J. I.   A normal human ovum in a stage preceding the primitive streak. Amer J Anat 61:429, 1937.

———— A human embryo in the bilaminar blastodisc stage (the Edwards-Jones-Brewer Ovum). Contrib Embryol 27:85, 1938.

Bryce, T. H., and Teacher, J. H.   Contribution to the Study of Early Development and Imbedding of the Human Ovum. Glasgow, J. Maclehouse & Sons, 1908.

Bryson, D. L.   Development of mouse eggs in diffusion chambers. Science 144:1351. 1964.

Chang, M. C.   Fertilization of rabbit ova in vitro. Nature (London) 184:466, 1959.

———— Effects of certain antifertility agents on the development of rabbit ova. Fertil Steril 15:97, 1964.

Clermont, Y.   Spermatogenesis in man. A study of the spermatogonial population. Fertil Steril 17:705, 1966.

Dickmann, Z., and Noyes, R. W.   Zona pellucida at the time of implantation. Fertil Steril 12:310, 1961.

Doyle, L. L., Gates, A. H., and Noyes, R. W.   Asynchronous transfer of mouse ova. Fertil Steril 14:215, 1963.

Edwards, R. G., Bavister, B. D., and Steptoe, P. C.   Early stages of fertilisation in vitro of human oocytes matured in vitro. Nature (London) 221:632, 1969.

———— and Fowler, R. E.   Human embryos in the laboratory. Scientific America 223:40, 1970.

Enders, A. C., and Schlafke, S.   Cytological aspects of trophoblast-uterine interaction in early implantation. Amer J Anat 125:1, 1969.

Freund, M., Saphier, A., and Wiederman, J.   In vitro studies of the effect of semen on the motility of the vagina, uterus and uterine horns in the guinea pig. Fertil Steril 15:188, 1964.

Greenwald, G. S.   In vivo recording of intraluminal pressure changes in the rabbit oviduct. Fertil Steril 14:666, 1963.

Hartman, C. G., and Ball, J.   On the almost instantaneous transport of spermatozoa through the cervix and the uterus in the rat. Proc Soc Exp Biol Med 28:312, 1930.

———— and Leathem, J. H.   Oogenesis and ovulation, in Hartman, C. G. (ed.), Conference on Physiological Mechanisms Concerned with Conception. New York, Macmillan Co., 1963, Ch. 5, p. 205.

Hertig, A. T., and Rock, J.   On the development of the early human ovum with special reference to the trophoblast of the previllous stage: a description of 7 normal and 5 pathologic human ova. Amer J Obstet Gynec 47:149, 1944.

———— and Rock, J.   Two human ova in the previllous stage, having a developmental age of about 7 and 9 days respectively. Contrib Embryol 31:65, 1945.

———— Rock, J., Adams, E. C., and Mulligan, W. J.   On the preimplantation stages of the human ovum. Contrib Embryol 35:199, 1954.

Heuser, C., Hertig, A. T., and Rock, J.   Two human embryos showing early stages of the definitive yolk sac. Contrib Embryol 31:85, 1945.

Hotchkiss, R. S.   Fertility in Men. Philadelphia, J. B. Lippincott Co., 1944.

Kendle, K. E., and Bennett, J. P.   Studies upon the mechanism of reserpine-induced arrest of egg transport in the mouse oviduct. J Reprod Fertil 20:429; 435, 1969.

Kirby, D. R. S., and Malhotra, S. K.   Cellular nature of the invasive mouse trophoblast. Nature (London) 201:520, 1964.

Krishnan, R. S., and Daniel, J. C.   "Blastokinin": inducer and regulator of blastocyst development in the rabbit uterus. Science 158:490, 1967.

Lanman, J. T.   Delays during reproduction and their effects on the embryo and fetus. New Eng J Med 278:993, 1047, 1092, 1968.

Lewis, W. H., and Gregory, P. W.   Cinematographs of living developing rabbit-eggs. Science 69:226, 1929.

———— and Hartman, C. G.   Early cleavage stages of the egg of the monkey, *Macaca* (*Pithecus*) *rhesus*. Contrib Embryol 24:187, 1933.

MacLeod, J.   Current reviews: Human semen. Fertil Steril 7:368, 1956.

Marston, J. H., and Kelly, W. A.   Time relationships of spermatozoon penetration into the egg of the rhesus monkey. Nature (London) 217:1073, 1968.

Mastroianni, L.   Discussion of tubal transport of ova, in Wynn, R. M. (ed.), First Conference on Fetal Homeostasis. New York, New York Academy of Sciences, 1965, p. 65.

Mattner, P. E.   The survival of spermatozoa in bovine cervical mucus and mucus fractions. J Reprod Fertil 20:193, 1969.

Miller, O. J.   Sex determination: The sex chromosomes and the sex chromatin pattern. Fertil Steril 13:93, 1962.

Moghissi, K. S.   Human and bovine sperm migration. Fertil Steril 19:118, 1968.

Mossman, H. W.   Comparative morphogenesis of the fetal membranes and accessory uterine structures. Contrib Embryol 26:129, 1937.

Nishimura, H., Takano, K., Tanimura, T., and Yasuda, M.   Normal and abnormal development of human embryos: first report of the analysis of 1,213 intact embryos. Teratology 1:281, 1968.

Noyes, R. W.   The capacitation of spermatozoa. A review. Obstet Gynec Survey 14:785, 1959.

———— and Dickmann, Z.   Survival of ova transferred into the oviduct of the rat. Fertil Steril 12:67, 1961.

———— Dickmann, Z., Clewe, T. H., and Bonney, W. A.   Pronuclear ovum from a patient using an intrauterine contraceptive device. Science 147:744, 1965.

Pinkerton, J. H. M., McKay, D. G., Adams, E. C., and Hertig, A. T.   Development of the human ovary: Study using histochemical technics. Obstet Gynec 18:152, 1961.

Platt, L. I., and Karling, E. W.   Sex chromatin frequency. JAMA 187:182, 1964.

Raven, C. P.   Oogenesis: The Storage of Developmental Information. Oxford, Pergamon Press, 1961.

Shelesnyak, M. C., and Tic, L.   Studies on the mechanism of decidualization, IV. Acta Endocr 42:465, 1963.

Sherman, J. K.   Research on frozen human semen—past, present, and future. Fertil Steril 15:485, 1964.

Streeter, G. L.   A human embryo (Mateer) of the presomite period. Contrib Embryol 9:389, 1920.

————   The "Miller" ovum—the youngest normal human embryo thus far known. Contrib Embryol 18:31, 1926.

Tachi, S., Tachi, C., and Lindner, H. R.   Ultrastructural features of blastocyst attachment and trophoblastic invasion in the rat. J Reprod Fertil 21:37, 1970.

Teacher, J. H.   On the implantation of the human ovum and the early development of the trophoblast. J Obstet Gynaec Brit Emp 31:166, 1924.

Tesh, J. M., and Glover, T. D.   Aging of rabbit spermatozoa in the male tract and its effect on fertility. J Reprod Fertil 20:287, 1969.

Thiede, H. A., and Salm, S. B.   Chromosome studies of human spontaneous abortions. Amer J Obstet Gynec 90:205, 1964.

Vickers, A. D.   Delayed fertilization and chromosomal anomalies in mouse embryos. J Reprod Fertil 20:69, 1969.

Westman, A. A.   Investigations into the transit of ova in man. J Obstet Gynaec Brit Emp 44:821, 1937.

Winter, G. F.   (Follicle counts in the ovaries of healthy nonpregnant female subjects). Zbl Gynaek 84:1824, 1962.

Wynn, R. M. (ed.)   First Conference on Fetal Homeostasis. New York, New York Academy of Sciences, 1965, p. 220.

Zaneveld, L. J. D., Srivastava, P. N., and Williams, W. L.   Relationship of a trypsin-like enzyme in rabbit spermatozoa to capacitation. J Reprod Fertil 20:337, 1969.

6

THE PLACENTA AND ITS HORMONES

Scientific interest in the placenta derives not only from its enormous diversity of form and function but from the unique biologic properties of its trophoblast. For purposes of comparative morphology, the definition of a placenta must be expanded to include *any union between fetal and parental tissues for the purpose of physiologic exchange.* As the major agent of nutrition and homeostasis, the placenta is vital to survival of the fetus. Zoologically the evolution of the placenta may be considered the prime factor in the adaptation to viviparity. The placenta develops wide anatomic diversity, unlike the kidney, for example, which maintains relative histologic similarity in most vertebrate groups. The applicability of results of animal experiments to the human being is thus related to the comparative morphology of the placenta. For this reason, as well as to provide the interested reader an introduction to the fascinating field of comparative placentation, the comparative anatomy of the placenta and some of the new developments are summarized at the close of this chapter. Especially recommended for an elegant pictorial description of human placentation is the extensively illustrated recent treatise *The Human Placenta* by Boyd and Hamilton.

DEVELOPMENT OF THE HUMAN PLACENTA

In the discussion of the earliest stages of human placentation in Chapter 5, the wall of the primitive blastodermic vesicle was described as consisting of a single layer of ectoderm. As early as 72 hours after fertilization, the 58-celled blastula was observed by Hertig to have differentiated into 5 embryo-producing cells and 53 cells destined to form the trophoblast. Although no definitive trophoblast has been seen before nidation of the ovum, the earliest implanted blastocyst of the monkey reveals both cellular and syncytial trophoblast. Soon after implantation, the trophoblast proliferates rapidly and invades the surrounding decidua. In its invasive and cytolytic behavior, its histologically characteristic cytoplasmic vacuolization, and its ultrastructure, the early trophoblast resembles choriocarcinoma (p. 578). As invasion of the endometrium proceeds, maternal blood vessels are tapped and cytoplasmic vacuoles coalesce to form larger lacunae (Fig. 1), which are soon filled with maternal blood. As the lacunae join, they form a complicated labyrinth with partitions of solid trophoblastic columns. The tro-

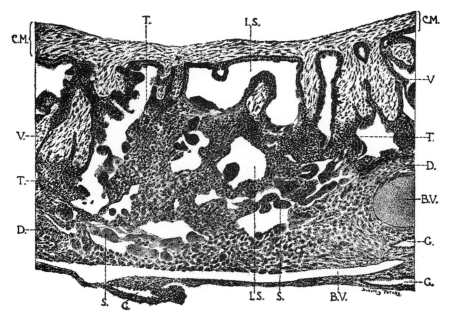

Fig. 1. Drawing of section through three weeks' human placenta, showing chorion, decidua, and intervillous spaces. B.V., maternal blood vessel; C.M., chorionic membrane; D., decidua; G., uterine gland, I.S., intervillous space; S., syncytium; T., trophoblast; V., villus.

phoblast-lined labyrinthine channels and the solid cellular columns form the inter-villous space and primary villous stalks, respectively. Most of our knowledge of the formation of the intervillous space of both man and the macaque is based on the classic study of Wislocki and Streeter.

Villi may first be easily distinguished in the human placenta on about the twelfth day after fertilization, when the solid trophoblast is invaded by a mesen-chymal core, presumably derived from cytotrophoblast, to form secondary villi. After angiogenesis occurs in situ from the mesenchymal cores, the resulting villi are termed tertiary. Maternal venous sinuses are tapped early, but until the fourteenth or fifteenth day no arterial maternal blood enters the intervillous space. Finally, by about the seventeenth day after fertilization, both fetal and maternal blood vessels are functional, and a true placental circulation is established. The fetal circulation is completed when the blood vessels of the embryo are con-nected with chorionic blood vessels, possibly formed in situ from the cytotropho-blast. Some villi, in which absence of angiogenesis leads to lack of a circulation, may distend with fluid to form vesicles. An exaggeration of this process may be operative in the development of hydatidiform mole (p. 564).

Proliferation of cellular trophoblast at the tips of the villi produces the cytotro-phoblastic cell columns, which are not invaded by mesenchyme but are anchored to the decidua at the basal plate. The floor of the intervillous space thus consists of cytotrophoblast from the cell columns, peripheral syncytium of the tropho-blastic shell, and decidua of the basal plate. The chorionic plate, comprising trophoblast externally and fibrous mesoderm internally, forms the roof of the intervillous space.

Between the eighteenth and nineteenth days of development the blastocyst, including the chorionic shell, measures 6 by 2.5 mm in diameter. The embryo is then in the primitive-streak stage with a maximal length of 0.6 to 0.7 mm. The trophoblastic shell is very thick, with villi formed of cytotrophoblastic projections, a central core of chorionic mesoderm in which blood vessels are developing, and an external covering of syncytium. The blastocyst lies buried in the decidua, separated from the myometrium by the decidua basalis and from the uterine epithelium by the decidua capsularis. The embryo itself is trilaminar, its endoderm continuous with the lining of the yolk sac. An intermediate layer of intraembryonic mesoderm may be traced in continuity with the extraembryonic mesoderm, which later forms part of the walls of the amnion and yolk sac and connects the embryonic structures to the chorionic mesoderm by the body stalk, or abdominal pedicle, the forerunner of the umbilical cord. At this stage the secondary or definitive yolk sac is completely lined by endoderm. External to the yolk sac is the fluid-filled exocelomic cavity, the early formation of which prevents approximation of the yolk sac and trophoblast in man, and hence precludes formation of a choriovitelline placenta.

At about three weeks after fertilization the relations of chorion to decidua are clearly seen in the human ovum (Fig. 2). The chorionic membrane consists

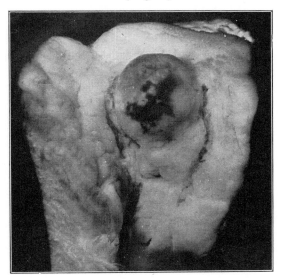

Fig. 2. Early ovum in situ. (Carnegie Collection No. 5960.) Note blood beneath decidua capsularis. (From Heuser. Contrib Embryol 23:253, 1932.)

of an inner connective tissue layer and an outer epithelium, from which rudimentary villi project. The connective tissue itself comprises spindly cells with protoplasmic processes within a loose intercellular matrix. The trophoblast differentiates into cuboidal or nearly round cells with clear cytoplasm and light-staining vesicular nuclei (Langhans cells) and an outer syncytium containing irregularly scattered, dark-staining nuclei within a coarsely granulated cytoplasm (syncytiotrophoblast).

In early pregnancy the villi are distributed over the entire periphery of the chorionic membrane; an ovum dislodged from the endometrium at this stage of development appears grossly shaggy (Fig. 3). The villi in contact with the decidua basalis proliferate to form the leafy chorion, or *chorion frondosum,* the fetal component of the placenta, whereas those in relation to the decidua capsu-

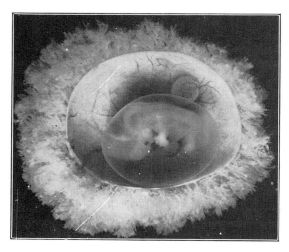

Fig. 3. Human chorionic vesicle. (Carnegie Collection No. 8537.) Ovulatory age, 40 days.

laris cease to grow, undergoing almost complete degeneration. The greater part of the chorion, thus denuded of villi, is designated the smooth or bald chorion or the *chorion laeve.* It is formed, according to Hertig, by a combination of direct pressure and interference with its vascular supply. It is generally more opaque than the amnion but rarely exceeds 1 mm in thickness. The chorion laeve contains ghost villi and, clinging to its surface, a few shreds of decidua. Bourne has described four layers, consisting, from within outward, of a cellular layer, a reticular layer, a pseudobasement membrane, and trophoblast. Electron micros-

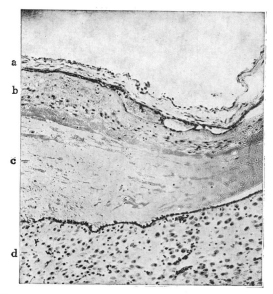

Fig. 4. Unfused decidua vera and capsularis. Section through uterus at 10 weeks' gestation, showing that the decidua vera and capsularis have not yet fused. a, amnion and chorionic membrane; b, degenerating decidua capsularis; c, uterine cavity; d, decidua vera.

copy of the human chorion laeve, however, has not revealed these layers to be so well defined (Wynn). The chorion laeve is separated from the amnion by the exocelomic cavity until about the end of the third month, when the amnionic and chorionic mesoderms fuse (Fig. 4). In man, the chorion laeve and amnion form an essentially avascular amniochorion, which may be an important site of transfer, corresponding to the paraplacental chorion of animals, such as the carnivores. Battaglia and Hellegers have reported considerable diffusion of carbohydrates across the human chorion laeve in vitro. The membrane offered very little resistance to the molecules, which crossed according to Fick's law governing transfer by simple diffusion rather than by carrier systems, such as those operative in transplacental passage of some carbohydrates in vivo. French, MacLennan, and Wynn, nevertheless, have recently shown that the human amnion is rich in membrane nucleoside phosphatases, which are often related to active transport.

Certain villi of the chorion frondosum extend from the chorionic plate to the decidua as anchoring villi. Most villi, however, arboresce and end freely in the intervillous space without reaching the decidua. As the placenta ages, the short, thick, early stem villi branch repeatedly, forming progressively finer subdivisions and greater numbers of increasingly small villi (Fig. 5). Each of the main stem villi and its ramifications constitute a *fetal cotyledon.*

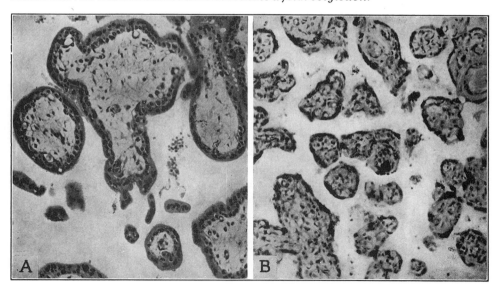

Fig. 5. Comparison of chorionic villi in early and late pregnancy. A, two months' gestation. Note inner Langhans cells and outer syncytial layer. B, term placenta. Syncytial layer is obvious, but Langhans cells are difficult to recognize at low magnification in light micrographs.

The origin and exact composition of the placental septa continue to stimulate controversy. They appear to consist of decidual tissue in which trophoblastic elements are encased and thus are very likely of dual origin, according to Boyd and Hamilton, Brosens and Dixon, and Wynn, among others. Brosens and Dixon believe that most spiral arteries bear a topographic relation to the septa, the distribution of which appears to be haphazard. Boyd and Hamilton state that septa are demonstrable from the 80 mm stage on and that they are more attenuated and irregular than is generally recognized. Since the septa therefore cannot serve as effective partitions between placental cotyledons, they are unlikely to play a significant role in the circulation of maternal blood within 'and from the intervillous space (p. 159).

The steady increase in size and weight of the placenta throughout pregnancy is shown in Table 1. The data obtained from weighing the placenta vary con-

Table 1. Growth of the Placenta

Duration (days)	Diameter (cm)	Volume (ml)	Surface (cm²)	Weight (g)	Fetal Weight / Placental Weight	Fetal Weight / Placental Surface
105–135	10.0	115	62	120	2.50	4.83
135–165	12.0	235	167	245	3.22	4.73
165–195	14.0	230	145	245	4.17	7.01
195–225	15.0	349	199	365	4.84	9.19
225–240	16.0	394	219	407	6.67	12.80
240–296	18.0	430	243	464	7.29	13.98

* Data from Snoeck. Le Placenta Humain, Masson et Cie; and from Crawford. J. Obstet Gynaec Brit Emp 66:885, 1959.

siderably, depending upon how the placenta is prepared. If membranes and most of the cord are left attached and adherent maternal blood clot is not removed, the weight is increased by nearly 50 per cent (Thomson and co-workers). Crawford indicates that the total number of cotyledons remains the same throughout gestation, but individual cotyledons continue to grow until term, although less actively in the final weeks. Although the concentration of capillary vessels may decline, growing buds continue to produce daughter villi, even at term. Further support for the concept of continuing metabolic activity of the placenta is provided by phase microscopy and electron microscopy, which suggest that syncytial "knots" may, sometimes at least, represent proliferating trophoblast rather than degenerative contraction of nuclear material.

Placental Aging.   As the villi continue to branch and the terminal ramifications become more numerous and smaller, the volume and prominence of cytotrophoblast (Langhans cells) in the villi decrease, although cellular trophoblast remains obvious in the placental floor. As the syncytium thins and forms knots, the vessels become more prominent and lie closer to the surface. The stroma of the villi also exhibits changes associated with aging. In early placentas the branching connective tissue cells are separated by an abundant loose intercellular matrix; later the stroma becomes denser, and the cells more spindly and more closely packed. Another change in the stroma involves the so-called Hofbauer cells, still of somewhat uncertain nature, origin, and significance. They are nearly round cells with vesicular, often eccentric nuclei and very granular or vacuolated cytoplasm. In a correlative study employing histochemistry, electron microscopy, and analysis of sex chromatin, Wynn concluded that the Hofbauer cells were of exclusively fetal origin in both normal and abnormal states. They were histochemically characterized by intracytoplasmic lipid and readily distinguished from plasma cells; their vacuolar cytoplasm, furthermore, was distinct ultrastructurally. Although Hofbauer cells may arise from several different elements in the placental mesenchyme, some of them are most likely to be phagocytic, although others appear to be degenerative.

As the placenta grows and ages, certain of the histologic changes suggest an increase in the efficiency of transport to meet the metabolic requirements of the growing fetus. Such changes involve a decrease in thickness of the syncytium, partial disappearance of Langhans cells, decrease in the stroma, and increase in the number of capillaries and their approximation to the syncytial surface. By four months the apparent continuity of the Langhans layer is broken, and the synctium forms knots on the more numerous, smaller villi. At term the villous covering may be focally reduced to a thin layer of syncytium with minimal connective tissue and fetal capillaries apparently abutting the trophoblast. The villous stroma, Hofbauer cells, and Langhans cells are markedly reduced, and the villi appear filled with thin-walled capillaries. Other changes, however, appear to decrease the efficiency for placental exchange, as, for example, the thickening of basement membranes of endothelium and trophoblast, obliteration of certain vessels, deposition of fibrin on the surface of the villi, deposits of fibrin in the basal and chorionic plates and elsewhere in the intervillous space, and calcification in the septa and elsewhere.

HISTOCHEMICAL AGING. The histochemical changes during aging of the placenta have been shown by McKay and others to involve primarily alkaline phosphatase, glycogen, and ribonucleoproteins. In their classic studies of the chemical cytology of the placenta, Wislocki and his associates showed that the trophoblast was entirely dependent upon the endometrium for nourishment, at first by destruction and absorption of decidua and its products and later by metabolism of constituents of the maternal blood in the intervillous space. The enzymes that mediate the varied lytic, secretory, and excretory functions of the trophoblast have been compiled by Page.

The high content of cytoplasmic ribonucleoprotein is correlated with both the basophilia of the syncytium and its extensive synthesis of proteins. Glycogen, though widely distributed throughout the placenta, was formerly thought to be associated with relative avascularity, since it is generally absent from the syncytium and other metabolically active areas. More extensive deposition of glycogen occurs in the stroma and the glandular epithelium of the decidua.

In a study of the oxidative enzymes of the placenta, Boss and Craig found histochemical reactions strongest for DPN-diaphorase and glucose-6-phosphate dehydrogenase, and weakest for α-glycerophosphatase and succinic dehydrogenase. The reactions for all the enzymes, furthermore, were most striking in the trophoblast, although considerable enzymatic activity was found in the amnion. No conspicuous decline in enzymatic reactions in the later stages of pregnancy was found. The pattern of distribution of the dehydrogenases of the amnion and syncytium paralleled those of the proximal renal tubules, where too there is rapid transfer of water and electrolytes.

Curzen and Morris found that circulating heat-stable alkaline phosphatase is of exclusively placental origin. Its increase, according to these authors, is a manifestation of placental aging. Measurements of heat-stable alkaline phosphatase in serum may perhaps be most useful when correlated with the results of maternal chorionic somatomammotropin and urinary estriol (p. 175).

In preeclampsia-eclampsia certain changes associated with histochemical aging of the placenta may appear prematurely. Accompanying the early diminution in ribonucleoprotein are a decrease in cytoplasmic basophilia and a concomitant increase in alkaline and acid phosphatases and affinity for acidic dyes. Thinning of the trophoblast may be followed by degeneration of its nuclei and eventually complete necrosis of both stroma and syncytium. The decrease in cytoplasmic basophilia may well be related directly to the breakdown of nucleic acids resulting from an increase in activity of phosphatases. The changes may reflect a disturbance in the placental metabolism of nucleoproteins.

THE DECIDUA

The Decidual Reaction. The decidua is the endometrium of the pregnant uterus, so named because much of it is shed following parturition. The decidual reaction encompasses the changes in the endometrium that begin in response to progesterone following ovulation and prepare the uterus for implantation and nutrition of the blastocyst. In human pregnancy the decidual reaction is not completed until several days after nidation. It first appears locally around maternal blood vessels, spreading in waves throughout the uterus. During development of the decidual reaction the endometrial stromal cells enlarge and form polygonal or round *decidual cells*. The nuclei become round and vesicular, and the cytoplasm becomes clear, slightly basophilic, and surrounded by a translucent membrane.

During pregnancy the decidua thickens, eventually attaining a depth of 5 to 10 mm. With a magnifying glass, furrows and numerous small openings representing the mouths of uterine glands can be detected. Since a true decidual reaction normally does not extend beyond the internal os, decidua is ordinarily confined to the corpus uteri. The portion of the decidua directly beneath the site of implantation forms the decidua basalis; overlying the developing ovum and separating it from the rest of the uterine cavity is the *decidua capsularis* (Figs. 6 and 7). The remainder of the uterus is lined by *decidua vera*, or *decidua parietalis*.

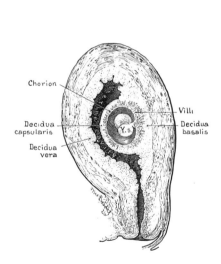

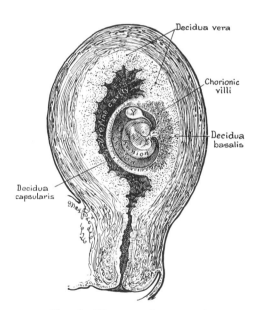

Fig. 6. Diagram showing chorion frondosum and chorion laeve of early pregnancy. Three portions of the decidua (basalis, capsularis, and parietalis, or vera) are also illustrated. (From Williams. Amer J Obstet Gynec, 13:1, 1927.)

Fig. 7. Diagram of more advanced stage of pregnancy, showing atrophic chorion laeve and chorion frondosum (chorionic villi) proliferating into decidua basalis. (From Williams. Amer J Obstet Gynec 13:1, 1927.)

Since during the early months of pregnancy the ovum does not occupy the entire uterine cavity, there is a space between the decidua capsularis and the decidua parietalis. By the fourth month, the growing ovum fills the uterine cavity; with fusion of the capsularis and parietalis, the endometrial cavity is obliterated. The decidua capsularis is most prominent around the second month of pregnancy, consisting of decidual cells covered by a single layer of flattened epithelial cells without traces of glands; internally it contacts the chorion laeve.

The decidua parietalis and the decidua basalis each comprise three layers (Fig. 8): a surface, or compact zone (*zona compacta*); a middle portion, or

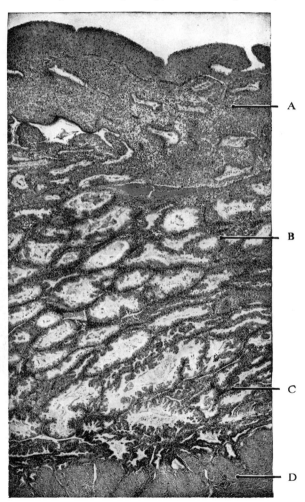

Fig. 8. Early decidua vera (parietalis). A, compact layer (see Fig. 9); B, spongy layer; C, uterine glands just above the basal layer; D, myometrium. (Compare with Figs. 1 through 4 in Ch. 4.)

spongy zone (*zona spongiosa*), with glands and numerous small blood vessels; and a basal zone (*zona basalis*). The compacta and the spongiosa together form the functional zone (*zona functionalis*). The basal zone remains after delivery and, except at the placental site, gives rise to new endometrium. As pregnancy advances, the glandular epithelium of the decidua parietalis changes from cylindric to cuboidal or flattened, at times even resembling endothelium. After the fourth month, because of uterine distention, the decidua parietalis gradually thins from its maximal height of 1 cm in the first trimester to 1 to 2 mm at term.

Histology.   The compact layer comprises large, closely packed, epithelioid, polygonal, lightly staining cells with round, vesicular nuclei (Fig. 9). Particularly when the decidua is edematous, many stromal cells appear stellate, with long protoplasmic processes that anastomose with those of adjacent cells. Scattered among typical decidual cells, especially early in pregnancy, are numerous small round cells with very little cytoplasm. Formerly considered to be lymphocytes, these cells are now regarded as precursors of new decidual elements. In the early months of pregnancy, ducts of uterine glands are found in the decidua compacta, but they become less obvious toward term.

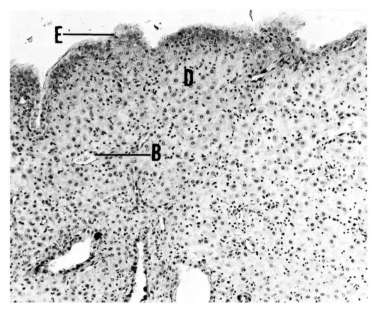

Fig. 9. Decidua parietalis, showing epithelium (E), decidualized stromal cells (D), and blood vessel (B). (Courtesy of Dr. Ralph M. Wynn.)

The spongy layer consists of large distended glands, often exhibiting marked hyperplasia and separated by minimal stroma. At first the glands are lined by typical cylindric uterine epithelium with abundant secretory activity. The glandular secretion contributes to the nourishment of the ovum during its histotrophic phase, before establishment of a placental circulation. The epithelium gradually becomes cuboidal or even flattened, later degenerating and sloughing to a great extent into the lumens of the glands. The interglandular stroma of the spongy zone undergoes little change during pregnancy.

From the basal zone of the decidua parietalis (not to be confused with decidua basalis) some of the endometrium regenerates during the puerperium (Ch. 18, p. 466). In comparing the decidua parietalis at four months' gestation with the nonpregnant, early proliferative endometrium (Fig. 1, Ch. 4), it becomes clear that during decidual transformation of the endometrial stroma there is marked hypertrophy but only slight hyperplasia.

The decidua basalis enters into formation of the basal plate of the placenta and differs from the decidua parietalis histologically in two respects (Fig. 10). First, the spongy zone consists mainly of arteries and widely dilated veins; by

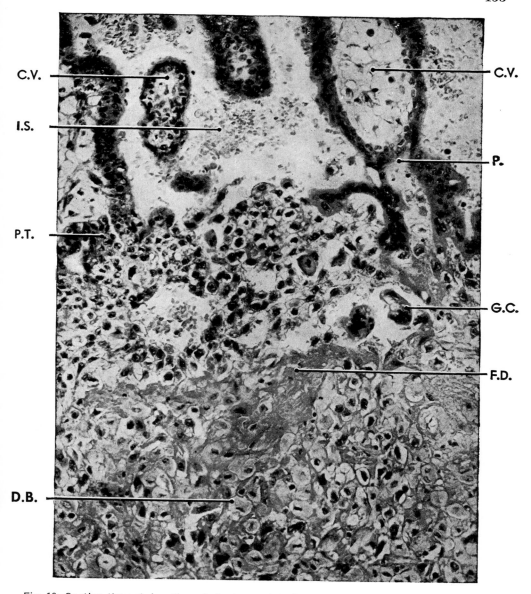

C.V.

I.S.

P.T.

D.B.

C.V.

P.

G.C.

F.D.

Fig. 10. Section through junction of chorion and decidua basalis. Fourth month of gestation. C.V., chorionic villi; D.B., decidua basalis; F.D., fibrinoid degeneration; G.C., giant cell; I.S., intervillous space containing maternal blood; P., fastening villus; P.T., proliferating trophoblast.

term, glands have virtually disappeared. Second, the decidua basalis is invaded extensively by trophoblastic giant cells (Fig. 11), which first appear as early as the time of implantation. The number and depth of penetration of the giant cells vary greatly. Although generally confined to the decidua, they have been shown by Boyd and Hamilton to penetrate the myometrium. In such circumstances their number and invasiveness may be so extensive as to suggest choriocarcinoma to the inexperienced observer.

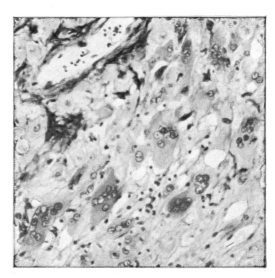

Fig. 11. Photomicrograph of giant cells in a uterus from the second half of pregnancy. (From Boyd and Hamilton. J Obstet Gynaec Brit Emp 67:208, 1960.)

Aging of the Decidua.   Changes similar to some of those described in the placenta occur also in the decidua. Where invading trophoblast meets the decidua, there is a zone of fibrinoid degeneration, *Nitabuch's layer.* Whenever the decidua is defective, as in placenta accreta (Ch. 33, p. 963), Nitabuch's layer may be absent. There is also an inconstant deposition of fibrin, *Rohr's stria,* at the bottom of the intervillous space and surrounding the fastening villi. McCombs and Craig have shown that decidual necrosis is a normal phenomenon in the first and probably the second trimester. The presence of necrotic decidua in endometrial curettings following spontaneous abortion in the first trimester should not, therefore, be interpreted necessarily as either a cause or an effect of the abortion.

   Histochemistry and Ultrastructure.   In their fundamental studies of placental histochemistry Wislocki and his associates indicated the difficulty of distinguishing, with conventional stains, trophoblast from decidua in the basal plate. They demonstrated, however, differences in the distribution of RNA and mitochondria, and characteristic "capsules" surrounding individual decidual cells. Wynn's electron microscopic study of the human basal plate indicates that this complex region of the placenta comprises intimately related fetal and maternal cells. Well-preserved trophoblastic and endometrial cells are rarely in direct contact, however, but remain separated by degenerating tissue and fibrinoid. The giant cells in the region are derived from the syncytium or arise from differentiation of cytotrophoblast in situ. These syncytial masses may be hormonally active late in pregnancy. Moe has recently confirmed these findings in showing that there is no intimate contact between apparently viable cytotrophoblast and decidua. The immunologic implications of these cellular relations are discussed on page 169.

BIOLOGY OF THE TROPHOBLAST

Origin of the Syncytium.   Of all placental components the trophoblast is the most variable in structure, function, and development. Its invasiveness mediates attachment of the blastocyst to the uterus; its role in nutrition of the conceptus is reflected in its name; and its function as an endocrine organ is requisite to main-tenance of pregnancy. Morphologically the trophoblast may be cellular or syncy-tial or it may appear as uninuclear or multinuclear giant cells. The true syncytial character of the human syncytiotrophoblast has been confirmed by electron mi-croscopy. The mechanism of growth of the syncytium, however, remained a mys-tery, in view of the discrepancy between increase in the number of nuclei in the syncytiotrophoblast and only equivocal evidence of intrinsic nuclear replication. Mitotic figures are completely absent from the syncytium and confined to the cytotrophoblast. To distinguish amitotic nuclear proliferation within the syncy-tium from cytotrophoblastic origin of the syncytiotrophoblast, Galton employed microspectrophotometry, based on the Feulgen method for measuring DNA. He noted a diploid, unimodal distribution of DNA in the syncytium at a time of rapid placental growth, whereas a high proportion of cytotrophoblastic nuclei contained DNA in excess of the diploid amount, reflecting synthesis of DNA in interphase nuclei preparatory to division (Ch. 5, p. 113). Galton concluded that the rapid accumulation of nuclei in the syncytiotrophoblast is explained by cellular prolif-eration within the cytotrophoblast, followed by coalescence of daughter cells in the syncytium.

Further evidence was provided by Richart, who noted the early incorporation of tritiated thymidine in the cytotrophoblast but not in the syncytium. Midgley and co-workers subsequently extended the idea and found that although tritiated thymidine appeared at first only in the nuclei of the cytotrophoblast, the label could be detected 22 hours later also in the syncytiotrophoblast, indicating that the syncytium is derived from cytotrophoblast and is itself a mitotic end stage (Fig. 12).

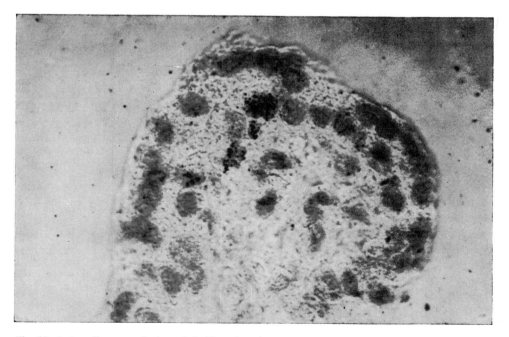

Fig. 12. Autoradiogram of placental villus. Langhans and stromal cells are labeled with triti-ated thymidine, indicating synthesis of deoxyribonucleic acid (DNA). (Courtesy of Drs. Ben Peckham and William Kiekhofer.)

Ultrastructure.   The electron microscopic studies of Wislocki and Dempsey provided the basic data upon which the functional interpretation of placental fine structure is based. The prominent microvilli of the syncytial surface, corresponding to the so-called brush border of light microscopy, and their associated pinocytotic vacuoles and vesicles are related to the absorptive and secretory functions of the placenta. The Langhans cells, which persist to term although often compressed against the trophoblastic basal lamina, retain their ultrastructural simplicity. They possess few specialized organelles, with abundant free ribosomes but scant ergastoplasm. Desmosomes connect individual Langhans cells with one another and with the syncytium, from which complete plasma membranes are absent. Ultrastructurally the syncytium is relatively complex, containing abundant endoplasmic reticulum, Golgi bodies, and mitochondria, as well as numerous secretory droplets, lipid granules, and highly convoluted plasma membranes. The electron density of the syncytial nuclei is related to their high content of deoxyribonucleoprotein, and the abundant ribosomes and granular endoplasmic reticu-

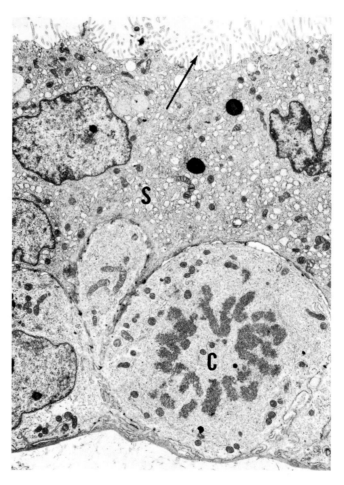

Fig. 13. Electron micrograph of human placenta at six weeks of gestation. Note prominent border of microvilli (arrow), syncytium (S), and mitotic figure in cytotrophoblast (C). (Courtesy of Dr. Ralph M. Wynn.)

lum of the syncytial cytoplasm are correlated with high content of the ribonucleo-protein and deep basophilia. As the syncytium matures, the fine structural changes reflect functional maturation. Early syncytiotrophoblast often exhibits a micro-vesicular endoplasmic reticulum; later, at the height of active synthesis of pro-teins, flattened ergastoplasmic channels assume prominence; and still later, asso-ciated with storage and transport of proteins, there appear dilated cisternae of endoplasmic reticulum, the largest of which are visible with the light microscope. Secretory granules, at least those thought to be glycoproteins, and osmiophilic lipid granules correspond to PAS-positive and sudanophilic droplets, respectively (Figs. 13, 14, and 15).

As the placenta matures, the collagen-rich stromal connective tissue de-creases, as do the numbers of fibroblasts and Hofbauer cells. The human placental membrane may be reduced anatomically to a thin covering of trophoblast, capil-lary endothelium, and trophoblastic and endothelial basement membranes sepa-rated by mere wisps of connective tissue. Although there is focal villous degenera-tion at term, morphologic evidence of activity in all layers persists. Since not only the trophoblast but the endothelium and even the basal laminas may show evi-dence of pinocytosis and other metabolic activity, it is hardly reasonable to equate the number of layers in the histologic "barrier" with the functional efficiency of the placenta. Reduction of the number of layers may result in more rapid trans-

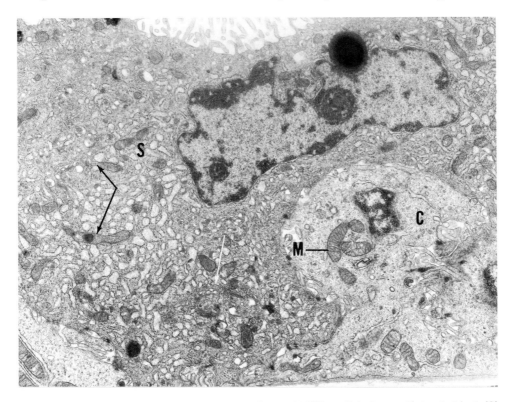

Fig. 14. First-trimester human placenta, showing well-differentiated syncytiotrophoblast (S) with numerous mitochondria (black arrows) and Golgi complexes (white arrow). Cytotropho-blast (C) has large mitochondria (M) but few other organelles. (Courtesy of Dr. Ralph M. Wynn.)

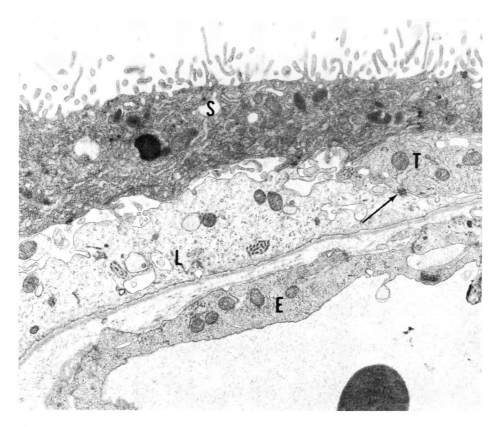

Fig. 15. Term human placenta, showing electron-dense syncytium (S), Langhans cell (L), transitional cytotrophoblast (T), and capillary endothelium (E). Arrow points to desmosome. (Courtesy of Dr. Ralph M. Wynn.)

placental passage of substances to which the laws governing simple diffusion apply, but metabolites regulated by "carrier systems" are not proportionally affected. As for pinocytosis, a virtually continuous system of vesicles and vacuoles may be found extending from the syncytial surface to the capillary endothelium. Boyd and co-workers describe a direct connection of some of these vacuoles with the perinuclear space, which receives tubular communications with the endoplasmic reticulum. The term "barrier" as applied to placental physiology should therefore be replaced by the more accurate term "placental membrane." The number of layers, furthermore, is a poor indication of the true approximation of the circulations, since in the six-layered epitheliochorial placenta of the pig, for example (p. 187), the indentation of both fetal and maternal epithelium by the respective capillaries results in a rather close vascular relation. Comparative ultrastructure has thus posed an apparently insurmountable obstacle to the acceptance of the Grosser classification (p. 187) as a basis for comparative functional placentology.

Localization of Placental Hormones.   That the syncytium is a source of placental steroids has not seriously been questioned since Wislocki's histochemical localization in the syncytiotrophoblast of sudanophilic droplets, which he associated with estrogens and progesterone. The origin of chorionic gonadotropin, however, has engendered considerable controversy. A third of a century ago Gey, Jones, and Hellman extracted from placental tissue cultures of gonadotropin that they assumed to originate from cytotrophoblast. Several years later Wislocki localized PAS-positive material, thought to represent the glycoprotein gonadotropin, in the Langhans cells. Further support for the origin of chorionic gonadotropin from cytotrophoblast was provided by the temporal coincidence of maximal cytotrophoblastic proliferation with the highest titers of human chorionic gonadotropin in the urine and serum.

Thiede and Choate have localized chorionic gonadotropin by immunofluorescent technics to the syncytium. A much smaller amount appeared in the amnion, but no specific fluorescence was detected in the cytotrophoblast. In combined ultrastructural and immunofluorescent studies, Pierce and Midgley, working with human choriocarcinoma, likewise detected the chorionic gonadotropin in the syncytium but not in the cytotrophoblast. In similar studies of transplanted human choriocarcinoma and hydatidiform mole, Wynn and Davies demonstrated by electron microscopy that the benign and malignant trophoblastic growths maintain the fine structural features of their normal counterparts (pp. 581 and 582). They indicated that only the syncytium contained the subcellular organelles required for synthesis of proteins, particularly abundant endoplasmic reticulum and well-developed Golgi complexes, whereas the cytotrophoblast was ultrastructurally simple.

In the demonstration of a spectrum of transitional cells, moreover, some of the more differentiated of which may begin to produce hormones, an explanation was provided for the simultaneous ultrastructural and endocrinologic differentiation of the trophoblast. Endocrine activity of these transitional cells, which were generally classified as cytotrophoblast by light microscopy, could explain the slight specific fluorescence noted in some so-called Langhans cells. Sciarra and co-workers noted the protein hormone (chorionic somatomammotropin) to be in the syncytium but absent from Langhans cells (p. 175).

On ultrastructural grounds Wynn and others regard the syncytium as the differentiated form of trophoblast, capable of synthesis of complex molecules and responsible for the production of all placental hormones, relegating to the ultrastructurally simple cytotrophoblast a role primarily in cellular growth and differentiation. Although there is impressive evidence from several fields of investigation that the syncytium is the source of these placental hormones, the anatomic localization of a hormone cannot necessarily be equated with its origin in a particular site. In simplest terms, the more complex the trophoblast, the more capable it is of producing protein hormones. As Langhans cells differentiate ultrastructurally, their endocrine potential increases simultaneously. Although the typical Langhans cell in the mature chorionic villus is an unlikely source of protein hormones, transitional cells and ultrastructurally complex forms of cytotrophoblast elsewhere in the normal placenta and in chorionic neoplasms may be endocrinologically active.

CIRCULATION IN THE MATURE PLACENTA

Since the placenta functionally represents a rather intimate presentation of the fetal capillary bed to maternal blood, its gross anatomy primarily concerns

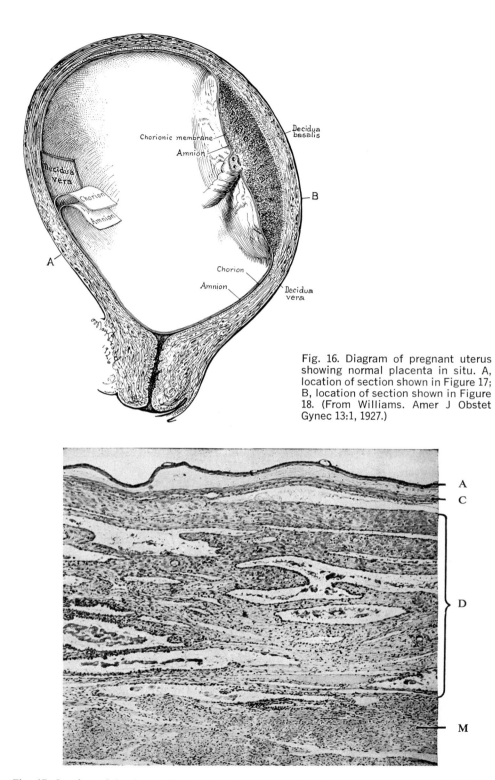

Fig. 16. Diagram of pregnant uterus showing normal placenta in situ. A, location of section shown in Figure 17; B, location of section shown in Figure 18. (From Williams. Amer J Obstet Gynec 13:1, 1927.)

Fig. 17. Section of fetal membranes and uterus opposite placental site at A in Figure 16. A, amnion; C, chorion; D, decidua parietalis; M, myometrium.

vascular relations. The human placenta at term is a discoid organ measuring approximately 15 to 20 cm in diameter and 2 to 3 cm in thickness. It weighs approximately 500 g and is generally located in the uterus anteriorly or posteriorly near the fundus. The fetal side is covered by transparent amnion beneath which the chorionic vessels course, with the arteries passing over the veins. A section through the placenta in situ (Figs. 16, 17, and 18) includes amnion, chorion, ramifying villi, decidual plate, and myometrium. The maternal surface of the placenta (Fig. 19) is divided into irregular lobes by furrows produced by septa, which consist of fibrous tissue with sparse vessels confined mainly to their bases. The broad-based

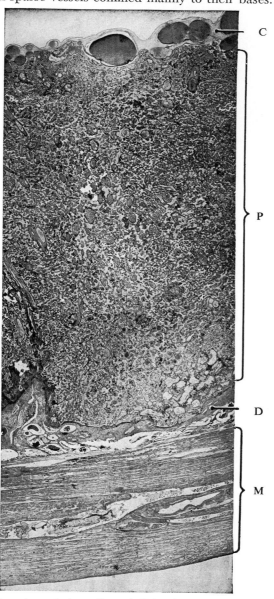

Fig. 18. Section of placenta and uterus through B in Figure 16. C, chorionic plate; P, placental villi; D, decidua basalis; M, myometrium.

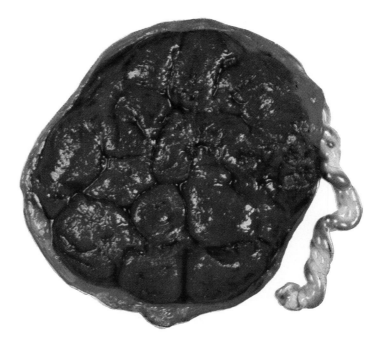

Fig. 19. Maternal surface of normal mature placenta.

septa do not ordinarily reach the chorionic plate, thus providing only incomplete partitions.

Fetal Circulation.   Fetal blood flows to the placenta through the two umbilical arteries, which carry deoxygenated, or "venous," blood. The vessels branch repeatedly beneath the amnion and again within the dividing villi, forming capillary networks in the terminal divisions (Figs. 20 and 21). Blood with a significantly higher oxygen content returns to the fetus from the placenta through the single umbilical vein (Ch. 7, p. 211).

Maternal Circulation.   Only relatively recently has the mechanism of the maternal placental circulation been explained in physiologic terms. Insofar as fetal homeostasis is dependent on efficient placental circulation, the extensive efforts of researchers and clinicians to elucidate the factors regulating the flow of blood into and from the intervillous space have led to important practical applications in obstetrics. An adequate theory must explain how blood may actually leave the maternal circulation, flow into an amorphous space lined by trophoblastic syncytium rather than capillary endothelium, and return through maternal veins, without effecting short circuits, which would prevent the blood from remaining in contact with the villi long enough for adequate exchange.

It was not until Ramsey's objective studies that a "physiologic" mechanism of placental circulation, consistent with both experimental and clinical findings, was available (Fig. 22). Discarding the crude corrosion technics of her predecessors, Ramsey, by careful slow injections under low pressure that avoid disruption of the circulation, proved that the venous exits as well as the arterial entrances are scattered at random over the entire base of the placenta. The arterial blood entering through the basal plate is driven by the head of maternal pressure high up toward the chorionic plate before lateral dispersion occurs. After bathing the

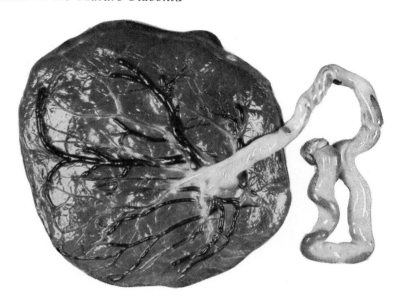

Fig. 20. Fetal surface of placenta, shown in Figure 19.

chorionic villi, the blood drains through venous orifices in the basal plate and enters the maternal placental veins. The maternal blood thus traverses the placenta randomly without preformed channels, propelled by the maternal arterial pressure. The spiral arteries are generally perpendicular and the veins parallel to the uterine wall, an arrangement that facilitates closure of the veins during a uterine contraction and prevents squeezing of essential maternal blood from the intervillous space. According to Brosens and Dixon, there are 120 spiral arterial entries into the intervillous space of the human placenta at term, discharging blood in spurts that displace the adjacent villi, as described by Borell and coworkers.

Ramsey and Harris compared the uteroplacental vasculature and circulation of the rhesus monkey and of women. The most significant morphologic variation is the greater dilation of human uteroplacental arteries. In the woman, particularly in early pregnancy, there may be multiple openings from a single arterial stem into the intervillous space. The force of the spurts is eventually dissipated with the creation of a small lake of blood roughly 5 mm in diameter about halfway toward the chorionic plate. The closeness of the villi slows the flow of blood, providing adequate time for exchange.

Ramsey's concept is supported by numerous arteriographic studies that clearly show the spiral arterial spurts associated with the "lakes" and by many pressure studies, which demonstrate clearly the closure of uteroplacental veins at the beginning of uterine contractions. Recent corroboration has been provided by cineradioangiography, which shows how, in the macaque, debouching streams from the spiral arteries connect with and develop into the small lakes, which then disperse in a general effusion of blood throughout the intervillous space (Fig. 23).

In Ramsey's motion pictures the effect of myometrial contractions upon placental circulation is unequivocally shown to involve diminution of arterial inflow and cessation of venous drainage. Continued observation of the contrast medium by televised fluoroscopy indicates that myometrial contractions cause a slight

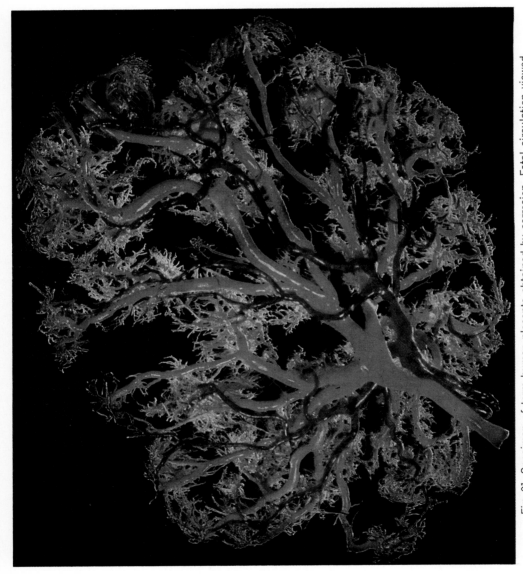

Fig. 21. Specimen of term human placenta obtained by corrosion. Fetal circulation viewed from the fetal side. (Prepared by Rudolph Skarda; courtesy of Abbott Laboratories.)

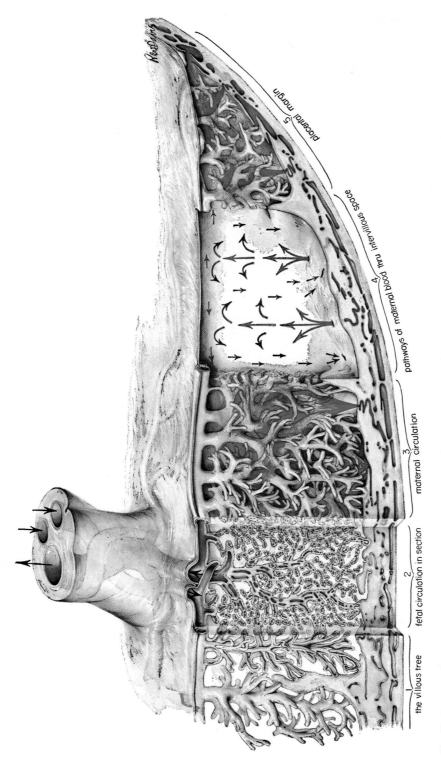

Fig. 22. A composite drawing of the placenta to show its structure and circulation: Maternal blood enters the intervillous space under the head of maternal arterial pressure. The entering blood is driven in funnel-shaped streams ("spurts") through the intervillous space where the pressure is low. As the maternal pressure dissipates, lateral dispersion of blood occurs. Metabolic exchange takes place as the blood flows around the chorionic villi. Inflowing arterial blood pushes venous blood out into the endometrial veins. (Drawing by Ranice W. Davis, Department of Art as Applied to Medicine of The Johns Hopkins University, for Dr. Elizabeth M. Ramsey. Reproduced by courtesy of Carnegie Institution of Washington.)

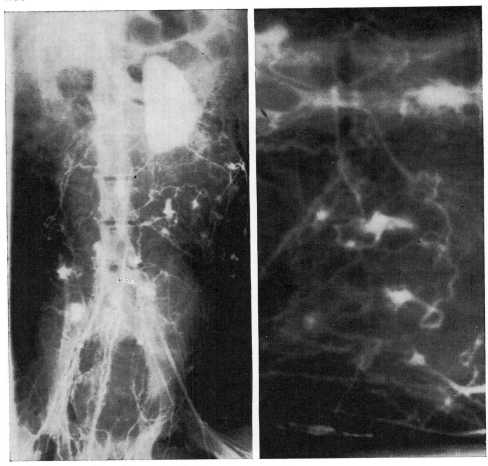

Fig. 23. Left, radiogram six seconds after injection of a radiopaque contrast medium into the right femoral artery of a monkey on day 111 of pregnancy. The primary placenta is below on the left; the secondary placenta is above on the right. Right, high magnification of an artery at the center of the secondary placenta in the same monkey. (Courtesy of Dr. Elizabeth M. Ramsey.)

delay in appearance of the contrast medium in the veins of the uterine wall when injection occurs during a strong contraction. The pressure in the intervillous space may be decreased to the point at which blood cannot be expressed against the prevailing myometrial pressure. Ramsey has provided further evidence of independent activity of the spiral arterioles, as indicated by the appearance of "spurts" in different locations even when injections are performed under conditions of minimal myometrial pressure. Not all endometrial spiral arteries are continuously patent, nor do they all necessarily discharge blood into the intervillous space simultaneously.

In summary, Ramsey's concept holds that the maternal blood enters the intervillous space in spurts produced by the maternal blood pressure. The *vis a tergo* forces blood in discrete streams toward the chorionic plate until the head of pressure is reduced. Lateral spread then occurs. Continuing influx of arterial blood exerts pressure on the contents of the intervillous space, pushing the blood toward the exits in the basal plate, from which it is drained through uterine and other pelvic veins. During uterine contractions, both inflow and outflow are curtailed, although the volume of blood in the intervillous space is maintained, thus providing for continual, though reduced, exchange.

Freese added support to older anatomic studies that showed that in both rhesus monkey and man, each placental cotyledon is supplied by one spiral artery, which is located beneath a central empty space. He believes that this relatively hollow central portion of the cotyledon, which he calls the intracotyledonary space, is the preferential site of entry of blood. Wigglesworth suggests that the structure of the fetal cotyledon may determine, in part, the pattern of maternal blood flow through the placenta and that fetal cotyledons develop around the spiral artery. Variations in histologic structure of the villi show that growth occurs around the center of the cotyledon, since the villi in this region are less mature than those in the vicinity of the intracotyledonary veins. The intervillous space thus has arterial, capillary, and venous zones. In this connection, Reynolds and co-workers showed that the blood pressure was highest around the central cavity of the cotyledon, the gradient diminishing radially and toward the subchorial lake. They postulate that Braxton-Hicks contractions (p. 241) enhance the movement of blood from the center of the cotyledon through the intervillous space.

The principal factors regulating the flow of blood in the intervillous space are thus shown to include intrauterine pressure, the pattern of uterine contractions including the contour of the individual contraction wave, and factors acting specifically upon the arteriolar walls. The lack of homogeneity of blood throughout the intervillous space has been emphasized by Fuchs, Spackman, and Assali, who measured blood samples thought to be from the intervillous space and found considerable variations in the pO_2, pCO_2, pH, and standard bicarbonate. Some samples resembled arterial and others uterine venous blood. They stress, furthermore, the difficulty of ascertaining the source of blood obtained by transuterine puncture of the placenta.

Studies of the placental circulation provide no evidence of countercurrent flow, a system by which fetal blood of low oxygen content as it enters the villous capillaries would flow first close to maternal blood of low oxygen content and then move in close proximity to progressively more oxygenated maternal blood. In the hemochorial villous placenta of man, strict countercurrent flow is precluded by the random distribution of villi, in the capillaries of which the direction of fetal to maternal flow can bear no fixed relationship.

Harris and Ramsey have published a summary of their anatomic studies of the uteroplacental vasculature. They note that cytotrophoblastic elements are initially confined to the terminal portions of the uteroplacental arteries but later extend proximally. By the sixteenth week, cytotrophoblast is found in many of the arteries of the inner layer of myometrium. Intraarterial accumulation of trophoblast may ultimately stop circulation through some of these vessels. The number of arterial openings into the intervillous space is gradually reduced by cytotrophoblast and by breaching of the walls of the more proximal parts of the arteries by deeply penetrating trophoblast. After the thirtieth week a prominent venous plexus separates the decidua basalis from the myometrium, thus providing a plane of cleavage for separation of the placenta. Brosens and co-workers have shown that the cytotrophoblast not only breaches the maternal spiral vessels but plays a major role in their progressive conversion to large tortuous channels by replacement of the normal muscular and elastic tissue of the wall by fibrous tissue and fibrinoid.

PLACENTAL IMMUNOLOGY

The early investigators assumed that an anatomic separation of arterial entrances and venous exits was required. In Bumm's scheme, for example, the arterial blood entered the intervillous space high along the sides and at the summits of the placental septa, and all venous exits were located along the basal plate. The villi were thus bathed by arterial blood flowing back from the septal arteries to the basal veins, with each cotyledon an independent circulatory unit. Bumm's theory is invalidated, however, by the absence of major arterial entrances high in the septa.

According to Spanner, arterial blood entered the intervillous space at the base of the placenta centrally, and venous drainage occurred exclusively at the placental margin. The villi were thus bathed by arterial blood rising between the septa toward the "subchorial lake," whence it flowed to the so-called marginal sinus. The cotyledons, functionally interconnected by "overflow filling," rendered the entire placenta a circulatory unit.

In Stieve's view the human placenta was essentially labyrinthine, comprising an interconnecting network formed by the fusion of villous tips, with fetal vessels running uninterruptedly from one villus to another. Except for the intervillous capillary anastomosis recently illustrated by Boyd and Hamilton, however, such vascular interconnections have been very rarely described.

Breaks in the Placental "Barrier."　　The failure of the placenta to maintain absolute integrity of the fetal and maternal circulations is documented by numerous studies of the passage of cells in both directions between mother and fetus, and best exemplified clinically by the occurrence of erythroblastosis. In the study by Zarou, Lichtman, and Hellman, maternal erythocytes tagged with radioactive chromium-51 were detected in the fetal circulation in some apparently normal

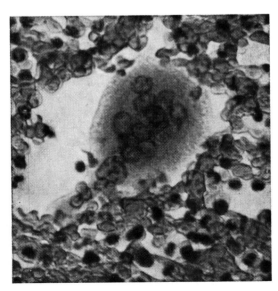

Fig. 24. Trophoblast in blood from vein in broad ligament, 26 weeks' gestation. (From Douglas et al. Amer J Obstet Gynec 78:960, 1959.)

pregnancies. Desai and Creger labeled maternal leukocytes and platelets with atabrine and found that they too crossed the placenta from mother to fetus. Lymphocytes passing into the fetus create the possibility of *chimerism*, the subject of a recent review by Benirschke. If the maternal cells then colonize, a "graft-versus-host" reaction or autoimmune disease may result. Zipursky and colleagues, furthermore, have shown that there may be 0.1 to 3.0 ml of fetal blood in the maternal circulation normally, and much more in cases of fetal anemia; with quantitative technics they demonstrated passage from mother to fetus also.

Fetal cells other than constituents of the blood have also been identified in the maternal circulation. Douglas and colleagues have found cells morphologically identical with trophoblast in the uterine venous blood (Fig. 24). The immunologic significance of continuous release of fetal elements into the maternal circulation remains to be explained. Salvaggio and co-workers, furthermore, report the occurrence of syncytiotrophoblast in blood from the umbilical vessels in 32 of their 53 cases.

Immunologic Considerations. Except in parthenogenesis or situations in which both parents are genetically identical, the fetus confronts the mother with foreign antigens. A fertilized egg transplanted to a recipient's uterus may, furthermore, result in a pregnancy with immunologic characteristics of a homograft. Interspecific hybrids, analogous to heterografts represent even more flagrant violations of the laws of immunology. Attempts to explain the survival of the "homograft" have occupied the attention of several of the world's outstanding biologists. An explanation based on antigenic immaturity of the fetus must be discarded in light of Billingham's demonstration that transplantation antigens appear very early in life. A second explanation, based on diminished immunologic reactivity of the mother during pregnancy, provides only an ancillary factor in the prevention of the development of maternal isoimmunization during pregnancy in a few species. If the uterus were an immunologically privileged site, as in a third explanation, advanced ectopic pregnancies could never occur. Since transplantation immunity can be evoked and expressed in the uterus as elsewhere, the survival of the homograft must be related to a peculiarity of the fetus rather than the uterus. A fourth explanation involves a physiologic barrier between fetus and mother. Lanman and colleagues have provided indirect support for the last hypothesis in their experiments in which fertilized rabbit's ova were transferred to a recipient's uterus. Neither prior exposure of the foster mother to skin grafts from the parents nor reexposure to homografts from these donors at the time of egg transfer or at midpregnancy adversely affected the pregnancy.

The only reasonable explanation for the survival of the homograft appears to be a fairly complete anatomic separation of maternal and fetal circulations. Comparative electron microscopy of the placenta has supported the concept of the prime role of the trophoblast in maintaining the immunologic barrier. In all placentas examined with the electron microscope, at least one layer of trophoblast has been shown to persist essentially throughout gestation (p. 190). If the trophoblast fails to express histocompatibility antigens, as described in Wynn's most recent papers, an immunologic barrier would be created.

The suggestion by Kirby and co-workers that deposition of fibrinoid was a general phenomenon of mammalian placentation rekindled interest in these amorphous deposits. We have used the term "fibrinoid" in the restricted conventional sense of the histopathologist to refer to a group of substances recognized with the light microscope. Although fibrinoids are not demonstrable in all mammalian placentas, a submicroscopic glycocalyx may be found with the electron microscope to coat most trophoblastic plasma membranes. It is still not clear whether these polysaccharide barriers serve as mechanical barriers to the passage of transplantation antigens from fetus to mother.

The interesting hypothesis of Currie and Bagshawe holds that pericellular sialomucins present a chemical barrier to immunologically competent cells. They reported that maternal lymphocytes respond in vitro to trophoblast as they do to other allogeneic tissues and suggested originally that trophoblast escapes attack in vivo by electrochemical repulsion of maternal lymphocytes, since the sialomucin confers a high electronegative surface charge. It now seems more likely that the sialic acids act by steric hindrance to prevent contact with underlying antigenic groups. More recently, Currie and co-workers showed that attacking the mucopolysaccharide coat with neuraminidase, which disrupts the sialomucin, results in the ability of the treated trophoblastic cells to express histocompatibility antigens on transplantation. It now seems reasonable to conclude that the immunologic protection of the placental homograft depends on the trophoblast and its pericellular sialomucins. The moot question is whether the protection is afforded by factors that are primarily cellular or extracellular.

Billingham suggests that the degenerative changes that occur normally in the placenta as gestation proceeds might be ascribed to sensitization of the mother to a special organ-specific antigen, possibly occurring rather late in maturation of the tissue. Parturition might thus represent an immunologic reaction similar to rejection of a homograft. Transplantation antigens, however, cannot be implicated in the process or placentas would never separate in pregnancies resulting from the mating of animals of identical genetic constitution.

The Amnion

According to the prevalent school of thought, the human amnion probably develops by delamination from the cytotrophoblast about the seventh or eighth day of development of the normal ovum. The other school of thought holds that the human amnion is essentially an extension of the fetal ectoderm. Initially a minute vesicle (Ch. 5, Fig. 20), the amnion develops into a small sac that covers the dorsal surface of the embryo. As the amnion enlarges, it gradually surrounds the growing embryo, which prolapses into its cavity. Distention of the amniotic sac eventually brings it into contact with the interior of the chorion; apposition of the mesoblasts of chorion and amnion about the middle of the third month results in obliteration of the extraembryonic celom. The amnion and chorion, though slightly adherent, are never intimately connected and can be separated easily even at term.

The normal amnion is 0.02 to 0.5 mm in thickness. The epithelium normally consists of a single layer of nonciliated, cuboidal cells. According to Bourne, there are five layers, comprising, from within outward, epithelium, basement membrane, the compact layer, the fibroblastic layer, and the spongy layer. Electron microscopic studies of amnion by Wynn and French and by Hoyes have not, however, revealed such sharply defined layers (Fig. 25).

Bourne was unable to find blood vessels or nerves in the amnion at any stage of development and, despite suggestive spaces in the fibroblastic and spongy layers, could not identify distinct lymphatic channels.

The ultrastructure of the amnion suggests that it is adapted to facilitation of transfer of fluid rather than to secretion. In an electron microscopic study of human amniotic epithelium, Hoyes found that the cells were capable of active reabsorption of fluid passing between the epithelial cells. Wynn and French also showed that the large "vacuoles" noted by light microscopists were actually dilated intercellular spaces.

At term, small rounded plaques are often found on the amnion, particularly near the attachment of the umbilical cord. These *amniotic caruncles* consist of stratified squamous epithelium that histologically resembles skin (Ch. 22, p. 604).

The normally clear fluid that collects within the amnionic cavity increases in quantity as pregnancy advances. An average of somewhat less than 1,000 ml is found at term, although the volume may vary widely in abnormal conditions (oligohydramnios and hydramnios, p. 599) from a few milliliters to many liters. The origin, composition, and function of the amniotic fluid are discussed further in Chapter 7 (p. 226).

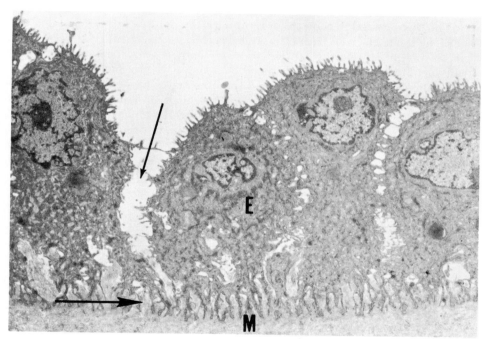

Fig. 25. Electron micrograph of human amnion at term obtained at time of cesarean section. Epithelium (E) and mesenchyme (M) are shown. Thin arrow indicates intercellular space. Thick arrow points to specializations of basal plasma membranes. (Courtesy of Dr. Ralph M. Wynn.)

UMBILICAL CORD AND RELATED STRUCTURES

Development of the Cord and Related Structures. The yolk sac and the umbilical vesicle into which it develops are quite prominent at the beginning of pregnancy. The embryo at first is a flattened disc interposed between amnion and yolk sac (p. 145). As the dorsal surface grows faster than the ventral, associated with the elongation of the neural tube, the embryo bulges into the amniotic sac, and the dorsal part of the yolk sac is incorporated into the body of the embryo to form the gut. The allantois projects into the base of the body stalk from the caudal wall of the yolk sac or, later, from the anterior wall of the hindgut. As pregnancy advances, the yolk sac becomes smaller and its pedicle relatively longer. By approximately the middle of the third month, the expanding amnion obliterates the exocelom, fuses with the chorion laeve, and covers the bulging placental disc and the lateral surface of the body stalk, which is then called the umbilical cord. Remnants of the exocelom in the anterior portion of the cord may contain loops of intestine, which continue to develop outside the embryo. Although the loops are later withdrawn, the apex of the midgut loop retains its connection with an attenuated vitelline duct, which terminates in a crumpled, highly vascular sac 3 to 5 cm in diameter lying on the surface of the placenta between amnion and chorion or in the membranes just beyond the placental margin, where it may occasionally be identified at term.

In an electron microscopic study of the human yolk sac, Hoyes confirmed that its endoderm is the origin of fetal blood cells. The epithelium of the yolk sac has ultrastructural features usually associated with those of a tissue that serves as a site of transfer of metabolites.

The three vessels in the cord at term normally are two arteries and one vein. The right umbilical vein usually disappears early, leaving only the original left vein. Section of any portion of the cord frequently reveals, near the center, the small duct of the umbilical vesicle, lined by a single layer of flattened or cuboidal epithelial cells. In sections just beyond the umbilicus, but never at the maternal end of the cord, another duct representing the allantoic remnant is occasionally found. The intraabdominal portion of the duct of the umbilical vesicle, which extends from umbilicus to intestine, usually atrophies and disappears, but occasionally remains patent, forming Meckel's diverticulum. The most common vascular anomaly in man is the absence of one umbilical artery, a condition associated with other fetal anomalies in 15 to 20 per cent of cases. Benirschke states that a single umbilical artery is found in about 1 per cent of singletons and up to about 6 per cent in at least one of each pair of twins. The subject is discussed further in Chapter 22 (p. 598).

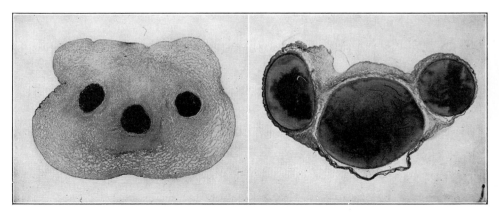

Fig. 26. Cross section of umbilical cord fixed after blood vessels had been emptied. The umbilical vein, carrying oxygenated blood to the fetus, is in the center; on either side are the two umbilical arteries carrying deoxygenated blood from the fetus to the placenta. (From Reynolds. Amer J Obstet Gynec 68:69, 1954.)

Fig. 27. Cross section of same umbilical cord shown in Figure 26, but through a segment from which the blood vessels had not been emptied. This photograph probably represents more accurately the conditions in utero. (From Reynolds. Amer J Obstet Gynec 68:69, 1954.)

Structure and Function of the Cord.   The umbilical cord, or funis, extends from the fetal umbilicus to the fetal surface of the placenta. Its exterior is dull white, moist, and covered by amnion, through which the three umbilical vessels may be seen. Its diameter is 1 to 2.5 cm, with an average length of 55 cm and a usual range of 30 to 100 cm. Folding and tortuosity of the vessels, which are longer than the cord itself, frequently create nodulations on the surface, or *false knots,* which are essentially varices. The matrix of the cord consists of Wharton's jelly (Figs. 26 and 27). After fixation the umbilical vessels appear empty, but Figure 27 represents more accurately the situation in vivo, when the vessels are not emptied of blood. The two arteries are smaller in diameter than the vein. When fixed in its normally distended state, the umbilical artery exhibits transverse intimal *folds of Hoboken* across part of its lumen (Chacko and Reynolds). The mesoderm of the cord, which is of allantoic origin, fuses with that of the amnion.

The egress of blood is via two routes, the ductus venosus, which empties directly into the inferior vena cava, and numerous smaller openings into the fetal hepatic circulation and thence into the inferior vena cava by the hepatic vein (Ch. 7, Fig. 8). The blood takes the path of least resistance through these alternate routes. Resistance in the ductus venosus is controlled by a sphincter, which is situated at the origin of the ductus at the umbilical recess and innervated by a branch of the vagus nerve.

Ellison and co-workers studied the innervation of the umbilical cord of the rat by means of localization of acetylcholinesterase and catecholamines. Cholinesterase-positive nerves were confined to periarterial plexuses, and adrenergic nerves were entirely absent from the cord. By these technics certain nerves could be traced to the placenta but not into it. Although several recent investigators, relying on histochemical methods, have reported nerves in placenta and amnion, ultrastructural confirmation is lacking. The question of innervation of the placenta and membranes thus remains open. Humoral stimuli, however, may well be transmitted across the placenta.

The Placental Hormones

The human placenta produces in abundance the protein hormones *chorionic gonadotropin* and *chorionic somatomammotropin* as well as the steroid hormones *progesterone* and *estrogens.* Quite recently considerable evidence has accumulated that trophoblast also synthesizes a substance with thyroid-stimulating properties. Odell and associates in 1963 first identified thyroid-stimulating activity in choriocarcinoma; subsequently Hennen and also Hershman and Starnes extracted from the normal placenta a substance with distinct thyrotropic properties. Whereas the human placenta was once believed to form corticotropin, critical analysis of the evidence indicates that it probably does not.

CHORIONIC GONADOTROPIN

Chorionic gonadotropin is produced almost certainly by syncytiotrophoblast rather than cytotrophoblast, as pointed out on page 159. The apparent function of chorionic gonadotropin in women is to maintain the corpus luteum during early pregnancy. In the human ovary that has been appropriately primed by follicle-stimulating hormone, the injection of chorionic gonadotropin induces ovulation and is sometimes so used to treat anovulation. In the immature albino rat, chorionic gonadotropin causes follicular growth, ovulation, and formation of the corpus luteum. In the hypophysectomized animal, however, it stimulates growth only of the interstitial cells of the ovary. It induces ovulation and prolongs pseudopregnancy in the adult albino rat.

The original demonstration by Aschheim and Zondek in 1927 of the "pregnancy hormone" in urine formed the basis for consideration of the placenta as an endocrine organ. Not until 1938, however, when Gey, Jones, and Hellman demonstrated production of chorionic gonadotropin by trophoblastic cells growing in tissue culture, was the placental source of the hormone verified. The hormone was finally crystallized in 1948 by Cleasson and co-workers.

The molecular weight of chorionic gonadotropin varies with the technic used (Bahl). By gel filtration its weight is $59,000 \pm 4,000$; with ultracentrifugation $46,600 \pm 3,000$; and reduced and carboxamidomethylated chorionic gonadotropin has a molecular weight of $30,000 \pm 2,000$. One international unit of chorionic gonadotropin is the amount of hormone equivalent in activity to that of 0.1 mg of the international standard powder of chorionic gonadotropin prepared under the auspices of the League of Nations Committee for Biological Standards.

The methods for assaying chorionic gonadotropin are of considerable clinical interest, since they form the basis for the majority of tests for pregnancy. Unfortunately neither the immunoassays nor bioassays are absolutely specific for chorionic gonadotropin. Recently it has been shown that the chorionic gonadotropin molecule is comprised of specific peptide chains and thus is analogous structurewise to the globin moiety of hemoglobin. The peptide chain designated as the alpha chain of chorionic gonadotropin is very similar to the alpha chain of pituitary follicle stimulating hormone, luteinizing hormone, and thyroid stimulating hormone. The similarity of the immunologic determinants in the alpha chains of these various hormones accounts for their cross reactivity when immunoassay is used. Moreover, the apparent chorionic gonadotropin activity in biologic fluids at times differs appreciably, depending upon whether immunoassay or bioassay is used. Wide and Hobson, and also Bridson and associates have demonstrated that chorionic gonadotropin synthesized in vitro by cloned choriocarcinoma cells yielded values twice as great by bioassay as by immunoassay. Their observations suggest that the reduction in material active in bioassay compared with immunoassay of urinary chorionic gonadotropin occurs as the result of alterations in the hormone molecule after it is secreted by the trophoblast. Some of the technics in current use for detecting chorionic gonadotropin are considered further in Chapter 9 (p. 283).

The excretion of chorionic gonadotropin in the urine during pregnancy is first detectable as early as the twenty-sixth day of pregnancy; the level gradually increases, reaching its peak between the sixtieth and seventieth days of gestation. The titer then begins to fall, although more slowly than it rose, reaching its low level between the one-hundredth and one-hundred-thirtieth days. The low level is maintained throughout the remainder of human pregnancy. The levels of chorionic gonadotropin in the serum closely parallel those in the urine, rising rapidly from approximately 1 international unit per milliliter at the time of the first missed period to about 100 IU per milliliter between the sixtieth and eightieth days after the last menstrual period (Fig. 28). Although most published curves constructed from mean values for chorionic gonadotropin in serum or urine are quite similar, the curves do not emphasize the considerable variations

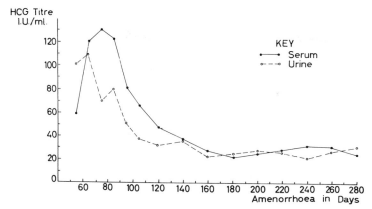

Fig. 28. Mean serum and urine chorionic gonadotropin levels in 600 normally pregnant women; the technic of hemagglutination-inhibition was used. (From Teoh. J Obstet Gynaec Brit Comm 74:77, 1967.)

in the hormone levels among individual subjects at the same duration of gestation, as demonstrated in the data presented in Figure 29.

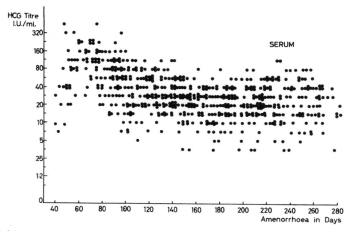

Fig. 29. Individual serum chorionic gonadotropin levels used to construct the curve in Figure 28. Note the scale along the ordinate of the graph is logarithmic. (From Teoh. J Obstet Gynaec Brit Comm 74:75, 1967.)

Significantly higher titers of chorionic gonadotropin may be found in pregnancies with multiple fetuses and pregnancies with a single erythroblastotic fetus resulting from maternal isoimmunization, as well as in hydatidiform mole and choriocarcinoma (Bradbury and Goplerud). Chorionic gonadotropin normally disappears rapidly from the urine after parturition and, in the absence of retained placental tissues, is below the level of detection within four days.

CHORIONIC SOMATOMAMMOTROPIN

Human chorionic somatomammotropin is detectable in the trophoblast as early as the third week after ovulation. It was first described by Ito and Higashi and subsequently isolated by Josimovich and MacLaren, who characterized it as a polypeptide hormone found in extracts of human placenta and retroplacental blood. Since it has both potent lactogenic activity and an immunochemical resemblance to human growth hormone, it was first called *human placental lactogen* or *chorionic growth hormone*. Chorionic somatomammotropin consists of a single polypeptide chain with a molecular weight of about 20,000 (Li and associates). It contains 184 amino acid residues compared to 188 in human growth hormone (pituitary somatomammotropin); the amino acid sequence in each hormone is also quite similar. Grumbach and Kaplan have shown by immunofluorescence that this hormone, like chorionic gonadotropin, is localized in the syncytiotrophoblast. Authoritative recent reviews have been published by Villee and by Saxena and co-workers.

Chorionic somatomammotropin can be detected in the serum of pregnant women as early as the sixth week of gestation, and it rises steadily during the first and second trimesters, with its concentration in maternal blood approximately proportional to placental mass. The concentration of chorionic somatomammotropin in maternal serum, as measured by radioimmunoassay in late pregnancy, reaches levels higher than those of any other known protein hormone. These high levels coupled with very short half-life in the circulation attest to a rate of production by the placenta of considerable magnitude, which has been estimated to be 1 to 2 g per day, practically none of which is found in the fetal circulation or in the urine of the mother or newborn. The concentration of the hormone in amniotic fluid is somewhat lower than that in the maternal plasma. Since chorionic somatomammotropin is secreted primarily into the maternal circulation with only small amounts found in cord blood, it appears that the role of the hormone in pregnancy is mediated by the mother rather than by the fetus.

Chorionic somatomammotropin participates in a number of profound metabolic actions. It induces lipolysis and elevation of circulating free fatty acids, thereby providing a source of energy for maternal metabolism, and it inhibits both the uptake of glucose and gluconeogenesis in the mother, thereby sparing both glucose and protein. The insulinogenic action of chorionic somatomammotropin leads to high maternal levels of insulin, which favors protein synthesis and, in turn, ensures a mobilizable source of amino acids for transport to the fetus. Additional metabolic effects are discussed by Samaan and co-workers. Villee postulates that although the growing fetus has its own supply of growth hormone, it is not unreasonable to assume that there are one or more placental hormones the function of which is to maintain a steady flow of chemical energy from mother to fetus to ensure unhampered fetal growth.

Although the indications in clinical obstetrics for assaying chorionic somatomammotropin are not clearly evident at this time, they should be clarified in the near future as several groups of investigators continue their vigorous studies of this problem. Spellacy and co-workers believe that the level of chorionic gonadotropin in the maternal serum may serve in some circumstances as a sensitive and practical index of placental function. Having observed that chorionic somatomammotropin levels in the maternal serum of some complicated pregnancies differ from those of normal pregnancies, they are carrying out a controlled study of the value of the hormonal assay to identify pregnancies in which the fetus is in jeopardy. Their preliminary observations indicate that in hypertensive pregnant women, any time the level of hormone falls below 4 μg per ml after the thirtieth week of gestation the fetus will succumb in about one half of the cases unless delivery is accomplished promptly. If, however, the level is more than 4 μg per ml, according to Spellacy and associates, the fetus is not in jeopardy from the effects of the hypertension, at least.

The observations of Samaan and associates and Josimovich and co-workers provide a note of caution concerning the value of serum chorionic somatomammotropin assays for monitoring the integrity of the placenta and the fetus. They have observed death in utero in instances of pregnancy-induced hypertension although the level of chorionic somatomammotropin in maternal serum was normal or even high.

Our own clinical observations indicate that from the standpoint of preventing death during the perinatal period, delivery is advantageous whenever the mother is clearly hypertensive, irrespective of whether the hypertension is pregnancy-induced or chronic, and the gestation has passed the thirty-third week. Similarly, the liveborn infant whose mother is hypertensive has an excellent chance for survival whenever the birth weight is 1,800 g or higher (Stone and Pritchard). Unfortunately, one of the most difficult and perplexing problems in clinical obstetrics is how to ascertain with reasonable precision the duration of gestation or the weight of the fetus. Assay of chorionic somatomammotropin in the mother's serum might allow the obstetrician to select those pregnancies complicated by hypertension in which the fetus is not in jeopardy and therefore not in need of premature delivery.

According to Saxena and co-workers, in some women with double-ovum twins, diabetes without hypertension, or a fetus with erythroblastosis, the serum level of chorionic somatomammotropin is high, whereas in subjects with fetal growth retardation and a small placenta, the level is below the normal range. When the period of gestation exceeds 40 weeks, the serum level of the hormone may fall, but as long as the drop is gradual and not in excess of 50 per cent of the initial value, watchful waiting is permissible, according to Saxena and co-workers. Further decrease in chorionic somatomammotropin requires prompt delivery.

Spellacy and Buhi could not detect chorionic somatomammotropin and noted a deficient output of pituitary somatomammotropin in the early postpartum period. They suggest that this relative lack of insulin antagonists is associated with low fasting levels of blood glucose during this period.

Chorionic somatomammotropin has been detected by direct radioimmunoassay of sera from patients with various malignancies other than those originating in trophoblast or gonad, including bronchogenic carcinoma, hepatoma, lymphoma, and pheochromocytoma (Weintraub and Rosen). Thus, production of chorionic somatomammotropin is not restricted to trophoblastic tissue.

ESTROGENS

Normal human pregnancy represents a hyperestrogenic state of continually increasing proportions that terminates abruptly after expulsion of the products of conception. Plasma level of 17β-estradiol, for example increase from about 2 ng per ml early in pregnancy to 12 ng per ml at term; they fall abruptly after delivery (Munson and co-workers). There is little doubt that the principal site of origin of the increased amounts of estrogen is the placenta. As early as the seventh week of gestation, more than 50 per cent of the estrogens entering the maternal circulation can be ascribed to placental production (MacDonald and Siiteri). Indeed, Diczfalusy and Borell have demonstrated that bilateral oophorectomy performed on the seventy-eighth day of gestation failed to result in reduction in the urinary excretion of estrogens. Similar results have been obtained in multiple studies of urinary excretion of estrogen by women after the surgical removal of the corpus luteum. It is thus evident that the ovary is not a quantitatively important source of estrogen after the first few weeks of human pregnancy.

The source of estrogens in normal pregnant women differs from that in the nonpregnant woman in other respects. As pointed out in Chapter 3, the principal product of estrogenic secretion in the nonpregnant woman is estradiol, from which the multiple urinary estrogenic metabolites are derived. In nonpregnant women the ratio of urinary estriol to estrone plus estradiol is approximately unity. During pregnancy, however, this ratio increases to ten or more near term (Brown). It is likely that the disproportionate increase in estriol during pregnancy results from the placental formation of estriol rather than from an alteration in the maternal metabolism of estrone-estradiol.

The biosynthetic pathways of estrogens in the placenta, furthermore, differ considerably from those in other endocrine organs. Although in vitro studies indicate clearly that ovarian estrogens may arise de novo from acetate or cholesterol (Ch. 3, Fig. 18), it has not been possible to demonstrate that acetate or cholesterol or even progesterone can serve as a precursor of placental estrogens. The classic experiments of Ryan have demonstrated the exceptionally high capacity of placental tissue to convert certain C_{19} compounds to estrone and estradiol. Dehydroisoandrosterone, Δ^4-androstenedione, and testosterone are efficiently converted to estrone, estradiol, or both by placental preparations in vitro. These findings led to an investigation of the role of circulating C_{19} steroids in maternal or fetal blood as precursors for the placental synthesis of estrogens.

Amoroso concluded that the placenta, although not directly secreting these estrogens, might, through its abundant enzymatic activity, bring about the conversion of inactive materials derived from elsewhere in the body. Support for this deduction was provided by Frandsen and Stakemann, who showed that women pregnant with an anencephalic fetus excrete very small amounts of estrogens in the urine, approximately one tenth that of the woman pregnant with a normal fetus at the same stage of gestation. Pointing to the characteristic absence of the fetal zone of the adrenal cortex in anencephaly, Frandsen and Stakemann postulated that the adrenal fetal zone is the site of origin of substances that serve as precursors of placental estrogens.

The first proof that the placenta utilizes plasma-borne precursors was provided by the demonstration that dehydroisoandrosterone sulfate in the maternal plasma is efficiently converted to estrogens by the placenta (Siiteri and MacDonald; Baulieu and Dray). It was shown too that other C_{19} steroids—namely, dehydroisoandrosterone, Δ^4-androstenedione, and testosterone—introduced into the maternal circulation are also converted to estrogens. The abundance of dehydroisoandrosterone sulfate in the plasma, however, and its much longer half-life uniquely qualify it as the principal circulating precursor of placental estrone-estradiol. The arrival of dehydroisoandrosterone as the sulfate at the site of conversion does not preclude its utilization in the synthesis of estrogen, since the placenta is a rich source of sulfatase (Pulkkinen; Warren and Timberlake). Using isotope-labeled dehydroisoandrosterone sulfate, it has been shown that as early as the seventh week of gestation there is readily demonstrable utilization of circulating maternal dehydroisoandrosterone sulfate for estrogen synthesis. By the thirtieth week of pregnancy, moreover, 35 per cent or more of dehydroisoandrosterone sulfate circulating in the maternal plasma is converted to estrone-estradiol by the placenta; additionally, maternal dehydroisoandrosterone sulfate is ultimately converted by the placenta to estriol via an estrone-estradiol independent pathway, to be described (MacDonald and Siiteri). The utilization of circulating maternal dehydroisoandrosterone sulfate undoubtedly accounts, in part, for the decrease in its concentration in the plasma of pregnant women (Migeon, Keller, and Holmstrom), as well as the decrease of the 11-deoxy-17-ketosteroids excreted in the urine.

As pregnancy advances, however, utilization of dehydroisoandrosterone sulfate in the maternal plasma can account for only a fraction of the estrogens produced by the placenta. The observation by Frandsen and Stakemann of lower excretion of estrogens in women pregnant with an anencephalic fetus, in which the fetal zone of the adrenal cortex is absent, together with the finding of high levels of dehydroisoandrosterone sulfate in the cord blood (Colás and co-workers), indicated the likelihood that precursors arising in the fetus also serve in the synthesis of placental estrogens. Confirmation of this hypothesis was provided by the experiments of Bolté and co-workers, who demonstrated that dehydroisoandrosterone sulfate introduced into the umbilical artery and perfused through the placenta in situ is converted to estrone-estradiol.

Although dehydroisoandrosterone sulfate circulating in both fetal and maternal plasmas is utilized for the production of estrone-estradiol, an explanation is still required for the inordinately large amounts of estriol in the urine of pregnant women. Estriol in the urine of nonpregnant women can be accounted for on the basis of catabolism of secreted estradiol. In the gravid woman, however, there is excreted in the urine a disproportionately large amount of estriol, which cannot be ascribed to a change in the metabolism of estradiol in the mother. Pearlman, Pearlman, Pearlman and Rakoff, as well as Fishman and co-workers, have demonstrated that the metabolism of estradiol in the pregnant woman is not significantly different from that in the nonpregnant woman. It has been impossible, however, to demonstrate conversion of more than trace amounts of estradiol to estriol in the placenta, indicating that the critical step of 16-hydroxylation is not efficiently performed by placental tissue. Consequently several other explanations have been offered to account for the origin of estriol in pregnancy.

One hypothesis holds that placental estrone-estradiol is circulated to the fetus and therein converted to estriol, which then reenters the maternal circulation (Fishman and co-workers; Gurpide and associates). Another explanation advanced by Bolté and co-workers, is that placental estrone is converted to 16α-hydroxyestrone by the fetus and circulated back to the placenta, where reduction to estriol occurs. A third explanation requires a 16α-hydroxyneutral steroid arising in the fetus or mother as a circulating precursor for placental synthesis of estriol. Although all three explanations are supported by data, quantitatively, the third mechanism is the most important. Ryan has demonstrated that 16α-hydroxylated neutral compounds, such as 16α-hydroxydehydroisoandrosterone, 16α-hydroxy-Δ^4-androsterone, and 16α-hydroxytestosterone, are efficiently converted to estriol by placental preparations in vitro. In addition, the presence of large amounts of 16α-hydroxydehydroisoandrosterone sulfate in umbilical cord blood has been demonstrated (Colás and co-workers). Finally, the conversion of 16α-hydroxydehydroisoandrosterone, introduced into the maternal circulation, to urinary estriol has been shown to occur (Siiteri and MacDonald).

The adrenal cortex of both mother and fetus is a site of origin of precursors of placental estrogens, especially estriol. In the absence of the fetal zone of the adrenal cortex, as in anencephaly, production of placental estrogens is severely diminished because of the lack of fetal precursors.

Verification of the lack of precursors has been provided by the absence of dehydroisoandrosterone sulfate in cord blood of anencephalic monsters (Nichols). In addition it has been shown that the total production of estrogens in women 33 to 40 weeks pregnant with an anencephalic fetus can be accounted for by the placental utilization of dehydroisoandrosterone sulfate circulating in the maternal plasma. The production of estrogens, furthermore, can be increased by the administration of ACTH, which raises the level of precursors produced by the maternal adrenal, dehydroisoandrosterone sulfate. Finally, placental production of estrogens can be decreased in pregnancies with an anencephalic fetus by the administration of a potent glucocorticoid, which decreases the availability of dehydroisoandrosterone sulfate from the maternal adrenal cortex (MacDonald and Siiteri).

Addisonian women have decreased excretion of estrogens during pregnancy (Baulieu, Bricaire, and Jayle), although the decrease is principally in the urinary estrone and estradiol fractions, since the fetal contribution to the synthesis of estriol, particularly in the latter part of pregnancy, is paramount, probably through the fetal production of the precursor of estriol, 16α-hydroxydehydroisoandrosterone sulfate. The synthesis of estrogen by the placenta is illustrated diagrammatically in Figure 30.

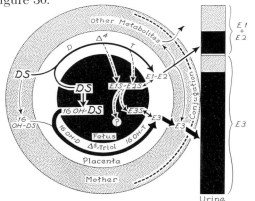

Fig. 30. Schematic representation of the origin of placental estrogens. Estrone and estradiol are derived from the utilization of dehydroisoandrosterone sulfate (DS) of maternal and fetal origin; approximately one half of maternal urinary estrone and estradiol ultimately arises from the utilization of maternal DS and one half from fetal DS. Estriol is synthesized principally through the placental conversion of 16-OH-dehydroisoandrosterone sulfate (16-OH-DS) of fetal and maternal origin; however, at term, approximately 90 per cent of maternal urinary estriol arises from the fetal contribution of 16-OH-DS precursor. (From Siiteri and MacDonald. J Clin Endocr 26:751, 1966.)

In summary, the evidence indicates (1) that the placenta is the site of origin of estrogens during human pregnancy; (2) that placental biosynthesis of estrogen results from the utilization of externally supplied precursors transported in the maternal and fetal plasmas, and (3) that the disproportionately elevated urinary estriol in pregnancy results from the independent synthesis of estriol in the placenta, principally derived from a 16α-hydroxylated neutral precursor arising in the fetus.

EXCRETION OF URINARY ESTRIOL DURING PREGNANCY AS A TEST OF PLACENTAL FUNCTION

Since the discovery that urine of pregnant women contains large amounts of estrogens (Aschheim and Zondek) originating in the placenta, measurements of the urinary excretion of the metabolites of these hormones have been performed in an attempt to provide an index of placental function. In the past, such work was generally limited by the cumbersome, expensive, and somewhat unreliable methods for measuring urinary estrogens. In recent years, however, new methods have been developed, providing accurate, rapid estimations of the levels of urinary estrogens.

Since the principal estrogen in the urine during pregnancy is estriol, most investigators have concentrated on developing reliable methods for its measurements. The discovery that the fetus plays an important role in contributing precursors for the synthesis of estriol fortuitously strengthens the possibility that pathologic pregnancies may be recognized by abnormal patterns of urinary excretion of estriol.

It has long been known that fetal death is accompanied by a marked reduction in the levels of urinary estrogens. Cassmer has supported that concept by demonstrating that ligation of the umbilical cord with the fetus and placenta in situ causes an acute and marked decrease in production of placental estrogens. These findings are subject to at least two interpretations, both of which are probably valid in part.

The first explanation, that maintenance of the fetal circulation is essential to the functional endocrine integrity of the placenta, is substantiated by the fact that in Cassmer's preparation the placental production of estrogens was maintained at "preligation" levels by perfusion of the placenta in situ through the fetal vessels with maternal blood after disconnecting the fetus. Further substantiation of the concept is afforded by the demonstration that fetal death may be associated with a marked reduction in the placental utilization of dehydroisoandrosterone sulfate circulating in the maternal plasma (Siiteri and MacDonald).

A second explanation of the marked decrease in urinary estrogens following fetal death is the elimination of one source of precursors of placental estrogens, the fetus. The quantitative importance of fetal precursors of placental estriol in normal pregnancy is amply demonstrated by the low levels of urinary estriol found in pregnancies with anencephalic fetuses.

Levels of estriol in the urine in pregnancy, therefore, may be influenced not only by the biosynthetic integrity of the placenta, but also by the availability of precursors of placental estrogens, and probably by other factors as yet unknown. The clinical usefulness of these measurements as corroborative evidence of fetal death is well established, but whether a clinically useful index of placental function or condition of the fetus is provided by estimations of urinary estriol remains to be proved. The value of these tests can be established only by proof of increased infant salvage resulting directly from therapeutic regimens predicated upon their results. The development of this aspect of obstetric endocrinology is thoroughly discussed by Frandsen, who reviewed the development of methods for measuring urinary estriol and described reliable procedures developed in his laboratories for the estimation of urinary estriol throughout normal human pregnancy. His measurements in early and late pregnancy are illustrated in Figures 31 and 32, respectively. The range of variation in levels of urinary estriol among different normal pregnant women is great. With reliable urinary collections and accurate

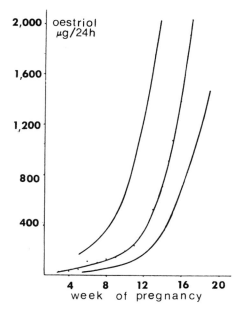

Fig. 31. Urinary excretion of estriol in normal pregnancy. The middle line represents the average excretion, and inside the area between the two other lines fall 95 per cent of the values found. (From Frandsen and Stakemann. Acta Endocr 44:196, 1963.)

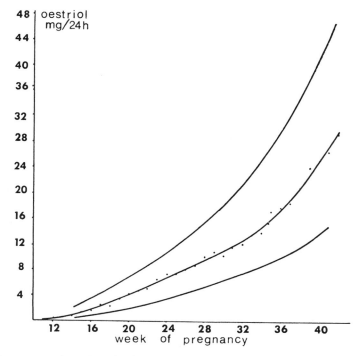

Fig. 32. Urinary excretion of estriol in normal pregnancies. The middle line represents the average excretion. In the area between the two other lines fall 95 per cent of the values found. (From Frandsen and Stakemann. Acta Endocr 44:183, 1963.)

chemical methods, however, Frandsen found that the day-to-day variation of estriol excretion by the same woman was relatively small, four fifths of his subjects exhibiting less than 20 per cent day-to-day variation during the last 30 weeks of pregnancy.

The interpretation of "abnormal" levels of urinary estriol, however, associated with possibly or definitely abnormal pregnancies must be made with caution and understanding of the following factors:

1. The wide range of normal values for excretion of estriol severely restricts the significance of a single measurement that falls in the "normal range."
2. In view of the difficulties of accurately ascertaining both duration of gestation and completeness of the collection of urine, and of eliminating technical error, *a single measurement considerably outside the "normal range" must be verified.*
3. Restriction of the supply of placental precursors of estriol, as in anencephaly or during the administration of potent glucocorticoids to the mother, will result in decreased synthesis of placental estriol, independently of placental function.
4. Factors apparently unrelated to the fetoplacental unit may be associated with decreased urinary estriol. For example, Taylor and colleagues found low levels of urinary estriol in women with acute pyelonephritis, who subsequently recovered and delivered a healthy infant.
5. Low levels of urinary estriol have been observed resulting apparently from a placental deficiency of sulfatase (France and Liggins), a situation that would preclude the utilization of the sulfurylated precursors of placental estrogen.

For these reasons there is general agreement that a single measurement of the urinary level of estriol may not reliably or accurately reflect the status of the fetoplacental unit. Repeated measurements to confirm the results or to identify a pattern are therefore essential.

High excretion of estriol occurs in multiple pregnancies and in some sensitized Rh-negative women carrying an erythroblastotic fetus (Greene and Touchstone; Taylor and associates). It is also theoretically possible that women pregnant with a fetus affected by congenital adrenal hyperplasia will have elevated levels of urinary estriol as a result of the increased production of C_{19} steroids by the affected fetal adrenal cortex.

Except in pregnancy with an anencephalic fetus, urinary excretion of estriol of less than 3 or 4 mg a day during the third trimester of pregnancy indicates fetal death or severe difficulty. In a study of 66 cases of suspected fetal death, Frandsen and Stakemann, on the basis of values of urinary estriol of less than 3 mg per day, correctly predicted fetal death in all 49 cases in which it had occurred.

One of the greatest problems in obstetric management today is the proper timing of delivery in complications that threaten the life of the fetus. The difficult common problem is to choose between prematurity and the high fetal risk of continued intrauterine existence. In such situations, notably diabetes, pregnancy-induced or chronic hypertension, poor previous obstetric history, and suspected postmaturity, the need for an index of fetal well-being is urgent. Current studies may substantiate the value of measurements of urinary estriol as a guide to obstetric management in these difficult situations. Barnes points out, however, that there is still little evidence that therapy based on levels of urinary estriol has improved infant salvage beyond that accomplished by sound clinical judgment alone.

PROGESTERONE

Although much more progesterone than estrogen is produced during normal human pregnancy, relatively much less is known about its biosynthesis. The placenta produces massive amounts of progesterone during pregnancy, as documented in the review by Diczfalusy and Troen, for a relatively small fraction of the total production of progesterone takes place in the ovary after the first few weeks of gestation. Surgical removal of the corpus luteum or even bilateral oophorectomy performed during the seventh to tenth weeks of pregnancy fails to produce a decrease in the urinary excretion of pregnanediol, the principal metabolite of progesterone. During normal human pregnancy there is a gradual increase in the urinary excretion of pregnanediol, until a plateau is reached at about 32 weeks of gestation, as shown in Figure 33, and of plasma progesterone, as indicated in Figure 34.

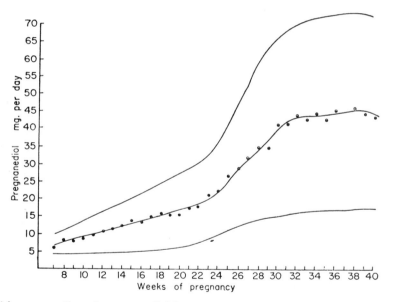

Fig. 33. Urinary excretion of pregnanediol in normal pregnancy. Filled circles represent observed means; the central line, fitted means. The upper and lower lines show the limit of 95 per cent probability. (From Shearman. J Obstet Gynaec Brit Emp 66:1, 1959.)

Isotope dilution technics for the measurement of endogenous rates of hormonal secretion were first applied to the study of progesterone secretion in pregnancy. These studies, performed by Pearlman in 1957, indicated that the daily production of progesterone in late pregnancy is about 250 mg. Studies by other methods agree with that figure. The biosynthetic origin of placental progesterone is not so clear as that of estrogen. Solomon and colleagues demonstrated that in vitro perfusion of the placenta with radioactive cholesterol resulted in the formation of isotope-labeled progesterone. In addition, incubation of Δ^5-pregnenolone with placental preparations by Wissim and Robson also resulted in formation of progesterone; and an "exceedingly great" capacity of the placenta to convert Δ^5-pregnenolone to progesterone has been demonstrated by in situ placental perfusion in Diczfalusy's laboratories.

In vivo studies by Bloch and by Werbin and co-workers have demonstrated the appearance of isotope-labeled urinary pregnanediol after the intravenous administration of isotope-labeled cholesterol to pregnant women. Recent studies by Hellig and associates also strongly suggest that maternal plasma cholesterol is the principal precursor (up to 90 per cent) of progesterone production in pregnancy. Production of placental progesterone, like that of placental estrogens, may thus occur through the utilization of circulating precursors; but unlike the production of estriol principally from fetal adrenal precursors, placental progesterone production arises through the utilization of maternal cholesterol.

The intimate relations between the fetus and placenta in the production of estrogen cannot be demonstrated in the case of progesterone. Fetal death, ligation of the umbilical cord in situ, and anencephaly are all associated with very low urinary excretion of estrogens, but a concomitant decrease in excretion of pregnanediol to anywhere near the same extent does not occur in these situations. Placental tissue cultures, as well as placental implantation experiments, have

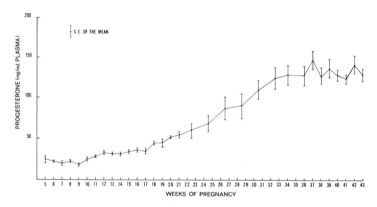

Fig. 34. Plasma progesterone levels during normal pregnancy. (From Johansson. Acta Endocr 61:607, 1969.)

failed to demonstrate significant elaboration of progesterone, indicating thereby a lack of de novo synthesis. The evidence, in summary, suggests that production of progesterone is accomplished by the placental utilization of precursors supplied by the mother.

ADRENOCORTICOSTEROIDS

Berliner and co-workers have isolated and characterized cortisol, cortisone, 11-dehydrocorticosterone, aldosterone, and corticosteroid metabolites in high concentration from the placenta. These findings, coupled with reports of increased blood levels of cortisol in pregnancy and increased urinary levels of "corticosteroids," have raised the question whether the placenta produces cortisol or related compounds. An alternate explanation, however, is provided by the combination of concentration of cortisol by the placenta and sequestration of blood (Berliner and co-workers). The large amounts of cortisol in the placenta can thus be explained without recourse to increased secretion of adrenocorticosteroids. In accord with the view that the placenta does not produce these corticoids, Baulieu and associates found no cortisol in the blood or urine of pregnant women with Addison's disease. The increase in free cortisol in the urine of gravid women is explained by alterations in the metabolism of cortisol in pregnancy. In both pregnancy and the course of treatment of nonpregnant patients with estrogen there is increased excretion of unconjugated corticosteroids, such as cortisol and 6β-hydroxycortisol (Frantz and associates). The increase is a response to the hyperestrogenic state of pregnancy and not necessarily the result of increased secretion of cortisol. At the same time the increased blood levels of cortisol in pregnancy are best explained by an estrogen-induced increase in protein binding and consequent delay in the metabolism of cortisol. The findings, again, are not necessarily associated with an increased secretion of hydrocortisone (see Ch. 8).

The reported increase in the levels of urinary corticosteroids is of questionable significance in supporting the concept of increased adrenal secretion of cortisol during pregnancy. The elevated glycogenic activity of the urine in pregnancy can be explained on the basis of the alteration in the metabolism of cortisol, resulting in increased amounts of free cortisol in the urine, a substance more active biologically than its reduced metabolites. The measurements of urinary "corticosteroids" by most chemical methods are subject to error during pregnancy, since falsely high values may be reported because of interfering substances produced in pregnancy (Baulieu and co-workers).

In summary, there is no direct evidence indicating production of adrenocorticosteroids by the placenta. Whether there is increased adrenal secretion of hydrocortisone during pregnancy, furthermore, remains to be proved. The accumulated evidence indicates that alterations in the metabolism of cortisol resulting from the hyperestrogenic state of pregnancy, coupled with the lack of validity of many of the chemical methods used to assay urinary corticosteroids, have led to the erroneous conclusion that during pregnancy there is increased production of cortisol.

COMPARATIVE ANATOMY

Types of Placentation. The debt of all comparative placentologists to George B. Wislocki, late Professor of Anatomy at Harvard University, and Harland W. Mossman, Professor Emeritus of Anatomy at the University of Wisconsin, can scarcely be overemphasized, as amply demonstrated by reference to the writings of Amoroso, Enders, Wimsatt, Wynn, and others. In this brief discussion only generalizations and some new developments are outlined, insofar as they focus attention on fundamental problems in human placentology.

The application of electron microscopy to study of placentation shows promise of elucidating many of its basic biologic features. Jollie and Jollie have shown, for example, that the ultrastructural changes following fertilization in the ovarian follicle of the common guppy represent conversion of the structure into the maternal portion of a site for respiratory exchange. Certain membranes of the developing intrafollicular embryo thus fulfill the criteria for "pseudoplacentation" in a viviparous fish.

Placentation in the higher mammals, or Eutheria, comprises several fundamentally distinct varieties of fetomaternal union. The basic fetal component of the placenta is the chorion, which is vascularized by either vitelline or allantoic vessels. In the absence of a vesicular allantois, the chorionic vessels arise from allantoic mesoderm, as in man. Whenever the chorion is vascularized by the allantois or its derivatives, *chorioallantoic* placentation is established. If the chorion is vascularized by vitelline vessels, the fetal component of the placenta develops from the trilaminar choriovitelline membrane, and *choriovitelline* placentation results. In formation of the *inverted yolk sac,* the fetal component is the vascularized splanchnopleuric wall of the yolk sac everted against the bilaminar omphalopleure. In man, the precocious formation of the exocelom results in failure of the yolk sac to establish intimate contact with the peripheral trophoblast, precluding the development of a yolk-sac placenta. In many animals, however, the endoderm of the yolk sac and the trophoblast of the blastocystic wall form the bilaminar omphalopleure, which may function as the fetal component of a yolk-sac placenta. Invasion of mesoblast and vitelline vessels converts the bilaminar omphalopleure into a vascular trilaminar omphalopleure, the fetal component of a true choriovitelline placenta. The vascular trilaminar omphalopleure of the embryonic hemisphere may split, as in the rodents, to form the splanchnopleure of the yolk sac wall and the somatopleure of the true chorion. Where the split separates vascularized from true chorion, the choriovitelline placenta as such is destroyed. The splanchnopleuric vascular derivative is added to the invaginated roof of the yolk sac, forming, with the abembryonic omphalopleure, the *inverted yolk-sac* placenta. When the abembryonic omphalopleure persists, as in certain of the lower rodents, the incompletely inverted yolk sac results. If, as in many of the common higher rodents, the bilaminar omphalopleure degenerates, the yolk sac becomes completely inverted and exposed to the endometrial lumen.

Numerous investigators have demonstrated the importance of the yolk sac in transfer of certain large molecules and proteins of immunologic significance. Since the yolk sac ceases to function early in human development but remains a prominent organ of transfer throughout gestation in the mouse, rat, guinea pig, and rabbit, upon which many physiologic studies are based, it provides a striking example of the danger of deriving conclusions regarding human placental function from laboratory animals (Fig. 35).

Although the true chorion is avascular, it may theoretically form, in conjunction with the amnion, a paraplacental organ or "chorioamnionic" placenta. The chorion laeve in man may serve such a function. In summary, all mammals, except the egg-laying Prototheria (monotremes) have a well-developed placenta. In most Metatheria (marsupials), except the bandicoot *Perameles,* which has a chorioallantoic placenta, the yolk sac forms the definitive and sole placenta. In the Eutheria (true "placental" mammals), the chorioallantoic placenta is the definitive organ, although a functionally important yolk sac may precede or coexist with it.

Chorioallantoic Placentation. Since the chorioallantoic placenta is the principal organ of fetomaternal exchange in most higher mammals, including man, it has been subjected to numerous attempts at classification. In dealing with biologic variation, however, overclassification reflects gaps in detailed knowledge rather than scholarly perfection. The well-known scheme of Grosser, in which placentas are classified according to the number of layers separating fetal and maternal blood, has proved progressively less useful in proportion to the increasing knowledge of placental structure and function. In Grosser's original classification the minimal placental "barrier" comprised the three fetal components (trophoblast, connective tissue, and endothelium), forming a *hemochorial* placenta, in which trophoblast was directly exposed to maternal blood. The persistence of maternal endothelium added a fourth layer to form an *endotheliochorial* placenta. If, in addition, endometrial connective tissue remains, a *syndesmochorial* placenta results. When the epithelium of the endometrium enters into formation of a six-layered placenta, an *epitheliochorial* condition obtains (Fig. 36).

The inadequacies of the Grosser classification involve its failure to account for anatomic variations within the placenta, changes accompanying placental aging, and accessory placental organs. Its basic deficiency, however, is the implication that a reduction in the number of layers in the placental "barrier" is equivalent to increased placental efficiency. Whereas the transfer of substances that cross the placenta by simple diffusion may be influenced directly by the thickness of the barrier, the Grosser scheme fails to consider the physiologic activity of the highly complex placental membrane, particularly with respect to active transport of metabolites.

Although attempts to modify the Grosser classification have been generally unsuccessful, the introduction of the term *"vasochorial"* by Wislocki represents an improve-

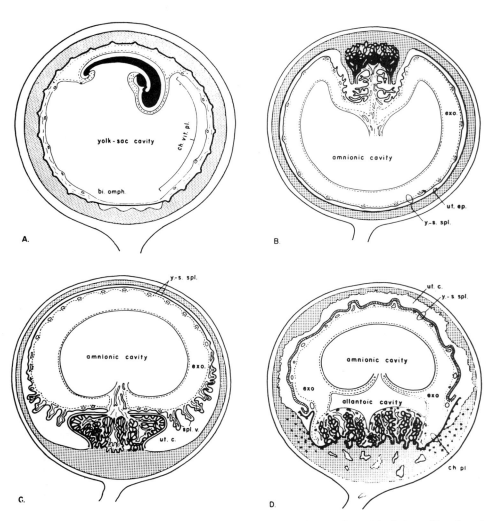

Fig. 35. A, schematic cross section of an early gestational sac of the black bear (Carnivora), illustrating central implantation and the early extensive vascular choriovitelline placenta (ch. vit. pl.). B, definitive arrangement of the placenta and fetal membranes in Solenodon (Insectivora), showing the discoidal chorioallantoic placenta antimesometrially, and the extensive completely inverted yolk-sac placenta over the remaining area of contact between fetal and maternal tissues. Key: exo., exocelom; ut. ep., uterine epithelium; y-s. spl., yolk-sac splanchnopleure.

C, definitive arrangement of placenta and membranes in the guinea pig. The discoidal chorioallantoic placenta lies mesometrially. The bilaminar omphalopleure has degenerated over the entire antimesometrial area, and the everted yolk-sac splanchnopleure is in contact with the endometrium, forming a completely inverted yolk-sac placenta over the antimesometrial hemisphere. In the paraplacental area the splanchnopleure has numerous villi (spl. v.) that project into the uterine cavity (ut. c.). D, fetal membranes and placenta in the rabbit, showing the surviving chorionic placenta (ch. pl.) at the margin of the placental disc and the extensive inverted yolk-sac placenta. The discoidal chorioallantoic placenta is situated mesometrially. The black dots in the decidua within the paraplacental zone represent free trophoblastic giant cells. (From Wimsatt. Amer J Obstet Gynec 84:1570, 1962.)

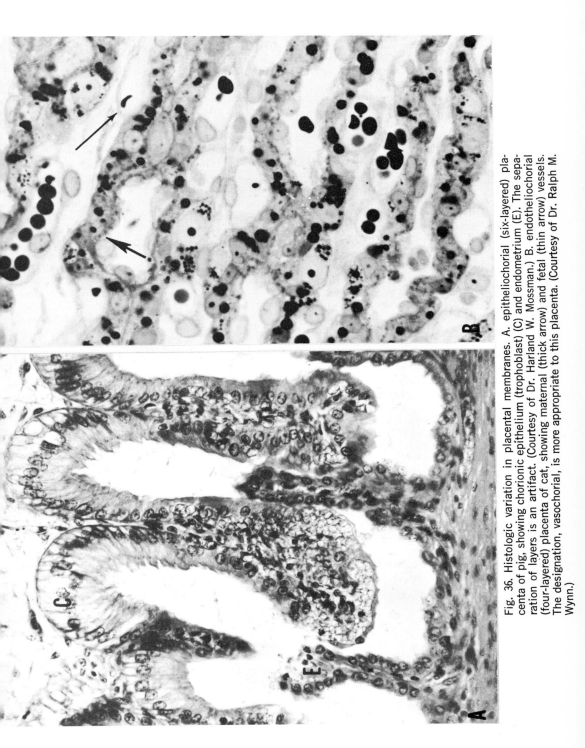

Fig. 36. Histologic variation in placental membranes. A. epitheliochorial (six-layered) placenta of pig, showing chorionic epithelium (trophoblast) (C) and endometrium (E). The separation of layers is an artifact. (Courtesy of Dr. Harland W. Mossman.) B. endotheliochorial (four-layered) placenta of cat, showing maternal (thick arrow) and fetal (thin arrow) vessels. The designation, vasochorial, is more appropriate to this placenta. (Courtesy of Dr. Ralph M. Wynn.)

189

ment, inasmuch as the occurrence of entirely unsupported endothelium, as implied in the term "endotheliochorial," is most unlikely. In the lamellae of the cat's "vasochorial" placenta, furthermore, decidualike cells persist, in an almost syndesmochorial relation. Rigid classifications, moreover, neglect the transitions between various histologic types within the same placenta and the fundamental differences in origin and function of numerous placental specializations that appear superficially homologous. In the "hematoma" of the typical carnivore's placenta, for example, stagnant blood extravasates between the chorion and the endometrial surface. Such a structure is *"histotrophic,"* a term used to describe nutrition obtained for the trophoblast from sources other than circulating blood, such as glandular secretions and extravasated blood. In contrast, the hemochorial placenta of man represents a true *"hemotrophic"* condition in that nutrition is derived from the circulating blood. The two conditions, though superficially similar histologically, are basically different in origin and function.

Mossman originally described placentas allegedly more intimate than the hemochorial types and postulated that even the trophoblast may disappear focally to produce hemoendothelial and endothelioendothelial placentas. Comparative electron microscopic studies, however, have consistently demonstrated at least one layer of trophoblast in all placentas studied thus far (Enders; Mossman; Wynn). Enders has suggested a most useful classification of hemochorial placentas based on the number of complete layers of trophoblast. The placentas of man and the guinea pig, for example, are *hemomonochorial;* that of the rabbit is *hemodichorial;* and that of the mouse is *hemotrichorial.* The immunologic significance of the persistence of trophoblast is discussed on page 168.

Additional factors of importance in the classification of chorioallantoic placentas are gross shape and presence or absence of true decidua. In general, placentas may be grossly divided into diffuse, cotyledonary, zonary, and discoid types. The definitive shape is usually determined by the initial distribution of villi over the chorionic surface, although it is occasionally secondarily derived. In the pig and horse the distribution of villi over almost the entire chorionic surface produces a diffuse placenta. In the ruminants (sheep, cow, deer, and antelope) the villi are restricted to separate tufts of cotyledons, widely scattered over the chorion to form a cotyledonary, or multiplex, placenta. In most carnivores, the Sirenia, and the Tubulidentata (aardvark), the grouping of villi in bands around the equator of the chorioallantoic sac results in a zonary placenta. In anthropoids, rodents, bats, and most insectivores, the placenta consists of a single disc, as in man, or a double disc, as in certain monkeys and primitive tree shrews. The definitive shape of the human placenta is a result of the disappearance of villi from all but a circumscribed locus on the chorion. Finally, placentas may be classified as deciduate (man, guinea pig), adeciduate (ungulates), or contradeciduate allegedly (some insectivores).

Interesting attempts have been made to assign evolutionary significance to the Grosser classification. One school held that the epitheliochorial placenta was the most primitive and the hemochorial the most advanced. Taxonomic evidence, however, conflicts with that concept. First, the epitheliochorial placenta is found in such diverse, specialized groups as the pig, horse, deer, whale, the mole *Scalopus*, and the lemur, which is usually classified as a primate. Typical "syndesmochorial" placentas, furthermore, have been shown by Björkman, with the electron microscope, to be at least partially epitheliochorial. The endotheliochorial (vasochorial) condition is widely distributed among some insectivores and bats, most carnivores, the sloth, the aardvark, and the Indian elephant. The hemochorial condition is common to such diverse groups as the higher primates, most higher rodents, some insectivores, the armadillo, and possibly the hyena. Since it is clearly impossible to establish phylogenetic relations among such divergent groups on the basis of similar placentas, and since the most "advanced" placentas (hemochorial and endotheliochorial) are found among the most primitive modern mammals (insectivores) and those nearer the mainstream of evolution (some primates and the carnivores), principles of convergent evolution must be operative. Mossman thus seems entirely justified in his contention that the modern epitheliochorial placenta is secondarily derived from a primitive endotheliochorial labyrinth. The absence of a fossil record, however, renders the fascinating question of placental evolution unanswerable by conventional paleontologic technics.

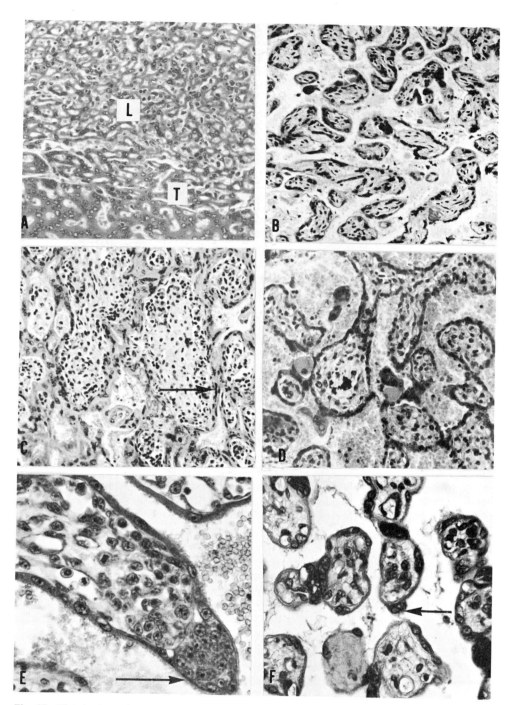

Fig. 37. Histologic variants of the hemochorial placenta. A. completely labyrinthine placenta of guinea pig, showing syncytiotrophoblastic lamellae (L) and trophospongium (T). B. villous placenta of rhesus monkey, showing free villi resembling those of human placenta. C. pseudolabyrinth of placenta of New World squirrel monkey, showing trophoblastic trabecula (arrow). D. semivillous placenta of spotted hyena, showing resemblance to that of platyrrhine monkey. This placenta may be partially endotheliochorial. E. villus of nine-banded armadillo, showing cytotrophoblast (arrow) restricted to tip. F. term human placenta, showing completely free villi with syncytial "knot" (arrow). (Courtesy of Dr. Ralph M. Wynn.)

The Hemochorial Villous Placenta. Hemochorial placentas, which are of special interest because they include the human placenta, comprise both labyrinthine and villous forms. In the hemochorial labyrinth, the trophoblast forms lamellae between blood-filled spaces. The villous condition results from the initial rupture by the trophoblast of the maternal vessels, with escape of blood to form large sinusoids and trabeculae across the blood-filled spaces. In studies based on both light and electron microscopy, Wynn and Davies and also Enders have demonstrated the villous condition in a variety of taxonomically unrelated animals, such as the scaly-tailed squirrel, the armadillo, and a variety of primates including man. They confirmed, furthermore, the presence of transitions from villous to labyrinthine forms, seen particularly well in the New World monkeys. In the human placenta the villi are almost entirely free; the apparent intervillous connections are formed not by syncytiotrophoblast, as Stieve believed, but rather by fibrinous adhesions resulting from the organization of minute hematomas. The breakdown of syncytium in the placentas of certain new world monkeys, for example, converts the trabeculae in these areas to villi, and the labyrinthine to the villous condition (Fig. 37).

It is reasonably clear that the hemochorial condition arose independently in several mammalian orders, as a result of extensive erosion of maternal vessels, associated with ontogenetic recapitulation of postulated phylogenetic development. Since the prospective placenta of man achieves a hemochorial status long before fetal vessels and mesenchyme appear—that is, before formation of a definitive placenta—there are no recognized intermediate stages of development. The varieties of placentation among the anthropoids are related to the differential activity of the ectoplacental trophoblast. In the platyrrhine (New World) monkeys, such as *Saimiri*, there is less freedom of individual villi, as a result of the initially broad attachment to the endometrium, with early and massive proliferation of trophoblast. In the catarrhine (Old World) monkeys, such as the macaque, there is earlier and more extensive trophoblastic invasion. The most highly invasive trophoblast occurs in the early human blastocyst, with the result that the chorionic villi lie free in the intervillous space in contact with maternal blood almost as soon as they are formed. Placental villi may arise as primary outgrowths of the chorionic membrane or secondarily, as in the case of man, as protrusions of cytotrophoblast that grow into a preformed mantle of syncytium. Although the deferred formation of villi usually leads to a labyrinthine condition, as indicated by Wimsatt, villi of the human placenta, according to Hamilton and Boyd, may arise in that manner from an antecedent previllous labyrinthine stage.

REFERENCES

Amoroso, E. C.   Placentation, in Marshall's Physiology of Reproduction, 3rd ed., A. S. Parkes (ed.). London, Longmans, 1952, Vol. 2, Ch. 15, p. 127.
———— Comparative aspects of the hormonal functions, in The Placenta and Fetal Membranes, C. A. Villee (ed.). Baltimore, Williams & Wilkins, 1960, p. 3.
Aschheim, S., and Zondek, B.   (Anterior pituitary hormone and ovarian hormone in the urine of pregnant women). Klin Wschr 6:248, 1927.
Bahl, O. P.   Human choronic gonadotropin I. Purification and physiochemical properties. J Biol Chem 244:567, 1969.
Barnes, A. C.   Discussion of paper by J. W. Greene. Amer J Obstet Gynec 91:688, 1965.
Battaglia, F. C., and Hellegers, A. E.   Permeability to carbohydrates of human chorion laeve in vitro. Amer J Obstet Gynec 89:771, 1964.
Baulieu, E. E., Bricaire, H., and Jayle, M. F.   Lack of secretion of 17-hydroxycorticosteroids in a pregnant woman with Addison's Disease. J Clin Endocr 16:690, 1956.
———— Desgrez, P., and Jayle, M. F.   Urinary corticosteroids during pregnancy, in Meeting on Biological and Clinical Aspects of Placental Steroidogenesis, F. Polvani and A. Bompiani (eds.). Baltimore, Williams & Wilkins, 1964, p. 43.
———— and Dray, F.   Conversion of H^3-dehydroisoandrosterone (3β-hydroxy-Δ^5-androsten-17-one) sulfate to H^3-estrogens in normal pregnant women. J Clin Endocr 23:1298, 1963.
Beck, J. S.   Time of appearance of human placental lactogen in the embryo. New Eng J Med 283:189, 1970.

Benirschke, K. Discussion of placental morphogenesis, in First Conference on Fetal Homeostasis, R. M. Wynn (ed.). New York, New York Academy of Sciences, 1965, p. 223.

——— Spontaneous chimerism in mammals—A critical review, in Current Topics in Pathology. Berlin, Springer-Verlag, 1970, p. 1.

Berliner, D. L., Jones, J. E., and Salhanick, H. A. The isolation of adrenal-like steroids from the human placenta. J Biol Chem 223:1043, 1956.

Billingham, R. E. Transplantation immunity and the maternal-fetal relation. New Eng J Med 270:667, 720, 1964.

Björkman, N. Ultrastructural features of placentae in ungulates. Fifth Internat Cong Anim Reprod 5:259, 1964.

Bloch, K. The biological conversion of cholesterol to pregnanediol. J Biol Chem 157:661, 1945.

Bolté, E., Mancuso, S., Eriksson, G., Wiqvist, N., and Diczfalusy, E. Studies on the aromatisation of neutral steroids in pregnant women. 1. Aromatisation of C-19 steroids by placentas perfused in situ. Acta Endocr 45:535, 1964.

——— Mancuso, S., Eriksson, G., Wiqvist, N., and Diczfalusy, E. Studies on the aromatisation of neutral steroids in pregnant women. 2. Aromatisation of dehydroisoandrosterone and of its sulphate administered simultaneously into a uterine artery. Acta Endocr 45:560, 1964.

——— Mancuso, S., Eriksson, G., Wiqvist, N., and Diczfalusy, E. Studies on the aromatisation of neutral steroids in pregnant women. 3. Over-all aromatisation of dehydroisoandrosterone sulphate circulating in the foetal and maternal compartments. Acta Endocr 45:576, 1964.

Borell, U., Fernström, I., and Westman, A. (An arteriographic study of the placental circulation). Geburtsh Frauenheilk 18:1, 1958.

Boss, J. H., and Craig, J. M. Histochemical distribution patterns of oxidative enzymes in the human placenta. Obstet Gynec 20:572, 1962.

Bourne, G. L. The Human Amnion and Chorion. Chicago, Year Book Medical Publishers, 1962.

Bourrillon, R., Got, R., and Marcy, R. (Action of enzymes on the biological activity of human chorionic gonadotropin). Acta Endocr 31:553, 1959.

Boyd, J. D. and Hamilton, W. J. The giant cells of the pregnant human uterus. J Obstet Gynaec Brit Comm 67:208, 1960.

——— and Hamilton, W. J. Placental septa. Z Zellforsch 69:613, 1966.

——— and Hamilton, W. J. Development and structure of the human placenta from the end of the 3rd month of gestation. J Obstet Gynaec Brit Comm 74:161, 1967.

——— and Hamilton, W. J. The Human Placenta. Cambridge, England, W. Heffer & Sons, Limited, 1970.

——— Boyd, C. A. R., and Hamilton, W. J. Observations on the vacuolar structure of the human syncytiotrophoblast. Z Zellforsch 88:57, 1968.

Bradbury, J. T., and Goplerud, C. P. Serum chorionic gonadotropin studies in sensitized Rh-negative patients. Obstet Gynec 21:330, 1963.

Bridson, W. E., Ross, G. T., and Kohler, P. O. Immunologic and biologic activity of chorionic gonadotropin synthesized by cloned choriocarcinoma cells in tissue culture. Clin Res 18:356, 1970.

Brody, S., and Carlstrom, G. Estimation of human chorionic gonadotropin in biological fluids by complement fixation. Lancet 2:99, 1960.

Brosens, I., and Dixon, H. G. The anatomy of the maternal side of the placenta. J Obstet Gynaec Brit Comm 73:357, 1966.

——— Robertson, W. B., and Dixon, H. G. The physiological response of the vessels of the placental bed to normal pregnancy. J Path Bact 93:569, 1967.

Brown, J. B. Urinary excretion of oestrogens during pregnancy, lactation, and the re-establishment of menstruation. Lancet 1:704, 1956.

Brown, W. E., and Bradbury, J. T. A study of the physiologic action of human chorionic hormone: the production of pseudopregnancy in women by chorionic hormone. Amer J Obstet Gynec 53:749, 1947.

Browne, J. S. L., and Venning, E. H. The effect of intramuscular injection of gonadotrophic substances on the corpus luteum phase of the human menstrual cycle. Amer J Physiol 123:26, 1938.

Bumm, E. (On the development of the maternal circulation in the human placenta). Arch Gynaek 43:181, 1893.

———— See English translation, Wynn, R. M. Amer J Obstet Gynec 87:829, 1963.

Cassmer, O. Hormone production of the isolated human placenta. Acta Endocr 32, Suppl. 45, 1959.

Chacko, A. W., and Reynolds, S. R. M. Architecture of distended and nondistended human umbilical cord tissues, with special references to the arteries and veins. Contrib Embryol 35:135, 1954.

Claesson, L., Högberg, B., Rosenberg, T., and Westman, A. Crystalline human chorionic gonadotrophin and its biological action. Acta Endocr 1:1, 1948.

Colás, A., Heinrichs, W. L., and Tatum, H. J. Pettenkofer chromogens in the maternal and fetal circulations: Detection of 3β, 16a-dihydroxyandrost-5-en-17-one in umbilical cord blood. Steroids 3:417, 1964.

Crawford, J. M. A study of human placental growth with observations on the placenta in ertyhroblastosis foetalis. J Obstet Gynaec Brit Emp 66:885, 1959.

Currie, G. A., and Bagshawe, K. D. The masking of antigens on trophoblast and cancer cells. Lancet 1:708, 1967.

———— Van Doorninck, W., and Bagshawe, K. D. Effect of neuraminidase on the immunogenicity of early mouse trophoblast. Nature (London) 219:191, 1968.

Curzen, P., and Morris, I. Heat-stable alkaline phosphatase in maternal serum. J Obstet Gynaec Brit Comm 75:151, 1968.

Delfs, E. An assay method for human chorionic gonadotrophin. Endocrinology 28:196, 1941.

Desai, R. G., and Creger, W. P. Maternofetal passage of leukocytes and platelets in man. Blood 21:665, 1963.

Diczfalusy, E. An improved method for the bioassay of chorionic gonadotrophin. Acta Endocr 17:58, 1954.

———— Endocrine functions of the human fetoplacental unit. Fed Proc 23:791, 1964.

———— and Borell, U. Influence of oophorectomy on steroid excretion in early pregnancy. J Clin Endocr 21:1119, 1961.

———— and Troen, P. Endocrine functions of the human placenta. Vitamins Hormones 19:229, 1961.

Douglas, G. W., Thomas, L., Carr, M., Cullen, N. M., and Morris, R. Trophoblast in the circulating blood during pregnancy. Amer J Obstet Gynec 78:960, 1959.

Ellison, J. P., Hibbs, R. G., Ferguson, M. A., Mahan, M., and Blasini, E. J. The innervation of the umbilical cord. Anat Rec 166:302, 1970.

Enders, A. C. A comparative study of the fine structure of the trophoblast in several hemochorial placentas. Amer J Anat 116:29, 1965.

Fishman, J., Brown, J. B., Hellman, L., Zumoff, B., and Gallagher, T. F. Estrogen metabolism in normal and pregnant woman. J Biol Chem 237:1489, 1961.

France, J. T., and Liggins, G. C. Placental sulfatase deficiency. J Clin Endocr 29:138, 1969.

Frandsen, V. A. The excretion of oestriol in normal human pregnancy. Copenhagen, Denmark, Bogtrykkeritet Forum, 1963.

———— and Stakemann, G. The site of production of oestrogenic hormones in human pregnancy. Hormone excretion in pregnancy with anencephalic foetus. Acta Endocr 38:383, 1961.

———— and Stakemann, G. The clinical significance of oestriol estimations in late pregnancy. Acta Endocr 44:183, 1963.

———— and Stakemann, G. The urinary excretion of oestriol during the early months of pregnancy. Acta Endocr 44:196, 1963.

Frantz, A. G., Katz, F. H., and Jailer, J. W. 6β-hydroxy-cortisol: High levels in human urine in pregnancy and toxemia. Proc Soc Exp Biol Med 105:41, 1960.

Freese, U. E. The uteroplacental vascular relationship in the human. Amer J Obstet Gynec 101:8, 1968.

French, G. L., MacLennan, A. H., and Wynn, R. M. Localization of nucleoside phosphatases in human amnion. Obstet Gynec, in press, 1971.

Fuchs, F., Spackman, T., and Assali, N. S. Complexity and nonhomogeneity of the intervillous space. Amer J Obstet Gynec 86:226, 1963.

Galton, M. DNA content of placental nuclei. J Cell Biol 13:183, 1962.

Gemzell, C. A. Blood levels of 17-hydroxycorticosteroids in normal pregnancy. J Clin Endocr 13:898, 1953.

Gey, G. O., Jones, G. E. S., and Hellman, L. M. The production of a gonadotrophic substance (prolan) by placental cells in tissue culture. Science 88:306, 1938.

Got, R., and Bourrillon, R. (New physical data concerning human chorionic gonadotropin). Biochim Biophys Acta 39:241, 1960.

Greene, J. W., and Touchstone, J. C. Urinary estriol as an index of placental function. Amer J Obstet Gynec 85:1, 1963.

Greer, M. A. Tropic hormones of the placenta: failure to demonstrate thyrotrophin or adrenocorticotrophin production in the hypophysectomized pregnant rat. Endocrinology 45:178, 1949.

Grosser, O. Frühentwicklung, Einautbildung und Placentation des Menschen und der Säugetiere, Dt. Frauenheilke, Vol. 5, Bergmann 1927.

Grumbach, M. M., and Kaplan, S. L. On placental origin and purification of chorionic growth hormone-prolactin and its immunoassay in pregnancy. Trans NY Acad Sci 27:167, 1964.

Gurin, S. Carbohydrates of gonadotropic hormones. Proc Soc Exp Biol Med 49:48, 1942.

Gurpide, E., Angers, M., Vande Wiele, R., and Lieberman, S. Determination of secretory rates of estrogens in pregnant and nonpregnant women from the specific activities of urinary metabolites. J Clin Endocr 22:935, 1962.

Hamilton, W. J., and Boyd, J. D. Development of the human placenta in the first three months of gestation. J Anat 94:297, 1960.

Harris, J. W. S., and Ramsey, E. M. The morphology of human uteroplacental vasculature. Contrib Embryol 38:43, 1966.

Hellig, H. D., Gattereau, D., Lefevre, Y., and Bolté, E. Steroid production from plasma cholesterol. I. Conversion of plasma cholesterol to placental progesterone in humans. J Clin Endocr 30:624, 1970.

Henne, G. Detection and study of a human-chorionic-thyroid-stimulating factor. Arch Int Physiol 73:689, 1965.

Hershman, J. M., and Starnes, W. R. Extraction and characterization of a thyrotropic material from the human placenta. J Clin Invest 48:923, 1969.

——— and Starnes, W. R. Placental content and purification of human chorionic thyrotropin. J Clin Invest 49:43a, 1970.

Hertig, A. T. The placenta: Some new knowledge about an old organ. Obstet Gynec 20:859, 1962.

Hoyes, A. D. Fine structure of human amniotic epithelium in early pregnancy. J Obstet Gynaec Brit Comm 75:949, 1968.

——— The human foetal yolk sac. An ultrastructural study of four specimens. Z Zellforsch 99:469, 1969.

Ito Y., and Higashi, K. Studies on prolactin-like substance in human placenta. II. Endocr Jap 8:279, 1961.

Jollie, W. P., and Jollie, L. G. The fine structure of the ovarian follicle of the ovoviviparous poeciliid fish, *Lebistes reticulatus*. II. Formation of follicular pseudoplacenta. J Morphol 114:503, 1964.

Josimovich, J. B., and MacLaren, J. A. Presence in human placenta and term serum of highly lactogenic substance immunologically related to pituitary growth hormone. Endocrinology 71:209, 1962.

——— Kosor, B., Bocella, L., Mintz, R. H., and Hutchinson, D. L. Placental lactogen in maternal serum as an index of fetal health. Obstet Gynec 36:244, 1970.

Kirby, D. R. S., Billington, W. D., Bradbury, S., and Goldstein, D. J. Antigen barrier of the mouse placenta. Nature (London) 204:548, 1964.

Lanman, J. T., Dinerstein, J., and Fikrig, S. Homograft immunity in pregnancy: Lack of harm to fetus from sensitization of mother. Ann NY Acad Sci 99:706, 1962.

Li, C. H., Grumbach, M. M., Kaplan, S. L., Josimovich, J. B., Friesen, H., and Cati, K. J. Human chorionic somatomammotropin (HCS), proposed terminology for designation of a placental hormone. Experimenta 24:1288, 1968.

MacDonald, P. C., and Siiteri, P. K. Utilization of circulating dehydroisoandrosterone sulfate for estrogen synthesis during human pregnancy (abstract). Clin Res 12:67, 1964.

——— and Siiteri, P. K. The conversion of isotope-labeled dehydroisoandrosterone and dehydroisoandrosterone sulfate to estrogen in normal and abnormal pregnancy, in Estrogen Assays in Clinical Medicine, C. A. Paulsen (ed.). Seattle, Univ. of Washington Press, 1965, p. 251.

——— and Siiteri, P. K.   Origin of estrogen in women pregnant with an anencephalic fetus. J Clin Invest 44:465, 1965.

Magendantz, H. G., and Ryan, K. J.   Isolation of the new estriol precursor (abstract). Fed Proc 23:275, 1964.

McCombs, H. L., and Craig, J. M.   Decidual necrosis in normal pregnancy. Obstet Gynec 24:436, 1964.

McKay, D. G., Hertig, A. T., Adams, E. C., and Richardson, M. V.   Histochemical observations on the human placenta. Obstet Gynec 12:1, 1958.

Midgley, A. R., Jr., Pierce, G. B., Jr., Deneau, G. A., and Gosling, J. R. S.   Morphogenesis of syncytiotrophoblast in vivo: an autoradiographic demonstration. Science 141:349, 1963.

Migeon, C. J., Keller, A. R., and Holmstrom, E. G.   Dehydroisoandrosterone, androsterone and 17-hydroxycorticosteroid levels in maternal and cord plasma in cases of vaginal delivery. Bull Johns Hopkins Hosp 97:415, 1955.

Mishell, D. R., Jr., Wide, L., and Gemzell, C. A.   Immunologic determination of human chorionic gonadotropin in serum. J Clin Endocr 23:125, 1963.

Moe, N.   The deposits of fibrin and fibrin-like materials in the basal plate of the normal human placenta. Acta Path Microbiol Scand 75:1, 1969.

Mossman, H. W.   Comparative morphogenesis of the fetal membranes and accessory uterine structures. Contrib Embryol 26:129, 1937.

——— Comparative biology of the placenta and fetal membranes, in Fetal Homeostasis, R. M. Wynn (ed.). New York, New York Academy of Sciences, 1967, Vol. 2, p. 13.

Munson, A. K., Mueller, J. R., and Yannone, M. E.   Free plasma 17B-estradiol in normal pregnancy, labor, and the puerperium. Amer J Obstet Gynec 108:340, 1970.

Nichols, J., Lescure, O. L., and Migeon, C. J.   Levels of 17-hydroxycorticosteroids and 17-ketosteroids in maternal and cord plasma in term anencephaly. J Clin Endocr 18:444, 1958.

Nissim, J. A., and Robson, J. M.   The conversion of pregnenolone to a more active progestational substance by incubation with endocrine tissues in vitro. J Endocr 8:329, 1952.

Odell, W. D., Bates, R. W., Revlin, R. S., Lipsett, M. B. and Hertz, R.   Increased thyroid function without clinical hyperthyroidism in patients with choriocarcinoma. J Clin Endocr 23:658, 1963.

Page, E. W.   Enzymes of the human placenta, in First Conference on Gestation, L. B. Flexner (ed.). New York, Josiah Macy, Jr., Foundation, 1955.

Pearlman, W. H.   [16-^{3}H] Progesterone metabolism in advanced pregnancy and in oophorectomized-hysterectomized women. Biochem J 67:1, 1957.

——— and Cerceo, E.   The isolation of progesterone from human placenta. J Biol Chem 198:791, 1952.

——— Pearlman, M. R. J., and Rakoff, A. E.   Estrogen metabolism in human pregnancy: A study with the aid of deuterium. J Biol Chem 209:803, 1954.

Pierce, G. B., Jr., and Midgley, A. R., Jr.   The origin and function of human syncytiotrophoblastic giant cells. Amer J Path 43:153, 1963.

Pulkkinen, M. O.   Arylsulphatase and the hydrolysis of some steroid sulphates in developing organism and placenta. Acta Physiol Scand 52, Suppl. 180, 1961.

Ramsey, E. M., and Davis, R. W.   A composite drawing of the placenta to show its structure and circulation. Anat Rec 145:366, 1963.

——— and Harris, J. W. S.   Comparison of uteroplacental vasculature and circulation in the rhesus monkey and man. Contrib Embryol 38:59, 1966.

Reynolds, S. R. M., Freese, U. E., Bieniarz, J., Caldeyro-Barcia, R., Mendez-Bauer, C., and Escarcena, L.   Multiple simultaneous intervillous space pressures recorded in several regions of the hemochorial placenta in relation to functional anatomy of the fetal cotyledon. Amer J Obstet Gynec 102:1128, 1968.

Richart, R. M.   Studies of placental morphogenesis. I. Radioautographic studies of human placenta utilizing tritiated thymidine. Proc Soc Exp Biol Med 106:829, 1961.

Riley, G. M., Smith, M. H., and Brown, P.   Rapid rat test for pregnancy: Ovarian hyperemia response as routine diagnostic procedure. J Clin Endocrinol 8:233, 1948.

Ryan, K. J.   Aromatization of steroids. J Biol Chem 234:268, 1959.

——— Metabolism of C-16-oxygenated steroids by human placenta: The formation of estriol. J Biol Chem 234:2006, 1959.

Salvaggio, A. T., Nigogosyan, G., and Mack, H. C.   Detection of trophoblasts in cord blood and fetal circulation. Amer J Obstet Gynec 80:1013, 1960.

Samaan, N., Yen, S. C. C., Gonzales, D., and Pearson, O. H.   Metabolic effects of placental lactogen (HPL) in man. J Clin Endocr 28:485, 1968.

Saxena, B. N., Emerson, K., Jr., and Selenkow, H. A.   Serum placental lactogen (HPL) levels as an index of placental function. New Eng J Med 281:225, 1969.

Sciarra, J. J., Kaplan, S. L., and Grumbach, M. M.   Localization of anti-human growth hormone serum within the human placenta: Evidence for a human chorionic-growth-hormone—Prolactin. Nature (London) 199:1005, 1963.

Simmer, H. H., Easterling, W. E., Jr., Pion, R. J., and Dignam, W. J.   Neutral C_{19}-steroids and steroid sulfates in human pregnancy.   I. Identification of dehydroepiandrosterone sulfate in fetal blood and quantification of the hormone in cord arterial, cord venous and maternal peripheral blood in normal pregnancies at term. Steroids 4:125, 1964.

Siiteri, P. K., and MacDonald, P. C.   The utilization of circulating dehydroisoandrosterone sulfate for estrogen synthesis during human pregnancy. Steroids 2:713, 1963.

———— and MacDonald, P. C.   The biogenesis of urinary estriol during human pregnancy (abstract). Clin Res 12:44, 1964.

Snoeck, J.   Le Placenta Humain—Aspects Morphologiques et Fonctionnels. Paris, Masson et Cie, 1958.

Solomon, S., Lenz, A. L., Vande Wiele, R. L., and Lieberman, S.   Pregnenolone and Intermediate in the Biogenesis of Progesterone and the Adrenal Hormones. Proc Amer Chem Soc New York, 29, 1954.

Spanner, R.   (Maternal and fetal circulation of the human placenta and their pathways). Z Anat 105:163, 1935.

———— See English translation, Harris, B. Amer J Obstet Gynec 71:350, 1956.

Spellacy, W. N., and Buhi, W. C.   Pituitary growth hormone and placental lactogen levels measured in normal term pregnancy and at the early and late postpartum periods. Amer J Obstet Gynec 105:888, 1969.

———— Cohen, W. D., and Carlson, K. L.   Human placental lactogen levels as a measure of placental function. Amer J Obstet Gynec 97:560, 1967.

———— Teoh, E. S., and Buhi, W. C.   Human chorionic somatomammotropin (HCS) levels prior to fetal death in high-risk pregnancies. Obstet Gynec 35:685, 1970.

Stieve, H.   (The intervillous space of the human placenta in the fourth and fifth months and at the end of pregnancy). Arch Gynaek 174:452, 1942.

Stone, S. R., and Pritchard, J. A.   Effect of maternally administered magnesium sulfate on the neonate. Obstet Gynec 35:574, 1970.

Stran, H. M., and Jones, G. E. S.   Some properties of human urinary gonadotrophins as elaborated by filter paper electrophoresis. Bull Johns Hopkins Hosp 95:162, 1954.

Taylor, E. S., Hassner, A., Bruns, P. D., and Drose, V. E.   Urinary estriol excretion of pregnant patients with pyelonephritis and Rh isoimmunization. Amer J Obstet Gynec 85:10, 1963.

Thiede, H. A., and Choate, J. W.   Chorionic gonadotropin localization in the human placenta by immunofluorescent staining II. Demonstration of HCG in the troploblast and ammon epithelium of immature and mature placentas. Obstet Gynec 22:433, 1963.

Thomson, A. M., Billewicz, W. Z., and Hytten, F. E.   The weight of the placenta in relation to birthweight. J Obstet Gynaec Brit Comm 76:865, 1969.

Velardo, J. T.   Hormonal actions of chorionic gonadotrophin. Ann NY Acad Sci 80:65, 1959.

Venning, E., and Browne, J. S. L.   Urinary excretion of sodium pregnanediol glucuronidate in the menstrual cycle (an excretion product of progesterone). Amer J Physiol 119:417, 1937.

Villee, D. B.   Development of endocrine function in the human placenta and fetus. New Eng J Med 281:473, 533, 1969.

Warren, J. C., and Timberlake, C. E.   Steroid sulfatase in the human placenta. J Clin Endocr 22:1148, 1962.

Weintraub, D., and Rosen, S. W.   Ectopic production of human chorionic somatomammotropin (HCS) in patients with cancer. Clin Res 18:375, 1970.

Werbin, H., Plotz, E. J., LeRoy, G. V., and David, M. E.   Cholesterol—a precursor of estrone in vivo. J Amer Chem Soc 79:1012, 1957.

Wide, L.   An immunological method for the assay of human chorionic gonadotropin. Acta Endocr 41, Suppl. 70, 1962.

———— and Gemzell, C. A.   An immunological pregnancy test. Acta Endocr 35:261, 1960.

———— and Hobson, B.   Immunological and biological activity of human chorionic gonadotropin in urine and serum of pregnant women and women with a hydatidiform mole. Acta Endocr 54:105, 1967.

Wigglesworth, J. S. Vascular anatomy of the human placenta and its significance for placental pathology. J Obstet Gynaec Brit Comm 76:979, 1969.

Wimsatt, W. A. Some aspects of the comparative anatomy of the mammalian placenta. Amer J Obstet Gynec 84:1568, 1962.

Wislocki, G. B., and Bennett, H. S. The histology and cytology of the human and monkey placenta with special reference to the trophoblast. Amer J Anat 73:335, 1943.

——— and Dempsey, E. W. The chemical histology of human placenta and decidua with reference to mucoproteins, glycogen, lipids and acid phosphatase. Amer J Anat 83:1, 1948.

——— and Dempsey, E. W. Electron microscopy of the human placenta. Anat Rec 123:133, 1955.

——— and Streeter, G. L. On the placentation of the macaque (*Macaca mulatta*), from the time of implantation until the formation of the definitive placenta. Contrib Embryol 27:1, 1938.

Wynn, R. M. Comparative morphogenesis and vascular relationships of the hemochorial placenta. Amer J Obstet Gynec 90:758, 1964.

——— Derivation and ultrastructure of the so-called Hofbauer cell. Amer J Obstet Gynec 97:235, 1967.

——— Fetomaternal cellular relations in the human basal plate: an ultrastructural study of the placenta. Amer J Obstet Gynec 97:832, 1967.

——— Comparative electron microscopy of the placental junctional zone. Obstet Gynec 29:644, 1967.

——— Morphology of the placenta, in Biology of Gestation, N. S. Assali (ed.). New York, Academic Press, 1968, Vol. 1, Ch. 3, p. 93.

——— Noncellular components of the placenta. Amer J Obstet Gynec 103:723, 1969.

——— Immunological implications of comparative placental ultrastructure, in Blastocyst Biology, R. J. Blandau (ed.). Chicago, University of Chicago Press, 1971, Ch. 29, p. 495.

——— and Davies, J. Comparative electron microscopy of the hemochorial villous placenta. Amer J Obstet Gynec 91:533, 1965.

——— and French, G. L. Comparative ultrastructure of the mammalion amnion. Obstet Gynec 31:759, 1968.

Zarou, D. M., Lichtman, H. C., and Hellman, L. M. The transmission of chromium-51 tagged maternal erythrocytes from mother to fetus. Amer J Obstet Gynec 88:565, 1964.

Zipursky, A., Pollack, J. Chown, B., and Israels, L. G. Transplacental foetal haemorrhage after placental injury during delivery or amniocentesis. Lancet 2:493, 1963.

7

THE MORPHOLOGIC AND FUNCTIONAL
DEVELOPMENT OF THE FETUS

Since World War II, and especially in the last decade, knowledge of the fetus and his environment has increased remarkably. As an important consequence the fetus has acquired status as a patient to be cared for by the physician as he long has been accustomed to caring for the mother. Undoubtedly investigations of human life in utero will continue to be among the most rewarding in all of biology and of great clinical importance. These studies will lead to better ways for ascertaining the maturity and the well-being of the fetus, for identifying abormalities directly affecting the fetus, and, it is hoped, for successfully treating these abnormalities. Several excellent monographs devoted to the fetus have been published recently. For more extensive analyses of fetal development and of some of the disorders that afflict the fetus the reader is referred especially to those edited by Adamsons, Assali, Barnes, Fuchs and Cederqvist, Klopper and Diczfalusy, and Wynn.

The Fetus at Various Times in Pregnancy.   The different terms commonly used to indicate the duration of pregnancy and fetal age are somewhat confusing. *Menstrual age* or *gestational age* commences on the first day of the last menstrual period before conception, or about 2 weeks before ovulation and fertilization, or nearly 3 weeks before implantation of the fertilized ovum. As pointed out in Chapter 8 (p. 236), about 280 days, or 40 weeks, elapse, on the average, between the first day of the last menstrual period and delivery of the infant. Two hundred eighty days correspond to nine and one-third calendar months or 10 units of 28 days each. The unit of 28 days has been commonly but imprecisely referred to as a lunar month of pregnancy, since the time from one new moon to the next is actually 29½ days. It is the usual practice for the obstetrician to calculate the duration of pregnancy on the basis of menstrual age. Embryologists, however, cite events in days or weeks from the time of ovulation (*ovulation age*) or conception (*conception age*), the two being nearly identical. Occasionally it is of some value to divide the period of gestation into three units of three calender months each, or three *trimesters,* since some important obstetric events may be conveniently categorized by trimesters. For example, the possibility of spontaneous abortion is limited almost entirely to the first trimester of pregnancy, whereas the likelihood of survival of the prematurely born infant is confined to pregnancies that reach the third trimester.

The following short description of various periods of development of the ovum and embryo is included. For a more detailed description, based on Streeter's timetables of human development ("Horizons"), the reader is referred to the text by Davies.

The Ovum.   During the first two weeks after ovulation the products of conception are usually designated as the ovum. The successive stages of development during this period are as follows: (1) unfertilized single-cell ovum; (2) fertilized single-cell ovum; (3) free blastocyst; (4) implanting blastocyst; (5) blastocyst implanted but still avillous. Primitive villi are formed after implantation. It is conventional to refer to the products of conception after the development of chorionic villi not as an ovum but as an embryo. The early stages of preplacental development are discussed in Chapter 5, and the formation of the placenta itself in Chapter 6.

The Embryo.   The beginning of the embryonic period is taken as the beginning of the third week after ovulation, or about 5 weeks after the onset of the last menstrual period. The embryonic disc is well defined and the body stalk is differentiated. At this stage the chorionic sac measures approximately 1 cm in diameter (Figs. 1 and 2). The chorionic villi at this time are distributed equally around the circumference of the chorionic sac. There is a true intervillous space containing maternal blood and villous cores with angioblastic chorionic mesoderm.

By the end of the fourth week after ovulation the chorionic sac measures 2 to 3 cm in diameter, and the embryo about 4 to 5 mm in length. The heart and pericardium are very prominent because of the dilatation of the chambers of the heart. Arm and leg buds are present, and the amnion is beginning to ensheath the body stalk, which becomes the umbilical cord (Figs. 3 and 4).

At the end of the sixth week from the time of ovulation, or about 8 weeks after the onset of the last menstrual period, the embryo measures 22 to 24 mm in length, and the head is quite large compared with the trunk. Fingers and toes are present, and the external ears form definitive elevations on either side of the head.

The end of the embryonic period and the beginning of the fetal period are arbitrarily considered by most embryologists to occur about 8 weeks after ovulation. At that time the embryo measures nearly 4 cm. Few, if any, new major structures are formed thereafter; subsequent development consists in the growth and maturation of existing structures.

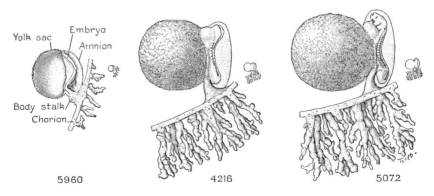

Fig. 1. Early human embryos. Small outline to right of each embryo gives its actual size. Ovulation ages: No. 5960, Carnegie Collection (presomite), 19 days; No. 4216 (7 somites), 21 days; No. 5072 (17 somites), 22 days. (After drawings and models in the Carnegie Institution.)

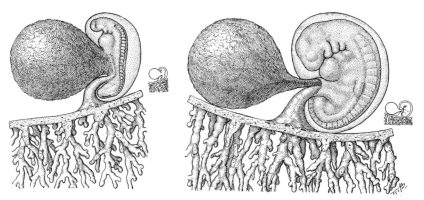

Fig. 2. Early human embryos. Small outline to right of each embryo gives its actual size. Ovulation ages: No. 2053, Carnegie Collection, 22 days; No. 836, 23 days. (After drawings and models in the Carnegie Institution.)

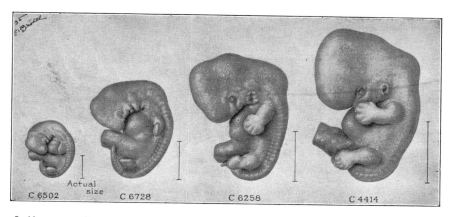

Fig. 3. Human embryos. Ovulation ages: No. 6502, Carnegie Collection, 28 days; No. 6728, 31 days; No. 6258, 38 days; No. 4414, 39 days.

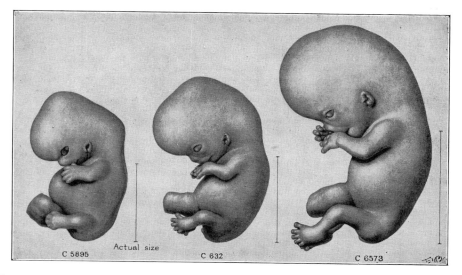

Fig. 4. Human embryos, 6 to 7 weeks ovulation age. (Numbers refer to embryos in the Carnegie Collection.)

Third Lunar Month. By the end of the twelfth week following the last menstrual period, or 10 weeks since ovulation, the fetus is 7 to 9 cm in length. Centers of ossification have appeared in most bones; the fingers and toes have become differentiated and are provided with nails; the external genitalia are beginning to show definite signs of male or female sex. A fetus born at this time may make spontaneous movements if still within the amniotic sac or if immersed in warm saline.

Fourth Lunar Month. By the end of the sixteenth week of postmenstrual age the fetus is from 13 to 17 cm long and weighs about 100 g. Careful examination of the external genital organs now definitely reveals the sex.

Fifth Lunar Month. The end of the fifth lunar month, or the twentieth week, is the midpoint of pregnancy if gestation is calculated from the time of the last normal menstrual period. The twentieth week is especially important clinically for confirming the duration of gestation. At this time the uterine fundus is normally at the level of the mother's umbilicus, fetal movement (quickening) has been felt by the mother for 2 to 4 weeks, and often, but not always, the fetal heartbeat may be heard by careful auscultation with a fetoscope. The fetus now weighs somewhat more than 300 g. The skin has become less transparent, and a downy lanugo covers its entire body, while some scalp hair is evident.

Sixth Lunar Month. The fetus now weighs about 600 g. The skin is characteristically wrinkled, and fat is first deposited beneath it; the head is still comparatively quite large. A fetus born at this period will attempt to breathe but almost always dies shortly after birth.

Seventh Lunar Month. By the end of the twenty-eighth week after the onset of the last menstrual period the fetus has attained a length of about 37 cm and weighs slightly more than 1,000 g. The thin skin is red and covered with vernix caseosa. The pupillary membrane has just disappeared from the eyes. An infant born at this period moves his limbs quite energetically and cries weakly. Usually the infant succumbs, but occasionally, with expert care he may survive.

Eighth Lunar Month. At the end of the eighth lunar month the fetus has attained a length of about 42 cm and a weight of about 1,700 g. The surface of the skin is still red and wrinkled. Infants born at this period may survive with proper care, although their chances are not excellent.

Ninth Lunar Month. At the end of the ninth lunar month the average fetus is about 47 cm long and weighs about 2,500 g. Because of the deposition of subcutaneous fat the body has become more rotund and the face has lost its previous wrinkled appearance. Children born at this time have an excellent chance of survival if given proper care.

Tenth Lunar Month. Term is reached 10 "lunar" months, or 40 weeks, after the last menstrual period. The fetus at this time is fully developed, with the characteristic features of the newborn child to be described here.

Because of the variability in the length of the legs and the difficulty of maintaining them in extension, measurement of the sitting height (crown-rump) is more accurate than that of the standing height. The average sitting height and weight of the fetus at the end of the various lunar months, as ascertained by Streeter from 704 specimens, are shown in Table 1. Such values are approximate, and generally the length is a more accurate criterion of the age of a fetus than is the weight. Although the measurements of Streeter were made a half-century ago, Gruenwald has pointed out that they represent by far the best study of fetal

Table 1. Average Sitting Height and Weight of the Fetus at the End
of Various Weeks of Pregnancy (Streeter)

Weeks from Last Menstrual Period	Sitting Height (Centimeters)	Weight (Grams)
8	0.23	1
12	6	14
16	12	108
20	16	316
24	21	630
28	25	1,045
32	28	1,680
36	32	2,478
40	36	3,405

growth during the first half of pregnancy. Moreover, the data obtained by Streeter for the latter half of pregnancy are quite comparable with those collected in much more recent times.

Haase suggested that for clinical purposes the length in centimeters of the embryo measured from crown to heel may be approximated during the first 5 months by squaring the number of the lunar month to which the pregnancy has advanced and, in the second half of pregnancy, by multiplying the month by 5.

The Fetus at Term. The average fetus at term is about 50 cm, or 20 inches, long (36 cm, or 14 inches sitting height) and weighs approximately 3,300 g with the variations to be discussed subsequently. The skin is smooth and lacking in lanugo except occasionally about the shoulders. The entire surface is covered by widely varying amounts of yellowish-white, greasy vernix caseosa, which is composed of sebaceous material, epithelial cells, and lanugo. The scalp is usually covered by dark hairs 2 to 3 cm in length, and the cartilages of the nose and ears are well developed. The fingers and toes possess well-developed nails, which project beyond their tips. In male fetuses the testes are usually found within the scrotum. In females the labia majora are well developed and in contact with each other, usually concealing the rest of the genitalia. The bones of the head are well ossified and are in close contact at the various sutures. The eyes usually have a uniform slate color, often different from their definitive color.

Black babies at birth differ slightly in appearance from white infants. Their skin is dusky, bluish red, but does not at all suggest the darker color that it will assume after a few weeks.

Weight of the Newborn. The average infant at birth weighs about 3,100 to 3,400 g depending upon race, economic status, size of the parents, and parity of the mother, with boys roughly 100 g (3 ounces) heavier than girls. The average weights of white and black infants born at the Kings County Hospital were 3,226 g and 3,153 g respectively, whereas the average weight of a random sample of white newborns taken from all the births in Hartford, Connecticut, was 3,350 g (Kohl). The higher average birth weight of the Hartford infants is probably related to the better economic status of the parents. This explanation is supported by the observations of Gruenwald and other investigators, which establish that during the second half of pregnancy the fetal weight increases linearly with time until about the thirty-seventh week of gestation and then decreases in rate. Gruenwald emphasizes that the principal determinants of the extent to which fetal growth late in pregnancy departs from the previously linear pattern are related in large part to the socioeconomic status of the mothers. In general, the greater the socioeconomic deprivation, the slower the growth late in pregnancy.

Apparently healthy term children may vary from 2,500 to 5,000 g (5.5 to 11 pounds) in weight. It is customary, however, to designate an infant weighing more than 4,500 g (10 pounds) as excessively large.

Birth weights over 5,000 g are occasionally reported, but most tales of huge babies vastly exceeding this figure are based on hearsay and inaccurate measurements at best. Presumably the largest baby recorded in the literature is that described by Belcher, a stillborn female weighing 11,340 g (25 pounds). In spite of these exceptional cases of macrosomia, extreme skepticism is justified in accepting reports concerning phenomenally heavy children. Term children, however, frequently weigh less than 3,200 g and sometimes as little as 2,250 g (5 pounds). When the birth weight is 2,500 g or less, however, the child is usually classified as premature even though in some instances the low birth weight is caused not by prematurity but rather by intrauterine growth retardation.

The many factors intimately involved in fetal growth are considered further in this chapter in the sections on placental transfer and fetal nutrition (pp. 206 and 224) as well as in Chapter 37 (p. 1029) on prematurity.

The Head.   Since, obstetrically, the head of the fetus is the most important part, insofar as an essential feature of labor is an adaptation between the head and the bony pelvis, knowledge of the characteristics and size of the head of the fetus is important.

Only a comparatively small part of the head of the fetus at term is represented by the face; the rest is composed of the firm hard skull, which is made up of two frontal, two parietal, and two temporal bones along with the upper portion of the occipital bone and the wings of the sphenoid. These bones are not firmly united but are separated by membranous spaces, the *sutures*. The most important sutures are the *frontal*, between the two frontal bones; the *sagittal*, between the two parietal bones; the two *coronal*, between the frontal and parietal bones; and the two *lambdoid*, between the posterior margins of the parietal bones and upper margin of the occipital bone. All of the sutures are palpable during labor, except the *temporal* sutures, which are situated on either side between the inferior margin of the parietal and the upper margin of the temporal bones, covered by soft parts, and cannot be felt in the living child.

Where several sutures meet there forms an irregular space, closed by a membrane and designated a *fontanel* (Fig. 5). Four such structures are usually distinguished: the greater, the lesser, and the two temporal fontanels. The *greater*, or *anterior, fontanel* is a lozenge-shaped space situated at the junction of the sagittal and the coronal sutures. The *lesser, or posterior, fontanel* is represented by a small triangular area at the intersection of the sagittal and lambdoid sutures. The *temporal, or casserian, fontanels*, are situated at the junction of the lambdoid and temporal sutures. The first two are readily felt during labor and their recognition gives important information concerning the presentation and position of the fetus. The temporal fontanels, however, have no diagnostic significance.

The *sagittal fontanel*, a lozenge-shaped space sometimes found in the sagittal suture at a point about halfway between the greater and lesser fontanels, may give rise to error in diagnosis whenever it is large enough to be felt and confused with either the posterior or anterior fontanel.

It is customary to measure certain critical *diameters* and *circumferences* (Figs. 5 and 6) of the infant's head. The diameters most frequently used and

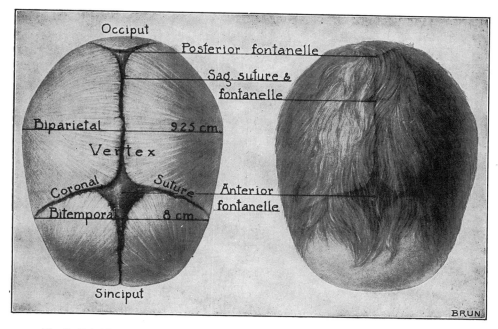

Fig. 5. Fetal head at term showing various fontanels (fontanelles) and diameters.

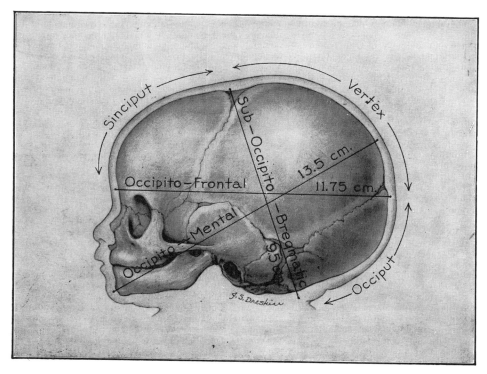

Fig. 6. Diameters of the fetal head at term.

their average lengths are (1) the *occipitofrontal* (11.75 cm), which follows a line extending from a point just above the root of the nose to the most prominent portion of the occipital bone; (2) the *biparietal* (9.25 cm), the greatest transverse diameter of the head, which extends from one parietal boss to the other; (3) the *bitemporal* (8.0 cm), the greatest distance between the two temporal sutures; (4) the *occipitomental* (13.5 cm), from the chin to the most prominent portion of the occiput; and (5) the *suboccipitobregmatic* (9.5 cm), which follows a line drawn from the middle of the large fontanel to the undersurface of the occipital bone just where it joins the neck.

The greatest circumference of the head, which corresponds to the plane of the occipitofrontal diameter, averages 34.5 cm, and the smallest circumference, corresponding to the plane of the suboccipitobregmatic diameter, is 32 cm. As a rule, white infants have larger heads than do nonwhite infants, boys somewhat larger than girls, and the fetuses of multiparas larger heads than those of nulliparas.

Because of the widely varying mobility at the sutures between the bones of the skull, fetal heads differ appreciably in their ability to adapt to the maternal pelvis by molding. The bones of one may be soft and readily molded, whereas those of another are firmly ossified, only slightly mobile, and therefore incapable of significant reduction in size.

Pʟᴀᴄᴇɴᴛᴀʟʟᴛʟ Tʀᴀɴsꜰᴇʀ

General Concepts   A major function of the placenta is to transfer oxygen and a great variety of nutrients from the mother to the fetus and, conversely, to convey carbon dioxide and other metabolic wastes from fetus to mother. To appreciate the complexity of the placenta as an organ of transfer, it is necessary only to reflect on the fact that the placenta, and to a limited extent the attached membranes, supply all material for fetal growth and energy production while removing all products of fetal catabolism.

There are no direct communications between the fetal blood in the vessels of the chorionic villi and the maternal blood in the intervillous space. Throughout most of pregnancy nearly all of the red blood cells in the fetal circulation can be shown, by their resistance to acid elution, to be rich in fetal hemoglobin, whereas only rarely does an erythrocyte in the maternal circulation display this property (Kleihauer, Braun, and Betke). The one exception to this generalization regarding the independence of the circulations is the development of an occasional break in the chorionic villi, permitting the escape of varying numbers of fetal erythrocytes into the maternal circulation (Ch. 6, p. 168). This leakage is the clinically significant mechanism by which some Rh-negative women become sensitized by the red blood cells of the Rh-positive fetus. Fetal hemorrhage into the maternal circulation is an uncommon cause of severe fetal anemia and, rarely, even of fetal death. These occasional leaks, however, do not controvert the basic principle that no gross intermingling of the macromolecular constituents of the two circulations occurs. The transfer of substances from mother to fetus and from fetus to mother, therefore, depends primarily on mechanisms that permit the transport of such substances through the intact chorionic villus.

At least nine variables determine the effectiveness of the human placenta as an organ of transfer: (1) The concentration in the maternal plasma of the substance under consideration and in some instances the extent to which it is bound to another compound. (2) The rate of maternal blood flow through the inter-villous space. (3) The area available for exchange across the villous epithelium. (4) In case the substance is transferred by diffusion, the physical properties of the tissue barrier interposed between blood in the intervillous space and blood in the fetal capillaries. (5) For any substance actively transported, the capacity of the biochemical machinery of the placenta for effecting active transfer. (6) The amount of the substance metabolized by the placenta during transfer. (7) The area for exchange across the fetal capillaries in the placenta. (8) The concentration in the fetal blood of the substance, exclusive of any that is bound. (9) The rate of fetal blood flow through the villous capillaries. Unfortunately in human pregnancy many of these processes, including blood flow, cannot be measured quantitatively in either the mother or the fetus. In recent years, however, technics have been developed for doing so in some experimental animals, as shown in Figure 7 and discussed in a current review by Battaglia.

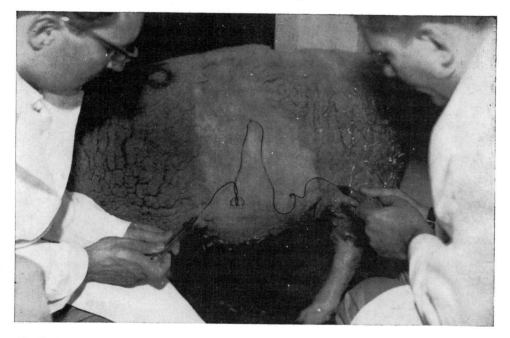

Fig. 7. The withdrawal of blood simultaneously from the uterine and fetal circulation in the pregnant, intact sheep. The right catheter is in a uterine vein and the left catheter in a fetal placental vein. (Courtesy of Dr. Donald Barron.)

The Intervillous Space.   The intervillous space functions as the depot from which materials are transferred, either passively or actively, through the chorionic epithelium to the fetal vessels, and where substances from the fetus enter the maternal circulation. Since this process of transfer supplies the fetus with oxygen as well as nutriment and provides for elimination of metabolic waste products in addition, the chorionic villi and the intervillous space, together, function for the fetus as a lung, gastrointestinal tract, and kidney.

The circulation of maternal blood within the intervillous space has been considered in detail in Chapter 6. The residual volume of the intervillous space of the delivered term placenta measures about 140 ml; however, the normal volume of the intervillous space before delivery is probably twice this value (Aherne and Dunnill). Uterine blood flow near term has been estimated at about 600 ml per minute with most of the blood apparently going through the intervillous space. Although much more remains to be learned about the hemodynamics of the intervillous space even in normal pregnancy, on the basis of a variety of animal studies and by using technics such as demonstrated in Figure 7, as well as clinical observations made in women, the following conclusions may be drawn: Uterine contractions reduce blood flow through the intervillous space, the degree of reduction depending in large part upon the intensity of the contraction. Blood pressure within the intervillous space is significantly less than uterine arterial pressure but somewhat greater than uterine venous pressure. Uterine venous pressure, in turn, varies depending upon several factors including posture. For example, when the mother is supine, pressure in the inferior vena cava is elevated; consequently, in this circumstance pressure in the uterine and ovarian veins and, in turn, the intervillous space is elevated. An even greater increase in intervillous pressure must occur when the mother stands.

The hydrostatic pressure in the capillaries of the chorionic villi is probably not grossly different from that in the intervillous space. During normal labor the rise in fetal blood pressure must parallel the pressure in the amniotic fluid and the intervillous space. Otherwise the capillaries in the chorionic villi would collapse and fetal blood flow through the placenta would cease.

The Chorionic Villus.   Substances that pass from the maternal blood to the fetal blood must traverse trophoblast, stroma, and capillary wall. These layers have a minimal aggregate thickness of 3 to 6 microns according to Wislocki. Although the histologic "barrier" separates the maternal and fetal circulations, it does not behave uniformly like a simple physical barrier, because throughout pregnancy it either actively or passively permits, facilitates, and adjusts the amount and rate of transfer of a wide range of substances to the fetus. Certain histologic alterations in the villus with advancing pregnancy appear to enhance placental permeability. As the prominence of Langhans cells decreases, the villous epithelium consists predominantly of syncytiotrophoblast. The walls of the villous capillaries likewise become thinner, and the relative number of fetal vessels increases in relation to the villous connective tissue. Flexner and colleagues attempted to correlate these changes with the amount of sodium that the placenta transfers. The amount transferred increases during gestation until near term, when the placenta transfers about 12 times as much sodium per gram per hour as at the third month.

Several attempts have been made to estimate the total surface area of chorionic villi in the human placenta at term. The planimetric measurements made by Aherne and Dunnill of the villous surface area of the placenta demonstrate a close correlation with fetal weight. According to their results, the total surface area at term is approximately 10 square meters.

Transfer by Diffusion.   Simple diffusion appears to be the mechanism involved in the transfer of oxygen, carbon dioxide, and water, and most but not all electrolytes. Anesthetic gases also pass through the placenta rapidly and apparently by simple diffusion. Practically all therapeutic agents that exert a systemic effect in the mother—for example, meperidine and atropine—cross the placenta to the fetus but not necessarily at the same rate.

Insulin, steroid hormones from the adrenal, and hormones from the thyroid pass through the placental membrane, but at slow rates. The hormones synthesized by the placenta enter both the maternal and fetal circulations but not necessarily to the same degree. For example, the concentrations of chorionic gonadotropin and chorionic somatomammotropin are appreciably lower in fetal than in maternal plasma.

Most substances with a molecular weight under 500 can readily diffuse through the placental tissue interposed between the maternal and fetal circulations. Diffusion, however, is by no means the only mechanism of transfer of compounds with a low molecular weight. The placenta actually facilitates the transfer of a variety of such compounds, especially those in low concentration in maternal plasma but essential for the rapid growth of the fetus. Molecular weight clearly has a bearing on the rate of transfer by diffusion; the smaller the molecule, the more rapid is the rate. Substances of very high molecular weight do not usually traverse the placenta, but there are pronounced exceptions, such as immune gamma globulin G with a molecular weight of about 160,000.

Transfer of Oxygen and Carbon Dioxide. Since even brief curtailment of the transfer of oxygen may cause sublethal injuries, the transfer of this gas across the placenta has received special attention. Because of the continuous passage of oxygen from the maternal blood in the intervillous space to the fetus, the oxygen saturation of this blood resembles that in the maternal capillaries, and is less than that of the mother's arterial blood. The average oxygen saturation of intervillous space blood is estimated to be 65 to 75 per cent with a partial pressure of oxygen of about 30 to 40 mm Hg. The oxygen saturation of the umbilical vein blood is approximately 60 per cent with an oxygen partial pressure in the general range of 20 mm Hg. Because of multiple sources of error, these data must be regarded as approximations only. In the estimations reported for the partial pressure of oxygen in the blood of the intervillous space, inconsistently high or low figures are often encountered, suggesting that this blood is not thoroughly mixed. If the needle or electrode happens to be at a point where it is bathed by a jet of arterial blood into the intervillous space, the estimate of oxygen saturation becomes falsely high, whereas the reverse obtains if the needle or electrode is placed at a location where the circulation is relatively sluggish or is mistakenly placed in an adjacent uterine vein. The collection of umbilical venous or arterial blood that is truly representative of the oxygenation in utero is fraught with even greater errors.

Despite relatively low partial pressure of oxygen and hemoglobin saturation, the fetus normally does not suffer from lack of oxygen. The human fetus probably behaves like the lamb fetus and, therefore, has a cardiac output considerably greater per unit of weight than does the adult. The high cardiac output and, late in pregnancy, the increased oxygen carrying capacity of fetal blood as the consequence of a higher hemoglobin concentration compensate effectively for the low oxygen tension. Both of these mechanisms are considered further in this chapter under Fetal Circulation and Fetal Blood. Additional evidence that the fetus does not normally experience lack of oxygen is supplied by measurement of the lactic acid content of fetal blood, which is only slightly higher than that of the mother.

Makowski and associates have studied the effects, on pregnant ewes and their fetuses, of relatively acute hypoxia produced by high altitude. Serially collected samples of umbilical vein blood demonstrated initially a significant decrease in their oxygen content, but with continuous exposure to high altitude the oxygen content of the umbilical vein blood soon rose toward normal values. The mechanisms of adaptation that were identified include an increase in maternal uteroplacental blood flow and in umbilical vein hemoglobin concentration.

Assali and co-workers were able to raise the partial pressure of oxygen in the umbilical vein of the lamb fetus by 10 to 15 mm Hg when the mother breathed 100 per cent oxygen at atmospheric pressure. They detected no fall in uteroplacental or umbilical blood flow in response to 100 per cent oxygen, although some workers had previously suggested that a fall did take place to the detriment of the fetus. When the ewe breathed hyperbaric oxygen that raised the maternal arterial oxygen partial pressure to 1,300 mm Hg, uteroplacental blood flow did not change and umbilical flow decreased only slightly, although the oxygen partial pressure in umbilical blood rose to nearly 600 mm Hg. Therefore, with intact maternal and fetal circulations oxygen can be delivered across the placenta, at least to the fetus of the sheep, under significantly increased tension.

There are no precise measurements of the ability of the human fetus to withstand severe hypoxia. Myers has recently measured the tolerance of the brain of the monkey fetus to hypoxia induced by cord compression causing complete cessation of flow. The rates at which bradycardia, hypotension, and acidosis developed varied with gestational age, so that the more mature the fetus, the more rapid the rate of deterioration.

In general, the transfer of carbon dioxide from the fetus to the mother obeys the same laws as those described for oxygen. This gas, however, traverses the chorionic villus more rapidly than does oxygen. Near term the partial pressure of carbon dioxide in the umbilical arteries is estimated to be about 45 mm Hg or about 5 mm more than in the maternal blood in the intervillous space. For several reasons fetal blood has somewhat less affinity for carbon dioxide than does the blood of the mother, thereby favoring the transfer of carbon dioxide from the fetus to the mother.

Selective Transfer.   Although diffusion is an important method of placental transfer, the chorionic villus exhibits enormous selectivity in transfer, maintaining different concentrations of a variety of metabolites on the two sides of the villus. One example of this selectivity is in the transfer of the two isomers of histidine, as demonstrated by Page. D-Histidine, the unnatural isomer, traverses the placenta more slowly, coming to equilibrium with the fetal blood within three or four hours. If only passive transfer by simple diffusion were involved, L-histidine, the natural isomer, would be expected to behave similarly, but in the case of this isomer, equilibrium is attained within a few minutes. The concentrations of a number of substances that are not synthesized by the fetus are several times higher in fetal than in maternal blood. Ascorbic acid is a good example of this phenomenon. This crystalline substance of relatively low molecular weight chemically resembles the pentose and hexose sugars and might be expected to traverse the placenta by simple diffusion. The concentration of ascorbic acid, however, is regularly two to four times higher in fetal than in maternal plasma (Braestrup; Manahan and Eastman). These two examples indicate that molecular weight alone does not necessarily determine the manner in which substances are transferred. The unidirectional transfer of iron across the placenta provides another example of the unique capabilities of the human placenta for transport. Typically the mineral is present in the plasma at a lower concentration in the mother than in the fetus, and, at the same time, the iron-binding capacity of the plasma is much greater in the mother than in the fetus. Nonetheless, iron is actively transported from maternal to fetal plasma, and in the human fetus the amount transferred appears to be independent of maternal iron status (Pritchard).

Intrauterine infections caused by viruses, bacteria, and protozoa are occasionally encountered. Many viruses, including those responsible for rubella, chickenpox, measles, mumps, smallpox, vaccinia, poliomyelitis, cytomegalic inclusion disease, coxsackie virus disease, and western equine encephalitis, may cross the placenta and infect the fetus. *Treponema pallidum* also may cross the placenta during the latter half of pregnancy and produce congenital syphilis. Toxoplasma, the malaria parasite, and the tubercle bacillus may similarly produce intrauterine infection. With protozoal and bacterial, but not necessarily viral, infections there is almost always histologic evidence of involvement of the placenta.

PHYSIOLOGY OF THE FETUS

Fetal Circulation.   Since the fetal lungs do not function and practically all materials needed for growth and maintenance are brought to the fetus from the placenta by the umbilical vein, the fetal circulation must differ fundamentally from that of the adult (Figs. 8 and 9). The single umbilical vein in the umbilical cord carries oxygenated, nutriment-bearing blood from the placenta to the fetus. The umbilical vein enters the fetus through the umbilical ring and ascends along the anterior abdominal wall to the liver. The vein then divides, with some branches carrying blood to the hepatic veins primarily of the left side of the liver, while others deliver umbilical vein blood to the intrahepatic portal circulation. The major "branch" of the umbilical vein, the *ductus venosus*, traverses the liver to enter directly the inferior vena cava. The blood flowing to the fetal heart from the inferior vena cava, therefore, consists of an admixture of "arterial" blood that passes through the ductus venosus and less well oxygenated blood that collects from most of the veins below the level of the diaphragm. As a consequence the oxygen content of blood delivered to the heart from the inferior cava is decreased with respect to that which leaves the placenta but is greater than that from the superior vena cava.

As emphasized by Dawes, the *foramen ovale* opens directly off the inferior vena cava so that blood from the inferior vena cava is, for the most part, immediately deflected by the *crista dividens* through the foramen ovale into the left atrium. Little or none of the less well oxygenated blood from the superior vena cava normally passes through the foramen ovale. The preferential flow of blood from the inferior vena cava through the foramen ovale to the left atrium bypasses the right ventricle and pulmonary circulation and permits delivery to the left ventricle of more highly oxygenated blood than if complete admixture had occurred in the right atrium. The more highly oxygenated blood that passes through the foramen ovale and is ejected from the left ventricle perfuses two vital organs, the heart and the brain. The blood that is typically venous in character, coming from the superior vena cava and ejected from the right ventricle into the pulmonary trunk, is, for the most part, shunted through the *ductus arteriosus* into the descending aorta. Only a small volume of blood goes through the lungs before the onset of respiration.

The lamb fetus has been intensively studied by several groups of investigators who believe that the circulatory function of the mature lamb fetus is similar in

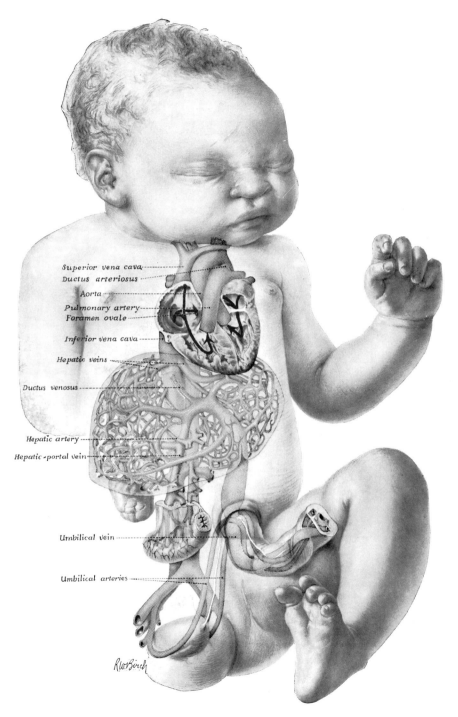

Fig. 8. Cardiovascular system of fetus.

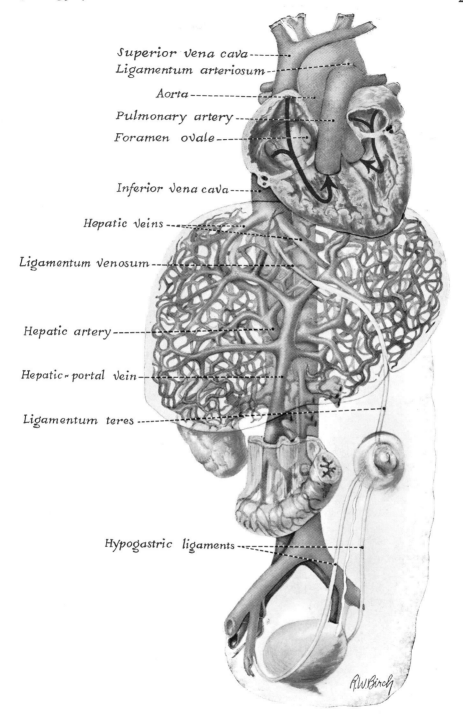

Superior vena cava

Ligamentum arteriosum

Aorta

Pulmonary artery

Foramen ovale

Inferior vena cava

Hepatic veins

Ligamentum venosum

Hepatic artery

Hepatic-portal vein

Ligamentum teres

Hypogastric ligaments

Fig. 9. Cardiovascular system of infant after birth.

many ways to that of the mature human fetus. Before birth in man and in sheep, both ventricles of the heart, as the consequence of the shunts just described, work in parallel rather than in series. Attempts to measure cardiac output in the lamb fetus have yielded somewhat variable results. Assali and associates, for example, have ascertained a mean value of about 200 ml per kg per minute but with considerable individual variation. Such a high fetal cardiac output, which per unit of weight is about three times that of an adult at rest, would compensate for the low oxygen content of fetal blood. The high cardiac output is accomplished in part by the fast heart rate of the fetus.

Before birth and expansion of the lungs the high pulmonary vascular resistance accounts for the high pressure and the low blood flow in the fetal pulmonary circuit. At the same time, resistance to flow through the ductus arteriosus and the umbilicoplacental circulation is low, probably accounting for the overall low fetal systemic vascular resistance. It is estimated that in the fetal lamb about one half the combined output of the two ventricles goes to the placenta. Rudolph and Heymann, by injecting isotopically labeled plastic microspheres into the fetal lamb circulation at various sites, have ascertained the distribution of cardiac output during the last third of gestation to be roughly as follows: placenta, 41 per cent; carcass, 35 per cent; brain, 5 per cent; heart, 5 per cent; gastrointestinal tract, 5 per cent; lungs, 4 per cent; kidneys, 2 per cent; spleen, 2 per cent; liver (hepatic artery only), 2 per cent.

After birth the umbilical vessels, the ductus arteriosus, the foramen ovale, and the ductus venosus constrict or collapse and the hemodynamics of the fetal circulation consequently undergo pronounced changes. According to Assali and associates, clamping of the umbilical cord and expansion of the fetal lungs, either through spontaneous breathing or artificial respiration, promptly induce a variety of hemodynamic changes in sheep. The systemic arterial pressure initially falls slightly, apparently the result of the reversal in the direction of blood flow in the ductus arteriosus, but it soon recovers and then rises above the control value. They conclude that several factors play a role in regulating the flow of blood through the ductus arteriosus, including the difference in pressure between the pulmonary artery and aorta and especially the oxygen tension of the blood passing through the ductus arteriosus. They were able to influence flow through the ductus arteriosus by altering the pO_2 of the blood. When the lungs were ventilated with oxygen and the pO_2 rose above 55 mm Hg, ductus flow dropped, but ventilation with nitrogen, initially at least, returned ductus flow to the original pattern. The oxygen tension of the blood passing through the ductus thus affected its patency, with the constricting effect of oxygen appearing to act directly on the walls of the ductus rather than through neurogenic or humoral mediation.

With expansion of the lungs, pressures in the right ventricle and pulmonary arteries fall because of the marked decrease in pulmonary vascular resistance. Theoretically, at least, an increase in the left atrial pressure above that of the right atrium would close the foramen ovale. There is some disagreement, however, as to when closure actually occurs. The experiments of Barclay and co-workers indicate that functional closure of the foramen ovale occurs within several minutes of birth. Arey, however, states that anatomic fusion of the two septa of the foramen ovale is not completed until about one year after birth, and that in 25 per cent of cases perfect closure is never attained. When the foramen ovale remains functionally patent, circulatory disturbances of variable gravity result.

The more distal portions of the hypogastric arteries, which course from the level of the bladder along the abdominal wall to the umbilical ring and into the cord as umbilical arteries, undergo atrophy and obliteration within three to four days after birth to become the *umbilical ligaments*. The intraabdominal remnants of the umbilical vein form the *ligamentum teres,* and those of the ductus venosus become the *ligamentum venosum,* whereas the obliterated ductus arteriosus is the *ligamentum arteriosum.*

Fetal Blood. Hematopoiesis is demonstrable first in the yolk sac of the very early embryo. The next major site of erythropoiesis is the liver and finally the bone marrow. The contributions made by each site throughout the growth and development of the embryo and fetus are demonstrated graphically in Figure 10.

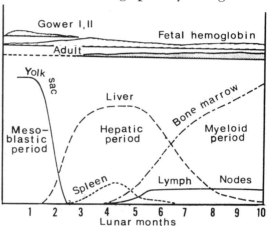

Fig. 10. Sites of hematopoiesis and kinds of hemoglobin synthesized at various stages of fetal development. (From Brown. Biology of Gestation, Vol. II, The Fetus and Neonate, p. 361. New York, Academic Press, 1968.)

The first red cells formed are nucleated, but as fetal development progresses, more and more of the circulating red cells are nonnucleated. As the fetus grows, not only does the volume of blood in the common circulation of the fetus and placenta increase but the hemoglobin concentration rises as well. As shown by the studies of Walker and Turnbull, the hemoglobin of fetal blood rises to the adult male level of about 15.0 g per 100 ml at midpregnancy, and at term it is somewhat higher. Fetal blood at or near term is characterized, therefore, by a hemoglobin concentration that is high by maternal standards. The reticulocyte count falls from a very high level in the very young fetus to about 5 per cent at term. Red blood cells in the fetus at the time of birth have a life-span that is significantly shorter than that of erythrocytes formed subsequently. These data support the concept that fetal erythrocytes are "stress erythrocytes." Pearson, using a variety of technics, has found the life-span of red cells from more mature fetuses to be approximately two thirds that of erythrocytes of normal adults, but red cells of less mature fetuses have an even shorter life-span. The red cells of the fetus differ metabolically from those of the adult; several enzymes, for example have appreciably different activities. The fetus is capable of making erythropoietin in increased amounts when severely anemic and of excreting it into the amniotic fluid (Finne).

Precise measurements of the volume of blood contained in the human fetoplacental circulation are lacking. Usher, Shepard, and Lind, however, have carefully measured the volume of blood of term normal infants very soon after birth and noted an average of 78 ml per kg when immediate cord clamping was carried out. Gruenwald found the volume of blood of fetal origin contained in the placenta after prompt cord clamping to average 45 ml per kg of fetus. These combined results suggest that the fetoplacental blood volume at term is approximately 125 ml per kg of fetus. Pritchard and co-workers have measured the volumes of blood in the infant with erythroblastosis fetalis and in the placenta and the cord immediately after delivery. The "fetoplacental" blood volume in these circumstances is very close to 125 ml per kg of infant weight. According to Creasy and associates, the volume of blood in the undelivered, intact ovine fetoplacental unit is quite similar to this value.

In the embryo and fetus the globin moiety of much of the hemoglobin differs from that of the normal adult. In the embryo three major forms of hemoglobin may be found (Pearson). The most primitive forms are Gower-1 and Gower-2. The globin moiety of Gower-1 consists of four epsilon peptide chains per molecule of protein, whereas in Gower-2 there are two alpha and two epsilon chains. All normal hemoglobins elaborated after Gower-1 contain a pair of alpha chains, but the other pair of peptide chains differs for each kind of hemoglobin. Hemoglobin F (so-called fetal hemoglobin or alkaline resistant hemoglobin) contains a pair of alpha peptide chains and a pair of gamma chains per molecule of hemoglobin. Actually, two varieties of gamma chains have been identified in hemoglobin F, their ratios changing steadily as the fetus and infant mature (Huisman and co-workers).

As shown in Figure 10, hemoglobin A, or A_1, the fourth hemoglobin to be formed by the fetus and the major hemoglobin formed after birth in normal people, is present in progressively greater amounts as the fetus matures. Its globin is made up of a pair of alpha chains and a pair of beta chains. Hemoglobin A_2, the globin of which contains a pair of alpha chains and a pair of delta chains, is present in only very small concentrations in the mature fetus but increases after birth. Thus, as growth proceeds, the embryo and fetus demonstrate a shift not only in the amounts but also in the kinds of globin synthesized.

The oxygen dissociation curve of fetal red blood cells rich in hemoglobin F has been described as lying to the left of that of normal adult red blood cells, which contain primarily hemoglobin A. As demonstrated in Figure 11, at any given oxygen tension and at identical pH, fetal red blood cells that contain mostly hemoglobin F bind more oxygen than do red blood cells containing nearly all hemoglobin A. Hemoglobin F in solution outside of the red blood cells, however, combines with the same amount of oxygen as does a similar solution of hemoglobin A (Allen, Wyman, and Smith). The greater affinity for oxygen ascribed to fetal erythrocytes is therefore not the result simply of the greater quantity of hemoglobin F. Mathew and co-workers, and Novy and associates have recently reported that the lower oxygen affinity of adult red cells compared with that of fetal red cells persists for several weeks, at least, after their intrauterine transfusion into the fetus. These studies indicate that whatever the cause of the differences in oxygen affinity between fetal and adult red cells, the responsible mechanism is most likely operative before release of the erythrocyte from the marrow. Kirschbaum and associates have questioned whether so large a difference exists in vivo between the oxygen dissociation curves of adult and fetal red blood cells. When the dissociation curves were constructed from measurements carried out within two minutes after drawing the blood, the dissociation curves for fetal and adult whole blood were quite similar. Kirschbaum reasons that in the human being the slightly lower pH in fetal

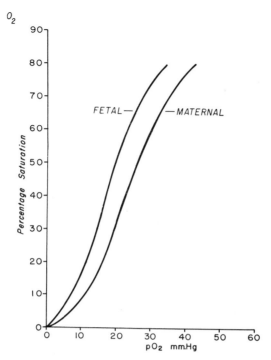

Fig. 11. Dissociation curves of fetal and maternal human bloods prepared at pH 7.40. (Courtesy of Dr. André Hellegers.)

blood compared with that in maternal blood shifts the oxygen dissociation curve of fetal blood enough to the right to make trivial the difference identified in Figure 11.

Since fetal erythrocytes formed late in pregnancy contain less hemoglobin F and more hemoglobin A than do the cells formed earlier, the content of hemoglobin F of the fetal red blood cells falls somewhat during the latter weeks of pregnancy. At term about three fourths of the total hemoglobin normally is hemoglobin F. During the first 6 to 12 months after delivery the proportion of hemoglobin F continues to fall eventually to reach the low level found in erythrocytes of normal adults (Schulman and Smith).

The kinds and numbers of white blood cells in the fetus are highly variable, depending upon the degree of maturity and the impact of labor.

The concentrations of several coagulation factors in the fetus are appreciably below the levels that develop within a few weeks after birth. The low factors in cord blood are II, VII, IX, X, XI, and XII. Without prophylactic vitamin K, most of these coagulation factors usually decrease even further during the first few days after birth and may lead to hemorrhage in the newborn infant (Chapter 37, p. 1049). Fibrinogen levels and platelet counts in cord blood are in the low-normal range for nonpregnant adults. The time for conversion of fibrinogen in plasma to fibrin clot when thrombin is added (thrombin time) is somewhat prolonged compared with that of older children and adults. Measurements of factor VIII have proved of value in accurately making or excluding the diagnosis of hemophilia in male infants (Kasper and associates). Nielsen has described low plasminogen levels but somewhat increased fibrinolytic activity in cord plasma as compared with maternal plasma.

In the mature fetus the concentration of albumin measured immunologically has been reported to average 2.7 g per 100 ml using cord serum collected at the time of cesarean section in the absence of any labor; at the same time the serum albumin in the mother was 2.9 g per 100 ml (Mendenhall). When measured by the same technic the concentration of albumin in nonpregnant women averaged 4.3 g per 100 ml. Near term the immunoglobulin IgG is present in approximately the same concentrations in cord and maternal sera; the concentrations of IgA and IgM immunoglobulins, however, are considerably lower in cord than in maternal serum. Although immunoglobulins IgA and IgM of maternal origin are effectively excluded from the fetus, IgG crosses the placenta with considerable efficiency by both simple diffusion and enzymatic transport. Increased amounts of IgM are found in the fetus only after the fetal immune mechanism has been provoked into antibody response by an infection in the fetus.

Urinary System.   Two primitive urinary systems, the pronephros and the mesonephros, precede the development of the metanephros. Embryologic failure of either of the first two may result in anomalous development of the definitive urinary system.

By the end of the first trimester the nephrons have some capacity for excretion through glomerular filtration, although the kidneys are functionally immature throughout fetal life. The ability to concentrate and to modify the pH of urine is quite limited even in the mature fetus. Fetal urine is hypotonic with respect to fetal plasma because of low concentrations of electrolytes. In the lamb fetus, and most likely in the human fetus, the fraction of the cardiac output perfusing the kidneys is low, and renal vascular resistance is high, compared with the values later in life (Assali and associates; Rudolph and Heymann). In the lamb fetus, urine flow varies considerably in response to stress. Transient marked fetal polyuria postoperatively has been noted by Gresham and co-workers.

Some urine is usually found in the bladder even in quite small fetuses. After obstruction of the urethra the bladder, ureters, and renal pelves may become quite dilated; the bladder may become sufficiently distended that dystocia results. The kidneys in these circumstances seem capable of excreting urine until back pressure ultimately destroys the renal parenchyma. Kidneys are not essential for survival in utero, but they play a role in the control of the composition and volume of amniotic fluid.

Respiratory System.   Within a very few minutes after birth the respiratory system must be able to provide oxygen as well as eliminate carbon dioxide if the neonate is to survive (Ch. 19, p. 477). Development of air ducts and alveoli, pulmonary vasculature, muscles of respiration, and coordination of their activities through the central nervous system to a degree that allows the fetus to survive, at least for a time, may be demonstrated as early as the end of the second trimester of pregnancy. The great majority of fetuses born at this time, however, succumb immediately or during the next few days from respiratory insufficiency.

From the beginning of the fourth month the fetus is capable of respiratory movement sufficiently intense to move amniotic fluid in and out of the respiratory tract. The roentgenogram in Figure 12, obtained 26 hours after injection of Thorotrast into the amniotic sac, clearly demonstrates the contrast medium in the lungs of the very immature fetus. The lungs of stillborn infants commonly contain histologically identifiable particulate matter found in amniotic fluid.

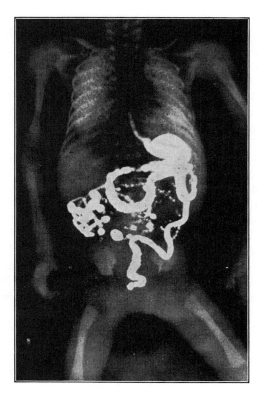

Fig. 12. X-ray of 115 g fetus in which Thorotrast is present in the lungs, esophagus, stomach, and entire intestinal tract following injection of Thorotrast into the amniotic cavity 26 hours before delivery. It demonstrates not only intrauterine respiration of the fetus but also active swallowing of amniotic fluid by the fetus. (From Davis and Potter. JAMA 131: 1194, 1946.)

Whether respiratory movements in utero sufficient to cause a tidal flow of amniotic fluid normally occur is not settled despite many investigations. There is evidence that in the lamb, for example, submersion of the neonate, except for the head, in warm water markedly depresses ventilation. Quite likely the warm fluid environment of the uterus inhibits respiratory activity before birth in similar fashion. This observation also lends credence to the clinical practice of applying warm, wet towels to the body of the infant during breech delivery to minimize aspiration of material from the uterus and birth canal.

Windle and associates rightfully doubt the validity of any experiment to demonstrate intrauterine respiration when the mother is traumatized or the fetus is manipulated. Windle is convinced that respiration does not occur normally in utero. It seems unlikely, however, that muscular coordination and force sufficient to establish respiratory exchange immediately after birth could be accomplished without some previous conditioning. In this regard, Milles and Dorsey report three pertinent cases in which certain fetal malformations, including absence of the trachea, made intrauterine respiration impossible. The fetuses demonstrated diminished pulmonary vascular development in association with a pronounced enlargement of the ductus arteriosus, suggesting that intrauterine respiratory excursions are essential to the appropriate development of the pulmonary vascular system. Moreover, hypoplasia of the lungs is common when amniotic fluid has been persistently scant or absent, as for example in renal agenesis (Potter). Finally, the classic study of Davis and Potter in which Thorotrast was injected into the amniotic sac at times varying from 15 minutes to 48 hours before surgical removal of the fetus avoids the objections raised by Windle. That study showed that the longer the exposure in utero after a single injection of Thorotrast, the greater the concentration in the lungs. Thorotrast was not identified in the lungs of the infant if it was injected into the amniotic fluid just before hysterotomy, but after 18 hours or more, the concentration of the contrast medium in the infant's lungs was higher than in the amniotic fluid.

In sheep and goat fetuses, the fluid filling the trachea is not simply inhaled amniotic fluid, for it has a composition somewhat different from that of surrounding amniotic fluid. Goodlin and Rudolph have recently reported detailed studies designed to measure the rate of formation of the tracheal fluid and to identify any significant excretory function of the lung through the formation of such fluid. They conclude that the tracheal fluid is not formed rapidly and that the lung in utero does not serve as an excretory organ of any importance. Further studies are needed to clarify the functions of the respiratory system in utero as well as immediately after birth.

Digestive System.   As early as the eleventh week of gestation the small intestine demonstrates peristalsis and is capable of actively transporting glucose (Koldovský and co-workers). By the fourth month of gestation gastrointestinal function is sufficiently developed to allow the fetus to swallow amniotic fluid, absorb much of the water from it, and, as shown in Figure 12, propel unabsorbed matter as far as the lower colon. Hydrochloric acid and some of the digestive enzymes characteristic of the gastrointestinal tract of the adult are demonstrable in the early fetus but in very small amounts compared with those in postnatal life.

Fetal swallowing at various stages of pregnancy has been measured by introducing a small volume of maternal red cells labeled with isotopic chromium into the amniotic sac and subsequently measuring the chromium that accumulated in the gastrointestinal tract either directly in fetuses that succumbed from immaturity after delivery or in the meconium and feces passed after birth by more mature fetuses (Pritchard). Term-size fetuses swallow approximately 450 ml of amniotic fluid per 24 hours, an amount that, according to Davidson, is very similar to the volume of breast milk ingested by healthy newborn infants. Although the volume of amniotic fluid swallowed daily early in pregnancy is quite small, nonetheless it amounts to 5 to 10 per cent of the weight of the fetus. Fetal swallowing appears to have little effect on amniotic fluid volume early in pregnancy, since the volume swallowed is slight compared with the total volume of amniotic fluid present. Late in pregnancy, however, the volume of amniotic fluid surrounding the fetus appears to be regulated to a significant degree by fetal swallowing, and when swallowing is inhibited, hydramnios is common.

The act of swallowing may enhance growth and development of the alimentary canal and condition the fetus for alimentation after birth, although anencephalic fetuses, which usually swallow very little amniotic fluid, have gastrointestinal tracts that appear grossly normal. In the latter part of pregnancy, swallowing serves to remove some of the insoluble debris that is normally shed into the amniotic sac and sometimes abnormally excreted into it. The undigested portions of the swallowed debris can be identified in meconium collected at birth. The amount of amniotic fluid swallowed probably contributes little to the caloric requirements of the fetus. Page, however, has considered the possibility of feeding fetuses suffering from intrauterine growth retardation by adding vital nutrients to the amniotic fluid through a chronically indwelling catheter. The risks to both fetus and mother inherent in the prolonged use of an indwelling catheter, however, seem excessive compared with any benefits that might accrue to the fetus.

Meconium consists not only of undigested debris from swallowed amniotic fluid, but to a larger degree of various products of secretion, excretion, and desquamation by the gastrointestinal tract. The dark greenish black appearance is caused by pigments, especially biliverdin. Intense hypoxia commonly leads to the evacuation of meconium from the large bowel into the amniotic fluid.

Liver and Pancreas.   Hepatic function differs in several ways from that of the adult. Many enzymes of the fetal liver are present in considerably reduced amounts compared with those in later life. The liver has a very limited capacity for converting free bilirubin to bilirubin diglucuronoside because of low activities of the enzymes uridine diphosphoglucose dehydrogenase and glucuronyl transferase. The more immature the fetus, the more deficient is the system for conjugating bilirubin.

As mentioned in the discussion on fetal blood, the life-span of the red cell of the fetus is shorter than that of the normal adult; as the result, relatively more bilirubin is produced. Only a small fraction of the bilirubin is conjugated by the fetal liver and excreted through the biliary tract into the intestine where, for the most part, it is oxidized to biliverdin. Biliverdin, in turn, causes the greenish-black color of meconium. Elegant studies of the fate of bilirubin in the fetus have been performed in the monkey and the dog by Bashore and associates and by Bernstein and co-workers. They demonstrated that labeled unconjugated bilirubin is promptly cleared from the fetal circulation by the placenta to be conjugated by the maternal liver and excreted through the maternal biliary tract. The transfer of the unconjugated bilirubin across the placenta, however, is bidirectional. This observation is supported by the rarely encountered case of fetal hyperbilirubinemia as the consequence of high levels of unconjugated bilirubin in maternal plasma. Conjugated bilirubin is not exchanged to any significant degree between mother and fetus, however.

Glycogen appears in low concentration in the fetal liver during the second trimester of pregnancy, but near term there is a rapid and marked increase in glycogen content to levels two to three times higher than those in adult liver. After delivery the glycogen content falls precipitously. If the rabbit fetus is decapitated by the technic developed by Jost, the rest of the body subsequently grows in utero to the same extent as the nondecapitated control fetus, but large amounts of glycogen do not accumulate in the liver of the decapitated fetus. Thus, decapitation in some way impairs the development of the hepatic enzymes involved in the formation of glycogen. These observations have led to the suggestion that the intrauterine development of some hepatic enzymes might be controlled by pituitary and adrenal hormones (Beuding and Colacci).

The exocrine function of the fetal pancreas appears to be limited but not necessarily absent. For example, iodine-labeled human albumin injected into the amniotic sac and swallowed by the fetus is digested to the extent that most of the iodine label is absorbed from the fetal intestine. It is not absorbed as undigested protein, however, and the iodine is promptly excreted in the maternal urine (Pritchard).

In the human fetus as early as the thirteenth week of gestation, insulin has been identified in the pancreas; the amount increases with age (Rastogi and associates). The fetal pancreas responds to hyperglycemia by increasing plasma insulin (Obenshain and co-workers). Although the precise role played by insulin of fetal origin is not clear, fetal growth must be determined to a considerable extent by the amounts of basic nutrients transferred from the mother and, through the action of insulin, the anabolism of these materials by the fetus. Proof that insulin of fetal origin helps meet the needs of the mother is lacking. The characteristic intense islet cell hypertrophy in the fetus whose mother has diabetes suggests that it may do so.

Other Endocrine Glands.   Corticotropin (ACTH) has been detected in the human *fetal pituitary* as early as the tenth week of gestation. Corticotropin from the fetal pituitary appears to be essential for maintenance of the fetal adrenals. Jost and co-workers, for example, have demonstrated that decapitation of the fetus causes the adrenals to atrophy even though the fetus continues to grow in utero; moreover, anencephalic human fetuses with very little pituitary tissue have atrophic adrenals. Lanman in one instance administered corticotropin to an anencephalic infant for 18 days after birth and found the adrenals hypertrophic, indicating that in the anencephalic fetus they are responsive to corticotropin. These observations in animals and man support the view that the relatively large adrenals of the fetus are dependent upon corticotropin derived primarily from the fetal pituitary.

The levels of pituitary somatomammotropin (growth hormone) are rather high in cord blood. There is additional evidence that the human fetus produces pituitary growth hormone, although the hormone's role in fetal growth and development is not clear. Decapitation in utero does not appreciably impair the growth of the rest of the fetus, as shown in animals by Bearn as well as others. Furthermore, human anencephalic fetuses with little or no pituitary tissue are not remarkably different in size from normal fetuses.

Little is known about gonadotropin production by the human fetal pituitary; however, if pituitary gonadotropins are produced, the levels must be very low.

Identification of thyroid stimulating hormone (thyrotropin) as early as the tenth week of human gestation has been reported (Mizusawa). Probably very little thyrotropin crosses the placenta from mother to fetus whereas the pathologic long-acting thyroid stimulator, or LATS, almost certainly does (Sunshine and co-workers).

By 10 to 14 weeks of gestation the fetal thyroid concentrates iodine and synthesizes thyroxine (Shepard). At the same time thyrotropin is present in the fetal pituitary and plasma. It increases appreciably during the second trimester suggesting rapid maturation of the fetal hypothalamic-pituitary unit (Fisher and associates.

Since the human placenta actively concentrates iodide on the fetal side and the fetal thyroid concentrates iodide throughout most of pregnancy, the hazard to the fetus of administering to the mother either radioiodide or large amounts of ordinary iodide is obvious.

Most evidence indicates that thyroid hormones of maternal origin cross the placenta to a limited degree, with triiodothyronine crossing more readily than thyroxin. The fetus, however, is probably dependent for the most part upon hormone produced by his own thyroid gland. The fact that athyreotic cretins generally have euthyroid mothers implies that a normal rate of maternal thyroid secretion cannot compensate completely for inadequate fetal glandular synthesis.

Lack of antidiuretic hormone production by the fetus has been suggested to account for the lack of urine concentrating ability in the newborn infant. The significance of such a deficiency continues to be debated, since the extent to which the kidney of the neonate can respond to exogenous antidiuretic hormone is not clear.

The *adrenal* of the human fetus is very much larger in relation to total body size than is that of the adult; the bulk of the enlargement is made up of the central, or so-called, fetal zone of the adrenal cortex. The fetal zone is scant to absent in rare instances where the fetal pituitary is missing. The normally hypertrophied fetal zone involutes rapidly after birth.

Bloch and Benirschke have demonstrated through incubation in vitro that the fetal adrenal cortex can synthesize many steroids from acetate. More recently, several groups have perfused the immature human fetus just after delivery with labeled progesterone and recovered a variety of labeled steroids including cortisol. As pointed out in Chapter 6 (p. 185), the human fetal adrenal normally produces from pregnenolone progressively greater amounts of dehydroisoandrosterone and its sulfate, which are, in turn, for the most part hydroxylated in position 16 by the fetal liver and then converted to estriol by the placenta. The estriol is subsequently excreted in the maternal urine, forming the basis for fetal monitoring through the measurement of urinary estriol.

Aldosterone, normally present in considerably elevated concentrations in maternal plasma, crosses the placenta with apparent ease. Studies carried out with labeled aldosterone administered to the mother strongly suggest, on the basis of isotope dilution in cord blood, that the fetal adrenal secretes aldosterone (Bayard and co-workers). Catecholamines are present in the adrenal medulla very early in fetal life.

The *testes* of the human fetus are capable of synthesizing androgens. Both testosterone and androstenedione have been isolated from immature fetal testes after perfusing the intact fetoplacental unit with 17-alpha-hydroxyprogesterone (Macnaughton). Little is known of the ability of the fetal *ovaries* to synthesize sex steroids.

Nervous System and Sensory Organs. Synaptic function is sufficiently developed by the eighth week of gestation to demonstrate flexion of neck and trunk (Temiras and associates). If the fetus is removed from the uterus during the tenth week, spontaneous movements may be observed, although movements in utero usually are not evident until several weeks later. At 10 weeks, local stimuli may evoke squinting, opening the mouth, incomplete finger closure, and plantar flexion of the toes. Complete finger closure is achieved during the fourth month. Swallowing and respiration are also evident during the fourth month, as demonstrated in Figure 12, but the ability to suck is not present until the sixth month.

During the third trimester of pregnancy integration of nervous and muscular function proceeds rapidly, so that the majority of fetuses delivered after the thirty-second week of gestation survive.

By the seventh lunar month the eye is sensitive to light, but perception of form and color is not complete until long after birth.

The internal, middle, and external components of the ear are well developed by midpregnancy. The fetus apparently hears some sounds in utero as early as the twenty-fourth to twenty-sixth week of gestation (Westin).

Taste buds are evident histologically in the third lunar month; by the seventh month of gestation the fetus is responsive to variations in the taste of ingested substances.

Immunology. Infections in utero have provided an excellent opportunity to examine some of the mechanisms for immune response by the human fetus.

Sterzl and Silverstein performed a retrospective analysis of aborted human fetuses with syphilitic infection. They concluded from the presence of plasmacytosis in sites of inflammation that the fetus can make antibody to treponema antigen by the twentieth week of gestation. Smith has colligated the considerable evidence that the human fetus by the fifth or sixth month of gestation has the capacity for producing the various immunoglobulins found in the adult. Therefore, the opinion that the fetus is immunologically incompetent is no longer tenable.

In the absence of a direct antigenic stimulus in the fetus, such as infection, the immunoglobulins in the fetus consist almost totally of species of immune globulin G(IgG) synthesized by the mother and subsequently transferred across the placenta by both diffusion and active transport. Therefore, the antibodies in the fetus and the newborn infant most often reflect the immunologic experiences of the mother. Not all species of IgG present in adults, however, are able to cross the placenta into the fetal circulation. Wang and associates were unable to identify in sera of normal newborns some of the heavy peptide chains of IgG that are present in pooled sera of adults. Moreover, sera of newborns contain a heavy chain that is not found in sera of adults, indicating that neonatal IgG is not made up entirely of IgG molecules passively transferred from the mother. They believe that the gene responsible for synthesis of the heavy chain unique to fetal sera is probably operational only in the fetus. The production of this heavy chain is therefore somewhat analogous to that of synthesis of beta chains in the formation of fetal hemoglobin. Differing from many animals, the human newborn infant does not acquire any passive immunity from the absorption of antibodies ingested in colostrum. Nonetheless, IgA ingested in colostrum may provide some protection against enteric infections, since the antibody resists digestion and is effective on mucosal surfaces.

In the adult, production of immune globulin M (IgM) in response to antigen is superseded in a week or so predominantly by production of IgG. In contrast, the IgM response remains the dominant one for weeks to months in the fetus and newborn. IgM serum levels in umbilical cord blood and identification of specific florescent antibodies offer promise in the diagnosis of intrauterine infection.

The transfer of some IgG antibodies from mother to fetus is harmful rather than protective to the fetus. The classical clinical example of antibodies of maternal origin that are dangerous to the fetus is hemolytic disease of the fetus and newborn. In this disease maternal antibody to fetal red cell antigen crosses the placenta to destroy the fetal red cells (Ch. 37, p. 1036).

Nutrition of the Fetus.   During the first two months of pregnancy the embryo consists almost entirely of water; in later months relatively more solids are added. The amounts of water, fat, nitrogen, and certain minerals in the fetus at successive weeks of pregnancy are shown in Table 2, adapted from Widdowson. Because of the small amount of yolk in the human ovum, growth of the fetus from the very early stage of development depends on nutrition obtained from the mother. During the first few days after implantation the nutrition of the fertilized ovum is derived directly from the interstitial fluid of the endometrium and from the surrounding maternal tissue, which has undergone proteolysis as the result of trophoblastic invasion. Within the next week the forerunners of the intervillous space arise, comprising at first simply lacunae filled with maternal blood. During the third week after ovulation blood vessels appear in the chorionic villi. During the fourth week after ovulation a cardiovascular system has formed, and thereby

Table 2. Total Amounts of Fat, Nitrogen, and Minerals in the Body of the Developing Fetus

Body Weight (g)	Approximate fetal age (weeks)	Water (g)	Fat (g)	N (g)	Ca (g)	P (g)	Mg (g)	Na (mEq)	K (mEq)	Cl (mEq)	Fe (mg)	Cu (mg)	Zn (mg)
30	13	27	0.2	0.4	0.09	0.09	0.003	3.6	1.4	2.4	—	—	—
100	15	89	0.5	1.0	0.3	0.2	0.01	9	2.6	7	5.1	—	—
200	17	177	1.0	2.8	0.7	0.6	0.03	20	7.9	14	10	0.7	2.6
500	23	440	3.0	7.0	2.2	1.5	0.10	49	22	33	28	2.4	9.4
1,000	26	860	10	14	6.0	3.4	0.22	90	41	66	64	3.5	16
1,500	31	1,270	35	25	10	5.6	0.35	125	60	96	100	5.6	25
2,000	33	1,620	100	37	15	8.2	0.46	160	84	120	160	8.0	35
2,500	35	1,940	185	49	20	11	0.58	200	110	130	220	10	43
3,000	38	2,180	360	55	25	14	0.70	240	130	150	260	12	50
3,500	40	2,400	560	62	30	17	0.78	280	150	160	280	14	53

From Widdowson, E. M. *Growth and composition of the fetus and newborn*, in *Biology of Gestation*, Vol. II, The Fetus and Neonate, N. S. Assali (ed.). New York, Academic Press, 1968.

a true circulation, both within the embryo and between the embryo and the chorionic villi.

The maternal diet is the ultimate source of the nutrients supplied to the fetus. Typically, the mother eats varying amounts and kinds of food several times a day. In turn, the food is digested, its constituents are absorbed, and, for the most part, they are immediately stored. The storage forms are then made continuously available in an orderly way to meet the demands for energy, tissue repair, and new growth including pregnancy. Three major storage depots—namely, the liver, muscle, and adipose tissue—and one principle storage hormone, insulin, are intimately involved in the metabolism of the nutrients absorbed from the maternal gut. Insulin is released from the maternal islands of Langerhans in response to various materials liberated from food during digestion and absorption. The secretion of insulin is sustained by rising levels of blood glucose and amino acids. The net effect is to store glucose as glycogen (primarily in the liver and muscle), to retain some amino acids as protein, and to store the excess as fat.

During the fasting state glucose is released from glycogen, but glycogen stores are not large in the mother and cannot in themselves provide an adequate amount of glucose to meet the requirements of the mother and fetus for energy and growth. The cleavage of stored triglycerides in adipose tissue, however, can provide the mother with energy in the form of free fatty acids. The process of lipolysis is activated directly or indirectly by a number of hormones including glucagon, norepinephrine, chorionic somatomammotropin, glucocorticoids, and thyroid hormone. Neutral fat does not cross the placenta. The extent of transport of free fatty acids is not known, although Szabo and associates have noted the active transfer of palmitic acid from the maternal to the fetal side of the human placenta perfused in vitro. Portman and co-workers, furthermore, have demonstrated rapid transfer of palmitic and linoleic acids from mother to fetus in subhuman primates. Glucose and the naturally occurring forms of amino acids, of course, readily cross the placenta to the fetus. Therefore, as emphasized by

Freinkel, since glucose is a major nutrient for growth and energy in the fetus, it is advantageous for mechanisms to be operational during pregnancy that minimize glucose utilization by the mother and thereby make the limited maternal supply available to the fetus. One metabolic action of chorionic somatomammotropin, a hormone present in abundance in the mother but not the fetus, is blocking the utilization of glucose by the mother while promoting the mobilization and utilization of free fatty acids.

For obvious reasons, a great deal of investigative effort continues to be focused on maternal nutrition and its effect on the growth and development of the fetus. Fetal size is not just a function of fetal age. For example, in maternal diabetes mellitus without significant vascular disease, the fetus typically is much larger than normal, but if severe maternal vascular disease further complicates the diabetes, the fetus may be appreciably smaller than normal (Ch. 27, p. 791). Page, in an interesting theoretical discussion of fetal growth, analyzed the factors known to control the delivery of a primary nutrient, glucose, to the fetus. Since maternal hyperglycemia leads to increased transfer of glucose across the placenta, he suggests that hyperglycemia and hyperinsulinemia in the fetus together accelerate fetal growth. Factors leading to growth retardation in the human fetus, however, are more complex. Growth retardation might result from insufficient concentration of a nutrient in the maternal arterial plasma, inadequate uterine blood flow and placental perfusion, reduced functional surface area of the chorionic villi, impairment of placental transport mechanisms, inadequate vascularity of the chorionic villi, or insufficient umbilical blood flow to transfer the nutrient in appropriate amounts from the placenta to the fetus. Maternal dietary deficiencies among species in which the weight of the fetus is relatively large compared with the mother's weight, and in which the duration of gestation is short, commonly cause fetal growth retardation. In women, however, in whom fetal size is slight compared with that of the mother and the duration of gestation is long, it has been difficult to demonstrate a clear-cut correlation between maternal nutritional deficiency and fetal growth retardation (Ch. 12, p. 336). It is possible that subtle but nonetheless deleterious changes in the human fetus may be induced by faulty maternal nutrition, but they may be difficult to recognize with the various analytical technics that have been applied thus far. Further critical analyses of the effects of variations in maternal nutrition on the human fetus are imperative.

AMNIOTIC FLUID

The fluid filling the amniotic sac serves several important functions. It provides a medium in which the fetus can readily move, cushions him against possible injury, and helps him maintain an even temperature. During labor, if the presenting part of the fetus is not closely applied to the lower uterine segment, the hydrostatic action of the amniotic fluid may be of importance in dilating the cervical canal.

By the twelfth day after fertilization of the ovum, a cleft enclosed by primitive amnion has formed adjacent to the embryonic plate (Fig. 20, Ch. 5, p. 134). Rapid enlargement of the cleft and fusion of the surrounding amnion first with the body stalk, and later with the chorion, creates the amniotic sac, which fills with an essentially colorless fluid. The amniotic fluid increases rapidly to an average volume of 50 ml at 12 weeks' gestation and 400 ml at midpregnancy; it reaches a maximum of about a liter at 36 to 38 weeks' gestation. The volume then decreases as term approaches; and if the pregnancy is prolonged, amniotic fluid may become relatively scant. There are rather marked individual differences in amniotic fluid volume, however, as reported by Fuchs and as the data of Gillibrand, plotted in Figure 13, clearly show. The physician performing amniocentesis for diagnostic purposes soon appreciates the considerable variability in the volume of amniotic fluid present at the same time in different pregnancies as well as at different times in the same pregnancy.

The composition and volume of amniotic fluid change as pregnancy advances. In the first half of pregnancy the fluid has essentially the same composition as maternal plasma except for a much lower protein concentration, and it is nearly devoid of particulate matter. As gestation advances, variable amounts of particulate matter in the form of desquamated fetal cells, lanugo and scalp hair, and vernix caseosa are shed into the fluid. The concentrations of various solutes also change significantly and, as a consequence, the osmolality decreases on the average about 20 to 30 milliosmoles, or about 10 per cent, as shown in Figure 13.

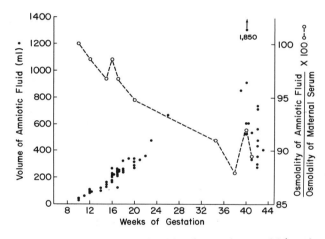

Fig. 13. Amniotic fluid volume and osmolality. The first and second trimesters are characterized by a rather orderly increase in volume, but at term the volume is quite variable. The osmolality decreases in approximately linear fashion as pregnancy advances. (From data of Gillibrand. J Obstet Gynaec Brit Comm 76:527 and 898, 1969.)

The forces responsible for the changes in volume and composition of amniotic fluid are not well understood. Ions and small molecules rapidly move into and out of amniotic fluid but at rates that are specific for each substance. In contradistinction to mass movement of amniotic fluid, this process involves simply molecular or ionic trade across a membrane without necessarily inducing changes in volume or concentration (Plentl).

There is no single mechanism that will account for all of the variations in composition and volume of amniotic fluid that have been observed during the course of a normal pregnancy. One relatively simple explanation is that amniotic fluid in early pregnancy is a product primarily of the amniotic membrane covering the placenta and cord. It is likely that fluid also passes across the fetal skin at this time. As the pregnancy advances, the surface of the amnion expands and the volume of fluid formed increases, but from about the fourth month the fetus is capable of modifying amniotic fluid composition and volume by both urinating and swallowing progressively larger amounts of fluid.

Changes in osmolality indicate that as gestation advances, the fetal urine makes an increasingly important contribution to the amniotic fluid. Fetal urine is quite hypotonic compared with maternal or fetal plasma, because of the lower electrolyte concentration in the urine, but it contains more urea, creatinine, and uric acid than does plasma. These observations have been made repeatedly on amniotic fluid and urine obtained at the time of delivery and have been shown to exist in utero as early as the twenty-fourth week of pregnancy. Mandelbaum and Evans have examined urine obtained inadvertently from the fetal bladder at the time of attempted intrauterine transfusion and compared the concentrations of several of the constituents of the urine with those of amniotic fluid. Even at 24 weeks' gestation the urea and creatinine concentrations were two to three times higher in the urine, whereas the concentrations of sodium, potassium, and chloride were only about one third to one fifth as great as those in the amniotic fluid. The admixture of sizable volumes of fetal urine with the amniotic fluid, therefore, would logically be expected to lower the osmolality, as demonstrated in Figure 13, and, at the same time, raise the concentration of urea, creatinine, and uric acid. Indeed, late in pregnancy, amniotic fluid normally differs from plasma in precisely these ways.

The fetus undoubtedly swallows amniotic fluid during much of pregnancy. As discussed earlier in this chapter, under Digestive System, the volume swallowed late in pregnancy amounts on the average to nearly 500 ml per day. If allowance is made for the difference in weight, this amount is quite similar to the volume of urine formed near term by the fetus of the rhesus monkey as well as by sheep, according to the studies of Chez and associates and of Gresham and co-workers. Often, but not always, a great excess of amniotic fluid (hydramnios) develops whenever fetal swallowing is greatly impaired (Ch. 22, p. 599). Classic examples of lesions in which fetal swallowing cannot or usually does not take place and thereby leads to hydramnios are esophageal atresia and anencephaly. Conversely, when urination in utero cannot take place, as in instances of renal agenesis or atresia of the urethra, the volume of amniotic fluid surrounding the fetus typically is extremely limited (oligohydramnios), as discussed in the section dealing with the urinary system.

Although lack of fetal swallowing with continuous production of normal amounts of fluid by the amnion and the fetal kidneys may lead to hydramnios, this mechanism is certainly not the sole cause of hydramnios. Progressive hydramnios has been observed in instances in which the normal fetus was known to ingest relatively large amounts of amniotic fluid, but in which maternal diseases known to predispose to hydramnios, such as diabetes, were not identified (Pritchard). Presumably in these instances, increased production by the amnion or possibly intense fetal polyuria, or even both, cause the increase in amniotic fluid volume.

The extent to which the fetal tracheobronchial tree participates in amniotic fluid exchange and volume control is not clear. It has been suggested that in the lamb fetus, fluid from the trachea contributes significantly to amniotic fluid, but recent studies by Goodlin and Rudolph do not support this idea.

Fetal Monitoring.   Analyses of several of the constituents in amniotic fluid obtained by amniocentesis have been recommended as means of monitoring the well-being of the fetus in complicated pregnancies. Some of the technics that use amniotic fluid for fetal monitoring are tabulated here. Some are quite useful whereas others appear to be of much more limited value. They are also discussed in more detail in the chapters that deal with the complication under consideration.

A. Examination of Cells in Amniotic Fluid
1. *Sex-linked disease,* for example, hemophilia, by identifying the nuclear sex chromatin (Barr) body as described below.
2. *Chromosomal abnormalities* detected by culturing and karyotyping cells of fetal origin, for example, mongolism.
3. *Fetal maturity* by demonstrating an abundance of cells that stain orange when treated with Nile blue sulfate.
4. *The presence of A or B blood group,* since these antigens may be identified on the desquamated fetal cells in the amniotic fluid. The Rh type can be identified, however, only if fetal red cells are obtained at the time of amniocentesis.
5. *Diseases with characteristic enzyme deficiencies.* Tay-Sachs disease has been predicted correctly by demonstrating very low levels of hexosaminidase-A activity in amniotic fluid cells and liquor itself (Schenck and co-workers). Other heritable diseases have been detected through the application of tissue culture technics to cells from amniotic fluid, including Lesch-Nyhan's syndrome, and galactosemia.

B. Measurement of Substances Dissolved in Amniotic Fluid
1. *Fetal maturity* by measuring in amniotic fluid the absorption of light by bilirubin or by its product formed with the diazo reaction, the creatinine or urea concentration, and the osmolality.
2. *Hemolytic disease* in the fetus by demonstrating an elevated bilirubin concentration. The bilirubin level may be more significant if the concentration of protein in the amniotic fluid is also measured. A low amniotic fluid estriol level is usually found when the fetus is severely affected even though maternal urinary estriol excretion may be normal.
3. *Congenital disease.* The utilization of amniotic fluid analyses to detect congenital disease is considered in detail in the publications of Fuchs and Cederqvist and of Nadler and Gerbie.

Sex of the Fetus

The accepted secondary sex ratio, that is, the sex ratio of human fetuses reaching viability is approximately 106 males to 100 females. This figure has been obtained by the examination of term and premature infants. Many attempts have been made to establish a sex ratio for fetuses of earlier gestational age. In general, such studies have been misleading, for as Wilson has shown, external genitals are an unreliable index of sex before the 50 mm stage.

Since, theoretically, there should be as many Y-bearing as X-bearing sperm, the primary sex ratio, or the ratio at the time of fertilization, should be 1 to 1. If so, the secondary sex ratio of 106 to 100 suggests that more females than males are lost during the early months of pregnancy. Until recently, however, there was no means of ascertaining sex in the absence of a fetus or embryo or on the basis of undifferentiated gonadal tissue. The discovery by Barr and Bertram of the *sex chromatin* body has proved of considerable help in identifying sex by microscopic examination of the resting nuclei of somatic tissues. The Barr body is not found in male somatic cells, and studies of chromosomal karyotypes in patients with anomalous sexual development indicate that in nuclei with the diploid autosomal set, the number of Barr bodies in a nucleus is one less than the number of X chromosomes. Particularly pertinent is the extension of Barr's work by Glenister, who noted the sex chromatin body in the trophoblastic cells of an implanting human blastocyst and in 6 of 13 human embryos with still undifferentiated gonadal tissue. Therefore, assignment of sex according to the presence of the sex chromatin body in resting nuclei is possible in the absence of an embryo, although formal karyotyping is, of course, more reliable.

Since sex may be ascertained by study of the nuclear sex chromatin of the fetal portion of the placenta, an estimate of the ratio of male-to-female embryos in abortions may·thus be obtained theoretically. Syncytiotrophoblast is not suitable for this purpose, however, and decidual tissue must be carefully excluded. The best cells from the placenta to use for analysis of sex chromatin are villous cyto-trophoblast (Langhans cells) and fibrocytes. Chromosomal studies by Carr and others, however, have shown that sex ratios in early pregnancy obtained by analysis of nuclear sex chromatin are unreliable.

Establishment of the primary sex ratio in man is at present impracticable, for it requires the recovery and assignment of zygotes that fail to cleave and blastocysts that fail to implant. Carr's studies, nevertheless, suggest that the primary human sex ratio may be unity.

Prediction of Sex of Fetus.   Cells promptly separated from freshly collected amniotic fluid can be concentrated by centrifugation, spread and fixed on a slide, appropriately stained as with the Feulgen reaction, and examined for the presence or absence of the Barr sex chromatin body (Serr). Only cells with well-preserved nuclei are reliable for identifying the Barr body, and such cells may be quite uncommon (Fuchs). Moreover, errors in predicting sex have been made and, infrequently, trauma and infection have resulted from the amniocentesis (Riis and Fuchs). More recently identification of the X and Y chromosomes of fetal cells grown in tissue culture have added precision to the prediction of the sex of the fetus.

REFERENCES

Abel, S., and Windle, W. F.   Relation of the volume of pulmonary circulation to respiration at birth. Anat Rec 75:451, 1939.

Acheson, G. H., Dawes, G. S., and Mott, J. C.   Oxygen consumption and arterial oxygen saturation in fetal and newborn lambs. J Physiol 135:623, 1957.

Adair, F. L., and Scammon, R. E.   A study of the ossification centers of the wrist, knee and ankle at birth. Amer J Obstet Gynec 2:35, 1921.

Adamsons, K.   Diagnosis and Treatment of Fetal Disorders. New York, Springer-Verlag, 1968.

Aherne, W., and Dunnill, M. S.   Morphometry of the human placenta. Brit Med Bull 22:1, 1966.

Allen, D. W., Wyman, J., and Smith, C. A.   The oxygen equilibrium of fetal and adult human hemoglobin. J Biol Chem 203:81, 1953.

Annual Report of the Registrar-General for Scotland (104th). Edinburgh, Her Majesty's Stationery Office, 1958.

Arey, L. B.   Developmental Anatomy: A Textbook and Laboratory Manual of Embryology, 5th ed. Philadelphia, W. B. Saunders Co., 1946.

Assali, N. S.   Biology of Gestation, Vol. II, The Fetus. New York, Academic Press, 1968.

———— Bekey, G. A., and Morrison, L. W.   Fetal and neonatal circulation, in Assali, N. S. (ed.), Biology of Gestation, Vol. II, The Fetus and Neonate. New York, Academic Press, 1968.

———— Kirschbaum, T. H., and Dilts, P. V.   Effects of hyperbaric oxygen on uteroplacental and fetal circulation. Circ Res 22:573, 1968.

———— and Morris, J. A. Maternal and fetal circulations and their interrelationships. Obstet Gynec Survey 19:923, 1964.

Bangham, D. R., Hobbs, K. R., and Terry, R. J. Selective placental transfer of serum-proteins in the *Rhesus.* Lancet 2:351, 1958.

Barclay, A. E., Barcroft, J., Barron, D. H., and Franklin, K. J. X-ray studies of closing of ductus arteriosus. Brit J Radiol 11:570, 1938.

———— Barcroft, J., Barron, D. H., and Franklin, K. J. Radiographic demonstration of circulation through heart in adult and in foetus, and identification of ductus arteriosus. Brit J Radiol 12:505, 1939.

Barcroft, J. Researches on Prenatal Life. Oxford, Blackwell, 1946.

Barnes, A. C. Intra-Uterine Development. Philadelphia, Lea & Febiger, 1968.

Barr, M. L., and Bertram, E. G. A morphological distinction between neurones of the male and female, and the behavior of the nucleolar satellite during accelerated nucleoprotein synthesis. Nature, London 163:676, 1949.

Barron, D. H. The changes in the fetal circulation at birth. Physiol Rev 24:277, 1944.

Bashore, R. A., Smith, F., and Schenker, S. Placental transfer and disposition of bilirubin in the pregnant monkey. Amer J Obstet Gynec 103:950, 1969.

Battaglia, F. C. Placental clearance and fetal oxygenation. Pediatrics 45:563, 1970.

Bayard, F. J., Ances, I. G., Topper, A. J., Weldon, V. V., Kowarski, A., and Migeon, C. J. Placental passage and fetal secretion of aldosterone. Presented before Society for Pediatric Research, Atlantic City, May 1, 1970.

Bearn, J. G. Role of fetal pituitary and adrenal glands in the development of the fetal thymus of the rabbit. Endocrinology 80:979, 1967.

Becker, R. F., Windle, W. F., Barth, E. E., and Schultz, M. D. Fetal swallowing, gastrointestinal activity and defecation in amnio. Surg Gynec Obstet 70:603, 1940.

Belcher, D. P. A child weighing 25 pounds at birth. JAMA 67:950, 1916.

Bernstein, R. B., Novy, M. J., Piasecki, G. J., Lester, R., and Jackson, B. T. Bilirubin metabolism in the fetus. J Clin Invest 48:1678, 1969.

Beuding, E., and Colacci, A. V. Enzymes of glycogen metabolism in mammalian fetal liver, in Barnes, A. C. (ed.), Intra-Uterine Development. Philadelphia, Lea & Febiger, 1968.

Bloch, E., and Benirschke, K. Synthesis in vitro of steroids by human fetal adrenal gland slices. J Biol Chem 234:1085, 1959.

Braestrup, P. W. Studies of latent scurvy in infants. II. Content of ascorbic (cevitamic) acid in the blood serum of women in labor and in children at birth. Acta Paediat 19: Suppl 1, 328, 1937.

Cantarow, A., Stuckert, H., and Davis, R. C. Chemical composition of amniotic fluid: a comparative study of human amniotic fluid and maternal blood. Surg Gynec Obstet 57:63, 1933.

Carr, D. Chromosome studies in abortuses and stillborn infants. Lancet 2:603, 1963.

Chez, R. A., Smith R. G., and Hutchinson, D. L. Renal function in the intrauterine primate fetus. Amer J Obstet Gynec 90:128, 1964.

Christie, A. Prevalence and distribution of ossification centers in the newborn infant. Amer J Dis Child 77:335, 1949.

Creasy, R. K., Drost, M., Green, M. V., and Morris, J. A. Methods of determination of fetal and neonatal blood volume and influence of respiration ond placental-neonatal transfusion. Circ Res, in press.

Davidson, M. Digestion and assimilation, in Barnett, H. L. (ed.), Pediatrics. New York, Appleton-Century-Crofts, 1968.

Davies, J. Human Developmental Anatomy. New York, Ronald Press, 1963.

Davis, M. E., and Potter, E. L. Intrauterine respiration of the human fetus. JAMA 131:1194, 1946.

Dawes, G. S. The umbilical circulation. Amer J Obstet Gynec 84:1634, 1962.

———— Foetal and Neonatal Physiology. Chicago, Year Book Medical Publishers, 1968.

Donald, I. Sonar in obstetrics and gynecology, in Greenhill, J. P. (ed.), Year Book of Obstetrics and Gynecology. Chicago, Year Book Medical Publishers, 1967-1968 Series.

Elliott, P. M., and Inman, W. H. Volume of liquor amnii in normal and abnormal pregnancy. Lancet 2:835, 1961.

Fehling, H. (Contribution to the physiology of placental transfer). Arch Gynaek 11:523, 1877.

Finne, P. H.   Antenatal diagnosis of the anemia in erythroblastosis. Acta Paediat Scand 55:609, 1966.

Fisher, D. A., Hobel, C. J., Garza, R., and Pierce, C. A.   Thyroid function in the preterm fetus. Pediatrics 46:208, 1970.

Flexner, L. B., Cowie, D. B., Hellman, L. M., Wilde, W. S., and Vosburgh, G. J.   The permeability of the human placenta to sodium in normal and abnormal pregnancies and the supply of sodium to the human fetus as determined with radioactive sodium. Amer J Obstet Gynec 55:469, 1948.

———— and Gellhorn, A.   Comparative physiology of placental transfer. Amer J Obstet Gynec 43:965, 1942.

Freinkel, N.   Homeostatic factors in fetal carbohydrate metabolism, in Wynn, R. M., (ed.), Fetal Homeostasis, Vol. IV. New York, Appleton-Century-Crofts, 1969.

Fuchs, F.   Volume of amniotic fluid at various stages of pregnancy. Clin Obstet Gynec 9:449, 1966.

———— Genetic information from amniotic fluid constituents. Clin Obstet Gynec 9:565, 1966.

———— and Cederqvist, L. L.   Recent advances in antenatal diagnosis by amniotic fluid analysis. Clin Obstet Gynec 13:178, 1970.

Gillibrand, P. N.   Changes in amniotic fluid volume with advancing pregnancy. J Obstet Gynaec Brit Comm 76:527, 1969.

Glenister, T. W.   Determination of sex in early human embryos (letter to the editor). Nature, London 177:1135, 1956.

Goodlin, R. C., and Rudolph, A. M.   Tracheal fluid flow and function in fetuses in utero. Amer J Obstet Gynec 106:597, 1970.

Gordon, H., and Brosens, I.   Cytology of amniotic fluid: A new test for fetal maturity. Obstet Gynec 30:652, 1967.

Gresham, E. L., Rankin, J. H. G., Makowski, E. L., Meschia, G., and Battaglia, F. C.   Fetal renal function in unstressed pregnancies. Presented before Society for Pediatric Research, Atlantic City, May 1, 1970.

Gruenwald, P.   Growth of the human foetus, in McLaren, A. (ed.), Advances in Reproductive Physiology. New York, Academic Press, 1967.

———— The amount of fetal blood remaining in the placenta at birth. Proc Soc Exp Biol Med 130:326, 1969.

Haase, W.   (Maternity Annual Report for 1875). Charité Annalen 2:669, 1875.

Hellman, L. M., Flexner, L. B., Wilde, W. S., Vosburgh, G. J., and Proctor, N. K.   The permeability of the human placenta to water and the supply of water to the human fetus as determined with deuterium oxide. Amer J Obstet Gynec 56:861, 1948.

———— Johnson, H. L., Tolles, W. E., and Jones, E. H.   Some factors affecting the fetal heart rate. Amer J Obstet Gynec 82:1055, 1961.

———— Kobayashi, M., Fillisti, L., and Lavenhar, M.   Sources of error in sonographic fetal mensuration and estimation of growth. Amer J Obstet Gynec 99:662, 1967.

———— Kobayashi, M., Tolles, W. E., and Cromb, E.   Ultrasonic studies on the volumetric growth of the human placenta. Amer J Obstet Gynec 108:740, 1970.

Huisman, T. H. J., Schroeder, W. A., and Brown, A. K.   Changes in the nature of human fetal hemoglobin during the first year of life. Presented before Society for Pediatric Research, Atlantic City, May 1, 1970.

Hutchinson, D. L., Gray, M. J., Plentl, A. A., Alvarez, H., Caldeyro-Barcia, R., Kaplan, B., and Lind, J.   The role of the fetus in the water exchange of the amniotic fluid of normal and hydramniotic patients. J Clin Invest 38:971, 1959.

———— Hunter, C. B., Neslen, E. D., and Plentl, A. A.   The exchange of water and electrolytes in the mechanism of amniotic fluid formation and the relationship to hydramnios. Surg Gynec Obstet 100:391, 1955.

Johnson, J. W. C.   Cardio-respiratory systems, in Barnes, A. C. (ed.), Intra-Uterine Development. Philadelphia, Lea & Febiger, 1968.

Jost, A., Jacquot, R., and Cohen, A.   The pituitary control of the foetal adrenal cortex, in Currie, A. R., Symington, T., and Grant, J. K. (eds.), The Human Adrenal Cortex. Edinburgh, Livingstone, 1962.

Kasper, C. K., Hoag, M. S., Aggeler, P. M., and Stone, S.   Blood clotting factors in pregnancy: Factor VIII concentrations in normal and AHF-deficient women. Obstet Gynec 24:242, 1964.

Kirschbaum, T. H., DeHaven, J. C., Shapiro, N., and Assali, N. S. Oxyhemoglobin dissociation characteristics of human and sheep maternal and fetal blood. Amer J Obstet Gynec 96:741, 1966.

Kleihauer, E., Braun, H., and Betke, K. (Demonstration of fetal hemoglobin in the erythrocytes of a blood smear). Klin Wschr 35:637, 1957.

Klopper, A., and Diczfalusy, E. (eds.). Foetus and Placenta. Oxford, Blackwell Scientific Publications, 1969.

Kohl, S. G. Perinatal Mortality in New York City: Responsible Factors. Study of 955 Deaths by Subcommittee on Neonatal Mortality, Committee on Public Health Relations, New York Academy of Medicine, Cambridge, Mass., 1955, published for the Commonwealth Fund by Harvard University Press.

Koldovský, O., Heringová, A., Jirsová, U., Jirasek, J. E., and Uher, J. Transport of glucose against a concentration gradient in everted sacs of jejunum and ileum of human fetuses. Gastroenterology 48:185, 1965.

Lanman, J. T. An interpretation of human foetal adrenal structure and function, in Currie, A. R., Symington, T., and Grant, J. K. (eds.), The Human Adrenal Cortex. Edinburgh, Livingstone, 1962.

Lea, A. W. W. The sagittal fontanelle in the heads of infants at birth. Trans Obst Soc London 40:263, 1898.

Macnaughton, M. C. Endocrinology of the foetus, in Klopper, A., and Diczfalusy, E. (eds.), Foetus and Placenta. Oxford, Blackwell Scientific Publication, 1969.

Makowski, E. L., Battaglia, F. C., Meschia, G., Behrman, R. E., Schruefer, J., Seeds, A. E., and Bruns, P. D. Effect of maternal exposure to high altitude upon fetal oxygenation. Amer J Obstet Gynec 100:852, 1968.

Manahan, C. P., and Eastman, N. J. The cevitamic acid content of fetal blood. Bull Hopkins Hosp 62:478, 1938.

Mandelbaum, B., and Evans, T. N. Life in the amniotic fluid. Amer J Obstet Gynec 104:365, 1969.

Mathers, N. P., James, G. B., and Walker, J. The oxygen affinity of the blood of infants treated by intrauterine transfusion. J Obstet Gynaec Brit Comm 77:648, 1970.

Mendenhall, H. W. Serum protein concentrations in pregnancy. II. Concentrations in cord serum and amniotic fluid. Amer J Obstet Gynec 106:581, 1970.

——— Serum protein concentrations in pregnancy. III. Analysis of maternal-cord serum pairs. Amer J Obstet Gynec 106:718, 1970.

Milles, G., and Dorsey, D. B. Intra-uterine respiration-like movements in relation to development of the fetal vascular system. Amer J Path 26:411, 1950.

Myers, R. E. Fetal brain tolerance to umbilical cord compression according to gestational age. Presented at the seventeenth annual meeting of the Society for Gynecologic Investigation, New Orleans, April 2, 1970.

Nadler, H. L., and Gerbe, A. B. Amniocentesis in the intrauterine detection of genetic disorders. New Eng J Med 282:596, 1970.

Necheles, T. F., and Snyder, L. M. Malabsorption of folate polyglutamates associated with oral contraceptive therapy. New Eng J Med 282:858, 1970.

Nielsen, N. C. Coagulation and fibrinolysin in normal women immediately postpartum and in newborn infants. Acta Obstet Gynec Scand 48:371, 1969.

Novy, M. J., Frigoletto, F. D., Easterday, C. L., and Nelson, N. M. Cord blood O_2 affinity following intrauterine transfusion for erythroblastosis. Presented at the seventeenth annual meeting of the Society for Gynecologic Investigation, New Orleans, April 2, 1970.

Obenshain, S. S., Adam, P. A. J., King, K. C., Teramo, K., Raivio, K. O., Räihä, N., and Schwartz, R. Human fetal insulin response to sustained maternal hyperglycemia. New Eng J Med 283:566, 1970.

Page, E. W. Transfer of materials across the human placenta. Amer J Obstet Gynec 74:705, 1957.

——— Glendening, M. B., Margolis, A., and Harper, H. A. Transfer of D- and L-histidine across the human placenta. Amer J Obstet Gynec 73:589, 1957.

Pearson, H. A. Recent advances in hematology. J Pediat 69:466, 1966.

Pitkin, R. M., and Zwirek, S. J. Amniotic fluid creatinine. Amer J Obstet Gynec 98:1135, 1967.

Plentl, A. A. Physiology of the placenta. III. Dynamics of amniotic fluid, in Assali, N. S.

(ed.), Biology of Gestation, Vol. I, The Maternal Organism. New York, Academic Press, 1968.

Portman, O. W., Behrman, R. E., and Soltys, P.   Transfer of free fatty acids across the primate placenta. Amer J Physiol 216:143, 1969.

Potter, E. L.   Pathology of the Fetus and Infant, 2nd ed. Chicago, Year Book Publishers, 1961.

Pritchard, J. A.   Deglutition by normal and anencephalic fetuses. Obstet Gynec 25:289, 1965.

———— Fetal swallowing and amniotic fluid volume. Obstet Gynec 28:606, 1966.

———— Unpublished observations.

———— Kay, J. L., Taylor, W. W., and Scott, D. E.   Fetoplacental blood volume in erythroblastosis fetalis. (To be published).

Prystowsky, H., Hellegers, A., and Bruns, P. D.   Fetal blood studies. XV. The carbon dioxide concentration gradient between fetal and maternal blood of humans. Amer J Obstet Gynec 81:372, 1961.

Ramsey, E. H.   The Placenta and Fetal Membranes, Villee, C. A. (ed.). Baltimore, Williams & Wilkins, 1960, pp. 36-62.

———— Corner, G. W., Long, W. N., and Stran, H. M.   Studies of amniotic fluid and intervillous space pressures in the rhesus monkey. Amer J Obstet Gynec 77:1016, 1959.

Rastogi, G. K., Letarte, J., and Fraser, T. R.   Proinsulin content of pancreas in human fetuses of healthy mothers. Lancet 1:7, 1970.

Reynolds, S. R. M.   Circulatory adaptations to birth. Sci Month 77:205, 1953.

———— Hemodynamic characteristics of the fetal circulation. Amer J Obstet Gynec 68:69, 1954.

———— Ardran, G. M., and Prichard, M. M. L.   Observations on regional circulation times in the lamb under fetal and neonatal conditions. Contrib Embryol 35:73, 1954.

Riis, P., and Fuchs, F.   Sex chromatin and antenatal sex diagnosis, in Moore, K. L. (ed.), The Sex Chromatin. Philadelphia, W. B. Saunders, 1966.

Rudolph, A. M., and Heymann, M. A.   The fetal circulation. Ann Rev Med 19:195, 1968.

Russell, J. G. B.   Radiological assessment of fetal maturity. J Obstet Gynaec Brit Comm 76:208, 1969.

Schenck, L., Valenti, C., Amsterdam, D., Friedland, J., Adachi, M., and Volk, B. W.   Prenatal diagnosis of Tay-Sachs disease. Lancet 1:582, 1970.

Schindler, A. E., Ratanasopa, V., Lee, T. Y., and Herrmann, W. L.   Estriol and Rh isoimmunization: A new approach to the management of severely affected pregnancies. Obstet Gynec 29:625, 1967.

Schulman, I., and Smith, C. H.   Fetal and adult hemoglobins in premature infants. Amer J Dis Child 86:354, 1953.

Serr, D. M., Sachs, L., and Danon, M.   The diagnosis of sex before birth using cells from the amniotic fluid. Bull Res Counc Israel 5B2:137, 1955.

Smith, R. T.   Development of fetal and neonatal immunological function, in Assali, N. S. (ed.), Biology of Gestation, Vol. II, The Fetus and Neonate. New York, Academic Press, 1968.

Snyder, F. F.   The rate of entrance of amniotic fluid into the pulmonary alveoli during fetal respiration. Amer J Obstet Gynec 41:224, 1941.

———— and Rosenfeld, M.   Intra-uterine respiratory movement of the human fetus. JAMA 108:1946, 1937.

Sterzl, J., and Silverstein, A. M.   Developmental aspects of immunity. Advances Immunol 6:337, 1967 (786 references).

Streeter, G. L.   Weight, sitting height, head size, foot length, and menstrual age of the human embryo. Contrib Embryol 11:143, 1920.

Sunshine, P., Kusumoto, H., and Kriss, J. P.   Survival time of circulating long-acting thyroid stimulator in neonatal thyrotoxicosis: Implications for diagnosis and therapy of the disorder. Pediatrics 36:869, 1965.

Szabo, A. J., Grimaldi, R. D., and Jung, W. F.   Palmitate transport across perfused human placenta. Metabolism 18:406, 1969.

Taylor, E. S., Thompson, H. E., Gottesfeld, K. R., and Holmes, J. H.   Clinical use of ultrasound in obstetrics and gynecology. Amer J Obstet Gynec 99:671, 1967.

Temiras, P. S., Vernadakis, A., and Sherwood, N. M.   Development and plasticity of the nervous system, in Assali, N. S. (ed.), Biology of Gestation, Vol. II, The Fetus and Neonate. New York, Academic Press, 1968.

Usher, R., Shepard, M., and Lind, J.   The blood volume of the newborn infant and placental transfusion. Acta Paediat 52:497, 1963.

Vosburgh, G. J., and Flexner, L. B.   Maternal plasma as a source of iron for the fetal guinea pig. Amer J Physiol 161:202, 1950.

———— Flexner, L. B., Cowie, D. B., Hellman, L. M., Proctor, N. K., and Wilde, W. S.   The rate of renewal in woman of the water and sodium of the amniotic fluid as determined by tracer techniques. Amer J Obstet Gynec 56:1156, 1948.

Walker, J., and Turnbull, E. P. N.   Haemoglobin and red cells in the human foetus and their relation to the oxygen content of the blood in the vessels of the umbilical cord. Lancet 2:312, 1953.

Wang, A-C., Faulk, W. P., Stuckey, M., and Fudenberg, H. H.   Chemical differences between adult, fetal, and hypogammaglobulinemic IgG's. Clin Res 18:178, 1970.

Westin, B.   Maternal factors in intrauterine growth: Acoustic response of the fetus, in Wynn, R. M. (ed.), Fetal Homeostasis, Vol. III. New York, Appleton-Century-Crofts, 1968.

Widdowson, E. M.   Growth and composition of the fetus and newborn, in Assali, N. S. (ed.), Biology of Gestation, Vol. II, The Fetus and Neonate. New York, Academic Press, 1968.

Wilson, K. M.   Correlation of external genitalia and sex-glands in the human embryo. Contrib Embryol 18:23, 1926.

Windle, W. F.   Physiology of the Fetus. Philadelphia, W. B. Saunders Co., 1940.

———— Circulation of blood through the fetal heart and lungs and changes occurring with respiration at birth. Quart Bull Northwest Univ Med Sch 14:31, 1940.

———— Becker, R. F., Barth, E. E., and Schulz, M. D.   Aspiration of amniotic fluid by the fetus. Surg Gynec Obstet 69:705, 1939.

Wislocki, G. B.   Gestation, Transactions of the First Conference. The Josiah Macy Jr. Foundation, New York, 1955.

Wynn, R. M.   Fetal Homeostasis, Vols. I–IV. New York, Appleton-Century-Crofts, 1965–1969.

8

MATERNAL PHYSIOLOGY IN PREGNANCY

DURATION OF PREGNANCY

The average duration of human pregnancy, counting from the first day of the last menstrual period, is about 280 days or 40 weeks. Kortenoever, in an analysis of 7,504 pregnancies, found the average duration to be 282 days. Data from the Obstetrical Statistical Cooperative are in close agreement; for 77,300 women who underwent spontaneous labor and whose infants weighed 2,500 g or more, the mean duration was 281 days.

It is customary to estimate the expected date of delivery by counting back 3 months from the first day of the last menstrual period and adding 7 days (Naegele's rule). For example, if the patient's last menstrual period began on September 10, the expected date of confinement (often abbreviated EDC) would be June 17. The calculation can be simplified by designating the month by numbers. Then, the foregoing example becomes 9/10 minus 3 months equals 6/10 plus 7 days, or 6/17. This method of calculation yields only an approximation, although about 40 per cent of women go into labor within 5 days of the calculated date and nearly two thirds do so within 10 days, as shown in Table 1.

Table 1. Deviation from Calculated Date of Confinement (According to Naegele's Rule) of 4,656 Births of Mature Infants

Deviation in Days	Early Delivery	Delivery on Calculated Date	Late Delivery
0	—	189 (4.1)	—
1–5	860 (18.5)		733 (16.6)
6–10	610 (13.1)		570 (12.2)
11–20	733 (15.7)		459 (9.9)
21–30	211 (4.5)		134 (2.9)
31 and over	75 (1.6)		42 (0.9)

The menstrual cycles of the mothers were 28 ± 5 days. The infants were at least 47 cm in length and 2,600 g in weight. (From Burger and Korompai. Zbl Gynaek, 63:1290, 1939.)

Since the interval between ovulation and the next menstrual period is more constant than the preovulatory phase of the cycle, the duration of pregnancy, when calculated from the first day of the last period, is related to the length of the cycle. In other words, a patient with a long cycle will ovulate later with respect to the previous period than will a woman with a short cycle. Hence, any pregnancy will begin later with respect to the last menstrual period from which the calculation is made and therefore, on the average, will end later. The data of McKeown and co-workers for 716 women indicate that the calculated period of gestation increases by about one day for each additional day of the cycle.

Henderson and Kay have demonstrated a racial difference in duration of gestation, which averaged eight days less in Negroes than in Caucasians. Socioeconomic factors recognized to influence the duration of pregnancy were taken into account.

Prolongation of pregnancy by as much as two to three weeks beyond the expected date of confinement calculated by Naegele's rule is fairly common, as shown in Table 1. Beischer, Evans, and Townsend noted, as part of an extensive study of the problems of postmaturity, that 12 per cent of women do not begin labor until 294 days or more after the start of the last menstrual period. Numerous cases are on record in which the duration of pregnancy is said to have exceeded 320 days from the onset of the last menstrual period—that is, extended more than 40 days beyond the calculated date. Such cases are usually questionable, either because of menstrual irregularity or because the woman may have been mistaken about the date of her last period. Nonetheless, Wells has documented a case in which the duration of pregnancy appeared to have been 334 days from the first day of the last menstrual period. Prolongation of pregnancy by two to perhaps three weeks is generally regarded in this country as physiologic and of no concern; however, several investigators have submitted evidence indicating that so-called postmaturity may be associated with higher perinatal mortality and morbidity, as discussed on page 1057.

The upper limit of the duration of pregnancy is of great medicolegal importance in cases in which the husband has been away for ten months or more and the legitimacy of the child is in question. Numerous legal decisions implicating the duration of pregnancy vary widely in their interpretations. In recent years pregnancies of 331 days and 346 days were ruled legitimate by English courts; and in the United States, a New York Supreme Court accepted as legitimate a pregnancy of 355 days (*Lockwood* v. *Lockwood*). In the famous *Preston-Jones* v. *Preston-Jones* peerage case conducted in the House of Lords in England in 1949, the husband petitioned divorce on the grounds of adultery, since the date of last coitus with the defendant required an extension of the total length of gestation to 360 days. The divorce commissioner dismissed the husband's petition, and the Court of Appeals directed two rehearings before judgment was rendered in favor of the husband, granting a divorce. The extensive legal literature on alleged prolongation of pregnancy has been reviewed by Perr.

A special problem noted by many clinicians is the association of prolonged gestation with anencephalic infants. One of the most interesting cases was a pregnancy associated with an anencephalic infant reported by Higgins. The pregnancy was terminated by cesarean section 1 year and 24 days after the last menstrual period. The patient was first examined when she was only 10 days past her missed menstrual period. Fetal movements were present until the moment of birth.

Occasionally, especially in nursing women, conception may take place during a period of amenorrhea. In such circumstances Naegele's rule is of no value, and other, unfortunately less satisfactory, means of estimation are required, as discussed in Chapter 9.

Precocious and Late Pregnancy.   The youngest mother whose history is authenticated is Lina Medina, who was delivered by cesarean section in Lima, Peru, on May 15, 1939. It was claimed that she was 4 years and 8 months old, but a careful review of the birth records indicates that she may have been 5 years and 8 months of age. In either event it is a record.

Although true precocious puberty, as demonstrated by Lina Medina, is still very uncommon, the average age of menarche and ovulation is appreciably lower than it was several decades ago. The mean age of menarche in the United States is now estimated to be 12.3 years. As a consequence of earlier menarche, and perhaps of greater sexual freedom, most obstetric services, especially those serving socioeconomically deprived populations, have witnessed a marked increase in the number of extremely young pregnant women.

Pregnancy after the age of 47 years is rare. According to the United States Vital Statistics for the year 1963 there were approximately 4,098,000 births, of which 82 were recorded in women 50 years or older. These reports have been discontinued because of the high degree of error. Greenhill reports that both he and DeLee have each delivered a woman of 52 without complications, and Natter reported pregnancies in a woman at 50 and again at 52 years of age, both resulting in liveborn infants. In a careful review of the literature from 1860 to 1964 on this subject, Wharton cited 26 women over the age of 50 with normal pregnancy; the oldest was said to be 63. The paucity of reports of pregnancy in women of advanced age is probably an underestimate of the prevalence, but it nevertheless indicates the rarity of pregnancy in the sixth decade of life. In New York City pregnancy beyond the age of 50 occurs approximately only once in every 50,000 births. Although it has been predicted by some that long-term suppression of ovulation by oral contraceptives could theoretically result in continued ovulation for years after the usual time of menopause, there is no evidence thus far of such a phenomenon.

UTERUS

One of the several unique features of the uterus is its profound ability to increase in size and capacity in a few months and then to return essentially to its original state within a few weeks. As the consequence of normal intrauterine pregnancy the almost solid uterus, approximately 7 cm in length, is converted into a thin-walled muscular sac of sufficient capacity to contain the fetus, placenta, and amniotic fluid. The total volume of the contents averages about 5 liters but may be as much as 10 liters or more. By the end of pregnancy the uterus is about 35 cm long and 500 to 1,000 times greater in capacity. A corresponding increase in weight converts the body of the uterus at term to an organ weighing approximately 1,100 g, as compared with about 60 g in the nonpregnant state. Hytten noted the weight of the uterus at term to range from 800 to 1,200 g, without precise correlation between the weight of the uterus and the weight of the contained fetus, however.

Uterine enlargement during pregnancy involves both stretching and marked hypertrophy of preexisting muscle cells; the contribution of new muscle cells is probably quite limited. At parturition a single myometrial cell is about 500 microns in length, with the nucleus eccentrically placed in the thickest part of the cell. The cell is surrounded by an irregular array of collagen fibrils. The force of contraction is transmitted from the contractile protein of the muscle cell to the surrounding connective tissue via the reticulum of collagen (Carsten). Accompanying the increase in size of the muscle cells is the accumulation of fibrous tissue, particularly in the external muscular layer, and a considerable increase in elastic tissue. The network thus formed adds materially to the strength of the uterine wall. There is concomitantly a great increase in the size of the blood vessels and lymphatics, particularly the veins, which, at the placental site, are converted into the large uterine sinuses. Hypertrophy of the nerve supply of the uterus also takes place, exemplified by the increase in size of Frankenhäuser's cervical ganglion from 2 by 2.5 cm to 3.5 by 6 cm.

During the first few months of pregnancy, hypertrophy of the uterine wall is probably stimulated chiefly by estrogen and perhaps progesterone (Fig. 1).

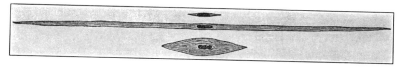

Fig. 1. Schematic drawing showing relative sizes and shapes of muscle cells from non-pregnant, and puerperal uterus. (From Stieve. Z Mikr Anat Forsch 6:351, 1926.)

That the early hypertrophy is not the direct mechanical result of the products of conception within the uterus is shown by the occurrence of similar uterine changes when the ovum is implanted in the fallopian tube or ovary. After the third month, however, the increase in size is in part mechanical, the effect of pressure exerted by the expanding products of conception.

During the first few months of pregnancy the uterine walls are considerably thicker than in the nonpregnant state, but as gestation advances they gradually thin. At term the walls of the uterine corpus are rarely greater than 5 mm in thickness. Early in pregnancy the organ loses the firmness and resistance characteristic of the nonpregnant condition; in the later months it changes into a muscular sac with thin, soft, readily indentable walls, as demonstrated by the ease with which the fetus may usually be palpated through the abdominal wall in the later months and by the readiness with which the uterine walls yield to the movements of the fetal extremities.

The enlargement of the uterus is not symmetric but is most marked in the fundus. The differential growth is readily appreciated by observing the relative positions of the attachments of the fallopian tubes and ovarian ligaments. In the early months of pregnancy they are only slightly below the level of the fundus, whereas in the later months they are inserted slightly above the middle of the uterus. The position of the placenta also influences the extent of the hypertrophy, since the portion of the uterus surrounding the placental site enlarges more rapidly.

Arrangement of the Muscle Cells. The musculature of the pregnant uterus is arranged in three strata: an external hoodlike layer, which arches over the fundus and extends into the various ligaments; an internal layer consisting of sphincter-like fibers around the orifices of the tubes and the internal os; and lying between the two a dense network of muscle fibers perforated in all directions by blood vessels. The main portion of the uterine wall is formed by this middle layer, which consists of an interlacing network of muscle fibers between which extend the blood vessels. Each cell in this layer has a double curve, so that the interlacing of any two gives approximately the form of the figure 8. As a result of such an arrangement, when the cells contract after delivery they constrict the vessels and thus act as living ligatures.

The muscle cells composing the uterine wall in pregnancy, especially in its lower portion, overlap one another like shingles on a roof (Fig. 2). One end of each fiber arises beneath the serosa of the uterus and extends obliquely downward and inward toward the decidua, forming a large number of muscular lamellae, which are interconnected by short muscular processes. When the tissue is slightly spread apart, it appears sievelike and, on closer examination, is seen to comprise innumerable rhomboidal spaces (Fig. 3).

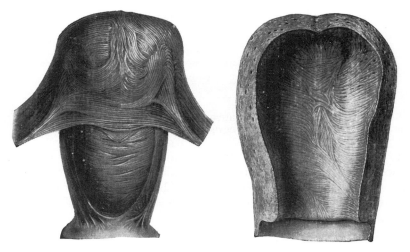

Fig. 2. External and internal muscular layers of pregnant uterus. (From Helie. Recherches sur la disposition des fibres musculaires de l'utérus developpés par la grossesse, Mellinet.)

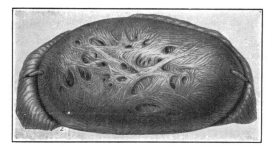

Fig. 3. Median muscular layer of pregnant uterus. (From Helie. Recherches sur la disposition des fibres musculaires de l'utérus developpés par la grossesse, Mellinet.)

Changes in Size and Shape of the Uterus.   As the uterus increases in size it also undergoes important modifications in shape. For the first few weeks its original pear-shaped outlines are retained, but the corpus and fundus soon assume a more globular form, becoming almost spherical at the third month. Thereafter, however, the organ increases more rapidly in length than in width and assumes an ovoid shape.

By the fourth lunar month the uterus is too large to remain wholly within the pelvis, its upper border reaching midway between the symphysis pubis and the umbilicus. As the uterus continues to enlarge, it contacts the anterior abdominal wall, displacing the intestines laterally and superiorly, and gradually rises, reaching ultimately almost to the liver. As the uterus rises, tension is exerted upon the broad ligaments, which partly unfold in their median and lower portions.

The pregnant uterus is rather mobile. With the woman standing, its longitudinal axis corresponds to an extension of the axis of the pelvic inlet; the abdominal wall supports the uterus and, unless quite relaxed, maintains this relation between the long axis of the uterus and the axis of the pelvic inlet. When the woman is supine, the uterus falls back to rest upon the vertebral column.

As the uterus rises out of the pelvis it usually rotates somewhat to the right, thereby directing its left margin more anteriorly. Much less often rotation may occur in the opposite direction. Dextrorotation has been considered to result in large measure from the presence of the rectosigmoid in the left side of the pelvis.

Changes in Contractility. The pregnant uterus manifests two different patterns of increased contractility:

1. From the first trimester of pregnancy onward the uterus undergoes irregular, painless contractions, which in the second trimester may be detected by bimanual examination and, later, by the abdominal hand alone. The previously relaxed uterus transiently becomes firm and then returns to its original state. Since attention was first called to the phenomenon by Braxton Hicks, the contractions have been known by his name. They appear sporadically and are usually nonrhythmic. Their intensity, according to Alvarez and Caldeyro-Barcia, is more than 8 cm of water. Until the last month of gestation *Braxton Hicks* contractions are infrequent. Their frequency increases during the last week or two, when they may occur as often as every 10 to 20 minutes and assume some degree of the rhythmicity. The partly rhythmic Braxton Hicks contractions account for most cases of so-called false labor (pp. 281 and 402).

2. Throughout pregnancy there are very frequent rhythmic contractions of such low intensity that they are not noticed by the pregnant woman or detectable by abdominal palpation. The mechanisms involved in the increased contractility of the uterus as pregnancy progresses are poorly understood. The increase is probably the result of a combination of stretch, increased concentration of actomyosin in the muscle cells (Csapo), and changes in estrogen, progesterone, and electrolytes (p. 450).

Changes in the Spiral Arteries. During the progestational phase of the cycle, the endometrial coiled arteries grow rapidly toward the uterine lumen, at the same time becoming increasingly coiled. Ramsey finds in the monkey that at the time of implantation the arterial tips are still several millimeters below the surface of the endometrium, but approximately a week later the continued growth of the ovum and trophoblastic invasion effect an opening of the maternal arteries into the developing intervillous space of the placenta. Beyond the fifty-third day the spiral arteries fail to increase materially in length, and there is no further significant alteration in their coiling for another five to seven weeks. At the end of that time the vessels undergo an abrupt transition, in the course of which two major qualitative changes occur. First, the coils of the arteries are paid out, and, second, the number of vessels communicating with the intervillous spaces is decreased. After these transformations have been effected, the remaining placental arteries continue unchanged to term, in a smooth, straight, direct course interrupted only by an occasional right-angle bend. It thus appears that the coiling of the arteries is a mechanism that permits the vessels, when they uncoil, to cover the greater distances presented by the enlarged pregnant uterus. Further details of the anatomic changes in uterine blood vessels are found in Chapter 2, p. 37.

Uterine Blood Flow.   The delivery of all substances essential for the growth and metabolism of the fetus and placenta, as well as the removal of all metabolic wastes, is dependent to a very large degree upon adequate perfusion of the placental intervillous space. Placental perfusion by maternal blood depends, in turn, upon blood flow to the uterus through the uterine and ovarian arteries. Assali and associates, as well as Metcalfe and co-workers, used the nitrous oxide method to estimate uterine blood flow in human pregnancy and found that at term the total flow varied between 500 and 700 ml per minute. Browne and Veall arrived at approximately the same values using the rate of disappearance of Na^{24}. Subsequently Assali and his group measured the uterine blood flow between 10 and 28 weeks of gestation in patients undergoing therapeutic abortion. They used, in the same patient, the nitrous oxide technic as well as an electromagnetic flowmeter attached to the uterine artery and found that the total uterine blood flow increased from 50 ml per minute at 10 weeks to 185 ml per minute at 28 weeks. When expressed in terms of unit weight of the uterus, fetus, and placenta, the uterine blood flow remains fairly constant throughout the course of gestation, averaging between 10 and 15 ml per 100 g per minute, depending on the method used. Similar findings have been reported in monkeys (Peterson and Behrman).

Although there is no question, in general terms, about the progressive augmentation of uterine blood flow in pregnancy, Barron has emphasized repeatedly that reported values must be viewed as approximations only, because of inherent errors in the methods of measurement.

The *oxygen consumption* of the pregnant uterus (calculated from the blood flow and the arteriovenous oxygen difference) follows a parallel course, increasing from 5 cc per minute at 10 weeks to 22 cc per minute at 28 weeks. When expressed per unit weight, it remains constant throughout gestation, averaging about 1 cc per 100 g per minute. After delivery of the fetus and the placenta, uterine blood flow falls to an average of 9 ml per 100 g per minute, and oxygen consumption falls to less than 1 cc per 100 g per minute. The blood flow decreases mainly because of an increase in uterine vascular resistance from an average of 6 mm Hg per 100 g per minute during pregnancy to an average of 9 mm postpartum.

Assali and co-workers, as well as others, have studied the effects of spontaneous and oxytocin-induced labor on uteroplacental blood flow in sheep and in dogs at term using electromagnetic flowmeters. They noted that uterine contractions, either spontaneous or induced, result in a decrease in uterine blood flow roughly proportional to the intensity of the contraction. A tetanic contraction caused a precipitous fall in uterine blood flow. Harbert and associates have made similar observations in gravid monkeys.

Obviously a great deal remains to be learned about factors controlling uterine blood flow and effective perfusion of the placenta, including not only the effects of maternal posture, physical activity, and emotional state, but also the impact of maternal diseases and, in turn, the treatment employed. On the basis of very limited studies in animals and even fewer observations in women, it appears that, as a general rule, the pattern of response of uterine blood flow to changes in cardiac output and systemic arterial blood pressure is similar to that of renal blood flow.

Changes in the Cervix.   During pregnancy there are pronounced softening and cyanosis of the cervix, often demonstrable as early as a month after conception, comprising two of the very earliest physical signs of pregnancy. The factors responsible for these changes are increased vascularity and edema of the entire cervix and hypertrophy and hyperplasia of the cervical glands.

As shown in Figures 4 and 5, the glands of the cervical mucosa undergo such marked proliferation that at the end of pregnancy the mucosa occupies approximately one half of the entire mass of the cervix, rather than a small fraction, as in the nonpregnant state. The septa separating the glandular spaces, moreover, become progressively thinner, resulting in the formation of a structure resembling a honeycomb, the meshes of which are filled with tenacious mucus; as a consequence, when the so-called mucous plug is expelled at the onset of labor, much of the endocervix is carried away with it. Furthermore, the glands near the external os proliferate beneath the stratified squamous epithelium of the portio vaginalis, giving the cervix the velvety consistency characteristic of pregnancy.

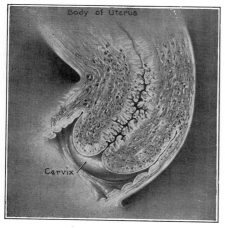

Fig. 4. Cervix in the nonpregnant woman.

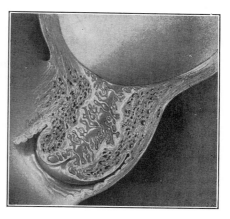

Fig. 5. Cervix in pregnancy. Note the elaboration of the mucosa into a honeycomb-like structure, the meshes of which are filled with a tenacious mucus—the so-called mucous plug.

The abundant endocervical tissue may protrude from the endocervical canal, producing a physiologic *eversion of the cervix.* To cover this exposed glandular epithelium there is often a rapid growth by squamous epithelium over the exposed tissue. This very common process of epidermidization, though by no means specific for pregnancy, is believed to occur more frequently at that time than in the nonpregnant state. There is, furthermore, a change in the pattern of the cervical mucus. In the great majority of pregnant women, cervical mucus spread and dried on a glass slide demonstrates fragmentary crystallization, or "beading," typical of the effect of progesterone (Ch. 4, p. 100). Arborization of the crystals, or "ferning," however, is not necessarily associated with a poor outcome of pregnancy (Salvatore).

So-called *erosions of the cervix* are common during pregnancy. An erosion is customarily defined as a red velvety lesion covered by columnar epithelium and spreading from the external os to involve the portio vaginalis to a varying extent. Although the term "erosion" implies an "eating out" or ulceration of the covering epithelium, the cause in pregnancy is rarely inflammatory. The term refers loosely to the gross manifestation of several different histologic conditions. The high frequency of cervical erosions in pregnancy is best explained on the basis that they represent an extension, or eversion, of the proliferating endocervical glands and the columnar endocervical epithelium.

During pregnancy, basal cells near the squamocolumnar junction of the cervix are likely to be prominent in size, shape, and staining qualities. These changes are considered to be estrogen-induced by most authorities (Hellman and others).

Although the cervix contains a little smooth muscle, its major component is connective tissue. The profound changes that the cervix undergoes during pregnancy, especially during labor, must therefore involve this collagen-rich connective tissue. Danforth and Buckingham have demonstrated an appreciable decrease in the hydroxyproline content of the cervix as pregnancy advances, as well as a marked decrease in the compactness and cohesiveness of the collagen fibers immediately after vaginal delivery. Unfortunately, however, the mechanisms responsible for the orderly effacement and dilatation of the cervix are still poorly understood.

OVARIES AND OVIDUCTS

Ovulation ceases during pregnancy and the maturation of new follicles is suspended. As a rule, only a single large corpus luteum of pregnancy can be found in one of the ovaries. Yoshima and associates noted the level of plasma progesterone to reach a nadir by the eighth week of pregnancy and then to rise again. By contrast, plasma 17-hydroxyprogesterone levels continued to decline to a level only somewhat higher than during the luteal phase. These observations indicate that corpus luteum of pregnancy most likely functions maximally during the first four weeks after ovulation.

In 1963 Sternberg described a solid ovarian tumor that developed during pregnancy and was composed of large acidophilic luteinized cells. The observations of Krause and Stembridge, as well as others, indicate that *luteoma of pregnancy* represents an exaggeration of the luteinization reaction of normal pregnancy and is not a true neoplasm. They noted that the enlargement regressed after delivery, and normal ovarian function returned.

A decidualike reaction on and beneath the surface of the ovaries, similar to that seen in the endometrial stroma, is common in pregnancy and may easily be

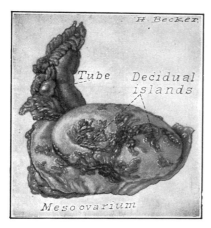
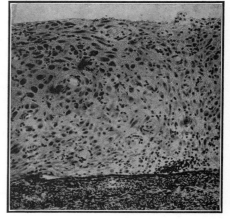

Fig. 6. Left, gross specimen. Right, drawing of the histologic appearance of decidual formation on surface of ovary.

demonstrated at cesarean section (Fig. 6). These elevated patches bleed easily and may on first glance resemble freshly torn adhesions. Similar decidual reactions are occasionally noted on the posterior uterine serosa and upon or within other pelvic and sometimes even extrapelvic abdominal organs.

Simple inspection of the *ovarian veins* at cesarean section reveals their enormous caliber. By actual measurement Hodgkinson has shown that the diameter of the ovarian vascular pedicle increases during pregnancy from 0.9 cm to approximately 2.6 cm at term.

The musculature of the fallopian tubes probably undergoes little or no hypertrophy during pregnancy. The epithelium of the tubal mucosa is flattened during gestation, as compared with the nonpregnant state. Decidual cells may develop in the stroma of the endosalpinx, but a continuous decidual membrane is not formed.

Vagina and Perineum

Increased vascularity prominently affects the vagina. The copious secretion and the characteristic violet color of pregnancy (*Chadwick's sign*), similar to that of the pregnant cervix, probably result chiefly from hyperemia. The vaginal walls undergo striking changes in preparation for the distention during labor, with a considerable increase in thickness of the mucosa, loosening of the connective tissue, and hypertrophy of the smooth muscle cells nearly as great as in the uterus. These changes may combine to produce an increase in length of the vaginal walls to such an extent that sometimes in parous women the lower portion of the anterior wall protrudes slightly through the vulvar opening. The papillae of the vaginal mucosa also undergo considerable hypertrophy, creating a fine hobnailed appearance.

The considerably increased vaginal secretion is normally represented by a thick, white discharge. Its pH varies from 3.5 to 6, as a result of increased production of lactic acid from glycogen in the vaginal epithelium by *Lactobacillus acidophilus*. The acidic pH probably plays a significant role in keeping the vagina relatively free of pathogenic bacteria.

The vaginal epithelial cells early in pregnancy are similar to those in the luteal phase of the menstrual cycle (Ch. 4, p. 103), but as pregnancy advances two patterns of response are seen: (1) Small intermediate cells, called navicular cells by Papanicolaou, are found in abundance in small dense clusters. The ovoid navicular cells contain a vesicular, somewhat elongated nucleus. (2) Vesicular nuclei without cytoplasm, or so-called naked nuclei, are evident along with an abundance of *Lactobacillus vaginalis*, a normal organism in the vagina. Evaluation of the epithelial cells identified in scrapings from the lateral walls of the upper vagina has been considered by some investigators, but certainly not all, to be of value in prognosticating the outcome of pregnancy (Meisels; McLennan and McLennan).

There is increased vascularity and hyperemia involving the skin and muscles of the perineum as well as softening of the abundant connective tissue.

Abdominal Wall

In the later months of pregnancy, reddish, slightly depressed streaks often develop in the skin of the abdomen and sometimes of the breasts and thighs.

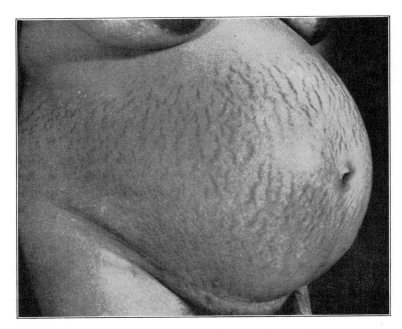

Fig. 7. Primigravida at term, showing striae of abdomen.

These *striae gravidarum* occur in about one half of all pregnancies (Fig. 7). In multiparas, in addition to the reddish striae of the present pregnancy, there are frequently glistening, silvery lines that represent the cicatrices of previous striae.

Occasionally the muscles of the abdominal walls are unable to withstand the tension to which they are subjected, and the recti separate in the midline, creating a *diastasis* of varying extent. In severe cases a considerable portion of the anterior uterine wall is covered by only a thin layer of skin, fascia, and peritoneum. In rare extreme instances herniation of the gravid uterus may occur.

BREASTS

During pregnancy marked changes occur in the breasts. In the early weeks the woman often complains of tenderness and tingling. After the second month the breasts increase in size and become nodular as a result of hypertrophy of the mammary alveoli; as they increase further in size delicate veins become visible just beneath the skin (Figs. 8 and 9). The changes in the nipples and areolae are even more characteristic. The nipples themselves soon become considerably larger, more deeply pigmented, and more erectile. After the first few months a thick, yellowish fluid, *colostrum,* may be expressed from them by gentle massage. At that time the areola becomes broader and more deeply pigmented; the depth of pigmentation varies with the patient's complexion. Scattered through the areola are a number of small elevations, the so-called *glands (follicles) of Montgomery,* representing hypertrophic sebaceous glands. If the increase in size of the breasts is very extensive, striations similar to those observed in the abdomen may develop. Histologic and functional changes induced by pregnancy are discussed further in Chapter 19 (p. 468).

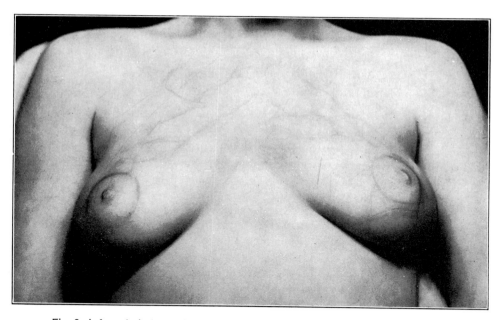

Fig. 8. Infrared photograph of a nonlactating breast in a nonpregnant woman.

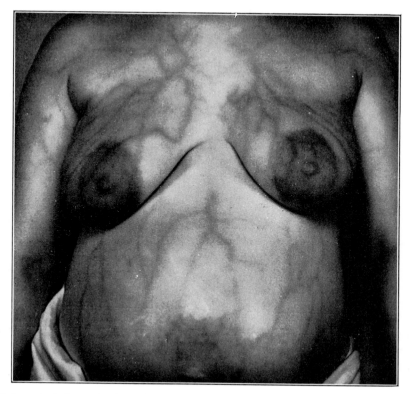

Fig. 9. Infrared photograph of gravida one month before term, showing accentuated venous pattern over breasts and abdomen.

METABOLIC CHANGES

In response to the rapidly growing fetus and placenta with their increasing demands, the mother undergoes metabolic changes that are numerous and intense. Certainly no other physiologic event in postnatal life induces such profound metabolic alterations.

Weight Gain.   One of the most notable alterations in pregnancy is weight gain. Part of the increase in weight is attributable to the weight of the products of conception (fetus, placenta, uterus, and amniotic fluid) and the hypertrophy of the uterus; a smaller fraction of the increase is the result of metabolic alterations, especially retention of water and deposition of some fat and protein. In an exhaustive survey Chesley found that the average total weight gain in pregnancy was 24 pounds. During the first trimester the average gain was only 2 pounds, compared with about 11 pounds during each of the last two trimesters. The individual rates of weight gain varied widely even in completely normal patients, especially in the last trimester; toward term the variability was quite marked.

In the average case at term the fetus weighs 7½ pounds, the placenta a little over 1 pound, the amniotic fluid 2 pounds, and the uterus 2½ pounds. The uterus and its contents thus account for more than half of the increase in weight. The breasts probably increase about 2 pounds, and the blood volume is expanded by about 1,500 ml, or 3½ pounds, leaving only about 5 pounds of the usual total weight gain not readily explained.

Water Metabolism.   Increased retention of water has long been regarded as a characteristic biochemical alteration of late pregnancy. Inasmuch as an exaggeration of this phenomenon to the extent of gross edema is commonly associated with one of the principal complications of gestation, preeclampsia-eclampsia, water metabolism is of importance.

At term the water content of the fetus, placenta, and amniotic fluid amounts to about 3.5 liters. Approximately 3.0 liters more of water accumulate as a result of increases in the maternal blood volume and in the size of the uterus and the breasts. Thus, the minimum of extra water that the average woman could be expected to retain during a normal pregnancy is about 6.5 liters. This value agrees quite well with the results obtained by Hytten and associates, who measured the changes in body water during and after 93 clinically normal pregnancies. They found that in women with no evidence of edema the increase in body water averaged 6.8 liters; in those with edema of the legs it was 7.2 liters. Therefore, as stressed by Chesley and co-workers, it is quite unlikely that normal pregnancy is accompanied by a significant hydration of the maternal tissues.

In considering the retention of water in normal pregnancy it is necessary to differentiate dependent edema of the ankles and legs from generalized edema, latent or manifest. Clearly demonstrable pitting edema of the ankles and legs occurs in a substantial proportion of pregnant women, especially at the end of the day, prior to retiring. It is caused by an increase in venous pressure in the lower extremities, which is a regular accompaniment of gestation, as discussed on page 258. Generalized retention of water, however, is usually not demonstrable clinically except by an increase in weight, although occasionally the patient's fingers will swell and her wedding ring will become tight.

Not all the causes of water retention in pregnancy are definitely known, but the following factors play a role:

1. The Effective Intracapillary Hydrostatic Pressure.   This factor favors filtration from the vascular bed. There is no evidence that increased capillary pressure is a cause of generalized edema in pregnancy. However, in the lower part of the body, below the level of the uterus, venous pressure is appreciably elevated when the patient is erect or supine, but not when lying on her side. The common finding of slight to moderate pedal edema by evening—representing, of course, the accumulation of extracellular fluid—is probably caused chiefly by elevated venous pressure and, in turn, capillary pressure, throughout the day.

2. The Effective Colloidal Osmotic (Oncotic) Pressure of the Plasma.   This factor limits filtration and effects reabsorption of filtered water. Pregnancy is characterized by a diminution in albumin of about 1 g per 100 ml of plasma. As a consequence, the colloidal osmotic pressure of the plasma is diminished by about 20 per cent. As Chesley has noted, although the changes in proteins in normal pregnancy are not sufficiently great to cause edema, they may well lead to some retention of water that would not appear as visible edema.

3. Increased Capillary Permeability.   Capillary permeability may be ascertained either indirectly by measuring the amount of protein in the edema fluid, or directly by the pressure plethysmograph. Using the former method, Dexter and Weiss found that the protein content of the edema fluid in normal pregnancy is less than 0.40 g per 100 ml and concluded that such very low concentrations of protein in the edema fluid indicate conclusively that the permeability of the capillaries to protein is not increased either in the edema of normal pregnancy or in the hypertensive toxemias. Using the pressure plethysmograph, McLennan found, in a small series of patients, that the rate of filtration through the capillary wall is somewhat increased above the normal in the latter weeks of pregnancy. He points out that this may be the result of an increase in permeability of the capillary wall or may possibly be attributable to other factors.

4. Sodium Retention.   Gray and Plentl measured the exchangeable sodium using radioactive sodium (Na^{24}) as a tracer and found that the average increment in exchangeable sodium in the second and third trimesters of nine normal pregnancies was 12 g. That entire amount can be accounted for in the products of conception and in the expanded plasma volume.

On the basis of the predisposing factors just listed, an increase in extracellular water in pregnancy is to be expected, and several studies by various technics indicate an augmentation in extracellular water of about 6 liters by the end of pregnancy (Chesley and co-workers; Seitchik and Alper).

Protein Metabolism.   The products of conception, as well as the uterus and maternal blood, are relatively rich in protein rather than fat or carbohydrate. Nonetheless, their protein content is rather small compared with the total body protein of the mother. The term fetus and placenta weighing about 4 kg contain approximately 500 g of protein or about one half of the total increase normally induced by pregnancy (Hytten and Leitch; Widdowson). Approximately 500 g more of protein are added to the maternal blood in the form of hemoglobin and plasma proteins, to the uterus as contractile and structural protein, and to the breasts, primarily in the glands. Several extensive balance studies carried out in the past seem to indicate that large amounts of protein were stored during pregnancy. It now appears doubtful, however, that any significant maternal storage of protein takes place, apart from what is accounted for by the products of conception, uterus, maternal blood, and breasts (Hytten and Thomson). Dietary protein requirements during pregnancy and lactation are discussed in Chapter 12 (p. 337).

Carbohydrate and Insulin Metabolism.   It has long been recognized that diabetes mellitus may be aggravated by pregnancy and that clinical diabetes may appear in some women only during pregnancy. Consequently, considerable attention has long been focused on the metabolism of carbohydrates and insulin. The concentration of fasting blood sugar is very slightly, but significantly, lower during pregnancy. Silverstone and co-workers noted the average fasting blood sugars of normal women to be as follows: nonpregnant, 66 mg per 100 ml; first trimester, 61 mg; second trimester, 59 mg; third trimester, 60 mg. Quite likely there is increased circulating insulin during pregnancy. Burt, Spellacy and co-workers, and Bleicher and associates have reported that plasma insulin in pregnancy is increased slightly while fasting and that the insulinogenic response to glucose administered intravenously is even greater than when not pregnant, as shown in Figure 10. Although the circulating insulin levels appear to be higher in normal pregnant women, the fall in blood sugar concentration produced by injected insulin is somewhat less than in nonpregnant women, perhaps in part as

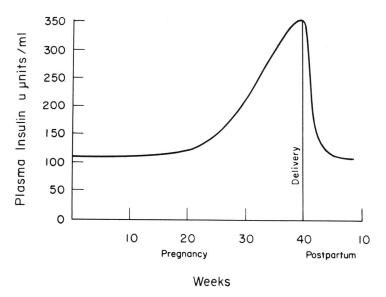

Fig. 10. Diagrammatic summary of the normal pattern of plasma insulin levels measured serially during normal pregnancy using a radioimmunoassay technic and an intravenous glucose stimulus. (From Spellacy, W., in Fetal Homeostasis, Vol. IV, Wynn, R. (ed.). New York, Appleton-Century-Crofts, 1969, p. 108.)

a result of the more rapid enzymatic destruction of insulin by the placenta, as well described by Freinkel and Goodner. Obviously, if during normal pregnancy the levels of plasma insulin are higher and the destruction of insulin is more rapid, the secretion of insulin during pregnancy is increased. Consequently, pregnancy can tax the maternal economy of insulin to the extent that diabetes may first become manifest during pregnancy in women with marginal pancreatic reserve.

Bleicher and associates presented the concept that the lower fasting glucose levels and the higher concentration of plasma free fatty acids normally found in pregnancy result from a state of "accelerated starvation" brought about by the "host-parasite" relation between mother and conceptus. During pregnancy there are safeguards that spare utilization of glucose by maternal tissues while "parasitization" of glucose and gluconeogenic precursors by the fetus continues. The placenta is known to synthesize and secrete a growth-hormonelike substance, chorionic somatomammotropin (p. 175). This hormone promotes lipolysis, brings about an increase in plasma free fatty acids, and provides alternative substrates for the mother. The ability of chorionic somatomammotropin to oppose the action of insulin, coupled with the accelerated degradation of insulin by placental insulinase, leads to increased maternal requirements for insulin during pregnancy.

The effects of the hyperestrogenemia and hyperprogesteronemia of normal pregnancy on metabolism of carbohydrate and insulin are not clear. Progesterone given to monkeys has been shown by Beck to produce a marked increase in the plasma insulin response to intravenous glucose similar to that noted in human pregnancy. Moreover, according to Beck and Wells, the potent synthetic estrogen, mestranol (ethynyl estradiol-3-methyl ether), causes not only an increased plasma insulin response to intravenous glucose but also a decreased sensitivity to the hypoglycemic action of exogenous insulin. Only subjects with limited ability to increase insulin production demonstrated decreased glucose tolerance after mestranol treatment, however, presumably because of failure to compensate for insulin resistance induced by mestranol.

Intravenous glucose tolerance tests commonly used by the clinician fail to demonstrate any distinct differences in the magnitude and duration of the induced hyperglycemia between normal pregnant and nonpregnant women. In oral glucose tolerance tests the hyperglycemia may persist somewhat longer than in normal nonpregnant women, probably because of slower and therefore more prolonged absorption of glucose, although this explanation may be an oversimplification of the problem. The hypoglycemic effect of tolbutamide is not nearly so great in normal pregnant women as in nonpregnant women even though insulin release detectable by immunoassay is appreciably greater (Spellacy and associates). Thus the decreased hypoglycemic effect of tolbutamide in pregnancy results mainly from the increased peripheral resistance to insulin that is induced by pregnancy.

The frequent occurrence during pregnancy of glucosuria is apparently the result, for the most part, of increased glomerular filtration without a comparable increase in tubular reabsorption.

Fat Metabolism.   It has long been recognized that the plasma lipids increase appreciably during the latter half of pregnancy. This increase involves total lipids, esterified and unesterified cholesterol, phospholipids, neutral fat, beta:alpha lipoprotein ratios, and free fatty acids. The magnitude of some of the changes is illustrated in Table 2. The reasons for the hyperlipemia of advanced pregnancy are not known. Starvation induces much more intense ketonemia and ketonuria, moreover, than in nonpregnant women.

Hytten and Thomson have concluded that extensive storage of fat takes place during early and mid pregnancy, the fat being deposited mostly in central rather

Table 2. Changes in Fasting Serum Lipids Induced by Pregnancy*

	Nonpregnant	37–40 Weeks	Per Cent Change
Serum total lipids (mg/100 ml)	711	1039	+46
Serum total cholesterol (mg/100 ml)	178	249	+40
% Esterified cholesterol	74	77	—
Serum phospholipids (mg/100 ml)	256	350	+37
Free fatty acids (µeq/L)	768	1226	+60

* *Data from deAlvarez and from Burt.*

than peripheral sites. They cite some evidence that progesterone may act to reset a "lipostat" in the hypothalamus; at the end of pregnancy the "lipostat" returns to its previous nonpregnant level and the added fat is lost. Such a mechanism for energy storage early in pregnancy, theoretically at least, might protect the mother and fetus at times of prolonged starvation or hard physical exertion. Otherwise, according to some current thinking, such deposition of fat might be undesirable.

Mineral Metabolism.   The requirements for iron during pregnancy are considerable, and often exceed the amounts available (p. 337). With respect to most other minerals, pregnancy induces little change in their metabolism other than their retention in amounts equivalent to those utilized for growth of fetal and, to a lesser extent, maternal tissues (Ch. 7, p. 225; Ch. 12, p. 338). Copper and ceruloplasmin in the plasma increase considerably early in pregnancy, probably because of increased availability of estrogen, which produces the same change when administered to nonpregnant subjects (Russ and Raymunt).

Acid-Base Equilibrium and Blood Electrolytes.   Normally the pregnant woman hyperventilates, compared with the nonpregnant subject, and so causes a respiratory alkalosis by lowering the pCO_2 of the blood. A moderate reduction in plasma bicarbonate from about 25 millimoles to about 22 millimoles per liter effectively compensates for the respiratory alkalosis. As a result there is only a minimal increase in blood pH (Sjöstedt). The concentration of some of the electrolytes and of total protein in the plasma is decreased slightly during pregnancy. The serum osmolality and the concentration of potassium and sodium are reduced about 3 per cent.

The calcium and magnesium levels are reduced very slightly, the reduction probably reflecting for the most part the lowered plasma protein concentration and the consequent decrease in the amount of each electrolyte that is bound to protein. Serum phosphorus levels are within the nonpregnant range.

HEMATOLOGIC CHANGES ASSOCIATED WITH NORMAL PREGNANCY

Blood Volume and Iron Metabolism.   The maternal blood volume increases markedly during pregnancy. In a study of 50 normal women their blood volumes at or very near term averaged about 45 per cent above their nonpregnant levels (Pritchard). The magnitude of this increase is similar to that described by Caton and associates and by Dahlström and Ihrman but is somewhat greater than the increase reported by several earlier investigators. The degree of expansion varies considerably, some women demonstrating only a modest increase and others nearly doubling their blood volume. A fetus is not essential for the development of hypervolemia during pregnancy, for increases in blood volume identical with those found commonly during normal pregnancy have been demonstrated also in some cases of hydatidiform mole (Pritchard). The pregnancy-induced hypervolemia serves to meet the demands of the enlarged uterus with its greatly hypertrophied vascular system, to help protect the mother and, in turn, the fetus against the deleterious effects of impaired venous return in the supine and erect positions, and to help safeguard the mother against the adverse effects of blood loss associated with parturition. The maternal blood volume starts to increase during the first trimester, expands most rapidly during the second trimester, and then rises at a much slower rate during the third trimester, essentially to reach a plateau during the last several weeks of pregnancy. The decrease in late pregnancy described in some earlier studies has not been confirmed (McLennan; Pritchard).

The increase in blood volume results from an increase in both plasma and erythrocytes. The usual pattern is an initial rise in the plasma volume, followed by an increase in the volume of circulating red blood cells. Although more plasma than erythrocytes is usually added to the maternal circulation, the increase in the volume of circulating erythrocytes is considerable, averaging, in the 50 women previously mentioned, about 450 ml of red blood cells, or an increase of about 33 per cent. The importance of this increase in creating a demand for iron is discussed in the following paragraphs. The increase in the volume of circulating red blood cells is accomplished by accelerated production rather than by prolongation of the life-span of the erythrocyte (Pritchard and Adams). Moderate erythroid hyperplasia is evident in the bone marrow, and the reticulocyte count is elevated slightly during normal pregnancy. Manasc and Jepson have identified increased levels of erythropoietin in maternal plasma and urine during pregnancy. They conclude that a major stimulus to erythropoiesis during human pregnancy is increased production of erythropoietin. Jepson and Friesen have reported that chorionic somatomammotropin purified from human placenta increases the incorporation of iron into erythrocytes of polycythemic mice, an effect that was abolished by its incubation with antichorionic somatomammotropin but not with antisheep erythropoietin. The precise roles of these substances in augmenting erythropoiesis during pregnancy await further clarification.

In spite of the augmented erythropoiesis the concentrations of hemoglobin and erythrocytes, as well as the hematocrit, commonly decrease slightly during normal pregnancy. In Sturgeon's careful study, for instance, in which iron was readily available to the mother for erythropoiesis, the hemoglobin concentration at term averaged 12.1 g, as compared with a nonpregnant level of 13.3 g per 100 ml. In a similar study the hemoglobin concentration at term averaged 12.5 g, with a level below 11.0 g per 100 ml in only 6 per cent of the pregnant subjects (Pritchard and Hunt). A hemoglobin concentration much below 11.0 g per 100 ml, especially late in pregnancy, suggests a pathologic process, usually iron deficiency, rather than the mere effect of the hypervolemia of pregnancy (Ch. 27, p. 761).

It is commonly stated that the *total body iron* content averages about 4 g, or slightly more, in the adult. The value, however, applies to normal males. In healthy young women of average size, the body iron content is probably not much more than half that amount. The hemoglobin mass of a woman weighing 60 kilograms with a hemoglobin concentration of 14.0 g per 100 ml is about 450 g (Table 3). Since 1 g of hemoglobin contains 3.4 mg of iron, the total iron in the

Table 3. **Measurements of Hemoglobin Iron and Iron Stores in Ten Healthy Young Women (Never Pregnant and Never Experienced Abnormal Blood Loss)**

	Age	Weight (kg)	Height (inches)	Hgb. Conc. (g/100 ml)	Serum Iron Conc. (µg/ 100 ml)	Hgb. Mass (g)	Hgb. Iron (mg)	Iron Stores* (mg)
Average	23	60	65	14.1	105	443	1,505	347
Range	21–26	49–72	60–68	13.0–15.6	76–132	358–492	1,210–1,670	150–629

* *Iron converted to hemoglobin in response to repeated phlebotomy.*
From Pritchard and Mason. JAMA 190:897, 1964.

circulating hemoglobin is about 1.5 g. Iron stores of normal young women are commonly only about 0.5 g or less (Scott and Pritchard; Pritchard and Scott). As in the male, heme iron in myoglobin and enzymes, and transferrin-bound circulating iron, together total only a few hundred milligrams. The total iron content of normal adult females, therefore, is probably in the range of 2.0 to 2.5 g.

An average increase in the total volume of circulating red blood cells of about 450 ml during pregnancy results in a need for nearly 500 mg of iron, for 1 ml of normal red blood cells contains 1.1 mg of iron. The iron content of the fetus at birth is close to 300 mg (Widdowson and Spray). As shown in Figure 11, about

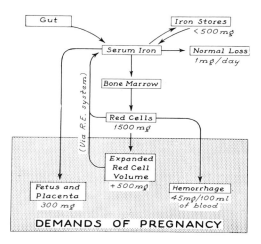

Fig. 11. The iron requirements of normal pregnancy. The 300 mg of iron transferred to the fetus are permanently lost from the mother. The 500 mg incorporated into maternal hemoglobin usually are not all lost; the amount recovered for storage depends upon the amount of blood lost at and after delivery.

800 mg of iron are needed during the antepartum period to meet the fixed iron demands of the fetus and placenta as well as to allow optimal expansion of maternal hemoglobin mass. Practically all of the iron for these purposes is utilized during the latter half of pregnancy. Throughout pregnancy, in the absence of hemorrhage, the pregnant woman probably excretes iron in an amount comparable to that of the male, or about 0.5 to 1.0 mg per day or 200 mg during all of pregnancy. Therefore, although the iron requirements during the first half of pregnancy are slight, they become quite large during the second half, averaging 6 to 7 mg per day. Since these amounts of iron cannot be mobilized from body stores by most women, the desired increase in maternal red blood cell volume and hemoglobin mass will not develop unless exogenous iron is made available in adequate amounts. Instead, as the maternal blood volume increases, the hemoglobin concentration and hematocrit fall appreciably. Hemoglobin production in the fetus, however, probably will not be impaired, since the placenta obtains iron from the mother in amounts sufficient for the fetus to establish normal hemoglobin levels even when the mother has severe iron-deficiency anemia. Iron stores in these newborns, however, might be low.

The amounts of iron absorbed from diet, together with that mobilized from stores, not infrequently fail to supply sufficient iron to meet the demands imposed by pregnancy, even though iron absorption from the gastrointestinal tract appears to be moderately increased during pregnancy (Hahn and associates). Supplemental iron during the latter half of pregnancy, therefore, is valuable, and for several weeks after delivery if the infant is to be breast-fed (Ch. 12, p. 338). Without iron therapy the maternal plasma iron concentration often decreases during pregnancy. Undoubtedly, in most instances, iron deficiency contributes significantly to the fall. The plasma iron-binding capacity (transferrin) increases during pregnancy even in those instances in which iron deficiency has been eliminated by appropriate treatment (Sturgeon). The administration of estrogen to nonpregnant women has been reported by some, but not all, investigators to produce an increase in serum transferrin levels comparable with that of pregnancy (Laurell and associates; Seal and Doe).

Not all of the iron added to the maternal circulation in the form of hemoglobin is lost from the mother. During usual vaginal delivery and through the next few days nearly half of the red blood cells added to the maternal circulation during pregnancy are lost by way of the placental site, the placenta itself, the episiotomy wound and lacerations, and the modest amount in the lochia. On the average, when precisely measured, maternal red cells corresponding to about 600 ml of predelivery blood are lost during and after the vaginal delivery of a single fetus (Newton; Pritchard and associates). The loss associated with the vaginal delivery of twins, however, is about 1 liter, or nearly twice that accompanying delivery of a single fetus. In delivery by cesarean section the loss of red blood cells from the maternal circulation is appreciably greater than in vaginal delivery of a single fetus. In elective repeated cesarean section the loss of red cells and hemoglobin averages nearly twice that in vaginal delivery, or the amount in nearly 1 liter of maternal blood before delivery (Wilcox, Hunt, and Owen; Pritchard). Therefore, depending upon the route of delivery and the number of fetuses, on the average nearly one half to two thirds of the red blood cells added to the maternal circulation during pregnancy will be lost. It is not rare, moreover, for the quantity of red cells lost to equal or even exceed the added volume accumulated during pregnancy.

The general pattern of change in maternal blood volume during labor, vaginal delivery, and the puerperium is as follows: (1) some hemoconcentration during labor, varying with the degree of muscular activity and dehydration; (2) further reduction in volume closely paralleling the amount of blood lost during and soon after delivery; (3) during the first few days of the puerperium little change or slight increase in blood volume, especially if hemoconcentration during labor or blood loss at delivery had been sizable; (4) further reduction in plasma volume to the extent that the maternal blood volume by one week after delivery is only slightly greater than several months later (McLennan and others; Pritchard).

Any excess circulating hemoglobin above the amount normally present in the pregnant state ultimately yields iron for storage. The mechanism is most likely not acceleration of the rate of erythrocyte destruction during the late puerperium, but rather reduced production of new erythrocytes. A similar process follows after a normal nonanemic subject receives transfused cells or when a normal person with polycythemia, induced by high altitude, returns to sea level. There is no evidence of an increased rate of erythrocyte destruction in normal postpartum women with a moderate excess of red blood cells after delivery.

Leukocytes. The blood leukocyte count varies considerably during normal pregnancy (Efrati and associates). It usually ranges from 5,000 to 12,000 per mm³, but during labor and the early puerperium it may become markedly elevated to levels of 25,000 or more. The cause for this marked increase is not known, but the same response is noted during and after strenuous exercise. It probably represents the reappearance in the circulation of leukocytes previously shunted out of the active circulation (Wintrobe). Beginning quite early in pregnancy, activity of alkaline phosphatase in the leukocytes is definitely increased. This observation has resulted in attempts to use measurements of this enzyme in leukocytes as the basis for a pregnancy test. Unfortunately, elevated leukocyte phosphatase activity is not peculiar to pregnancy but occurs in a wide variety of conditions, including most inflammatory states. There is a neutrophilia during pregnancy, consisting predominantly of mature forms; close examination of smears of the peripheral blood, however, not uncommonly reveals an occasional myelocyte.

Blood Coagulation. Several blood coagulation factors are increased during pregnancy. The plasma fibrinogen (factor I) concentration, measured as thrombin-clottable protein in normal nonpregnant women, averages very close to 300 mg and ranges from about 200 to 400 mg per 100 ml. During normal pregnancy the fibrinogen concentration increases about 50 per cent, averaging about 450 mg late in pregnancy, with a range from approximately 300 to 600 mg per 100 ml. The increase in the concentration of fibrinogen undoubtedly contributes greatly to the marked increase in the blood sedimentation rate in normal pregnancy. The increased sedimentation rate, therefore, has no diagnostic or prognostic value when employed for the usual clinical purposes in pregnancy, such as the assessment of the activity of rheumatic heart disease.

Other clotting factors, the activities of which are increased appreciably during normal pregnancy, are factor VII (proconvertin), factor VIII (antihemophiliac globulin), factor IX (plasma thromboplastin component or Christmas factor), and factor X (Stuart factor). Factor II (prothrombin) usually is increased only slightly, whereas factor XIII (fibrin stabilizing factor) is decreased during pregnancy (Kasper and associates; Talbert and Langdell; Coopland and co-workers). The Quick one-stage prothrombin time and the partial thromboplastin time are both shortened slightly as pregnancy progresses. Platelets during normal pregnancy show little change in number per unit volume, appearance, or function. The clotting times of whole blood in either plain glass tubes (wettable surface) or silicone-coated or plastic tubes (nonwettable surface) do not differ significantly in normal pregnant and nonpregnant women. Some, but not all, of the pregnancy-induced changes in the levels of coagulation factors can be induced in part by several of the progestin-estrogen contraceptive tablets currently used (Fletcher and Alkjaersig).

During normal pregnancy maternal plasminogen (profibrinolysin) increases considerably; however, fibrinolytic or clot lytic activity, measured either as the time for clotted whole plasma to dissolve or as the time for the clotted euglobulin fraction from plasma to undergo lysis, is distinctly prolonged compared with that in the normal nonpregnant state. Symptomatic thrombosis is uncommon, however, despite the reduction in blood fibrinolytic activity, the increase in several blood procoagulants, and the increase in stasis of blood in the lower half of the body imposed by pregnancy. Paradoxically, after delivery, at a time when these changes are undergoing reversal, thrombosis and thromboembolism are much more likely to occur (Ch. 35, p. 1001).

Labor and delivery, in common with most physical activity, results in an increase in plasma fibrinolytic activity (Margulis and associates; Ratnoff and co-workers).

There are many important changes involving the heart and the circulation during pregnancy.

Heart. As the diaphragm is progressively elevated during pregnancy, the heart is displaced to the left and upward, while at the same time it is rotated somewhat on its long axis. As a result the apex of the heart is moved somewhat laterally from its position in the normal pregnant state, and an increase in the size of the cardiac silhouette is noted radiologically (Fig. 12). The extent of these changes is affected by the size and position of the uterus, the strength of the abdominal muscles, and the configurations of the abdomen and thorax. Their variability renders difficult the identification of moderate degrees of cardiomegaly by physical examination or simple roentgenographic studies. The physician must, therefore, be cautious in making a diagnosis of pathologic cardiomegaly during pregnancy.

The question whether the heart enlarges at all during normal pregnancy

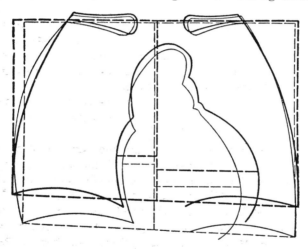

Fig. 12. Change in cardiac outline that occurs in pregnancy. The light lines show the relations between the heart and thorax in the nonpregnant woman, and the heavy lines show the conditions existing in pregnancy. This diagram, which is based on teleoroentgenograms, shows the average findings in 33 women. (From Klaften and Palugyay. Arch Gynaek 131:347, 1927.)

has been debated for over a century. A newer approach to the problem has been the calculation of cardiac volume from frontal and sagittal roentgenograms. The heart is considered to be an ellipsoid, the length, breadth, and depth of which are ascertained from the films, and its volume calculated from these measurements. In several studies the cardiac volume has been found to increase normally by about 75 ml, or a little more than 10 per cent, between early and late pregnancy (Ihrman). Such an increase in cardiac volume might involve slight hypertrophy or dilatation or both.

Some of the cardiac sounds during pregnancy may be altered to the extent that they would be considered pathologic in the absence of pregnancy. Pulmonic systolic murmurs are very common, and apical systolic murmurs are detactable in about one half of normal pregnant women (Burwell and Metcalfe). These murmurs are probably created by the lowered blood viscosity together with the displacement of the heart with resulting torsion of the great vessels. The physician must obviously be cautious in his interpretation of systolic murmurs during pregnancy; diastolic murmurs, however, are pathologic just as in nonpregnant patients. Normal pregnancy produces no changes in the electrocardiogram other than slight deviation of the electrical axis to the left, as a result of the altered position of the heart.

Resting cardiac output varies considerably in pregnancy, depending upon the duration of pregnancy and especially the position of the mother at the time of measurement (Kerr; Lees and co-workers; Ueland and associates). When cardiac output is measured in the lateral recumbent rather than supine position, venous return is not significantly affected by the uterus and its contents, and maternal cardiac output is not reduced. More striking effects of the supine position are described in connection with "postural shock" (p. 689).

Even though cardiac output at rest in the supine position late in pregnancy is only slightly greater than in the nonpregnant condition, identical physical activity late in pregnancy requires more cardiac work than in the nonpregnant state. The pregnancy-induced increase in weight of 20 to 25 pounds, which the pregnant woman must carry, in itself provides an explanation. During the first stage of labor in the supine position maternal cardiac output increases moderately (Ueland and Hansen). During the second stage of labor with vigorous expulsive efforts, the cardiac output is appreciably greater.

The resting pulse rate is moderately increased in pregnancy. During the period when the cardiac output is increased, the stroke volume is appreciably larger than in the nonpregnant condition.

Circulation.   In normal pregnancy the brachial arterial blood pressure shows little change. In Andros' study of 300 cases of normal pregnancy the 661 prepregnancy systolic and diastolic readings averaged 114.6 and 72.6 mm Hg, respectively (pulse pressure 42). In pregnancy the average systolic pressure for the group remained unchanged, and the diastolic pressure was only slightly (3 to 4 mm Hg) below the prepregnancy figure. There is general agreement that normal pregnancy causes no increase in systolic and diastolic blood pressures; any rise of 30 mm or more above preexisting levels, under basal conditions, is therefore indicative of an abnormality, usually preeclampsia (Ch. 26, p. 686).

Several investigators have reported an alteration in the circulation time in normal pregnancy. Cohen and Thomson found the arm-to-carotid time to average 17 seconds in early pregnancy, with a drop to 14 seconds at 24 weeks, and a gradual increase to 16 seconds at term. Manchester and Loube measured the arm-to-tongue, arm-to-lung, and lung-to-tongue circulation times throughout pregnancy and found slight decreases during the third trimester.

As shown by McLennan, the antecubital venous pressure remains constant in pregnancy, but the femoral venous pressure, in the supine position, shows a steady rise from 8 to 24 cm of water pressure at term (Fig. 13). By means of radioactive tracer substances, Wright and co-workers have demonstrated a retardation of blood flow in the legs during pregnancy. This tendency toward stagnation of blood in the lower extremities during the latter part of pregnancy is attributable entirely to the pressure of the enlarged uterus on the pelvic veins and inferior vena

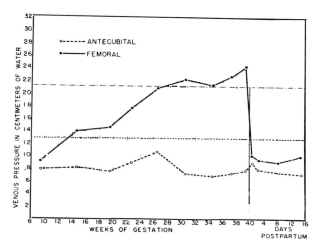

Fig. 13. Plotted are the serial changes in antecubital and femoral venous blood pressure throughout normal pregnancy and early puerperium. These measurements were made on supine subjects. (From McLennan. Amer J Obstet Gynec 45:568, 1943.)

cava, as shown by the fact that the elevated venous pressure returns to normal if the patient lies on her side or immediately after delivery of the infant by cesarean section (McLennan). From a clinical viewpoint the retarded blood flow and increased venous pressure in the legs, which are demonstrable in the latter months of pregnancy, are of great importance. They contribute to the dependent edema frequently experienced by women as they approach term and to the development of varicose veins in the legs and vulva during gestation.

It is now firmly established that in the supine position the large uterus of pregnancy rather consistently compresses the venous system that returns blood from the lower half of the body to the extent that cardiac filling is reduced and cardiac output is decreased. Bieniarz and associates have observed significant changes in arterial pressure caused by compression of the aorta by the enlarged uterus in the supine position. Their studies demonstrate that the usual sphygmomanometric measurement of blood pressures in the brachial artery does not provide a reliable estimate of the pressures in the uterine arteries or others that lie distal to the compression exerted on the aorta by the gravid uterus and its contents. When the mother is supine, uterine arterial pressure is significantly lower than that in the brachial artery. In the presence of systemic hypotension the decrease in uterine arterial pressure is even more marked than in arteries above the level of compression of the aorta. Their observations provide further evidence that the supine position can be deleterious to the mother and the fetus, especially in the presence of other physiologic disturbances, such as those induced by hemorrhage or conduction anesthesia.

Burwell pointed out some similarity between the circulatory changes in arteriovenous fistulas and certain circulatory alterations in pregnancy, which he believed to be caused mainly by the "arteriovenous shunt" created by the placenta and by obstruction of venous return by the enlarged uterus. The circulatory changes in pregnancy similar to those associated with an arteriovenous fistula include the elevated pulse rate, the slightly decreased arterial blood pressure, the elevated venous pressure in the pelvis and legs, the increased blood volume and cardiac output, and the placental murmur or bruit. Current research on placental circulation, however, furnishes no evidence of significant arteriovenous shunts.

Increased cutaneous blood flow in pregnancy serves to dissipate the excess heat generated by the increased metabolism. Burt and more recently Spetz found the blood flow in the hand (chiefly skin) to increase remarkably during pregnancy.

Respiratory Tract

The primary function of the respiratory apparatus, in conjunction with the maternal and fetal circulatory systems, is maintenance of optimal partial pressures of oxygen and carbon dioxide throughout the tissues. Although this balance is usually maintained quite satisfactorily, several aspects of pulmonary function are somewhat modified during normal pregnancy. Since the respiratory rate and the *tidal volume* (the amount of air breathed with an ordinary respiration) are both increased somewhat, the *minute volume* (amount of air ordinarily breathed per minute) is definitely increased. In other words, pregnancy induces a certain degree of hyperventilation. The exact cause is not known, but it probably involves more than increased consumption of oxygen and production of carbon dioxide by the products of conception, for the increase in minute volume is greater than that needed to deliver the extra oxygen, and the maternal pCO_2 is actually lower than in the nonpregnant state. Progesterone has been shown to lower blood pCO_2, possibly by increasing the sensitivity of the respiratory center to stimulation by carbon dioxide.

The diaphragm is elevated during pregnancy, chiefly by the enlarging uterus. At the same time the thoracic cage expands through flaring of the ribs, its transverse diameter increasing about 2 cm and its circumference about 6 cm. The expansion is presumably a result of increased mobility of the rib attachments, similar to the condition elsewhere in the skeletal system during pregnancy. The elevation of the diaphragm causes a decrease in pulmonary *functional residual capacity* (the volume occupied by the lungs at the end of a normal expiration). This change is quite similar to that produced by pneumoperitoneum, a procedure formerly used extensively in the treatment of pulmonary tuberculosis. The *vital capacity* and the *maximum breathing capacity*, a more important index of ventilatory function, are not significantly altered by normal pregnancy. Gee and associates have investigated several aspects of pulmonary mechanics during pregnancy and have obtained the following results: *lung compliance* was unaffected by pregnancy; *total pulmonary resistance* was reduced about 50 per cent during pregnancy; and *airway conductance* was increased during pregnancy. The mechanism responsible for the increase in airway conductance during pregnancy was not identified by Gee and associates; they speculated that progesterone might modify bronchomotor tone.

Gastrointestinal Tract

As pregnancy progresses, the stomach and intestines are displaced by the enlarging uterus. As the result of the positional changes in these viscera the physical findings in certain diseases are altered. The appendix, for instance, is usually moved upward and somewhat laterally as the uterus increases in size.

The gastric secretions and gastrointestinal motility are altered to a variable extent. Strauss and Castle noted a frequent reduction in free hydrochloric acid and pepsin secretion during pregnancy, but Clark and Tankel found no such reduction in free hydrochloric acid. Gryboski and Spiro, furthermore, detected no reduction in blood pepsin, an index of pepsin secretion. Heartburn, common during pregnancy, is most likely caused by reflux of acidic secretions into the lower esophagus, the altered position of the stomach probably contributing to its frequent occurrence. There are usually decreased tone and motility of the gastrointestinal tract, which lead to prolongation of the times of gastric emptying and intestinal transit. The large amounts of progesterone produced by the placenta contribute to the generalized relaxation of smooth muscle characteristic of pregnancy. The gastrointestinal tract is affected, as well as the uterus, ureters, and blood vessels.

The gums may become hyperemic and softened during pregnancy to the extent that they bleed when mildly traumatized, as with a toothbrush. A focal, highly vascular swelling of the gums, the so-called epulis of pregnancy (Fig. 14),

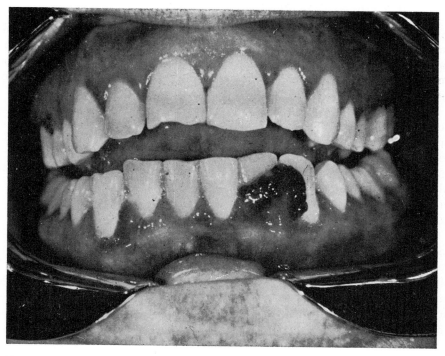

Fig. 14. Pregnancy epulis, a benign vascular lesion that may bleed vigorously if traumatized. After pregnancy it usually regresses spontaneously. (Courtesy of Dr. Robert Walker.)

occasionally develops but typically regresses spontaneously after delivery. Hemorrhoids are fairly common during pregnancy; they are caused in large measure by the elevated pressure in veins below the level of the enlarged uterus.

LIVER AND GALLBLADDER

Histologic studies of liver obtained by biopsy, including examination with the electron microscope, have demonstrated no distinct changes as the consequence of normal pregnancy (Ingerslev and Teilum; Adams and Ashworth). The very few measurements of hepatic blood flow during pregnancy are in conflict, although there may perhaps be a slight increase. Some of the laboratory tests commonly used to evaluate hepatic function, however, yield appreciably different results during normal pregnancy. Moreover, the changes induced by pregnancy often occur in the same direction as those found in patients with hepatic disease.

Nonspecific alkaline phosphatase activity in serum approximately doubles during normal pregnancy and commonly reaches levels that would be considered abnormal in the nonpregnant woman. Much of the increase is attributable to alkaline phosphatase isozymes from the placenta (Birkett and associates). Whether all of the increase is due to enzymes of placental origin is not clear, since nonpregnant women given estrogen in amounts comparable with those found in pregnancy frequently demonstrate increased serum alkaline phosphatase activity (Song and Kappas). Serum cholinesterase activity is reduced during normal pregnancy, as it is in certain liver diseases. The magnitude of the decrease is about the same as that of the concentration of albumin in the serum, namely, about 25 per cent (Pritchard). Recently Mendenhall, as part of a study of the effects of pregnancy on several serum proteins, confirmed the decrease in serum albumin concentration, showing it to average 3.0 g per 100 ml late in pregnancy compared with 4.3 g in nonpregnant women. The reduction in serum albumin, combined with a slight increase in globulins that occurs normally during pregnancy, results in a decrease in the albumin-globulin ratio similar to that in certain hepatic diseases.

Leucine aminopeptidase activity is markedly elevated in serum from pregnant women; at term it reaches a level approximately three times the nonpregnant value. The increase in total serum leucine aminopeptidase activity during pregnancy results from the appearance of a pregnancy-specific enzyme (or enzymes) with distinct substrate specificities (Song and Kappas). The pregnancy-induced aminopeptidase has oxytocinase activity and has been called cystine aminopeptidase by Page and co-workers. The site of origin of the enzymes with high activity for oxytocin is not clear.

Combes and associates have demonstrated that the capacity of the liver for secreting sulfobromophthalein into bile is somewhat decreased during normal pregnancy, while, at the same time, the ability of the liver to extract and store sulfobromophthalein is increased. The administration of estrogens to nonpregnant women induces comparable changes (Mueller and Kappas). Spider nevi and palmar erythema, both of which occur in patients with liver disease, are commonly found in normal pregnant women, most probably as a result of the increased circulating estrogens during pregnancy, but they disappear soon after delivery (Bean and associates).

Gallbladder function is altered during pregnancy. Potter noted that quite often the gallbladder at the time of cesarean section is distended but hypotonic; moreover, aspirated bile was quite thick. It is commonly accepted that pregnancy predisposes to formation of gallstones.

URINARY SYSTEM

Striking changes in both structure and function take place in the urinary tract during normal pregnancy.

Kidney. Glomerular filtration (GFR) and renal plasma flow (RPF) increase early in pregnancy, the former as much as 50 per cent by the beginning of the second trimester, and the latter not quite so much (Chesley; Sims). The elevated GFR has been found by most investigators to persist almost to term, whereas the RPF decreases toward the nonpregnant range during the third trimester. Most studies of renal function carried out during pregnancy, however, have been performed while the subjects were supine, a position that late in pregnancy can produce marked systemic hemodynamic changes and alter several aspects of renal function, as described on page 258. Late in pregnancy, for instance, urinary flow and sodium excretion are grossly affected by posture, averaging less than half the rate of excretion in the supine, as compared with the lateral recumbent, position (Hendricks and Barnes; Pritchard and associates; Chesley and Sloan). The release of antidiuretic hormone (ADH) has been suggested by some as playing a role, but ADH is not essential, since postural changes have produced similar reductions in a pregnant woman with severe diabetes insipidus (Whalley and co-workers). Nor is aldosterone essential, since women late in pregnancy with either severe Addison's disease or bilateral adrenalectomy also develop marked oliguria with a comparable decrease in sodium excretion when supine (Whalley and co-workers). The GFR and RPF, moreover, commonly are somewhat lower if measured in the same patient in the supine rather than the lateral recumbent position (Chesley and Sloan). In the standing position, urinary flow, sodium excretion, GFR, and RPF may be reduced even further. The major cause of these changes in function in the supine position is most likely the reduced venous return to the heart, the result of obstruction of the inferior vena cava and iliac veins by the large pregnant uterus and the consequent reduction in cardiac output and, in turn, lowering of RPF and GFR.

The results of several of the tests of renal function used clinically may be altered by normal pregnancy. The concentrations of creatinine and urea in pregnancy decrease as a consequence of the increased GFR. At times the urea concentration may be so low as to suggest impaired hepatic synthesis, as sometimes occurs with severe liver disease. Urine concentration tests may yield misleading results. During the day pregnant women tend to accumulate water in the form of dependent edema (see p. 258), and at night, while recumbent, they mobilize this fluid and excrete it via the kidneys. This reversal of the usual nonpregnant diurnal pattern of urinary flow causes not only nocturia but the excretion of urine more dilute than in the nonpregnant state. Failure, therefore, to excrete a concentrated urine after withholding fluids for approximately 18 hours does not mean renal damage. The kidney, in fact, in these circumstances functions perfectly normally by excreting mobilized extracellular fluid of relatively low osmolality.

Dye excretion tests, such as the timed measurement of the amount of injected phenolsulfonphthalein (PSP) excreted in the urine, may yield grossly misleading results. At low rates of urinary flow the dye may very well be excreted by the kidney but not collected and measured because of stagnation of urine in the considerably dilated renal pelves and ureters. The dead space of the urinary tract has been estimated to be doubled in the latter half of pregnancy (Longo and Assali). For the same reason all measurements of renal clearance should be carried out only when the urinary flow is relatively constant.

Anatomic changes in the kidney during normal pregnancy are limited to hydronephrosis, as described subsequently.

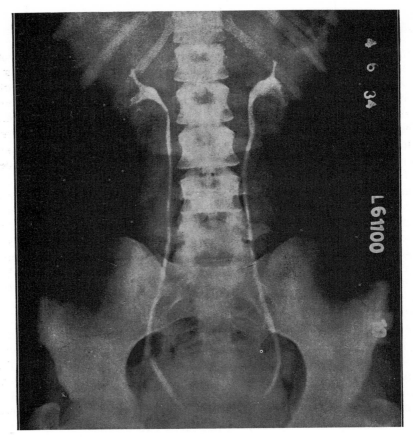

Fig. 15. Pyeloureterogram following intravenous injection of contrast material; normal nulligravida.

Glucosuria during pregnancy is not necessarily pathologic. The appreciable increase in glomerular filtration without an increase in tubular reabsorptive capacity for filtered glucose accounts in most cases for the glucosuria. Chesley has calculated that for these reasons alone about one sixth of all pregnant women should spill glucose in the urine. Even though glucosuria is common during pregnancy, the possibility of diabetes mellitus cannot be ignored. Patients with glucose in the urine should therefore be evaluated for abnormal glucose metabolism. Proteinuria does not normally occur during pregnancy except occasionally in slight amounts during or soon after vigorous labor. If not the result of contamination during collection, blood cells in the urine during pregnancy indicate disease somewhere in the urinary tract. Difficult labor and delivery, of course, can cause hematuria as the consequence of trauma to the lower urinary tract.

Ureters. Various theories have been advanced to explain the long-known dilatation of the ureters and renal pelves during pregnancies (Figs. 15 and 16). The predominating factor was formerly believed to be compression of the ureter at the pelvic brim by the pregnant uterus, with damming back of urine; that theory, however, did not explain why dilatation usually commences about the fourth month, at which time the uterus cannot exert much pressure. It did not, moreover, account for the observations of Van Wagenen, who demonstrated that in the monkey the ureters continued to dilate after removal of the fetus with the placenta remaining in situ. A major causative mechanism therefore seems to be hormonal, predominantly an effect of progesterone, with ureteral compression, especially at the pelvic brim, enhancing the dilatation. Typically, ureteral dilatation is more marked on the right side. The unequal degrees of dilatation may result from a cushioning provided the left ureter by the sigmoid and perhaps from some compression of the right ureter as the consequence of dextrorotation of the uterus.

In women, as the uterus and its contents begin to fill much of the abdomen and rest upon the ureters, especially at the pelvic brim, ureteral compression can be demonstrated. Rubi and Sala, for example, demonstrated increased intraureteral tonus above the level of the pelvic rim compared with that of the pelvic portion of the ureter. Moreover, when pregnant women lie in the lateral recumbent position, the tonus of the dependent ureter beneath the pregnant uterus is appreciably higher than on the other side. No such differences were demonstrable in nonpregnant women.

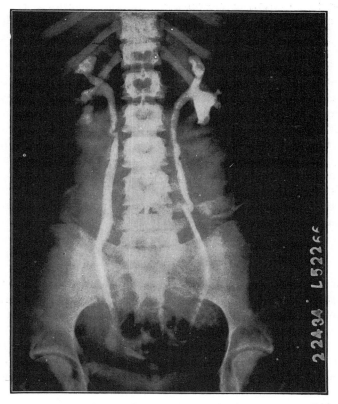

Fig. 16. Intravenous pyelogram illustrating the changes in the ureter usually associated with pregnancy. The kidneys are normal. Both ureters are dilated and elongated, the right more than the left. They are also displaced laterally. These changes may be considered normal during the latter half of pregnancy.

Elongation accompanies distention of the ureter, which is frequently thrown into curves of varying size, the smaller of which may be sharply angulated, producing, at least theoretically, partial or complete obstruction. These so-called kinks are poorly named, since the term connotes obstruction. They are in fact, in a large majority of cases, merely single or double curves, which when viewed in the roentgenogram taken in the same plane as the curve appear as more or less acute angulations of the ureter. Another exposure at right angles nearly always reveals them to be more gentle curves rather than kinks. The ureter, in both its abdominal and pelvic portions, undergoes not only elongation but frequently lateral displacement by the pressure of the enlarged uterus.

After delivery, resolution occurs so rapidly in normal women that in four to six weeks the urinary tract has returned to pregestational dimensions. The stretching and dilatation do not continue long enough to impair permanently the elasticity of the ureter unless infection supervenes or the pregnancies follow in such rapid succession that involutional changes are not completed before the process is repeated. These changes induced by pregnancy have been reviewed by Fainstat.

Bladder. There are few significant changes in the bladder before the fourth month of pregnancy. From that time onward, however, the increase in size of the uterus, together with the hyperemia affecting all pelvic organs and the definite hyperplasia of the muscle and connective tissue, elevates the trigone and causes thickening of its posterior, or interureteric, margin. Continuation of the process to the end of pregnancy produces a marked deepening and widening of the trigone. The vesical mucosa undergoes no change other than an increase in the size and tortuosity of its blood vessels. Toward the end of pregnancy, particularly in primigravidas in whom the presenting part often engages before the onset of labor, the entire base of the bladder is pushed forward and upward, converting the normal convex surface into a concavity, as viewed through the cystoscope. As a result, difficulties in diagnostic and therapeutic procedures are greatly increased. In addition, the pressure of the presenting part impairs the drainage of blood and lymph from the base of the bladder, often rendering the area edematous, easily traumatized, and more susceptible to infection. Normally there is no residual urine in primigravidas, but occasionally it develops in the multipara with relaxed vaginal walls and cystocele. Incompetence of the ureterovesical valve may supervene, with the consequent probability of vesicoureteral reflux of urine, as Lund and co-workers have demonstrated with cinefluoroscopy.

ENDOCRINE GLANDS

Some of the most important endocrine changes of pregnancy have already been discussed—namely, the production of estrogens, progesterone, chorionic gonadotropin, and chorionic somatomammotropin by the placenta (Ch. 6, pp. 173 to 177).

Pituitary. The pituitary enlarges somewhat during pregnancy. There are suggestions that it may increase in size sufficiently to compress the optic chiasma and reduce the visual fields. Such visual changes during normal pregnancy are either absent or minimal.

Although chorionic somatomammotropin is abundant in the pregnant woman's blood, the level of pituitary somatomammotropin (growth hormone) is decreased markedly. After delivery, the hormone of chorionic origin rapidly disappears, but the pituitary hormone remains quite low for some time (Spellacy and Buhi). The relative lack of these hormones with the loss of their "anti-insulin" effects may account in part for the usually abrupt and rather marked reduction in insulin requirements of women with diabetes during the early puerperium. The pituitary gland is not essential for the maintenance of pregnancy, however (Little and associates; Kaplan). Women who have undergone hypophysectomy have successfully completed pregnancy and undergone spontaneous labor while receiving corticosteroids along with thyroid hormone and vasopressin. Extensive destruction of both the maternal and the fetal pituitary glands carried out on monkeys during the second trimester by Hutchinson and co-workers failed to interrupt gestation. The absence of marked maternal adrenal atrophy suggests that in these primates the placenta might be the source of an adrenal weight-maintaining hormone, perhaps chorionic somatomammotropin. Although it has been long known that extracts of human placenta injected into hypophysectomized rats will maintain the animal's adrenal weight, there is no good evidence that the extract increases the adrenal secretion of corticosteroids (Cater and Stack-Dunn).

Thyroid. During pregnancy there is moderate enlargement of the thyroid, usually detected by palpation. It is caused by hyperplasia of the glandular tissue and increased vascularity. The *basal metabolic rate* (BMR) progressively increases during normal pregnancy to as high as +25 per cent. Most of this increase in oxygen consumption, however, is the result of the metabolic activity of the products of conception. As shown by Sandiford and Wheeler, if the body surface of the fetus is considered along with that of the mother, the predicted and the measured basal metabolic rates are quite similar.

Beginning as early as the second month of pregnancy the concentration of thyroid hormone, measured as either protein-bound iodine (PBI), butanol-extractable iodine (BEI), or thyroxin, rises sharply in the mother's plasma to a plateau, which is maintained until after delivery. The plateau is reached at from 7 to 12 μg per 100 ml of PBI, as compared with 4 to 8 μg in nonpregnant euthyroid women (Man and associates; Singh and Morton). Such an elevation of circulating thyroid hormone incorrectly suggests an overtly hyperthyroid state during pregnancy. During pregnancy the *thyroxin-binding proteins* of plasma, principally an alpha globulin, are considerably increased. Although the total concentration of hormone is therefore elevated, the amount of unbound, or effective, hormone is not appreciably higher. As shown by Russell and co-workers, the augmentation in the thyroid-binding capacity of maternal serum proteins is approximately 100 per cent, whereas the increase in PBI is only about 50 per cent. The increase in circulating estrogen during pregnancy presumably is the major cause of these changes in circulating thyroxin and binding capacity, for they can be reproduced by administering estrogen, including most oral contraceptives, to a nonpregnant woman. Although the early increase in PBI and thyroid-binding globulin is sometimes absent in women destined to abort, the abortion almost certainly is not the result of failure of the PBI and binding protein to increase, but rather is the consequence of low estrogen production by a faulty conceptus.

During pregnancy there is increased uptake of ingested radioiodide by the maternal thyroid gland, again suggesting a hyperthyroid state. Aboul-Khair and associates, however, claim that although the clearance of inorganic iodine is increased by the thyroid gland during pregnancy, the absolute uptake is not increased. They conclude that the goiter of pregnancy simply reflects and compensates for the lower concentration of circulating iodide available for synthesis of thyroxin. Hershman and Starnes, however, have recently identified a thyrotropic substance obtained from human placenta; its role in thyroid function during pregnancy is not clear at this time (Ch. 6, p. 173).

In 1957 Hamolsky and associates reported that the in vitro uptake of radioactive triiodothyronine by red blood cells was increased during incubation with serum from hyperthyroid subjects but was decreased if the serum came from hypothyroid or pregnant patients; furthermore, the administration of estrogen lowered the uptake of radioactive iodine. The decreased uptake by the red blood cells both in pregnancy and following administration of estrogen is clearly the result of increased binding of the triiodothyronine to serum proteins. The change in uptake is similar in its time of appearance to that of the PBI, but in the opposite direction. In Table 4 the pregnancy-induced changes are compared with

Table 4. Comparison of Effects of Pregnancy and of Estrogen Administration on Tests Used to Evaluate Thyroid Function

	Normal Pregnancy	Estrogen Administration	Hyperthyroidism
Basal metabolic rate	Increased	Not increased	Increased
Protein-bound iodine	Increased	Increased	Increased
Thyroxin-binding globulin	Increased	Increased	Not increased
Unbound thyroxin	Not increased	Not increased	Increased
% Radioiodine uptake	Increased	Not increased	Increased
Absolute iodine uptake	Not increased	Not increased	Increased
RBC triiodothyronine uptake	Decreased	Decreased	Increased
Serum cholesterol level	Increased	Variable	Decreased

those found in hyperthyroidism and those induced by administration of estrogen. PBI, thyroxin-binding capacity, and red cell triiodothyronine uptake values in cord serum are less than those in maternal serum but greater than the nonpregnant levels (Russell).

Parathyroids.   Little is known about parathyroid function during pregnancy, and the status of parathormone secretion is not clear. In general, the level of ionized calcium in the blood provides a basis for a feedback mechanism regulating the secretion of the hormone. When the level of ionized calcium is reduced, hormone secretion is increased; but during normal pregnancy, the level of maternal circulating ionized calcium is not appreciably lower than in the nonpregnant state. However, in pregnant women on quite low intakes of calcium, secondary hyperparathyroidism is an important physiologic adjustment for maintaining homeostasis in the mother and the fetus. Hyperparathyroidism is more common in women than in men, but whether pregnancy in some way predisposes to its development is not known.

Adrenal.   In normal pregnancy there is probably very little morphologic change in the maternal adrenal. There is a considerable increase in the concentration of circulating *cortisol,* but much of it is bound by the protein *transcortin.* Nonetheless, according to Doe and associates, the amounts of nonprotein-bound, physiologically active hormone is somewhat greater during pregnancy. The rate of secretion of cortisol by the maternal adrenal is not greater and is probably even lower than in the nonpregnant state. The rate of metabolism of cortisol is lower during pregnancy, as indicated by a half-life of intravenously injected labeled cortisol nearly twice as long as in nonpregnant women (Migeon, Bertrand, and Wall). Administration of estrogen, including that in most oral contraceptives, causes changes in levels of cortisol and transcortin similar to those of pregnancy.

The adrenal as early as the fifteenth week of normal pregnancy secretes considerably increased amounts of *aldosterone.* By the third trimester about 1 mg per day is secreted. If sodium intake is restricted, aldosterone secretion is even further elevated (Watanabe and co-workers). At the same time, levels of renin,

renin substrate, and angiotensin are appreciably increased, especially during the latter half of pregnancy (Geelhoed and Vander; Massani and associates). The augmented renin-angiotensin system appears to account for the markedly elevated secretion of aldosterone. It has been suggested that the elevated secretion of aldosterone during normal pregnancy affords protection against the natriuretic effect of progesterone (Landau and Lugibihl). Progesterone administered to nonpregnant women promptly causes a marked increase in aldosterone excretion (Laidlaw, Ruse, and Gornall).

As discussed in Chapter 6 (p. 186), the levels of 11-deoxy-17-ketosteroids circulating in maternal blood and excreted in the urine may not be increased during normal pregnancy.

SKIN

The formation of striae and the pigmentation of the nipple and areola are described on pages 246-247. In many cases the midline of the abdominal skin becomes markedly pigmented, assuming a brownish black color to form the *linea nigra*. Occasionally, irregular brownish patches of varying size appear on the face and neck, giving rise to *chloasma* or the "mask of pregnancy," which, fortunately, usually disappears or at least regresses considerably after delivery. Oral contraceptives tend to cause chloasma in these same women. There is very little basic knowledge of the nature of these pigmentary changes, although *melanocyte-stimulating hormone* has been shown to be elevated from the end of the second month of pregnancy until term. Estrogen and progesterone, moreover, are reported to exert a melanocyte-stimulating effect (Diczfalusy and Troen).

Vascular spiders develop in about two thirds of white and approximately 10 per cent of black women during pregnancy, as demonstrated by Bean and colleagues. They are minute, red elevations of the skin, particularly common on the face, neck, upper chest, and arms, with radicles branching out from a central body. The condition is often designated as nevus, angioma, or telangiectasis. Palmar erythema is also frequently encountered in pregnancy, having been observed by Bean and his associates in about two thirds of white and one third of nonwhite women. The two conditions frequently occur together but are of no clinical significance, disappearing in most cases shortly after the termination of pregnancy. The high incidence of vascular spiders and palmar erythema in pregnancy may possibly be related to the hyperestrogenemia.

MUSCULOSKELETAL SYSTEM

Progressive lordosis is a characteristic feature of normal pregnancy. Compensating for the anterior position of the enlarging uterus, it shifts the center of gravity back over the lower extremities. There is increased mobility of the sacroiliac, sacrococcygeal, and pubic joints during pregnancy, presumably as a result of hormonal changes. Their mobility contributes to the alteration of maternal posture, which, in turn, may cause discomfort in the lower portion of the back, especially late in pregnancy. During the last trimester of pregnancy, aching, numbness, and weakness are occasionally noted in the upper extremities, presumably as a result of the marked lordosis with anterior flexion of the neck and slumping of the shoulder girdle, which, in turn, produces traction on the ulnar and median nerves (Crisp and DeFrancesco).

EMOTIONAL CHANGE

Mild emotional changes are common in pregnancy, including the craving for unusual or abnormal articles of diet (pica) (Ch. 12, p. 345). Many women also undergo changes in disposition; in fact, multiparas sometimes recognize the onset of pregnancy by the appearance of changes in personality. In patients with psychopathic tendencies the emotional equilibrium may be disrupted, leading to excitability, depression, or anxiety, and in extreme cases to frank psychosis.

REFERENCES

Aboul-Khair, S. A., Crooks, J., Turnbull, A. C., and Hytten, F. E.   The physiological changes in thyroid function during pregnancy. Clin Sci 27:195, 1964.

Adams, R. H., and Ashworth, C. T.   Personal communications.

Alvarez, H., and Caldeyro-Barcia, R.   Contractility of the human uterus recorded by new methods. Surg Gynec Obstet 91:1, 1950.

Andros, G. J.   Blood pressure in normal pregnancy. Amer J Obstet Gynec 50:300, 1945.

Assali, N. S., Dignam, W. J., and Dasgupta, K.   Renal function in human pregnancy. II. Effect of venous pooling on renal hemodynamics and water, electrolytes and aldosterone excretion during normal gestation. J Lab Clin Med 54:395, 1959.

——— Dilts, P. V., Plentl, A. A., Kirschbaum, T. H., and Gross, S. J.   Physiology of the placenta, in Assali, N. S. (ed.). Biology of Gestation, The Maternal Organism. New York, Academic Press, 1968, Vol. I.

——— Douglass, R. A., Baird, W. W., Nicholson, D. B., and Suyemoto, R.   Measurement of uterine blood flow and uterine metabolism. IV: Results in normal pregnancy. Amer J Obstet Gynec 66:248, 1953.

——— Rauramo, L., and Peltonen, T.   Measurement of uterine blood flow and uterine metabolism. VIII. Uterine and fetal blood flow and oxygen consumption in early human pregnancy. Amer J Obstet Gynec 79:86, 1960.

Barron, D.   First International Conference on Congenital Malformations. Philadelphia, J. B. Lippincott Co., 1961.

Bean, W. B., Cogswell, R., Dexter, M., and Embick, J. F.   Vascular changes of the skin in pregnancy—vascular spiders and palmar erythema. Surg Gynec Obstet 88:739, 1949.

Beck, P.   Effects of gonadal hormones and contraceptive steroids on glucose and insulin metabolism, in Salhanick, H. A., Kipnis, D. M., and Vande Wiele, R. L. (eds.). Metabolic Effects of Gonadal Hormones and Contraceptive Steroids. New York, Plenum Press, 1969.

——— and Wells, C.   Comparison of mechanisms underlying carbohydrate intolerance in subclinical diabetic women during pregnancy and during post-partum oral contraceptive steroid treatment. J Clin Endocr 29:807, 1969.

Beischer, N. A., Evans, J. H., and Townsend, L.   Studies in prolonged pregnancy. I. The incidence of prolonged pregnancy. Amer J Obstet Gynec 103:476, 1969.

Bieniarz, J., Branda, L. A., Maqueda, E., Morozovsky, J., and Caldeyro-Barcia, R.   Aortocaval compression by the uterus in late pregnancy.   III. Unreliability of the sphygmomanometric method in estimating uterine artery pressure. Amer J Obstet Gynec 102:1106, 1968.

Birkett, D. J., Done, J., Neale, F. C., and Posen, S.   Serum alkaline phosphatase in pregnancy: An immunological study. Brit Med J 1:1210, 1966.

Bleicher, S. J., O'Sullivan, J. B., and Freinkel, N.   Carbohydrate metabolism in pregnancy. V. The interrelations of glucose, insulin, and free fatty acids in late pregnancy and postpartum. New Eng J Med 271:866, 1964.

Browne, J. C. M., and Veall, N.   The maternal placental blood flow in normotensive and hypertensive women. J Obstet Gynaec Brit Emp 60:142, 1953.

Burger, K., and Korompai, I.   (The value of the calculation of the end of gestation according to Naegele's rule in light of our present knowledge.) Zbl Gynaek 63:1290, 1939.

Burt, C. C.   Forearm and hand blood flow in pregnancy, in Toxaemias of Pregnancy. Ciba Foundation Symposium, Philadelphia, The Blakiston Co., 1950, p. 151.

Burt, R. L.   Reactivity to tolbutamide in normal pregnancy. Obstet Gynec 12:447, 1958.
———   Plasma nonesterified fatty acids in normal pregnancy and the puerperium. Obstet Gynec 15:460, 1960.
———   Glucose tolerance in pregnancy. Diabetes 11:227, 1962.
Burwell, C. S.   The placenta as a modified arteriovenous fistula, considered in relation to the circulatory adjustments to pregnancy. Amer J Med Sci 195:1, 1938.
——— and Metcalfe, J.   Heart Disease and Pregnancy. Boston, Little, Brown & Co., 1958.
Carsten, M. E.   Regulation of myometrial composition, growth, and activity, in Assali, N. S. (ed.). Biology of Gestation, The Maternal Organism. New York, Academic Press, 1968, Vol. I.
Cater, D. B., and Stack-Dunn, M. P.   Mitotic activity in the adrenal cortex studied in the rat, in Ciba Foundation Colloquia on Endocrinology, London, J. & A. Churchill, 1955, Vol. 8, p. 31.
Caton, W. L., Roby, C. C., Reid, D. E., and Gibson, J. G.   Plasma volume and extravascular fluid volume during pregnancy and the puerperium. Amer J Obstet Gynec 57:471, 1949.
Chesley, L. C.   Weight changes and water balance in normal and toxic pregnancy. Amer J Obstet Gynec 48:565, 1944.
———   Renal function during pregnancy, in Carey, H. M. (ed.), Modern Trends in Human Reproductive Physiology. London, Butterworth, 1963.
——— and Sloan, D. M.   The effect of posture on renal function in late pregnancy. Amer J Obstet Gynec 89:754, 1964.
——— Valenti, C., and Uichanco, L.   Alterations in body fluid compartments and exchangeable sodium in the early puerperium. Amer J Obstet Gynec 77:1054, 1959.
Clark, D. H., and Tankel, H. I.   Gastric acid and plasma-histaminase during pregnancy. Lancet 2:886, 1954.
Cohen, M. E., and Thomson, K. J.   Studies on the circulation in pregnancy. JAMA 112:1556, 1939.
Combes, B., Shibata, H., Adams, R., Mitchell, B. D., and Trammell, V.   Alterations in sulfobromophthalein sodium-removal mechanisms from blood during normal pregnancy. J Clin Invest 42:1431, 1963.
Coopland, A., Alkjaersig, N., and Fletcher, A. P.   Reduction in plasma factor XIII (fibrin stabilizing factor) concentration during pregnancy. J Lab Clin Med 73:144, 1969.
Crisp, W. E., and DeFrancesco, S.   The hand syndrome of pregnancy. Obstet Gynec 23:433, 1964.
Csapo, A. I.   Actomyosin content of the uterus. Nature (London) 162:218, 1948.
Dahlström, H., and Ihrman, K.   A clinical and physiological study of pregnancy in a material from Northern Sweden.   IV. Observations on the blood volume during and after pregnancy. Acta Soc Med Upsal 65:295, 1960.
Danforth, D. N., and Buckingham, J. C.   Connective tissue mechanisms and their relation to pregnancy. Obstet Gynec Survey 19:715, 1964.
deAlvarez, R. R., Afonso, J. F., and Sherrard, D. J.   Serum protein fractionation in normal pregnancy. Amer J Obstet Gynec 82:1096, 1961.
——— Gaiser, D. F., Simkins, D. M., Smith, E. K., and Bratvold, G. E.   Serial studies of serum lipids in normal human pregnancy. Amer J Obstet Gynec 77:743, 1959.
Dexter, L., and Weiss, S.   Preeclamptic and Eclamptic Toxemia, Boston, Little, Brown & Co., 1941.
Diczfalusy, E., and Troen, P.   Endocrine functions of the human placenta. Vitamins Hormones 19:229, 1961.
Doe, R. P., Dickinson, P., Zinneman, H. H., and Seal, U. S.   Elevated nonprotein-bound cortisol (NPC) in pregnancy, during estrogen administration, and in carcinoma of the prostate. J Clin Endocr 29:757, 1969.
Efrati, P., Presentey, B., Margalith, M., and Rozenszajn, L.   Leukocytes of normal pregnant women. Obstet Gynec 23:429, 1964.
Fainstat, T.   Ureteral dilatation in pregnancy. A review. Obstet Gynec Survey 18:845, 1963.
Fletcher, A. P., and Alkjaersig, N.   Thromboembolism and contraceptive medications: incidence and mechanism, in Salhanick, H. A., Kipnis, D. M., Vande Wiele, R. L. (eds.)., Metabolic Effects of Gonadal Hormones and Contraceptive Steroids. New York, Plenum Press, 1969.
Freinkel, N., and Goodner, C. J.   Carbohydrate metabolism in pregnancy.   I. The metabolism of insulin by human placental tissue. J Clin Invest 39:116, 1960.

Gee, J. B. L., Packer, B. S., Millen, J. E., and Robin, E. D.   Pulmonary mechanics during pregnancy. J Clin Invest 46:945, 1967.

Geelhoed, G. W., and Vander, A. J.   Plasma renin activities during pregnancy and parturition. J Clin Endocr 28:412, 1968.

Gray, M. J., and Plentl, A. A.   The variations of the sodium space and the total exchangeable sodium during pregnancy. Amer J Obstet Gynec 71:1165, 1956.

Greenhill, J. P.   Obstetrics, 12th ed. Philadelphia, W. B. Saunders, 1960, p. 108.

Gryboski, W. A., and Spiro, H. M.   The effect of pregnancy on gastric secretion. New Eng J Med 225:351, 1958.

Hahn, P. F., Carothers, E. L., Darby, W. J., Martin, M., Sheppard, C. W., Cannon, R. O., Beam, A. S., Densen, P. M., Peterson, J. C., and McClellan, G. S.   Iron metabolism in human pregnancy as studied with the radioactive isotope Fe^{59}. Amer J Obstet Gynec 61:477, 1951.

Hamolsky, M. W., Stein, M., and Freedberg, A. S.   The thyroid hormone–plasma protein complex in man. II. A new in vitro method for study of "uptake" of labelled hormonal components by human erythrocytes. J Clin Endocr 17:33, 1957.

Harbert, G. M., Cornell, G. W., Littlefield, J. B., Kayan, J. B., and Thornton, W. N.   Maternal hemodynamics associated with uterine contraction in gravid monkeys. Amer J Obstet Gynec 104:24, 1969.

Hélie, Th.   Recherches sur la disposition des fibres musculaires de l'utérus développés par la grossesse.   Nantes, Mellinet, 1864.

Hellman, L. M., Rosenthal, A. H., Kistner, R. W., and Gordon, R.   Some factors influencing the proliferation of the reserve cells in the human cervix. Amer J Obstet Gynec 67:899, 1954.

Henderson, M., and Kay, J.   Differences in duration of pregnancy. Negro and white women of low socio-economic class. Arch Environ Health 14:904, 1967.

Hendricks, C. H., and Barnes, A. C.   Effect of supine position on urinary output in pregnancy. Amer J Obstet Gynec 69:1225, 1955.

Hershman, J. M., and Starnes, W. R.   Extraction and characterization of a thyrotropic material from the human placenta. J Clin Invest 48:923, 1969.

Higgins, L. G.   Prolonged pregnancy. Lancet 2:1154, 1954.

Hodgkinson, C. P.   Physiology of the ovarian veins in pregnancy. Obstet Gynec 1:26, 1953.

Hutchinson, D. L., Plentl, A. A., and Taylor, H. C.   The total body water and the water turnover in pregnancy studied with deuterium oxide as isotopic tracer. J Clin Invest 33:235, 1954.

——— Westover, J. L., and Will, D. W.   The destruction of the maternal and fetal pituitary glands in subhuman primates. Amer J Obstet Gynec 83:857, 1962.

Hytten, F. E., and Cheyne, G. A.   The size and composition of the human pregnant uterus. J Obstet Gynaec Brit Comm 76:400, 1969.

——— and Leitch, I.   The Physiology of Human Pregnancy. Philadelphia, F. A. Davis, 1964.

——— Thomson, A. M., and Taggert, N.   Total body water in normal pregnancy. J Obstet Gynaec Brit Comm 73:553, 1966.

——— and Thomson, A. M.   Maternal physiological adjustments, in Assali, N. S. (ed.), Biology of Gestation. The Maternal Organism. New York, Academic Press, 1968. Vol. I.

Ihrman, K.   A clinical and physiological study of pregnancy in a material from northern Sweden. VII. The heart volume during and after pregnancy. Acta Soc Med Upsal 65:326, 1960.

Ingerslev, M., and Teilum, G.   Biopsy studies on the liver in pregnancy. II. Liver biopsy on normal pregnant women. Acta Obstet Gynec Scand 25:352, 1946.

Jepson, J. H., and Friesen, H. G.   The mechanism of action of human placental lactogen on erythropoiesis. Brit J Haemat 15:465, 1968.

Kaplan, N. M.   Successful pregnancy following hypophysectomy during the twelfth week of gestation. J Clin Endocr 21:1139, 1961.

Kasper, C. K., Hoag, M. S., Aggelar, P. M. and Stone, S.   Blood clotting factors in pregnancy: Factor VIII concentrations in normal and AHF-deficient women. Obstet Gynec 24:242, 1964.

Kerr, M. G.   The mechanical effects of the gravid uterus in late pregnancy. J Obstet Gynaec Brit Comm 72:513, 1965.

Kortenoever, M. E.   Pathology of pregnancy: pregnancy of long duration and postmature infant. Obstet Gynec Survey 5:812, 1950.

Krause, D. E., and Stembridge, V. A.   Luteomas of pregnancy. Amer J Obstet Gynec 95:192, 1966.

Laidlaw, J. C., Ruse, J. L., and Gornall, A. G. The influence of estrogen and progesterone on aldosterone excretion. J Clin Endocr 22:161, 1962.

Landau, R. L., and Lugibihl, K. The catabolic and natriuretic effects of progesterone in man. Recent Progr Hormone Res 17:249, 1961.

Laurell, C. B., Kullander, S., and Thorell, J. Effect of administration of combined estrogen-progestin contraceptive on the level of individual plasma proteins. Scand J Clin Lab Invest 21:337, 1968.

Lees, M. M., Scott, D. B., Slawson, K. B., and Kerr, M. G. Haemodynamic changes during caesarean section. J Obstet Gynaec Brit Comm 75:546, 1968.

Little, B., Smith, O. W., Jessiman, A. G., Selenkow, H. A., Van't Hoff, W., Eglin, J. M., and Moore, F. D. Hypophysectomy during pregnancy in a patient with cancer of the breast. J Clin Endocr 18:425, 1958.

Longo, L. D., and Assali, N. S. Renal function in human pregnancy. IV. The urinary tract "dead space" during normal gestation. Amer J Obstet Gynec 80:495, 1960.

Lund, C. J., Fullerton, R. E., and Tristan, T. A. Cinefluorographic studies of the bladder and urethra in women. II. Stress incontinence. Amer J Obstet Gynec 78:706, 1959.

Man, E. B., Heinemann, M., Johnson, C. E., Leary, D. C., and Peters, J. P. Precipitable iodine of serum in normal pregnancy and its relation to abortions. J Clin Invest 30:137, 1951.

Manasc, B., and Jepson, J. Erythropoietin in plasma and urine during human pregnancy. Canad Med Ass J 100:687, 1969.

Manchester, B., and Loube, S. D. Velocity of blood flow in normal pregnant women. Amer Heart J 32:215, 1946.

Margulis, R. R., Luzadre, J. H., and Hodgkinson, C. P. Fibrinolysis in labor and delivery. Obstet Gynec 3:487, 1954.

Massani, Z. M., Sanguinetti, R., Gallegos, R., and Raimondi, D. Angiotensin blood levels in normal and toxemic pregnancies. Amer J Obstet Gynec 99:313, 1967.

McKeown, T., Gibson, J. R., and Dougray, T. Association between period of gestation and length of menstrual cycle. Brit Med J 2:253, 1953.

McLennan, C. E. Antecubital and femoral venous pressure in normal and toxemic pregnancy. Amer J Obstet Gynec 45:568, 1943.

——— Rate of filtration through capillary walls in pregnancy. Amer J Obstet Gynec 46:63, 1943.

——— Lowenstein, J. M., Sayler, C. B., and Richards, E. M. Blood volume changes immediately after delivery. Stanford Med Bull 17:152, 1959.

——— and Thouin, L. G. Blood volume in pregnancy. Amer J Obstet Gynec 46:63, 1943.

McLennan, M. T., and McLennan, C. E. Failure of vaginal wall cytologic smears to predict abortion. Amer J Obstet Gynec 103:228, 1969.

Meisels, A. Hormonal cytology in pregnancy. Clin Obstet Gynec 11:1121, 1968.

Mendenhall, H. W. Serum protein concentrations in pregnancy. I. Concentrations in maternal serum. Amer J Obstet Gynec 106:388, 1970.

Metcalfe, J., Meschia, G., Hellegers, A., Prystowsky, H., Huckabee, W., and Barron, D. Transfer of oxygen across the sheep placenta at high altitude. Fed Proc 18:104, 1959.

——— Romney, S. L., Ramsey, L. H., Reid, D. E., and Burwell, C. S. Estimation of uterine blood flow in normal human pregnancy at term. J Clin Invest 34:1632, 1955.

Migeon, C. J., Bertrand, J., and Wall, P. E. Physiological disposition of 4-C^{14}-cortisol during late pregnancy. J Clin Invest 36:1350, 1957.

Mueller, M. N., and Kappas, A. Estrogen pharmacology. I. The influence of estradiol and estriol on hepatic disposal of sulfobromophthalein (BSP) in man. J Clin Invest 43:1905, 1964.

Natter, E. C. Pregnancy after fifty. Obstet Gynec 24:641, 1964.

Newton, M. Postpartum hemorrhage. Amer J Obstet Gynec 94:711, 1966.

Page, E. W., Glendening, M. B., Dignam, W., and Harper, H. A. The causes of histidinuria in normal pregnancy. Amer J Obstet Gynec 68:110, 1954.

——— Titus, M. A., Mohun, G., and Glendening, M. B. The origin and distribution of oxytocinase. Amer J Obstet Gynec 82:1090, 1961.

Perr, I. N. Paternity and prolonged pregnancy. Cleveland-Marshall Law Review 8:234, 1959.

Peterson, E. N., and Behrman, R. E. Changes in cardiac output and uterine blood flow of the pregnant *Macaca mulatta*. Amer J Obstet Gynec 104:988, 1969.

Potter, M. G. Observations of the gallbladder and bile during pregnancy at term. JAMA 106:1070, 1936.

Pritchard, J. A.   Changes in the blood volume during pregnancy and delivery. Anesthesiology 26:393, 1965.

———   Plasma cholinesterase activity in normal pregnancy and in eclamptogenic toxemias. Amer J Obstet Gynec 70:1083, 1955.

———   Unpublished observations.

———   and Adams, R. H.   Erythrocyte production and destruction during pregnancy. Amer J Obstet Gynec 79:750, 1960.

———   Barnes, A. C., and Bright, R. H.   The effect of the supine position on renal function in the near-term pregnant woman. J Clin Invest 34:777, 1955.

———   and Hunt, C. F.   A comparison of the hematologic responses following the routine prenatal administration of intramuscular and oral iron. Surg Gynec Obstet 106:516, 1958.

———   and Mason, R. A.   Iron stores of normal adults and their replenishment with oral iron therapy. JAMA 190:897, 1964.

———   and Scott, D. E.   Iron demands during pregnancy, in Iron Deficiency–Pathogenesis, Clinical Aspects and Therapy, London, Academic Press (in press).

Ramsey, E. M.   The vascular pattern of the endometrium of the pregnant rhesus monkey (*Macaca mulatta*). Contrib Embryol 33:113, 1949.

Ratnoff, O. D., Colopy, J. E. and Pritchard, J. A.   The blood-clotting mechanism during normal parturition. J Lab Clin Med 44:408, 1954.

Rubi, R. A., and Sala, N. L.   Ureteral function in pregnant women.   III. Effect of different positions and of fetal delivery upon ureteral tonus. Amer J Obstet Gynec 101:230, 1968.

Russ, E. M., and Raymunt, J.   Influence of estrogens on total serum copper and caeruloplasmin. Proc Soc Exp Biol Med 92:465, 1956.

Russell, K. P., Rose, H., and Starr, P.   Further observations on thyroxine interactions in the newborn at delivery and in the immediate neonatal period. Amer J Obstet Gynec 90:682, 1964.

———   Tanaka, S., and Starr, P.   Thyroxin-binding capacity of serum of mothers and newborn infants after normal pregnancies. Amer J Obstet Gynec 79:718, 1960.

Salvatore, C. A.   Cervical mucus crystallization in pregnancy. Obstet Gynec 32:226, 1968.

Sandiford, I., and Wheeler, T.   Basal metabolism before, during, and after pregnancy. J Biol Chem 62:329, 1924.

Scott, D. E., and Pritchard, J. A.   Iron deficiency in healthy young college women. JAMA 199:897, 1967.

Seal, U. S., and Doe, R. P.   Effects of gonadal and contraceptive hormones on protein and amino acid metabolism, in Salhanick, H. A., Kipnis, D. M., and Vande Wiele, R. L. (eds.). Metabolic Effects of Gonadal Hormones and Contraceptive Steroids, New York, Plenum Press, 1969.

Seitchick, J., and Alper, C.   The estimation of changes in body composition in normal pregnancy by measurement of body water. Amer J Obstet Gynec 71:1165, 1956.

Silverstone, F. A., Solomons, E., and Rubricius, J.   The rapid intravenous glucose tolerance test in pregnancy. J Clin Invest 40:2180, 1961.

Sims, E. A. H.   The kidney in pregnancy, in Strauss, M. B., and Welt, L. G. (eds.). Diseases of the Kidney, Boston, Little, Brown & Co., 1963.

Singh, P. B., and Morton, D. G.   Blood protein-bound iodine determinations as a measure of thyroid function in normal pregnancy and threatened abortion. Amer J Obstet Gynec 72:607, 1956.

Sjöstedt, S.   Acid-base balance of arterial blood during pregnancy, at delivery, and in the puerperium. Amer J Obstet Gynec 84:775, 1962.

Song, C. S., and Kappas, A.   The influence of estrogens, progestins and pregnancy on the liver. Vitamins Hormones 26:147, 1968.

Spellacy, W. N.   Plasma insulin measurements, in Wynn, R. M. (ed.). Fetal Homeostasis. New York, Appleton-Century-Crofts, 1969, Vol. IV.

———   and Buhi, W. C.   Pituitary growth hormone and placental lactogen levels measured in normal term pregnancy and at the early and late postpartum periods. Amer J Obstet Gynec 105:888, 1969.

———   and Goetz, F. C.   Plasma insulin in normal late pregnancy. New Eng J Med 268:988, 1963.

———   Goetz, F. C., Greenberg, B. Z., and Schoeller, K. L.   Tolbutamide response in normal pregnancy. J Clin Endocr 25:1251, 1965.

Spetz, S. Peripheral circulation during normal pregnancy. Acta Obstet Gynec Scand 43:309, 1964.

Sternberg, W. H. Non-functioning ovarian neoplasms, in Grady, H. G., and Smith, D. E. (eds.). International Academy of Pathology Monograph, No. 3, The Ovary, Baltimore, Williams & Wilkins, 1963.

Stieve, H. (The regular alterations of the musculature and connective tissue of the human uterus.) Z Mikr Anat Forsch 6:351, 1926.

Strauss, M. B., and Castle, W. B. Studies of anemia in pregnancy. Amer J Med Sci 184:655, 1932; 185:539, 1933.

Sturgeon, P. Studies of iron requirements in infants. III. Influence of supplemental iron during normal pregnancy on mother and infant. A. The mother. Brit J Haemat 5:31, 1959.

Talbert, L. M., and Langdell, R. D. Normal values of certain factors in the blood clotting mechanism in pregnancy. Amer J Obstet Gynec 90:44, 1964.

Ueland, K., Gills, R. E., and Hansen, J. M. Maternal cardiovascular dynamics. I. Cesarean section under subarachnoid block anesthesia. Amer J Obstet Gynec 100:42, 1968.

———— and Hansen, J. M. Maternal cardiovascular dynamics. II. Posture and uterine contractions. Amer J Obstet Gynec 103:1, 1969.

Van Wagenen, G., and Jenkins, R. H. An experimental examination of factors causing ureteral dilatation of pregnancy. J Urol 42:1010, 1939.

Watanabe, M., Meeker, C. I., Gray, M. J., Sims, E. A. H., and Solomon, S. Secretion rate of aldosterone in normal pregnancy. J Clin Invest 42:1619, 1963.

Wells, S. M. A case of prolonged pregnancy. Guys Hosp Gaz 62:299, 1948, abstracted in Obstet Gynec Survey 4:378, 1949.

Whalley, P. J., Roberts, A. D., and Pritchard, J. A. The effects of posture on renal function during pregnancy in a patient with diabetes insipidus. J Lab Clin Med 58:867, 1961.

———— MacDonald, P. C., and Pritchard, J. A. Unpublished observations.

Wharton, L. R. Normal pregnancy with living children in women past the age of fifty. Amer J Obstet Gynec 90:672, 1964.

Widdowson, E. M. Growth and composition of the fetus and newborn, in Assali, N. S. (ed.). Biology of Gestation, The Fetus and Neonate. New York, Academic Press, 1968, Vol. II.

———— and Spray, C. M. Chemical development in utero. Arch Dis Child 26:205, 1951.

Wilcox, C. F., Hunt, A. B., and Owen, C. A. The measurement of blood lost during cesarean section. Amer J Obstet Gynec 77:772, 1959.

Wintrobe, M. M. Clinical Hematology. Philadelphia, Lea & Febiger, 1961.

Wright, H. P., Osborn, S. B., and Edmonds, D. G. Measurement of the rate of venous blood-flow in the legs of women at term and in the puerperium, using radioactive sodium. J Obstet Gynaec Brit Emp 56:36, 1949, abstracted in Obstet Gynec Survey 4:476, 1949.

———— Osborn, S. B., and Edmonds, D. G. Changes in rate of flow of venous blood in the leg during pregnancy, measured with radioactive sodium. Surg Gynec Obstet 90:481, 1950.

Yoshima, T., Strott, C. A., Marshall, J. R., and Lipsett, M. D. Corpus Luteum function early in pregnancy. J Clin Endocr Metab 29:225, 1969.

9

DIAGNOSIS OF PREGNANCY

The diagnosis of pregnancy ordinarily offers little or no difficulty, and the patient most often is aware of the probability of pregnancy before she consults a physician. In some instances, the task is by no means easy, and a certain diagnosis is occasionally impossible despite all clinical and laboratory aids.

Mistakes in diagnosis are most frequently made in the first few months while the uterus is still a pelvic organ. Although it is possible to mistake a pregnant uterus even at term for a tumor of some other nature, such errors are usually the result of hasty or careless examination. There is hardly a gynecologist of experience who has not opened the abdomen on one or more occasions with the expectation of removing a tumor of the uterus or its appendages only to find a pregnancy.

It is often a matter of considerable importance that a diagnosis be made in the early months of pregnancy, but unfortunately it is just at this period that diagnostic ability is most restricted. It follows therefore that in cases in which a diagnosis of pregnancy might affect the reputation or interests of the patient, a positive expression of opinion should be deferred until the diagnosis is beyond all doubt.

The diagnosis is based upon certain subjective symptoms, certain signs noted on careful physical examination, and laboratory procedures. The signs and symptoms are usually classified into three groups: the positive signs, which cannot usually be detected until after the fourth month; the probable signs, which can be appreciated earlier; and the presumptive evidence, which is usually subjective and may be experienced at varying periods.

Positive Signs of Pregnancy.   These three signs comprise (1) hearing and counting the fetal heartbeat separately and distinctly from that of the mother; (2) perception of active fetal movements by the examiner; (3) recognition of the fetus, radiologically or by sonographic examination.

1. *Fetal Heart.*   Hearing and counting the pulsations of the fetal heart, of course, assure the diagnosis of pregnancy. This sign cannot usually be detected by ordinary auscultation with a head stethoscope until about the twentieth to twenty-second week of gestation. The fetal heart rate normally ranges from 120 to 140 beats a minute and is a double sound resembling the tick of a watch under

a pillow. It is not sufficient merely to hear the fetal heart; it must be proved distinctly different from the maternal pulse. In the early months the fetal heart tones are best heard just over the symphysis pubis, but later the most favorable location varies according to the position and presentation of the fetus.

In recent years several instruments to detect action of the fetal heart have become available that make use of the Doppler principle of a shift in the frequency of sound whenever sound strikes a moving object. Ultrasound is directed toward the moving blood cells; as the sound is reflected by the moving cells it undergoes a shift in frequency, which is detected by a receiving crystal immediately adjacent to the transmitting crystal. Because of the difference in heart rates pulsatile flow in the fetus is easily differentiated from that in the mother. Fetal cardiac action has been detected by the end of the first trimester of pregnancy with commercially available instruments that use the Doppler principle.

The fetal electrocardiogram sometimes can be detected quite early in pregnancy and when clearly identified offers proof of a living fetus. Failure to detect fetal cardiac electrical activity, however, does not exclude pregnancy nor does it necessarily prove that the fetus is dead.

Auscultation of the abdomen in the later months of pregnancy often reveals sounds other than the fetal heart tones, the most important of which are (1) the funic (umbilical cord) souffle, (2) the uterine souffle, (3) sounds resulting from movement of the fetus, (4) the maternal pulse, and (5) the gurgling of gas in the intestines of the mother.

The *funic*, or *umbilical cord*, *souffle* is a sharp, whistling sound, synchronous with the fetal pulse and can be heard in about 15 per cent of all cases. It is inconstant, being recognizable distinctly at one examination and absent on other occasions. It is caused by the rush of blood through the umbilical arteries.

The *uterine souffle* is a soft, blowing sound, synchronous with the maternal pulse, and is usually most distinctly heard upon auscultating the lower portion of the uterus. It is produced by the passage of blood through the dilated uterine vessels and is characteristic not only of pregnancy but of any condition in which the blood supply to the uterus is markedly increased; accordingly, it may be heard in nonpregnant women with large myomas of the uterus or large tumors of the ovaries.

Certain movements of the fetus also may be recognized on auscultation. The maternal pulse can frequently be distinctly heard on auscultating the abdomen, and in some instances the pulsation of the aorta is unusually loud. Occasionally the pulse of the mother may become so rapid during examination as to simulate the fetal heart sounds. In addition to the sounds just mentioned it is not unusual to hear certain others produced by the passage of gases or liquids through the mother's intestines.

2. *Movements of the Fetus.* The second positive sign of pregnancy is detection by the physician of spontaneous movements of the fetus.

After the fifth lunar month the active movements may be felt at intervals by placing the examining hand over the mother's abdomen. They vary from a faint flutter in the early months to brisk motions at a later period, which are sometimes visible as well. Occasionally somewhat similar sensations may be produced by contractions of the intestines or the muscles of the abdominal wall, although they should not deceive an experienced examiner.

3. *Roentgenographic Examination.* Whenever the fetal skeleton can be

distinguished radiologically, the diagnosis of pregnancy is certain. Unfortunately, like the other positive signs, this method of diagnosis is usually not applicable until after the fourth lunar month. By this means Bartholomew and co-workers were able to make a positive diagnosis in one third of their patients at the fifth lunar month, in one half at the sixth lunar month, and in almost all later. Just how early the fetal skeleton will show in the roentgenogram depends, for the most part, upon the thickness of the abdominal wall and the radiologic technic. Foci of ossification in the fetus have been demonstrated as early as the fourteenth week by Elward and Belair (Fig. 1). Roentgenography is of especial value in differentiating the pregnant uterus from other abdominal tumors, particularly when the fetus is dead.

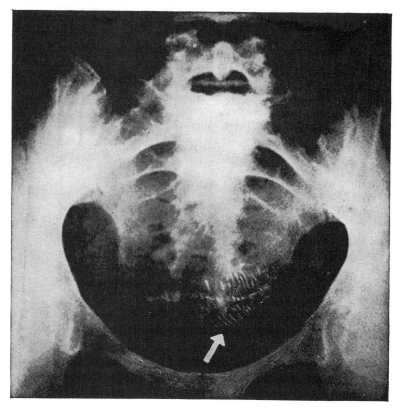

Fig. 1. Roentgenogram of pregnancy of 95 days' duration. (From Elward and Belair. Radiology 31:678, 1938.)

4. *Sonographic Examination.* In the majority of cases pregnancy can be diagnosed between the fifth and sixth week of gestation (Donald). The gestational sac appears as a white ring in the fundus of the uterus (Fig. 2). Pregnancy can be diagnosed earlier than with roentgenographic technics with the additional advantage of avoiding harm to the products of conception (Hellman and associates).

Probable Evidence of Pregnancy. These signs include (1) enlargement of the abdomen; (2) changes in the shape, size, and consistency of the uterus; (3) changes in the cervix; (4) the detection of intermittent contractions of the uterus;

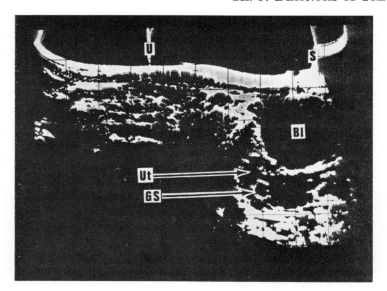

Fig. 2. Sonogram at 5 weeks' gestation (menstrual age). Bl, Bladder; V, vagina; S, symphysis pubis; U, umbilicus; Ut, uterus; Gs, gestational sac.

(5) ballottement; (6) outlining the fetus; and (7) positive hormonal test for pregnancy.

    1. *Enlargement of the Abdomen.* Near the end of the third lunar month the uterus usually can be felt through the abdominal wall as a tumor that gradually increases in size up to the end of pregnancy (Fig. 3). In general, any enlargement of the abdomen during the childbearing period strongly suggests pregnancy.

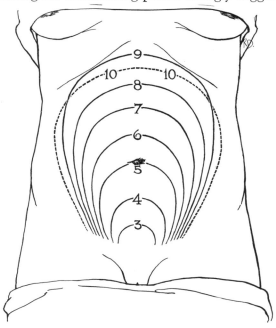

Fig. 3. Relative height of the fundus at the various lunar months of pregnancy.

The abdominal enlargement is less pronounced in nulliparas than in multiparas whose abdominal walls have lost a great part of their tone and are sometimes so flaccid that the uterus sags forward and downward, producing a pendulous abdomen. This difference is so obvious that it is not rare for women in the latter part of a second pregnancy to suspect twins because of the increased size of the abdomen, as compared with that in the corresponding month of the previous pregnancy. The abdomen, moreover, undergoes significant changes of shape depending on the woman's position. It is, of course, much less prominent when she is in the supine position.

2. *Changes in Size, Shape, and Consistency of Uterus.* In the first three months these are the only physical signs detectable. During the first few weeks the increase in size is limited almost entirely to the anteroposterior diameter, but at a little later period the body of the uterus becomes almost globular, attaining at the third month an average diameter of 8 cm. During the first two months the pregnant uterus remains an entirely pelvic organ, whereas during the third lunar month it begins to rise above the symphysis. At the same time the anteflexion of the corpus on the cervix increases.

More characteristic than the changes in shape are those in consistency. On bimanual examination the uterine body feels doughy or elastic and sometimes becomes exceedingly soft. At about the sixth week after the last period another very important sign, *Hegar's sign,* becomes manifest. As shown in Figures 4 and 5, with one hand on the abdomen and two fingers of the other hand in the vagina, the firm, hard cervix is felt, with the elastic body of the uterus above the compressible soft isthmus, which lies between the two. Occasionally the change in consistency at the isthmus is so marked that the cervix and corpus appear to be separate; the inexperienced examiners may therefore mistake the cervix for a small uterus, and the softened body for a tumor of the tubes or ovaries. Hegar's sign is not, however, positively diagnostic of pregnancy, since it may occasionally be elicited when the walls of the nonpregnant uterus are excessively soft.

3. *Cervix.* Beginning at the second month of pregnancy the cervix becomes considerably softened; in primigravidas the consistency of the portion surrounding the external os resembles that of the lips, more than the more resistant nasal cartilage, as at other times. As pregnancy advances the cervical canal may often become sufficiently patulous to admit the tip of the examining finger. Occasionally, however, the softening does not occur until much later in pregnancy, and in certain inflammatory conditions, as well as in carcinoma, the cervix may remain firm, yielding only with the onset of labor, if at all.

4. *Braxton Hicks Contractions.* The pregnant uterus produces painless palpable contractions at irregular intervals from an early stage in gestation. These Braxton Hicks contractions, however, are not positive signs of pregnancy, since similar contractions are sometimes noted in cases of hematometra and occasionally with soft myomas, especially the pedunculated submucous variety. Braxton Hicks contractions may be of aid in ruling out abdominal pregnancy (p. 241).

5. *Ballottement.* During the fourth and fifth months of pregnancy the fetus is small in relation to the volume of amniotic fluid; a sudden tap on the uterus consequently causes the fetus to sink in the amniotic fluid, rebound to its original position, and tap the examining finger.

6. *Outlining the Fetus.* In the second half of pregnancy the fetal outlines may be palpated through the abdominal wall; the procedure becomes easier the

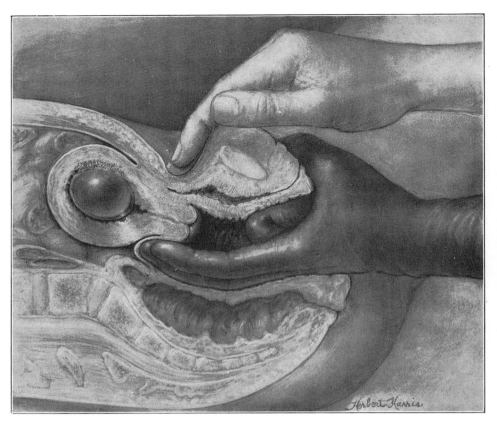

Fig. 4. Method of detecting Hegar's sign. (Compare with Fig. 5.)

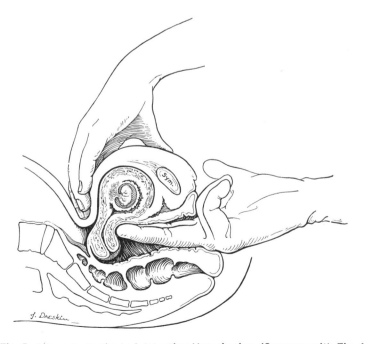

Fig. 5. Alternate method of detecting Hegar's sign. (Compare with Fig. 4.)

nearer that term is approached. Subserous myomas, however, may occasionally simulate the fetal head or small parts, or both, thus causing serious diagnostic errors; a diagnosis of pregnancy should, therefore, not be made on this sign alone.

7. *Endocrine Tests.* The presence of chorionic gonadotropin in maternal plasma and its excretion in urine provide the basis for the endocrine tests for pregnancy. Chorionic gonadotropin may be identified in body fluids by any one of a variety of immunoassays or bioassays. Hormonal tests, as they are actually run in the physician's office or clinic or in the clinical laboratories, do not absolutely identify the presence or absence of pregnancy. In fact, Hobson emphasizes that the degree of accuracy attained by some laboratories with commonly used pregnancy tests is not greater than might be achieved by tossing a coin.

One basic problem in most assay procedures arises from the immunologic and biologic similarities between chorionic gonadotropin formed by the trophoblast and luteinizing hormone secreted by the pituitary. In practically all test systems using immunoassay, luteinizing hormone cross-reacts with antibody to chorionic gonadotropin; moreover, luteinizing hormone may induce a response similar to that of chorionic gonadotropin in most methods of bioassay (Ch. 6, p. 174). If the test used is so sensitive as to detect very slight amounts of chorionic gonadotropin, it may yield a positive test for pregnancy, especially in problem cases, because of the reactivity of circulating or excreted luteinizing hormone. At the time of menopause, for example, amenorrhea not infrequently causes considerable fear of a possible pregnancy. At the same time the levels of pituitary gonadotropins usually are elevated and may be the cause of a falsely positive pregnancy test. If, however, the sensitivity of the pregnancy test is reduced in order to exclude a falsely positive result from luteinizing hormone, some pregnancies will not be identified because the levels of chorionic gonadotropin are too low to be detected. The falsely negative test is most likely to be encountered after the fourth month, although with pathologic early pregnancies, such as a tubal pregnancy, chorionic gonadotropin may be present only in small amounts and therefore not be identified by the less sensitive methods of testing.

IMMUNOASSAY. Kerber and associates have recently compared several of the

Table 1. **Immunologic Tests for Pregnancy**[*]

1. *Latex Inhibition Slide Tests*

Name	*Source*	*Minimal Detectable Levels of HCG*[†]*/liter of Urine*
HCG Test	Hyland Laboratories	2,000–8,000 IU/liter
Gravindex	Ortho Diagnostics	3,500 IU/liter
Pregnosticon Slide	Organon Inc.	1,000–2,000 IU/liter

2. *Hemagglutination-Inhibition Tube Tests*

Name	*Source*	*Minimal Detectable Levels of HCG/liter of Urine*
UCG	Wampole Laboratories	1,000 IU/liter
Pregnosticon Tube	Organon Inc.	700–750 IU/liter
Pregnosticon Accuspheres	Organon Inc.	750–1,000 IU/liter

3. *Direct Latex Agglutination Slide Test*

Name	*Source*	*Minimal Detectable Levels of HCG/liter of Urine or Serum*
DAP	Wampole Laboratories	2,000–3,000 IU/liter

[*] *Data obtained from Kerber and associates.*
[†] *HCG = human chorionic gonadotropin.*

commercially available immunologic tests for identifying chorionic gonadotropin (Table 1). They found some methods of testing, at least, which use the technic of hemagglutination-inhibition (Pregnosticon tube test or UCG test) to be quite sensitive and therefore very unlikely to yield a falsely negative result. The assay takes about two hours to complete. As a general all-purpose rapid pregnancy screening test, Kerber and associates found one of the latex inhibition slide tests, the Pregnosticon slide test, which take only a few minutes to perform to offer the greatest number of advantages and the fewest disadvantages. Some of the other commercially available latex inhibition slide tests, however, were found often to be relatively insensitive and, therefore, to yield a high incidence of false results.

It is evident that no one immunologic test for chorionic gonadotropin is foolproof, primarily because of the cross-reactivity of chorionic gonadotropin and luteinizing hormone. Hobson, however, reports an accuracy of 99.2 per cent in 19,887 instances in which the hemagglutination-inhibition technic (Pregnosticon tube test) was used. To achieve this degree of accuracy he urges that personnel be especially trained to recognized atypical reactions and that the test be repeated whenever the result is doubtful.

BIOASSAY. Few of the many technics that have been used in the past to bioassay chorionic gonadotropin are still employed. Of these the *rat ovarian hyperemia test* is probably the most satisfactory for general pregnancy testing. Several of the bioassay methods previously used widely and of some historical

Table 2. **Biologic Tests for Pregnancy**

Name	Test Animal	End Point	Time of Test
Aschheim-Zondek	*Mice or rats*	Corpus luteum formation	5 days
Friedman	*Rabbits*	Corpus luteum formation	48 hours
Ovarian hyperemia (Beck and co-workers)	*Rats*	Hyperemia	12–18 hours
Frog test (Wiltberger and Miller)	*Female*	Extrusion of eggs	24 hours
Toad test (Galli Mainini, Shapiro)	*Male*	Extrusion of sperm	2–5 hours

importance are listed in Table 2. This test depends upon the detection of gross hyperemia in the ovary of the immature rat 16 to 24 hours after the subcutaneous injection of 3 ml of centrifuged, untreated urine or 0.5 ml of serum. Most investigators report the accuracy of the test to be 95 per cent or higher. Beck and co-workers record excellent agreement between a hemagglutination-inhibition reaction and the rat ovarian hyperemia test.

OTHER PREGNANCY TESTS. Recently the technic of *radioimmunoassay* has been applied to the measurement of chorionic gonadotropin. Its advantages and disadvantages are basically the same as those of other highly sensitive methods of assay.

Progesterone-induced and synthetic progestin-induced withdrawal bleeding have been used in an attempt to differentiate pregnancy from other causes of amenorrhea. In the absence of pregnancy, bleeding usually occurs four or five days after the last dose of the progestin. This response, of course, requires an estrogen-primed endometrium. Withdrawal of the progestin results in uterine bleeding if there is little or no endogenous progesterone. If there is sufficient production of endogenous progesterone in the absence of pregnancy or if the endometrium is not estrogen-primed, no bleeding occurs, resulting in a falsely positive test. In general, this method offers little that could not be accomplished by evaluating carefully the patient's history and by ascertaining at the time of pelvic examination whether there is any cervical mucus and, if so, whether the spread and dried mucus crystallizes to form a fern or a cellular pattern (Ch. 4, p. 100). If an intact fern develops, early pregnancy is very unlikely and the patient almost certainly will demonstrate withdrawal bleeding after a progestin. If a highly cellular pattern forms, she may or may not be pregnant. If not pregnant, she may or may not develop withdrawal bleeding after receiving progestin depending upon her own supply of endogenous progesterone.

In summary, none of these tests is of sufficient accuracy to provide positive proof of pregnancy. In most instances the low rate of error is of little significance; unfortunately, however, falsely negative or falsely positive results are often obtained in the particular cases in which the clinical data are inconclusive.

Presumptive Evidences of Pregnancy. The presumptive evidences of pregnancy largely comprise subjective symptoms and signs appreciated by the patient herself. The signs include cessation of the menses, changes in the breasts, alteration of the color of the mucous membranes, and increased pigmentation. The symptoms include nausea with or without vomiting, disturbances in urination, fatigue, and the sensation of fetal movement.

1. *Cessation of the Menses.* In a healthy woman who has previously menstruated regularly, abrupt cessation of menstruation strongly suggests pregnancy. Not until ten days or more after the missed period, however, is the absence of menses a reliable indication of pregnancy. When the second period is missed the probability is stronger.

Although cessation of menstruation is an early and very important indication of pregnancy, gestation may begin without prior menstruation, and uterine bleeding that simulates menstruation is occasionally noted after conception. In certain Oriental countries where girls marry at a very early age and in sexually promiscuous groups, pregnancy sometimes occurs before the menstrual periods are established. Nursing mothers who usually do not menstruate during lactation sometimes conceive at that time and, more rarely, women who think they have passed the menopause become pregnant. Conversely, one or two incidents of bloody discharge, simulating menstruation, during the first half of pregnancy are not uncommon, but almost without exception they are brief and scant. In a series of 225 consecutive patients who did not abort, Speert and Guttmacher reported that macroscopic vaginal bleeding was noted by 22 per cent between conception and the one hundred and ninety-sixth day of pregnancy. In 8 per cent bleeding began on or before the fortieth day in the absence of any cervical lesion and was interpreted as physiologic response to implantation. Bleeding was three times as frequent among multiparas as among primigravidas. Of 83 multiparas, 25 per cent observed bleeding. Cases in which women are said to have "menstruated" every month throughout pregnancy are of questionable authenticity and are probably caused by some abnormality of the reproductive organs. Vaginal bleeding at any time during pregnancy should be regarded as abnormal and investigated at once.

Absence of menstruation may result from a number of conditions other than pregnancy. Probably one of the most common causes of delay in the onset of the period is emotional, particularly fear of pregnancy. Environmental change and certain chronic diseases may also suppress the menstrual flow.

2. *Changes in the Breasts.*   Generally the changes in the breasts (Ch. 8) are quite characteristic in primigravidas but are less so in multiparas, whose breasts may contain a small amount of milk or colostrum for months or even for years after the last delivery. Occasionally, changes in the breasts similar to those produced by pregnancy may be observed in women with ovarian or intracranial tumors and in those taking certain tranquilizers. Instances have also been reported of such breast changes occurring in cases of spurious or imaginary pregnancy (pseudocyesis).

3. *Nausea and Vomiting.*   Pregnancy is frequently characterized by disturbances of the digestive system, particularly nausea and vomiting. The so-called morning sickness of pregnancy usually comes on in the early part of the day and passes off in a few hours, although it occasionally persists longer or may occur at other times. It usually appears soon after the end of the first month and disappears spontaneously 6 to 12 weeks later.

4. *Quickening.*   Sometime between the sixteenth and the nineteenth weeks after the last period the pregnant woman usually becomes conscious of slight fluttering abdominal movements that gradually increase in intensity. They result from fetal activity and their first appearance is designated "quickening," or the perception of life. This sign provides only corroborative evidence of pregnancy and in itself is of little value.

5. *Discoloration of the Mucosa and Skin of Vagina and Vulva.*   Under the influence of pregnancy the vaginal mucosa frequently appears dark bluish or purplish-red and congested. Attention was first called to this sign by Jacquemier, but particular stress was laid upon its significance by Chadwick of Boston; in America, therefore, it is known as *Chadwick's sign.* It provides presumptive evidence but is not conclusive, since it may be observed in any condition leading to intense congestion of the pelvic organs.

6. *Pigmentation of the Skin and Abdominal Striae.*   These cutaneous manifestations are common but not absolutely diagnostic of pregnancy; they may be absent in gestation and, conversely, may be associated with tumors of different origin.

7. *Urinary Disturbances.*   In the early weeks of pregnancy the enlarging uterus, by exerting pressure on the bladder, may cause frequent micturition. It continues for the first few months and gradually disappears as the uterus rises up into the abdomen, to reappear at or near the end of pregnancy when the head descends into the pelvis.

8. *Fatigue.*   Easy fatigability is such a frequent concomitant of early pregnancy that it affords a noteworthy diagnostic clue.

Differential Diagnosis of Pregnancy.   The pregnant uterus is often mistaken for other tumors occupying the pelvis or abdomen; less frequently the opposite error is made. The early periods of pregnancy may be simulated by enlargement of the uterus caused by interstitial or submucous myomas, hematometra, and certain pelvic inflammatory lesions. As a rule, the uterus in these circumstances is firmer than in pregnancy and less elastic and boggy. Except in hematometra, moreover, such conditions are not attended by apparent cessation of the menses. If, however, uncertainty remains, a delay of a few weeks usually confirms the diagnosis.

The early pregnant uterus is occasionally mistaken for a small ovarian or tubal tumor. This error is minimized, however, by careful bimanual examination under an anesthetic, if necessary. As the tumor becomes larger and rises up into the abdomen, the differential diagnosis is simplified, particularly by the positive signs of pregnancy and the intermittent contractions of Braxton Hicks.

The diagnosis of pregnancy in a uterus that also contains myomas is often very difficult and for a time may be impossible. Soon, however, there is a more rapid increase in the size of the tumor than occurs in uncomplicated myoma; variations in the consistency of its different parts, moreover, also suggest pregnancy.

Occasionally an ovarian cystoma is complicated by pregnancy. In the early stages the diagnosis, as a rule, is easily made, since careful bimanual examination helps to differentiate between the two tumors; in the later months, however, it may become extremely difficult and sometimes impossible because of the increased distention of the abdomen. If the positive signs cannot be elicited, the pregnancy is usually overlooked and a simple cystoma diagnosed, whereas if the heart sounds are heard and the radiologic findings are positive, the cystoma may escape recognition and the excessive abdominal enlargement be attributed to hydramnios.

Spurious Pregnancy.　　Imaginary pregnancy, or *pseudocyesis,* is usually observed in patients nearing the menopause or in young women who intensely desire to be pregnant. Such patients may present all the subjective symptoms of pregnancy, associated with a considerable increase in the size of the abdomen, caused either by an abdominal and rapid deposition of fat, by gas in the intestinal tract, or by abdominal fluid. When pseudocyesia occurs in the earlier years of life, the menses do not as a rule disappear, but they may become irregular.

Changes in the breasts, such as enlargement, the appearance of secretion, and increased pigmentation, sometimes occur. They are probably related to endocrine disturbances, involving the ovary, anterior pituitary, or hypothalamus adrenals. In a majority of these cases, there is morning sickness, probably psychogenic.

The supposed fetal movements usually result from contractions of the intestines or the muscles of the abdominal wall and occasionally are so marked as to deceive even physicians. Careful examination of the patient usually leads to a correct diagnosis without great difficulty, since the small uterus can be demonstrated on bimanual examination—if necessary, under anesthesia. The greatest difficulty in these cases is to convince the patient of the correct diagnosis. Psychotic women may persist for years in the delusion that they are pregnant.

Distinction Between First and Subsequent Pregnancies.　　Occasionally it is of practical importance to decide whether a patient is pregnant for the first time or has previously borne children. Ordinarily, but not always, there are indelible traces of a former pregnancy.

In a nullipara the abdomen is usually tense and firm, and the uterus is felt through it only with difficulty. The characteristic old striae and the distinctive changes in the breasts are absent. The labia majora are usually in close apposition and the frenulum is intact. The vagina is usually narrow and marked by well-developed rugae. The cervix is softened but does not usually admit the tip of the finger until the very end of pregnancy. During the last four to six weeks of pregnancy the presenting part often has descended through the pelvic inlet to be fixed in the pelvis or actually engaged, unless, of course, there is disproportion.

In multiparas the abdominal wall is usually lax and frequently pendulous and the uterus is readily palpated through it. In addition to the pink striae associated with the present condition, the silvery cicatrices of past pregnancies may also be noted. The breasts are usually not so firm as in the first pregnancy and frequently present striae similar to those on the abdomen. The vulva usually gapes to some extent, the frenulum has disappeared, and the hymen is transformed into the myrtiform caruncles. The external os even in the early months of pregnancy usually manifests lacerations and a little later readily admits the tip of the finger, which can be carried up to the internal os. In the majority of cases the presenting part does not pass through the pelvic inlet into the true pelvis until the onset of labor.

Identification of Fetal Life or Death.   In the early months of pregnancy the diagnosis of fetal death presents considerable difficulty; most often it can be made only after repeated examinations show that the uterus has remained stationary or has actually decreased in size over a number of weeks. Since the placenta may continue to produce chorionic gonadotropin for several weeks after death of the embryo or fetus, a positive endocrine test for pregnancy is not necessarily an indication that the fetus is alive. A negative test early in pregnancy, however, points to fetal death, especially if further tests continue to be negative.

In the later months of pregnancy the disappearance of fetal movements usually directs the attention of the mother to the possibility of fetal death, but if fetal cardiac action can be identified distinct from that of the mother, the fetus certainly is alive. If the fetal heart tones are not recognized by careful auscultation or by electrocardiography, the fetus is probably dead. Both of these methods are somewhat imprecise, however, especially in pregnancies in which the fetal heart is remote from the examiner, for example, in maternal obesity or hydramnios. Instruments using the Doppler shift principle, as described on page 278, may be of considerable value in instances in which the fetal heart cannot be heard by auscultation with a heart stethoscope. Barton reports no inaccuracies in diagnosing fetal life or death in 40 pregnancies beyond the twentieth week in which the fetal heart tones could not be detected by auscultation. Brown, using the Doppler principle in 64 pregnancies in which the fetus was considered to be dead, was in error once; one fetus thought to be dead was subsequently found to be viable. Therefore, an instrument that uses the Doppler principle is most likely from midpregnancy on to identify correctly fetal cardiac action but infrequently it fails to do so.

If the fetus has succumbed, careful investigations show that the uterus does not correspond in size to the estimated duration of pregnancy or actually has become smaller than previously, while at the same time retrogressive changes have occurred in the breasts. With the death of the fetus maternal weight gain usually ceases, and not infrequently there is even a slight decrease in weight. The diagnosis of fetal death cannot usually be made at a single examination, but certainly must be considered when the signs just mentioned are identified and fetal cardiac action and fetal movement cannot be detected.

Occasionally a positive diagnosis of fetal death can be made by palpating the collapsing skull through the partially dilated cervix; in that event the loose bones of the fetal head feel as though they were contained in a flabby bag.

In instances in which the fetus has been dead for several days, at least, the amniotic fluid is red or brown and usually turbid rather than clear and nearly colorless. Demonstration of such amniotic fluid is not absolutely diagnostic of fetal death, however, since prior hemorrhage into the amniotic sac, as sometimes occurs with amniocentesis, may lead to similar discoloration of the amniotic fluid even though the fetus is alive.

There are three principal radiologic signs of fetal death: (1) *Spalding's sign.* This is the best-known sign which consists of an overlapping of the fetal skull bones. It is based on liquefaction of the brain and hence requires several days to develop. A similar sign may result occasionally with a living fetus, when the fetal head is compressed in the pelvis. (2) *Exaggerated curvature of the fetal spine.* Since development of this sign depends on maceration of the spinous ligaments, it also requires several days to become evident; mild degrees of curvature, moreover, may be misleading. (3) *Demonstration of gas in the fetus* is considered by Holm to be the most reliable of the roentgenologic signs of fetal death.

REFERENCES

Aschheim, S., and Zondek, B. (The diagnosis of pregnancy from urine by demonstration of anterior pituitary hormone). Klin Wschr 7:1404, 1928.

Bartholomew, R. A., Sale, B. E., and Calloway, J. T. Diagnosis of pregnancy by the roentgen ray. JAMA 76:912, 1921.

Barton, J. J. Evaluation of the Doppler shift principle as a diagnostic aid in obstetrics. Amer J Obstet Gynec 102:563, 1968.

Beck, P., Shagan, B. P., Cutler, A., and Kupperman, H. S. Comparison of an immunologic pregnancy test with the rat ovarian hyperemia test. Obstet Gynec 25:528, 1965.

Brown, R. E. Detection of intrauterine death. Amer J Obstet Gynec 102:965, 1968.

Chadwick, J. R. Value of the bluish coloration of the vaginal entrance as a sign of pregnancy. Trans Amer Gynec Soc 11:399, 1886.

Donald, I. Practical Obstetric Problems, 4th ed. Philadelphia, J. B. Lippincott Co., 1969, p. 934.

Elward, J. F., and Belair, J. F. Roentgen diagnosis of pregnancy. Radiology 31:678, 1938.

Friedman, M. H. Mechanism of ovulation in the rabbit. II. Ovulation produced by the injection of urine from pregnant women. Amer J Physiol 90:617, 1929.

Galli Mainini, C. Pregnancy test using male toad. J Clin Endocr 7:653, 1947.

Hellman, L. M., Duffus, G. M., Donald, I., and Sundén, B. The safety of diagnostic ultrasound in obstetrics. Lancet 1:1133, 1970.

Hicks, J. B. On the contraction of the uterus throughout pregnancy. Trans Obstet Soc London 13:216, 1871.

Hobson, B. M. Pregnancy diagnosis. Lancet 2:56, 1969.

Holm, O. F. The roentgenologic signs of intra-uterine foetal death. Acta Obstet Gynec Scand 36:58, 1957.

Jacquemier, J. M. Manuel des accouchements et des maladies des femmes grosses et accouchées contenant les soins à donner aux nouveaux-nés. Paris, Germer-Baillière, 1846.

Johnson, W. L., Stegall, H. F., Lein, J. N., and Rushmer, R. F. Detection of fetal life in early pregnancy with an ultrasonic Doppler flowmeter. Obstet Gynec 26:305, 1965.

Kerber, I. J., Inclan, A. P., Fowler, E. A., Davis, K., and Fish, S. A. Immunologic tests for pregnancy: a comparison. Obstet Gynec 36:37, 1970.

Shapiro, H. A., and Zwarenstein, H. Rapid test for pregnancy on *Xenopus laevis.* Nature 133:762, 1934.

Spalding, A. B. A pathognomonic sign of intra-uterine death. Surg Gynec Obstet 34:754, 1922.

Speert, H., and Guttmacher, A. F. Frequency and significance of bleeding in early pregnancy. JAMA 155:712, 1954.

Wiltberger, P. B., and Miller, D. F. The male frog, *Rana pipiens,* a new test animal for early pregnancy. Science 107:198, 1948.

Zondek, B. (On the theory of the pregnancy reaction from the urine by demonstration of anterial pituitary hormone; rapid precipitation reaction; eliminating the effects of poisons from the urine. Improvement of the pregnancy reaction). Klin Wschr 9:964, 1930.

10

THE NORMAL PELVIS

Since the mechanism of labor is essentially a process of accommodation of the fetus to the bony passage through which it must pass, the size and the shape of the pelvis are of extreme importance in obstetrics. In both sexes the pelvis forms the bony ring through which the body weight is transmitted to the lower extremities, but in the female it assumes a special form that adapts it to childbearing (Fig. 1).

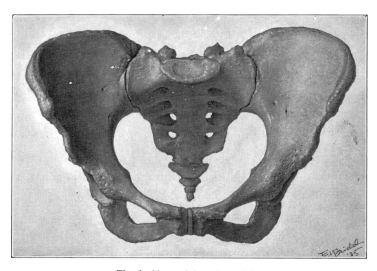

Fig. 1. Normal female pelvis.

The adult pelvis is composed of four bones: the sacrum, the coccyx, and the two innominate bones. Each innominate bone is formed by the fusion of the ilium, the ischium, and the pubis. The innominate bones are firmly joined to the sacrum at the sacroiliac synchondroses, and to each other at the symphysis pubis. Consideration will be limited to those pecularities of the female pelvis of importance in childbearing.

Pelvic Anatomy from an Obstetric Point of View

The linea terminalis demarcates the false pelvis from the true pelvis. The false pelvis lies above the linea terminalis and the true pelvis below this anatomic boundary. The *false pelvis* is bounded posteriorly by the lumbar vertebrae and laterally by the iliac fossae; in front the boundary is formed by the lower portion

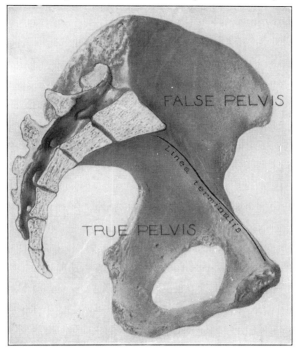

Fig. 2. Sagittal section of pelvis showing false and true pelvis.

of the anterior abdominal wall (Fig. 2). It is of no particular obstetric significance. It varies considerably in size in different women according to the flare of the iliac bones.

The *true pelvis* lies beneath the linea terminalis and is the portion important in childbearing. It is bounded above by the promontory and alae of the sacrum, the linea terminalis, and the upper margins of the pubic bones and below by the pelvic outlet. Its cavity may be compared with an obliquely truncated, bent cylinder with its greatest height posteriorly, since its anterior wall at the symphysis pubis measures 4.5 to 5 cm and its posterior wall 10 cm. With the woman in the upright position, the upper portion of the pelvic canal is directed downward and backward, and in its lower course it curves and becomes directed downward and forward.

The walls of the true pelvis are partly bony and partly ligamentous. Its posterior boundary is furnished by the anterior surface of the sacrum, and its lateral limits are formed by the inner surface of the ischial bones and the sacrosciatic notches and ligaments. In front it is bounded by the obturator foramina, the pubic bones, and the ascending rami of the ischial bones.

The side walls of the true pelvis of the normal adult female converge somewhat. If, therefore, the planes of the ischial bones of a normal adult female pelvis were extended downward, they would meet near the knee. Extending from the middle of the posterior margin of each ischium are the *ischial spines*, which are of great obstetric importance, inasmuch as a line drawn between them typically represents the shortest diameter of the pelvic cavity; moreover, since they can be readily felt on vaginal or rectal examination, they serve as valuable landmarks in ascertaining the extent to which the presenting part of the fetus has descended into the pelvis.

The sacrum forms the posterior wall of the pelvic cavity. Its upper anterior margin, corresponding to the body of the first sacral vertebra and designated as the promontory, can be felt on vaginal examination and therefore provides a landmark for internal pelvimetry. Normally the sacrum presents a marked vertical and a less pronounced horizontal concavity, which, in abnormal pelves, may undergo important variations. A straight line drawn from the promontory to the tip of the sacrum usually measures 10 cm, whereas the distance along the concavity averages 12 cm.

In the female the appearance of the pubic arch is characteristic. The descending rami of the pubic bones unite to an angle of 90 to 100 degrees to form a rounded arch under which the fetal head may readily pass (Fig. 1).

Planes and Diameters of the Pelvis.   Because of the peculiar shape of the pelvis it is difficult to describe the exact location of an object therein. For convenience the pelvis has long been described as having four imaginary planes: (1) the plane of the pelvic inlet (superior strait, Fig. 3); (2) the plane of the pelvic outlet (inferior strait); (3) the plane of greatest pelvic dimensions; and (4) the plane of the midpelvis (least pelvic dimensions) (Fig. 4).

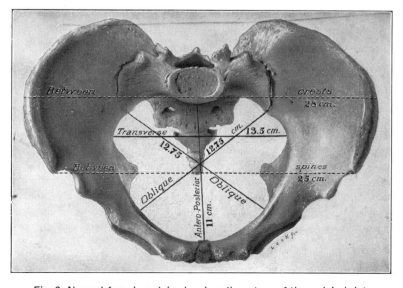

Fig. 3. Normal female pelvis showing diameters of the pelvic inlet.

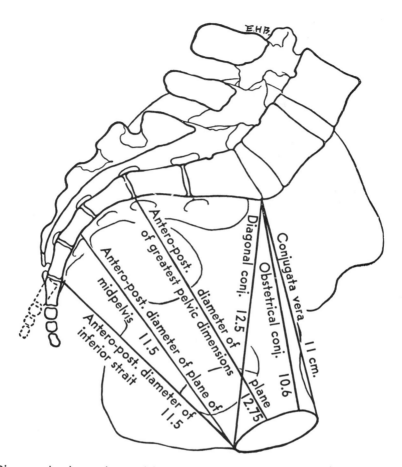

Fig. 4. Diagram showing various pelvic planes and diameters. Conjugata vera = true conjugate.

The superior strait represents the upper boundary of the true pelvis and is frequently designated as the pelvic inlet. In the past it has been described as somewhat oval with a depression on its posterior border corresponding to the promontory of the sacrum. Thoms, however, found the oval type in only one third of a series of 800 white women, whereas the round type was encountered in nearly one half. Caldwell and Moloy have described the typical female or "gynecoid" pelvis as one in which the inlet is more rounded than oval or heart-shaped. Their incidence of 50 per cent for the round, or gynecoid, pelvis compares closely with the above figure of Thoms. These investigations, based upon roentgenologic studies of large series of cases, lead to the conclusion that the typical female pelvis has an inlet that is more nearly round than oval. Thomas has described a *"round inlet"* as one in which the transverse diameter is equal to, or slightly greater (not more than 1 cm) than, the anteroposterior diameter.

The pelvic inlet is bounded posteriorly by the promontory and alae of the sacrum, laterally by the linea terminalis, and anteriorly by the horizontal rami of the pubic bones and the upper margin of the symphysis pubis. Its lateral margins, represented by the linea terminalis, are at a lower level than its central portion between the promontory and the upper border of the symphysis, as clearly seen in the sagittal section through a normal pelvis (Fig. 2).

Four diameters of the pelvic inlet are usually described: the anteroposterior, the transverse, and two obliques. The anteroposterior diameter extends from the middle of the promontory of the sacrum to the upper margin of the symphysis pubis and is designated the *true conjugate*. Normally the true conjugate measures 11 cm or more, but it may be markedly shortened in abnormal pelves. The transverse diameter is constructed at right angles to the true conjugate and represents the greatest distance between the linea terminalis on either side; it usually intersects the conjugata vera at a point about 5 cm in front of the promontory. In the oval pelvis it measures about 13 cm, whereas in the round type it is somewhat shorter. Each of the oblique diameters extends from one of the sacroiliac synchondroses to the iliopectineal eminence on the opposite side of the pelvis. They average just under 13 cm and are designated right and left, respectively, according to whether they originate at the right or left sacroiliac synchondrosis.

The anteroposterior diameter of the pelvic inlet, identified as the true conjugate, does not represent the shortest distance between the promontory of the sacrum and symphysis pubis. The shortest distance is the line from the sacral promontory to the inner surface of the symphysis somewhat below its upper margin. The latter line, which in most pelves is the shortest diameter through which the head must pass in descending through the pelvic inlet, was called by Michaelis the *obstetric conjugate*.

In the living woman the obstetric conjugate cannot be measured directly with the examining fingers. Various instruments have therefore been designed in an effort to obtain such a measurement, but none gives satisfactory results. For clinical purposes, therefore, it is sufficient to estimate the length of the obstetric conjugate indirectly by measuring the distance from the lower margin of the symphysis to the promontory of the sacrum—that is, the *diagonal conjugate*—and subtracting 1.5 to 2 cm from the result, according to the height and inclination of the symphysis pubis. The importance of the diagonal conjugate was first emphasized by Smellie.

The outlet of the pelvis consists of two approximately triangular areas not in the same plane but having a common base, which is a line drawn between the two ischial tuberosities. The apex of the posterior triangle is at the tip of the sacrum; the lateral boundaries are the sacrosciatic ligaments and the ischial tuberosities. The anterior triangle is formed by the area under the pubic arch (Fig. 5). Three diameters of the pelvic outlet are usually described: the anteroposterior, the transverse, and the posterior sagittal. The anteroposterior diameter extends from the lower margin of the symphysis pubis to the tip of the sacrum (11.5 cm). The transverse diameter is the distance between the inner edges of the ischial tuberosities (11.0 cm). The posterior sagittal diameter extends from the tip of the sacrum to a right-angled intersection with a line between the ischial tuberosities (7.5 cm).

The *plane of greatest pelvic dimensions*, as its name implies, represents the roomiest portion of the pelvic cavity. It extends from the middle of the posterior surface of the symphysis pubis to the junction of the second and third sacral vertebrae and laterally passes through the ischial bones over the middle of the acetabulum. Its anteroposterior and transverse diameters average about 12.5 cm. Since its oblique diameters terminate in the obturator foramina and the sacrosciatic notches, their length is indeterminate. This plane has no obstetric significance.

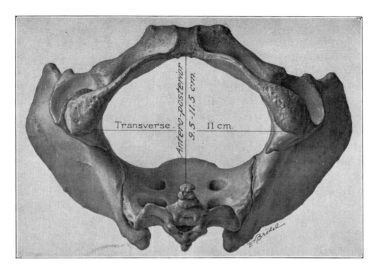

Fig. 5. Pelvic outlet.

The midpelvis at the level of the ischial spines (midplane, or plane of least pelvic dimensions) is of particular importance in obstructed labor following engagement of the fetal head. The shortest anteroposterior diameter at the level of the ischial spines normally measures at least 11.5 cm. The interspinous diameter of 10.0 cm or somewhat more is usually the smallest diameter of the pelvis except for the posterior sagittal diameter, which is the portion of the anteroposterior diameter between the sacrum and its intersection with the interspinous diameter. The posterior sagittal diameter is usually at least 4.5 cm.

Pelvic Inclination.   The normal position of the pelvis, in the erect woman, can be reproduced by holding a specimen with the incisures of the acetabula pointing directly downward. The same result is achieved when the anterior superior spines of the ilium and the pubic tubercles are placed in the same vertical plane (Figs. 2, 4, and 6).

The Pelvic Joints.   Anteriorly, the pelvic bones are held together by the symphysis pubis, which consists of fibrocartilage, and by the superior and inferior pubic ligaments, the latter frequently designated the arcuate ligament of the pubis (Fig. 7). The symphysis has a certain degree of mobility, which increases during pregnancy, particularly in multiparas. This fact was demonstrated by Budin, who showed that if a finger were inserted into the vagina of a pregnant woman and she were to walk, the ends of the pubic bones could be felt moving up and down with each step. The articulations between the sacrum and innominate bones also have a certain degree of mobility (Fig. 8).

Relaxation of the pelvic joints during pregnancy is probably the result of hormonal changes. Abramson and co-workers noted relaxation of the symphysis pubis in women, beginning in the first half of pregnancy and increasing during the last three months. These authors observed that retrogression begins immediately after parturition and is complete within three to five months. Further observations confirm these findings and show that the symphysis pubis increases in width during pregnancy, more in multiparas than in primigravidas, and returns

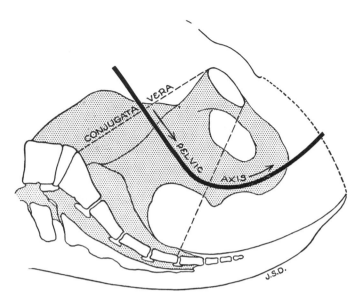

Fig. 6. Diagram showing the pelvic axis.

to normal soon after delivery. Careful roentgenographic studies of Borell reveal rather marked mobility of the pelvis at term caused by an upward gliding movement of the sacroiliac joint. The displacement, which is greatest in the dorsal lithotomy position, may cause an increase in the diameter of the outlet of 1.5 to 2 cm.

Because of the elasticity of the pelvic joints in pregnancy it was formerly

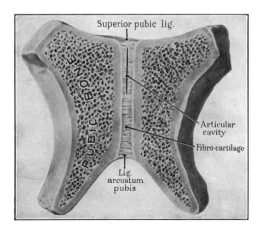

Fig. 7. Frontal section symphysis pubis. Lig. arcuatum pubis = arcuate pubic ligament (From Spalteholz. Hand-Atlas of Human Anatomy, Vol. I, J. B. Lippincott.)

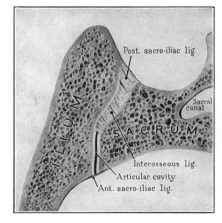

Fig. 8. Sacroiliac synchondrosis. (From Spalteholz. Hand-Atlas of Human Anatomy, Vol. I, J. B. Lippincott.)

thought that positioning the patient in extreme hyperextension increased the obstetric conjugate. To obtain this objective the patient was placed on her back with her buttocks extending slightly over the edge of the delivery table and with her legs hanging down by their own weight, the so-called Walcher position. The roentgenologic studies of Young and of Brill and Danelius show clearly that this concept is erroneous and that no appreciable increase in pelvic size results from the Walcher position. The position is both useless and very uncomfortable for the patient.

Sexual Differences in the Adult Pelvis.   The pelvis presents marked sexual differences. Generally, the male pelvis is heavier, higher, and more conical than the female. In the male the muscular attachments are much more strongly marked, and the iliac bones flare less than in the female. The male pubic arch is more angular and presents an aperture of 70 to 75 degrees, as compared with 90 to 100 degrees in the female. In the male pelvis the pelvic inlet is smaller and more nearly triangular, and the pelvic cavity is deeper and more conical; the sacrosciatic notch is narrower and the distance between the lower border of the sacrum and the ischial spine smaller than in the female pelvis.

Pelvis of the Newborn Child. The mechanism by which the pelvis of the fetus is converted into the adult form is of interest from both scientific and practical points of view, since it affords important information about the mode of production of certain varieties of deformed pelves.

The pelvis of the child at birth is partly bony and partly cartilaginous (Fig. 9).

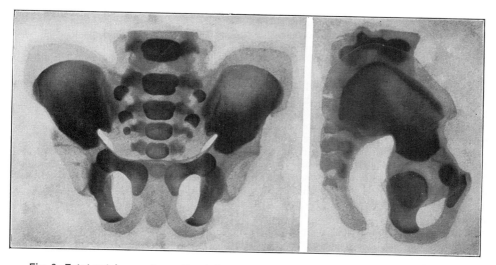

Fig. 9. Fetal pelvis near term. Frontal and lateral views showing extent of ossification.

The innominate bone does not exist as such, but is represented by the ilium, ischium, and pubis, which are united by a large Y-shaped cartilage, the three bones meeting in the acetabulum. The iliac crests and the acetabula, as well as the greater part of the ischiopubic rami, are entirely cartilaginous.

The cartilaginous portions of the pelvis gradually give place to bone, but complete union in the acetabulum does not occur until about puberty, and occasionally even later. The innominate bones may not, in fact, become completely ossified until between the twentieth and twenty-fifth years.

Transformation of Fetal into Adult Pelvis. The evolution of the form of the pelvis is generally thought to involve two sets of factors: developmental and inherent tendencies, and mechanical influences. That the process is not entirely the result of mechanical forces is manifested by the existence of sexual and racial differences in the adult pelvis. The mechanical influences that come into play after birth are identical in both sexes, but the sexual differences are, nevertheless, established as puberty approaches.

The part played by developmental and hereditary influences was clearly demonstrated by Litzmann, who showed that the female sacrum is markedly wider than that of the male. At birth, in both sexes, the body of the first sacral vertebra is twice as broad as the alae (100 to 50), but in the adult the ratio becomes 100 to 76 in the female, and 100 to 56 in the male, indicating a much more rapid growth of the alae in the female. Early investigators held that all the changes in the developing pelvis are similarly caused and that the influence of mechanical factors is merely accessory. The growth and development of that portion of the ilium forming the upper boundary of the great sacrosciatic notch profoundly affect the shape and size of the pelvic inlet.

Three mechanical forces take part in bringing about the final shape of the pelvis: the body weight, the upward and inward pressure exerted by the heads of the femurs, and the cohesive force exerted by the symphysis pubis. So long as the child remains constantly in the recumbent position these forces are not operative, but as soon as she sits up or walks, the body weight is transmitted through the vertebral column to the sacrum. Inasmuch as the center of gravity is anterior to the sacral promontory, the transmitted force is resolved into two components. One force is directed downward, and the other forward. The two together thus tend to force the promontory of the sacrum downward and forward toward the symphysis pubis, a process that can be accomplished only by the sacrum's rotating about its transverse axis. Its tip tends to become displaced both upward and backward. The strong sacrosciatic ligaments, however, resist this displacement and therefore permit only slight extension, with the result that the partly cartilaginous sacrum becomes bent upon itself just in front of its axis—that is, about the middle of its third vertebra—so that its anterior surface becomes markedly concave from above downward, instead of flat, as previously. At the same time the body weight forces the bodies of the sacral vertebrae forward so that they project slightly beyond the alae, thereby diminishing the transverse concavity of the sacrum.

Since the anterior surface of the sacrum is wider than the posterior, the bone tends to sink into the pelvic cavity under the influence of the body weight and would prolapse completely into it were it not held in place by the strong posterior iliosacral ligaments that suspend it, as it were, from the posterior superior spines of the ilium. As the sacrum is pushed downward into the pelvic cavity it exerts traction upon these ligaments, which in turn drag the posterior superior spines inward toward the midline and consequently tend to rotate the anterior portions of the innominate bones outward. Excessive outward rotation is prevented, however, by the cohesive force exerted at the symphysis but particularly by the upward and inward pressure exerted by the heads of the femurs. Practically, then, the iliac bone becomes converted into a two-armed level with the articular surface of the sacrum as a fulcrum; as a consequence, it bends at its point of least resistance, which is just anterior to the articulation, and thus gives the pelvis a greater transverse and a lesser anteroposterior diameter. At the same time, much of the transverse widening is more apparent than real and is caused by the relative shortening of the true conjugate by the downward and forward displacement of the promontory of the sacrum.

It is evident that the forces just mentioned must act in the same manner in the two sexes, so that whereas they may explain many points in the transformation of the fetal into the adult pelvis, they fail to explain satisfactorily its sexual differences.

The cohesive force exerted at the symphysis pubis cannot act by itself, since it is manifested only when the force exerted by the body weight causes a tendency toward gaping of the pubic bones. The effect of the upward and inward force exerted by the femurs cannot be observed by itself, since it comes into play only when it has to react against the body weight; nor has the action of the body weight alone ever been observed, though theoretically it might be noted in an individual presenting a split pelvis (congenital lack of union at the symphysis pubis) who has never walked. The action of the body weight, however, has been studied experimentally by Freund, who suspended a cadaver by the iliac crests after cutting through the symphysis and found that the innominate bones gaped widely.

The effect of the combined action of the body weight and the force exerted by the femurs has been studied by Litzmann in cases of congenital absence of the symphysis pubis. In such circumstances, there is a marked transverse widening of the posterior portion of the pelvis, while the force exerted by the femurs causes the anterior portions of the innominate bones to become almost parallel.

The action of the body weight and the cohesive force exerted at the symphysis without the upward and inward pressure exerted by the femurs can be studied in people whose lower extremities are absent and occasionally in cases of congenital dislocation of the hips. Holst has described a case in which the lower extremities were congenitally absent and the pelvis was characterized by a marked increase in width and a marked decrease in its anteroposterior diameter. Because of the excessive pressure exerted upon the tubera ischii in the absence of the counteracting force exerted by the femurs, the innominate bones are inwardly rotated so as to turn their crests inward and the tubera ischii outward, thus producing a considerable transverse widening of the inferior strait. More or less similar changes may be observed in cases of congenital dislocation of the hip in patients who have never walked. The effect of the various mechanical influences is exaggerated in pelves softened by diseases such as rickets and osteomalacia.

PELVIC SIZE AND ITS ESTIMATION

The Diagonal Conjugate Measurement.   In many abnormal pelves the shortest anteroposterior diameter of the pelvic inlet, or the obstetric conjugate, is considerably affected. It is therefore important to ascertain its length, but this measurement can be obtained only by roentgenologic technics. The distance from the sacral promontory to the lower margin of the symphysis pubis (the diagonal conjugate), however, can be measured clinically. **The diagonal conjugate measurement is most important, and every practitioner of obstetrics should be thoroughly familiar with its technic and interpretation.**

For this purpose the patient should be placed upon an examining table with her knees drawn up and her feet supported by suitable stirrups. If such an examination cannot be conveniently arranged, she should be brought to the edge of the bed where a firm pillow should be placed beneath her buttocks. Two fingers are introduced into the vagina; before measuring the diagonal conjugate, the mobility of the coccyx is ascertained and the anterior surface of the sacrum is palpated. The mobility of the coccyx is tested by seizing it between the fingers in the vagina and the thumb externally and attempting to move it to and fro. The anterior surface of the sacrum is then methodically palpated from below upward and its vertical and lateral curvatures are noted. In normal pelves only the last three sacral vertebrae can be felt without indenting the perineum, whereas in markedly contracted varieties the entire anterior surface of the sacrum is usually readily accessible. Frequently the mobility of the coccyx and the anatomic features of the lower sacrum may be more easily ascertained by rectal examination.

Except in extreme degrees of contraction, in order to reach the promontory of the sacrum the elbow must be depressed and the perineum forcibly indented by the knuckles of the third and fourth fingers. The index and the second fingers, held firmly together, are carried up over the anterior surface of the sacrum, where by sharply depressing the wrist the promontory is felt by the tip of the second finger as a projecting bony margin at the base of the sacrum. With the finger

closely applied to the most prominent portion of the upper sacrum, the vaginal
hand is elevated until it contacts the pubic arch, and the immediately adjacent
point on the index finger is marked, as shown in Figure 10. The hand is withdrawn and the distance between the mark and the tip of the second finger is

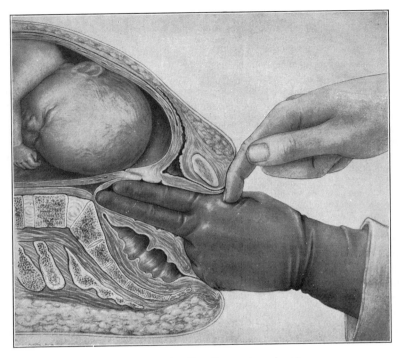

Fig. 10. Measuring the diagonal conjugate.

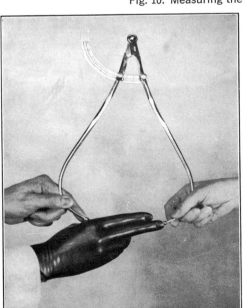

Fig. 11. Estimating the length of diagonal conjugate with pelvimeter.

measured. Because measurement using the pelvimeter, as demonstrated in Figure 11, often introduces an error of 0.5 to 1 cm, it is better to employ a rigid measuring scale attached to the wall, as shown in Figure 12. The diagonal conjugate is thus determined and the obstetric conjugate is estimated by deducting 1.5 to 2.0 cm, depending upon the height and inclination of the symphysis pubis, as illustrated in Figure 13.

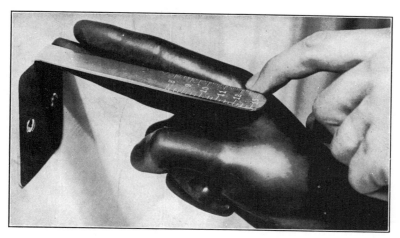

Fig. 12. Metal scale fastened to wall for measuring the diagonal conjugate diameter as ascertained manually.

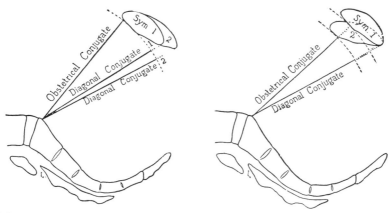

Fig. 13. Diagrams showing variations in length of diagonal conjugate dependent on height and inclination of the symphysis pubis.

If the diagonal conjugate is greater than 11.5 cm, it is justifiable to assume that the pelvic inlet is of adequate size for childbirth. As shown in Figure 14, in 61 consecutive cases in which the diagonal conjugate measured in excess of 11.5 cm, there was not a single instance in which the obstetric conjugate fell below 10.0 cm.

Objection to measurement of the diagonal conjugate is sometimes raised on the basis that it is painful to the patient. It probably causes mild momentary

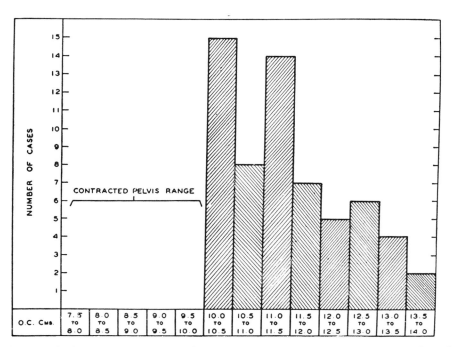

Fig. 14. The distribution of the obstetric conjugate measurement (x-ray) in 61 cases in which the diagonal conjugate was greater than 11.5 cm. Mean length of obstetric conjugate was 11.4 cm; shortest length, 10.0 cm; greatest length, 13.7 cm. (From Dippel. Surg Gynec Obstet 68:642, 1939.)

discomfort, but if properly performed and deferred until the latter half of pregnancy, when the distensibility of the vagina is greater, patients object to it no more than to a venipuncture.

Transverse contraction of the inlet can be measured only by x-ray pelvimetry. Transverse contractions have been recognized even in the presence of an adequate anteroposterior diameter.

Engagement.   Engagement is the descent of the biparietal plane of the fetal head to a level below that of the pelvic inlet. In other words, when the biparietal or largest diameter of the normally flexed head has passed *through* the inlet, engagement has taken place, and the head is *engaged*. Although engagement is usually regarded as a phenomenon of labor (and will be discussed later in that connection), in primigravidas it frequently occurs during the last few weeks of pregnancy. When it does so, it is confirmatory evidence that the pelvic inlet is adequate for that particular head. When engagement has occurred the fetal head has served as an internal pelvimeter to demonstrate that the inlet is ample for that particular infant.

Whether the head is engaged may be ascertained either by rectal or vaginal examination or by abdominal palpation. After a little experience with rectal or vaginal examination it becomes relatively easy to locate the station of the lowermost part of the head in relation to the level of the ischial spines. **If the lowest part of the occiput is at or below the level of the spines, the head usually, but not always, is engaged, since the distance from the biparietal plane of the pelvic inlet** to the level of the ischial spines approximates 5 cm in most pelves, whereas the distance from the biparietal plane of the unmolded fetal head to the vertex is only about 3 to 4 cm. In these circumstances the vertex cannot possibly reach the level of the spines unless the biparietal diameter has passed the inlet or unless there has been considerable elongation of the head because of molding and formation of caput succedaneum (p. 384 and also Figs. 15 and 16).

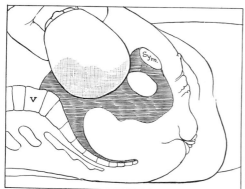 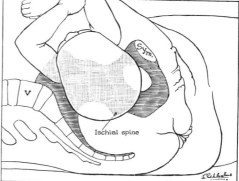

Fig. 15. When the lowermost portion of the head is several centimeters above the ischial spines it is not engaged.

Fig. 16. When the lowermost portion of the head is at or below the ischial spines it is engaged. Exceptions may occur with a huge caput succedaneum.

Engagement may be ascertained somewhat less satisfactorily by abdominal examination. If in a mature infant the biparietal plane has descended through the inlet, that plane so completely fills the inlet that the examining fingers (Fig. 17) cannot reach the lowermost part of the head. Hence, when pushed downward over the lower abdomen the examining fingers will slide over that portion of the head proximal to the biparietal plane (nape of the neck) and diverge. Conversely,

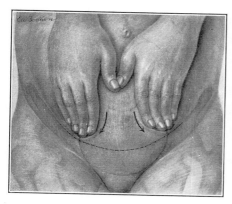 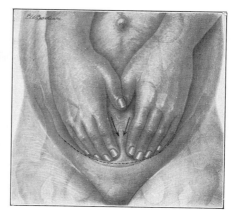

Fig. 17. If the fingers diverge when palpating the lateral aspects of the fetal head, it is engaged.

Fig. 18. If the fingers converge when palpating the lateral aspects of the fetal head, it is not engaged.

if the head is not engaged the examining fingers can easily palpate the lower part of the head and will hence converge, as shown in Figure 18.

Fixation of the fetal head is descent of the head through the pelvic inlet to a depth that prevents its free movement in any direction when pushed by both hands placed over the lower abdomen; it is not necessarily synonymous with engagement. Although a head that is freely movable on abdominal examination cannot be engaged, fixation of the head is sometimes seen when the biparietal plane is a centimeter or more above the pelvic inlet. In our experience the maneuver based on divergence or convergence of the examining fingers is more reliable than fixation in ascertaining engagement of the fetal head.

Engagement occurs before the onset of labor in over 90 per cent of primigravidas. Data on the frequency of engagement in primigravidas ten days to two weeks before the expected date of confinement are meager, but on the basis of our experience it is probably of the order of 75 per cent. In multiparas, however (in whom there is usually less concern about pelvic contraction because of the record of previous childbearing), engagement will have occurred before the onset of labor in only a minority of cases.

Although engagement is conclusive evidence of an adequate pelvic inlet for the baby concerned, its absence is by no means always indicative of pelvic contraction. For instance, in Bäder's study, labor was entirely normal in 87 per cent of the 499 primigravidas with unengaged heads at the onset of labor. Nevertheless, the incidence of contraction of the inlet is decidedly higher in this group than in the female population at large.

Outlet Measurements.   The other important dimension of the pelvis accessible for clinical measurement is the diameter between the ischial tuberosities, variously called the bisischial diameter, the intertuberous diameter, and the transverse diameter of the outlet. With the patient in lithotomy position the measure-

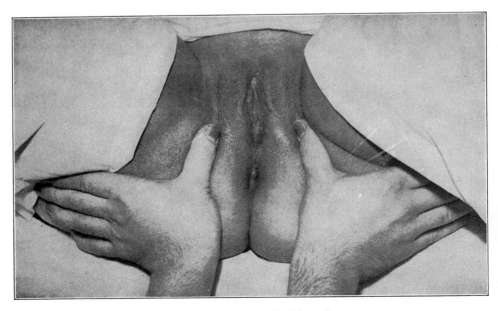

Fig. 19. Palpation of pubic arch.

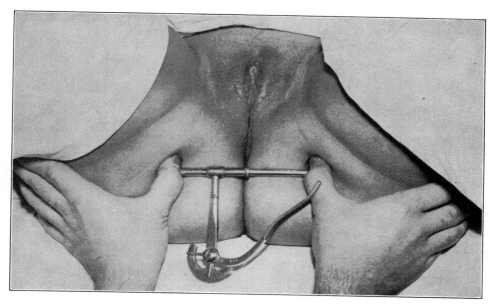

Fig. 20. Mensuration of transverse diameter of outlet with Thoms' pelvimeter.

ment is made from the inner and lowermost aspect of the ischial tuberosities, as shown in Figures 19 and 20. A measurement over 8 cm is considered to be normal. For measuring that diameter the pelvimeter devised by Thoms can be used.

The shape of the subpubic arch can be best appreciated if the pubic rami are palpated from the subpubic region to the ischial tuberosities.

Clinical Estimation of Midpelvic Size. Clinical estimation of midpelvic capacity by any direct form of measurement is not possible. If the ischial spines are quite prominent, or if the side walls of the pelvis are felt to converge, or if the concavity of the sacrum is very shallow, suspicion of contraction in this region is aroused, but only by roentgenologic studies can the midpelvis be precisely measured.

X-RAY PELVIMETRY

Status of X-Ray Pelvimetry. Considerable difference of opinion about the value of x-ray pelvimetry remains. Some obstetricians consider it superfluous and even misleading. Others regard it as the solution to all problems in the management of pelvic contraction. The logical view is something between these two extremes. The prognosis for successful labor in any given case cannot be established on the basis of x-ray pelvimetry alone, since the pelvic capacity is but one of several factors that determine the outcome. As enumerated by Mengert, there are at least five factors concerned: (1) size and shape of the bony pelvis; (2) size of the fetal head; (3) force of the uterine contractions; (4) moldability of the head; and (5) presentation and position. Only the first of these factors is amenable to precise roentgenologic measurement, and it is the object of x-ray pelvimetry simply to eliminate this one factor from the category of the unknown. X-ray pelvimetry must hence be regarded merely as a valuable adjunct in the management of patients suspected of having a contracted pelvis.

X-ray pelvimetry has the following advantages over manual estimation of pelvic size:

1. It provides precision of mensuration to a degree otherwise unobtainable. The clinical importance of such precision becomes evident when the shortcomings of the diagonal conjugate measurement are considered. In our experience when the diagonal conjugate exceeds 11.5 cm, the anteroposterior dimension of the inlet (the obstetric conjugate) is very rarely contracted (Fig. 14). When the diagonal conjugate is under 11.5, however, it is not always a reliable index of the obstetric conjugate, since the difference between these two diameters, usually about 1.5 cm, may range between 0.1 and 3.1 cm, as shown in Figure 21. For ex-

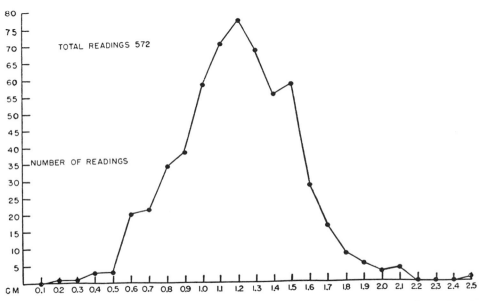

Fig. 21. The extent to which the diagonal conjugate is greater than the obstetric conjugate by x-ray. Mean 1.19 cm; median 1.30 cm; mode 1.20 cm; range 0.1 to 2.5 cm. (Modified from Kaltreider. Amer J Obstet Gynec 61:1075, 1951.)

ample, two primigravidas may have conjugates of 10.5 cm, but in one the obstetric conjugate may be 10.2 cm and easy vaginal delivery follows, whereas in the other it may be 8.2 cm, in which case cesarean section is obligatory.

2. It provides exact mensuration of diameters not otherwise obtainable: the transverse diameter of the inlet, the interischial spinous dimension, and the anteroposterior diameters of the midpelvis and the outlet. These measurements of the lower pelvis are receiving merited recognition as important causes of midpelvic arrest and of difficult forceps operations.

.3. By the stereoscopic technic, x-ray pelvimetry permits visualization of the general architecture of the pelvis. In experienced hands, that information is almost as valuable as actual mensuration.

4. In the course of labor, if roentgenograms are obtained with the mother standing, precise information about the descent or lack of descent of the biparie-

tal plane of the head is provided. This information is sometimes difficult to obtain by palpating the presenting part, because elongation of the head as a result of molding and caput succedaneum may make such digital findings misleading.

Indications for X-Ray Pelvimetry. Because of the expenses involved, as well as radiologic hazards (p. 316), radiographic pelvic measurement is not feasible for all pregnant women, nor is it necessary in the great majority of cases. In some populations, however, the incidence of contracted pelvis approaches 4 to 5 per cent. Such a frequency of pelvic contractions equals the incidence of ante-partum hemorrhage and exceeds that of tuberculosis, syphilis, and erythroblasto-sis, for the detection of which these same clinics carry out routine procedures on all patients. There are, however, certain clinical circumstances that point to the probability of pelvic contraction or potential dystocia and often make x-ray pel-vimetry an integral part of good obstetric practice:

A. Obstetric history
    1. Severe trauma or unexplained death of infant of average size or greater
    2. Previous cesarean section, if vaginal delivery is contemplated
    3. Previous injury or disease likely to affect the bony pelvis
B. Manual mensuration
    1. Inlet
        a. Ability to touch sacral promontory easily on vaginal examination (diagonal conjugate less than 11.5 cm)
    2. Midplane
        a. Unusually prominent ischial spines with converging pelvic side walls or flattened sacrum
    3. Outlet
        a. Markedly narrowed intertuberous diameter with narrow subpubic angle
C. Failure to progress in labor
D. Breech, face, and other abnormal presentations

The characteristics and measurements of the pelvis, combined with consid-eration of the fetal size, presentation, and position, will aid the obstetrician in reaching his clinical decisions before or during labor. X-ray pelvimetry is a valu-able aid to the obstetrician, but it is not a substitute for his clinical judgment. X-ray pelvimetry is of greatest value to the patient and the obstetrician when the films are interpreted by someone qualified in clinical obstetrics. *Only in occa-sional instances is a trial of labor not justified.* Not infrequently the size of the infant is overestimated and the forces of labor defy prognostication. When the obstetrician is forewarned and forearmed with accurate knowledge of the pelvis, his patient is unlikely to receive unwarranted oxytocin or to suffer from a trial of labor if properly supervised. Vaginal delivery may often follow without in-creased maternal or fetal risk.

Technics of X-Ray Pelvimetry. It is essential to correct for distortion of the image produced by the divergence of the x-rays (Fig. 22). The amount of distortion depends upon (1) the distance of an object (or a pelvic diameter) from the x-ray film and (2) the distance from the x-ray tube to the film. The latter can be eliminated as an unknown by establishing a standard tube-film distance. The farther above the film an object is, the greater will be the distortion of its image. Unfortunately, in some diameters of the pelvis the exact distance above the x-ray film is unknown. A great variety of mechanical and mathematical methods have been devised to correct for this variable image distor-tion of the different pelvic diameters.

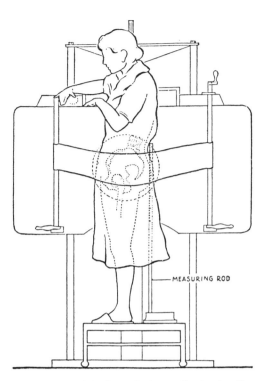

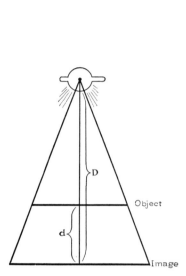

Fig. 22. Principle of divergent distortion. Size of the image depends on object-film distance (d) and tube-film distance (D).

Fig. 23. Positioning of the patient, standing, for lateral x-ray of pelvis to cbtain anteroposterior diameters by Thoms' technic. (Courtesy of Dr. Herbert Thoms.)

Lateral Positioning

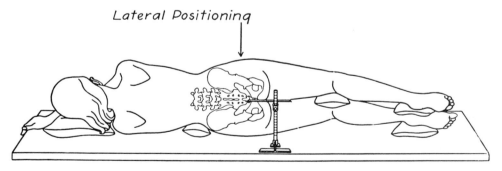

Fig. 24. Positioning of the patient, reclining, for lateral x-ray of pelvis to obtain anteroposterior diameters by Thoms' technic. (Courtesy of Dr. Herbert Thoms.)

Lateral (Isometric) Film. Technic For Anteroposterior Measurements. The problem of correction for distortion here is simple. The measurement to be obtained from this view, such as the anteroposterior diameters of the inlet, midplane, and outlet, as well as the posterior sagittal diameters of these planes, are all located in the midsagittal plane of the patient. This plane is readily located by anatomic landmarks. A metal ruler placed in this plane will be subject to the same distortion as the pelvic diameters, and its image may be used to measure these diameters directly (isometric scale).

OBTAINING THE LATERAL FILM. The patient stands with one side against a vertical Bucky diaphragm in symmetric profile position. A canvas binder is helpful in preventing motion (Fig. 23). The tube is centered just above the trochanter at a tube-film distance of 36 inches. A metallic ruler with centimeter notches supported on a standard is placed close to the sacrum or symphysis pubis in the midsagittal plane of the patient and parallel to the film. The exposure varies with the thickness of the patient.

If a standing film is inconvenient, the patient may be positioned lying on the side with the table horizontal. A head pillow, lateral lumbar pad, and pads between knees and ankles are necessary for good positioning (Fig. 24). The marker is positioned between the buttocks or directly in front of the symphysis pubis and parallel to the table top. Other factors are the same as for the standing film.

The above-described laeral film and measurements, or slight variations thereof, are universal in almost all varieties of x-ray pelvimetry. The major variation in accepted methods of pelvimetry is the manner in which the transverse diameters are measured.

MEASURING THE LATERAL FILM. The end points of each diameter are located. Each diameter is then spanned by a caliper, and that distance is transferred directly to the image of the centimeter scale on the film, giving the corrected diameter. Diameters that may be measured are the obstetric conjugate; posterior sagittal of the inlet, midpelvis, and outlet; and anteroposterior diameter of midpelvis and outlet. Observation should be made of the curvature and inclination of the sacrum and of the appearance of the sacrosciatic notch (Fig. 25).

The lateral isometric film with its exact measurement of the important obstetric conjugate is the most valuable single tool in the commonest type of serious pelvic contraction, that is, of the inlet. Such a film can be obtained by any physician with access to a standard x-ray machine. The only special equipment needed is a metal ruler with centimeter notches or perforations. A review of the contours and bony anatomy of the lateral view of the pelvis will facilitate location of the symphysis, sacrum, and ischial spines, which can be easily accomplished with a little practice.

Anteroposterior Film. Technic For Transverse Measurements. Correction for divergent distortion in this view is more complicated because the diameters of interest (the transverse of the inlet, interspinous, and intertuberal diameters) are at somewhat different levels. The locations of these levels, moreover, are not clearly marked anatomically as is the midline. Hence the use of isometric scales is more difficult.

THOMS' METHOD. The patient is placed on the x-ray table in a semirecumbent position. Back rests have been especially designed to support the patient at an angle such that the inlet of the pelvis is parallel to the x-ray plate. This positioning of the inlet should be checked by adjusting the patient so that the perpendicular distance from the junction of the fourth and fifth lumbar interspace to the table top and the distance from a point 1 cm below the upper border of the symphysis to the table top are equal. This measurement is recorded so that the perforated grid may later be properly placed. The x-ray tube is centered about 6 cm cephalad to the symphysis and at a tube-film distance of 36 inches. The intensity of the exposure is varied according to the girth of the patient.

The patient is removed from the table, leaving the tube and exposed film in place. The centimeter grid, a special lead plate with perforations along one edge, is placed in the same plane as that previously occupied by the pelvic inlet, as ascertained by the measurements (Fig. 26). A second (flash) exposure is made on the edge of the previously exposed film; for this purpose the tube is positioned over the perforated region in the grid at the distance of 36 inches.

The top row of centimeter perforations as they appear on the film is the correction for the plane of the pelvic inlet (Fig. 27). The lower rows are correction scales for 5, 6, 7, 8, and 9 cm below the plane of the outlet.

MEASURING THE ANTEROPOSTERIOR FILM. The transverse diameter of the inlet is spanned by a caliper and measured on the top row of perforations. The levels below the inlet at which the midplane and outlet are placed can be ascertained from the lateral film. The caliper measures the interspinous and transverse outlet diameters, and these measurements are read directly from the appropriate correction scales.

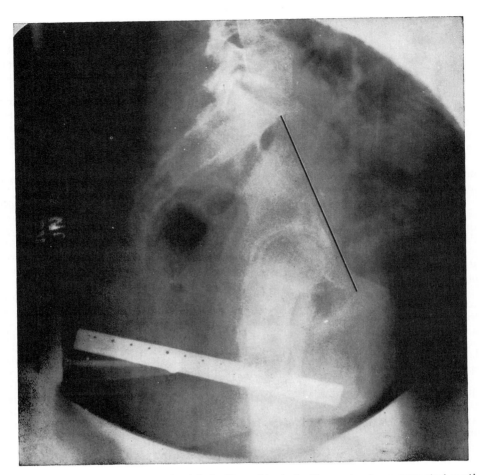

Fig. 25. Lateral roentgenogram of pelvis by Thoms' technic. The scale shows corrected centi-meters in the sagittal plane.

COLCHER-SUSSMAN METHOD.   This is a greatly simplified method of obtaining the transverse diameters of the pelvis by a single scale method that depends upon position-ing the patient so that the transverse diameters of the inlet, midplane, and outlet occupy the same plane. A single isometric scale is placed in this plane. Unfortunately, these diameters cannot always be brought into the same plane, causing considerable error in some pelves, the greatest of which appears to be underestimation of the interspinous diameter.

STEREOSCOPIC METHOD.   This technic is a parallax type of pelvimetry. Two films are taken under the same conditions. Between exposures the x-ray tube is shifted a standard predetermined distance. The distortion may be corrected either by the use of a precision stereoscope or by geometric calculations or construction of a nomogram.

Caldwell and Moloy developed a precision stereoscope in which the factors used in taking the films were duplicated in the optical systems. A centimeter rule applied to the image, in space, gives the measurements directly. The subjective factor is large in this technic, and special equipment is needed. It is, furthermore, almost impossible to purchase such equipment at the present time.

Hodges has applied to the pair of stereoscopic films geometric calculations that produced accurate measurements of the transverse diameters of the pelvis. This variation

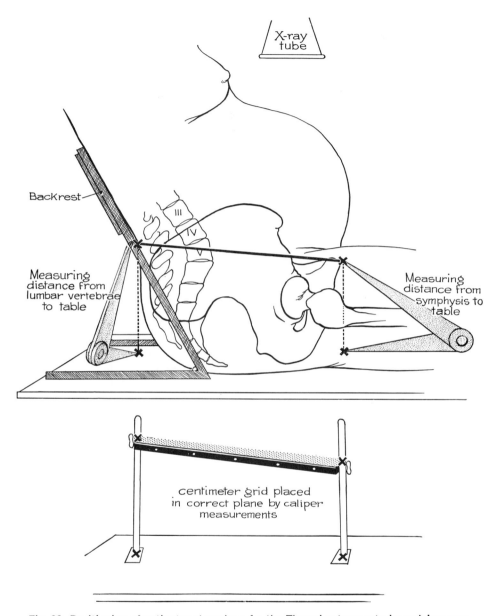

Fig. 26. Positioning of patient and markers for the Thoms' anteroposterior pelvic x-rays.

of the Caldwell-Moloy technic permits the use of standard roentgen equipment. The films may be studied in standard stereoscopic viewers for interpretation of morphology. This method has been used satisfactorily in our clinics and several other teaching hospitals for many years.

Taking Stereoscopic Films for Geometric Calculation: The patient is placed in the recumbent position with a small lumbar pad. There must be no movement between the two exposures. Centering is at the level of the anterior iliac spines. Tube-film distance is constant at 36 inches, and tube shift between exposures is *exactly* 10 cm. The tray and cassettes must occupy a fixed position for the two exposures. A perforated lead

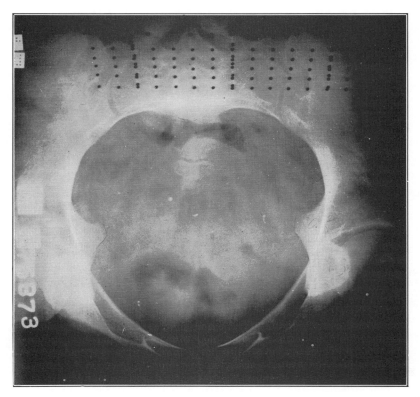

Fig. 27. Anteroposterior roentgenogram of pelvis by Thoms' technic. (Courtesy of Dr. Herbert Thoms.)

marker is centered over one side of the cassette to register on each film and allow accurate superimposition of the two films.

Measuring the Films: End points of the diameters to be measured (the transverse of the inlet, interspinous, and intertuberal diameters) are perforated with a stylet and each distance measured. The two films are then superimposed over a view-box using the register markers for alignment. The parallax shift (P) of each end point is measured. A correction factor for *each* diameter is calculated using the parallax shift for that diameter:

$$\text{Factor} = \frac{\text{Tube Shift}}{\text{Parallax} + \text{Tube Shift}} = \frac{10}{P + 10}$$

This factor is derived from the geometric setup used in taking the films. Each diameter measured on the film is multiplied by its own correction factor.

SNOW'S METHOD. The transverse measurements of the pelvis are obtained by taking a film with the patient in the same position as that used in Thoms' method. The tube-film distance is 36 inches. Instead of using a distortion scale, a special ruler has been constructed that automatically allows for the distortion. Both the anteroposterior and lateral films are used for ascertaining distortion. There are assumptions concerning distortion that may or may not pertain. The measurements achieved are not of the same order of accuracy as those obtained by the stereoscopic method. This method is relatively simple, however.

There are certain critical measurements at or below which the pelvic plane is con-

Table 1. Critical Measurements in X-Ray Pelvimetry

Planes	Anteroposterior	Diameters in Centimeters Transverse	Posterior-Sagittal
Inlet	10.0	12.0	—
Midplane	11.5	9.5	4.0
Outlet	11.5	10.0	7.5

sidered technically contracted (Table 1). These numbers by no means imply that a cesarean section is necessary. They do indicate caution, however, in the use of oxytocin if the fetus is of normal size (Ch. 28, p. 845).

PELVIC SHAPE

As described in the foregoing section, x-ray pelvimetry not only provides greater precision of mensuration but makes possible the measurement of many important diameters that cannot be obtained manually. Pelvic roentgenography has also afforded an understanding of the general architecture or configuration of the pelvis, apart from its size. The classical studies of Caldwell and Moloy have produced a classification of the pelvis according to shape that is now widely used.

Familiarity with such a classification contributes to the understanding of the mechanism of labor and the intelligent management of labor in pelvic contraction. In that connection, study of pelvic shape has pointed up the importance of the pelvic space actually available to the fetal head, as opposed to the total space indicated by absolute dimensions. For example, a spherical object can pass through a circular opening of smaller area than that occupied by the smallest rectangle that it could traverse, because all the area is utilized by the object.

The Caldwell-Moloy classification is based on the type of the posterior and anterior segments of the inlet (Figs. 28 and 29). A line drawn through the greatest transverse diameter of the inlet divides the inlet into anterior and posterior segments. The posterior segment determines the type, whereas the anterior segment may show variations. Many pelves are not pure but mixed types—as, for example, a gynecoid pelvis with android "tendency," meaning that the hindpelvis is gynecoid and the forepelvis is android. The pelvic characteristics upon which the Caldwell-Moloy classification is based are considered in the following paragraphs.

The Inlet.   The pelvic inlet is divided into anterior and posterior segments by the widest transverse diameter. The posterior sagittal diameter of the inlet is that portion of the anteroposterior diameter posterior to the point of intersection with the transverse diameter. The first question concerns the length of the posterior sagittal diameter. Whether the transverse diameter of the pelvis is very close to the promontory of the sacrum or some distance removed determines whether the posterior segment is flattened anteroposteriorly or elongated. It is also important to know whether the sides of the posterior segment are well rounded or form a wedge. The anterior segment should then be examined to ascertain whether it forms a fairly good semicircle, a flattened semicircle, or a wedge-shaped triangular area. The length of the anterior sagittal diameter, moreover, must be noted. Finally, the relation of the transverse to the anteroposterior diameter of the pelvis as a whole must be ascertained. If the transverse diameter is greater than the anteroposterior, the inlet will naturally be ovoid transversely; if the reverse is true,

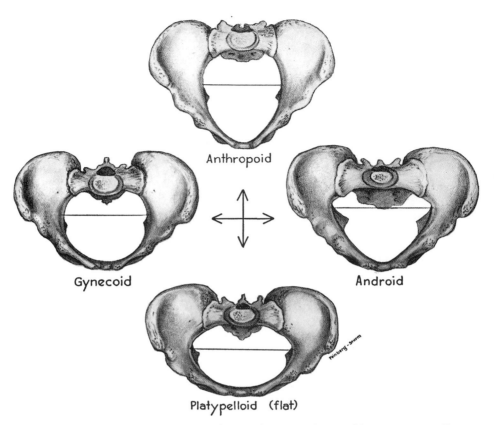

Fig. 28. The four parent pelvic types. A line passing through the widest transverse diameter divides the inlet into anterior and posterior segments. (From Moloy and Swenson. Diagnostic Roentgenology. Courtesy Thos. Nelson & Sons.)

the ovoid will be anteroposterior; if the measurements are approximately equal, the inlet will, of course, be circular.

The Sacrosciatic Notch.   The size and width of the sacrosciatic notch must be ascertained, for capacity of the posterior inlet is determined largely by the size of the sacrosciatic notch. If the notch is large, the posterior sagittal diameter of the inlet is usually large, whereas if it is small, that diameter will be short. This relation holds because the width or narrowness of the sacrosciatic notch affects the ilium and consequently the length of the posterior iliac portion of the inlet. When the sacrum has been rotated backward to a considerable extent with forward rotation of the sacral promontory, the reverse may obtain; that is, the sagittal diameter of the inlet may be short and the sacrosciatic notch wide.

Splay of Side Walls.   Whether the side walls are divergent, straight, or convergent is of clinical importance, since it is important to know whether the width at the inlet is preserved throughout the pelvis. When the splay is actually divergent the pelvis always has a very wide subpubic arch, although the angle of the forepelvis may be either wide or narrow. Convergent side walls are usually found in conjunction with a narrow subpubic arch, but the angle of the forepelvis may be either wide or narrow.

Character of the Ischial Spines.   It is important to know whether the ischial spines project into the pelvic cavity or are barely visible or invisible when the inlet is viewed from above. Since prominent ischial spines are located in the plane of least pelvic dimensions, they may cause great difficulty in labor; they indicate, furthermore, the possibility

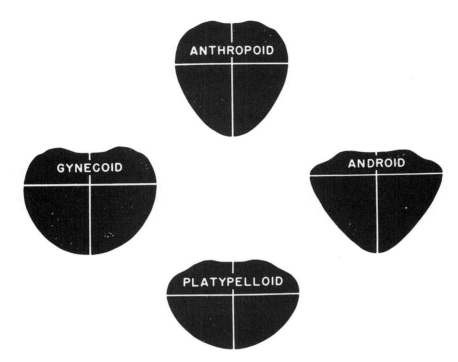

Fig. 29. The pelvic inlets of the parent types, showing anterior and posterior segments. (From Steele. Amer J Obstet Gynec 44:783, 1942.)

of definite convergence of the side walls of the pelvis, another unfavorable prognostic sign.

The Sacrum. The inclination of the sacrum as a whole is the fixed position of the anterior sacral surface in relation to the true pelvis. It determines the anteroposterior diameter of the bony pelvis, from symphysis to sacrum, at any level. The sacrum may be forward in the pelvis, parallel to the symphysis, or sloping backward to approach an almost horizontal position. The length, width, curvature, and number of sacral segments are important data. An increase in length of the sacrum is usually the result of partial or complete fusion of the fifth lumbar vertebra with the first sacral segment above or of bony union of the last sacral segment with the first coccygeal vertebra below.

Subpubic Arch. The subpubic arch may be wide, moderate, or narrow. Roentgenograms of the subpubic arch afford an opportunity to estimate its width as well as to judge the character of the bones, which may be delicate, average, or heavy.

Caldwell, Moloy, and Swenson consider it most advisable for the obstetrician to note the characteristics of the inlet, the sacrum, the ischial spines, and the pubic arch while viewing the stereoroentgenograms or even when estimating pelvic shape and size by vaginal examination. It then becomes easier to judge the obstetric capacity of any pelvis, even if it is difficult to classify.

Gynecoid Pelvis. This pelvis displays the anatomic characteristics ordinarily associated with the human female. The posterior sagittal diameter at the inlet is only slightly shorter than the anterior sagittal. The sides of the posterior segment are well rounded, and the forepelvis is also well rounded and wide. Since the transverse diameter of the inlet is either slightly greater than or about the same as the anteroposterior diameter, the inlet as a whole is either slightly oval or round. The side walls of the pelvis are straight; the spines are not prominent; and the pubic arch is wide, with a transverse diameter at the spines of 10 cm or more. The sacrum is inclined neither anteriorly nor posteriorly. The sacrosciatic notch is well rounded and never narrow. Caldwell, Moloy, and Swenson ascertained the frequency of the four parent types by study of Todd's collection of pelves of known sex. They found the gynecoid pelvis the most common type, occurring in 41 to 42 per cent of women.

Android Type.   The posterior sagittal diameter at the inlet is much shorter than the anterior sagittal, precluding use of the posterior space by the fetal head. The sides of the posterior segment are not rounded but tend to form, with the corresponding sides of the anterior segment, a wedge at their point of junction. The forepelvis is narrow and triangular. The side walls are usually convergent; the ischial spines are prominent; and the subpubic arch is narrowed. The bones are characteristically heavy. The sacrosciatic notch is narrow and high-arched. The sacrum is set forward in the pelvis and is usually straight, with little or no curvature, and the posterior sagittal diameter is decreased from inlet to outlet by the forward inclination. Not infrequently there is considerable forward inclination of the tip.

The extreme android pelvis presages a very poor prognosis for delivery by the vaginal route; the frequency of difficult forceps operations and stillbirths increases substantially in the small android pelvis. The android type makes up 32.5 per cent of pure-type pelves encountered in white women and 15.7 per cent in nonwhite women in the Todd collection.

Anthropoid Pelvis.   This pelvis is characterized essentially by an anteroposterior diameter of the inlet greater than the transverse, forming more or less an oval anteroposteriorly, with the anterior segment somewhat narrow and pointed. The sacrosciatic notch is large. The side walls are often somewhat convergent, and the sacrum is inclined posteriorly, thus increasing the posterior space at all levels. The sacrum usually has six segments and is straight, making the anthropoid pelvis deeper than the other types.

The ischial spines are likely to be prominent. The subpubic arch is frequently somewhat narrow but well shaped. The anthropoid pelvis is said to be more common in nonwhite races, whereas the android form is more frequent in the white race. Anthropoid types make up 23.5 per cent of pure-type pelves in white women, in comparison with 40.5 per cent in nonwhite women.

Platypelloid Type.   This pelvis is a flat gynecoid pelvis, with a short anteroposterior and a wide transverse diameter. The latter is set well in front of the sacrum, as in the typical gynecoid form. The angle of the forepelvis is very wide, and the anterior puboiliac and posterior iliac portions of the iliopectineal lines are well curved. The sacrum is usually well curved and rotated backward. Thus, the sacrum is short and the pelvis shallow, creating a wide sacrosciatic notch. The platypelloid pelvis is the rarest of the pure varieties, occurring in but 2.6 per cent of white and 1.7 per cent of nonwhite women.

Intermediate Types.   Intermediate or mixed types of pelves are much more frequent than the pure types. The character of the posterior segment determines the type, and that of the anterior segment the tendency.

HAZARDS OF X-RADIATION

An increasing awareness of the hazards of radiation has focused attention on the true value of diagnostic x-rays in obstetrics as compared with the potential damage to the mother, her infant, and generations yet unborn. Although no categorical answer to the complex questions is possible, the increasing data give the obstetrician and the radiologist the opportunity to weigh the dangers against the potential value to the patient of the proposed procedure.

In women there are three focal points of danger: (1) damage to the mother's genetic contribution to the particular infant and thereby to future generations; (2) damage to the fetus both immediate and subsequent (childhood leukemia, for example); (3) damage to the gonads of the fetus, producing an increase in incidence of congenital malformations in future generations.

Most geneticists firmly believe that the results of animal experimentation may be transferred to man and that the only entirely safe dose of irradiation is zero. Yet all of the projections for man are theoretical. In studying the reproductive histories of women from Hiroshima exposed at the time of the atom bomb to 200 roentgens or more of total body irradiation, Neel and Schull found no increase in congenital malformations, although the sex ratio was reversed. They believe that the strong tendency toward genetic homeostasis in man may invalidate some of the dire genetic predictions.

Stewart and associates reported an increase in leukemia in children of women x-rayed during pregnancy. Townsend found a real but minimal risk in Australia. Very carefully planned studies of MacMahon in the United States have indicated that the chances of cancer (including leukemia) are increased 40 per cent in the children of mothers who received abdominal or pelvic radiation during pregnancy.

The Genetics Committee of the National Academy of Sciences has set 10 roentgens as a permissible accumulated dose of medical radiation in the first 30 years of life. Although such a dose may be reasonable, the committee carefully points out that it cannot be considered harmless. At most this limit is of theoretical value, but it clearly points to a real concern with dosage. If x-ray pelvimetry is to be used at all, it is most important to know how much radiation the fetus and mother receive. The best available information from many sources (including the papers of Bewley, Laws, and Myddleton; Clayton, Farmer, and Warrick; Ardran and Crooks; and Berman and Sonnenblick) indicates that the mother's gonadal dose from pelvimetry is from 2 to 4 roentgens, and that of the fetus varies from 0.5 to 7 roentgens (Table 2). Walsh has suggested that the po-

Table 2. **Average Gonadal Dose in Milliroentgens per Exposure to Fetal Gonads and Maternal Ovaries in Pelvimetry**

Projection	Maternal Ovary	Fetal Gonads
1. Anteroposterior	460	630
2. Lateral	577	535
3. Subpubic arch and pelvic outlet	670	140
4. Superoinferior, pelvic inlet of Thoms	992	2,242

From the Second Report of the Committee on Radiologic Hazards to Patient, Ministry of Health Department of Health for Scotland. Her Majesty's Stationery Office, London, 1960.

tential hazard could be reduced by as much as 75 per cent if ultrafast films, lightening screens, shielding, and high milliamperage were employed.

It is clear that x-ray pelvimetry can no longer be justified as a routine procedure. It is equally clear that when indicated to reduce maternal or fetal damage from a host of obstetric complications, it should be employed, but only with all of the modern safety precautions.

References

Abramson, D., Roberts, S. M., and Wilson, P. D. Relaxation of the pelvic joints in pregnancy. Surg Obstet Gynec 58:595, 1934.

Ardran, G. M., and Crooks, H. E. Gonad radiation dose from diagnostic procedures. Brit J Radiol 30:295, 1957.

Bäder, A. (The significance of the unengaged head in primiparous labors). Abstracted in Ber ges Gynak u Geburtsh 31:395, 1936.

Baudelocque, J. R. 1775, L'Art des accouchements. Nou. ed., Paris, Des Prez Mequinon, 1789, T.I., pp. 76–90.

Berman, R., and Sonnenblick, B. P. Intravaginal measurement of radiation dose incident to x-ray pelvimetry and hysterosalpingography. Amer J Obstet Gynec 74:1, 1957.

Bewley, D. K., Laws, J. W., and Myddleton, C. J. Maternal and fetal radiation dosage during obstetric radiographic examinations. Brit J Radiol 30:286, 1957.

Borell, U., and Fernström, I. Movements at the sacro-iliac joints and their importance to changes in pelvic dimensions during parturition. Acta Obstet Gynec Scand 36:42, 1957.

Brill, H. M., and Danelius, G. Roentgen pelvimetric analysis of Walcher's position. Amer J Obstet Gynec 42:821, 1941.

Budin, R. C. (X-radiography of a Naegele pelvis). Obstetrique Par 2:499, 1897.

Caldwell, W. E., Moloy, H. C., and D'Esopo, D. A. A roentgenologic study of the mechanism of engagement of the fetal head. Amer J Obstet Gynec 28:824, 1934.

———— and Moloy, H. C. Anatomical variations in the female pelvis and their effect in labor with a suggested classification. Amer J Obstet Gynec 26:479, 1933.

———— Moloy, H. C., and D'Esopo, D. A. Studies on pelvic arrests. Amer J Obstet Gynec 36:928, 1938.

———— Moloy, H. C., and Swenson, P. C. The use of the roentgen ray in obstetrics. Part I. Roentgen pelvimetry and cephalometry; technic of pelvioroentgenography. Amer J Roentgen 41:305, 1939.

———— Moloy, H. C., and Swenson, P. C. The use of the roentgen ray in obstetrics. Part II. Anatomical variations in the female pelvis and their classification according to morphology. Amer J Roentgen 41:505, 1939.

———— Moloy, H. C., and Swenson, P. C. The use of the roentgen ray in obstetrics. Part III. The mechanism of labor. Amer J Roentgen 41:719, 1939.

Clayton, C. G., Farmer, F. T., and Warrick, C. K. Radiation doses to the foetal and maternal gonads in obstetrics radiography during late pregnancy. Brit J Radiol 30:291, 1957.

Colcher, A. E., and Sussman, W. A practical technique for roentgen pelvimetry with new positioning. Amer J Roentgen 51:207, 1944.

Dippel, A. L. The diagonal conjugate versus x-ray pelvimetry. Surg Gynec Obstet 68:642, 1939.

Eastman, N. J. Pelvic mensuration: a study in the perpetuation of error. Obstet Gynec Survey 3:301, 1948.

———— Editorial comment. Obstet Gynec Survey 12:848, 1957.

Eller, W. C., and Mengert, W. F. Recognition of midpelvic contraction Amer J Obstet Gynec 53:252, 1947.

Freund, W. A. (On the so-called kyphotic pelvis). Gynaek Klin Strassb I pp. 1–84, 1885.

Gurlt, E. F. Über einige Missgestaltungen des weiblichen Beckens. Berlin, G. Reimer, 1854.

Hanson, S. A new pelvimeter for the measurement of the bispinous diameter. Amer J Obstet Gynec 19:124, 1930.

———— Internal pelvimetry as a basis for the morphological classification of pelves. Amer J Obstet Gynec 35:228, 1938.

Hodges, P. C. An epiphyseal chart. Amer J Roentgen 30:809, 1933.

———— Roentgen pelvimetry and fetometry. Amer J Roentgen 37:644, 1937.

———— The role of x-ray pelvimetry in obstetrics. Minnesota Med 32:33, 1949.

———— and Dippel, A. L. Collective review. The use of x-rays in obstetrical diagnosis, with particular reference to pelvimetry and fetometry. Internat Abstr Surg 70:421, 1940.

———— and Hamilton, J. E. Pelvic roentgenography in pregnancy. Further experiments with 90° triangulation methods. Radiology 30:157, 1938.

———— Hamilton, J. E., and Pearson, J. W. Roentgen measurement of the obstetrical conjugate of the pelvic inlet. Amer J Roentgen 43:127, 1940.

Holst. (Description of the pelvis and the delivery of a 40-year-old female Amelus). Holst's Beiträge, Hef. 2 pp 145–148, 1869.

Javert, C. T. A combined isometric and steroscopic technic for radiographic examination of the obstetrical patient. N Carolina Med J 4:465, 1943.

Kaltreider, D. F. The diagonal conjugate. Amer J Obstet Gynec 61:1075, 1951.

———— Criteria of midplane contraction. Amer J Obstet Gynec 63:392, 1952.

Laughlin, J. S., and Pullman, I. Report of the Genetics Committee of the National Academy of

Sciences' Study of the Biological Effects of Atomic Radiation: Gonadal Dose Produced by the Medical Use of X-rays. Washington, National Academy of Sciences, 1957.

Litzmann, C.C.T. Die Formen des Beckens. Berlin, G. Reimer, 1861.

MacMahon, B. Prenatal x-ray exposure and childhood cancer. J Nat Cancer Inst 28:1173, 1962 (13 ref. cited).

Mengert, W. F. Estimation of pelvic capacity. JAMA 138:169, 1948.

———— and Eller, W. C. Graphic portrayal of relative pelvic size. Amer J Obstet Gynec 52:1032, 1946.

Morton, D. G., and Hayden, C. T. A comparative study of male and female pelves in children with a consideration of the etiology of pelvic conformation. Amer J Obstet Gynec 41:485, 1941.

Neel, J. V., and Schull, W. J. The effect of exposure to the atomic bomb on pregnancy termination in Hiroshima and Nagasaki, Washington, D.C., National Academy of Sciences, National Research Council Publication No. 461, 1956.

Report of the Committee on Genetic Effects of Atomic Radiation. Washington, D.C., National Academy of Sciences, 1956; Amer J Hum Genet 8:207, 1956.

Smellie Treatise on the Theory and Practice of Midwifery, with Collection of Cases, 8th ed., London, 1774.

Snow, W. Late extrauterine pregnancy diagnosed by soft tissue roentgenography. Amer J Roentgen 41:537, 1939.

———— Roentgenology in Obstetrics. Springfield, Ill., Charles C Thomas, 1952.

Stewart, A., Webb, J., Giles, D., and Hewitt, D. Malignant disease in childhood and diagnostic irradiation in utero. Lancet 2:447, 1956.

Thoms, H. Outlining the superior strait of the pelvis by means of the x-ray. Amer J Obstet Gynec 4:257, 1922.

———— The Obstetric Pelvis. Baltimore, The Williams & Wilkins Co., 1935.

———— The uses and limitations of roentgen pelvimetry. Amer J Obstet Gynec 34:150, 1937.

———— Routine roentgen pelvimetry in 600 primiparous white women consecutively delivered at term. Amer J Obstet Gynec 37:101, 1939.

———— The estimation of pelvic capacity. Amer J Surg 47:691, 1940

———— Roentgen pelvimetry as a routine prenatal procedure. Amer J Obstet Gynec 40:891, 1940.

———— The clinical application of roentgen pelvimetry and a study of the results in 1,100 white women. Amer J Obstet Gynec 42:957, 1941.

———— The relation of the sacral promontory to the pelvic inlet. Amer J Obstet Gynec 46:110, 1943.

———— Precision methods in cephalometry and pelvimetry. Amer J Obstet Gynec 46:753, 1943.

———— Foote, W. R., and Friedman, I. The clinical significance of pelvic variations. Amer J Obstet Gynec 38:634, 1939.

———— and Godfried, M. S. The suboccipitobregmatic circumference. Amer J Obstet Gynec 39:841, 1940.

———— and Greulich, W. W. A comparative study of male and female pelves. Amer J Obstet Gynec 39:56, 1940.

———— and Wilson, H. M. Lateral roentgenometry of the pelvis. A newly modified technic. Yale J Biol Med 9:305, 1937.

———— and Wilson, H. M. Roentgen methods for routine obstetrical pelvimetry. Yale J Biol Med 10:437, 1938.

———— and Wilson, H. M. Practical application of modern pelvimetric methods. Yale J Biol Med 11:179, 1939.

———— and Wilson, H. M. The roentgenological survey of the pelvis. Yale J Biol Med 13:831, 1941.

Townsend, L. Radiation hazards to the fetus. Med J Aust 2:289, 1958.

Walsh, J. W. Diagnostic x-ray procedures in obstetrics. Obstet Gynec 13:74, 1959.

Young, J. Relaxation of pelvic joints in pregnancy; pelvic arthropathy of pregnancy. J Obstet Gynaec Brit Emp 47:493, 1940.

11

PRESENTATION, POSITION, ATTITUDE, AND LIE OF THE FETUS

Irrespective of the relation that it may bear to the mother, the fetus in the later months of pregnancy assumes a characteristic posture, which is described as the *attitude* or *habitus* (Fig. 1), and which indicates the relations of the fetal

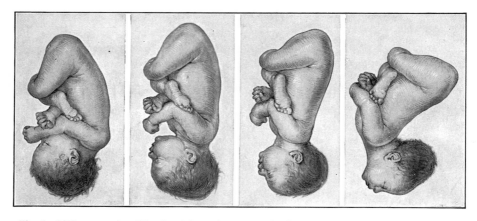

Fig. 1. Differences in attitude of fetus in vertex, sinciput, brow, and face presentations.

parts to one another. As a rule, the fetus forms an ovoid mass corresponding roughly to the shape of the uterine cavity and is folded or bent upon itself in such a way that the back becomes markedly convex; the head is sharply flexed so that the chin is almost in contact with the chest; the thighs are flexed over the abdomen; the legs are bent at the knee joints; and the arches of the feet rest upon the anterior surfaces of the legs. The arms are usually crossed over the thorax or are parallel to the sides, and the umbilical cord lies in the space between them and the lower extremities. This characteristic attitude results partly from the mode of growth of the fetus and partly from a process of accommodation to the uterine cavity.

Lie of the Fetus. The *lie* is the relation of the long axis of the fetus to that of the mother and is either *longitudinal* or *transverse*. Occasionally during pregnancy the fetal and the maternal axes may cross at a 45-degree angle, forming an *oblique lie,* which always become longitudinal or transverse during the course of labor. Longitudinal lies are noted in over 99 per cent of labors at term.

Presentation and Presenting Part. The presenting part is that portion of the fetus either foremost within the birth canal or in closest proximity to it and which is felt through the cervix on vaginal examination. The presenting part determines the *presentation.* Accordingly, in longitudinal lies the presenting part is either the head or the breech, creating *cephalic* and *breech presentations,* respectively. When the fetus lies with its long axis transversely, the shoulder is the presenting part, and a shoulder presentation obtains.

Cephalic presentations are classified according to the relation of the head to the body of the fetus. Usually, the head is sharply flexed, so that the chin is in contact with the thorax. In these circumstances the occipital region of the skull, or the *vertex,* is the presenting part (*vertex presentation*). Much less commonly the neck may be sharply extended so that the occiput and back come in contact and the face is foremost in the birth canal (*face presentation*). The head may assume a position between these extremes, partially flexed in some cases with the large fontanel presenting (*sincipital presentation*), or partially extended in other cases with the brow presenting (*brow presentation*). The last two should perhaps not be classified as distinct presentations, since they are usually transient; as labor progresses they become converted into vertex or face presentations by flexion or extension, respectively.

When the fetus presents by the breech, the thighs may be flexed and the legs extended over the anterior surfaces of the body (*frank breech presentation*); or the thighs may be flexed on the abdomen and the legs upon the thighs (*full breech presentation*); or one or both feet may be lowermost (*single or double foot or footling presentation*). When one or both feet, or one or both knees, are lowermost, an *incomplete breech presentation* results. Since the mechanism of labor is essentially the same in all breech presentations, the several types need not be considered separately here.

Position. Position refers to the relation of an arbitrarily chosen portion of the fetus to the right or left side of the maternal birth canal. Accordingly, with each presentation there may be two positions, right or left. The occiput, chin, and sacrum are the determining points in vertex, face, and breech presentations, respectively (Figs. 2–9).

Variety. For still more accurate orientation, the relation of a given portion of the presenting part to the anterior, transverse, or posterior portion of the mother's pelvis is considered. Since there are two positions, there must be six varieties for each presentation (Figs. 10–13).

Nomenclature. Since the presenting part in any presentation may be in either the left or right position, there are left and right occipital, left and right mental, and left and right sacral presentations, which in abbreviated form may be written LO and RO, LM and RM, LS and RS, respectively. Since the presenting part in each of the two positions may be directed anteriorly, transversely, or posteriorly, there are six varieties of each of these three presentations, as classified in Table 1.

In shoulder presentations the acromion (or the scapula) is the portion of the fetus arbitrarily chosen to orient it with the maternal pelvis; one example of the terminology sometimes employed for this purpose is illustrated in Figure 9. The acromion or back of the fetus may be directed either posteriorly, anteriorly, superiorly, or inferiorly (Ch. 29, p. 872). Since, however, it is impossible by clinical

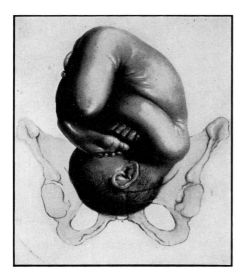

Fig. 2. Left occiput transverse (LOT), the most common position.

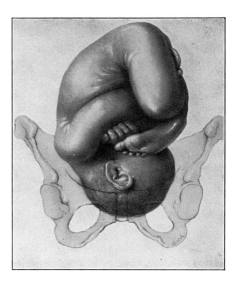

Fig. 3. Right occiput transverse (ROT), the second most common position.

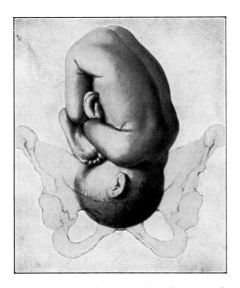

Fig. 4. Left occiput anterior (LOA) position.

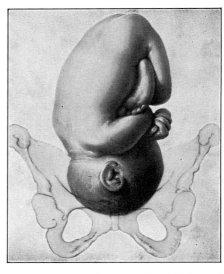

Fig. 5. Right occiput anterior (ROA) position.

examination to differentiate exactly the several varieties of shoulder presentation, and since such differentiation serves no practical purpose, it is customary to refer to all transverse lies of the fetus simply as shoulder presentations.

Frequency of the Various Presentations and Positions.   At or near term the incidence of the various presentations is approximately as follows: vertex, 95 per cent; breech, 3.5 per cent; face, 0.5 per cent; shoulder, 0.5 per cent. About two

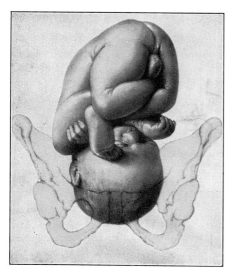

Fig. 6. Right occiput posterior (ROP) position.

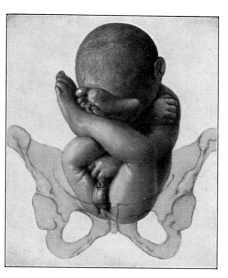

Fig. 7. Left sacrum posterior (LSP) position.

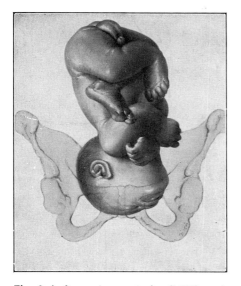

Fig. 8. Left mentum anterior (LMA) position.

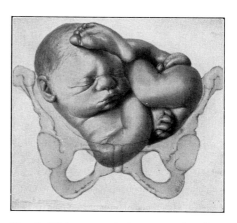

Fig. 9. Right acromiodorsoposterior (RA-DP) position. The acromium is to the mother's right and the back is posterior.

thirds of all vertex presentations are in the left position, and one third in the right. The occiput is usually directed transversely; the frequency of the various positions of the vertex is shown in Table 1 on page 324.

Although the incidence of breech presentation is only a little over 3 per cent at term, it is much greater earlier in pregnancy. White found the incidence of

Table 1. **Classification of Vertex, Face, and Breech Presentations**

	Position	*Presentation*	*Variety*	*Abbreviation*
Vertex presentations	Left	Occiput	Anterior	LOA
	"	"	Transverse	LOT
	"	"	Posterior	LOP
	Right	"	Anterior	ROA
	"	"	Transverse	ROT
	"	"	Posterior	ROP
Face presentations	Left	Mentum	Anterior	LMA
	"	"	Transverse	LMT
	"	"	Posterior	LMP
	Right	"	Anterior	RMA
	"	"	Transverse	RMT
	"	"	Posterior	RMP
Breech presentations	Left	Sacrum	Anterior	LSA
	"	"	Transverse	LST
	"	"	Posterior	LSP
	Right	"	Anterior	RSA
	"	"	Transverse	RST
	"	"	Posterior	RSP

breech presentation to be 7.2 per cent by x-ray examination at the end of the thirty-fourth week. In about one third of the nulliparas and two thirds of the multiparas the breech converted to vertex spontaneously before delivery. The same progressive decline in the incidence of breech presentation is seen when the weight of the infants delivered by the breech is analyzed (Table 2).

Table 2. **The Incidence of Breech Delivery by Fetal Weight Groups**

Weight (g)	*Breech Births*	*Total Births*	*Per Cent Breech*
401–1,000	251	682	36.8
1,001–1,500	167	613	27.2
1,501–2,000	196	1,235	15.9
2,001–2,500	337	4,197	8.0
2,501 and over	1,616	54,726	3.0
Total	2,567	61,453	4.2

From The Obstetrical Statistical Cooperative, courtesy of Schuyler Kohl.

Reasons for the Predominance of Cephalic Presentations. Of the several reasons advanced to explain why the fetus at term usually presents by the vertex, the most logical seems to be the piriform shape of the uterus. Although the fetal head at term is slightly larger than the breech, the entire podalic pole of the fetus— that is, the breech and its flexed extremities—is bulkier than the cephalic pole and more movable. The cephalic pole is represented by the head only, since the upper extremities are some distance removed and small and less protruding. Until about the thirty-second week the amniotic cavity is large in relation to fetal mass, and there is no crowding of the fetus by the uterine walls. At approximately that time, however, the ratio of amniotic contents to fetal mass alters by relative diminution of amniotic fluid. As a result, the uterine walls are more closely apposed to the fetal parts, and only then does the piriform shape of the uterus exert its effect. The fetus, if presenting by the breech, changes its polarity to make use of the roomier fundus for its bulkier and more movable podalic pole. The high

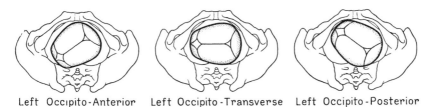

Left Occipito-Anterior   Left Occipito-Transverse   Left Occipito-Posterior

Fig. 10. Left positions in occiput presentations, with fetal head viewed from below.

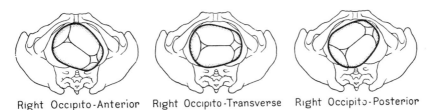

Right Occipito-Anterior   Right Occipito-Transverse   Right Occipito-Posterior

Fig. 11. Right positions in occiput presentations.

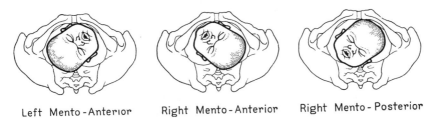

Left Mento-Anterior   Right Mento-Anterior   Right Mento-Posterior

Fig. 12. Left and right positions in face presentations.

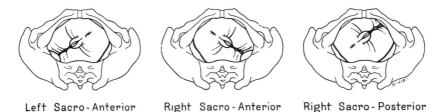

Left Sacro-Anterior   Right Sacro-Anterior   Right Sacro-Posterior

Fig. 13. Left and right positions in breech presentations.

incidence of breech presentation in hydrocephalic fetuses is in accord with this theory, since there the cephalic pole is definitely larger than the podalic. The relatively high frequency of breech presentations in anencephalic monsters is not inconsistent with the theory, since such fetuses are usually premature at delivery and hydramnios is the rule.

Vartan believes that the cause of breech presentation is some circumstance that prevents the normal version from taking place. Abnormal uterine shape must play a relatively small role, or breech presentations would recur much more commonly. A septum protruding into the upper uterine segment is such a factor, however. Vartan believes that a peculiarity of fetal attitude, particularly extension of the vertebral column in frank breeches, may prevent the fetus from turning; his series of roentgenograms in which the fetus did not turn and could not be turned affords convincing evidence of this contention. Another important factor, he points out, is a diminished volume of amniotic fluid.

Diagnosis of Presentation and Position of the Fetus

There are several diagnostic methods at our disposal: abdominal palpation, vaginal and rectal touch, combined examination and auscultation, and, in certain doubtful cases, roentgenography or ultrasonography.

Obstetric Palpation.   To obtain satisfactory results the examination should be performed systematically, following the four maneuvers suggested by Leopold and Sporlin. The mother should be on a firm bed or examining table, with her abdomen bared. During the first three maneuvers the examiner stands at the side of the bed most convenient to him and faces the patient, but he reverses his position and faces her feet for the last maneuver (Figs. 14 and 15).

First Maneuver.   After outlining the contour of the uterus and ascertaining how nearly its fundus approaches the xiphoid cartilage, the examiner gently palpates the fundus with the tips of the fingers of both hands to discover by which fetal pole it is occupied. The breech gives the sensation of a large, nodular body, whereas the head feels hard and round and is freely movable and ballottable.

Second Maneuver.   Having ascertained which pole of the fetus lies in the fundus, the examiner places the palms of his hands on either side of the abdomen and makes gentle but deep pressure. On one side he feels a hard resistant structure, the back, and on the other, numerous nodulations, the small parts. In women with thin abdominal walls the fetal extremities can readily be differentiated, but in obese patients only irregular nodulations can be felt. In the presence of obesity or considerable amniotic fluid, the back is more easily felt by making deep pressure with one hand while palpating with the other. By next noting whether the back is directed anteriorly, transversely, or posteriorly, a more accurate picture of the orientation of the fetus is obtained.

Third Maneuver.   The examiner grasps the lower portion of the abdomen, just above the symphysis pubis, between the thumb and fingers of one hand. If the presenting part is not engaged, a movable body will be felt, usually the head. The differentiation between head and breech is made as in the first maneuver. If the presenting part is not engaged, the examination is almost complete; with the situation of the head, breech, back, and extremities known, all that remains is to ascertain the attitude of the head. If careful palpation shows that the cephalic prominence is on the same side as the small parts, the head must be flexed, and the vertex is therefore the presenting part. When the cephalic prominence is on the same side as the back, the head must be extended. If, however, the presenting part is deeply engaged, this maneuver simply indicates that the lower pole of the fetus is fixed in the pelvis; the details are then ascertained by the last maneuver.

Fourth Maneuver.   The examiner faces the patient's feet and, with the tips of the first three fingers of each hand, makes deep pressure in the direction of

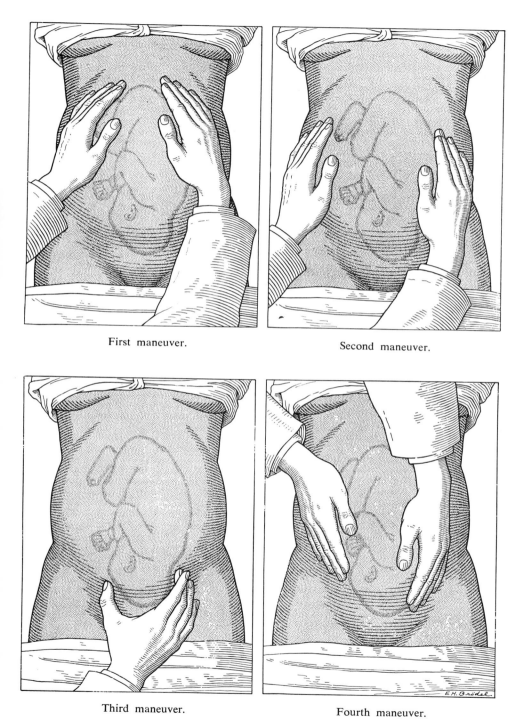

First maneuver.

Second maneuver.

Third maneuver.

Fourth maneuver.

Fig. 14. Palpation in left occiput anterior position (maneuvers of Leopold).

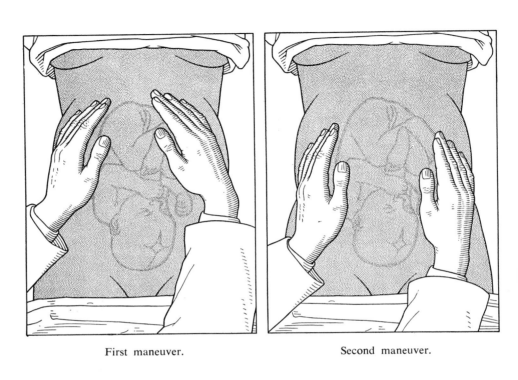

First maneuver.   Second maneuver.

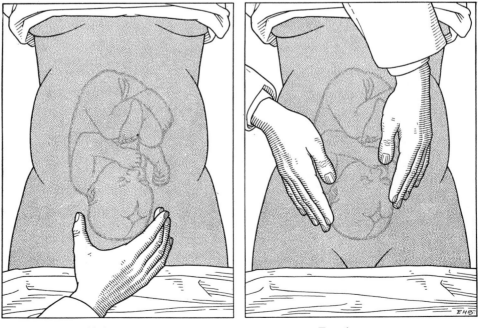

Third maneuver.   Fourth maneuver.

Fig. 15. Palpation in right occiput posterior position.

the axis of the superior strait. If the head presents, one hand is arrested sooner than the other by a rounded body, the cephalic prominence, while the other hand descends more deeply into the pelvis. In vertex presentations the prominence is on the same side as the small parts, and in face presentations on the same side as the back. The ease with which the prominence is felt indicates the extent to which descent has occurred. In many instances when the head has descended into the pelvis, the anterior shoulder of the fetus may be readily differentiated by the third maneuver. In breech presentations the information obtained from this maneuver is less precise.

Abdominal palpation may be performed throughout the later months of pregnancy and in the intervals between the contractions during labor. It provides information about the presentation and position of the fetus and the extent to which the presenting part has descended into the pelvis. For example, so long as the cephalic prominence is readily palpable, the vertex has not descended to the level of the ischial spines; when it can no longer be palpated from above, the head has descended so deeply that its most dependent part can be palpated through the pelvic floor. The degree of cephalopelvic disproportion, moreover, can be gauged by noting the extent to which the anterior portion of the head overrides the symphysis pubis. With practice, it is possible to estimate roughly the size of the fetus and even to map out the presentation of the second fetus in a twin gestation.

During labor, palpation also provides valuable information about the *lower uterine segment.* When there is obstruction to the passage of the fetus a *pathologic retraction* ring (p. 850) may be sometimes felt as a transverse or oblique ridge extending across the lower portion of the uterus. Even in normal cases, moreover, the contracting body of the uterus and the passive lower uterine segment may be distinguished by palpation. During a contraction the upper portion of the uterus is firm or hard, whereas the lower segment feels elastic or almost fluctuant.

Vaginal Examination.   Before labor the diagnosis of fetal presentation and position by vaginal examination is necessarily somewhat inconclusive, because the presenting part must be palpated through the lower uterine segment. During labor, however, after dilatation of the cervix, important information may be obtained. In vertex presentations the position and variety are recognized by differentiation of the various sutures and fontanels; in face presentations, by the differentiation of the portions of the face; and in breech presentations, by the palpation of the sacrum and ischial tuberosities.

In the most favorable circumstances the information derived from vaginal touch alone is not more accurate than that obtainable by abdominal palpation. In vertex presentations the fontanels are frequently mistaken for each other; and occasionally face and breech presentations are confused. Later in labor, moreover, after the formation of the *caput succedaneum*, detection of the various diagnostic landmarks often becomes impossible.

In attempting to ascertain presentation and position by vaginal examination, it is advisable to pursue a definite routine, comprising three maneuvers (Figs. 16 and 17): (1) After the patient is appropriately prepared, two fingers of either gloved hand are introduced into the vagina and carried up to the presenting part. The differentiation of vertex, face, and breech is then readily accomplished. (2) If the vertex is presenting, the fingers are carried up behind the symphysis pubis

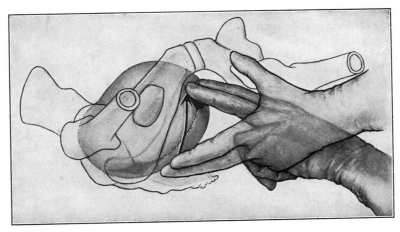

Fig. 16. Locating the sagittal suture on vaginal examination.

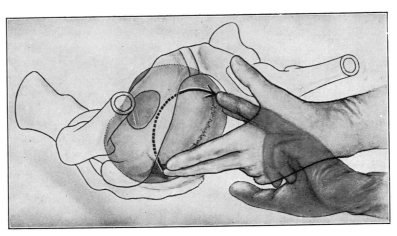

Fig. 17. Differentiating the fontanels on vaginal examination.

and are then swept backward over the head toward the sacrum. During this movement they necessarily cross the sagittal suture. When it is felt, its course is outlined, with small and large fontanels at the opposite ends. (3) The positions of the two fontanels are then ascertained. The fingers are passed to the anterior extremity of the sagittal suture, and the fontanel there encountered is carefully examined and identified; then by a circular motion the fingers are passed around the side of the head until the other fontanel is felt and differentiated. The various sutures and fontanels are thus readily located, and the possibility of error is considerably lessened; in face and breech presentations it is minimized, since the various parts are more readily distinguished.

Auscultation.   By itself auscultation does not yield very reliable information about the presentation and position of the fetus, but it sometimes reinforces the results obtained by palpation. Ordinarily the fetal heart sounds are transmitted through the convex portion of the fetus that lies in intimate contact with the uterine wall. They are therefore best heard through the back in vertex and breech and through the thorax in face presentation. The region of the abdomen in which the fetal heart tones are heard most clearly varies according to the presentation and the extent to which the presenting part has descended. In cephalic presentations the point of maximal intensity is usually midway between the umbilicus and the anterior superior spine of the ilium, whereas in breech presentations it is usually about level with the umbilicus. In occipitoanterior positions the heart sounds are usually best heard a short distance from the midline; in the transverse varieties they are heard more laterally, and in the posterior varieties well back in the patient's flank.

X-Ray and Sonar.   Improvements in roentgenographic technic have provided another diagnostic aid of particular value in doubtful cases. In obese women or those with rigid abdominal walls, an x-ray film may solve many diagnostic problems and lead to early recognition of a breech or shoulder presentation that might otherwise have escaped detection until late in labor. Ultrasonography locates the fetal head without hazards of ionizing radiation.

REFERENCES

Leopold and Sporlin.   (Conduct of normal births through external examination alone). Arch Gynaek 45:337, 1894.

Vartan, C. K.   Cause of breech presentation. Lancet 1:595, 1940.

——— The behavior of the foetus in utero with special reference to the incidence of breech presentation at term. J Obstet Gynaec Brit Emp 52:417, 1945.

White, A. J.   Spontaneous cephalic version in the later weeks of pregnancy and its significance in the management of breech presentation. J Obstet Gynaec Brit Emp 63:706, 1956.

12

PRENATAL CARE

The objective of prenatal care is to insure as far as possible that every pregnancy culminates in a healthy mother and a healthy baby.

Before the rise of present-day obstetrics the pregnant woman usually had but a single interview with a physician before he saw her in labor. At that interview he often merely sought to calculate the expected date of her confinement. When next seen by a physician she might have been in the throes of an eclamptic convulsion or striving futilely to overcome the resistance offered by a contracted pelvis. In the prevention of such calamities antepartum care has been of great value.

A priori pregnancy should be considered normal. Unfortunately the great variety and complexity of the functional and anatomic changes induced by gestation tend to stigmatize the pregnancy as an abnormal state if not actually a disease. The myriad changes in the maternal organism during pregnancy sometimes make demarcation between health and disease less distinct. Consequently, it is necessary to observe women closely throughout all of pregnancy to identify as early as possible any abnormality that might threaten the well-being of the mother and her fetus.

Examination before pregnancy undoubtedly would prove quite beneficial to the physical and emotional health of the mother-to-be and, in turn, her child-to-be. Ideally, prenatal care should be a continuation of a regimen of physician-supervised health care already established for the woman. As the consequence of such a program, acquired diseases and developmental abnormalities for the most part would be recognized before pregnancy with appropriate steps taken to eradicate them or, at least, to minimize their deleterious effects. In any event, the mother should be seen as early in pregnancy as possible and at least monthly thereafter until the seventh month; she should then visit her obstetrician at least every two weeks until the last month; thereafter she must be seen weekly. If an abnormality is discovered, the subsequent visits should be timed according to the severity of the situation.

GENERAL PROCEDURE

Definitions. A *gravida* is a woman who is or has been pregnant. With the first pregnancy she is a *primigravida* and with more than one a *multigravida*.

A *primipara* is a woman who has been delivered once of a fetus or fetuses that have reached the stage of viability. Therefore the completion of any pregnancy beyond the stage of abortion (Ch. 20, p. 493) bestows parity upon the mother. A *multipara* is a woman who has completed two or more pregnancies to the stage of viability. It is the number of *pregnancies* reaching viability and not the number of *fetuses* delivered that determines parity. Parity is not greater if a single fetus, twins, or triplets are delivered, and not less if the fetus or fetuses are stillborn.

In certain clinics it is customary to summarize the past obstetric history of a woman by a series of digits connected by dashes, thus: 6-1-2-6. The first digit refers to the number of term infants the patient has delivered, the second to the number of premature infants, the third to the number of abortions, and the fourth to the number of children currently alive. The example given indicates that the patient has had 6 term deliveries, 1 premature delivery, 2 abortions, and has 6 children alive at present. This series of digits obviously gives a more complete obstetric history than the mere designation para VII.

A *parturient* is a woman in labor.

A *puerpera* is a woman who has just given birth.

The History. For the most part the same essentials go into appropriate history taking from the pregnant woman as elsewhere in medicine. The history should be obtained unhurriedly in a reasonably private setting. This is the best time for the physician and those associated with him in providing care for the mother and her fetus to establish the good rapport that is important for a successful outcome of the pregnancy. It is undesirable for a patient to wait for protracted periods of time before interview, but it is far worse for her to be hurriedly and indifferently interrogated without having her answers appropriately evaluated. Moreover, it is mandatory that all data important to the care of the mother and fetus be recorded in such a way that all members of the obstetric team using the record can clearly understand them.

The *family history* is taken with special reference to diseases or events in which heredity appears to contribute, such as diabetes mellitus, pregnancy-induced hypertension, and twinning. The *past obstetric history* is reviewed in detail by both interrogating the mother and reviewing all available maternal and newborn records. Whenever the past history suggests that a complication had occurred elsewhere, an adequate summary of events should be obtained from the physician or clinic that provided the care. The *present pregnancy history* is then obtained, including a careful review of all systems. It is important to identify carefully the times of menstruation and other vaginal bleeding and the time of onset of fetal quickening in order to ascertain the duration of pregnancy with the greatest possible precision. A prenatal form often proves most satisfactory for recording these details.

Physical Examination A complete general examination must be performed in addition to the more specialized obstetric examination of the abdomen and pelvis. This antepartum physical examination sometimes proves to be the first reasonably thorough examination that the patient has ever had. The obstetric examination should include (1) palpation and auscultation of the uterus and its contents; (2) visualization and palpation of the cervix and vagina; (3) clinical evaluation of the bony pelvis, as described in Chapter 10; (4) palpation of the presenting part if the fetus is sufficiently large; and (5) examination of the vulva, perineum, anus, and rectum. If a Papanicolaou smear has not been evaluated recently, smears from the cervix should be obtained at the very beginning of the pelvic examination. In general, a gross lesion of the cervix should be promptly studied by punch biopsy and histologic examination.

Laboratory Tests.   Early in pregnancy the following laboratory studies are indicated: The *hemoglobin* concentration or the *hematocrit* should be ascertained at the time of the initial antepartum visit and should be repeated at about 32 weeks' gestation. If it is abnormally low at any time, further hematologic evaluation and appropriate therapy are indicated. A *serologic test for syphilis* is usually required by law. Maternal infection with the passage of spirochetes across the placenta may result in congenital syphilis, which can cause severe fetal morbidity and even death (p. 1053). Once detected, maternal syphilis is usually easy to treat, and congenital syphilis can be eradicated. In view of the current upsurge of contagious syphilis, it may be advisable to repeat the serologic test upon the patient's admittance in labor. The maternal *Rh* and *major blood type* should be ascertained. If the blood is Rh negative, detection of anti-Rh antibodies should be attempted (p. 1045). *Urine,* preferably clean voided midstream urine, should be examined for glucose and protein at the time of the initial antepartum visit and at least two or three additional times. It has long been customary to check for proteinuria at every antepartum visit, in an attempt to detect preeclampsia early. It is quite unusual, however, for proteinuria caused by preeclampsia to antedate both elevation of the blood pressure and edema. It is more important in the early detection of preeclampsia that the physician pay attention to any increase in blood pressure and to any sudden gain in weight. Bacteriuria should be searched for at least in women who have any symptoms that suggest the possibility of urinary tract infection or who had urinary tract infection previously. Technics for identifying significant bacteriuria and the diagnostic and therapeutic implications of such a finding are discussed in Chapter 27 (p. 748).

Chest X-Ray.   In many clinics a roentgenogram of the woman's chest is routinely obtained early in pregnancy. According to Schaefer this procedure leads to the detection of tuberculosis in about 1.5 to 2 per cent of patients. Because of the slight risk of radiation of the gonads of the fetus and those of the mother, as well as the very remote danger of subsequent leukemia in the child, routine chest x-ray of all pregnant women may not be warranted. In cases of disease involving the thorax, however, the benefits of roentgenographic examination of the chest far outweigh the very slight risks involved. During roentgenography the mother's abdomen should be shielded to protect the fetus, and a six-foot filtered x-ray beam should be used with the defining cone limiting the beam as nearly as possible to the thorax.

To avoid irradiation of the fetus, while continuing to search for unrecognized cases of tuberculosis, it may be of value to obtain a chest x-ray in the postpartum period before discharge from the hospital.

Return Visits.   In subsequent visits questions are asked about the general well-being of the patient and any untoward signs and symptoms, such as edema of the fingers or face, bleeding, constipation, and headache. The patient is weighed, and her blood pressure is estimated. Abdominal examinations are usually carried out at regular intervals to ascertain whether the pregnancy is progressing normally and to detect quickening and subsequent signs of fetal life. At each visit it is important to measure and record the size of the uterus, including the height of the fundus above the symphysis pubis. Failure to perform a pelvic examination on all pregnant women leads only to loss of valuable information, costly errors, and poor obstetric results.

Indicated rectal and vaginal examinations in the last month of pregnancy provide valuable information about the development of the lower uterine segment and especially the effacement and dilatation of the cervix. These data aid in estimating approach of the time of labor and in prognosticating the rapidity of labor.

Instruction to Patients. After completing the history and physical examination, the patient is instructed about diet, relaxation and sleep, bowel habits, exercise, bathing, clothing, recreation, general care, smoking, and drug ingestion. It is usually possible, and always desirable, to assure the patient that she may anticipate an uneventful pregnancy followed by an uncomplicated delivery. At the same time, however, she is tactfully instructed about the following danger signals, which must be reported immediately to the doctor:

1. Any vaginal bleeding
2. Swelling of the face or fingers
3. Severe or continuous headache
4. Dimness or blurring of vision
5. Abdominal pain
6. Persistent vomiting
7. Chills or fever
8. Dysuria
9. Escape of fluid from the vagina.

NUTRITION DURING PREGNANCY

Throughout most of this century the diets of pregnant women have been the subject of endless discussion, which has caused considerable confusion. Diet enthusiasts have urged pregnant women to adhere to a wide variety of diets, ranging from those that emphasize rigid caloric restriction to those that provide large amounts of protein, primarily of animal origin. These high-protein diets, if followed, often resulted in a relatively high caloric intake due to associated fat. The faulty reasoning that led to rigid caloric restriction stemmed primarily from the observation that the prominent feature of preeclampsia and eclampsia was excessive weight gain. That the weight gain in preeclampsia and eclampsia resulted from edema rather than excessive caloric intake was not generally appreciated.

Meaningful studies of nutrition and pregnancy in human beings are exceedingly difficult to design. Past experience suggests that a state of near starvation must be induced to establish clear differences in outcome; ethically, however, overt dietary deficiency cannot be reproduced experimentally in pregnant women. In instances in which severe nutritional deficiencies have been induced as a consequence of social, economic, or political disaster, coincidental events usually have created many variables, the effects of which are not amenable to quantitation. Examples are attempts to analyze the effects of near starvation imposed on pregnant women in World War II during the siege of Leningrad and late in the occupation of the Netherlands.

Considerable data have accumulated from experimental studies in a variety of species, especially the rat, indicating that marked restriction of the maternal diet leads to undesirable effects on the fetus and the neonate. The physical, biochemical, physiologic, and behavioral defects are usually intensified during the neonatal period, except perhaps when the newborn is nursed by a mother that has not been subjected to serious nutritional deprivation during pregnancy. Caution must be exercised, however, in applying observations made on one species to another. For example, severe protein deprivation of a few days' duration in the pregnant rat, in which gestation is only 21 days and in which total fetal weight represents 25 per cent of maternal weight, may lead to serious reproductive casualties. In human pregnancy, which lasts 280 days and in which fetal weight is only 5 per cent that of the mother, failure to ingest protein for the same number of days could hardly be expected to produce an insult of the same intensity.

The Committee on Maternal Nutrition of the Food and Nutrition Board, National Research Council, has recently reviewed the current status of our knowledge of the interrelation of maternal nutrition and reproductive performance. The deliberations and recommendations of this committee are summarized in the treatise Maternal Nutrition and the Course of Pregnancy.

During a normal pregnancy with a single fetus a weight gain of nearly 18 pounds can be accounted for on the basis of obvious pregnancy-induced physiologic changes. They include an increase of almost 11 pounds of intrauterine contents accounted for by fetus (7½ pounds), placenta (a little over 1 pound), and amniotic fluid (2 pounds), in addition to a maternal contribution of 7 pounds accounted for by increases in the weights of the uterus (2 pounds), blood (3½ pounds), and breasts (1½ pounds). The moderate expansion of the volume of interstitial fluid in the pelvis and lower extremities directly attributable to the increased venous pressure created by the large pregnant uterus is a normal event. In the ambulatory woman it most likely adds 2 to 3 pounds more. There is, therefore, a physiologic basis for a maternal weight gain of about 20 pounds.

For the woman whose weight is normal before pregnancy a gain of 20 to 25 pounds appears to be associated with the most favorable outcome of pregnancy. In most pregnant women this result may be achieved by eating according to appetite a well-balanced diet—that is, a diet that includes an ample amount of meat and other foods containing animal protein, fresh vegetables (especially the green leafy variety), and fruits. Seldom, if ever, should maternal weight gain be restricted deliberately below this level.

Eastman and Jackson have carefully evaluated the relation between maternal weight gain and birth weight in term pregnancies and noted that, in general, birth weight parallels maternal weight gain. The full significance of this relation is best appreciated when the fate of low-birth-weight infants is considered. Neonatal mortality for chronologically mature white newborns weighing 2,500 g or less was 45.1 per 1,000 live births, in contrast to 6.1 per 1,000 live births for those whose weight exceeded 2,500 g.

Undoubtedly, failure of the mother to gain weight was caused in some instances by associated maternal disease rather than just imposed caloric restriction. Nonetheless, observations such as those of Eastman and Jackson, coupled with several well-controlled animal studies demonstrating deleterious effects on the offspring when severe maternal caloric restriction is imposed, point out that rigid caloric restriction during pregnancy might be dangerous to the fetus.

Eastman and Jackson found that the incidence of low birth weight was greatest in pregnant women with both low weight before pregnancy and low weight gain during gestation. They therefore recommend that women whose weight before pregnancy is less than 120 pounds be urged to eat according to appetite, at least during the first half of pregnancy. At about the twentieth week weight gain should be reviewed. If less than 10 pounds, someone who possesses nutritional expertise should evaluate the diet and make appropriate corrections so that weight gain approaches a pound a week. Pregnancies in women in this category should be regarded as high risk and be closely followed, especially in regard to weight gain.

Periodically, the Food and Nutrition Board of the National Research Council after careful review recommends dietary allowances for women, including those who are pregnant or lactating. Their most recent guidelines are summarized in Table 1. These values are applicable to women who have completed their own growth—that is, those who are in their late teens or older and are of average

Table 1. **Food and Nutrition Board, National Research Council, Recommended Daily Dietary Allowances for Women 18 to 35 Years Old, 64 Inches Tall and Weighing 128 Pounds When Not Pregnant (Revised 1968)**

| | | Increase | |
Nutrient	*Nonpregnant*	*Pregnant*	*Lactating*
Kilocalories	2,000	200	1,000
Protein (g)	55	10	20
Vitamin A (IU)	5,000	1,000	2,000
Vitamin D (IU)	400	none	none
Vitamin E (IU)	25	5	5
Ascorbic Acid (mg)	55	5	5
Folacin* (mg)	0.4	0.4	0.1
Niacin† (mg)	13.0	2	7
Riboflavin (mg)	1.5	0.3	0.5
Thiamin (mg)	1.0	0.1	0.5
Vitamin B6 (mg)	2.0	0.5	0.5
Vitamin B12 (μg)	5.0	3.0	1.0
Calcium (g)	0.8	0.4	0.5
Phosphorus (g)	0.8	0.4	0.5
Iodine (μg)	100	25	50
Iron (mg)	18	none	none
Magnesium (mg)	300	150	150

* *Refers to dietary sources ascertained by* Lactobacillus casei *assay; pteroylglutamic acid may be effective in smaller doses.*
† *Includes dietary sources of the vitamin plus 1 mg equivalent for each 60 mg of dietary tryptophan.*

build. In the case of the very young mother who is not fully grown or the mother who is significantly taller than 64 inches, the recommended nutritional allowance should be increased. This recommendation applies as well to women who are underweight.

Very rigid caloric restriction even for the overtly obese pregnant woman may not necessarily be in the best interest of the fetus. For example, such a dietary regimen might precipitate maternal ketoacidosis. There is some evidence that ketoacidosis during pregnancy can result in neuropsychologic defects in the offspring (Churchill and Berendes). As a minimum, if a reducing regimen were to be imposed during pregnancy, the danger of ketosis caused by starvation should be kept in mind and a system for careful monitoring established so as to minimize the likelihood of ketoacidosis developing.

Protein.   The requirements for protein are increased during pregnancy. To the basic needs of the nonpregnant woman for repair of her tissues are added the demands for growth and repair of the fetus, placenta, uterus, and breasts, and increased maternal blood volume. The Food and Nutrition Board recommends for the nonpregnant woman of average size a protein intake per day of 0.9 g per kg or about 55 g per day. The addition of 10 g of protein per day is recommended during pregnancy. It has been estimated that during the last six months of pregnancy about 950 g of protein or about 5 g per day are deposited. Therefore 10 g per day of additional protein should readily cover this need. It is desirable that the majority of the protein be supplied from animal sources such as meat, milk, eggs, cheese, poultry, and fish, since they furnish amino acids in optimal combinations.

Minerals.   The requirements for calcium, phosphorus, iron and iodine have been studied the most extensively. It appears that if these minerals are adequately provided, the others are almost certain to be present in sufficient quantities. An adequate dietary intake of protein simultaneously provides enough phosphorus. The use of iodized salt is recommended during pregnancy.

Since the calcium content of the fetus at term is about 25 g, an average utilization of about 0.8 g daily throughout pregnancy is required. More than half of the fetal calcium, however, is deposited during the last month; considerable storage of calcium therefore must take place in the earlier months of gestation to minimize depletion of maternal stores during the last month. The Food and Nutrition Board of the National Research Council recommends that the normal nonpregnant woman ingest at least 0.8 g of calcium a day. During pregnancy an ample excess over these combined requirements should be provided; the amount recommended is 1.2 g daily. One quart of cow's milk supplies approximately 1 g of calcium.

The reasons for increased iron requirements during pregnancy are discussed in Chapter 8 (p. 252). Of the approximately 800 mg of iron transferred to the fetus and placenta or incorporated into the expanding maternal hemoglobin mass, nearly all is utilized during the latter half of pregnancy. During that time, therefore, the average iron requirements are about 6 mg a day imposed by the pregnancy itself in addition to nearly 1 mg to compensate for maternal excretion, or a total of about 7 mg of iron per day. Very few women have sufficient iron stores to supply this amount of iron; moreover, the diet seldom contains enough iron to meet this demand. The recommendations by the Food and Nutrition Board of the National Research Council (Table 1) of 18 mg of dietary iron per day for women, pregnant as well as nonpregnant, represents the ceiling imposed by caloric requirements. To ingest any more iron from dietary sources would simultaneously provide an undesirable excess of calories. The Board acknowledges that because of small iron stores the pregnant woman often will be unable to meet the iron requirements imposed by pregnancy.

Supplementation with medicinal iron is commonly practiced in the United States. Scott and Pritchard have recently shown that 30 mg of iron supplied in the form of a simple iron salt such as ferrous gluconate or ferrous fumarate and taken regularly once each day throughout the latter half of pregnancy will provide sufficient iron to meet requirements of pregnancy and will protect any preexisting iron stores. The Committee on Iron Deficiency of the Council on Foods and Nutrition of the American Medical Association recommends supplementation at this level. Furthermore, 30 mg of supplemental iron daily should be adequate during lactation. The mother should be warned to keep iron-containing medications out of reach of small children lest they ingest a large number of the usually quite attractive tablets or capsules.

The value of supplemental fluoride during pregnancy is not proved. The studies of Horowitz and Heifetz indicate that the prenatal exposure to fluoride is of no practical value in reducing decay in the child's deciduous or permanent teeth.

Vitamins.   Most evidence concerning the essentiality of various vitamins for successful reproduction has been obtained from animal experiments. Typically, severe deficiency has been produced in the animal either by withholding the vitamin completely, beginning long before the time of pregnancy, or by giving a very potent vitamin antagonist. The administration of some vitamins in great excess to animals can also exert deleterious effects on the fetus and newborn. Excessive ingestion of vitamin D by pregnant women may possibly cause the development in their offspring of the "supravalvar syndrome," with supravalvar pulmonic and aortic stenosis and physical and mental retardation (Neill).

The practice of supplying vitamin supplements prenatally is a deeply ingrained habit of many obstetricians, at least in the United States, even though scientific evidence is quite meager to show that the usual vitamin supplements are of benefit to either the mother or her fetus. The Committee on Maternal Nutrition of the National Research Council has pointed out that in the majority of cases routine pharmaceutical supplementation of vitamin and mineral preparations to pregnant women is of doubtful value except for iron and possibly folic acid. Such vitamin and mineral preparations should not be regarded as substitutes for food.

The advantages to be gained from supplemental iron during pregnancy are quite straightforward, namely, protection against maternal iron deficiency and anemia. Benefits to be derived from folic acid supplementation are not nearly so distinct. Hibbard and associates in Great Britain, Fraser and Watt in Canada, and Streif and Little as well as Stone and associates in the United States have implicated maternal folate deficiency in a variety of reproductive casualties, including placental abruption, pregnancy-induced hypertension (toxemia of pregnancy), and fetal anomalies. However, their studies have not been confirmed by Giles and Varadi and colleagues in Great Britain, or by either Alperin and associates or Whalley, Scott, Pritchard, and their co-workers in the United States. To date no one has significantly reduced the frequency of these complications simply by administering folic acid during pregnancy.

Evidence is abundant, however, that maternal folate requirements are increased significantly during pregnancy. Not infrequently in the mother this increase leads to lowered plasma folate levels, less often to hypersegmentation of neutrophils, infrequently to overt megaloblastic erythropoiesis, and seldom to megaloblastic anemia. The amount of folic acid supplement that will prevent these changes varies considerably, depending primarily on the diet consumed by the pregnant woman. Since 1 mg of folic acid orally per day produces a vigorous hematologic response in pregnant women with severe megaloblastic anemia, this amount would almost certainly provide very effective prophylaxis. Chanarin and associates have noted that as little as 0.1 mg of folic acid per day raised the blood folate level to at least the normal nonpregnant range. Food and Drug Administration regulations require that vitamin preparations providing more than 0.1 mg of folic acid per day be dispensed only on prescription.

GENERAL HYGIENE

Exercise.   In general, it is not necessary for the pregnant woman to limit exercise, provided she does not become excessively fatigued. For the many American women who are sports enthusiasts, marked restriction of such activities shifts the emphasis during pregnancy from a normal physiologic experience toward an abnormal state bordering on illness. Regarding pregnancy as a malady that necessitates abandoning of an habitual sport is obviously undesirable; however dangerous activities that carry a risk of bodily injury should be prohibited.

Employment.   It is estimated that nearly one third of all women of childbearing age in the United States are now in the labor force and even larger proportions of socioeconomically less fortunate women are working. Although most studies have not found work in itself to be deleterious to the outcome of pregnancy, certain safeguards are recommended. Any occupation that subjects the pregnant woman to severe physical strain should be avoided. Ideally, no work or play should be continued to the extent that fatigue develops. Adequate periods of rest should be provided during the working day. Women with previous complications of pregnancy that are likely to be repetitive (for example, low-birth-weight infants) should minimize physical work.

Travel.   The restriction of travel to short trips had been a rule for obstetric patients until World War II, when many women found it necessary to follow their husbands regardless of distance or mode of travel. The data compiled during that era show that travel, virtually irrespective of distance and type of conveyance, has no deleterious effect on pregnancy (Guilbeau and Turner). Travel in properly pressurized aircraft offers no unusual risk. About every two hours during travel by automobile a ten-minute break should be taken to allow the pregnant woman to walk about.

Bathing.   There is no objection to shower or sponge baths at any time during pregnancy or the puerperium. During the last trimester of pregnancy the heavy uterus usually upsets the balance of the pregnant woman and increases the likehood of her slipping and falling in a bathtub. For that reason alone, tub baths at the end of pregnancy may be inadvisable. The statement that wash water readily enters the vagina and thereby carries infection to the uterus is not true.

Clothing.   Clothing during pregnancy should be practical, attractive, and nonconstricting. Intricate, expensive supporting girdles and brassieres are rarely used today; constricting garters should be avoided during pregnancy because of the interference with venous return and the aggravation of varicosities.

The increasing mass of the breasts may make them pendulous and painful. In such instances well-fitting supporting brassieres are indicated.

Backache and pressure associated with lordotic posture and a pendulous abdomen may be relieved by a properly fitted maternity girdle. Unless the pregnant woman develops backache from the increased lordosis as a result of shoes with high heels or is unable to maintain good balance, there is no real reason for insisting that she wear only low-heeled shoes.

Bowel Habits.   During pregnancy, bowel habits tend to become more irregular because of generalized relaxation of smooth muscle and compression of the lower bowel by the enlarging uterus early in pregnancy or by the presenting part of the fetus late in pregnancy. In addition to the discomfort caused by the passage of hard fecal material, bleeding and painful fissures in the edematous and hyperemic rectal mucosa may develop. There is also greater frequency of hemorrhoids and, much less commonly, of prolapse of the rectal mucosa.

Women whose bowel habits are reasonably normal in the nonpregnant state may prevent constipation during pregnancy by close attention to bowel habits, sufficient quantities of fluid, and reasonable amounts of daily exercise, supplemented when necessary by a mild laxative, such as prune juice, milk of magnesia, bulk-producing substances, or stool-softening agents. The use of nonabsorbable oil preparations has been discouraged because of their possible interference with the absorption of lipid-soluble vitamins. The use of harsh laxatives and enemas is not recommended, except perhaps when they are necessary to prevent fecal impaction.

Coitus.   When abortion or premature labor threatens, coitus should be avoided. Otherwise there is general agreement that in healthy pregnant women sexual intercourse usually does no harm before the last four to six weeks of pregnancy.

It has long been the custom of many obstetricians to recommend abstinence from intercourse during the last four to six weeks of pregnancy, a recommendation undoubtedly not carried out in many instances. Pugh and Fernandez, in one of the few detailed studies to ascertain the effect of coitus on pregnancy, could not implicate it as a cause of premature labor, rupture of the membranes, bleeding, or infection. They concluded that it is not necessary to abstain from coitus during the final weeks of gestation.

On occasion the couple's sexual drive in the face of the admonishment against intercourse late in pregnancy has led to unusual sexual practices with disastrous consequences. Aronson and Nelson, for instance, describe fatal cases of air embolism late in pregnancy as a result of air blown into the vagina during cunnilingus.

Douches.   Douching in pregnancy, which should be kept to a minimum, is unnecessary in most cases. If it is necessitated by excessive vaginal secretions the following precautions should be observed: (1) *Hand bulb syringes must be absolutely forbidden, since several deaths in pregnancy from air embolism have followed their use* (Forbes). (2) The douche bag should be placed not more than two feet above the level of the hips to prevent high fluid pressure. (3) The nozzle should not be inserted more than three inches into the vagina.

Care of Breasts and Abdomen.   Special care of the breasts during pregnancy is often advised to increase the ability to nurse, to toughen the nipples and thereby reduce the incidence of cracking, and to effect enlargement and eversion of the nipples. The available data suggest that ointments, massage, and traction on the nipples do not always improve these functions, but they are usually harmless. Massages and ointments do not alter significantly the incidence of striae on the breasts or abdomen. In general, the extent of striation is proportional to the weight gain of the patient.

Smoking.   Mothers who smoke during pregnancy frequently bear smaller infants than do nonsmokers. Underwood and associates, for instance, report that in private white patients the infants of heavy smokers—defined as women who smoke more than one pack of cigarettes per day—weighed 353 g, or about 12 oz, less than infants of nonsmokers. Yerushalmy noted not only an increase in the number of children of low birth weight born to smokers, but also a quantitative relation between the incidence of infants of low birth weight and the number of cigarettes smoked by the mother. However, the overall neonatal mortality rate for infants of mothers who smoke was not greater than that for infants of mothers who did not smoke. Underwood and co-workers found no increase in the number of stillbirths, major fetal anomalies, or maternal complications in the group of mothers who smoked during pregnancy. Mulcahy, Murphy, and Martin found no difference in weight and appearance of placentas from smoking and nonsmoking mothers, even though the birth weights of infants whose mothers smoked averaged 396 g less.

Previously, a limitation of smoking to no more than ten cigarettes per day during pregnancy was recommended. In view of the obvious dangers to people who smoke, many obstetricians now urge that cigarettes be avoided completely, irrespective of any deleterious effects on pregnancy.

Alcohol.   Although alcohol readily crosses the placenta, its use in moderation has not been shown to produce pathologic changes in the mother or fetus or to affect the course of pregnancy. However, a few cases of the syndrome of acute withdrawal of alcohol (delirium tremens) have been described in the newborn infants of mothers who consumed excessive amounts of alcohol (Nichols). The affected newborn is depressed at birth but soon becomes extremely hyperactive with sweating, tremors, and episodes of generalized twitching of the face and extremities. At the same time the mother suffers delirium tremens.

Maternal chronic alcoholism may lead to fetal underdevelopment. Ulleland and co-workers have recently reported that infants of alcoholic mothers are commonly undergrown for gestational age. Moreover, growth retardation is likely to persist after birth.

Care of the Teeth.   In general, pregnancy does not contraindicate required dental treatment. The concept that dental caries are aggravated by pregnancy is unfounded.

Immunization.   Pregnancy is not a contraindication to any of the standard procedures of immunization except that for *rubella*. At this time it is not absolutely clear whether the rubella vaccine will cause deleterious effects in the fetus and newborn; therefore it should not be given to pregnant women or to women who could become pregnant during the next two months (Ch. 27, p. 808).

In view of the apparent increase in susceptibility of pregnant women to poliomyelitis, as well as the increased gravity of the disease during pregnancy, all pregnant women should be vaccinated if they have not already been immunized. Whenever an epidemic of influenza is anticipated, pregnant women should receive suitable injections of vaccine, since pregnant women appear more susceptible to the effects of influenzal pneumonitis.

Medications.   All physicians should develop the habit of ascertaining the likelihood of pregnancy before prescribing drugs for any woman, since a number of medications in common use can be overtly deleterious to the embryo and the fetus. Some of them are listed in Table 2. If a drug is administered during pregnancy, the advantages to be gained should clearly outweigh any risks inherent in its use.

Table 2. Some Maternally Administered Drugs That Can Adversely Affect the Fetus and Newborn

Maternal Medication	*Effects on Fetus and Newborn*
Drugs to control epilepsy	Low levels of coagulation factors II, VII, IX, and X
Vitamin K analogues in excess	Hemolysis and kernicterus
Bishydroxycoumarin (Dicumarol)	Hemorrhage
Ethyl biscoumacetate (Tromexan)	Hemorrhage
Sodium warfarin (Coumadin)	Hemorrhage
Salicylates in large amounts	Neonatal bleeding
Sulfonamides	Kernicterus
Nitrofurantoin (Furadantin)	Hemolysis in susceptible fetuses, kernicterus
Tetracyclines	Inhibition of bone growth, staining of deciduous teeth
Potassium iodide	Goiter
Propylthiouracil	Goiter
Methimazole (Tapazole)	Goiter
Ammonium chloride	Acidosis
Reserpine	Stuffy nose, obstructed breathing
Morphine or heroin chronically	Addiction, withdrawal symptoms
Androgens	Masculinization
Some progestins	Masculinization
Tolbutamide (Orinase)	Neonatal hypoglycemia
Chlorothiazide	Thrombocytopenia
Quinine	Thrombocytopenia
Cephalothin (Keflin)	Positive direct Coombs test

COMMON COMPLAINTS

Nausea and Vomiting. Nausea and vomiting are common complaints during the first half of pregnancy. Typically they commence between the first and second missed menstrual period and continue until about the time of the fourth missed period. Nausea and vomiting are usually worst in the morning but may continue throughout the day.

The genesis of pregnancy-induced nausea and vomiting is not clear. Possibly the hormonal changes of pregnancy are the cause. Chorionic gonadotropin, for instance, has been implicated on the basis that its levels are rather high at the same time that nausea and vomiting are most common. Moreover, in cases of hydatidiform mole, in which levels of chorionic gonadotropin typically are very much higher than in normal pregnancy, nausea and vomiting are often prominent clinical features.

Emotional factors undoubtedly can contribute to the severity of the nausea and vomiting, which at times may become so intense or so protracted as to cause serious metabolic derangements in the mother and fetus. Fortunately, in most instances vomiting is usually not very severe, so that dehydration, electrolyte and acid-base disturbances, and starvation seldom become serious problems. Between one and five gravidas per 1,000 vomit so severely that they require hospitalization. The syndrome of nausea and vomiting of such intensity as to require hospitalization is referred to as *hyperemesis gravidarum.* Prompt correction of fluid and electrolyte imbalances usually relieves the symptoms. Nowadays therapeutic abortion is rarely required.

Seldom is the treatment of nausea and vomiting of pregnancy so successful that the mother is afforded complete relief. However, the unpleasantness and discomfort can usually be minimized. Eating small feedings at more frequent intervals but stopping short of satiation is of value. Since the smell of certain foods often precipitates or aggravates the symptoms, such foods should be avoided as much as possible.

In our experience, dimenhydrinate (Dramamine) often seems to reduce the intensity of the nausea and vomiting. Usually a satisfactory dosage is one 50 mg tablet upon arising, followed by 50 mg every four hours, depending upon how long the symptoms persist throughout the day.

Meclizine (Bonine) and meclizine with pyridoxine (Bonadoxin), which have been widely used in an effort to control nausea and vomiting, seem to provide some benefit. The suggestion has been made that meclizine might be teratogenic, but the evidence is not convincing (Yerushalmy and Milkovich).

A great variety of other agents have been recommended for treatment. Fairweather, for example, in his comprehensive review of nausea and vomiting in pregnancy, has tabulated such bizarre and diverse treatments as hibernotherapy, intravenously administered honey, husband's blood, and the husband's sex hormone (testosterone).

Fortunately, effective psychologic support can be offered in the form of reassurance to the pregnant woman that these symptoms nearly always will disappear by the fourth month and, moreover, that pregnancies in which nausea and vomiting occur are more likely to have a favorable outcome than are those without nausea and vomiting (Yerushalmy and Milkovich).

Backache.   Backache occurs to some extent in most pregnant women. Minor degrees follow excessive strain or fatigue and excessive bending, lifting, or walking. Mild backache usually requires little more than elimination of the strain and occasionally a light maternity girdle.

Severe backaches should not be dismissed as caused simply by pregnancy until a thorough orthopedic examination has been carried out. Muscular spasm and tenderness, which are often classified clinically as acute strain or "fibrositis," respond well to analgesics, heat, and rest.

In some women motion of the symphysis and lumbosacral joints and general relaxation of pelvic ligaments may be demonstrated. In severe cases the patient may be unable to walk or even remain comfortable without support furnished by a heavy girdle and prolonged periods of rest. Occasionally anatomic defects are found, either congenital or traumatic, which may precipitate the complaints. Pain caused by herniation of an intervertebral disc occurs during pregnancy with about the same frequency as at other times.

Varicosities.   Varicosities, generally resulting from congenital predisposition, are exaggerated by prolonged standing, pregnancy, and advancing age. Usually they become more prominent as pregnancy advances, as weight increases, and as the length of time spent on the feet is prolonged.

The symptoms produced by varicosities vary from cosmetic blemishes on the lower extremities and mild discomfort at the end of the day to severe pain that requires prolonged rest with the feet elevated.

The treatment of varicosities of the lower extremities is generally limited to periodic rest with elevation of the legs, or elastic stockings, or both. Surgical correction of the condition during pregnancy is usually not advised, although the symptoms may rarely be so severe that injection, ligation, or even stripping of the veins is necessary to allow the patient to remain ambulatory. In general, these operations should be postponed until after delivery. Varicosities of the vulva may be controlled by application of a foam rubber pad suspended across the vulva by a belt of the type used with a perineal pad. Rarely, large varicosities may rupture with resulting profuse hemorrhage.

Hemorrhoids. Varicosities of hemorrhoidal veins occasionally first appear during pregnancy; more often, pregnancy causes an exacerbation or recurrence of previous symptoms. The development or aggravation of hemorrhoids during pregnancy is undoubtedly related to increased pressure in the hemorrhoidal veins caused by obstruction of venous return by the large pregnant uterus, as well as the tendency toward constipation during pregnancy. Pain and swelling are usually relieved by topically applied anesthetics, warm soaks, and agents that soften the stool. Thrombosis of a hemorrhoidal vein can cause considerable pain, but the clot can usually be evacuated by incising the wall of the involved vein with a scalpel under topical anesthesia.

Bleeding from hemorrhoidal veins may occasionally result in loss of sufficient blood to cause iron-deficiency anemia. The loss of only 15 ml of blood results in the loss of 6 to 7 mg of iron, an amount equal to the daily requirements for iron during the latter half of pregnancy. If bleeding is persistent, hemorrhoidectomy may be required. In general, however, hemorrhoidectomy is not necessary during pregnancy, since most hemorrhoids become asymptomatic soon after delivery.

Heartburn. Heartburn, one of the most common complaints of pregnant women, is usually caused by reflux of acidic gastric contents into the lower esophagus. The increased frequency of regurgitation during pregnancy most likely results from the upward displacement and compression of the stomach by the uterus combined with decreased gastrointestinal motility. In some instances the cardia actually herniates through the diaphragm.

Antacid preparations usually provide considerable relief. Aluminum hydroxide, magnesium trisilicate, or magnesium hydroxide, alone or in combination (for example, Amphojel, Gelusil, Maalox, and milk of magnesia), should be used in preference to sodium-containing antacids such as sodium bicarbonate. The pregnant woman who tends to retain sodium can become edematous as the result of the ingestion of sodium bicarbonate. Antacids that contain magnesium and aluminum hydroxides impair absorption of iron somewhat but otherwise appear quite innocuous (Gant, Scott, and Pritchard).

Pica. Occasionally during pregnancy bizarre cravings develop for strange foods and at times for materials hardly considered edible, such as laundry starch, clay, and even dirt. For example, at Parkland Memorial Hospital interrogation of recently delivered mothers in a single day disclosed that the following items were craved and consumed by them during the current pregnancy: Argo Gloss Starch, flour, baking powder, baking soda, clay, baked dirt, powdered bricks, and frost scraped from the refrigerator.

The ingestion of starch (amylophagia) or clay (geophagia) or related items is practiced more often by socioeconomically less privileged pregnant women. It is quite unlikely, however, that the craving for these materials is simply the result of hunger but is rather, in part at least, a social custom. In this country pica involving lump laundry starch or clay appears to have long been prevalent among Negroes in the South; with their migration the custom spread throughout most of the country. Since young women are continually introduced to the practice by older women, the custom is not dying out. McGanity and co-workers, for instance, recently reported that one half of the teen-age pregnant women cared for in their clinic admitted to pica.

The desire for dry lump starch, clay, chopped ice, or even refrigerator frost has been considered by some to be triggered by severe iron deficiency. Although women with severe iron deficiency sometimes crave these items, and although the craving is ameliorated after correction of the iron deficiency, not all women with pica are necessarily iron-deficient.

Minnich and associates found that the ingestion of clay, especially Turkish clay and to a lesser extent clays from Georgia and Mississippi, impaired absorption of iron. In Dallas, however, we were unable to demonstrate that either of two Texas clays studied or Argo Gloss Starch reduced absorption of iron significantly (Talkington and co-workers).

The consumption of starch in sufficient quantities to provide a significant portion of the calories ingested or to cause ptyalism is not healthful nor is the ingestion of clay to the extent that the intestine is sufficiently filled to cause obstruction of labor or fecal impaction. Another complication of ingestion of clay, symptomatic hypokalemia, has been reported by Tyler and colleagues. The clay was thought to act in the manner of an ion-exchange resin and thereby remove potassium from the gastrointestinal tract. Nonetheless, it is quite unlikely that either lanudry starch or clay free of parasites is distinctly harmful to the pregnancy if consumed in moderation and if the diet is nutritionally adequate.

Ptyalism.   Women during pregnancy are occasionally distressed by profuse salivation. The cause of the ptyalism sometimes appears to be stimulation of the salivary glands by the ingestion of starch. This cause should be looked for and eradicated if found.

Fatigue and Somnolence.   Early in pregnancy most women complain of fatigue and desire excessive periods of sleep. The condition usually remits spontaneously by the fourth month of pregnancy and has no special significance.

Headache.   Headache early in pregnancy is a frequent complaint. A few cases may result from sinusitis or ocular strain caused by refractive errors. In the vast majority, however, no cause can be demonstrated. Treatment is largely symptomatic. By the middle of pregnancy most of these headaches decrease in severity or disappear.

Leukorrhea.   Pregnant women commonly note increased vaginal discharge, which in most instances has no pathologic cause. Increased formation of mucus by cervical glands is undoubtedly a contributing factor. If the secretion is troublesome, the patient should be advised to douche with water mildly acidified with vinegar. The precautions for douching listed on page 341 should be stressed.

Occasionally troublesome leukorrhea is the result of an infection caused by *Trichomonas vaginalis* or *Candida albicans*.

Trichomonas vaginalis.   This organism can be identified in about 20 to 30 per cent of women during prenatal examination; however, the infection is symptomatic in a much smaller percentage of patients. Trichomonal vaginitis is characterized by foamy leukorrhea with pruritus and irritation. Trichomonads are readily demonstrated in fresh vaginal secretions as flagellated, pear-shaped, motile organisms that are somewhat larger than leukocytes.

Metronidazole (Flagyl) has proved effective in eradicating *Trichomonas vaginalis*. The drug may be administered both orally and vaginally. When ingested by the mother it crosses the placenta and enters the fetal circulation; however, hundreds of women have received metronidazole during pregnancy without any reported adverse effects on the fetus (Perl).

Candida albicans. Candida (*Monilia*) can be cultured from the vagina in about 25 per cent of women approaching term. Asymptomatic vaginal moniliasis requires no treatment. Candidiasis may sometimes cause an extremely profuse irritating discharge, however. Gentian violet applied as a 1 per cent aqueous solution has been a dependable local therapeutic agent, although it may stain the skin and clothing and produce local edema. Nystatin (Mycostatin) is a fungicide that may prove more effective. Nystatin is applied locally to the vagina in the form of vaginal tablets. Candidiasis is likely to recur, thereby requiring repeated treatment during pregnancy, but it usually subsides at the end of gestation.

REFERENCES

Alperin, J. B., Haggard, M. E., and McGanity, W. J.   Folic acid, pregnancy, and abruptio placentae. Amer J Clin Nutr 22:1359, 1969.

Aronson, M. E., and Nelson, P. K.   Fatal air embolism in pregnancy resulting from an unusual sex act. Obstet Gynec 30:127, 1967.

Chanarin, I., Rothman, D., Ward, A., and Perry, J.   Folate status and requirements in pregnancy. Brit Med J 2:390, 1968.

Churchill, J., and Berendes, H.   Intelligence of children whose mothers had acetonuria during pregnancy. The Proceedings of the Eighth Meeting of the Pan American Health Organization Advisory Committee on Medical Research, Washington, D.C., June, 1969.

Eastman, N. J., and Jackson, E.   Weight relationships in pregnancy.   I. The bearing of maternal weight gain and pre-pregnancy weight on birth weight in full term pregnancies. Obstet Gynec Survey 23:1003, 1968.

Fairweather, D. V. I.   Nausea and vomiting in pregnancy. Amer J Obstet Gynec 102:135, 1968.

Forbes, G.   Air embolism as complication of vaginal douching in pregnancy. Brit Med J 2:529, 1944.

Fraser, J. L., and Watt, H. J.   Megaloblastic anemia in pregnancy and the puerperium. Amer J Obstet Gynec 89:532, 1964.

Gant, N. F., Scott, D. E., and Pritchard, J. A.   Unpublished observations.

Giles, C.   An account of 335 cases of megaloblastic anaemia of pregnancy and the puerperium. J Clin Path 19:1, 1966.

Guilbeau, J. A., and Turner, J. L.   The effect of travel on interruption of pregnancy. An analysis of 1,917 cases with minimum journeys of 300 miles. Amer J Obstet Gynec 66:1224, 1953.

Hibbard, B. M., Hibbard, E. D., and Jeffcoate, T. N. A.   Folic acid and reproduction. Acta Obstet Gynec Scand 44:375, 1965.

——— Hibbard, E. D., Hwa, T. S., and Tan, P.   Abruptio placentae and defective folate metabolism in Singapore women. J Obstet Gynaec Brit Comm 76:1003, 1969.

Horowitz, H. S., and Heifetz, S. B.   Effects of prenatal exposure to fluoridation on dental caries. Public Health Rep 82:297, 1967.

McGanity, W. J., Little, H. M., Fogelman, A., Jennings, L., Calhoun, E., and Dawson, E. B.   Pregnancy in the adolescent.   I. Preliminary summary of health status. Amer J Obstet Gynec 103:773, 1969.

Minnich, V., Okcuoglu, A., Tarcon, Y., Arcasoy, A., Cin, S., Yorukoglu, O., Renda, F., and Demirag, B.   Pica in Turkey.   II. Effect of clay upon iron absorption. Amer J Clin Nutr 21:78, 1968.

Mulcahy, R., Murphy, J., and Martin, F.   Placental changes and maternal weight in smoking and nonsmoking mothers. Amer J Obstet Gynec 106:703, 1970.

Neill, C. A.   Etiologic and hemodynamic factors in congenital heart disease, in Cheek, D. B. (ed.). Human Growth, Philadelphia, Lea & Febiger, 1968.

Nichols, M. M.   Acute alcohol withdrawal syndrome in a newborn. Amer J Dis Child 113:714, 1967.

Perl, G.   Metronidazole treatment of trichomoniasis in pregnancy. Obstet Gynec 25:273, 1965.

Pritchard, J. A.   Anemias complicating pregnancy and the puerperium, in Maternal Nutrition and the Course and Outcome of Pregnancy, A Report of the Committee on Maternal Nutrition, Food and Nutrition Board, National Research Council, Standard Book Number 309-01761. National Academy of Sciences, Washington, D.C., 1970.

———— Scott, D. E., and Whalley, P. J.   Folic acid requirements in pregnancy-induced megaloblastic anemia. JAMA 208:1163, 1969.

———— Scott, D. E., Whalley, P. J., and Haling, R. F.   The infants of mothers with megaloblastic anemia due to folate deficiency. JAMA 211:1982, 1970.

Pugh, W. E., and Fernandez, F. L.   Coitus in late pregnancy. Obstet Gynec 2:636, 1953.

Recommended Dietary Allowances, 7th rev. ed., A Report of the Food and Nutrition Board, National Research Council, Publication 1694, National Academy of Sciences, 1968.

Schaefer, G.   Clinical management of pregnant women with tuberculosis. New York J Med 55:1189, 1955.

Scott, D. E., and Pritchard, J. A.   Iron demands during pregnancy, in Iron Deficiency—Pathogenesis, Clinical Aspects, Therapy, London and New York (in press).

Streif, R. R., and Little, A. B.   Folic acid deficiency in pregnancy. New Eng J Med 276:776, 1967.

Talkington, K. M., Gant, N. F., Scott, D. E., and Pritchard, J. A.   Effect of ingestion of starch and some clays on iron absorption. Amer J Obstet Gynec 108:262, 1970.

Tyler, M., Johnson, B. B., Sledge, C., Mosey, L., and Lewis, C. J.   Pregnancy, pica, potassium depletion, and paralysis. Clin Research 16:398, 1969.

Ulleland, C., Igo, R. A., and Smith, N. J.   The offspring of alcoholic mothers. Pediat Research 4:474, 1970.

Underwood, P., Hester, L. L., Laffitte, T., and Gregg, K. V.   The relationship of smoking to the outcome of pregnancy. Amer J Obstet Gynec 91:270, 1965.

Varadi, S., Abbott, D., and Elwis, A.   Correlation of peripheral white cell and bone marrow changes with folate levels in pregnancy and their clinical significance. J Clin Path 19:33, 1966.

Whalley, P. J., Scott, D. E., and Pritchard, J. A.   Maternal folate deficiency and pregnancy wastage.   I. Placental abruption. Amer. J Obstet Gynec 105:670, 1969.

———— Scott, D. E., and Pritchard, J. A.   Maternal folate deficiency and pregnancy wastage. III. Pregnancy-induced hypertension. Submitted for publication.

Yerushalmy, J.   Mother's cigarette smoking and survival of infant. Amer J Obstet Gynec 88:505, 1964.

———— and Milkovich, L.   Evaluation of the teratogenic effect of meclizine in man. Amer J Obstet Gynec 93:553, 1965.

13

THE FORCES CONCERNED IN LABOR

Labor comprises the series of processes by which the mature, or nearly mature, products of conception are expelled by the mother. Childbirth, accouchement, confinement, and parturition are all synonyms. The word "delivery" refers to the actual birth of the baby.

CAUSE OF THE ONSET OF LABOR

In all species, whether the fetus weighs a few grams at the end of a 19-day pregnancy, as in the mouse, or whether it weighs several hundred pounds at the end of a 640-day pregnancy, as in the elephant, labor quite regularly begins at a specific time—namely, when the fetus is sufficiently mature to cope reasonably well with extrauterine conditions but not large enough to cause mechanical difficulties in delivery. The factors regulating this highly synchronized sequence of events are obscure. In fact, the old adage, "When the fruit is ripe it will fall," serves to summarize the extent of our knowledge of the causation of spontaneous labor.

The myometrium during pregnancy is made up of a large number of greatly hypertrophied smooth muscle cells, each of which may be likened to a contractile system surrounded by an excitable membrane (Ch. 8, p. 239). The capacity of each cell to perform work is a function of the actomyosin content and the ability of the metabolic machinery to generate adenosine triphosphate. A most fundamental question is what stimulates these myometrial cells at a rather precise time, in most pregnancies at least, to contract rhythmically in an exquisitely coordinated way and with sufficient force to dilate the cervix and expel the fetus. Of the many theories regarding the onset of labor none alone provides an adequate explanation. It appears that labor is initiated and maintained not by a single mechanism but by several; moreover, the contribution of each to the genesis of labor will vary depending upon individual circumstances.

1. Progesterone Deprivation Theory.   Heckel and Allen a third of a century ago demonstrated that progesterone administered to pregnant rabbits uniformly prolonged gestation. This finding, coupled with the observation that removal of the corpus luteum

of the rabbit at any time during pregnancy promptly resulted in evacuation of the products of conception, has served as the major basis for implicating withdrawal of progesterone in the genesis of labor in women. An attractive hypothesis, championed especially by Csapo and by Kumar and associates, holds that progesterone produced by the human placenta establishes a myometrial blocking effect that is greatest at the placental site; as production of progesterone drops, the block is removed and synchronous uterine contractions characteristic of labor develop.

No one has yet been able to demonstrate unequivocally either decreased levels of circulating progesterone or decreased excretion of its metabolite pregnanediol in women at or about the time of onset of labor. Furthermore, the administration of progesterone or some of the newer synthetic progestational compounds does not arrest labor once it is clinically evident. Kumar, Goodno, and Barnes were not able to diminish appreciably uterine activity in women with premature labor by intravenous administration of very large doses of progesterone dissolved in ethanol. Csapo and associates have administered as much as 500 mg of progesterone and 4,000 mg of medroxyprogesterone acetate (Depo-Provera) to women in early labor with at most only a very slight and transient damping effect on uterine activity. Paradoxically, medroxyprogesterone acetate given to patients with threatened abortion commonly results in prolonged retention of dead products of conception, or missed abortion (Ch. 20, p. 494). Obviously the precise role of progesterone in the control of myometrial activity during pregnancy is still far from clear.

2. Oxytocin Theory.   Since oxytocin, administered late in pregnancy, profoundly augments myometrial contractions, it appears logical to attempt to relate the spontaneous onset of labor to endogenously produced oxytocin. Caldeyro-Barcia and associates, and others, have clearly demonstrated the increasing sensitivity of the uterus to oxytocin as pregnancy advances (Fig. 1). Coch and associates have detected increasing oxytocin-

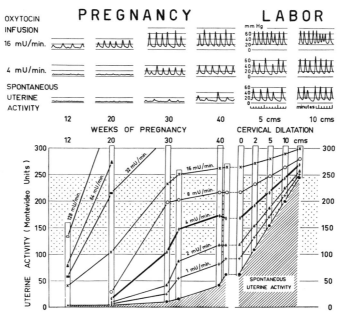

Fig. 1. Increased uterine sensitivity to oxytocin with the progression of pregnancy. (From Caldeyro-Barcia et al. Surg Gynec Obstet 91:641, 1950.)

like activity in maternal jugular vein blood as labor progresses, with the highest concentrations found during the second stage. Since surgical operations in males, as well as in females, cause a great increase in oxytocinlike activity of the blood, it is possible that any stress, of which labor is but one example, may release the neurohypophysial hormone.

Blood contains an oxytocinase that promptly inactivates oxytocin; although the activity of the enzyme in the blood has been reported by some to drop just prior to the onset of labor, most investigators have detected no decrease. Any theory that assigns to oxytocin a dominant role in the initiation and maintenance of labor faces the serious objection raised by the fact that in women, as well as in rats, rabbits, cats, and monkeys, in which the pars posterior and pars intermedia of the hypophysis have been removed or destroyed, normal labor may subsequently occur.

3. Uterine Stretch Theory.   Any hollow viscus tends to contract and empty itself when distended beyond a certain volume. The uterus is no exception. With multiple fetuses, for instance, labor usually occurs earlier than when the uterus is less distended by only one fetus. Uterine distention, however, cannot be the primary cause of labor, for pregnancies in which the fetus dies and the volume of the products of conception may actually decrease nearly always terminate in spontaneous labor at or even before the completion of the normal gestational period.

4. Fetal Endocrine Control Theory.   For many years it has been known that certain breeds of dairy cattle tend to have greatly prolonged gestations. The calves in these instances have either aplasia of the adenohypophysis or poorly granulated acidophils. This phenomenon is genetically determined for the affected cattle.

Veratrum californium fed to ewes at the end of the second week of pregnancy induces teratogenic effects that include absence of the fetal pituitary and greatly prolonged gestation. The fetus continues to grow, sometimes reaching such size as to cause death of the mother. Liggins and associates have recently performed a series of elegant experiments in pregnant sheep to elucidate the mechanisms involved in the prolongation of gestation and have made the following observations. Destruction of the fetal pituitary or hypothalamus markedly prolonged gestation unless there were twin fetuses; with twins the pituitary or hypothalamus had to be destroyed in both fetuses in order to prolong pregnancy. Conversely, administration of either corticotropin or cortisol directly into the fetus led to premature labor. In the case of twins, unless both fetuses received the injections the pregnancy continued to term. Administration of corticotropin or cortisol to the mother did not influence the duration of gestation. Moreover, the intravenous infusion of large doses of progesterone into the mother at the same time that corticotropin or cortisol was infused into the fetus or fetuses did not prevent premature delivery.

Typically in the anencephalic human fetus most or all of the hypophysis is lacking; as a result the adrenals are very small. It has long been observed that human gestation is sometimes considerably prolonged when the fetus is anencephalic. Milic and Adamsons, for example, noted that the onset of labor occurred past term in 40 per cent of pregnancies with anencephalic fetuses.

The importance, if any, of these several fascinating phenomena as critical determinants of the duration of normal human gestation is not yet clear.

THE THREE STAGES OF LABOR

Labor is conveniently divided into three distinct stages:

The first stage of labor, or the stage of cervical dilatation, **begins with the** first true labor pain and ends with the complete dilatation of the cervix.

The second stage of labor, or the stage of expulsion, **begins with the com-**plete dilatation of the cervix and ends with the birth of the baby.

The third stage of labor, or the placental stage, **begins with the delivery of** the baby and ends with the delivery of the placenta.

THE CHARACTERISTICS OF UTERINE CONTRACTIONS IN LABOR

Alone among physiologic muscular contractions, those of labor are painful. Therefore, the common designation in many languages for such a contraction is "pain." The cause of the pain is not definitely known, but the following hypotheses have been suggested: (1) hypoxia of the contracted muscle cells (as in angina pectoris); (2) compression of nerve ganglia in the cervix and lower uterine segment by the tightly interlocking muscle bundles; (3) stretching of the cervix during dilatation; and (4) stretching of the peritoneum.

Uterine contractions are involuntary and, for the most part, independent of extrauterine control. In fact, rhythmic changes in myometrial length and tension occur in completely denervated preparations and in the presence of neural blocking agents. Stimulation of the hypogastric plexus and the nervus erigens in the pregnant dog yields variable results according to Rudolph and Ivy, who concluded that the extrinsic nerves of the uterus play a subordinate role in parturition. In women, neural blockage from caudal or epidural anesthesia, if initiated quite early in labor, sometimes reduces the frequency and intensity of uterine contractions but not after labor is well established. Moreover, paraplegics have normal though painless contractions, as do women after bilateral lumbar sympathectomy. Thus far the attempts to initiate labor in women by electrical stimulation have been only partially successful (Theobald).

Ivy, Hartman, and Koff showed that the uterus has pacemakers that initiate uterine contractions and control their rhythmicity. As pointed out recently by Carsten, however, in a comprehensive review of myometrial composition, growth, and activity, the cells participating in the pacemaker activities, unlike those of the heart, do not differ anatomically from the surrounding myocytes. Furthermore, pacemaker activity is not confined to a specific site in the uterus; in fact, it requires only a group of highly excitable myometrial cells and it may start in a variety of sites. The contractile rhythm of one pacemaker may reinforce or block that of another. Since electric current does not flow easily from one myometrial cell to another, activation of individual myometrial cell membranes almost certainly serves to propagate the impulse throughout the myometrium. In women the pacemaker sites most often appear to be near the uterotubal junctions.

Mechanical stretching of the cervix enhances activity in several species, including man. This phenomenon has been referred to as the Ferguson reflex. The exact mechanism by which mechanical dilatation of the cervix causes increased myometrial contractility is not clear. Release of oxytocin was suggested as the cause by Ferguson but has not been proved. Spinal or epidural anesthesia effectively blocks this effect, according to Sala and associates.

The interval between the onset of contractions diminishes gradually from about 10 minutes early in labor to as little as 2 minutes in the second stage. Periods of relaxation between contractions are essential to the welfare of the fetus, since unremitting contractions may interfere with blood flow and placental transfer sufficiently to produce fetal hypoxia. The duration of each contraction ranges from 30 to 90 seconds, averaging about one minute. Each contraction comprises three phases: increment, acme, and decrement. The increment, or crescendo, phase is longer than the other two combined. Caldeyro-Barcia, Alvarez, and Reynolds have found that the intrauterine pressure during a contraction in normal labor is about 35 mm Hg, with occasional pressures as high as 50 mm.

Local Characteristics of Uterine Behavior in the Two Uterine Segments.   Under the influence of contractions in labor, the uterus gradually becomes differentiated into two distinct portions. The upper, actively contracting portion becomes thicker as labor advances. The lower portion, comprising the lower seg-

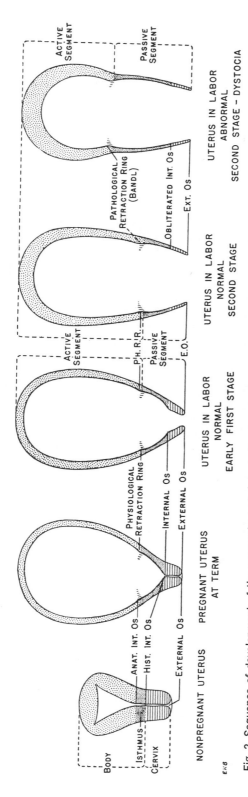

Fig. 2. Sequence of development of the segments and rings in the pregnant uterus. Note comparison between the nonpregnant uterus, uterus at term, and uterus in labor. The passive lower segment of the uterine body is derived from the isthmus; the physiologic retraction ring develops at the anatomic internal os. The pathologic retraction ring develops from the physiologic ring. (Anat. Int. os = anatomic internal os; Hist. Int. os = histologic internal os; Ph. R. R. = physiologic retraction ring; E.O. = external os.)

ment of the corpus and the cervix, is passive, developing into a thin-walled
muscular passage for the fetus. The *lower uterine segment* is the greatly expanded
and thinned-out isthmus of the nonpregnant uterus. Its formation is not solely a
phenomenon of labor; it develops gradually as pregnancy progresses and then
thins progressively during labor (Figs. 2 and 3). On abdominal palpation, even
before rupture of the membranes, two zones can be differentiated during a contraction; the upper is firm or hard, whereas the lower feels much softer. The
former represents the actively contracting portion of the uterus; the latter is the
distended, passive portion.

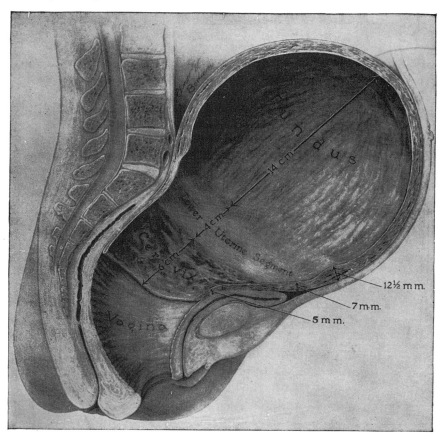

Fig. 3. The relations of the upper portion of the uterus, the lower uterine segment, and the
cervix as found in a patient dying in the second stage of labor with poliomyelencephalitis.
The twin pregnancy was about 28 weeks in duration.

Were the entire sac of uterine musculature, including the lower uterine segment and cervix, to contract simultaneously and with equal intensity, the net
expulsive force would be essentially zero; conditions after such a contraction
would be the same as before. Therein lies the importance of the division of the
uterus into upper and lower segments, which differ not only anatomically but
also physiologically. Briefly, the upper segment contracts, retracts, and expels the
fetus, while the lower segment and cervix dilate in response to the force of contractions of the upper segment. They thereby form a greatly expanded, thinned-out
muscular tube through which the baby can pass.

The musculature of the *upper uterine segment* undergoes a type of contraction in which the muscle, after contracting, does not relax to its original length but becomes relatively fixed at a shorter length, the tension, however, remaining the same as before the contraction. The ability of the musculature to retract— that is, to contract down on its diminishing contents with tension remaining constant—is designed to take up slack, to hold the advantage gained, and to maintain the uterine musculature in firm contact with the intrauterine contents. Without retraction, each individual contraction would start at the same point (in relation to uterine size) as its predecessor. With retraction, however, each successive contraction starts where its predecessor left off, the uterine cavity becoming permanently smaller with each successive contraction, thus preventing the fetus' slipping back. As a result of this successive shortening of its muscular fibers with each contraction, the upper segment becomes progressively thickened throughout the first and second stages of labor and tremendously thickened immediately after the birth of the baby. The phenomenon of retraction of the upper uterine segment is contingent upon a decrease in the volume of its contents. For its contents to be diminished, particularly early in labor when the entire uterus is virtually a closed sac with only a minute opening at the cervix, requires that the musculature of the lower segment relax, permitting increasingly more of the intrauterine contents to distend its walls. Indeed, the upper segment retracts only to the extent that the lower segment and cervix relax.

The relaxation of the lower uterine segment is by no means complete relaxation, but rather the opposite of retraction. The fibers of the lower segment become stretched with each contraction of the upper segment, after which they do not return to their previous length but remain relatively fixed at the longer length, the tension, however, remaining the same as before. The musculature still manifests tone, still resists stretch, and still contracts on stimulation. This phenomenon has been called "receptive" or "postural" relaxation.

The successive lengthening of the muscular fibers in the lower uterine segment as labor progresses is accompanied by thinning, normally to only a few millimeters in its thinnest part. As a result of the thinning of the lower uterine segment and the concomitant thickening of the upper, the boundary between them is marked by a ridge on the inner uterine surface, the *physiologic retraction ring*. When the thinning of the lower uterine segment is extreme, as in obstructed labor, the ring is very prominent, forming, in extreme cases, the *pathologic retraction ring (Brandl's ring)*, an abnormal condition discussed further on page 850.

Quantitative measurements of the difference in behavior of the upper and lower parts of the uterus during normal labor have disclosed a gradient of diminishing physiologic activity from the fundus to the lower uterine segment. Several ingenious devices have been used, including the tokodynamometer, intrauterine receptors, and intramyometrial catheters.

The tokodynamometer employs three strain gauges set in heavy brass ring mountings, which may be placed anywhere on the abdomen. When the uterus contracts, the increased convexity of the local arc of uterus underlying the ring pushes upward on the gauge and applies a strain to its elements proportional to the local force of the uterine contraction. A record is obtained electrometrically, an example of which is shown in Figure 4. It is at once evident from these tracings that the intensity of each contraction is greater in the upper zone than in the midzone, and greater in the midzone than lower down. Equally noteworthy is the differential in the duration of the contractions; those in the midzone are much

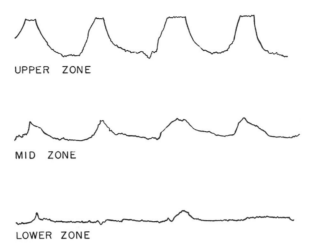

UPPER   ZONE

MID   ZONE

LOWER ZONE

Fig. 4. Tracings of uterine contractions in various parts of the uterus made by Reynolds' tokodynamometer. The lower zone probably corresponds roughly to the lower uterine segment. The patient was a primigravida in active labor, with cervix 5 cm dilated, and contractions about three minutes apart. The original tracings have been inked over for clearer reproduction. (From Reynolds, Hellman, and Bruns. Obstet Gynec Survey 3:629, 1948.)

briefer than those above, whereas the contractions in the lower zone are extremely brief and sometimes absent. This subsidence of contraction in the midzone while the upper zone is still contracting indicates that the upper part of the corpus, throughout a substantial portion of each contraction, exerts pressure caudally on the more relaxed parts of the uterus. Occasionally when labor is not progressing, this gradient is absent, and both the intensity and the duration of the contractions may be the same in all three zones.

These findings of Reynolds have been confirmed through use of an entirely different apparatus by Karlson. His technic measures the internal pressure in the uterus at any point by means of so-called receptors (metal capsules about 12 mm long with a diameter of 4.5 mm), in the middle of which is a small aperture. On

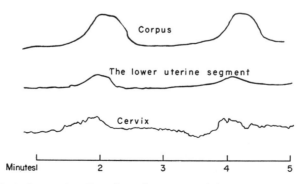

Corpus

The lower uterine segment

Cervix

Minutes| 2   3   4   5

Fig. 5. Tracings of uterine contractions in various parts of the uterus recorded by Karlson by means of intrauterine receptors. The patient was in early labor, but from the time this tracing was made, progress was rapid. To permit clearer reproduction the background of the original record has been eliminated and the tracings inked over. (Modified from Karlson. Acta Obstet Gynec Scand 28:209, 1949).

the inner side of this aperture is a membrane sensitive to pressure. Pressure exerted against the window is carried and registered electrometrically; an example of one of Karlson's tracings is shown in Figure 5. Here again there is a gradient of diminishing activity from the corpus to the lower uterine segment. Karlson's other tracings, like Reynolds', indicate that in the absence of this gradient—that is, when the intensity of contraction of the lower segment equals or exceeds that of the corpus—cervical dilatation may cease. Similar findings were obtained by Caldeyro-Barcia and Alvarez, who inserted either small intramyometrial balloons or open-ended catheters at various levels and recorded the pressures during contractions.

Ligamentous Action.   The round ligaments are not mere reduplications of the peritoneum but are composed principally of smooth muscle extending from the uterus. Therefore, whenever the uterine musculature contracts, they contract also. Because they are anchored, like guy ropes, to the lowermost part of the anterior abdominal wall, they may pull the parturient uterus forward with each contraction. With each contraction, in any event, the uterus pushes the anterior abdominal wall forward, as its long axis is aligned with that of the birth canal (Fig. 6).

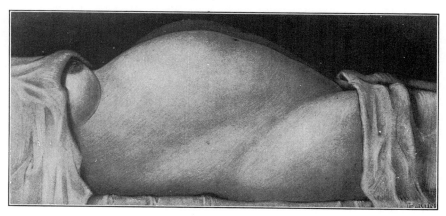

Fig. 6. Composite picture showing shape of abdomen before and during a uterine contraction, the shadowy outline indicating contraction.

Change in Uterine Shape.   Each contraction produces an elongation of the uterine ovoid with a concomitant decrease in the transverse and anteroposterior diameters. This change in shape has two important effects on the process of labor: (1) The decrease in lateral diameter produces a straightening of the fetal vertebral column, pressing its upper pole firmly against the fundus of the uterus, while the lower pole is thrust farther downward into the pelvis. The lengthening of the fetal ovoid thus produced has been estimated as between 5 and 10 cm. The pressure so exerted is known as *fetal axis pressure.* (2) With the lengthening of the uterus, the longitudinal fibers are drawn taut; and since the lower segment and cervix are the only parts of the uterus that give, they are pulled upward over the lower pole of the fetus. This effect on the musculature of the lower segment and on the cervix is an important factor in cervical dilatation.

OTHER FORCES CONCERNED IN LABOR

Intraabdominal Pressure.   After the cervix is fully dilated, particularly after the membranes have ruptured, the chief force that expels the fetus is contraction of the abdominal muscles and the respiratory diaphragm during inspiration with consequent increase in intraabdominal pressure. The force is similar to that in- volved in defecation but greatly intensified. The important role played by intra- abdominal pressure in fetal expulsion is most plainly attested by the labors of paraplegic women. Such patients suffer no pain, although the uterus may contract violently. Cervical dilatation, solely the result of uterine contractions, proceeds normally, but expulsion of the infant is rarely possible except when the patient is instructed to bear down at the time that the obstetrician palpates uterine con- tractions. Although increased intraabdominal pressure is required for the spon- taneous completion of labor, it is futile unless the uterus is contracted. In other words, it is a necessary auxiliary to uterine contractions in the second stage of labor, but accomplishes nothing in the first stage but fatigue of the mother.

Intraabdominal pressure is important not only in the second but also in the third stage of labor. After the placenta has separated, its expulsion is aided by the mother's bearing down—that is, by an increase in intraabdominal pressure.

Resistance.   Labor is work, and work mechanically is the generation of motion against resistance. The forces involved in labor are those of the uterus and ab- domen that expel the infant and that must overcome the resistance offered by the cervix to dilatation and the friction created by the birth canal during passage of the presenting part. In addition, forces are exerted by the muscles of the pelvic floor. The work involved in labor, according to Gemzell and others, is only a frac- tion of the maximal functional capacity of the normal woman.

Very little is known about the nature of the resistance of the cervix to dilata- tion, but the many hours required and the fact that almost all cervices suffer at least minor lacerations in labor indicate that substantial resistance must be over- come. The friction in the birth canal is sufficiently great to mold the fetal head, and the troughlike structure of the pelvic floor so resists descent of the head that internal rotation is usually effected, as described on page 377. The resistance of the perineum, moreover, may create so much obstruction that its surgical incision becomes necessary.

In short, labor may be regarded as a contest between the forces of expulsion and the resistances offered by the cervix and birth canal.

CHANGES OF THE UTERUS DURING THE FIRST STAGE OF LABOR

The forces concerned in the first stage of labor are (1) the uterine contrac- tions and (2) the resultant hydrostatic pressure of the membranes against the cervix and lower uterine segment or, in the absence of the membranes, the pres- sure of the presenting part against the cervix and lower uterine segment. As the result of the action of these forces, two fundamental changes are wrought in the cervix: *effacement* and *dilatation*.

The Mechanism of Cervical Effacement.   Effacement ("obliteration" or "taking up") is the shortening of the cervical canal from a structure approximately 2 cm in length to one in which the canal is replaced by a mere circular orifice with almost paper-thin edges. The process takes place from above downward; it oc- curs as the muscular fibers around the internal os are pulled upward, or "taken up," into the lower uterine segment, while the condition of the external os remains temporarily unchanged. As seen in Figures 7 through 10, the edges of the internal os are drawn several centimeters upward to become functionally part of the lower

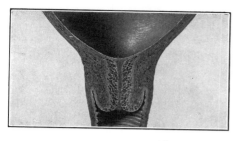

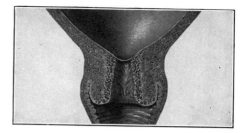

Fig. 7. Cervix at end of pregnancy.

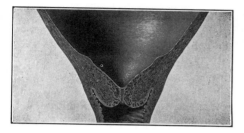

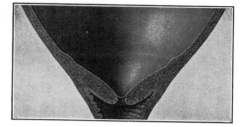

Fig. 8. Beginning effacement of cervix. Note dilatation of internal os and funnel-shaped cervical canal.

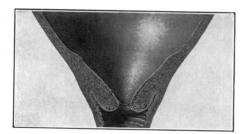

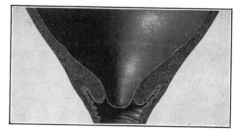

Fig. 9. Further effacement of cervix. Note higher position of internal os and bulging of membranes.

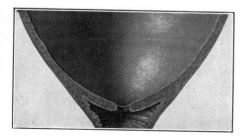

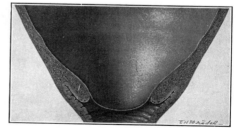

Fig. 10. Cervical canal obliterated. Left, primigravida; right, multigravida.

uterine segment. Effacement may be compared to a funneling process in which the whole length of a moldable tube is converted into a very obtuse flaring funnel with only a small circular orifice for an outlet. As the result of Braxton Hicks contractions, considerable effacement is sometimes attained before true labor begins. Such effacement usually facilitates expulsion of the mucous plug.

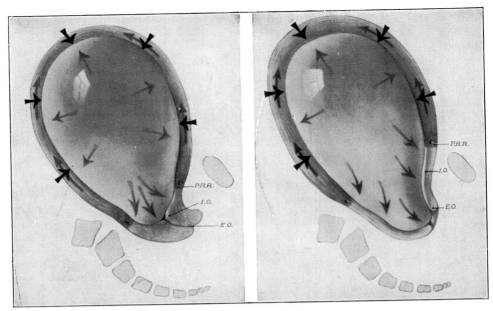

Fig. 11. Hydrostatic action of membranes in effecting cervical effacement and dilatation. In absence of intact membranes, the presenting part applied to the cervix and lower uterine segment (P.R.R.) acts similarly. In this and the next two illustrations note changing relations of external os (E.O.), internal os (I.O.), and physiologic retraction ring (P.R.R.).

Fig. 12. Hydrostatic action of membranes at completion of effacement.

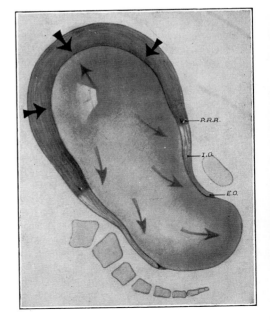

Fig. 13. Hydrostatic action of membranes at full cervical dilatation.

The Mechanism of Cervical Dilatation (Figs. 11–13).　　　Dilatation of the cervix is the enlargement of the external os from an orifice a few millimeters in diameter to an aperture large enough to permit passage of the baby. When dilatation has reached a diameter of 10 cm it is commonly said to be "complete" or "full."

Because the lower uterine segment and cervix are regions of least resistance, they are subjected to distention, in the course of which a centrifugal pull is exerted on the cervix. As the uterine contractions exert pressure on the membranes, the hydrostatic action of the amniotic sac in turn dilates the cervical canal in the manner of a wedge. In the absence of intact membranes, the pressure of the presenting part against the cervix and lower uterine segment is similarly effective. Rupture of the membranes does not retard cervical dilatation, so long as the presenting part exerts pressure against the cervix and lower uterine segment.

There is still controversy about the mechanism or mechanisms that transmit the uterine forces of labor to the amniotic fluid and fetus. When the fetus is floating free in fluid, throughout the contraction the amniotic sac behaves as one simple fluid-filled compartment and the force of the contraction is transmitted to the amniotic fluid equally in all directions. When the volume of amniotic fluid is rather small, however, as in late pregnancy and especially after rupture of the membranes, the contracting uterus is not necessarily separated from the fetus by fluid. In this circumstance the forces generated by different parts of the uterus might not be transmitted with uniform intensity to the fetus. Nonetheless, the dominant nature of the fundal force is quite appropriate for effecting cervical dilatation.

The decidua of the lower uterine segment is thin and poorly developed. Toward the end of pregnancy the spongiosa in that area consists of only a few filaments of thinned-out glandular walls. The slightest movement of the underlying muscle, therefore, might sever them and allow the fetal membranes to slip back and forth over the mucosa. This loosening of the membranes in the lower segment is a normal feature of early labor and a prerequisite to successful cervical dilatation. Membranes that slide readily over the lower segment and partly through the cervix are much more efficacious dilators than those attached to the surface. The observation that digital stripping of the membranes in the region of the cervix sometimes suffices to initiate labor in gravidas at term is in accord with those observations. The chemical changes accompanying cervical dilatation are discussed on page 244 (Ch. 8).

CHANGES IN THE UTERUS DURING THE SECOND STAGE OF LABOR

By the end of the first stage of labor the uterine contractions have resulted in the differentiation of the organ into two anatomically and functionally different parts. Above is the active, contractile portion, which becomes thicker as labor advances, and below, the thin-walled, passive, lower uterine segment and the completely dilated cervix (Fig. 14).

There may be no fetal descent during cervical effacement, but as a rule, the station of the presenting part descends somewhat as the cervix dilates. During the second stage, descent occurs rather slowly but steadily in nulliparas. In multiparas, however, particularly those of high parity, descent may be very rapid.

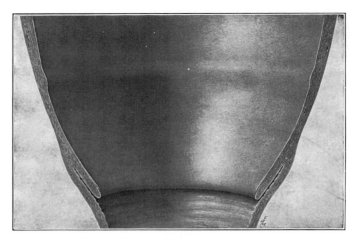

Fig. 14. Complete effacement and full dilatation of cervix.

During the course of labor, spontaneous rupture of the membranes usually occurs, manifested most often by a sudden gush of a variable quantity of clear or slightly turbid, nearly colorless fluid. Infrequently the membranes remain intact until the time of delivery of the infant. If by chance the membranes remain intact until completion of delivery, the fetus is born surrounded by them, and the portion covering its head is sometimes referred to as the *caul*.

The changes in shape of the uterus during contraction may be noticed in the first stage, but particularly in the second, when the organ increases considerably in length and at the same time diminishes in its transverse and anteroposterior diameters with each contraction. The increase in length results partly from stretching of the lower uterine segment and partly from straightening of the fetus. With the formation of the lower uterine segment, the upper portion of the uterus increases greatly in thickness and, as labor proceeds, covers a progressively smaller portion of the fetus. In neglected prolonged labors in which there is definite disproportion between the size of the presenting part and the pelvic canal, the lower uterine segment is subjected to excessive stretching; consequently, the retraction ring rises much higher and is sometimes palpable as a distinct transverse or oblique ridge at a variable level between the symphysis pubis and umbilicus. In such circumstances, rupture of the uterus is imminent unless labor is promptly terminated.

In addition, the contractions of the abdominal muscles play a significant part in expelling the child. Where abdominal contractions are absent or inadequate, labor is frequently delayed and forceps are often required.

Immediately after birth of the child a striking change occurs in the position and size of the uterus, which on palpation is firm and rounded and barely reaches the umbilicus. At that time its contracted body, freely movable above the collapsed lower uterine segment and cervix, can be readily moved in any direction.

CHANGES IN THE VAGINA AND PELVIC FLOOR DURING LABOR

The pelvic outlet, or birth canal, is supported and functionally closed by a number of layers of tissues that together form the pelvic floor. From within outward they are (1) peritoneum, (2) subperitoneal connective tissue, (3) internal pelvic fascia, (4) levator ani and coccygeus muscles, (5) external pelvic fascia, (6) superficial muscles and fascia, (7) subcutaneous tissue, and (8) skin.

Of these structures the most important are the levator ani and the fascia covering its upper and lower surfaces, which for practical purposes may be considered the pelvic floor (Figs. 15–18). This muscle (or group of muscles) closes the lower end of the pelvic

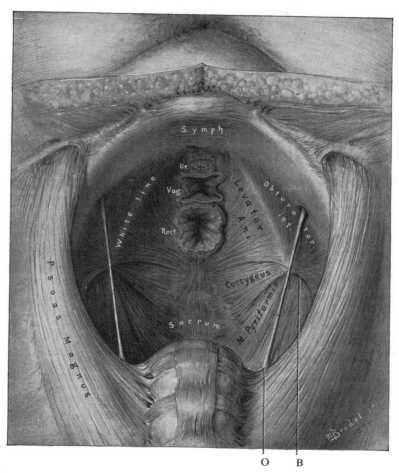

O   B

Fig. 15. The pelvic floor seen from above. O, obturator nerve; B, border of great sciatic foramen. (From Kelly. Operative Gynecology, D. Appleton & Co., 1906.)

cavity as a diaphragm and presents a concave upper and a convex lower surface. On either side it consists of a pubic and iliac portion. The former is a band 2 to 2.5 cm in width arising from the horizontal ramus of the pubis 3 to 4 cm below its upper margin and 1 to 1.5 cm from the symphysis pubis. Its fibers pass backward to encircle the rectum and possibly give off a few fibers that pass behind the vagina. The greater or iliac portion of the muscle arises on either side and from the white line, the tendinous arch of the pelvic fascia, and from the ischial spine at a distance of about 5 cm below the margin of the pelvic inlet. Its fibers are not uniformly arranged, but according to Dickinson, several portions can be distinguished. Passing from before backward, there is a narrow band that crosses the pubic portion and descends to the rectovaginal septum.

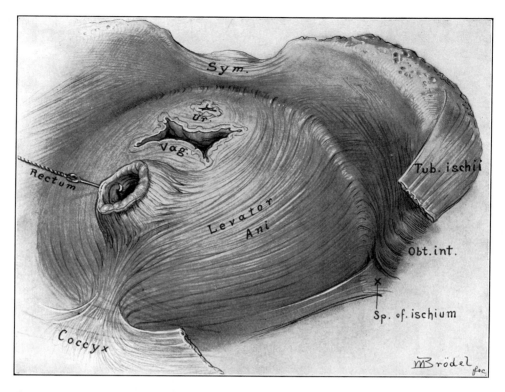

Fig. 16. The pelvic floor seen from below. (From Kelly. Operative Gynecology, D. Appleton & Co., 1906.)

The greater part of the muscle passes backward and unites with that from the other side of the rectum; the posterior portions meet in a tendinous raphe in front of the coccyx, with the most posterior fibers attached to the bone itself. The posterior and lateral portions of the pelvic floor, which are not filled out by the levator ani, are occupied by the piriformis and coccygeus muscles on either side.

The levator ani varies from 3 to 5 mm in thickness, though its margins encircling the rectum and vagina are somewhat thicker. It undergoes considerable hypertrophy during pregnancy. On vaginal examination its internal margin may be felt as a thick band extending backward from the pubis and encircling the vagina about 2 cm above the hymen. On contraction it draws both the rectum and vagina forward and upward in the direction of the symphysis pubis and is thus the real closer of the vagina, for the more superficial muscles of the perineum are too delicate to serve more than an accessory function.

The internal pelvic fascia, which forms the upper covering of the levator ani, is attached to the margin of the pelvic inlet, where it is joined by the fascia of the iliac fossa, as well as by the transverse fascia of the abdominal walls. It passes down over the piriformis and the upper half of the obturator internus and is firmly attached to the periosteum covering the lateral wall of the pelvis. The white line indicates its point of deflection from the latter, whence it spreads out over the upper surface of the levator ani and coccygeus muscles.

The inferior fascial covering of the pelvic diaphragm is divided into two parts by a line drawn between the ischial tuberosities. Its posterior portion consists of a single layer, which, taking its origin from the sacrosciatic ligament and the ischial tuberosity, passes up over the inner surface of the ischial bones and the obturator internus to the white line,

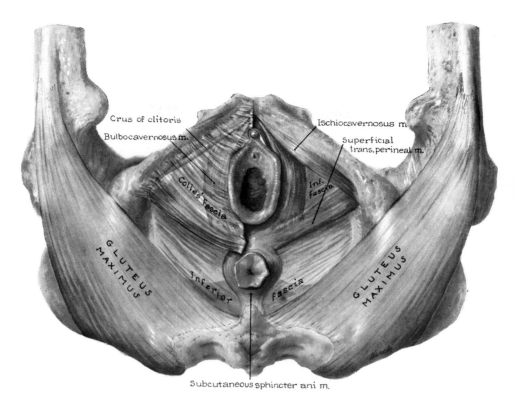

Fig. 17. Superficial muscles and fascia of pelvic floor.

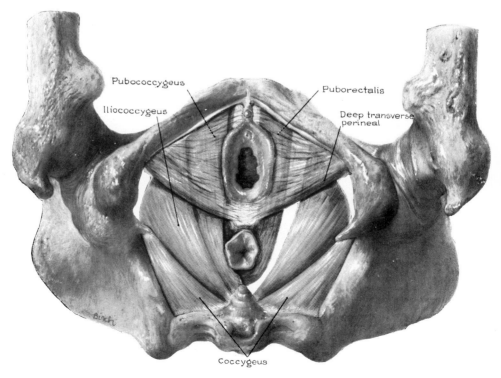

Fig. 18. Deep muscles of pelvic floor.

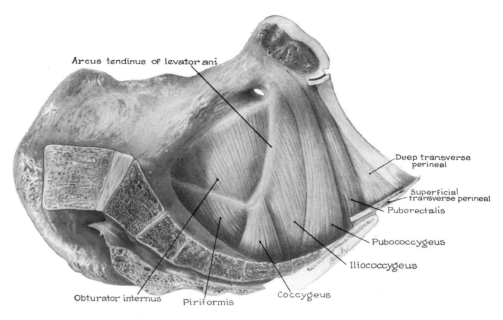

Arcus tendinus of levator ani

Deep transverse perineal

Superficial transverse perineal

Puborectalis

Pubococcygeus

Iliococcygeus

Coccygeus

Obturator internus   Piriformis

Fig. 19. Lateral view of muscles of pelvic floor.

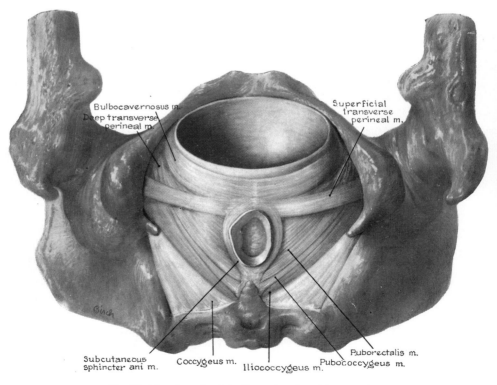

Bulbocavernosus m.
Deep transverse perineal m.

Superficial transverse perineal m.

Subcutaneous sphincter ani m.   Coccygeus m.   Iliococcygeus m.   Pubococcygeus m.   Puborectalis m.

Fig. 20. Muscles of pelvic floor when head is crowning.

in the formation of which it takes part. From this tendinous structure it is reflected at an acute angle over upon the inferior surface of the levator ani; the space included between the latter and the lateral pelvic wall forms the *ischiorectal fossa*. The structure filling out the triangular space between the pubic arch and a line joining the ischial tuberosities is known as the *urogenital diaphragm*, which, exclusive of skin and subcutaneous fat, consists principally of three layers of fascia: (1) the deep perineal fascia, which covers the anterior portion of the inferior surface of the levator ani muscle and is continuous with the fascia just described; (2) the middle perineal fascia, which is separated from the former by a narrow space in which are situated the pubic vessels and nerves; (3) the

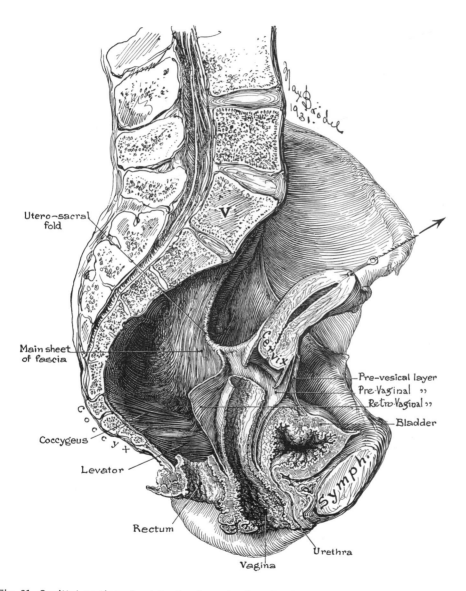

Fig. 21. Sagittal section of pelvic structures to show fascia surrounding vagina. (From Sears. Amer J Obstet Gynec 25:484, 1933.)

superficial perineal fascia, which, together with the layer just described, forms a compartment in which lie the superficial perineal muscles, with the exception of the sphincter ani, the rami of the clitoris, the vestibular bulbs, and the vulvovaginal glands (see Ch. 2, Fig. 3).

The superficial perineal muscles consist of the bulbocavernosus, the ischiocavernosus, and the superficial transverse perineal muscles. These structures are delicately formed and are of no obstetric significance except that the superficial transverse perineal muscles are always torn in perineal lacerations.

In the first stage of labor the membranes and presenting part of the fetus play a role in dilatation of the upper portion of the vagina, which has been prepared for the process by important changes in its mucosa and connective tissue and hypertrophy of its muscularis (Ch. 8, p. 245). Chemical changes similar to those in the cervix may also occur. After the membranes have ruptured, however, the changes in the pelvic floor are caused entirely by pressure exerted by the presenting part of the fetus. When the head distends the vulva, the vulvar opening is diverted upward and forward, and the birth canal follows a curve along the pelvic floor (Figs. 19–21).

The most marked change consists in the stretching of the fibers of the levator ani and the thinning of the central portion of the perineum, which becomes transformed from a wedge-shaped mass of tissue 5 cm in thickness to a thin, almost transparent membranous structure less than a centimeter in thickness. When the perineum is maximally distended, the anus becomes markedly dilated and presents an opening, varying from 2 to 3 cm in diameter, through which the anterior wall of the rectum bulges. The extraordinary increase in the number and size of the blood vessels supplying the vagina and pelvic floor allows for great compression, but at the same time greatly increases the danger of hemorrhage if the tissues are torn.

PHYSIOLOGY OF THE THIRD STAGE OF LABOR

The third stage of labor comprises the *phase of placental separation* and *the phase of placental expulsion.*

The Phase of Placental Separation.   As the baby is born, the uterus contracts down on its diminishing contents. Normally, by the time the infant is completely delivered, the uterine cavity is obliterated and the organ is represented by an almost solid mass of muscle, the walls of which are several centimeters thick and the fundus of which lies just below the level of the umbilicus. This sudden diminution in uterine size is inevitably accompanied by a decrease in the area of the placental site. To accommodate itself to this reduced area, the placenta increases in thickness, but because of its limited elasticity it is soon forced to buckle. The resulting tension causes the weakest layer of the decidua, the spongiosa, to give way, and cleavage takes place there. Separation of the placenta, therefore, is a result primarily of disproportion between the unchanged size of the placenta and the reduced size of the placental site.

Cleavage is greatly facilitated by the loose structure of the spongy decidua, which may be likened to the row of perforations between postage stamps. As separation proceeds, a hematoma forms between the separating placenta and the remaining decidua. Formation of the hematoma is usually the result rather than the cause of the separation, since in some cases bleeding is negligible. The hematoma may, however, accelerate the process.

Most investigators report that placental separation occurs within a very few minutes after delivery (Fig. 22). Brandt and others in combined clinical and roentgenologic studies have supported the idea that because the periphery of the placenta is probably the most adherent portion, separation usually begins elsewhere. Sometimes separation begins even before the third stage of labor, probably accounting for certain cases of fetal distress just before expulsion of the child.

After birth of the baby the contraction of the uterus causes a great decrease in the surface area of the cavity. Consequently, the fetal membranes and the decidua parietalis are thrown into innumerable folds that increase the thickness of the layer from less than a millimeter to 3 to 4 mm.

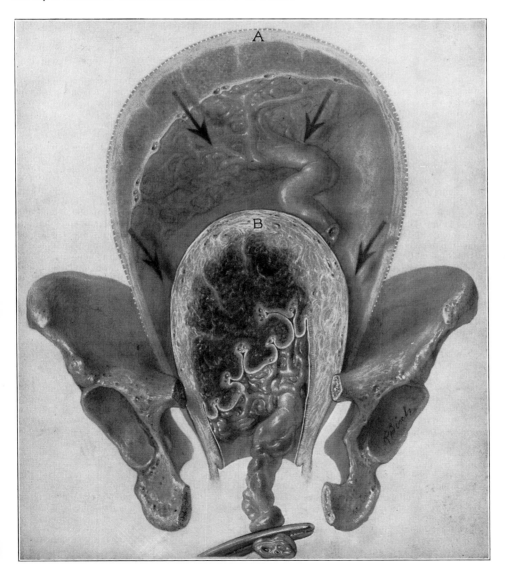

Fig. 22. Diminution in size of placental site after birth of baby. A, placental relations before birth of infant; B, placental relations after birth of infant.

Figures 23 and 24, which represent the lining of the uterus at the end of pregnancy and early in the third stage, respectively, indicate that much of the decidua parietalis is included between the folds of the festooned amnion and chorion laeve. Since the separation of the placenta is through the spongy layer of the decidua (Ch. 6, p. 151), part of the decidua is cast off with the placenta, while the rest remains attached to the myometrium (Figs. 25 and 26). The amount of decidual tissue retained at the placental site varies considerably.

The membranes usually remain in situ until the separation of the placenta is practically completed. They are then peeled off the uterine wall partly by the further contraction of the myometrium and partly by traction exerted by the

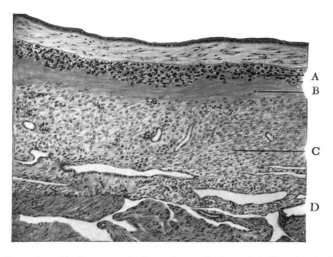

Fig. 23. Section through wall of pregnant uterus beyond placental site. A, chorion laeve; B, fibrin layer; C, decidua parietalis; D, myometrium.

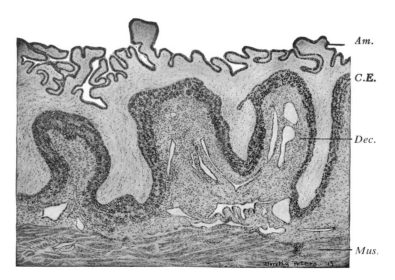

Fig. 24. Section through uterine wall beyond placental site during third stage, showing festooning of membranes. Am., amnion; C.E., epithelium of chorion laeve; Dec., decidua parietalis; Mus., muscularis (myometrium).

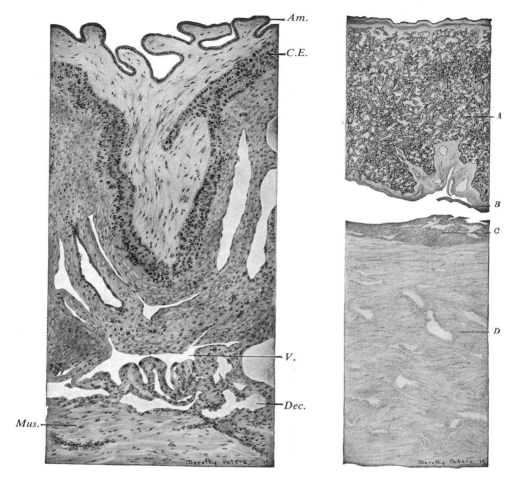

Fig. 25. Detail of portion of Figure 24 more highly magnified. Am., amnion; C.E., epithelium of chorion laeve; Dec., decidua parietalis; Mus., muscularis (myometrium); V., vascular spaces in decidua.

Fig. 26. Diagram showing separation of placenta through decidua basalis X 3. A, placenta; B, decidua cast off with placenta; C, decidua retained in utero; D, myometrium.

separated placenta, which lies in the flabby lower uterine segment or the upper portion of the vagina. The body of the uterus at that time forms an almost solid mass of muscle, the anterior and posterior walls of which, each measuring 4 to 5 cm in thickness, lie in such close apposition that the uterine cavity is practically obliterated.

The Phase of Placental Expulsion.   After the placenta has separated, the pressure exerted upon it by the uterine walls causes it to slide downward into the flaccid lower uterine segment or the upper part of the vagina. In some cases it may be expelled from those locations by increase in abdominal pressure, but women in the recumbent position frequently cannot expel the placenta spontaneously. An artificial means of terminating the third stage is therefore generally required. The usual method is pressure over the fundus by the hand of an attendant, employing the uterus as a piston to expel the placenta.

Mechanisms of Placental Extrusion.   When the central, or usual, type of placental separation occurs, the retroplacental hematoma is believed to push the placenta toward the uterine cavity, first the central portion and then the rest. The placenta, thus inverted and weighted with the hematoma, then descends. Since the surrounding membranes are still attached to the decidua, the placenta can do so only by dragging after it the membranes, which peel off its periphery. Consequently, the sac formed by the membranes is inverted, with the glistening fetal surface of the placenta presenting at the vulva. The retroplacental hematoma either follows the placenta or is demonstrable within the invered sac. In this process, known as *Schultze's mechanism* of placental expulsion, blood from the placental site pours into the inverted sac, not escaping externally until after extrusion of the placenta.

The other method of placental extrusion is known as the *Duncan mechanism,* according to which separation occurs first at the periphery, with the result that blood collects between the membranes and the uterine wall and escapes from the vagina. In that event, the placenta descends to the vagina sideways, and the maternal surface appears first at the vulva.

If the cord is severed immediately upon completion of the second stage and a radiopaque medium is injected through the umbilical vessels into the placenta, it appears that in about two thirds of all cases separation occurs after the first or second succeeding contraction. Furthermore, the placenta passes through the contraction ring by its margin, the retroplacental hematoma playing very little part in bringing about its separation. The mechanisms described by Duncan and Schultze, moreover, occur only in the vagina and consequently apply only as the placenta emerges from the vagina.

References

Brandt, M. L.   Mechanism and management of the third stage of labor. Amer J Obstet Gynec 25:662, 1933.

Caldeyro-Barcia, R., Alvarez, H., and Reynolds, S. R. M.   A better understanding of uterine contractility through simultaneous recording with an internal and a seven channel external method. Surg Gynec Obstet 91:641, 1950.

Carsten, M. E.   Regulation of myometrial composition, growth, and activity, in Assali, N. S. (ed.), Biology of Gestation, Vol. I, The Maternal Organism. New York, Academic Press, 1968.

Coch, J. A., Brovetto, J., Cabot, H. M., Fielitz, C. A., and Caldeyro-Barcia, R.   Oxytocin-equivalent activity in the plasma of women in labor and during the puerperium. Amer J Obstet Gynec 91:10, 1965.

Csapo, A.   Progesterone "block." Amer J Anat 98:273, 1956.

———— Function and regulation of the myometrium. Ann NY Acad Sci 75:790, 1959.

———— DeSousa-Filho, M. B., DeSouza, J. C., and DeSouza, O.   Effect of massive progestational hormone treatment on the parturient human uterus. Fertil Steril 17:621, 1966.

Dickinson, R. L.   Studies of the levator ani muscle. Amer J Obstet 22:897, 1889.

Ferguson, J. K. W.   A study of the motility of the intact uterus at term. Surg Gynec Obstet 73:359, 1941.

Gemzell, C. A., Robbe, H., Stern, B., and Ström, G.   Observation on circulatory changes and muscular work in normal labour. Acta Obstet Gynec Scand 36:75, 1957.

Heckel, G. P., and Allen, W. M.   Prolongation of pregnancy in the rabbit by the injection of progesterone. Amer J Obstet Gynec 35:131, 1938.

Ivy, A. C.   Functional anatomy of labor, with special reference to the human being. Amer J Obstet Gynec 44:952, 1942.

———— Hartman, C. G., and Koff, A.   The contractions of the monkey uterus at term. Amer J Obstet Gynec 22:388, 1931.

Karlson, S.   On the motility of the uterus during labour and the influence of the motility pattern on the duration of the labour. Acta Obstet Gynec Scand 28:209, 1949.

Kelly, H. A.   Operative Gynecology, 2nd rev. and enlarged edition. New York, D. Appleton & Co., 1909, 2 vols.

Kumar, D., Goodno, J. A., and Barnes, A. C.   In vivo effects of intravenous progesterone infusion on human gravid uterine contractility. Bull Hopkins Hosp 113:53, 1963.

Liggins, G. C.   Premature delivery of foetal lambs infused with glucocorticoids. J Endocr 45:515, 1969.

———— Premature parturition after infusion of corticotrophin or cortisol into foetal lambs. J Endocr 42:323, 1968.

———— Kennedy, P. C., and Holm, L. W.   Failure of initiation of parturition after electrocoagulation of the pituitary of the foetal lamb. Amer J Obstet Gynec 98:1080, 1967.

Lyon, R.   Pregnanediol excretion at the onset of labor. Amer J Obstet Gynec 51:403, 1946.

Milic, A. B., and Adamsons, K.   The relationship between anencephaly and prolonged pregnancy. J Obstet Gynaec Brit Comm 76:102, 1969.

Reynolds, S. R. M.   Physiology of the Uterus with Clinical Correlations, 2nd ed. New York, Paul B. Hoeber, 1949.

———— Heard, O. O., Bruns, P., and Hellman, L. M.   A multi-channel strain-gage tokodynamometer: an instrument for studying patterns of uterine contractions in pregnant women. Bull Hopkins Hosp 82:446, 1948.

———— Hellman, L. M., and Bruns, P.   Patterns of uterine contractility in women during pregnancy. Obstet Gynec Survey 3:629, 1948.

Rudolph, L., and Ivy, A. C.   The coordination of the uterus in labor. Amer J Obstet Gynec 21:65, 1931.

Sala, N. L., Schwarcz, R. L., Althabe, O., Fisch, L., and Fuente, O.   Effect of epidural anesthesia upon uterine contractility induced by artificial cervical dilatation in human pregnancy. Amer J Obstet Gynec 106:26, 1970.

Theobald, G. W.   Nervous control of uterine activity. Clin Obstet Gynec 11:15, 1968.

Watts, D. T.   Stimulation of uterine muscle by adenosinetriphosphate. Amer J Physiol 173:291, 1953.

14

THE MECHANISM OF LABOR IN VERTEX PRESENTATIONS

Vertex, or occiput, presentations occur in about 95 per cent of all labors. In the majority of cases the vertex enters the pelvis with the sagittal suture in the transverse pelvic diameter. The preponderance of transverse positions of the head at the onset of labor and the frequency of the various vertex positions are shown in Table 1, based on 1,040 cases studied roentgenologically by Steele and Javert.

Table 1. Position of the Fetal Head at the Onset of Labor
(per 100)

Station of Head	LOT	ROT	LOA	ROA	OA	ROP	LOP	OP	Number of Cases
Above or at inlet	39.9	23.5	13.2	9.6	1.8	7.3	3.0	0.6	763
At, above, or below spines	33.7	28.8	11.9	5.7	2.8	11.5	3.2	1.8	277

These findings indicate a transverse position of the head in over 60 per cent of patients at the onset of labor irrespective of whether the head is engaged.

MECHANISM IN OCCIPITOTRANSVERSE POSITIONS

The mechanism of labor will be discussed first in the transverse varieties of vertex presentations, since they are the most common.

Diagnosis. The presentation of the fetus is most commonly ascertained by abdominal palpation, which is useful not only during pregnancy but also during labor, provided it is performed in the intervals between contractions. Its accuracy, however, is greatly impaired in patients with markedly obese abdominal walls and in those in whom the uterus is overdistended by excess amniotic fluid or deformed by myomas, which may occasionally be mistaken for fetal parts.

For diagnosis the four maneuvers of Leopold are employed (Ch. 11, p. 326). With the fetus in the left occipitotransverse position, the following findings are obtained:

First maneuver:	Fundus occupied by the breech.
Second maneuver:	Resistant plane of the back felt directly to the left in the flank; small parts on the right, readily palpated through the flank.
Third maneuver:	Negative if the head is engaged; otherwise, the movable head detected above the superior strait or pelvic inlet.
Fourth maneuver:	Cephalic prominence on the right.

The left occipitotransverse position is somewhat more frequent than the right; in the right position palpation yields similar information, except that the fetal back is in the right flank and the small parts and cephalic prominence are on the left.

On vaginal or rectal examination the sagittal suture is found to occupy the transverse diameter of the pelvis, more or less midway between the sacrum and the symphysis. In left transverse positions the smaller posterior fontanel is directed toward a point midway between the iliopectineal and the sacroiliac synchondrosis on that side, and the larger anterior fontanel is directed toward the same point on the right side of the pelvis. In right transverse positions, the reverse holds true. The fetal heart is usually heard in the right or left flank of the mother, in right and left positions, respectively, at or slightly below the level of the umbilicus. The heart tones may sometimes be heard, though less clearly, also on the side opposite the fetal back, when for various reasons the sound is transmitted through the fetal thorax as well.

THE CARDINAL MOVEMENTS OF LABOR

Because of the irregular shape of the pelvic canal and the relatively large dimensions of the mature fetal head, it is evident that not all diameters of the head can necessarily pass through all diameters of the pelvis. It follows that a process of adaptation or accommodation of suitable portions of the head to the various segments of the pelvis is required for completion of childbirth. These positional changes of the presenting part constitute the *mechanism of labor*. The cardinal movements are (1) engagement, (2) descent, (3) flexion, (4) internal rotation, (5) extension, (6) external rotation, and (7) expulsion.

For purposes of instruction the various movements are often described as though they occurred separately and independently, whereas in reality the mechanism of labor consists of a combination of movements, several of which may be going on at the same time. It is manifestly impossible for the movements to be completed unless the presenting part descends simultaneously. Concomitantly the uterine contractions effect important modifications in the attitude, or habitus, of the fetus, especially after the head has descended into the pelvis. These changes consist principally in a straightening of the fetus, with loss of its dorsal convexity and closer application of the extremities and small parts to the body. As a result the fetal ovoid is transformed into a cylinder with the smallest possible cross section for passage through the birth canal.

Engagement.   As discussed on page 302, of Chapter 10, the mechanism by which the biparietal diameter, the greatest transverse diameter of the head in vertex presentations, passes through the pelvic inlet is designated engagement, a phenomenon that usually occurs in primigravidas with normal pelves during the last few weeks of pregnancy but does not ordinarily take place in multiparas until after the commencement of labor.

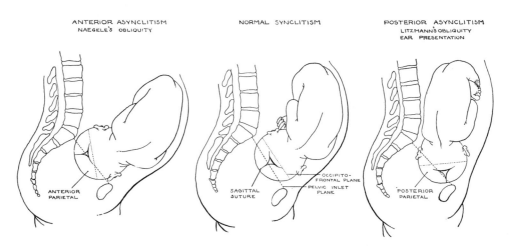

Fig. 1. Synclitism and asynclitism.

In most multiparas at the end of pregnancy the fetal head is freely movable above the pelvic inlet in one of the iliac fossae. A normal-sized head usually does not engage with its sagittal suture directed anteroposteriorly. It must therefore enter the pelvic inlet either in the transverse, as usually occurs, or in one of its oblique diameters.

Although the fetal head tends to accommodate to the transverse axis of the pelvic inlet, the sagittal suture, while remaining parallel to that axis, may not lie exactly midway between the symphysis and sacral promontory; it is frequently deflected either posteriorly toward the promontory or anteriorly toward the symphysis, as shown in Figure 1. Such deflection of the head anteriorly or posteriorly is called *asynclitism*. If the sagittal suture approaches the promontory, the anterior parietal bone presents itself to the examining fingers, in the condition called anterior parietal presentation or anterior asynclitism. If, however, it lies close to the symphysis, the posterior parietal bone will present and the condition

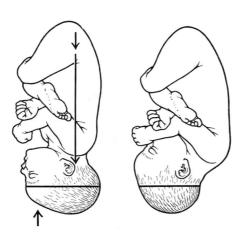

Fig. 2. Diagrams showing lever action producing flexion of head; conversion of occipitofrontal to suboccipitobregmatic diameter.

is called posterior parietal presentation or posterior asynclitism. Moderate degrees of asynclitism are the rule in normal labor; Javert and Steele noted posterior asynclitism in 75 per cent of cases in which the fetal head was at the pelvic brim, and anterior asynclitism in the same percentage of women in whom the head had descended into the pelvis. The findings of Caldwell and his associates are similar. Successive changes from posterior to anterior asynclitism facilitate descent by allowing the fetal head to take advantage of the roomiest areas of the pelvic cavity.

Descent.   The first requisite for the birth of the child is descent, the extent varying materially from primigravida to multipara. In the former, when there is no disproportion between the size of the head and the pelvis, engagement frequently occurs at or before the onset of labor, and further descent does not necessarily follow until the onset of the second stage of labor. In multiparas, descent usually begins with engagement. Descent is brought about by one or more of four forces: (1) pressure of the amniotic fluid; (2) direct pressure of the fundus upon the breech; (3) contraction of the abdominal muscles; and (4) extension and straightening of the child's body.

Flexion.   As soon as the descending head meets resistance, whether from the cervix, the walls of the pelvis, or the pelvic floor, flexion results. In this movement, as shown in Figure 2, the chin is brought into more intimate contact with the fetal thorax, and the shorter suboccipitobregmatic diameter is substituted for the longer occipitofrontal diameter.

The purely mechanical phenomenon of flexion by which a biparietal diameter of 9.5 cm replaces as the greatest diameter of the head an occipitofrontal of 11.75 cm may be a result of the manner in which the head is joined to the vertebral column. The head may be considered a two-armed lever, of which the short arm extends from the occipital condyles to the occipital protuberance, and the long arm from the condyles to the chin. When resistance is encountered, the long arm of the lever, following the ordinary laws of mechanics, ascends while the short arm descends, and flexion results.

According to D'Esopo, flexion of the head depends upon the relation between the line of force, transmitted in the direction of the fetal spine and foramen magnum, and the occipitofrontal plane rather than upon the lever action as just outlined. Rydberg, on the basis of extensive roentgenologic studies, believes that flexion usually takes place before engagement and is thus not a regular part of the mechanism of labor. He studied 53 gravidas near term but not in labor, in whom the head was neither floating nor engaged but just dipping into the inlet. In 31 cases the degree of flexion was found to be "advanced," and in 7 more it was "complete," as illustrated in Figure 3. It is possible, therefore, that flexion may occur before engagement and before the onset of labor. Regardless of when flexion takes place, it is an essential to descent, since it reduces greatly the presenting diameters of the fetal head, as shown in Figure 3.

Internal Rotation.   This movement is a turning of the head in such a manner that the occiput gradually moves from its original position anteriorly toward the symphysis pubis or, less commonly, posteriorly toward the hollow of the sacrum.

Internal rotation is essential for the completion of labor, except when the child is abnormally small. Regardless of the original position of the head, the occiput usually rotates to the front, although exceptionally in occipitoposterior positions it may turn toward the hollow of the sacrum (Figs. 4–8).

Internal rotation, which is always associated with descent of the presenting part, is usually not accomplished until the head has reached the level of the spines and therefore becomes engaged. Calkins studied more than 5,000 labors to ascertain when internal rotation occurs. He concluded that in approximately

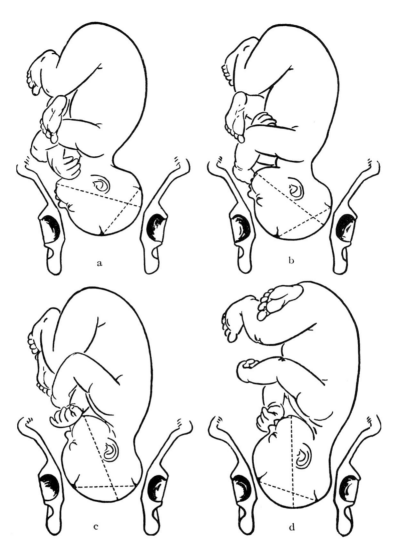

Fig. 3. Four degrees of positional flexion. Its relation to the fontanels. The dotted lines indicate the occipitomental diameter and the line connecting the center of the anterior fontanel with the posterior fontanel: a, positional flexion poor; b, positional flexion moderate; c, positional flexion advanced; d, positional flexion complete. (From Rydberg. The Mechanism of Labour. Charles C Thomas.)

two thirds of all patients internal rotation is complete by the time the head reaches the pelvic floor; in about one fourth, internal rotation is completed very shortly after the head reaches the pelvic floor; and in about 5 per cent, rotation to the anterior does not take place. When rotation fails to occur until the head reaches the pelvic floor, it takes place during the next one or two contractions in multiparas, and in primigravidas during the next three to five. Rotation before the head reaches the pelvic floor is definitely more frequent in multiparas than in primigravidas, according to Calkins.

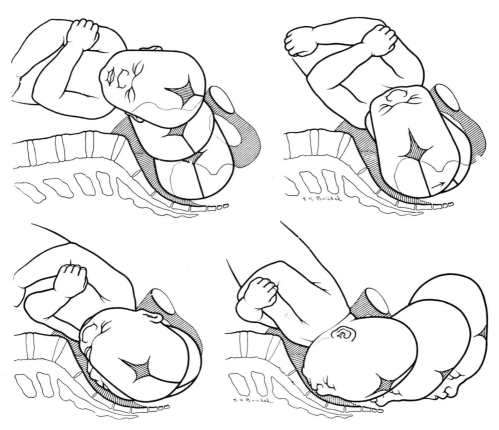

Fig. 4. Mechanism of labor for left occiput transverse position, lateral view. Posterior parietal presentation at the brim followed by lateral flexion, resulting in anterior parietal presentation after engagement, further descent, rotation, and extension. (From Steele and Javert. Surg Gynec Obstet 75:477, 1942.)

The factors responsible for internal rotation are as follows: (1) As shown in Chapter 13, Figure 15, the levator ani muscle forms a V-shaped sling with its attachments at the sides of the pubis and ischia. As shown also in that illustration and in Figure 20 of Chapter 13, the coccygeus and ileococcygeus muscles form another slinglike structure posteriorly. The musculature of the pelvic floor therefore makes up a V-shaped trough, the inclined sides of which diverge anteriorly and superiorly. (2) The ischial spines encroach on the pelvic cavity, creating the plane of the least pelvic dimensions, the greatest diameter of which is anteroposterior. (3) with flexion the occiput is lower than the bregma and sinciput (chin) as the head descends.

Extension. When, after internal rotation, the sharply flexed head reaches the vulva it undergoes another movement that is essential to its birth, namely, extension, which brings the base of the occiput into direct contact with the inferior margin of the symphysis pubis. This movement is brought about by two factors. First, as the vulvar outlet is directed upward and forward, extension must occur before the head can pass through it. If the sharply flexed head, on reaching the

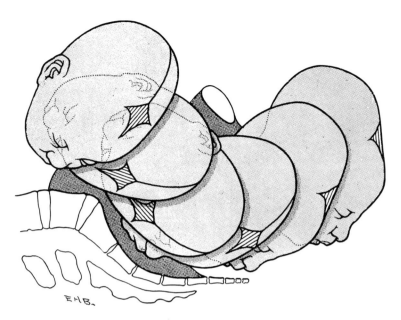

Fig. 5. Mechanism of labor for left occiput anterior position.

pelvic floor, were driven farther downward in the same direction, it would impinge upon the end of the sacrum and the posterior portion of the perineum and, if the vis a tergo were sufficiently strong, would eventually carry away the lowermost portion of the sacrum and be forced through the tissues of the perineum. When the head presses upon the pelvic gutter, however, two forces come into play: the first, exerted by the uterus, acts more posteriorly, and the second, supplied by the resistant pelvic floor, acts more anteriorly. The resultant force is in the direction of the vulvar opening, thereby causing extension.

After the suboccipital region has come in contact with the inferior margin of the symphysis pubis, the head can no longer be regarded as a two-armed lever. The occiput is the fulcrum with the single arm extending from it to the chin; any force exerted upon the head must necessarily lead to further extension. The vulvar opening gradually dilates as extension becomes marked and the scalp of the child becomes visible.

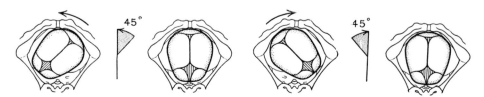

Fig. 6. Anterior rotation from LOA.   Fig. 7. Anterior rotation from ROA.

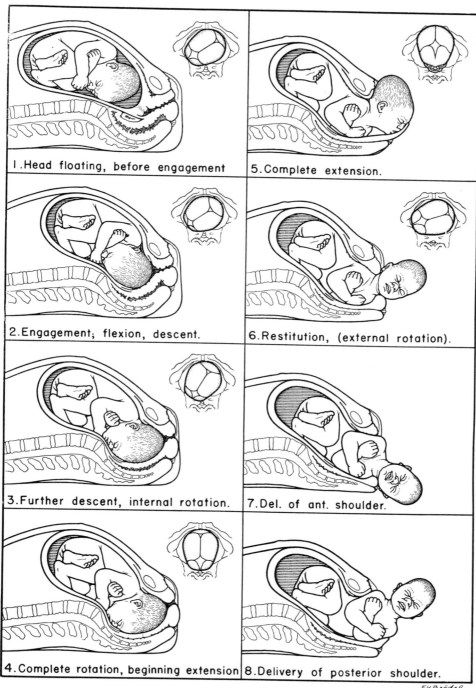

1. Head floating, before engagement
2. Engagement; flexion, descent.
3. Further descent, internal rotation.
4. Complete rotation, beginning extension
5. Complete extension.
6. Restitution, (external rotation).
7. Del. of ant. shoulder.
8. Delivery of posterior shoulder.

Fig. 8. Principal movements in the mechanism of labor and delivery; LOA position.

With increasing distention of the perineum and vaginal opening, an increasingly large portion of the occiput gradually appears. The head is born by further extension as the occiput, bregma, forehead, nose, mouth, and finally the chin pass successively over the anterior margin of the perineum. Immediately after its birth the head drops downward so that the chin lies over the maternal anal region (Fig. 8).

External Rotation.   The head next undergoes another movement: if the occiput was originally directed toward the left, it rotates toward the left ischial tuberosity, and in the opposite direction if originally directed toward the right. The return of the head to the oblique position (*restitution*) is followed by completion of *external rotation* to the transverse position, a movement that corresponds to rotation of the fetal body, serving to bring its bisacromial diameter into relation with the anteroposterior diameter of the pelvic outlet. This movement is brought about by essentially the same pelvic factors that effect internal rotation of the head.

Expulsion.   Almost immediately after external rotation the anterior shoulder appears under the symphysis pubis, and the perineum soon becomes distended by the posterior shoulder. After delivery of the shoulders the rest of the body of the child is quickly extruded.

Mechanism in Occiput Anterior Positions

In these positions the head enters the pelvis with the occiput rotated 45 degrees anteriorly from the transverse position. This degree of anterior rotation produces only slight differences on palpation and in the mechanism of labor from those in transverse positions of the occiput (Fig. 5).

Diagnosis.   For the left occiput anterior position the findings are as follows:

First maneuver: Irregular breech in fundus.
Second maneuver: Resistant plane of back on the left and anterior portion of the abdomen, with the small parts on the right side.
Third maneuver: If the head is not engaged, it is felt as a freely movable body over the superior strait; but if it is fixed or engaged, the anterior shoulder may be detected.
Fourth maneuver: Negative if the head is not engaged; otherwise the cephalic prominence is felt on the right side (Fig. 14 of Ch. 11).

For the right occiput anterior position the findings are as follows:

First maneuver: Irregular breech in fundus.
Second maneuver: Resistant plane of back on the right and anterior portion of the abdomen, with the small parts on the left side.
Third maneuver: As in LOA.
Fourth maneuver: Cephalic prominence on the left side.

Mechanism in Occiput Posterior Positions

The incidence of occipitoposterior positions is approximately 10 per cent; the ROP position is much more common than LOP or OP.

Evidence from radiographic studies indicates that a narrow forepelvis is often associated with posterior positions. D'Esopo found two different pelvic forms frequently encountered in these positions: in one, the transverse diameter is contracted at the brim or midpelvis, or both, with an ample anteroposterior diameter; in the other, the converse obtains, and the anteroposterior diameter is short because of a flat posterior segment at the inlet or a forward sacrum at the midpelvis, with an ample transverse diameter.

Whenever the back of the fetus is felt on the right side of the mother, the possibility of a right posterior position should always be borne in mind. Similarly, whenever the small parts are distinctly felt in the anterior portion of the abdomen, a posterior position is likely, especially in the rare instances in which the occiput has rotated into the hollow of the sacrum. In the less frequent left posterior positions palpation gives similar results, except that the back is felt in the left flank and the small parts and cephalic prominence are found on the right side of the abdomen.

Diagnosis. Palpation in a right occipitoposterior position provides the following data:

First maneuver:	The fundus is occupied by the breech.
Second maneuver:	The resistant plane of the back is felt well back in the right flank, with the small parts on the left side and in front and much more readily palpable than in anterior positions.
Third maneuver:	Negative if the head is engaged; otherwise the movable head is detected above the superior strait.
Fourth maneuver:	Cephalic prominence on the left side.

On vaginal or rectal examination in the right posterior position, the sagittal suture occupies the right oblique diameter; the small fontanel is felt opposite the right sacroiliac synchondrosis, and the large fontanel is directed toward the left iliopectineal eminence; in the left position, the reverse obtains. In many cases, particularly in the early part of labor, because of imperfect flexion of the head, the large fontanel lies at a lower level than in anterior positions and is more readily felt.

The fetal heart tones are heard in the right or left flank of the mother in right and left positions, respectively. In these positions the heart sounds are sometimes transmitted through the fetal thorax and are best heard either in the midline or slightly to one side of it, because of partial extension of the head and an altered relation of the body of the fetus, whereby the thorax comes in contact with the anterior uterine wall.

Mechanism. In the great majority of occipitoposterior positions the mechanism of labor is identical with that observed in the transverse and anterior varieties, except that the occiput has to rotate to the symphysis pubis through 135 degrees instead of 90 degrees and 45 degrees, respectively (Fig. 9).

With good contractions, adequate flexion, and a fetus of average size, the great majority of posterior occiputs rotate promptly as soon as they reach the pelvic floor. Consequently, neither the second stage nor the total length of labor is appreciably lengthened. In a small minority of cases, however, perhaps 5 to 10 per cent, these favorable circumstances do not obtain. For example, with poor contractions or faulty flexion, or both, especially if the fetus is large, rotation may be incomplete or may not take place at all. If rotation is incomplete, *transverse arrest* results. If rotation toward the symphysis does not take place at all, the occiput usually rotates to the direct occiput posterior position, a condition known as *persistent occiput posterior*. Both transverse arrest and persistent occiput pos-

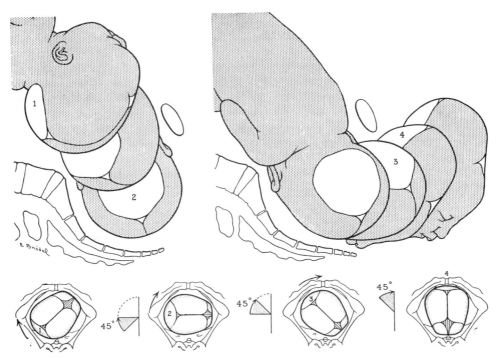

Fig. 9. Mechanism of labor for right occiput posterior position, anterior rotation.

terior represent deviations from the normal mechanisms of labor, which will be considered further in Chapter 29.

Changes in the Shape of the Head

In vertex presentations the fetal head undergoes important characteristic changes in shape as the result of the pressures to which it is subjected during labor. In prolonged labors before complete dilatation of the cervix, the portion of the fetal scalp immediately over the cervical os becomes edematous, forming a swelling known as the *caput succedaneum* (Fig. 10). It usually attains a thickness of only a few millimeters, but in prolonged labors it may be sufficiently extensive to prevent the differentiation of the various sutures and fontanels. More commonly the caput is formed when the head is in the lower portion of the birth canal and frequently only after the resistance of a rigid vaginal outlet is encountered. Since it occurs over the most dependent portion of the head, in left occipitotransverse position it is found over the upper and posterior extremity of the right parietal bone, and in right positions over the corresponding area of the left parietal bone. Hence it follows that often after labor the original position may be ascertained by noting the location of the caput succedaneum.

Of considerable importance is the degree of *molding* that the head undergoes. Because the various bones of the skull are not firmly united, movement may occur at the sutures. Ordinarily the margins of the occipital bone, and more rarely

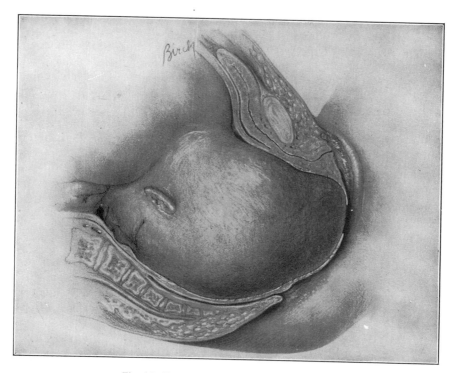

Fig. 10. Formation of caput succedaneum.

Fig. 11. Molding of head at birth.

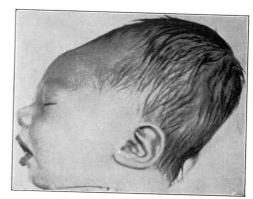

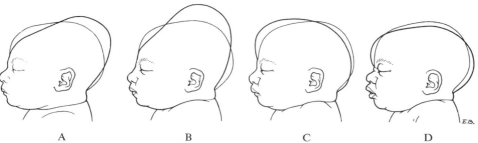

Fig. 12. Molding of head in cephalic presentations. A, occiput anterior; B, occiput posterior; C, brow; D, face.

those of the frontal bone, are pushed under those of the parietal bones; in many cases one parietal bone may overlap the other, the anterior parietal usually overlapping the posterior. These changes are of greatest importance in contracted pelves, when the degree to which the head is capable of molding may make the difference between successful vaginal delivery and a major obstetric operation (Figs. 11 and 12). Molding may account for a diminution in certain cephalic diameters of 0.5 to 1.0 cm, or even more in neglected cases of prolonged labor.

As a result of pressure the head also undergoes a marked change in shape, involving diminution of its suboccipitofrontal and occipitofrontal diameters, becoming lengthened from chin to occiput and compressed in other directions. In occipitoposterior positions, when the occiput has rotated into the hollow of the sacrum, the frontal bone is sometimes markedly overlapped by the anterior margins of the parietal bones, leading to a distinct depression in that part of the head. An estimate is thereby provided of the force with which the region of the large fontanel has been pressed against the lower margin of the symphysis. Such pressure changes are of much greater consequence than formerly believed, for they may play an important part in the production of fatal subdural hemorrhage. Holland's important work on cranial stresses during labor showed that they may subject the tentorium cerebelli or the falx to excessive tension. The hemorrhagic lesions that may result provide an explanation for certain fetal deaths that have no other obvious cause.

References

Caldwell, W. E., Moloy, H. C., and D'Esopo, D. A.   A roentgenologic study of the mechanism of engagement of the fetal head. Amer J Obstet Gynec 28:824, 1934.
———— Moloy, H. C., and D'Esopo, D. A.   The role of the lower uterine soft parts in labor. Amer J Obstet Gynec 32:727, 1936.
———— Moloy, H. C., and Swenson, P. C.   The use of the roentgen ray in obstetrics. Part I. Roentgen pelvimetry and cephalometry; technic of pelvioroentgenography. Amer J Roentgen 41:305, 1939.
———— Moloy, H. C., and Swenson, P. C.   The use of the roentgen ray in obstetrics. Part II. Anatomical variations in the female pelvis and their classification according to morphology. Amer J Roentgen 41:505, 1939.
———— Moloy, H. C., and Swenson, P. C.   The use of the roentgen ray in obstetrics. Part III. The mechanism of labor. Amer J Roentgen 41:719, 1939.
Calkins, L. A.   The etiology of occiput presentations. Amer J Obstet Gynec 37:618, 1939.
———— Occiput posterior presentation. Obstet Gynec 1:466, 1953.
D'Esopo, D. A.   The occipitoposterior position. Its mechanism and treatment. Amer J Obstet Gynec 42:937, 1941.
Holland, E.   Cranial stress in the foetus during labor. J Obstet Gynaec Brit Emp 29:549, 1922.
Javert, C. T., and Steele, K. B.   The transverse position and the mechanism of labor. A historical collective review. Internat Abstr Surg 75:507, 1942.
Litzmann, C. C. T.   (On posterior parietal presentation: a not uncommon abnormality of labor). Arch Gynaek 2:433, 1871.
Naegele, F. C.   (On the mechanism of labor). Deutsches Archiv Physiologie 5:483, 1819.
Rydberg, E.   The Mechanism of Labour. Springfield, Ill., Charles C Thomas, 1954.
Steele, K. B., and Javert, C. T.   Mechanism of labor for transverse positions of the vertex. Surg Gynec Obstet 75:477, 1942.

15

THE CLINICAL COURSE OF LABOR

Lightening.   A few weeks before the onset of labor the abdomen often undergoes a change in shape; its lower portion becomes more pendulous, whereas near the costal margin it looks decidedly less protuberant. The change results from descent of the fundus of the uterus from the position that it occupied at about 36 weeks to that of the month before. Concomitantly the head, which was previously freely movable, descends and becomes fixed in the pelvic inlet. These changes are most pronounced in nulliparas and frequently do not occur in multiparas until the onset of labor. The descent of the uterus that results from sinking of the fetal head into the pelvic inlet is termed "lightening."

After "lightening" the patient experiences considerably greater ease in respiration; at the same time, however, locomotion may become more difficult, and she may suffer from cramps in the lower extremities and more frequent micturition.

False Labor Pains.   For a varying period before the establishment of true, or effective, labor women often suffer from so-called false labor pains, which must be distinguished from effective uterine contractions. False labor pains may begin as early as three or four weeks before the termination of pregnancy. They are merely an exaggeration of the relatively painless intermittent uterine contractions that occur throughout the entire period of gestation. They occur at irregular intervals, are confined chiefly to the lower abdomen and groin, and rarely start in the fundal region and radiate over the uterus and through to the back, in the manner of true labor pains. The duration of a false labor pain is short, and unlike true labor, false labor is rarely intensified by walking; it may even be relieved by such activity. False labor pains, furthermore, do not increase progressively in intensity, duration, and frequency as in true labor. The only certain way to distinguish between false and true labor pains, however, is to ascertain their effect on the cervix. True labor pains in the course of a few hours produce a demonstrable degree of effacement and some dilatation of the cervix, whereas the effect of false labor pains on the cervix is minimal.

Show.   A rather dependable sign of the approach of labor (provided no rectal or vaginal examination has been done in the preceding 48 hours) is "show" or "bloody show," which is the discharge from the vagina of a small amount of blood-tinged mucus, representing the extrusion of the plug of mucus that has filled the cervical canal during pregnancy. "Show" is a late sign, for labor usually ensues during the next several hours to few days. Normally, only a few drops of blood escape with the mucous plug; *more substantial bleeding suggests a pathologic condition.*

First Stage of Labor.   At the beginning of the first stage the pains are short, mild, separated by intervals of 10 to 20 minutes, and not productive of great discomfort. The patient may walk about and remain confortable between pains. Early in the first stage the pain is usually located in the small of the back, but thereafter sweeps around to the anterior part of the abdomen. The pains recur at decreasing intervals and become stronger and longer. Indeed, the pains that immediately precede and accompany full dilatation are often of excruciating severity. At that time, furthermore, there is usually a marked increase in the amount of bloody show, caused by rupture of capillary vessels in the cervix and perhaps also by separation of the membranes from the decidua in the lower uterine segment.

The average duration of the first stage of labor in primigravidas is about 12 hours, and in multiparas about 7 hours, but there is marked individual variation, as pointed out on page 396.

Second Stage of Labor.   Uterine contractions at this time are long, lasting 50 to 100 seconds and occurring at intervals of two or three minutes. Spontaneous rupture of the membranes usually occurs during the early part of the second stage of labor and is accompanied by a gush of amniotic fluid from the vagina.

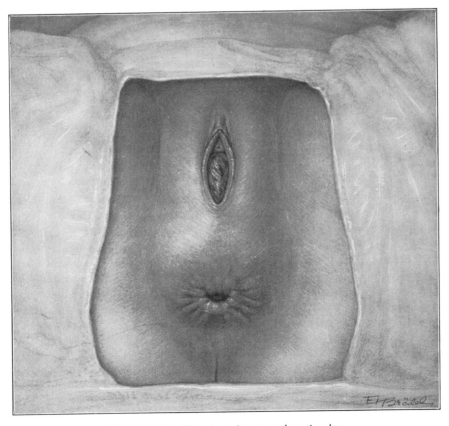

Fig. 1. Birth of head, scalp appearing at vulva.

Sometimes, however, the membranes rupture during the first stage and occasionally even before labor starts; rupture prior to the onset of labor is designated *premature rupture of the membranes.*

During the second stage, the muscles of the abdomen are brought into play.
During the pains the patient will strain, or "bear down" strenuously, her face
becoming flushed and the large vessels in her neck distending. At the onset of a
contraction the patient emits the grunt or groan characteristic of this stage of
labor and endeavors to expel the products of conception. As a result of the exertion she may perspire profusely.

Toward the end of the second stage, when the head is near the vaginal outlet, the pressure often causes the expulsion of small particles of fecal material
with each pain. As the head descends still farther, the perineum begins to bulge
and the overlying skin becomes tense and glistening. At that time the scalp of
the fetus may be detected through the slitlike vulvar opening (Fig. 1). With each
subsequent pain the perineum bulges increasingly and the vulvar opening becomes increasingly dilated by the head (Fig. 2), gradually forming an ovoid and
finally an almost circular opening. With the cessation of each contraction the
opening becomes smaller as the head recedes, to advance again with the next
pain. As the head becomes increasingly visible the vulva is stretched further until

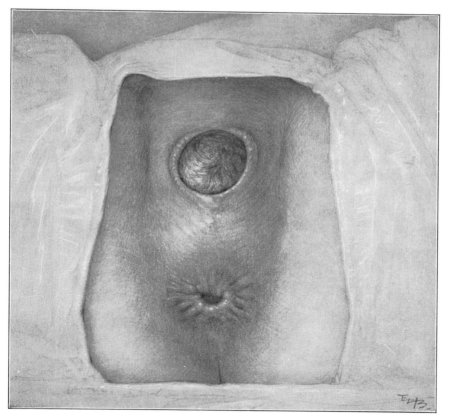

Fig. 2. Birth of head, vulva partially distended. Usually an episiotomy is made at this time
or earlier.

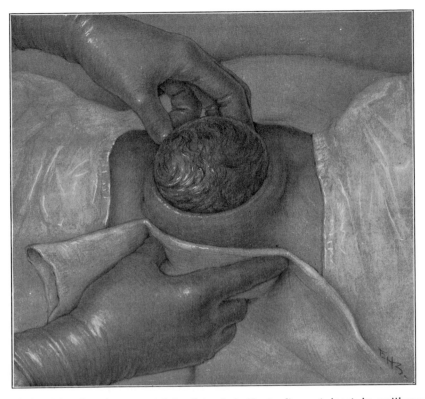

Fig. 3. Birth of head, vulva completely distended. Most often, at least in nulliparas, an episiotomy is made before this degree of perineal distention occurs.

it ultimately encircles the largest diameter of the baby's head (Fig. 3). This encirclement of the largest diameter of the fetal head by the vulvar ring is known as *crowning*. The perineum is then extremely thin, its frenulum paper-thin and almost at the point of rupture with each pain. At the same time the anus becomes greatly stretched and protuberant, and the anterior wall of the rectum may be easily seen through it. The perineum has become converted into a deep gutter 5 to 6 cm long, at the end of which is the vulvar opening, directed upward and distended by the fetal head, the occiput of which in the case of occiput anterior is firmly pressed against the symphysis pubis. The distention of the vulva is more marked at its perineal margin than at its upper and lateral portions.

The head advances a little with each pain and recedes between contractions until the engagement of the parietal bosses by the vulva prevents further recession. With the next two or three pains the head is rapidly expelled by extension (Fig. 4), the base of the occiput rotating around the lower margin of the symphysis pubis as a fulcrum, while the bregma, brow, and face successively pass over the fourchet (Fig. 5). In the majority of nulliparas the perineum is unable to withstand the strain to which it is subjected and tears in its anterior portion unless an episiotomy has been performed.

Immediately after its birth the head falls posteriorly, bringing the face almost

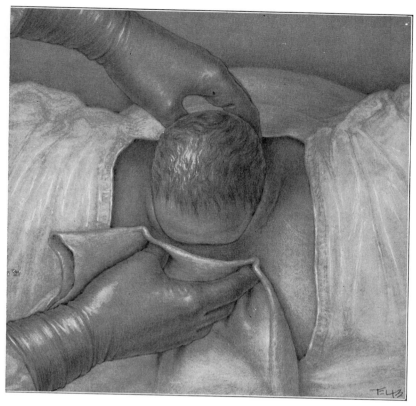

Fig. 4. Birth of head, showing delivery by extension.

into contact with the anus. Within a few moments the occiput turns toward one of the maternal thighs, the entire head eventually assuming a transverse position (Fig. 6). The successive movements of restitution and external rotation indicate that the bisacromial diameter of the infant has rotated into the anteroposterior diameter of the pelvis.

At this time the perineum has retracted around the neck of the infant; the next pain forces the anterior shoulder down under the symphysis pubis where it becomes fixed while the posterior shoulder emerges over the anterior margin of the perineum; the body of the child is then rapidly expelled by lateral flexion, following the curve of the birth canal. Occasionally the anterior shoulder is normally born first.

Immediately after extrusion of the child there is usually a gush of amniotic fluid, often tinged with blood, representing the fluid that did not escape when the membranes ruptured.

The median duration of the second stage is 50 minutes in nulliparas and 20 minutes in multiparas. In women of higher parity, two or three contractions may suffice to complete the expulsion.

Third Stage of Labor. Immediately following birth of the child there is usually a slight flow of blood. For a short time the patient experiences no pain, but

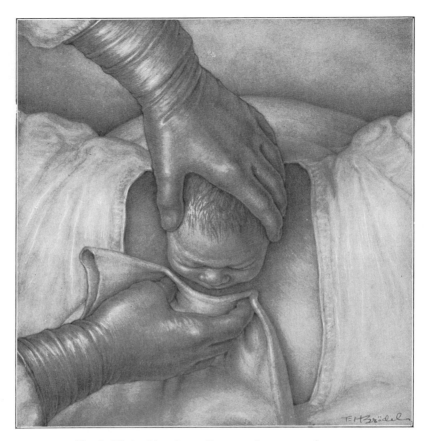

Fig. 5. Birth of head, mouth appearing over perineum.

after a few minutes uterine contractions resume at regular intervals until the placenta becomes separated and is expelled into the lower uterine segment.

Normally following delivery the uterus promptly becomes a firm discoid mass at or just below the level of the umbilicus. Shortly thereafter the uterus relaxes and assumes a globular shape. With each subsequent contraction the shape of the uterus changes from globular to discoid. After the placenta has separated, however, the globular shape persists.

If the placenta remains in the uterus after its separation, further clinical changes occur. Between 3 and 30 minutes after birth of the child, the fundus of the uterus rises to or above the umbilicus, while simultaneously a slight prominence appears immediately above the symphysis pubis. At the same time the portion of umbilical cord protruding from the vulva has increased by several centimeters. These changes indicate that the placenta has been extruded from the upper portion of the uterine cavity into the lower uterine segment, or even into the upper part of the vagina. The fundus rises because the lower uterine segment, which immediately after the birth of the child had collapsed upon itself, is distended by the placenta and mechanically lifts the tightly contracted body of the uterus to a higher level.

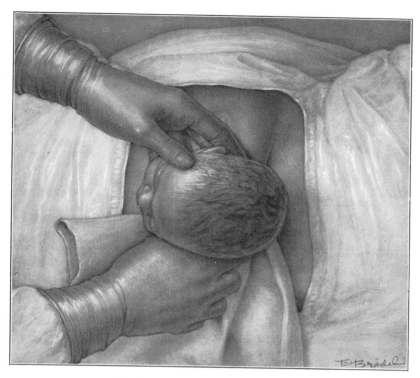

Fig. 6. Birth of head, external rotation.

In 4,000 deliveries studied by Halsey the duration of the third stage averaged about eight minutes. The phase of placental separation usually lasts only two or three minutes. The duration of the phase of expulsion varies with the management of the third stage.

It is important to differentiate clinically between separation of the placenta and its expulsion from the uterus. The four cardinal signs of placental separation are (1) change in the shape of the uterus from discoid to globular; (2) bleeding ranging from a trickle to a gush; (3) descent of the umbilical cord; and (4) rise of the fundus.

Blood Loss in Third Stage. The volume of maternal blood shed during and very soon after the third stage of labor is usually more than generally appreciated. With apparently uncomplicated vaginal delivery it commonly amounts to 500 ml or somewhat more (Ch. 33, p. 958).

Circulation. During the first stage of labor there is little change in blood pressure between pains, but during contractions an average increase of about 10 mm Hg is normal. In the second stage, elevations in both the systolic and diastolic pressures are more frequent and pronounced, especially during contractions. Brown found an average increase in this stage of about 10 mm Hg between pains in both systolic and diastolic pressures; during contractions the systolic pressure shows an average increment of 30 mm Hg, and the diastolic pressure about 25 mm Hg. During the work of labor there is an increase in maternal cardiac output. During the third stage both systolic and diastolic pressures fall to the previous normal levels or slightly below. Except in prolonged labors the maternal pulse rate ordinarily shows little change even during severe contractions, but Pardee and Mendelson have shown that it may occasionally go as high as 110 per minute.

Gastrointestinal Tract. Nausea and vomiting are common, especially near the time of complete cervical dilatation. Gastrointestinal motility and absorption are sluggish. Food ingested just before the onset of labor may remain in the stomach for many hours, a most important practical point if general anesthesia is to be administered, especially in view of the tendency to vomiting. Drugs administered orally during labor may be very slowly absorbed, again probably because of delayed gastric emptying.

Leukocytosis. The leukocyte count increases during labor to an average of about 15,000 per mm^3 at complete dilatation, but may be elevated to as high as 25,000 per mm^3 as the result of labor itself.

Proteinuria. Proteinuria, usually slight, occurs in about 30 per cent of normal paturients, as demonstrated by Morton and Chesley (Table 1). Proteinuria to the extent of 2-plus to 4-plus (1.0 to 4.0 g per liter) is uncommon (3 per cent) and should always suggest preeclampsia or renal disease. In prolonged labor the incidence of proteinuria is greater.

Table 1. **Incidence of Proteinuria in Labor, Based on 500 Normal Cases in Which Parturients with Any Other Evidence of Preeclampsia Had Been Excluded**

(Morton and Chesley)

Clinical Reading	Quantitative (g/liter)	Cases	Per Cent of 500
Trace	0.25	25	5.0
1	0.25–0.50	68	13.6
2	0.50–1.0	47	9.4
2–4	1.0–4.0	15	3.0

Fetal Heart Rate. The fetal heart can be monitored in a number of ways. The simplest, and still very effective, method is by frequent auscultation using a specialized head stethoscope. The widely used DeLee-Hillis stethoscope is quite satisfactory for this purpose. In recent years electronic equipment has been designed specifically to try to provide continuous monitoring of the fetal heart during labor, especially in circumstances in which the pregnancy is believed to be abnormal. One type of instrument utilizes the Doppler principle, in which low-intensity ultrasonic waves return to the transmitting source at a slightly altered frequency when reflected from a moving object such as blood cells in a vessel. The greater the velocity of the blood cells, the greater the shift in frequency and the higher the pitch of the audible signal emitted from the speaker. The sounds so generated in response to the alteration in the frequency usually can be identified as those of the fetal heart, umbilical cord, placenta, and major maternal vessels. Several different instruments that utilize the Doppler principle are available commercially, including the Doptone, Ultradop, and Magnaflux MD 500, as well as others manufactured abroad.

Fetal heart rate monitors have been developed to detect the fetal heart rate and exhibit it either by means of a meter or by continuous recording on paper strips. Fetal heart rate monitors are not successful in every case, however. Those that utilize an acoustical system for detecting the fetal heartbeat sometimes cannot

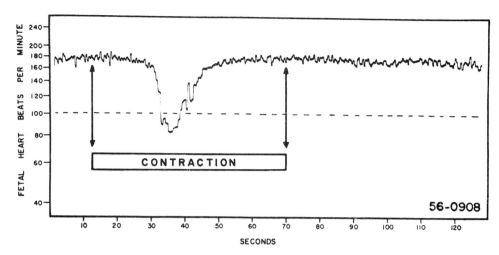

Fig. 7. Normal slowing of the fetal heart rate during uterine contraction. (From Hon. Amer J Obstet Gynec 77:1084, 1959.)

detect the level of sound that is generated by the fetal heart and transmitted to the site of the electronic pickup on the maternal abdominal wall. Those that detect the electrical activity of the fetal heart are uniformly satisfactory only when an electrode can be attached directly to the fetus. To accomplish this end trans-vaginally, the membranes must be ruptured, the cervix somewhat dilated, and the presenting part fixed in the pelvis. Paul and Hon have recently described their experiences with a commercially available fetal monitoring unit that displays the fetal heart rate by means of a meter and the fetal EKG complex on an oscilloscope, and records intrauterine pressures as well as fetal heart rate continuously on a moving paper strip. They claim that the use of the monitor resulted in a marked decrease in the incidence of cesarean section for fetal distress. The practical value of this monitoring unit cannot be evaluated completely at this time, as pointed out by Paul and Hon, but must await a sizable, carefully controlled study.

Auscultation of the fetal heart at the beginning of a contraction commonly reveals muffling of the heart tones followed by transient slowing. Hon, utilizing a fetal heart rate meter, has studied this type of bradycardia and found that in multiparas the fetal heart rate commonly falls from 140 to 110–120 beats per minute at the acme of a contraction. In nulliparas the drop is often more marked, sometimes to as low as 60 to 70 beats per minute for a few seconds during the contraction. This bradycardia begins soon after the onset of the contraction and terminates a few seconds before its end (Fig. 7). Hon and others believe that such bradycardia results not from fetal hypoxia but from compression of the fetal skull against the partially dilated cervix by the force of the contraction. Hon found it to be most common between 4 and 8 cm cervical dilatation and supported his argument by reproducing the results with application of pressure to the fetal skull.

From a clinical standpoint any slowing of the fetal heart detected by auscultation during or immediately after a contraction should alert the obstetrician to the possibility of fetal distress. Should the rate fall below 100 beats per minute and persist for more than a few seconds after termination of a contraction, the tentative diagnosis of fetal distress should be made (Ch. 36, p. 1009).

Duration of Labor. The mean duration of first labors is about 14 hours, although there is wide variation. In primigravidas carefully studied by Friedman the mean duration of labor was 14.4 hours. The corresponding figure cited by Busby in an analysis of first labors in white women at the Johns Hopkins Hospital was 13 hours. The average time for each of the three stages of labor is ordinarily divided as follows: first stage, 12½ hours; second stage, 1⅓ hours; and third stage, about 5 minutes.

The average duration of multiparous labors is about 6 hours shorter than first labors; Busby reported the figure of 8.3 hours. In multiparas labor is ordinarily divided among the three stages as follows: first stage, 7⅓ hours; second stage, ½ hour; and third stage, about 5 minutes. In general, after the fetal head has reached the perineal floor, most nulliparas will deliver during the next 20 contractions or so; the corresponding figure for multiparas is 10 contractions or fewer (Hellman and Prystowsky).

Even though dilatation of the cervix is not complete until it reaches approximately 10 cm in average diameter, the first stage of labor is usually more than two thirds over when cervical dilatation is 5 cm.

FACTORS AFFECTING THE PROGNOSIS OF LABOR

As discussed in Chapter 13, labor may be regarded as a contest between the forces of expulsion and the resistance. If the powers of expulsion are very strong and the resistance very weak, the duration of labor is usually only an hour or two; but if the reverse holds true, it may last for days unless aid is rendered. Most labors, of course, are intermediate in duration. Although other factors may play a role in the duration of normal labor, they do so only through their influence on either the powers of expulsion or the resistance.

The expulsive forces are measured largely in terms of the frequency, intensity, and duration of uterine contractions. In the second stage of labor the bearing-down efforts of the mother are the additional force affecting duration. The resistance is chiefly that of the cervix, but during the second stage the perineal floor poses additional resistance.

Parity. Once a cervix has been completely dilated in a previous labor, it offers less resistance to dilatation in subsequent parturition. In multiparas, moreover, the pelvic floor is generally more relaxed, offering less resistance than that of a nullipara.

Age of Mother. According to Marchetti and Menaker and also Morrison, labor in primigravidas, aged 12 to 16, is of average duration, but the incidence of toxemia of pregnancy is about twice that for primigravidas in general. Duenhoelter has recently reviewed the experiences in pregnancy of 372 girls who were 14 years of age or younger at the time of delivery at Parkland Memorial Hospital (unpublished data). Anemia, pregnancy-induced hypertension, and prematurity (birth weight 2,500 g or less) occurred one and a half to two times more often than in the older control group of comparable parity. The average duration of labor was 12 hours, the same as in the control group. Cesarean section was used to effect delivery in 6.3 per cent of these very young girls; the figure was only 2.5 per cent in the control patients. Although the obstetric problems of these adolescents were significant, the sociologic problems before, during, and after the obstetric event were much more profound.

It is evident that for a woman having her first baby, reproductive efficiency is at its maximum at 18 to 20 years of age (Baird and associates). Perinatal mortality, for example, is nearly twice as great in women who wait until age 35 or longer to conceive. The woman who undergoes her first pregnancy at or beyond the age of 35 years is customarily termed an "elderly primigravida." The frequency of prolonged labor is increased because of uterine dysfunction and apparent cervical rigidity. Hypertensive cardiovascular disease and other degenerative diseases are common in this age group. Skilled obstetric care is most valuable in dealing with these complications; nonetheless, the statistical evidence is clear that in elderly nulliparas, despite excellent care, there is a perinatal mortality rate of about 10 per cent, or more than three times the figure for primigravidas under 30 years of age (Davis and Seski).

Interval Between Births.   When the interval between births equals or exceeds ten years, pregnancy and labor may simulate those in elderly primigravidas. In an analysis of 200 such cases, Ballard showed that the incidence of prolonged labor was increased almost fourfold, with similar increases in placenta previa and abruptio placentae. There was also an elevated perinatal mortality rate in this group.

Size of Baby.   In primigravidas there is a considerable tendency to prolongation of both the first and second stages when the babies are large. Calkins found a difference in the first stage of nearly two hours between 3,000 and 4,000 g babies. In the second stage he found a difference of about 25 minutes between 2,500 and 4,000 g babies. The size of the baby apparently does not influence the duration of labor in multiparas to the same degree.

Posterior Position of Occiput.   The duration of the first stage of labor is not likely to be greatly affected by posterior positions of the occiput, but the second stage is often prolonged. The second stage of labor in posterior positions of the occiput may be increased by the increased expulsive forces required to rotate the head through the necessarily greater arc and by the increased resistance that is sometimes encountered because of incomplete flexion. Hellman and Prystowsky have shown that when the posterior position persists, the length of the second stage is more than doubled.

Spontaneous Premature Rupture of the Membranes.   Rupture of the membranes before the onset of labor (premature rupture of the membranes) occurs in about 12 per cent of all pregnancies. It is somewhat more frequent (17 per cent) in premature labor. The interval between rupture of the membranes and the onset of labor, usually called the "latent" or "lag" period, is less than 24 hours in 80 to 90 per cent of cases in which the woman is at or near term when the accident occurs. If the infant is premature, however (2,500 g or below), the lag is usually considerably longer. Premature rupture of the membranes is ordinarily followed by a labor that is shorter than usual. Calkins cites a figure for the average duration of labor in such cases of about 10 hours for primigravidas and about 6 hours for multiparas.

When the membranes rupture prematurely at or near term, the latent period exceeds 48 hours in about 5 to 10 per cent of the cases. Such prolonged latent periods affect the fetus adversely, as indicated in Table 2. Although most of these

Table 2. Effect of the Duration of the Latent Period on Perinatal Mortality of Mature Infants
(Unpublished Data of Guilbeau and Eastman)

Latent Period	Cases	Deaths	Per Cent	
0–6 hours	1,274	25		2.0
6–12 hours	426	4	1.7	0.9
12–24 hours	418	6		1.4
24–48 hours	234	4		1.7
48–72 hours	126	10		6.6
3– 7 days	106	6	6.8	7.9
7–14 days	16	1		5.6
14 days and over	15	1		6.2

perinatal deaths are caused by infection, they are by no means entirely prevented by antibiotics administered to the mother during the latent period. Lebherz and co-workers conducted an extensive collaborative study to ascertain whether a broad-spectrum antibiotic administered prophylactically to women with premature rupture of the membranes would decrease the perinatal mortality. It did not; the perinatal mortality was essentially the same in the treated and untreated groups, and about 25 per cent of the deaths were directly attributable to infection. Most obstetricians have had similar experience. Consequently, when labor fails to ensue soon after rupture of the membranes and the fetus is not premature, serious thought should be given to inducing labor. If the fetus is grossly premature, however, the dangers of prematurity outweigh the advantages of prompt delivery. Death related to prematurity increases markedly as the birth weight drops much below 2,000 g.

Our general plan of management consists of inducing labor with a dilute intravenous infusion of oxytocin if the fetus is not grossly premature and there is no contraindication to the use of oxytocin (Ch. 28, p. 845). When the fetus is grossly premature the patient is observed in the hospital; no further vaginal or rectal examinations are performed, and no antibiotics are administered prophylactically. If leakage of fluid ceases and there is no evidence of infection, the patient may be discharged from the hospital if the obstetrician is satisfied that such a course of action is safe; otherwise hospitalization is continued. If the mother becomes febrile or if the escaping amniotic fluid becomes foul, therapy with broad-spectrum antibiotics is begun. Delivery may be accomplished vaginally if an oxytocin infusion promptly induces labor; otherwise cesarean section or sometimes cesarean section followed by hysterectomy, especially in a multipara, is the safest course for both fetus and mother. The recent report by Wynn confirms the soundness of this general approach.

Contrary to widespread opinion, prolapse of the umbilical cord does not frequently accompany premature rupture of the membranes unless the fetus presents as footling breech or by the shoulder.

REFERENCES

Baird, D., Hytten, F. E., and Thomson, A. M.   Age and human reproduction. J Obstet Gynaec Brit Emp 65:865, 1958.

Ballard, M. B.   A statistical study of 200 cases of 10 or more years interval between pregnancies. Bull Sch Med Univ Maryland 38:66, 1953.

Brown, R. C.   A study of the maternal blood pressure; variations in 50 cases of normal labor with a consideration of the effects of analgesia. Anesthesia 6:66, 1951.

Busby, T.   The duration of labor: mean, median and mode. Amer J Obstet Gynec 55:846, 1948.

Calkins, L. A.   The length of labor. III. Amer J Obstet Gynec 27:349, 1934.

———   Premature spontaneous rupture of the membrane. Amer J Obstet Gynec 64:871, 1952.

Davis, M. E., and Seski, A.   Childbearing in the twilight of the reproductive period. Surg Gynec Obstet, 87:145, 1948.

Freidman, E. A.   Graphic appraisal of labor. A study of 500 premigravidas. Bull Sloan Hosp Women 1:42, 1955.

Halsey, H. H.   The duration of the third stage of labor. Amer J Obstet Gynec 65:97, 1953.

Hellman, L. M., and Prystowsky, H.   The duration of the second stage of labor. Amer J Obstet Gynec 63:1223, 1952.

Hon, E. H.   Electronic evaluation of the fetal heart rate. Amer J Obstet Gynec 75:1215, 1958.

———   Observations on "pathologic" fetal bradycardia. Amer J Obstet Gynec 77:1084, 1959.

Lebherz, T. B., Hellman, L. P., Madding, R., Anctil, A., and Arje, S. L.   Double-blind study of premature rupture of the membranes. Amer J Obstet Gynec 87:218, 1963.

Marchetti, A. A., and Menaker, J. S.   Pregnancy and the adolescent. Amer J Obstet Gynec 59:1013, 1950.

Morrison, J. H.   The adolescent primigravida. Obstet Gynec 2:297, 1953.

Morton, R. F., and Chesley, L. C.   Intrapartum proteinuria. Obstet Gynec 7:373, 1956.

Pardee, H.E.B., and Mendelson, C. L.   Pulse and respiratory variations in normal women during labor. Amer J Obstet Gynec 41:36, 1941.

Paul, R. H., and Hon, E. H.   A clinical fetal monitor. Obstet Gynec 35:161, 1970.

Wynn, R. M.   Premature rupture of the membranes. Chicago Med 72:39, 1969.

16

THE CONDUCT OF NORMAL LABOR AND DELIVERY

Because most infants in this country are born in hospitals, this chapter will deal with the management of normal labor in a hospital setting.

Psychologic Approach to Patients. Since the pains of childbirth have long been the subject of conversation among women, many young mothers approach childbirth in dread of the ordeal. It is not an easy task to dispel this age-old fear, but from the first prenatal visit the obstetrician must make a conscious effort to impart the point of view that labor and delivery are normal physiologic processes. He must instill not only confidence but also the feeling that he is a medically wise friend, sincerely desirous of sparing the mother all possible pain within the limit of safety for her and her child. The very presence of such a doctor is in itself an effective analgesic.

During the past two decades increasing emphasis has been placed on the emotional aspects of labor, which are as significant as their physical counterparts. There can be no doubt that the attitude of a woman toward her delivery has a major influence on the ease of her labor. These facts have been stressed for many years by the late British obstetrician, Read, and endorsed by various groups in this country. Read attempted to answer the questions: "Is labor easy because a woman is calm, or is she calm because her labor is easy?" and conversely: "Is a woman pained and frightened because her labor is difficult, or is her labor difficult and painful because she is frightened?" After scrutinizing many cases, Read concluded: "Fear is in some way the chief pain-producing agent in otherwise normal labor." Quite likely fear may exert a deleterious effect on the quality of uterine contractions and on cervical dilatation.

To eliminate the harmful influence of fear in labor, a school of thought has developed emphasizing the advantages of "natural childbirth" or "physiologic childbirth." As Thoms pointed out, natural childbirth is a broad concept that represents an attempt on the part of those who care for pregnant and parturient women to understand the physiology of pregnancy and labor, especially the emotional aspects, so that these important functions may be viewed with less apprehension and better understanding by patients, and greater skill in caring for them may be developed. Natural (physiologic) childbirth entails antepartum education designed to eliminate fear; exercises to promote relaxation, muscle control, and breathing; adroit management throughout labor with a nurse or physician skilled in reassurance of the patient constantly in attendance. Gaining the confidence of the patient is all important. To quote Read:

> Women demand of all things complete confidence in the dependability, personal strength and skill of the man who is with them during labor. They do not want soft words or sob stuff but explanation, instruction, and encouragement. They want to hear that all is going well, that the baby is well and that they are conducting their job in an admirable manner.

Most proponents of natural childbirth have never claimed that labor should be conducted without anesthetic aids or that it can be made devoid of pain. With natural childbirth most patients experience some pain, and analgesics and anesthetics are not withheld when they are indicated. As stated by Speck, the presence of the obstetrician is often worth more than analgesics. Physicians, medical students, and nurses should note especially that the morale of women in labor may sometimes be destroyed by careless remarks. Casual comments outside the room of patients are often overheard, and laughter is frequently interpreted by the patient as directed toward her. The medical staff and all others involved in the care of the woman and her fetus would do well to take these words of Oliver Wendell Holmes to heart:

> The woman about to become a mother, or with her newborn infant upon her bosom, should be the object of trembling care and sympathy wherever she bears her tender burden or stretches her aching limbs. . . . God forbid that any member of the profession to which she trusts her life, doubly precious at that eventful period, should hazard it negligently, unadvisedly, or selfishly!

Admittance Procedures.   The pregnant woman is urged to come to the hospital at the onset of labor rather than to delay until delivery is imminent. As a routine part of good antepartum care she will have been informed of the sequence of events that occur during hospitalization for labor and delivery.

The physician ascertains the general condition of the mother and fetus, including the frequency, intensity, and duration of the uterine contractions, as well as the amount of show, if any, the status of the membranes, and the character of fetal movements. The maternal temperature, pulse, respiratory rate, and blood pressure are recorded. By means of abdominal examination the approximate size, presentation, and heart rate of the fetus are ascertained. A voided urine specimen is examined for glucose and protein. The hematocrit or hemoglobin concentration is checked; at the same time blood is often drawn for routine serologic testing and a tube of clotted blood kept available for use by the blood bank to cross-match donor blood when necessary. A small microhematocrit centrifuge in the labor-delivery area can be used to obtain the hematocrit reading in about two minutes. The vulva and perineum are shaved, and unless labor is judged to be progressing rapidly, an enema is usually given.

PREPARATION OF VULVA AND PERINEUM.   The purpose in shaving and washing the vulva and perineum is to cleanse thoroughly the area without contaminating the vagina. First, the patient is placed on a bedpan with her legs widely separated. The hair is then removed either by shaving or by clipping. While washing the area, the attendant holds the sponge to the patient's introitus to prevent wash water from running into the vagina. Rubbing is directed from above downward and away from the introitus. Attention should be paid to the vulvar folds during the cleansing procedure. As the scrub sponge passes over the anal region it is immediately discarded.

Diagnosis of Labor.   False labor pains frequently are mistaken for true labor. Although the differential diagnosis is occasionally difficult, it can usually be made on the basis of the following features:

True Labor Pains	*False Labor Pains*
Occur at regular intervals	Occur at irregular intervals
Intervals gradually shorten	Intervals remain long
Intensity gradually increases	Intensity remains same
Located in back and abdomen	Located chiefly in lower abdomen
Usually intensified by walking	Not intensified by walking
Not affected by mild sedation	Usually relieved by mild sedation

MANAGEMENT OF FIRST STAGE

As soon as possible after admittance a general physical examination is carried out. The pulse and respiratory rates and temperature are recorded and repeated routinely at least every four hours. In febrile patients or in prolonged labor the temperature should be recorded at least every two hours. The blood pressure reading should be repeated at least every four hours in normal cases, but more frequently in the presence of hypertension.

Abdominal Examination.   The abdominal examination is similar to that carried out in the prenatal course, comprising estimation of the size and position of the fetus and auscultation of the fetal heart sounds. The character of the fetal heart sounds in labor is of great importance and should be noted during active labor at least once every half-hour during the first stage; in the second stage it should be noted every five or ten minutes. After rupture of the membranes the fetal heart rate should be auscultated during a contraction and immediately thereafter to detect compression of a prolapsed cord. The rate of the fetal heart normally ranges between 120 and 160, averaging about 140. At the acme of a contraction it slows, sometimes falling transiently to about 100 or even somewhat lower (Fig. 7, Ch. 16, p. 411). Provided the fetus is not compromised, however, as the intensity of the uterine contraction diminishes, the heart rate returns rapidly to its previous value. If the fetus is distressed from hypoxia, however, its heart rate remains slow, often around 80 per minute or even slower. Not infrequently the fetal hypoxia that causes the pathologic bradycardia also leads to the passage of meconium. *Frequent, careful auscultation of the fetal heart sounds is one of the most important features of the conduct of the first and second stages of labor.*

In the course of each abdominal examination attention should be directed to the bladder. The suprapubic region should be palpated frequently to detect a full bladder. If the mother is unable to empty her bladder by voiding, it is essential to perform catheterization.

Rectal and Vaginal Examinations.   Rectal examinations were once thought to be much safer than vaginal because they were less likely to carry bacteria from the introitus into the cervix and above. A vaginal examination, properly performed with appropriate preparation and care, is probably not much more likely than a rectal to carry pathogenic bacteria to the cervix. The major advantage of rectal examination is the limited preparation required of both the patient and the

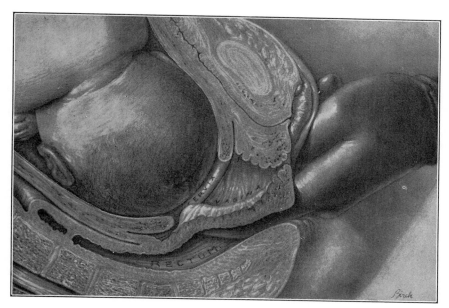

Fig. 1. Rectal examination. Note that the thumb is flexed into the palm of the hand so that it will not enter the vagina.

examiner. A clean glove is drawn over the unscrubbed hand. As shown in Figure 1, the thumb should be flexed into the palm of the hand to prevent its entry into the vagina. The well-lubricated index finger is carefully inserted through the anus. The presenting part and, if possible, its position are identified through the anterior wall of the rectum. The cervical opening is felt as a depression circumscribed by an elevated ridge of tissue. Intact membranes may commonly be felt bulging into the cervical opening. The softness of the cervix, the degree of cervical *effacement* and *dilatation,* and the *station* of the presenting part are noted.

EFFACEMENT. The degree of effacement of the cervix is usually expressed in terms of the length of the cervical canal, compared with that of an uneffaced cervix. When its length is only 1 cm, the cervix is said to be 50 per cent effaced, since the normal uneffaced cervix averages about 2 cm in length. When the cervix becomes as thin as the adjacent lower uterine segment, it is completely or 100 per cent effaced.

DILATATION. The amount of cervical dilatation is ascertained by estimating the average diameter of the cervical opening. The examining finger is swept from the margin of the cervix on one side to the opposite side, and the diameter traversed is expressed in centimeters. The cervix is said to be fully dilated when the diameter of the opening measures 10 cm, for the presenting part usually can pass through a cervix so widely dilated. The novice can quickly learn to estimate the extent of cervical dilatation with reasonable accuracy by practicing with a simple device. In a piece of heavy cardboard several circular holes of known diameter are made. The tip of the index finger then moves along the circumference of the hole, and an idea is obtained of the respective diameters.

STATION. When carrying out a rectal or vaginal examination it is valuable to identify the level of the presenting part in the birth canal. The ischial spines are about halfway between the pelvic inlet and the pelvic outlet. When the lowermost portion of the presenting part is at the level of the ischial spines, it is designated as being at zero station.

The long axis of the birth canal above the ischial spines is arbitrarily divided into thirds. If the presenting part is at the level of the pelvic inlet it is at −3 station; if it has descended one third the distance from the pelvic inlet to the ischial spines it is at −2 station; if it has reached a level two thirds the distance from the inlet to the spines it is at −1 station. The long axis of the birth canal between the level of the ischial spines and the outlet of the pelvis is similarly divided into thirds. If the level of the presenting part in the birth canal is one third or two thirds the distance between the ischial spines and the pelvic outlet, it is at +1 station or +2 station, respectively. When the presenting part is at the perineum its station is +3. Unless the head is unusually molded, or there is an extensive formation of caput, or both, if the vertex is at 0 station or below, engagement of the head has occurred—that is, the biparietal diameter of the head has passed through the pelvic inlet. Progressive cervical dilatation with no change in the station of the presenting part suggests fetopelvic disproportion.

Although rectal examinations have the advantage of considerably less preparation of the patient and the examiner, they are more likely to be inconclusive. It is now common practice to evaluate the pelvis and its contents thoroughly by means of a detailed vaginal examination when the patient is admitted to the labor area. This policy allows more adequate identification and evaluation of (1) the presenting part, including its position and station; (2) the extent of cervical effacement and dilatation; (3) the status of the membranes; (4) the architecture of the bony pelvis and its capacity in relation to the size of the presenting part; (5) the distensibility of the vagina; and (6) the rigidity of the perineum.

After the vulvar and perineal regions have been properly prepared, and the examiner has donned sterile gloves, the thumb and forefinger of one hand separate the labia widely to expose the vaginal opening and prevent the examining fingers from coming in contact with the inner surfaces of the labia and the margins of the hymen. The index and second fingers of the other hand are then introduced into the vagina (Fig. 2).

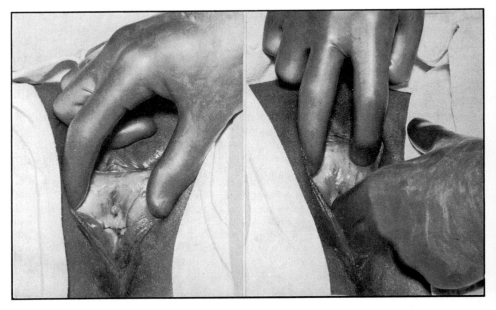

Fig. 2. Vaginal examination. Left, spreading labia apart. Right, insertion of fingers.

In this examination a definite routine should be followed. A very important consideration in the technic of the examination is avoidance of withdrawal of the fingers from the vagina until the examination is entirely completed. The fingers should be introduced along the anterior surface of the vaginal wall, and the shape and size of the pubic arch and the height of the symphysis noted. The cervix should then be examined to ascertain the length of the canal, the degree to which it is dilated, and the character of its margins. The status of the membranes is next noted, taking care to avoid inadvertently rupturing them. The presentation and position of the fetus should be noted, as well as the relation of the presenting part to the level of the ischial spines. The palmar surface of the fingers should then be directed posteriorly, and the perineum palpated between the two fingers in the vagina and the thumb outside, noting particularly its consistency, thickness, and resistance. The mobility of the coccyx should then be tested, and the fingers then passed upward over the anterior surface of the sacrum to feel its vertical and lateral curvature. If the presenting part is not low, the three lower sacral vertebrae are readily palpable in normal women, whereas the first and second can be felt only in contracted pelves. If the presenting part is neither engaged nor firmly fixed in the birth canal and if the membranes are intact, the diagonal conjugate can be measured. The head should not be dislodged if the membranes are ruptured, because of the danger of prolapse of the umbilical cord.

Subsequent examinations during labor may be either vaginal or rectal. After a thorough initial evaluation an occasional examination usually suffices. In the normal patient with adequate pelvic measurements and a fetus of normal size, the progress of labor can be followed to a great extent by careful and repeated evaluation of the patient's signs and symptoms. In the argument concerning the relative merits and dangers of vaginal and rectal examinations an important point often disregarded is the number of examinations performed. A few careful examinations usually supply all the necessary information. Numerous carelessly performed vaginal examinations undoubtedly are a source of danger, but a large number of rectal examinations are similarly dangerous. A comparison of routine vaginal and rectal examinations has been reported by several investigators, including Prystowsky, and Peterson and Richey; from these studies it can be concluded that properly performed vaginal examinations are safe for the patient.

After completing the examination the physician should discuss with the mother the probable course of events. If everything is normal he should assure her that all is well, but he should guard against making any precise statement as to the probable duration of labor. The obstetrician who ventures to make more precise statements will find that his predictions are often faulty, even when the head is on the perineum. It is not always wise to inform the mother of an abnormality, but the physician should be careful to impart the information to a responsible member of the family, if only for medicolegal reasons.

Methods of Detecting Rupture of the Membranes. The clinical detection of ruptured membranes may be surprisingly uncertain. Although several diagnostic tests have been recommended, none is completely reliable.

Perhaps the most widely employed procedures concern testing the acidity or alkalinity of the vaginal fluid. The basis for these tests is that normally the pH of the vaginal secretion ranges between 4.5 and 5.5, whereas that of the amniotic fluid is usually 7.0 to 7.5.

NITRAZINE TEST.   The use of the indicator nitrazine for the diagnosis of ruptured membranes was first suggested by Baptisti and is a simple and fairly reliable method. Test papers are impregnated with the dye, and the color of the reaction is interpreted by comparison with a standard color chart. The pH of the vaginal secretion is estimated by inserting a sterile cotton-tipped applicator deeply into the vagina and then touching it to a strip of the nitrazine paper and comparing the paper with the chart. Color changes are interpreted as follows:

Yellow	pH 5.0	}
Olive-yellow	pH 5.5	Intact membranes
Olive-green	pH 6.0	
Blue-green	pH 6.5	
Blue-gray	pH 7.0	Ruptured membranes
Deep blue	pH 7.5	

Baptisti points out that a false reading is likely to be encountered in patients with intact membranes who have an unusually large amount of bloody show, since blood, like amniotic fluid, is alkaline. A more extended study of the nitrazine test by a slightly different technic was made by Abe. He reported 176 cases in which the nitrazine test was found correct in 98.9 per cent of patients with known rupture of membranes and in 96.2 per cent of patients with intact membranes. We find the test easy to carry out and reasonably dependable. In ordinary clinical practice these tests will not, however, yield such accurate results as those just mentioned, because they are used in questionable cases in which the amount of fluid is small and often therefore more susceptible to a change in pH by admixed blood and vaginal secretions.

Smith and Callagan have applied to the detection of rupture of the membranes the phenomenon of fernlike crystallization of the sodium chloride in dried smears of amniotic fluid. Swabbings of the vaginal pool and of the cervical canal, made through a sterile unlubricated speculum, were applied to clean slides and allowed to dry, preferably by warming over the microscope light. Smith and Callagan noted that more than 1 part of blood mixed with 10 parts of amniotic fluid interfered with crystallization. Aqueous merthiolate formed a crystalline pattern when dried, and surgical soap formed granules. Even with these problems they concluded that the accuracy of this test was equal to that of other methods. Ferron and Bilodeau and others have reported similar experience. Unfortunately the factors that may invalidate the nitrazine test—namely, blood and normal or infected secretions of the vagina and cervix—interfere also with the fern test.

Kushner and associates have recommended the preparation of smears from swabbings of the posterior fornix and the cervix, which are then air-dried and stained with acridine orange. Anucleate fetal squamous cells are looked for under low magnification. They report an accuracy of 90 per cent in 126 patients with ruptured membranes and 87 per cent in 174 with intact membranes. False interpretation occurred chiefly when there was a paucity of cellular material. Microscopic examination to identify fat droplets from amniotic fluid in vaginal and cervical smears has been suggested by Numers.

Ferguson and associates have suggested a cytologic technic in which the cervix and posterior fornix are wiped with a sterile-gloved hand. The wipings are smeared on a glass slide, fixed, and stained with pinacyanol chloride solution. They have claimed, as features of the test, quickness and ease of performance, as well as reasonable accuracy.

Since a full bladder may be a serious impediment to labor, the patient should be asked to void at least every three or four hours. If she is unable to do so and if the distended bladder is palpable above the symphysis, catheterization may be required. Figure 1 in Chapter 31 illustrates a case in which overdistention of the bladder resulted in extreme delay in the progress of labor.

Since the median duration of labor is less than 10 hours, and since ingestion of food may create anesthetic difficulties at delivery, it is customary to withhold solid food during labor. In fact, patients in labor rarely desire food and are likely to vomit if fed solids. If vomiting or dehydration occurs or if labor is longer than 12 hours, glucose in water, and, at times electrolytes should be administered intravenously.

MANAGEMENT OF SECOND STAGE

Certain events herald the onset of the second stage of labor and should be watched for carefully: (1) The patient begins to bear down of her own accord as the head begins to press on the perineal floor. (2) There may be a sudden increase in bloody show. (3) The patient senses that she needs to defecate; this feeling also results from pressure of the fetal head on the perineal floor and rectum. (4) The perineum begins to bulge and the anal orifice begins to dilate. This sign occurs late, but should be watched for with every contraction after the first three signs have been noted. Only rectal or vaginal examination, however, can definitely confirm the suspicion. If these signs are overlooked, the delivery may occur without proper attention. In general, nulliparas should be transported to the delivery room when the cervix is fully dilated, and multiparas at 7 or 8 cm.

In most cases, bearing-down efforts are reflex and spontaneous in the second stage of labor, but occasionally the patient does not employ her expulsive forces to good advantage and coaching is desirable. In some hospitals straps or handles are placed in the patient's hands. These devices are firmly attached to the delivery table and so adjusted in length that she can reach them comfortably. Her legs should be half-flexed so that she can push with them against the floor of the table. Instructions should then be given the patient to take a deep breath as soon as the next uterine contraction begins and, with her breath held, to exert downward pressure exactly as though she were straining at stool. Pulling on the straps at this time is a helpful adjunct. The effort should be as long and sustained as possible, since grunts and short endeavors are of little avail. Usually these bearing-down efforts are rewarded by increasing bulging of the perineum—that is, by further descent of the head. The patient should be informed of such progress, for encouragement at this stage is very important. During this period of active bearing down, the fetal heart sounds should be auscultated immediately after each pain. The maternal pulse must be counted frequently also, since substantial increase in pulse rate indicates exhaustion and calls for means of meeting the situation other than the continuation of bearing-down efforts.

As the head descends through the pelvis, small particles of feces are frequently expelled; as they appear at the anus they should be sponged off with large fresh pledgets soaked in antiseptic solution. *Asepsis* and *antisepsis* are most

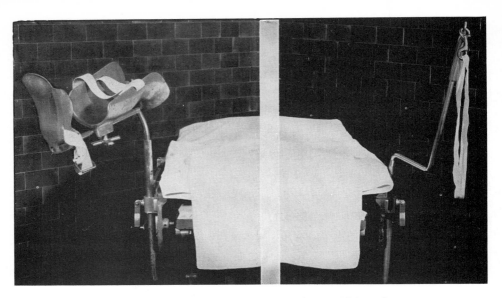

Fig. 3. Two types of leg holders. Left, knee rest. Right, stirrups.

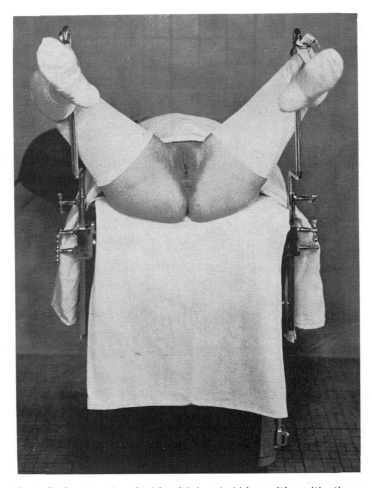

Fig. 4. Patient at edge of table with legs held in position with stirrups.

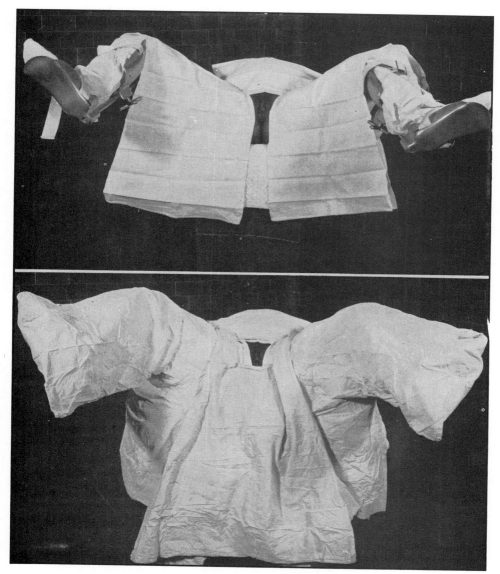

Fig. 5. Top, patient partly covered with sterile draping in leg holders. Bottom, patient completely draped for delivery.

important in the second stage of labor. No one should be permitted in the delivery room without a scrub suit, a mask covering both nose and mouth, and a cap that completely covers the hair. Preparation for actual delivery entails thorough vulvar and perineal scrubbing and draping with sterile towels and sheets in such a way that only the immediate region about the vulva is exposed (Figs. 3 through 5).

In placing the legs of the anesthetized patient in stirrups or leg holders, care should be taken not to separate the legs too widely and not to place one leg higher than the other.

Surgical Scrubbing and Gloving.   Because the hands cannot be rendered entirely free of bacteria, sterile rubber gloves are worn. Since the gloves tear occasionally, the necessity for meticulously cleansing the hands before putting them on is apparent. Their use, however, even in conjunction with other precautions, does not entirely eliminate the possibility of introducing bacteria into the genital tract, since the organisms may be carried up from the vaginal outlet by the sterile gloved finger. In all cases the hands should be cleansed as carefully as for a major surgical operation:

1. The fingernails are cut and cleaned before starting to scrub.
2. Using an antiseptic soap, both hands and forearms to 5 cm above the elbows are washed for one minute. The mixture is then rinsed off with running lukewarm water.
3. A sterile orangewood stick is next employed to clean thoroughly beneath the fingernails.
4. Utilizing a sterile hand brush and the antiseptic solution, each hand is then vigorously scrubbed for two minutes; each forearm to 5 cm above the elbow is

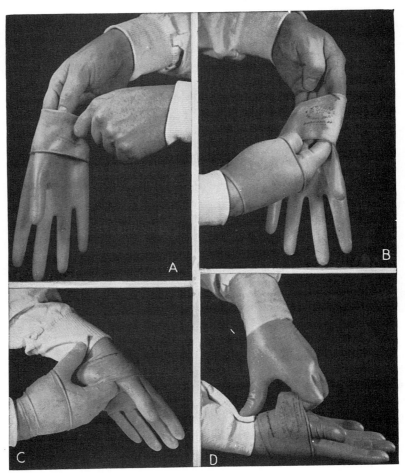

Fig. 6. Method of putting on sterile gloves so that the outsides of the gloves are never touched by the ungloved hand. Care must be exercised not to contaminate the gloved left thumb on the right cuff or wrist (see A and D).

then scrubbed for one minute. The hands followed by the forearms are now rinsed off with lukewarm water.

This technic thus involves a total of at least six minutes after the initial one-minute wash. When the birth of the baby becomes imminent or in any emergency the time is shortened accordingly.

After the hands are scrubbed, a sterile gown is donned in such a manner that the hands do not touch its outer surface. Likewise, the gloves are put on in such a manner that the ungloved hands never touch the outer surface of the gloves, as in the standard surgical method shown in Figure 6.

Delivery.   After the patient has been prepared for delivery, catheterization, only when indicated, is carried out by the physician.

Cramps in the leg are common in the second stage of labor because of pressure exerted by the baby's head on nerves in the pelvis. They are readily relieved by changing the position of the leg or brief massage, but should never be ignored, since they may sometimes cause excruciating pain.

As soon as the head distends the perineum to a diameter of 6 or 8 cm—that is, when crowning is about to occur (Fig. 7)—it is desirable to place a towel

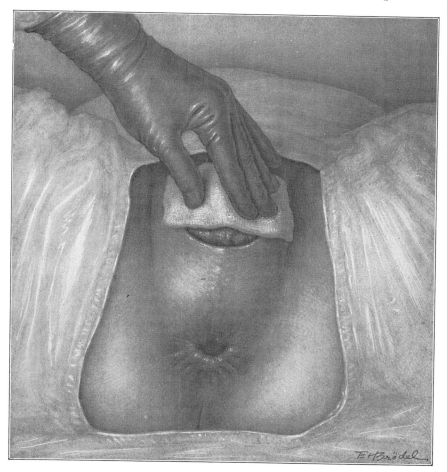

Fig. 7. Method of controlling head to increase flexion and protect perineum. Force must not be applied in any way that prevents delivery of the head. Often an episiotomy is performed somewhat before this time.

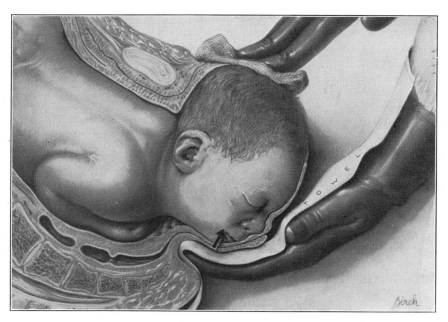

Fig. 8. Delivery by the modified Ritgen maneuver. The arrow indicates the direction of moderate pressure applied by the posterior hand.

over the hand to protect it from the anus and then exert forward pressure on the chin of the baby's head through the perineum while the other hand exerts pressure on the occiput (Fig. 8). Although this maneuver is simpler than that originally described by Ritgen, it is customarily designated *Ritgen's maneuver* or the *modified Ritgen maneuver*. It allows the physician to control the delivery of the head; it also favors extension so that the head is born with the smallest diameter presenting. The head is usually delivered between contractions, as slowly as possible. Ritgen's maneuver, gradual extension, and slow delivery between contractions all help to prevent lacerations, as does an episiotomy (p. 423). After delivery of the shoulders, the remainder of the body usually follows with ease. The posterior shoulder is often delivered first, but as shown in Figures 9 and 10, the anterior shoulder may be born first in entirely normal deliveries.

In most cases the shoulders appear at the vulva just after external rotation and are born spontaneously. Occasionally a delay occurs and immediate extraction may appear advisable. In that event the head should be held between the two hands and gentle downward traction applied until the anterior shoulder appears under the pubic arch; then by an upward movement, the posterior shoulder is delivered, and the anterior shoulder usually drops down from beneath the symphysis. An equally effective method entails completion of delivery of the anterior shoulder before that of the posterior (Figs. 9 and 10).

The body almost always follows the shoulders without difficulty, but in case of prolonged delay its birth may be hastened by moderate traction upon the head and by pressure upon the abdomen; hooking the fingers in the axillae should be avoided, however, since it may injure the nerves of the upper extremity, produc-

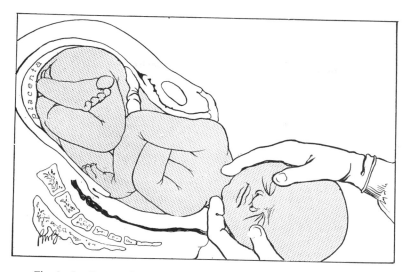

Fig. 9. Gentle traction to bring about descent of anterior shoulder.

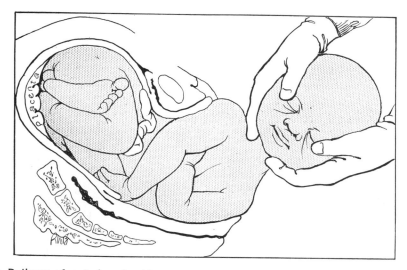

Fig. 10. Delivery of anterior shoulder completed; gentle traction to deliver the posterior shoulder.

ing a transient or possibly even a permanent paralysis. Traction, furthermore, should be exerted only in the direction of the long axis of the child, for if applied obliquely it causes bending of the neck and excessive stretching of the brachial plexus.

Immediately after birth of the head, the finger should be passed to the neck of the child to ascertain whether it is encircled by one or more coils of the umbilical cord. Coils occur in about every fourth case and ordinarily do no harm, but occasionally they may be so tight that constriction of the vessels and consequent hypoxia result. If a coil is felt it should be drawn down between the

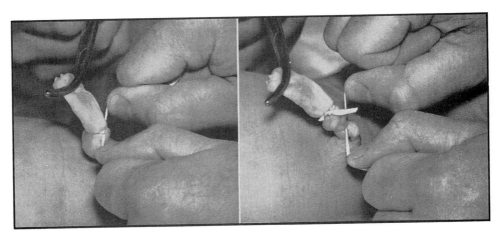

Fig. 11. Double ligation of umbilical cord with cord tie. If knuckles are kept together, as shown, sudden traction on the cord from slipping of the fingers is prevented.

fingers and, if loose enough, slipped over the infant's head; but if it is too tightly applied to the neck to be slipped over the head, it should be cut between two clamps and the infant delivered promptly.

Tying the Cord.   The cord is cut between two clamps placed 4 or 5 cm from the abdomen, and subsequently a sterile tape ligature, tightly tied not closer than about 2 cm from the abdomen (Fig. 11), or a clamp, is applied. A plastic clamp that is safe, efficient, easy to sterilize, and fairly inexpensive is shown in

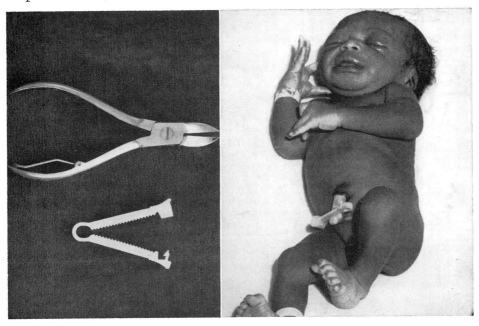

Fig. 12. Modern plastic cord clamp. These clamps lock in place and cannot slip. They are removed on the second or third day simply by cutting the plastic at the loop, or they can be allowed to drop off with the cord.

Figure 12. The cord should be clamped as soon as reasonably convenient. The optimal time for clamping the umbilical cord is not absolutely clear. If after delivery the infant is placed at the level of the introitus or below and the feto-placental circulation is not immediately occluded by clamping the cord, as much as 100 ml of blood may be shifted from the placenta to the infant. Yao and Lind, for example, have measured the residual volume of placental blood in response to positioning the infant at precisely measured distances above or below the introitus for varying periods of time before clamping the cord. They observed that placing the infant within 10 cm above or below the introitus for three minutes resulted in the shift of about 80 ml of blood from the placenta to the infant. Lowering to 40 cm below the introitus for only 30 seconds effected the same degree of transfer. If the infant was held 50 to 60 cm above the introitus, however, transfer of blood to the infant was negligible even after three minutes.

Although it is clear that a volume of blood equal to approximately one third of the entire fetal blood volume is added to the infant as a consequence of holding the infant at or below the level of the introitus and delaying clamping of the cord, the advantages and disadvantages of the procedure are still disputed. One benefit to be derived from placental transfusion is that the hemoglobin in 80 ml of placental blood adds about 50 mg of iron to the infant's stores and no doubt reduces the frequency of iron-deficiency anemia later in infancy. In the presence of accelerated destruction of erythrocytes, as occurs with isoimmunization, the bilirubin formed from the extra erythrocytes contributes further to the danger of hyperbilirubinemia. Although theoretically the risk of circulatory overloading from gross hypervolemia is formidable, especially in premature infants, the addition of placental blood to the infant's circulation does not ordinarily cause difficulty. Moss, Duffie, and Fagan, in fact, believe that early clamping of the cord before respirations are established may be a factor in the pathogenesis of the respiratory distress syndrome of the newborn, a fairly common complication. They therefore recommend delayed clamping. Taylor, Bright, and Birchard, however, have concluded that placental transfusion does not benefit premature infants.

MANAGEMENT OF THIRD STAGE

Immediately after delivery of the infant the height of the uterine fundus and its consistency are ascertained. As long as the uterus remains hard and there is no bleeding, watchful waiting until the placenta is separated is the usual practice. No massage is practiced, the hand simply resting on the fundus to make certain that the organ does not become atonic and fill up with blood.

Since attempts to express the placenta prior to its separation are futile and possibly dangerous, it is most important that the following signs of placental separation be recognized:

1. The uterus becomes globular and, as a rule, firmer. This sign is the earliest to appear.
2. There is often a sudden gush of blood.
3. The uterus rises in the abdomen because the placenta, having separated, passes down into the lower uterine segment and vagina where its bulk pushes the uterus upward.

4. The umbilical cord protrudes farther out of the vagina, indicating that the placenta has descended.

These signs sometimes appear within about a minute after delivery of the infant and usually within five minutes. When the placenta has separated, the physician first ascertains that the uterus is firmly contracted. He may then ask the patient, if she is not anesthetized, to bear down, and the intraabdominal pressure so produced may be adequate to expel the placenta. If such efforts fail or if spontaneous expulsion is not practicable because of anesthesia, the physician, again having made certain that the uterus is hard, exerts pressure with his hand on the fundus and propels the detached placenta into the vagina (Figs. 13 and 14).

Placental expression should never be attempted before placental separation, lest the uterus be turned inside out. Inversion of the uterus is one of the grave accidents associated with delivery (Ch. 33, p. 965). As pressure is applied to the fundus, the umbilical cord is kept moderately taut. Traction on the cord, however, must not be used to pull the placenta out of the uterus. As the placenta passes through the introitus, it is grasped and the fundal pressure is stopped. The placenta is then gently lifted away from the introitus. Care is taken to prevent the membranes from being torn off and left behind. If the membranes start to tear they are grasped with a clamp and removed by gentle traction. The placenta should be carefully examined to ascertain whether it has been delivered in its entirety from the uterine cavity.

In the belief that much unnecessary blood loss occurs between separation

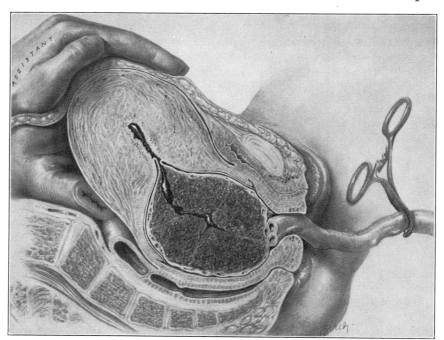

Fig. 13. Expression of placenta. The fundus should be massaged, but not squeezed, before carrying out this procedure to make certain that the uterus is firmly contracted.

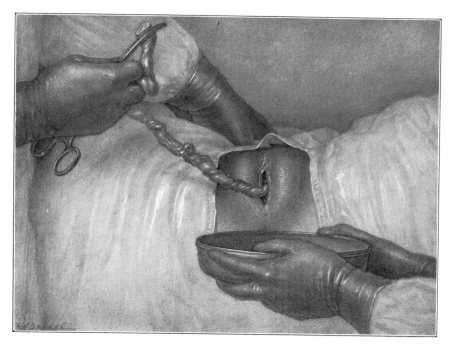

Fig. 14. Expression of placenta.

and expulsion as the result of the growing retroplacental hematona, Calkins recommended a technic for the conduct of the third stage that aims at earlier recognition of placental separation and earlier expulsion. His procedure embraces two departures from the standard method previously quoted: (1) constant application of the hand to the uterine fundus after birth of the child to detect the first signs of placental detachment; and (2) vigorous massage of the uterus immediately after separation, followed at once by efforts at expulsion.

If at any time there is brisk bleeding and the placenta cannot be delivered by these technics, manual removal of the placenta is indicated as described in Chapter 33 (p. 962).

Occasionally the placenta will not separate promptly. A question to which there is still no definite answer concerns the length of time that should elapse before the placenta is manually removed. If the placenta has not separated within about five minutes after birth of the baby, and if the patient is anesthetized, and if there has been no contamination of the operative field, manual removal of the placenta should probably be carried out. The principal advantage of this approach is the reduction of blood loss during the third stage, whereas the main disadvantage is the possibility of introducing infection into the uterine cavity.

The hour immediately following delivery of the placenta is a critical period. It has even been designated by some obstetricians as the "fourth stage of labor." At this time postpartum hemorrhage is most likely to occur as the result of uterine relaxation. It is mandatory that the uterus be watched constantly throughout this period by a competent attendant, who keeps a hand on the fundus and massages it at the slightest sign of relaxation. At the same time the vaginal and perineal region is frequently inspected to identify promptly any excessive bleeding.

Oxytocin, Ergonovine, and Methylergonovine. After the uterus is emptied and the placenta is delivered the primary mechanism by which hemostasis is achieved at the placental site is vasoconstriction produced by a well-contracted myometrium. Oxytocin (Pitocin, Syntocinon), ergonovine maleate (Ergotrate), and methylergonovine (Methergine) are employed in various ways in the conduct of the third stage of labor, principally to stimulate myometrial contractions and thereby reduce the blood loss.

OXYTOCIN. Oxytocin, an octapeptide, the amino acid composition of which is shown in Figure 15, is obtained from the posterior pituitary of domestic animals or is chemically synthesized. Only the synthetic form is now commercially available (Syntocinon, Pitocin). Each milliliter of injectable oxytocin solution contains 10 USP units of oxytocin. Each milligram of highly purified oxytocin has about 500 units of oxytocin activity. Oxytocin administered parenterally during late pregnancy and early in the puerperium can cause a marked increase in uterine contractility. After the fetus has been delivered, even doses greatly in excess of those that will induce vigorous uterine contractions produce few adverse effects.

One of the most important adverse effects of oxytocin is antidiuresis, caused primarily by reabsorption of free water. Abdul-Karim and Assali have clearly demonstrated in both pregnant and nonpregnant women that synthetic oxytocin, as well as oxytocin derived from mammalian posterior pituitary glands, possesses antidiuretic activity. Before synthetic oxytocin was available for study, any evidence of antidiuresis following administration of oxytocin was usually attributed to contamination of the oxytocin with vasopressin. In subjects who are undergoing diuresis in response to the administration of water, the continuous intravenous infusion of 20 milliunits of oxytocin per minute usually produces a demonstrable decrease in flow. When the rate of infusion is raised to 40 to 50 milliunits per minute, urinary flow is drastically reduced. With doses of this magnitude it is possible to produce water intoxication if the oxytocin is administered in a large volume of electrolyte-free aqueous dextrose solution (Liggins; Whalley and Pritchard). In general, if oxytocin is to be administered at a relatively high rate of infusion for a considerable period of time, increasing the concentration of the hormone is preferable to increasing the rate of flow of the more dilute solution. The antidiuretic effect of intravenously administered oxytocin disappears within a few minutes after the infusion is stopped. Oxytocin injected intramuscularly in doses of 5 to 10 units (0.5 to 1 ml) every 15 to 30 minutes also may cause intense antidiuresis, but the possibility of water intoxication is not nearly so great, since large volumes of electrolyte-free aqueous solution are not used as a vehicle (Whalley and Pritchard).

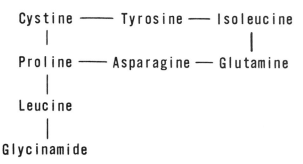

Fig. 15. Eight amino acids form the oxytocin peptide. Human vasopressin differs from oxytocin in the replacement of isoleucine by phenylalanine and leucine by arginine.

Oxytocin administered by continuous intravenous infusion in very high concentrations may cause hypertension. One subject with a fetus dead in utero for many weeks was observed to develop rather marked hypertension with frontal headache while receiving about 2,000 milliunits of oxytocin per minute by continuous intravenous infusion. The headache and hypertension promptly disappeared when the infusion was stopped but reappeared after it was restarted. When concentrated solutions of oxytocin are given intravenously as a single rapid injection, both the synthetic and natural hormone have been reported to produce transient hypotension, tachycardia, and electrocardiographic changes (Tipton and associates; Bergquist and Kaiser). When administered as a dilute intravenous infusion, however, oxytocin has little effect on the blood pressure or electrocardiogram.

Oxytocin causes milk ejection by inducing contractions of the myoepithelial cells of the mammary gland. This phenomenon is not seen in nonpregnant women, but from very early in pregnancy the gland becomes progressively more sensitive to the hormone; during the second half of pregnancy a demonstrable effect can be elicited with as little as 1 milliunit of oxytocin (Sala). The milk-ejecting effect induced by oxytocin is about 40 to 50 times greater than that of vasopressin. Measurements of milk-ejection pressure have been used for bioassay of oxytocin. The intravenous injection of 10 milliunits of oxytocin per kilogram is followed by an appreciable increase in the concentration of free fatty acids in the plasma and sizable decreases in the levels of blood glucose in very recently pregnant and nonpregnant subjects (Burt, Leake, and Dannenburg). The significance of these effects, however, is not clear. Oxytocin is without effect when taken orally because of its rapid destruction in the gastrointestinal tract. Slight oxytocic and milk-ejection effects can sometimes be induced by applying oxytocin to the nasal mucosa in the form of a pledget or a spray; a very small amount, moreover, may be absorbed when continuously applied to the buccal mucosa.

Posterior pituitary extract (Pituitrin) is a mixture of both the oxytocic and vasopressor-antidiuretic principles from the pituitary glands of domestic animals. It is mentioned only to condemn its use. Along with oxytocic action there is the potent vasopressor effect of vasopressin. If given in large doses parenterally, especially if administered intravenously, it can produce profound shock. Pituitrin shock probably results in large part from constriction of coronary arteries by the rapid injection of large amounts of vasopressin. Oxytocin should have long since completely replaced Pituitrin in all hospitals.

ERGONOVINE AND METHYLERGONOVINE.   Ergonovine is an alkaloid either obtained from ergot, a fungus that grows upon rye and some other grains, or synthesized in part from lysergic acid. Methylergonovine is a very similar alkaloid, also made from lysergic acid. These two alkaloids differ structurally only in that methylergonovine contains one more carbon radical in the side chain than does ergonovine (Fig. 16). The alkaloids are dispensed as the maleate (Ergotrate and Methergine, respectively) either in solution for parenteral use or in tablets for oral use.

There is no convincing evidence of any appreciable difference in the actions of ergonovine and methylergonovine; they will therefore be considered together. Whether

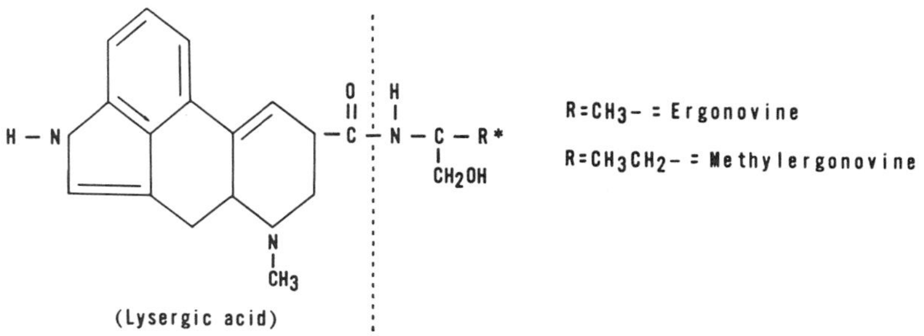

R=CH₃- : Ergonovine

R=CH₃CH₂- : Methylergonovine

(Lysergic acid)

Fig. 16. The basic structure of ergonovine and methylergonovine is shown. Methylergonovine contains one more methylene group in the side chain R than does ergonovine.

given intravenously, intramuscularly, or orally, ergonovine and methylergonovine are powerful stimulants of myometrial contraction, exerting an effect that may persist for several hours. The effect of oxytocin on the myometrium lasts only a few minutes after intravenous injection and probably an hour or less when given intramuscularly; it is without effect when given orally. The sensitivity of the uterus to ergonovine and methylergonovine is very great; in pregnant women an intravenous dose of as little as 0.1 mg or an oral dose of only 0.25 mg results in a tetanic contraction, which occurs almost immediately after intravenous injection of the drug and within a few minutes after intramuscular or oral administration. As shown in Figure 17, moreover, the response is sustained with little tendency toward relaxation. The tetanic effect of ergonovine and methylergonovine is ideal for the prevention and control of postpartum hemorrhage but is very dangerous for the fetus and the mother prior to delivery. The parenteral administration of these alkaloids, especially by the intravenous route, sometimes initiates transient but severe hypertension. Such a reaction is most likely to occur when conduction anesthesia is used for delivery. Nausea is another troublesome feature. Otherwise these alkaloids produce no serious side effects.

The history of ergot is fascinating. For centuries it has been recognized that ergot could cause severe pain, convulsions, extensive gangrene of the extremities, and death. Repeated epidemics of ergotism plagued Europe until ergot was proved to be their cause and they were then brought under control. A local outbreak, nevertheless, occurred in France about a decade ago. Centuries ago ergot was recognized as capable of producing uterine contractions, and early in the nineteenth century Pulvis Parturiens was introduced into medicine. A letter by John Stearns published in the *Medical Repository of New York* in 1808 is presented in part (quoted from Goodman and Gilman): "It expedites lingering parturition and saves to the accoucheur a considerable portion of time, without producing any bad effects on the patient. . . . Previous to its exhibition it is of the utmost consequence to ascertain the presentation . . . as the violent and almost incessant action which it induces in the uterus precludes the possibility of turning. . . . If the dose is large it will produce nausea and vomiting. In most cases you will be surprised with the suddenness of its operation; it is, therefore, necessary to be completely ready before you give the medicine. . . . Since I have adopted the use of this powder I have seldom found a case that detained me more than three hours."

After a flurry of widespread administration it became apparent that powdered ergot was capable of producing violent uterine contractions with fetal and maternal death.

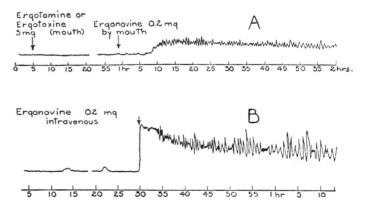

Fig. 17. Effects on the human uterus of various alkaloids of ergot. A, oral administration of 3 mg of ergotamine or ergotoxin as compared with 0.2 mg of ergonovine (B). This record, obtained by means of a balloon and manometer, is that of the uterine motility of a woman (para IV) seven days postpartum. B, intravenous administration of 0.2 mg of ergonovine. This record is that of a woman (para II) seven days postpartum. (After Davis, Adair, and Pearl. From Goodman and Gilman. The Pharmacological Basis of Therapeutics. The Macmillan Co.)

Moir has pointed out that such has been the history of most uterine stimulants. There was initial surprise and pleasure on discovering the uterine stimulating effect; the cautious employment of the drug clinically to initiate or stimulate labor followed. Favorable reports were soon followed by uncritical and dangerous use with extensive fetal and maternal injuries and deaths. Finally the way to safe use of the drug evolved or, if there was none, it was discarded.

Ergot as a powder or as the fluid extract was recognized until recently in official compendia of drugs. Attempts to standardize the oxytocic activity of ergot were based on assays that compared its ability to produce gangrene of a rooster's comb with that of a standard preparation. This bioassay measured the activity of the wrong constituents, since the alkaloids that produced the gangrene possessed little or no oxytocic activity, and vice versa.

The alkaloid with potent oxytocic properties, ergonovine, was isolated in 1935. Fortunately it has no direct vasoconstrictive action nor does it produce endothelial damage. Ergonovine and methylergonovine are now used in obstetrics to induce contractions of the myometrium either after delivery of the fetus or sometimes during an incomplete abortion; they are not used to induce or stimulate labor in this country.

Oxytocin, ergonovine, and methylergonovine are all employed widely in the conduct of the normal third stage of labor, but the timing of their administration differs in various clinics. In most cases following uncomplicated vaginal delivery the third stage can be conducted with reasonably small blood loss without their aid. A technic of administration of oxytocics that we consider very satisfactory for the management of the third stage, from the viewpoint of minimizing blood loss and general safety, is as follows. Ten units of oxytocin are injected intramuscularly immediately after birth of the baby, followed by ergonovine or methylergonovine, 0.2 mg intramuscularly, immediately after the delivery of the placenta. There are two important precautions with this regime. It is important to be sure that the uterus does not contain another fetus before injecting the oxytocin, and if the patient demonstrates any evidence of hypertension, the ergonovine or methylergonovine should not be given. Other methods of administering these oxytocic drugs are discussed in Chapter 28.

The obstetrician can often predict with considerable accuracy which patients are likely to have a hypotonic uterus with resulting gross hemorrhage during and after the third stage of labor. This complication can be anticipated in the following circumstances: (1) uterine atony during and after the third stage of labor in previous pregnancies; (2) prolonged first and second stages of labor; (3) very rapid labor; (4) labor induced and maintained with oxytocin; (5) older women of high parity; (6) uterus markedly distended by large fetus, multiple fetuses, or hydramnios; (7) preeclampsia-eclampsia; and (8) deep or prolonged general anesthesia used for delivery. In these situations an intravenous aqueous infusion should be begun before the onset of the third stage of labor and oxytocin then added to the infusion as soon as the infant is delivered. Twenty to forty units of oxytocin per liter of infusion administered at 30 to 60 drops per minute supply an adequate amount of the drug.

Lacerations of the Birth Canal. Lacerations of the vagina and perineum are classified as first, second, or third degree.

First-degree lacerations (Fig. 18) involve the fourchet, the perineal skin and vaginal mucous membrane but not the muscles.

Second-degree lacerations (Fig. 19) involve, in addition to skin and mucous membrane, the muscles of the perineal body but not the rectal sphincter. These

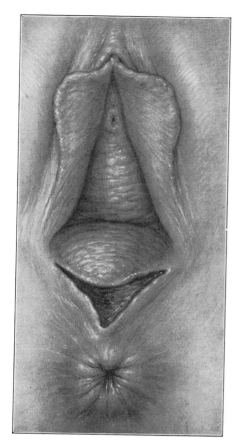

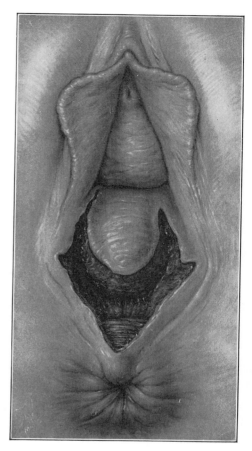

Fig. 18. First-degree perineal tear.   Fig. 19. Deep second-degree perineal tear.

tears usually extend upward on one or both sides of the vagina, forming an irregular triangular injury.

Third-degree lacerations extend completely through the skin, mucous membrane, and perineal body, and involve the anal sphincter. This type is often referred to as a complete tear. Not infrequently, these third-degree lacerations extend a certain distance up the anterior wall of the rectum.

In some clinics a so-called fourth-degree laceration is distinguished; this designation is applied to third-degree tears that extend through the rectal mucosa to expose the lumen of the rectum. The term "fourth-degree laceration" will not be used in the ensuing discussion; when third-degree lacerations with rectal wall extension are mentioned, they will be so designated.

The causes of perineal lacerations are rapid and sudden expulsion of the head; persistent occiput posterior positions; excessive size of the infant; difficult forceps deliveries and breech extractions; outlet contraction of the pelvis, forcing the head posteriorly; exaggerated lithotomy position; and friable maternal tissues. Some tears are unavoidable even in the most skilled hands. First- and second-degree lacerations are extremely common in nulliparas; for that reason, among others, episiotomy is widely employed. In addition to the types of perineal injury mentioned to here, lacerations of the vagina at higher levels occasionally occur, sometimes causing extensive hemorrhage. Tears in the region of the urethra are especially likely to bleed profusely.

Since the repair of perineal tears is virtually the same as that of episiotomy incisions, albeit often more difficult because of irregular lines of tissue cleavage, the technic of repairing them will be discussed in the following section.

EPISIOTOMY AND REPAIR

Episiotomy, in a strict sense, is incision of the pudenda. Perineotomy is incision of the perineum. In common parlance, however, episiotomy is often used synonymously with perineotomy, a practice that will be followed here. The in-

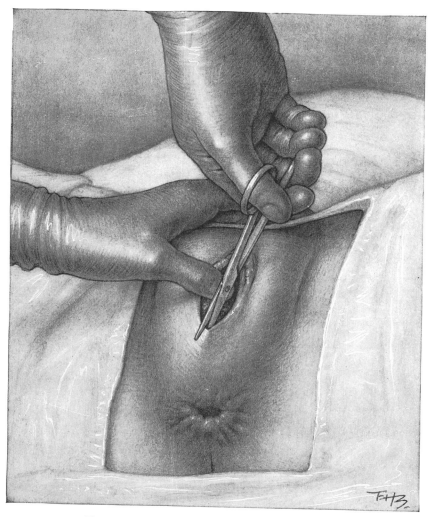

Fig. 20. Scissors placed for mediolateral episiotomy.

cision may be made in the midline (*median episiotomy*), or it may be begun in the midline and directed laterally and downward away from the rectum (*mediolateral episiotomy*).

Purposes of Episiotomy.   Except for cutting and tying the umbilical cord, episiotomy is the most common operation in obstetrics. The reasons for its popularity are clear. First, it substitutes a straight, clean surgical incision for the ragged laceration that otherwise frequently results. Furthermore, the episiotomy is easier to repair and heals better than a tear. Second, it spares the baby's head the necessity of serving as a battering ram against perineal obstruction. If prolonged, the pounding of the infant's head against the perineum may cause brain injury. Third, the operation shortens the second stage of labor. Finally, mediolateral episiotomy reduces the likelihood of third-degree lacerations.

The important questions concerning the episiotomy are (1) how soon before delivery it should be performed; (2) whether to choose the median or mediolateral operation; (3) whether the incision should be sutured before or after expulsion of the placenta; and (4) the best suture materials and technic to employ.

Timing of the Episiotomy.   If episiotomy is done unnecessarily early, bleeding from the gaping wound may be considerable during the interim between the incision and the birth of the baby. If episiotomy is done too late, the muscles of the perineal floor will have already undergone excessive stretching, and one of the objectives of the operation is defeated. It is our practice, as a compromise, to perform episiotomy when the head is visible to a diameter of 2 to 3 cm—that is, slightly sooner than shown in Figures 20 and 21.

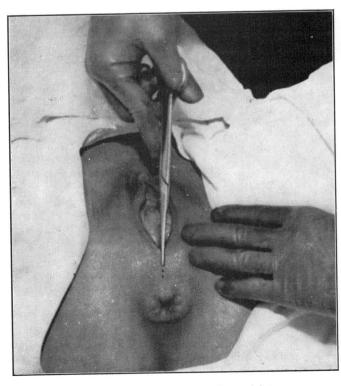

Fig. 21. Scissors placed for median episiotomy.

In this connection, the question arises whether episiotomy should be performed before or after the application of forceps. Although it is slightly more awkward to perform episiotomy with the forceps in place, blood loss from the episiotomy wound is less with this technic, since immediate traction on the forceps can be exerted, and the resultant tamponade of the perineal floor by the baby's head is effected earlier than could otherwise be achieved.

Median Versus Mediolateral Episiotomy. The advantages and disadvantages of the two types of episiotomy may be enumerated as follows:

Median Episiotomy	*Mediolateral Episiotomy*
1. Easy to repair	1. More difficult to repair
2. Faulty healing rare	2. Faulty healing more common
3. Rarely painful in puerperium	3. Pain in one third of cases for a few days
4. Dyspareunia rarely follows	4. Dyspareunia occasionally follows
5. Anatomic end results almost always excellent	5. Anatomic end results more or less faulty in some 10 per cent of cases (depending on operator)
6. Blood loss smaller	6. Blood loss greater
7. Third-degree extension in 2 to 5 per cent of cases (depending on operator)	7. Third-degree extension in less than 1 per cent of cases

With proper selection of cases it is possible to secure the advantages of median episiotomy and at the same time reduce to a minimum its one disadvantage, the greater likelihood of third-degree extension. The size of the perineal body is related to the likelihood of third-degree laceration, since the accident is naturally more likely to occur if it is short. The likelihood of extension of a median episiotomy into the rectal sphincter is also much greater when the baby is large, when the occiput is posterior, in midforceps deliveries, and, in our experience, in breech deliveries. It is our practice, in general, to use mediolateral episiotomy in the circumstances mentioned but to employ the median incision otherwise. Even with this selection of cases, however, the total number of third-degree lacerations sustained with this policy is probably greater than with routine mediolateral episiotomy.

In the days when most babies were born in the home it is understandable that a third-degree laceration was at times a major catastrophe. With poor lighting, inadequate exposure, poor choice of instruments, and no assistance, an inevitable sequel in most cases was a rectovaginal fistula, with consequent fecal incontinence. Such accidents carried with them a stigma that persists in the minds of most obstetricians today. Under conditions of hospital delivery a third-degree laceration, even though it extends up the rectum, is a much less serious accident than it was formerly. In a study by Kaltreider and Dixon of 710 third-degree lacerations, in which all the patients were managed under modern hospital conditions by competent personnel, repair of the laceration proved ultimately satisfactory in nearly 99 per cent of the cases. The most serious complication, rectovaginal fistula, occurred in 2 per cent. Of these fistulas, two thirds healed spontaneously. In other terms, a rectovaginal fistula that required repair occurred only once in 3,000 median episiotomies reported by these authors. Therefore, a third-degree laceration as the consequence of a median episiotomy is not a major catastrophe when properly repaired; and if all aspects of the question are considered, median episiotomy, despite its one drawback, is a satisfactory procedure in 9 out of 10 deliveries. Some authorities, however, employ mediolateral episiotomy routinely, especially in nulliparas.

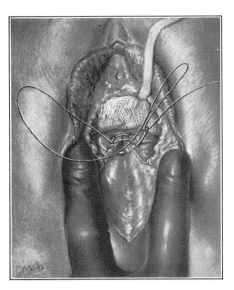

Fig. 22. Repair of median episiotomy. A half length of chromic catgut 00 or 000 is used as a continuous suture to close the vaginal mucosa.

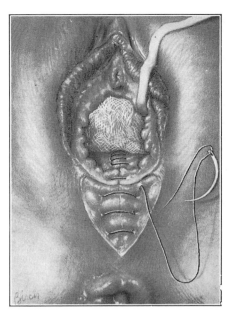

Fig. 23. Repair of median episiotomy. Following closure of the vaginal mucosa and fourchet, the continuous suture is laid aside, and three or four interrupted sutures of 00 or 000 catgut are placed in the fascia and muscle.

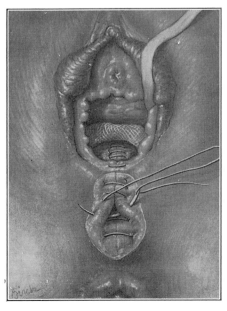

Fig. 24. Repair of median episiotomy. The continuous suture is now picked up and carried downward to unite the subcutaneous fascia.

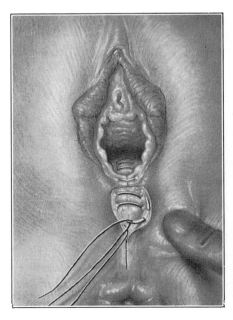

Fig. 25. Repair of median episiotomy. Finally, the continuous suture is carried upward as a subcuticular stitch. A few interrupted sutures of 000 chromic catgut placed through the skin and loosely tied are equally satisfactory for closure.

426

Timing of the Repair of Episiotomy.   The most common practice perhaps is to defer repair of the episiotomy until after the placenta has been delivered. That policy permits the obstetrician to give his undivided attention to the signs of placental separation and to expel the organ just as soon as it has separated. Early delivery of the placenta is believed to decrease the loss of blood, since it prevents the development of extensive retroplacental bleeding. A further advantage of this practice is that the episiotomy repair is not interrupted or disrupted by the obvious necessity of delivering the placenta.

Technic.   There are many ways to close the episiotomy incision, but hemostasis and anatomic restoration without excessive suturing are essential for success with any method. A technic that is commonly employed in episiotomy repair is shown in Figures 22 through 25. The suture material ordinarily employed is 00 or 000 chromic catgut.

The technic of repairing a third-degree laceration with extension into the wall of the rectum (Fig. 26) is shown in Figure 27. Here again various technics have been recommended, but all emphasize careful suturing of the rectal wall with stitches about 0.5 cm apart, covering this layer of sutures with a layer of fascia, and finally, careful isolation and suture of the anal sphincter with two or three

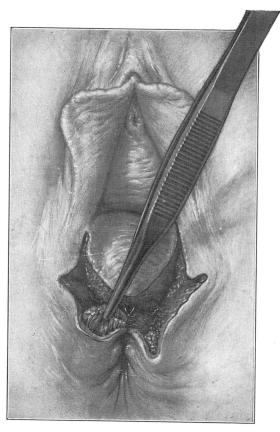

Fig. 26. Third-degree, or complete, tear through the perineum involving the anal sphincter. One end of the severed sphincter is identified.

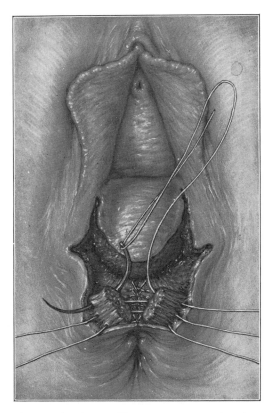

Fig. 27. Repair of complete perineal tear. The rectal mucosa has been repaired with inter-rupted, fine chromic catgut sutures. The torn ends of the sphincter ani are then approxi-mated with two or three interrupted chromic catgut sutures. The wound is then repaired, as in a second-degree laceration or an episiotomy.

interrupted stitches. The remainder of the repair is the same as for episiotomy. ***Pain After Episiotomy.*** For the relief of episiotomy pain, a heat lamp is the standard remedy, but during the summer months it may produce more discomfort than relief. An ice collar applied early tends to reduce swelling and allay dis-comfort. Analgesics such as codeine give considerable relief. Since pain may be a signal of a large vulvar, paravaginal, or ischiorectal hematoma or abscess, it is essential to examine these sites carefully if pain is severe and persistent. Manage-ment of these complications is discussed in Chapter 35.

REFERENCES

Abdul-Karim, R., and Assali, N. S.   Renal function in human pregnancy. V. Effects of oxytocin on renal hemodynamics and water and electrolyte excretion. J Lab Clin Med 57:522, 1961.
Abe, T.   The detection of the rupture of fetal membranes with the nitrazine indicator. Amer J Obstet Gynec 39:400, 1940.
Baptisti, A.   Chemical test for the determination of ruptured membranes. Amer J Obstet Gynec 35:688, 1938.
Bergquist, J. R., and Kaiser, I. H.   Cardiovascular effects of intravenous Syntocinon. Obstet Gynec 13:360, 1959.

Burt, R. L., Leake, N. H., and Dannenburg, W. N. Effect of synthetic oxytocin on plasma nonesterified fatty acids, triglycerides, and blood glucose. Obstet Gynec 21:708, 1963.

Calkins, L. A. Management of the third stage of labor. JAMA 101:1128, 1933.

Ferguson, J. H., Averette, H. E., and Hopman, B. C. Rupture of the membranes. JAMA 186:296, 1963.

Ferron, M., and Bilodeau, R. Amniotic fluid crystallization tests for ruptured membranes. Canad Med Ass J 89:1064, 1963.

Forman, J. B., and Sullivan, R. L. The effects of intravenous injections of ergonovine and Methergine on the postpartum patient. Amer J Obstet Gynec 63:640, 1952.

Goodman, L. S., and Gilman, A. The Pharmacological Basis of Therapeutics. New York, The Macmillan Co., 1965.

Goodrich, F. W., and Thoms, H. A clinical study of natural childbirth. Amer J Obstet Gynec 56:875, 1948.

Harris, R. E. An evaluation of the median episiotomy. Amer J Obstet Gynec 106:660, 1970.

Holmes, O. W. Medical Essays. Boston and New York, Houghton Mifflin & Co., 1891, p. 125.

Kaltreider, D. F., and Dixon, D. M. A study of 710 complete lacerations following central episiotomy. Southern Med J 41:814, 1948.

Kushner, D. H., Chang, I. W., and Vercruysse, J. M. Fluorescence microscopy for determination of ruptured fetal membranes by vaginal smear. Obstet Gynec 23:196, 1964.

Liggins, G. C. Treatment of missed abortion by high dosage syntocinon intravenous infusion. J Obstet Gynaec Brit Comm 69:277, 1962.

Lipton, B., Gittler, R. D., and Slotnik, H. O. Cardiovascular effects of oxytocin injection (USP), synthetic, prepared oxytocin, and ergot alkaloids. New York J Med 60:4006, 1960.

Moir, J. C. Clinical comparison of ergotoxine and ergotamine. Brit Med J 1:1022, 1932.

——— The obstetrician bids, and the uterus contracts. Brit Med J 2:1025, 1964.

——— and Dale, H. The action of ergot preparations on the puerperal uterus. Brit Med J 1:1119, 1932.

Moss, A. J., Duffie, E. R., and Fagan, L. M. Respiratory distress syndrome in the newborn. Study on the association of cord clamping and the pathogenesis of distress. JAMA 184:48, 1963.

Numers, C. (A new method of diagnosis of rupture of the membranes). Acta Obstet Gynec Scand 16:249, 1936.

Pastore, J. B. A study of the blood loss during the third stage of labor and the factors involved. Amer J Obstet Gynec 31:78, 1936.

——— and Stander, H. J. Hemorrhage in obstetrical patients. Texas J Med 35:390, 1939.

Peterson, W. F., and Richey, T. W. Routine vaginal examinations during labor: Comparative study with bacteriologic analysis. Illinois Med J 122:35, 1962.

Prystowsky, H. Is the danger of vaginal examination in labor overestimated? Amer J Obstet Gynec 68:639, 1954.

Read, G. D. Correlation of physical and emotional phenomena of natural labor. J Obstet Gynaec Brit Emp 53:55, 1946.

Ritgen, G. (Concerning his method for protection of the perineum. Monatschrift für Geburtskunde 6:21, 1855). See English translation, Wynn, R. M. Amer J Obstet Gynec 93:421, 1965.

Sala, N. L. The milk-ejecting effect induced by oxytocin and vasopressin during human pregnancy. Amer J Obstet Gynec 89:626, 1964.

Smith, R. W., and Callagan, D. A. Amniotic fluid crystallization test for ruptured membranes. Obstet Gynec 20:655, 1962.

Speck, G. Childbirth with dignity. Obstet Gynec 2:544, 1953.

Taylor, P. M., Bright, N. H., and Birchard, E. L. Effect of early versus delayed clamping of the umbilical cord on the clinical condition of the newborn infant. Amer J Obstet Gynec 86:893, 1963.

Thoms, H. The preparation for childbirth program. Obstet Gynec Survey 10:1, 1955.

Whalley, P. J., and Pritchard, J. A. Oxytocin and water intoxication. JAMA 186:601, 1963.

Yao, A. C., and Lind, J. Effect of gravity on placental transfusion. Lancet 11:505, 1969.

17

ANALGESIA AND ANESTHESIA

The relief of pain in labor presents special problems, which may best be understood by reviewing the several important differences between obstetric and surgical anesthesia and analgesia.

1. In surgical procedures there is but one patient to consider, whereas in parturition there are two, the mother and the baby. The respiratory center of the infant is highly vulnerable to sedative and anesthetic drugs; since these agents, if given systematically, regularly traverse the placenta, they may jeopardize the initiation of respiration at birth. This consideration is more than a mere theoretical possibility, since sluggish respiration is observed to some extent in the majority of infants whose mothers have received sedation during labor. Moreover, degrees of maternal hypoxemia so slight as to be innocuous to the mother may sometimes be lethal to the fetus, especially when associated with even transient maternal hypotension. The particular sensitivity of the fetus to the effects of almost all forms of maternal anesthesia poses one of the most difficult problems in obstetrics.

2. In major surgery, anesthesia is essential to the safe, satisfactory, and humane execution of the technical procedures. Whereas anesthesia is mandatory in many abnormal labors, it is not absolutely necessary in normal labor, because the baby can be born satisfactorily without any medication, albeit the mother may suffer severe pain. Hence, in a strict sense, an anesthetic death in obstetrics is usually an unnecessary death. When any form of pain relief is administered in labor, therefore, *safety is the* sine qua non.

3. Surgical anesthesia is administered for the duration of the operation, which lasts in most cases for not more than an hour or two. Efficient pain relief in labor must cover not only the delivery ("obstetric anesthesia") but also a preceding period of from 1 to 12 or even 24 hours ("obstetric analgesia").

4. In both obstetric analgesia and obstetric anesthesia it is important that the agents used exert little effect on uterine contractions. If they do, the progress of labor may stop. If uterine contractions are suppressed, postpartum hemorrhage may occur.

5. In the majority of surgical operations there is ample time to prepare the patient for anesthesia, especially by withholding food and fluids for 12 hours. Since most labors begin without warning, obstetric anesthesia is often administered within a few hours after a full meal. Vomiting with aspiration of gastric

430

contents is hence a frequent threat and sometimes a cause of death in obstetric anesthesia (Edwards and co-workers).

Because of these inherent difficulties, no completely safe and satisfactory method of pain relief in obstetrics has yet been developed. It is therefore sometimes falsely alleged that the hazards of pain relief in labor offset its advantages. On the contrary, vast experience has shown that obstetric analgesia and anesthesia, when judiciously employed, are in general beneficial rather than detrimental to both baby and mother. First, pain relief forestalls the importunities of the parturient and her family for premature operative interference. Formerly, premature and injudicious operative delivery, thus provoked, constituted the commonest cause of trauma to both mother and infant. Such injuries were occasionally fatal to the mother and frequently so to the baby. The relief of pain itself, although desirable, would not justify the methods that are not without danger, did they not permit more careful, gentler, and frequently easier deliveries, resulting in healthier mothers and more living babies.

General Principles. As stressed in another connection (p. 400), the proper psychologic management of the patient throughout the antepartum period and labor is a valuable basic sedative. A woman who is free of fear and who has complete confidence in her obstetrician and nurses usually enjoys a relatively comfortable first stage and requires a minimum of medication. This attitude toward parturition must be fostered as an important part of the relief of pain.

The optimal time for starting medicinal analgesia demands astute judgment, garnered only from experience. A common grave error is to initiate it too soon. In retrospect, some of our worst cases of prolonged labor may be charged to the premature use of sedative drugs or continuous conduction anesthesia. One rule should be absolute: such medication should never be started without positive proof that the cervix is progressively effacing and dilating. In general, primigravidas should not be given analgesic medication until the contractions are strong and the cervix is 3 cm dilated; in multiparas it is prudent to avoid it until the cervix is at least 4 cm dilated. It is a less costly error to begin medication too late than too early. When relief of pain is started appreciably later than the optimal time, its efficacy is obviously diminished, especially in rapid multiparous labors.

Patients under any form of analgesia require constant attention. If unattended, a patient under heavy sedation may throw herself out of bed or against a wall, or may vomit and aspirate the gastric contents. Numerous injuries and a few deaths as a result of such negligence are on record. Similarly, safe conduction anesthesia demands assiduous attention to the blood pressure and anesthetic levels.

For an obstetrician to master many of the various technics recommended for pain relief in labor is impossible. He should, however, master at least one program of obstetric analgesia and anesthesia, and should have at his disposal (1) a method of systemic analgesia, such as a barbiturate or meperidine (Demerol) and promethazine (Phenergan); (2) a method of general anesthesia, such as thiopental sodium (Pentothal), nitrous oxide-oxygen, and succinylcholine, if needed; and (3) a method of regional anesthesia, such as pudendal block, continuous caudal or epidural, low subarachnoid, paracervical block, or local infiltration.

THREE ESSENTIALS OF OBSTETRIC PAIN RELIEF:
FETAL HOMEOSTASIS, SIMPLICITY, AND SAFETY

Fetal homeostasis must not be impaired by the analgesic or anesthetic method. Most important is the transfer of oxygen, which is dependent on the concentration of inhaled oxygen, uterine blood flow, and the pO_2 gradient across the placenta, and the umbilical blood flow. The exact level to which inhaled oxygen can be reduced before fetal distress is produced is unknown, but a conservative estimate is about 15 per cent at normal atmospheric pressure. The principal factor impairing fetal oxygenation is not so often the concentration of the inhaled oxygen but prolonged or repeated falls in blood pressure, which reduce markedly the pO_2 gradient across the placenta. The maintenance of acid-base equilibrium may also be impaired during long labor and by pain-relieving agents. How maternal acidosis jeopardizes the fetus is not clear, but a drop in pH shifts the oxygen dissociation curves in the direction of less available oxygen to the fetus (see Fig. 11, Ch. 7). If they shift at unequal rates, as Hellegers thinks possible, the fetus may well lose an important protective mechanism.

Finally, fetal homeostatic mechanisms, remarkably efficient though they may be, are increasingly less competent during repeated or prolonged stress. In the face of maternal disease or complications of labor, therefore, great care should be exercised in the choice of pain-relieving agents and methods.

ANALGESIA, AMNESIA, AND SEDATION DURING LABOR

The search continues for drugs that singly or in combination produce effective analgesia, amnesia, and sedation during labor, but at the same time are completely safe for the mother and the fetus. Until rather recently, at least, a mainstay of most regimens has been scopolamine, used primarily for its amnesic effects and given in conjunction with narcotic drugs for their analgesic and euphoric effects. Barbiturates in combination with narcotic drugs or with scopolamine have also been widely used in the past.

Scopolamine, narcotics, and barbiturates all possess certain disadvantages. Although scopolamine in appropriate doses causes amnesia, in the presence of pain it is likely to cause varying degrees of restlessness, excitement, and even hallucinations and delirium. Patients so affected create difficult nursing problems and, if not observed closely, may inflict serious injury on themselves and the fetus. Therefore, if scopolamine is to be used, the laboring mother must be closely and continuously observed by a trained labor-room attendant. The narcotic analgesics, in doses comparable to those that produce satisfactory postsurgical analgesia and euphoria, are likely to cause respiratory depression in the newborn, especially the premature, and, in turn, all of the serious problems engendered by hypoxia. These untoward events are most likely to happen when delivery occurs within the hour after injection of the narcotic. The literature is replete with reports describing new compounds that produce excellent maternal analgesia without fetal depression. Unfortunately, in each instance once the aura of newness faded, it became evident that fetal depression closely paralleled maternal analgesia. Barbiturates, although providing sedation, suffer the disadvantages of negligible analgesic action and in larger doses cause disorientation in the mother and respiratory depression in the newborn.

In recent years the ataractic or "tranquilizer" drugs have been widely used in combination with a narcotic, especially meperidine, to produce analgesia and sedation. The "tranquilizer" drugs currently in common use include promethazine (Phenergan), hydroxyzine (Vistaril), and more recently diazepam (Valium). The amounts and the frequency of administration vary for these compounds. When given with meperidine the usual doses intramuscularly are promethazine 25 to no more than 75 mg, hydroxyzine 50 to 100 mg, and diazepam 10 to 15 mg. Friedman and associates, Flowers and co-workers, and Niswander described their experiences with diazepam given intravenously during labor. They noted the drug reduced the amount of meperidine that was necessary. Flowers and co-workers found the respiratory system of the infant not to be depressed, but the neonates were somewhat hypoactive and hypotonic. We have had extensive experience with promethazine and are impressed by its safety in doses of 25 to 50 mg intramuscularly once or twice during labor.

Once labor is established—i.e., the cervix is somewhat effaced and dilating, and the contractions are regular, firm, and cause discomfort—medication with a narcotic drug plus one of the tranquilizer drugs is usually indicated. Some still prefer scopolamine to an ataractic drug, whereas others use both in combination with a narcotic. Meperidine, 50 to 100 mg intramuscularly, may be administered. The smaller dose repeated more frequently usually is more advantageous than 100 mg at intervals of four hours or so. Moreover, if delivery occurs during the next hour or two, the infant will not be so depressed by the drug. The size of the mother should be taken into account in determining the size of the dose. It is not unusual on our large service, for example, to encounter patients as small as 90 pounds and as large as 300 pounds. A more rapid effect is achieved by giving meperidine intravenously, but not more than 50 mg should be injected at one time by this route. Whereas analgesia is maximal about 30 minutes to one hour after intramuscular injection of meperidine, it develops very rapidly when given intravenously. The times for the depressant effect to develop in the fetus and, in turn, the neonate do not lag far behind.

Morphine has been nearly abandoned after a period of popularity in which it was used with scopolamine to produce so-called twilight sleep. The combination produced excellent analgesia and anesthesia but the mother sometimes became quite excited, and even delirious and hallucinated. Moreover, at birth the newborn was apt to demonstrate apnea, which persisted dangerously long.

With a successful program of analgesia, amnesia, and sedation the patient rests quietly between contractions, and although some discomfort is felt at the acme of an effective uterine contraction, the pain is not unbearable. Finally, she does not recall labor as a horrifying experience. Appropriate drug selection and administration should accomplish these objectives for the great majority of laboring women without risk to them or their infants.

Nalorphine (Nalline). This synthetic compound is closely related to morphine. Pharmacologic data published in the early 1940's indicated that in animals it was capable of reducing the respiratory depression produced by morphine and that when given before morphine prevented the depression otherwise induced by the morphine. Several clinical reports indicate that in man, too, nalorphine counteracts the respiratory and circulatory depression caused by morphine, meperidine, Dilaudid, Pantopon, and methadone but is ineffective against barbiturates and general anesthetics. In fact, nalorphine may intensify respiratory depression resulting from nonnarcotic agents.

Apgar states that in two years at the Sloane Hospital there have been only 30 infants in whom the use of the drug seemed justified. It was successful in improving respiration in 75 per cent of them, although it was difficult to attribute the improvement to the drug alone because of the multiple factors in treatment. We agree with Apgar's conclusion that it is wiser to avoid large doses of opiates, rendering the antidote unnecessary.

Lerallorphan (Lorphan) is similar in action to rallorphine but per unit weight is approximately ten times as patent.

General Anesthesia

The placenta is not a barrier to general anesthetics. Without exception all anesthetic agents that depress the central nervous system of the mother cross the placenta and depress the central nervous system of the fetus. Another constant hazard with any general anesthetic is aspiration of gastric contents. Fasting before the time of anesthesia is not always an effective safeguard, since fasting gastric juice, free of particulate matter but strongly acidic can produce fatal aspiration pneumonitis. At many institutions general anesthesia is not induced until delivery can be accomplished immediately so as to minimize transfer of the anesthetic agent to the fetus and, in turn, depression of the newborn. At the same time endotracheal intubation is used routinely to minimize the risk of aspiration. Trained personnel and specialized equipment are mandatory for the safe use of general anesthesia.

Gas Anesthetics

Nitrous Oxide.   Nitrous oxide is the one gas that is commonly used to provide intermittent relief of pain during labor. This agent produces analgesia and altered consciousness but not true anesthesia. The concentration of nitrous oxide mixed with oxygen for analgesia should never exceed 80 per cent. Use of this gas in higher concentrations may result in maternal as well as fetal hypoxia, as shown by Eastman, Adriani, Hustead, and others. Many studies have shown that satisfactory hypalgesia can be obtained with concentrations of 40 to 70 per cent.

When the patient indicates that a uterine contraction has begun, the mask is placed on her face and she is encouraged to take three deep breaths of a 40 to 70 per cent mixture of nitrous oxide in oxygen. Frequently a higher concentration of oxygen and less nitrous oxide will suffice. The use of nitrous oxide in this method may be continued until the head crowns, when the anesthetic may be deepened by adding a little ether, halothone, or cyclopropane to aid in control of the head and for the performance of an episiotomy if necessary. Alternatively local or pudendal nerve block is used.

Nitrous oxide does not prolong labor or interfere with uterine contractions. Van Liere as well as Vasicka and Kretchmer observed little effect of nitrous oxide on the pattern of uterine contractions during the first and second stages of labor. Although satisfactory analgesia can be produced with nitrous oxide, its routine use is impractical from the standpoint of personnel, and it has been largely replaced by other types of analgesia in many institutions. Its greatest weakness is its lack of potency as an anesthetic agent in concentrations compatible with adequate fetal oxygenation.

Cyclopropane. Bourne and also Morgan and his associates have reported extensively on the use of cyclopropane for delivery and cesarean section. It is highly explosive and is always given with a closed system. Three to five per cent concentration in oxygen will produce analgesia, whereas 6 to 8 per cent will produce unconsciousness. Fifteen to twenty-five per cent concentration of the gas will maintain surgical anesthesia. Respiratory failure develops if concentrations reach 30 per cent or more.

Cyclopropane is a good anesthetic for delivery and for cesarean section, especially in cases in which rapid induction with good relaxation is desired. It presents advantages in certain bad-risk cases, particularly with hemorrhage, as in placenta previa and abruptio placentae. In spite of the excess oxygen administered to the mother with this gas, Smith and also Rovenstine and co-workers have shown that low fetal oxygenation sometimes occurs. Resuscitation is required in almost 30 per cent of infants born under this anesthetic. Maternal cardiac irregularities and ventricular fibrillation, furthermore, occasionally result when pituitary extract or vasopressors are used during cyclopropane anesthesia. Certainly, if this combination is used, it should be employed with great caution. Morris and others have shown that the combination of synthetic oxytocin and cyclopropane produces few instances of dysrhythmia, apparently because of the absence of vasopressin.

VOLATILE ANESTHETICS

Of the volatile anesthetics, ether, halothane (Fluothane), trichlorethylene (Trilene), and chloroform merit consideration. These agents cross the placenta readily and are capable of producing narcosis in the fetus. Ether, halothane, and chloroform inhibit uterine contractions. With the exception of trichlorethylene, these compounds are unsuitable for analgesia but sometime are appropriate for anesthesia for delivery or cesarean section.

Ether. In the hands of less experienced anesthetists the margin of safety is usually greater with ether than with any other anesthetic. Administered by the open-drop method with an adequate mixture of air to prevent any possibility of hypoxia, it is a relatively safe anesthetic. With the closed method of administration it is possible to complement or indeed supplement nitrous oxide anesthesia with ether when more relaxation or deeper anesthesia is required. As soon as the need for deeper anesthesia is removed the ether can be discontinued and anesthesia maintained with nitrous oxide plus oxygen. Because of its relative safety for the mother, ether has in the past been used extensively for cesarean section. Cole and Kimball, however, showed a striking increase in perinatal mortality from narcosis in elective cesarean sections done under ether as compared with those under spinal anesthesia. Hellman and others showed a similar higher perinatal mortality in infants delivered by cesarean section under ether anesthesia as compared with those under thiopental sodium (Pentothal). Ether frequently causes vomiting during the induction and recovery, which is often an underlying factor in death from aspiration. It is, moreover, conducive to uterine relaxation and bleeding.

Halothane (Fluothane). This is a potent, nonexplosive agent usually employed with nitrous oxide and oxygen for general anesthesia. It may be used in combination with soda lime, a feature that makes this gas more useful than other nonexplosive, volatile agents. Its place in obstetric anesthesia is still uncertain because of its propensity to produce marked uterine relaxation with subsequent postpartum hemorrhage as well as the possibility that it might cause serious liver damage. Therefore, its use should probably be limited to obstetric problems that require rapid relaxation of the uterus. Sheridan has shown that halothane readily passes the placenta; according to Montgomery, when used for cesarean section, there is greater fetal depression than with thiopental, nitrous oxide, and muscle relaxants.

Trichlorethylene (Trilene). This agent has found favor in Great Britain but has not been widely adopted in the United States despite good reports by Flowers, by Morgan and colleagues, and by others. Several difficulties have been encountered. In the first place, Trilene precludes the subsequent use of inhalation anesthetics requiring soda lime. Second, American women have rather consistently objected to the use of any self-administered method of analgesia such as the Minnitt gas machine or the various devices required to administer trichlorethylene. Third, trichlorethylene seems to prolong the second stage of labor.

Chloroform. Prolonged administration of this drug is occasionally followed by pronounced central necrosis of the hepatic lobules, which may cause death several days after delivery. In addition, there is an immediate danger of cardiac or respiratory arrest during anesthesia. Although chloroform is a superb anesthetic from the viewpoint of the fetus because of the oxygenation that it permits, its dangers have militated against its widespread use; nevertheless, it is employed successfully in a number of clinics. In fact Duncan and associates, as well as Belew and Wulff, have reported large series of deliveries conducted successfully under chloroform anesthesia.

The inhalation of the volatile anesthetics other than nitrous oxide may be contraindicated in the presence of upper respiratory infection. When diabetes and, perhaps, heart disease complicate labor, other methods of pain relief often yield better results. These volatile anesthetic agents are contraindicated in the presence of prematurity or anticipated fetal hypoxia.

Intravenous Anesthesia

Thiopental Sodium (Pentothal). Intravenous thiopental sodium (Pentothal) as an anesthetic agent in obstetrics offers the advantages of ease and extreme rapidity of induction, ample oxygenation, ready controllability, minimal postpartum bleeding, and promptness of recovery without vomiting. The first and last of these advantages make it very popular with patients. Originally, thiopental sodium and other short-acting barbiturates were employed in obstetrics as the sole anesthetic agent, administered intermittently during the entire course of the anesthesia. Very large series of vaginal deliveries and cesarean sections with minimal maternal and fetal complications were cited by Hellman and co-workers, as well as by many others. However, thiopental and similar compounds are poor analgesic agents, and the administration of enough of the drug to maintain anesthesia in the mother may cause appreciable depression of the newborn. The intravenous barbiturates are no longer employed as sole anesthetic agents but are now usually used in small single doses to induce sleep, with nitrous oxide or another analgesic agent in conjunction with a muscle relaxant as the mainstay of the anesthesia. A commonly used technic consists of a single rapid injection of thiopental intravenously, the inhalation of nitrous oxide–oxygen, and the injection of succinylcholine intravenously combined with endotracheal intubation. Intubation allows effective ventilation to be maintained and minimizes the possibility of aspiration of gastric contents.

Barbiturate crosses the placenta with great rapidity, raising the infant's blood level to that of the mother's after two or three minutes. The usual alertness of the infant at birth in these circumstances is difficult to explain without consideration of several other factors. Brand and colleagues have pointed out that blood levels bear little relation to tissue levels of barbiturate or to the depth of anesthesia. The maternal uptake of barbiturate, furthermore, is so rapid that it is incorrect to interpret similar maternal and fetal levels at the end of a given period of time as equilibrium. Much more study of this perplexing problem is needed.

Regional Anesthesia: Sensory Pathways Involved in Obstetric Anesthesia and Analgesia

Analgesia for Labor. Pain in the first stage of labor stems largely from the uterus, the sensory innervation of which is derived primarily from the sympathetic nervous system but also in part from the parasympathetics. The parasympathetic component is represented by the pelvic nerve, which consists of a few fibers derived from the second, third, and fourth sacral nerves. The sympathetic fibers emerge from the uterus, travel through Frankenhäuser's ganglion (posterior cervical) to the pelvic plexus and thence through the hypogastric nerves to the hypogastric plexus. The fibers then travel in the lumbar and lower thoracic sympathetic chains and enter the spinal cord through the white rami communicantes at the level of the eleventh and twelfth dorsal vertebrae. Any method of autonomic block that does not also block the motor pathways to the uterus, which enter the spinal cord at the level of the seventh and eighth thoracic vertebrae, may be used for obstetric analgesia (Fig. 1).

Anesthesia for Delivery. Although painful contractions of the uterus continue during the second stage of labor, most of the pain of delivery is transmitted through the pudenal nerve, the peripheral branches of which provide sensory innervation to the perineum, anus, and much of the vulva and clitoris. The pudendal nerve traverses the lateral wall of the ischiorectal fossa in Alcock's canal and crosses the spines of the ischium on their anterior and inferior surfaces before entering the pelvis through the greater sciatic foramen. The fibers of the pudendal nerve are derived from the ventral branches of the second, third, and fourth sacral nerves. Blocking this nerve at any of several sites with any of the drugs listed in Table 1 renders possible the conduct of painless delivery.

Local Infiltration. This technic is of no value for analgesia during labor but may be employed for either vaginal or abdominal delivery. From the standpoint of safety, local infiltration anesthesia is preeminent. Its advantages were summarized by Greenhill as follows:

1. There is practically no anesthetic mortality.
2. Fetal mortality or hypoxia from direct effect of the anesthetic agent is absent.
3. Simplicity of administration is obvious. It can be administered by the obstetrician and is suitable for home and hospital delivery.
4. Uterine contractions are not impaired.
5. There is no need to hurry through an operation.
6. The toxic effects are minimal.

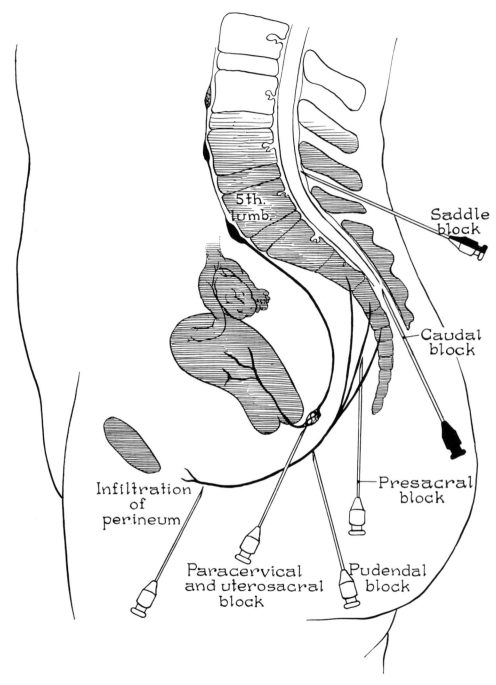

Fig. 1. Schematic diagram of the various methods of blocking obstetric pain.

Table 1. **Locally Acting Anesthetic Drugs**

Concentrations and doses used for local infiltration; paravertebral block of eleventh and twelfth thoracic somatic nerves; paravertebral block of second lumbar sympathetic ganglia; paracervical block; presacral block; and pudendal nerve block.

Chemical Name	Trade Name	Conc. (%)	Maximal Dosage (mg)	Onset of Surgical Analgesia (min)	Duration of Analgesia (hr)
Procaine	Novocain	0.5 to 2.0	1,000	1 to 10	¾–1½
Tetracaine	Pontocaine	0.1 to 0.25	200	1 to 15	2–6
Lidocaine	Xylocaine Lignocaine	0.5 to 2.0	500	1 to 10	1½–2½
Mepivacaine	Carbocaine	0.5 to 2.0	500	1 to 10	1½–2½
Piperocaine	Metycaine	0.5 to 1.5	1,000	1 to 10	1–1½
Hexylcaine	Cyclaine	0.5 to 2.0	500	1 to 10	1¼–2
Chloroprocaine	Nesacaine	0.5 to 2.0	1,000	1 to 10	¾–1
Prilocaine	Citanest	0.5 to 3.0	600	1 to 10	½–3

Modified from Moore. Anesthetic Techniques for Obstetrical Anesthesia and Analgesia. Charles C Thomas.

In spontaneous delivery the patient is placed in lithotomy position, a wheal is made as shown in Figure 2, and the fourchet and the adjoining region are infiltrated with a 5-cm-long No. 20 needle. The injection is made on the right side of the patient, as shown in Figure 2, moving the needle in a fan-shaped manner and following the lower border of the vulva on each side. The anesthesia may be begun when delivery is imminent. If more profound anesthesia is desired, additional wheals may be made at the upper portion of each labium and a line of infiltration directed downward to join the previously infiltrated areas. As a rule, not more than 20 ml of a 1 per cent solution of lidocaine (Xylocaine) should suffice. In using local anesthetic agents a more prolonged action may be obtained if epinephrine is added in a final dilution of between 1:100,000 and 1:200,000.

Transperineal Pudendal Block. In the event of operative delivery, more profound anesthesia may be obtained if the pudendal nerves are blocked. With the patient in lithotomy position, draped and prepared for delivery, bilateral wheals in the skin are made with a hypodermic needle midway between the anus and the tuberosity of the ischium. The index finger of the left hand is inserted into the rectum and the left ischial spine is palpated. A 20-gauge needle, 10 cm long, is passed horizontally through the wheal on the left side to a point just below and beyond the spine (Fig. 2, left side of patient). Injury to the rectum is prevented by the left index finger in the rectum. About 15 ml of solution are injected to anesthetize the internal pudendal nerve. The needle is withdrawn to a point just beneath the skin; the direction is then changed laterally and the needle is inserted directly toward the tuberosity of the ischium until the bone is reached, where 5 ml of solution are injected. The needle is again withdrawn to just beneath the skin, and the labia on the left side are infiltrated. With the right index finger in the rectum the procedure is repeated on the right side. Relaxation of the perineal muscles and anesthesia of the skin of the perineum follow in a few minutes. Since uterine contractions are not impaired, the cooperation of the patient, in voluntary expulsive efforts, may be utilized during the operation. In difficult forceps operations it is sometimes advisable to block the ilioinguinal nerve, which supplies a

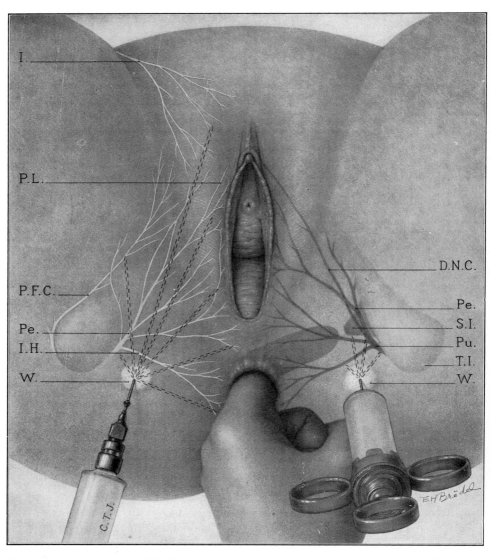

Fig. 2. Technic of local infiltration of the nerves of the female perineum. Superficial and deep innervation is shown on the right and left sides of the patient, respectively. I., Ilioinguinal nerve; P.L., posterior labial nerve; P.F.C., posterior femoral cutaneous nerve, perineal branch; Pe., perineal nerve; I.H., inferior hemorrhoidal nerve; D.N.C., dorsal nerve of clitoris; Pu., pudendal nerve; S.I., spine of ischium; T.I., tuberosity of ischium; W., wheal, intradermal. (From Griffen and Benson. Amer J Obstet Gynec 42:862, 1941.)

few fibers to the anterior portion of the vulva and clitoris. Since the nerve runs directly beneath the fascia along Poupart's ligament, the block is easily effected. **_Transvaginal Pudendal Block_**   The end of the needle is protected by the ball of the index finger and introduced into the vagina until the finger presses against the ischial spine, or, preferably, a tubular director that allows 1.5 cm of a 20- or

22-gauge, 15 cm needle to protrude from its tip is used to guide the needle into position. The needle is advanced just posterior and medial to the tip of the spine (Fig. 3). A submucosal wheal is made and the needle is then advanced until it touches the sacrospinous ligament, which is then infiltrated with 2 or 3 ml of solution. The needle is advanced, and as it pierces the loose areolar tissue behind the ligament, the resistance of the plunger decreases and the fluid flows easily. After aspiration, to guard against intravascular injection, the remainder of the fluid in the syringe is injected in the area. Wilds believes that the transvaginal

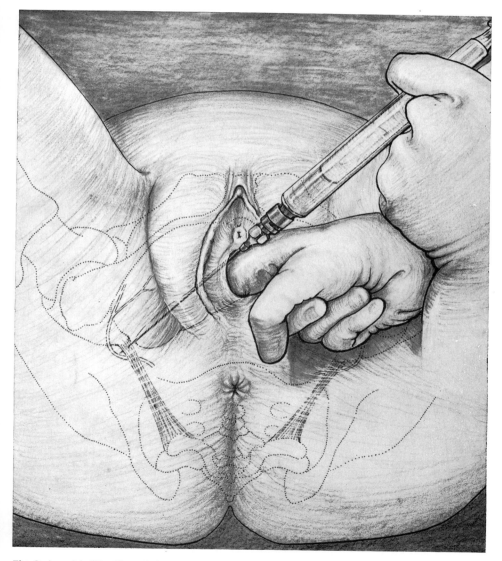

Fig. 3. Local infiltration of the pudendal nerve. Transvaginal technic showing needle passing through the sacrospinous ligament.

route is quicker and simpler than the transperineal route. In our experience the reliability of both has been satisfactory but not outstanding. Considerable experience is required to obtain a high incidence of successful nerve blocks.

With gentleness and care, patients can be delivered by these methods with little pain. In general, local technics of infiltration require larger amounts of anesthetic drugs than do direct regional blocks, but toxic manifestations are uncommon. Rare cases of death have, nevertheless, been reported in sensitive women. The extreme safety to the infant in vaginal delivery is shown in Table 2, based

Table 2. Perinatal Loss Under Local Anesthesia, 1951–1959

	Births	Stillbirths		Neonatal Deaths		Total Loss	
		No.	Per Cent	No.	Per Cent	No.	Per Cent
Premature*	1,793	47	2.62	101	5.62	148	8.24
Mature	13,309	64	0.48	57	0.43	121	0.91
Total	15,102	111	0.74	158	1.05	269	1.79

  * *1,001–2,500 g.*

on experience at the Kings County Hospital.

The few contraindications to the use of local anesthesia include drug sensitivity, apprehension on the part of the patient, and the need for relaxation during the operation.

Parasacral and Paravertebral Block.   Several attempts have been made to apply these technics in obstetrics, but certain disadvantages, particularly the short duration of the anesthesia and the need for multiple injections, have rendered them unsatisfactory. They have therefore been superseded by the continuous caudal and spinal methods.

Paracervical Block.   Sometimes known as uterosacral block, this technic places the anesthetic agent along the base of the broad ligaments and lateral walls of the lower uterine segment, thus blocking the afferent sympathetic pathways from the uterus (Kobak and colleagues). The technic serves best in relieving pain from the uterus during the latter half of labor, but inasmuch as the pudendal nerve is not blocked, additional anesthesia is required for delivery. Since the anesthetic is short-acting, it may have to be repeated.

A tubular director that allows 1.5 cm of a 20-gauge 15 cm needle to protrude from its tip is placed in the lateral vaginal fornix at the three o'clock position. The needle is then passed through the tube and vaginal mucosa (Fig. 4). After aspiration to see whether blood is obtained, 10 to 15 ml of local anesthetic solution are injected. We have found both 1 per cent lidocaine (Xylocaine) or mepivacaine (Carbocaine) to be quite satisfactory. Continuous technics with indwelling plastic catheters have been reported by Burchell and Sadove, as well as by Baggish, and by Tafeen, Freedman, and Harris (Figs. 5 and 6). There are numerous reports concerning this technic, nearly all of them favorable. Gomez, for example, cites his experience with 700 deliveries, in which 97 per cent of the mothers reported substantial relief of pain. The perinatal loss was 0.9 per cent and there were only 17 cases of delayed labor. A similar, although not quite so optimistic, report comes from Cooper and Moir in Great Britain.

Maternal complications, such as allergic or anaphylactic reactions and sacral neuritis, have been reported but are quite rare. All reports indicate a 1 to 20 (with an average of 10) per cent incidence of transitory fetal bradycardia, how-

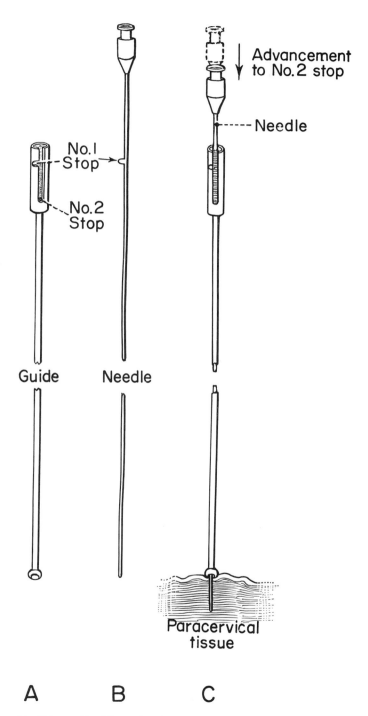

Fig. 4. The guide (A), needle (B), and guide and needle in place (C) for administration of single dose paracervical anesthesia.

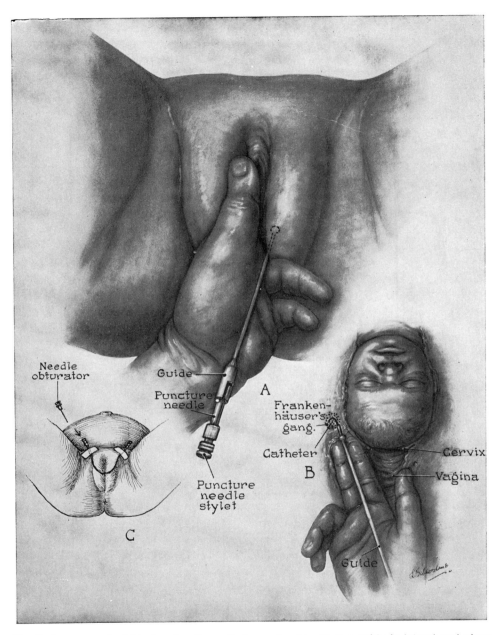

Fig. 5. A, paracervical block using the catheter and guide; B, the guide is lateral and close to the cervix; C, the inlying catheters strapped in place.

ever. Nyirjesy and his associates report death of one infant and 15 instances of low Apgar scores in 68 randomly selected deliveries under paracervical block. The incidence of transient fetal bradycardia was almost 25 per cent, but its cause is not clear. Hellman and co-workers have shown that it results from the action of the anesthetic, for it occurs without the addition of epinephrine, but not if

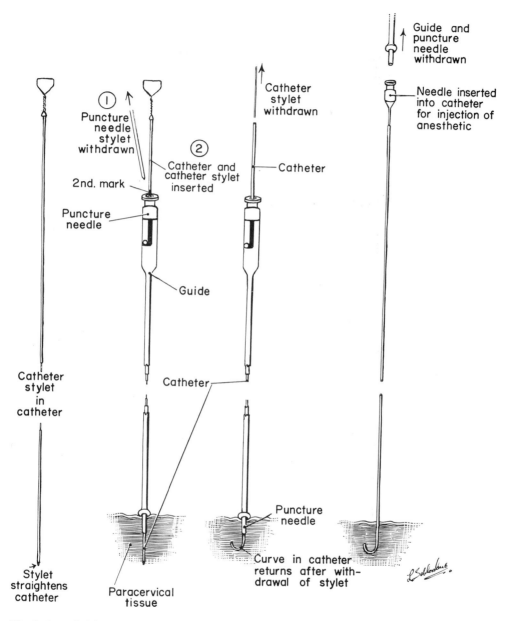

Fig. 5. (cont.). Diagrams showing the insertion of inlying catheters for paracervical analgesia.

physiologic saline alone is injected (Fig. 7). Gordon and others have shown that fetal bradycardia and acidosis are associated with significant fetal blood levels of the anesthetic. The fetal hazards of depression with occasional death associated with paracervical block have been clearly demonstrated by Rosefsky and Petersiel. According to Usubiaga and co-workers, the hazards may be lessened by using procaine rather than mepivacaine. In our experience serious fetal brady-

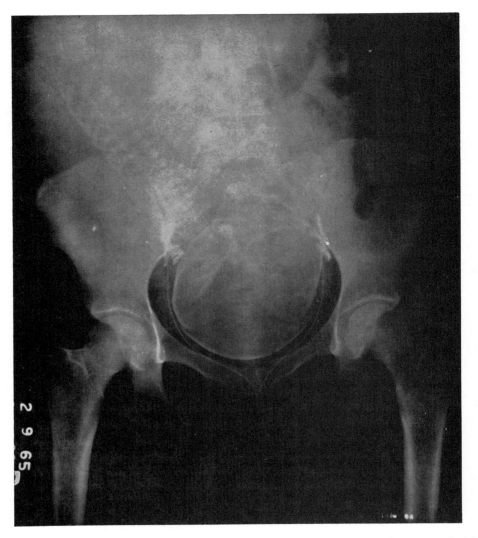

Fig. 6. Plastic catheters in the paracervical space with the injection of radiopaque material to demonstrate the dispersion of local anesthetic solutions in paracervical block. (Courtesy of Drs. C. Tafeen, H. Freedman, and H. Harris.)

cardia occurs quite rarely with the small intermittent dosage of local anesthetics that is used with the continuous technics.

Continuous Caudal Analgesia and Anesthesia.   At the lower end of the sacrum on its posterior surface there is a foramen resulting from the nonclosure of the laminae of the last sacral vertebra. It is screened by a thin layer of fibrous tissue. This foramen, called the sacral hiatus, leads to a space within the sacrum known as the caudal canal or caudal space, which is actually the lowest extent of the bony spinal canal. Through it a rich network of sacral nerves passes downward after having emerged from the dural sac a few inches higher. The dural sac separates the caudal canal below from the spinal cord and its surrounding fluid above.

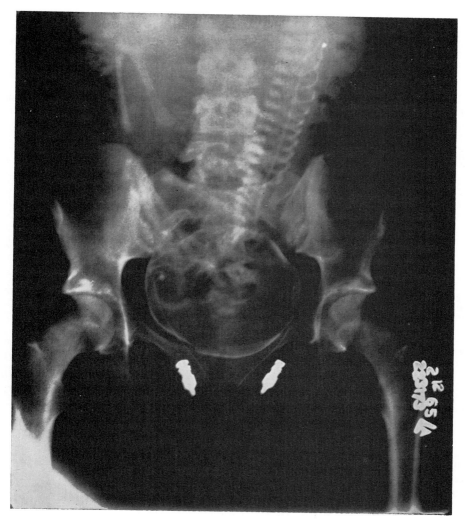

Fig. 6 (cont.). These catheters curl at the tip and are thus retained in place during labor. (Courtesy of Drs. C. Tafeen, H. Freedman, and H. Harris.)

A suitable anesthetic solution (Table 3) that fills the caudal canal may abolish the sensation of pain carried via the sacral nerves and anesthetize the pelvis, producing *caudal anesthesia*. If the procedure is successful the patient experiences no pain whatsoever in labor and is conscious of neither uterine contractions nor perineal distention. The continuous caudal technic provides both analgesia in the first and second stages and anesthesia for delivery.

Caudal anesthesia by the single-dose method is not new in obstetrics. The method never achieved great popularity, however, for several reasons, principal among which are short duration of the anesthesia, accidents resulting from inadvertent insertion of the needle into the spinal canal, and other technical difficulties. Hingson reported satisfactory relief of pain in 92 per cent of 3,000 patients

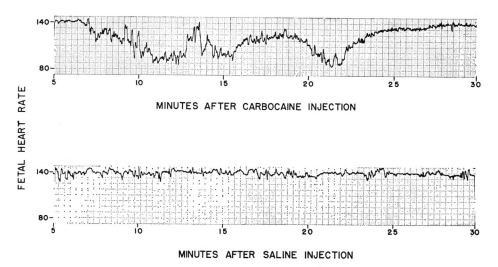

Fig. 7. Fetal bradycardia occurring after the paracervical injection of mepivacaine (Carbocaine) without norepinephrine. Physiologic saline injected into the paracervical area has no effect on the fetal heart rate.

by the continuous caudal technic, the climax of five years of work to improve caudal anesthesia. The importance of Hingson's contribution lay not only in the development of the continuous caudal technic but in the introduction of the principle of the test dose, which precludes the likelihood of introducing large and potentially lethal amounts of anesthetic solution into the spinal canal.

When the patient is in good labor with the cervix at least 3 to 4 cm dilated, she is placed on her side in the Sims position. The sacral and coccygeal areas are prepared with an antiseptic solution. Considerable experience under supervision is necessary for accurate palpation of the sacral hiatus. Once the sacral hiatus has been identified, a small skin wheal is made over the area with an anesthetic solution. Using a slightly longer needle, the solution is carried down and injected into the fascia over the sacral hiatus. A 16-gauge Love-Barker needle or a similar 16-gauge, 3 to 5 inch needle is directed toward the sacral hiatus. It is then depressed and inserted into the canal for a distance of approximately 1 cm. A polyethylene or polyvinyl catheter is then passed

Table 3. **Locally Acting Anesthetic Drugs**

Concentrations and Doses for Caudal Block and Lumbar Epidural Block

Chemical Name	*Trade Name*	*Conc. (%)*	*Maximal Single Dose (mg)*	*Onset of Surgical Analgesia (min)*	*Duration of Analgesia (hr)*
Procaine	Novocaine	2	1,000	8–15	¾–1¼
Piperocaine	Metycaine	1.5	1,000	8–15	¾–1¼
Lidocaine	Xylocaine	1 or 2	500	8–15	1¼–2
	Lignocaine	2			
Mepivacaine	Carbocaine	1 or 2	500	8–15	1¼–2
Chloroprocaine	Nesacaine	2	1,000	8–15	¾–1½

From Moore. Anesthetic Techniques for Obstetrical Anesthesia and Analgesia. Charles C Thomas.

through the needle and into the caudal canal for a distance of 3 to 5 cm. Once the catheter has passed the tip of the needle, care should be taken not to withdraw the catheter lest the end be severed. After placement of the catheter, the 16-gauge needle is withdrawn. The catheter is then attached to one of the closed systems currently in use for the administration of caudal anesthesia. Any of the local anesthetics may be used. The catheter is held in place with adhesive tape. The patient is then permitted free movement. A test dose of 8 ml of one of the anesthetic solutions is injected slowly. After five minutes the patient is tested for spinal anesthesia. If she can move both legs freely and there is no sensory impairment, the caudal is then administered. We commonly use an initial dosage of 22 ml, which with the test dose should produce anesthesia to the umbilicus in about 20 minutes. The dose is repeated as necessary. On the average, it is necessary to administer 20 ml doses every 40 minutes. For a more detailed description of these technics, the reader is referred to the textbook on the subject by Hingson and Hellman.

A summary of the results of 10,000 cases based on the questionnaire of Hingson and Edwards indicates that complete relief of pain may be achieved in 81 per cent of women and partial relief in 12 per cent, with failure in only 7 per cent. There is no question, however, that caudal analgesia impairs the frequency and intensity of uterine contractions. The alteration in uterine contractions is much more common if anesthesia is started very early in labor or if the level is raised to the seventh and eighth thoracic vertebrae. There is prolongation of the second stage, thereby increasing the incidence of forceps delivery. In most instances, however, the head will descend sufficiently to allow simple forceps delivery without danger to mother or child. In two studies carried out in different cities, Hingson compared caudal analgesia with other types of pain relief. In both studies there was a reduction of stillbirths and neonatal mortality rate in the caudal group, not only in term infants but in prematures as well. In the Memphis study, furthermore, there was a diminution in the term and premature neonatal mortality rates in the caudal analgesia group, as compared with a control group to whom no pain relief was administered. In these studies the validity of the control groups may be questioned, but there is little doubt that caudal anesthesia exerts the least possible effect on the baby, *provided the maternal systolic blood pressure does not fall below 100 mm Hg.* It is of particular advantage to the premature infant, since it tends to retard rapid and forceful labor and enables the operator to perform a gentle, controlled delivery. For the healthy mature infant the choice of sedation, general anesthesia, or local infiltration makes less difference. For the infant whose life is endangered by any of a number of obstetric hazards, caudal block presents many advantages. An uncommon complication of the technic is the accidental injection of the anesthetic into the infant's skull. Four such cases have been reported by Finster and associates.

One of the chief problems of caudal anesthesia is the fall in maternal blood pressure. A fall of more than 20 mm has been observed by Hingson in 20 per cent of patients. This hypotension can usually be controlled by prompt action by the physician, particularly the administration of vasopressors or often mere elevation of the patient's legs for a few minutes. The maintenance of anesthesia at or below the level of the umbilicus avoids many of the drops in pressure.

Hingson has reported 43 maternal deaths in the course of 200,000 cases of continuous caudal analgesia; 11 were definitely related to the method. These deaths do not necessarily militate against caudal analgesia but should call attention to the need for experience.

There are several contraindications to this method of analgesia. Infection of the skin over the sacral area, especially an old pilonidal sinus, should preclude its use. For patients who desire to remain asleep during the actual delivery, another form of analgesia is preferable. In prolonged labors caudal anesthesia is contraindicated because it may become troublesome and ineffective after six to eight hours. It should not be employed in the presence of hemorrhage or shock because of its vasodepression. For the same reason it should be used cautiously, if at all, in preeclampsia and eclampsia. Caudal analgesia may be the method of choice in prematurity, cardiac disease, pulmonary disease, or diabetes.

Continuous caudal anesthesia has never been popular abroad and now seems to have fewer exponents in this country, despite the inability to improve upon this form of anesthesia. Hingson has shown quite clearly in the Baltimore study that the acceptance of caudal anesthesia by the patients was exceedingly high. Only 6.6 per cent of 1,529 mothers considered the pain relief unsatisfactory. Similar results have been reported from other clinics where the majority of patients were delivered with this technic and where adequate facilities and personnel were available. The difficulty seems to be that both the success and safety of caudal anesthesia depend on the availability of trained nurses and doctors. There is, furthermore, a definite trend in this country to simplify analgesic technics. Despite the excellent results with certain of the more complicated procedures, most obstetricians feel safer with technically less difficult methods.

Continuous Lumbar Epidural Block for Vaginal Delivery.   With the decline in the use of caudal block in recent years, continuous lumbar epidural analgesia has become increasingly popular. The technic for placement of the epidural catheter is described on page 455. Lumbar epidural block is similar to caudal block but it has several distinct advantages. The approach is technically easier than the insertion of a caudal catheter. The failure rate in expert hands is about 3 per cent, as compared with 5 per cent for caudal.

Small amounts of drug are employed. The segmental control of labor pains is achieved by positioning the patient and by varying the amount of anesthetic used. Early in labor, only the fibers conducting uterine pain need be blocked (T11–T12). As the fetal head descends, the sacral fibers can be blocked as well to provide perineal anesthesia.

As with caudal block, maternal hypotension is the most common and potentially serious complication. The systolic pressure falls below 90 mm Hg in about 5 per cent of parturients (Bonica). The success of this method has been attested in many thousands of deliveries (Eisen and associates, Hellmann, and Kandel and colleagues). If proper technical assistance is provided, continuous epidural analgesia is a superior method of pain relief in obstetrics.

Spinal Anesthesia for Vaginal Delivery.   Low subarachnoid block, with a level below the tenth or twelfth thoracic dermatome, is a most popular method of anesthesia for delivery in the United States today. Nearly all the local anesthetic agents have been used, as shown in Table 4. By the addition of dextrose to the solution of dibucaine (Nupercaine) or similar anesthetic agent, localization and concentration of the drug in the conus of the dural sac are facilitated. Inasmuch as the anesthesia from the single injection is of relatively short duration, it is necessary to time its administration properly, anticipating delivery within approximately an hour of the onset of anesthesia. With the patient in the sitting position, spinal puncture is performed through the fourth lumbar interspace. A short-

Table 4. Technic of Low Subarachnoid Anesthesia with Various Drugs

Drugs	Dose* (mg)	Method of Preparation	Time Sitting Up (seconds)
1. (a) Dibucaine (Nupercaine) (buffered), 1:200 solution	2.5	Draw up 2 ml of 10% dextrose, then 2 ml of Nupercaine. Mix. Discard all but 1 ml.	30
(b) Dibucaine (Nupercaine) (unbuffered), 2.5 mg/ml in 5% dextrose		Draw up 1 ml of prepared solution. Use as such.	
2. Tetracaine (Pontocaine), 1% solution	5	Draw up 2 ml of 10% dextrose, then 2 ml of Pontocaine. Mix. Discard all but 1 ml.	30
3. Procaine (Novocaine) 20% solution	50	Draw up 2 ml of 10% dextrose, then 1 ml of Novocaine. Mix. Discard all but 1 ml.	35

* *The doses cited represent the maximal amounts to be given. Current trends are toward using about two thirds or even half of these doses. For instance, 35 mg of procaine are usually adequate for low forceps, episiotomy, and repair.*
From Andros et al. Amer J Obstet Gynec 55:806, 1948.

beveled 22- to 26-gauge needle is commonly used. When free flow of clear spinal fluid is obtained, a Luer-Lok syringe containing the properly prepared solution is attached to the needle, aspiration of 0.1 ml of spinal fluid is carried out, and solution is rapidly injected. After 10 seconds, the needle is removed, and at exactly the proper time indicated in Table 4 the patient is placed on her back with the upper portion of her body raised. The procedure should be carried out entirely between uterine contractions.

In a review of 2,016 vaginal deliveries under spinal anesthesia with lidocaine (Xylocaine), Phillips and colleagues report excellent relief of pain in 87 per cent, and partial relief in an additional 6 per cent. In only 1 per cent of cases was supplementary anesthesia necessary. Only one patient had any neurologic damage, which, moreover, was but transient with 95 per cent eventual recovery. In 3.3 per cent of patients a fall in blood pressure below 80 mm Hg occurred. Another troublesome complication of spinal anesthesia is headache. Franksson and Gordh indicate that headache results from continued leakage of spinal fluid through the site of puncture in the dura. The leakage can be largely prevented by the use of a small-gauge spinal needle, as evidenced by the low incidence of headache, 0.3 per cent, in Phillips' report.

Low subarachnoid block was first described by Adriani and Roman-Vega and by Parmley and Adriani. In a series of 136 women in whom injection was made when the cervix was 5 to 6 cm dilated, there was complete relief of pain during the remainder of labor and delivery in 81 per cent. A momentary fall in blood pressure, sometimes to as low as 80 mm Hg, occurred in one half the patients; in the other half, lowering of the blood pressure averaged 10 mm Hg. Little or no paralysis of the leg or thigh muscles or of the recti occurred. In general, the regions anesthetized corresponded to the parts of a horseback rider in contact with the saddle. The popular term "saddle block" is thus derived. Certain authorities prefer the designation "low subarachnoid block," however.

ANESTHESIA FOR CESAREAN SECTION

About half of the cesarean sections in the United States are performed electively as repeated procedures. These patients can be adequately prepared for anesthesia and for operation. The other half includes patients with failure of progress of labor, fetal distress, or serious and potentially lethal accidents of pregnancy and labor. Obviously, no single anesthetic agent or technic is safe and effective in such a variety of circumstances. In some, the operation may be performed slowly and deliberately, whereas in others the utmost speed is necessary. The anesthesiologist is faced with patients ranging from the well-prepared patient to the woman in shock, in danger of serious hemorrhage, or with a full stomach. The various technics presented here, if skillfully selected, may obviate most of these difficulties, but the prime desideratum is an experienced, capable anesthesiologist.

Spinal (Subarachnoid) Anesthesia.   The drawbacks of spinal anesthesia for cesarean section are the occasional high levels of neural blockade and the frequent precipitous drops in maternal blood pressure. Were it not for these complications, spinal anesthesia would be ideal for all cesarean sections, except those with hemorrhagic complications and potential shock. Doses of anesthetic drugs that are reasonably safe in surgical patients may lead to extremely high levels of spinal anesthesia in obstetric patients. MacCausland and Holmes have shown that, although the spinal fluid pressure is normal between contractions, it is slightly raised with each contraction. If the patient bears down, the pressure rises to 700 mm of water in about one third of the cases. According to Marx and colleagues and Vasicka and co-workers, the oscillations in pressure of the spinal fluid are caused not primarily by uterine contractions, but by the increased respiratory rate and bearing down that accompany them. In addition, "postural shock" may intensify spinal hypotension.

"Postural shock" is a misnomer for the hypotensive syndrome characterized by sweating, nausea, and tachycardia that occurs to some degree in 50 per cent of women near term when they assume the supine position; it is sometimes called the supine hypotensive syndrome. The condition has been extensively studied by Howard and associates and by Holmes, who believe the cause to be occlusion of the inferior vena cava by the pregnant uterus. More recently Kerr and his colleagues have shown by venograms and pressure measurements that such occlusion is the rule in supine pregnant women near term and that adequate venous return is secured by collateral circulation. Kerr has shown also that, although the cardiac output is diminished, the conscious patient can maintain her blood pressure. Under anesthesia, however, shock may be produced. The important point is that this type of hypotension is immediately relieved by placing the patient on her side.

Hypotension caused by spinal anesthesia must never be allowed to progress in severity or duration but must be controlled at its onset by intravenous hypertensive agents. There are two additional practical methods of preventing these unexpectedly high levels. One is to administer the drug in the smallest volume compatible with safety in a single dose. The other method is to give the drugs intermittently.

The spread of anesthetic drugs in the spinal fluid is related to the volume and specific gravity of diluent, to the method of injection, and to dose. Keeping to a small volume, adequate amounts of drug can be given to ensure successful anesthesia in a high percentage of cases. A suitable single-dose technic is as follows:

1. The patient is placed in the left lateral decubitus position while receiving an infusion of 5 per cent dextrose in water through an 18-gauge needle.

2. The table is adjusted so that the vertebral column is parallel to the floor, usually requiring placement of the patient in approximately five degrees of reverse Trendelenburg. A diminution of the lumbar spinal curvature is then effected by an assistant's holding the patient in complete flexion.

3. The lower back is then prepared with tincture of benzalkonium chloride (Zephiran) and draped in sterile fashion.

4. With a stock solution of 1 per cent procaine and a standard 26-gauge needle on a 2 ml syringe, a skin wheal is raised in the midline over the interspace between the third and fourth lumbar vertebrae.

5. Using a 22-gauge needle and the same syringe, the interspace is then infiltrated with the 1 per cent procaine to the depth of the ligamentum flavum.

6. A second injection with a 22-gauge 1¾-inch needle is then made through the original skin wheal and directed laterally into the paravertebral muscle group for the administration of 10 to 15 mg of methamphetamine hydrochloride (Methedrine) as a vasopressor agent.

7. A midline intrathecal puncture is then made with a 26-gauge 3-inch spinal needle with the bevel directed downward. Seven mg of tetracaine (Pontocaine) in a solution containing 10 per cent glucose are now administered in a steady stream with constant pressure in the absence of a uterine contraction.

8. The spinal needle is removed and the patient is immediately placed in the supine position. The desirable level of anesthesia, at T8, is obtained by manipulation of the table above or below the horizontal plane. Since fixation of the anesthetic agent occurs within 20 minutes, deep Trendelenburg is not advised before this time. During the period of fixation, blood pressure and pulse recordings should be made at frequent intervals, preferably every two minutes. A vasopressor agent in the form of 0.001 per cent phenylephrine hydrochloride (Neo-synephrine) solution (10 mg or 1 ml of 1 per cent phenylephrine HCl in 1,000 ml of 5 per cent dextrose in water) is kept immediately available to combat hypotension.

The continuous technic for preventing high levels is as follows:

With the patient lying on her side, a Tuohy needle is inserted into the second or third lumbar interspace and passed into the spinal canal. Once the flow of clear fluid is obtained, a small plastic catheter is passed through the needle 2 to 3 cm downward in the canal. The catheter is taped in place, and 15 to 25 mg of procaine or 10 to 25 mg of piperocaine (Metycaine) are injected slowly. Five-minute blood pressure readings should be obtained. If the systolic pressure remains at 100 mm Hg, the operator may proceed with small additional doses as necessary. When the level of anesthesia has reached approximately the area of the costal margin, the patient is ready for operation. Repeated small doses of the anesthetic agent will usually be necessary. An intravenous infusion of 0.1 per cent thiopental sodium (Pentothal) in glucose will maintain the patient in slight euphoria without producing any deleterious effect upon the fetus.

Intermittent Lumbar Epidural Block. To avoid the danger of high spinal anesthesia and to preclude the possibility of postspinal headache, epidural block has been recommended. Although caudal block has been successfully employed for cesarean section, the level of anesthesia is too uncertain to merit its extensive

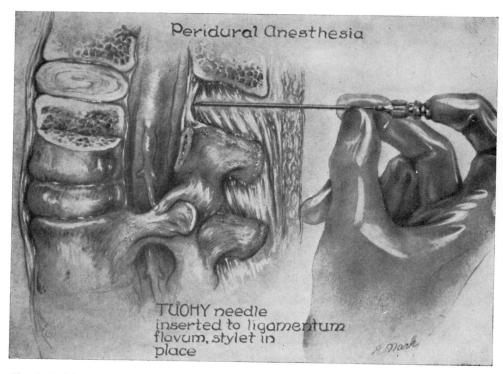

Fig. 8. Peridural anesthesia. Insertion of needle to ligamentum flavum. (From Pitkin. Conduction Anesthesia, 2nd ed. J. B. Lippincott Co.)

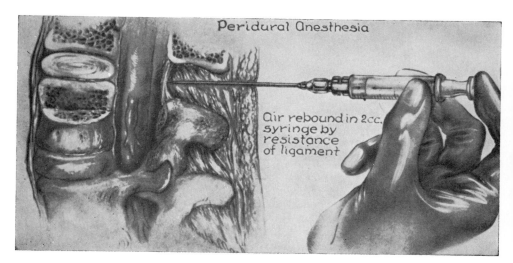

Fig. 9. Peridural anesthesia: air-rebound technic. When the bevel of the needle rests against the ligamentum flavum, air cannot be injected with ease. (From Pitkin. Conduction Anesthesia, 2nd ed. J. B. Lippincott Co.)

use. The recommended technic for epidural block is not more difficult than the method used for continuous caudal analgesia. The patient is placed on her left side, with shoulders parallel and legs partially flexed. No attempt is made to keep the spinal column convex, since that position reduces the peridural space and stretches the dura, rendering it more susceptible to puncture. If the interspaces of the patient are small, the sitting position is most advantageous.

The back is cleaned and draped as for a spinal puncture. The skin, the interspinous ligament, and the ligamentum flavum are successively infiltrated with the same anesthetic solution that is used for the continuous block. A 16-gauge Tuohy spinal needle is introduced into any of the lumbar interspaces. The needle is blunted, but has a sharp stylet in place to facilitate piercing the skin, subcutaneous tissue, and interspinous ligament. The site chosen is frequently the lumbar area, since the largest peridural spaces are found there. The needle should be placed directly into the center of the interspace without anterior or posterior deviation. The needle should engage the ligamentum flavum, which is the most important landmark for a peridural injection; unless the needle pierces the middle of the ligamentum flavum, the center of the peridural space will not be entered, and a catheter cannot be passed with ease. When the dense ligamentum flavum has been entered, after a pause, the ease with which 2 cc of air are introduced with a small syringe is tested. When an attempt is made to inject air into the ligamentum flavum, the plunger of the syringe rebounds quickly.

This "air-rebound" method for ascertaining the depth of insertion of the needle for peridural anesthesia is regarded by some anesthetists as the most reliable sign. The essential features are illustrated in Figures 8 and 9. The needle is inserted, guided by palpation into an interspace until the blunt bevel impinges on the ligamentum flavum. The location is then verified by injection of a small amount of air. If the needle is situated properly on the ligament, as shown in the figures, there is rebound of the plunger of the syringe, and the depth of the needle at the ligament is reasonably certain; its advancement approximately another millimeter results in entry into the extradural space. Air may then be injected with ease (Figs. 10 and 11), and no cerebrospinal fluid can be aspirated.

When air is injected into the peridural space, however, the plunger of the syringe actually falls into place. As the needle is advanced through the ligamentum flavum, frequent minute "air tests" are made with a small syringe to ascertain when the negative pressure in the peridural space is encountered. Entrance into the peridural space is often evidenced by the release of resistance as the blunt 16-gauge Tuohy needle passes through the dense ligamentum flavum.

When the Tuohy needle has been properly placed and no spinal fluid is aspirated, a plastic catheter is introduced through the needle into the peridural space. The catheter is directed either cephalad or caudad, depending upon the somatic segments involved in transmitting the painful impulses. The plastic catheter passes as easily into the peridural space as it does into the caudal canal. Its passage sometimes elicits a distinct hyperesthetic response in the leg, hip, or back, if the soft tip of the catheter touches a nerve in the peridural space. Indications of proper placement of the catheter in the peridural space include the following:

1. The ease with which air can be injected through the Tuohy needle after the ligamentum flavum has been penetrated.

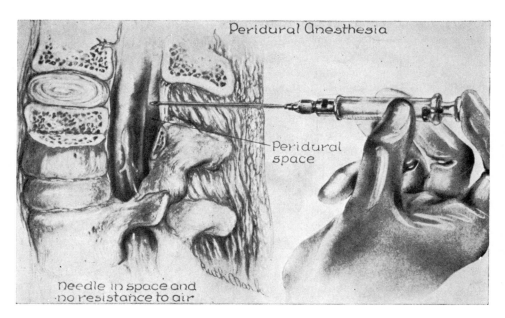

Fig. 10. Peridural anesthesia: air-rebound technic. When the needle has entered the extradural space, air can be injected with ease. (From Pitkin. Conduction Anesthesia, 2nd ed. J. B. Lippincott Co.)

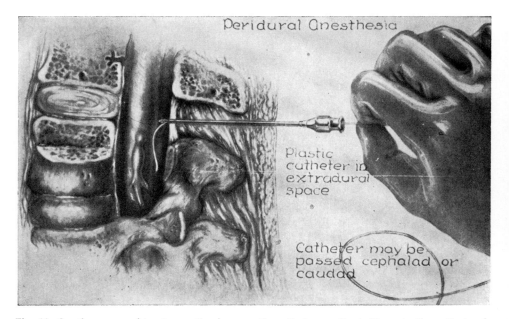

Fig. 11. Continuous peridural anesthesia: puastic-catheter method. The plastic catheter is passed through the needle and advanced into the extradural space. (From Pitkin. Conduction Anesthesia, 2nd ed. J. B. Lippincott Co.)

2. Hyperesthesia upon passage of the catheter into the peridural space in the absence of spinal fluid.
3. Easy passage of the catheter either up or down the peridural space in the absence of spinal fluid.
4. Absence of somatic anesthesia following a test with a dose of 2 ml of anesthetic agent to rule out spinal anesthesia.
5. Prompt somatic anesthesia after one 10 ml dose of anesthetic maintained one to two hours with short-acting agents.

Notwithstanding these signs of a proper placement of the catheter and needle, there are two safeguards of the utmost importance. The first is the use of two test doses of 2 ml of 1.5 per cent piperocaine (Metycaine), 1 per cent lidocaine (Xylocaine), 2 per cent procaine, or 0.15 per cent tetracaine (Pontocaine) five minutes apart to ensure absolutely the absence of spinal anesthesia. Either of these two test doses will produce safe low spinal anesthesia if the catheter is in the subarachnoid space but will not produce anesthesia if the solution enters the peridural space, as intended. The second safeguard is the ready availability of oxygen, vasopressors, and intravenous fluids.

Epidural block carries some of the dangers of subarachnoid block, particularly hypotension. It requires greater anesthesiologic skill, takes longer to initiate, and produces a less definite block. In spite of these objections, Bodell, Tisdall, and Ansbro, as well as many others, continue to find epidural block satisfactory. In Bodell's series of 800 cesarean sections, he obtained excellent anesthesia in all but 2 to 3 per cent. The mothers experienced no postanesthetic headaches and no neurologic sequelae, nor were any infants lost because of the anesthetic.

Both Stenger and associates and Ward and co-workers have demonstrated significant physiologic differences between subarachnoid and epidural block that indicate an advantage for the latter in cesarean section. The combined results of these two groups of investigators show less profound and less rapid falls in blood pressure with epidural block. In contradistinction to the sequelae of subarachnoid anesthesia, neither bradycardia nor reduction in cardiac output accompanied hypotension with epidural block. These differences should benefit the fetus.

Inhalation Anesthesia.　　Nitrous oxide and cyclopropane are the two common gaseous anesthetics. One of the safest and most satisfactory ways to employ nitrous oxide, especially for patients with little premedication and those in labor, is to supplement the gas with thiopental and a muscle relaxant. According to Cohen, sleep is induced with thiopental, and after intubation the anesthesia is maintained with light nitrous oxide–oxygen and muscle relaxant. In our experience, this method provides for rapid induction, and none of the anesthetic components is used in sufficient concentration to depress the fetus appreciably.

The most commonly employed muscle relaxants in obstetrics are *d*-tubocurarine (curare) and succinylcholine (Anectine, Quelicin). Although there is generally no need for such drugs in vaginal delivery, they are of inestimable value in cesarean section, during which relaxation may be increased without deepening the anesthetic, and smaller amounts of narcotizing drugs may be sufficient. The muscle relaxants do not affect smooth muscle, nor do they pass the placenta in sufficient quantity to affect the fetus (Pittinger and Morris). Moya has shown that after a single large dose of 300 mg of succinylcholine to the mother, small amounts of the drug are found in the umbilical vein, but these levels are too low to cause muscular relaxation in the fetus. Stenger and colleagues measured the maternal oxygen, carbon dioxide, pH, lactate, pyruvate, and glucose before opening the uterus and the comparable values in the infant's umbilical cord vessels after birth. Although they found marked variations, the mean results were compatible with their findings under conduction anesthesia. They cited the absence of hypotension as an advantage.

In cases of shock or potentially serious hemorrhage, as in abruptio placentae or placenta previa, nitrous oxide–oxygen plus succinylcholine or cyclopropane is probably the anesthetic agent of choice. Cyclopropane crosses the placenta, and after about ten minutes of anesthesia, the concentration in the baby's blood may be as high as 60 to 80 percent of that of the mother. Such levels may depress the newborn infant, rendering cyclopropane a less desirable agent. Stenger and associates mention an increased maternal arterial blood pressure and pO_2 and an unchanged pCO_2 as a measure of safety with this method.

Local Infiltration of the Abdominal Wall.   Two general principles must be followed to achieve success with this technic. First, extreme gentleness is essential in handling tissues; any manipulation that entails tugging on the peritoneum or uterine ligaments is particularly painful. Second, minute attention to detail in the injection of the anesthetic solution is necessary.

The solution most commonly employed is 1 per cent procaine. The amount required is about 100 ml. To prevent overly rapid absorption, 0.5 ml of a 1:1,000 solution of epinephrine is added to 100 ml of the procaine solution. The first step in the technic is production of an intradermal wheal in the lower midline of the abdomen after all other preparations have been made for cesarean section. The skin is then infiltrated from the umbilicus to the suprapubic region. Injection in a fan-shaped manner of the upper angle and particularly of the lower angle above the symphysis is important. It is well, at this point, to infiltrate the fascia on either side for several centimeters lateral to the incision. The parietal peritoneum is carefully infiltrated and incised. An alternate and equally satisfactory procedure is fascial infiltration up and down the lateral border of the rectus muscles. By blocking the nerves before they give off their terminal branches, these injections anesthetize the whole thickness of the abdominal wall from the skin to the perioneum, inclusive. The skin incision should be extensive enough to avoid retraction of the deeper margins of the incision. The uterine serosa may also be injected before the uterus is opened, especially the peritoneal reflection in low cervical sections. Morphine (15 mg) and scopolamine (0.4 mg) given hypodermically ten minutes before the baby is delivered add to the patient's comfort. Less anesthetic solution is required, and a more profound block of the abdominal wall may be obtained by the following technic: The tenth, eleventh, and twelfth intercostal nerves on each side are blocked with 3 to 5 ml of anesthetic solution just posterior to the lateral cutaneous branches. Blocking the ilioinguinal nerve point medial to the anterior superior spine of the pelvis adds to the efficacy of the block. Occasionally, slight infiltration of the skin makes the anesthesia more effective. For details of this procedure the reader is referred to Pitkin's *Conduction Anesthesia*.

Abdominal Decompression

In 1959, Heyns introduced a plastic shield that produced negative pressure when applied to the abdomen of the parturient. He claimed that the device reduced the pain and duration of labor and increased the oxygenation of the fetus, thus producing infants with high IQ's. These claims have not been substantiated. Castellanos and colleagues were unable to show that the decompression apparatus relieved the pains of labor. Liddicoat, in a controlled study, was unable to find a difference in intelligence quotients between children born to mothers who used the apparatus and those who did not.

Psychologic Methods of Pain Relief

Moderate interest in the psychologic methods of pain relief in labor has been maintained over the past two decades. Factual information is not easily elicited from the vast number of publications, many quite unscientific and far from dispassionate. Spiegel, a psychiatrist, and Gross and Posner have attempted to approach the subject in logical perspective. According to Gross, all the psychologic methods have as their common goal the elevation of the threshold of pain through physical and mental relaxation. These methods fall into five groups: (1) the Read method of "natural childbirth" (Buxton); (2) the psychoprophylactic method, based on the conditioning principles of Pavlov and advocated by Nicolaev in Russia; (3) the autogenous training of Schultz in Germany; (4) Lamaze's "l'accouchement sans douleur" in Belgium and France; and (5) hypnotic training by Kroger and others in the United States.

Pregnant women, especially those in labor with the accompanying anxiety, fear, and pain, represent uniquely circumscribed experiments of nature, particularly responsive to suggestive technics that alter the state of awareness. Most good obstetricians recognize this phenomenon intuitively, and each in his own way supports and conditions his patients to meet the situation. Such psychologic therapy by any other name is equally effective, and the widely varying technics of its application make little difference in the final result. In ordinary circumstances, about 60 per cent of women can go through labor with psychologic assistance and a minimum of pain-relieving drugs in a manner satisfactory to both them and their obstetricians. In the course of training, many of the psychologic methods contribute to the education for motherhood, a clearly desirable objective.

As Spiegel points out, it is doubtful that hypnosis or any other psychologic method is harmful to normal pregnant women in good mental health. For the emotionally abnormal woman, pregnancy and childbirth themselves are often traumatic. The psychiatrically unskilled or imperceptive obstetrician, whether employing psychologic methods of pain relief or analgesic drugs, is more than likely to compound the trauma. The crucial point is that pregnancy presents a unique situation in which the obstetrician and psychiatrist can work together to expand vastly, by both clinical and experimental methods, the present state of knowledge of psychic relief of stress.

Summary

It is evident that no single method is entirely satisfactory for the alleviation of pain during labor. At the same time there has been an increasing demand by the laity for relief of suffering associated with childbirth. Such relief of pain is desirable, provided it carries no danger to mother or child. The prime desideratum must remain safety.

Anesthesia is playing an increasing role in maternal mortality. It is the decisive factor in 5 per cent of such deaths and a contributing cause in another 5 per cent. Aspiration of vomitus with inhalation anesthesia and unusually high levels with spinal are the prime offenders. These deaths are doubly tragic insofar as they are largely preventable in the hands of experienced personnel who choose their anesthetics wisely.

A satisfactory physician-patient relationship will often enable the obstetrician to carry his patient for some time during the early stages of labor without pain-relieving agents. When well administered, all methods and most drugs yield between 85 and 90 per cent satisfactory results. Most well-trained obstetricians will attain the same rate of success with whatever method they choose. These sobering facts should lead to reduction of excessive doses of all drugs.

References

Adriani, J.   The Pharmacology of Anesthetic Drugs, 4th ed. Springfield, Ill., Charles C Thomas, 1960.
——— and Roman-Vega, D. A.   Saddle block anesthesia. Amer J Surg 71:12, 1946.
Andros, G. J., Dieckmann, W. J., Ouda, P., Priddle, H. D., Smitter, R. C., and Bryan, W. M. Spinal (saddle block) anesthesia in obstetrics. Amer J Obstet Gynec 55:806, 1948.
Apgar, V.   Anesthesia for Obstetrics, in Hingson, R. A. and Hellman, L. M. (eds.). Philadelphia, Lippincott, 1956.
——— Burns, J. J., Brodie, B. B., and Papper, E. M.   The transmission of meperidine across the human placenta. Amer J Obstet Gynec 64:1368, 1952.
——— Holaday, D. A., James, L. S., Prince, C. E., Weisbrot, I. M., and Weiss, I.   Comparison of regional and general anesthesia in obstetrics with special reference to transmission of cyclopropane across the placenta. JAMA 165:2155, 1957.
Baggish, M. S.   Continuous paracervical block. Amer J Obstet Gynec 88:968, 1964.
Batterman, R. C., and Himmelsbach, C. K.   Demerol—new synthetic analgesia; review of its present status and comparison with morphine. JAMA 122:222, 1943.
Belew, J. E., and Wulff, G. J.   Chloroform anesthesia for delivery. Obstet Gynec 16:372, 1960.
Benson, C., and Benson, R. C.   Hydroxyzine—meperidine analgesia and neonatal response. Amer J Obstet Gynec 84:37, 1962.
Bodell, B., Tisdall, L. H., and Ansbro, F. P.   Epidural anesthesia for cesarean section. A report of 800 cases. Anesth Analg 41:453, 1962.
Bonica, J. J.   Principles and Practice of Obstetric Analgesia and Anesthesia. Philadelphia, F. A. Davis Co., 1967, Vol. 1.
Bourne, A. W.   Cyclopropane anaesthesia in obstetrics. Lancet 2:20, 1934.
Brand, L., Mazzia, V. D., Van Poznak, A., Burns, J. J., and Mark, L. C.   Lack of correlation between electroencephalographic effects and plasma concentration of thiopentone. Brit J Anaesth 33:92, 1961.
Burchell, R. C., and Sadove, M. S.   Continuous paracervical block in obstetrics. Obstet Gynec 23:112, 1964.
Buxton, C. L.   A Study of the Psychoprophylactic Methods of the Relief of Childbirth Pain. Philadelphia, W. B. Saunders Co., 1962.
Castellanos, R., Aguero, O., and deSoto, E.   Abdominal decompression. A method of obstetric analgesia. Amer J Obstet Gynec 100:924, 1968.
Cohen, E. N.   Thiopental-curare-nitrous oxide anesthesia for cesarean section, 1950 to 1960. Anesth Analg 41:122, 1962.
Cole, W.C.C., and Kimball, D. M.   Relationship of maternal ether anesthesia to inauguration of fetal respiration. Nebraska Med J 28:200, 1943.
Cooper, K., and Moir, J. C.   Paracervical nerve block. A simple method of pain relief in labour. Brit Med J 1:1372, 1963.
Duncan, C., Hindman, J. F., and Mayberger, H. W.   Chloroform as an obstetrical anesthetic. A report of 18,302 cases. Amer J Obstet Gynec 72:1004, 1956.
Eastman, N. J.   Fetal blood studies: the role of anesthesia in the production of asphyxia neonatorum. Amer J Obstet Gynec 31:563, 1936.
Eckenhoff, J. E., Hoffman, G. L., and Funderberg, L. W.   N-allylnormorphine: an antagonist to neonatal narcosis produced by sedation of the parturient. Amer J Obstet Gynec 65:1269, 1953.

Edwards, G., Morton, H. J. V., Pask, E. A., and Wylie, W. D.   Deaths associated with anaesthesia—report on 1,000 cases. Anesthesia 11:194, 1956.

Eisen, S. M., Rosen, N., Winesanker, H., Hellmann, K., Axelrod, H. I., Rotenberg, M., Relle, A., and Sheffman, E.   The routine use of lumbar epidural anesthesia in obstetrics: A clinical review of 9,532 cases. Canad Anaesth Soc J 7:280, 1960.

Finster, M., Poppers, P. J., Sinclair, J. C., Morishima, H. O., and Daniel, S. S.   Accidental intoxication of the fetus with local anesthetic drug during caudal anesthesia. Amer J Obstet Gynec 92:922, 1965.

Flowers, C. E.   Trilene, an adjunct to obstetrical anesthesia and analgesia. Amer J Obstet Gynec 65:1027, 1953.

——— Rudolph, A. J., and Desmond M. M.   Diazepam (Valium) as an adjunct in obstetric analgesia. Obstet Gynec 34:68, 1969.

Franksson, C., and Gordh, T.   Headache after spinal anesthesia and technique for lessening its frequency. Acta Chir Scandinav 94:443, 1946.

Freidman, E. A., Niswander, K. R., and Sachtleben, M. R.   Effect of diazepam on labor. Obstet Gynec 34:82, 1969.

Gomez, D. F.   Hazards of paracervical block: Letter to the editors. Amer J Obstet Gynec 88:1099, 1964.

Gordon, H.   Fetal bradycardia after paracervical block. Correlation with fetal and maternal blood levels of local anesthetic (Mepivacaine). New Eng J Med 279:910, 1968.

Greenhill, J. P.   Use of local infiltration anesthesia in obstetrics and gynecology. S Clin N Amer 23:143, 1943.

Griffen, E. L., and Benson, R. C.   Gynecologic surgery under local anesthesia. Amer J Obstet Gynec 42:862, 1941.

Gross, H. N., and Posner, N. A.   An evaluation of hypnosis for obstetric delivery. Amer J Obstet Gynec 87:912, 1963.

Hellman, L. M.   Electronics in obstetrics and gynecology. J Obstet Gynaec Brit Comm 72:896, 1965.

——— and Hingson, R. A.   Continuous peridural anesthesia and analgesia for labor, delivery and cesarean section. Anesth Analg 28:181, 1949.

——— and Hingson, R. A.   The effect of various methods of obstetric pain relief on infant mortality. New York J Med 53:2767, 1953.

——— Shettles, L. B., Manahan, C. P., and Eastman, N. J.   Sodium pentothal anesthesia in obstetrics. Amer J Obstet Gynec 48:851, 1944.

Hellmann, K.   Epidural anaesthesia in obstetrics: a second look at 26,127 cases. Canad Anaesth Soc J 12:398, 1965.

Heyns, O. S.   Abdominal decompression in the first stage of labour. J Obstet Gynaec Brit Emp 66:220, 1959.

Hingson, R. A.   Contraindications and cautions in the use of continuous caudal analgesia. Amer J Obstet Gynec 47:718, 1944.

——— and Edwards, W. B.   Continuous caudal analgesia in obstetrics. JAMA 121:225, 1943.

——— and Hellman, L. M.   Eight thousand parturients evaluate drugs, techniques, and doctors during labor and delivery. Amer J Obstet Gynec 68:262, 1954.

——— and Hellman, L. M.   Anesthesia for Obstetrics. Philadelphia, Lippincott, 1956.

Holmes, F.   Incidence of the supine hypotensive syndrome in late pregnancy. A clinical study in 500 subjects. J Obstet Gynaec Brit Emp 67:254, 1960.

Howard, B. K., Goodson, J. M., and Mengert, W. F.   Supine hypotensive syndrome in late pregnancy. Obstet Gynec 1:371, 1953.

Hustead, R. F.   Nitrous oxide in obstetrics. Clin Anesth 1:97, 1964.

James, L. S.   The effect of pain relief for labor and delivery on the fetus and newborn. Anesthesiology 21:405, 1960.

Kandel, P. F., Spoerel, W. E., and Kinch, R. A.   Continuous epidural analgesia for labour and delivery: review of 1000 cases. Canad Med Ass J 95:947, 1966.

Kerr, M. G., Scott, D. B., and Samuel, E.   Studies of the inferior vena cava in late pregnancy. Brit Med J 1:532, 1964.

——— The mechanical effects of the gravid uterus in late pregnancy. J Obstet Gynaec Brit Comm 72:513, 1965.

Kobak, A. J., Sadove, M. S., and Mazeros, W. T.   Anatomic studies of transvaginal regional anesthesia, roentgenographic visualization of neural pathways. Obstet Gynec 19:302, 1962.

Kroger, W. S., and Freed, C. Psychosomatic Gynecology. Los Angeles, Wilshire Book Co., 1962.

Lamaze, F., and Vellay, P. Psychologic Analgesia in Obstetrics. New York, Pergamon Press, 1957.

Liddicoat, R. The effects of maternal antenatal decompression treatment on infant mental development. S Afr Med J 42:203, 1968.

MacCausland, A. M., and Holmes, F. Spinal fluid pressures during labor. Western J Surg 65:220, 1957.

Marx, G. F., Zemalis, M. T., and Orkin, L. R. Cerebrospinal fluid pressures during labor and obstetrical anesthesia. Anesthesiology 22:348, 1961.

Montgomery, J. B. The effect of halothane on the newborn infant delivered by caesarean section. Brit J Anaesth 33: 156, 1961.

Moore, D. C. Anesthesia Techniques for Obstetrical Anesthesia and Analgesia. Springfield, Ill. Charles C Thomas, 1964.

Morgan, H. S., Cole, F., and Gorthey, R. Trichlorethylene in obstetrics. Nebraska M J 38:119, 1953.

Morris, L. E., Noltensmeyer, M. H., and White, J. M. Epinephrine induced cardiac irregularities in the dog. Anesthesiology 14:153, 1953.

———— Thornton, M. J., and Harris, J. W. Comparison of the effect of pituitrin, pitocin and ergonovine on cardiac rhythm during cyclopropane anesthesia for parturition. Amer J Obstet Gynec 63:171, 1952.

Moya, F. Considerations in maternal and placental physiology. Anesth Analg 42:661, 1963.

———— and Kvisselgaard, N. Placental transmission of succinylcholine. Anesthesiology 22:1, 1961.

———— and Thorndike, V. Passage of drugs across the placenta. Amer J Obstet Gynec 84:1778, 1962.

———— and Thorndike, V. The effects of drugs used in labor on the fetus and newborn. Clin Pharmacol Ther 4:628, 1963.

Nikolaev, A. P. (Current status and perspectives of labor anesthesia in USSR). Vestn Akad Med Nauk SSSR 16:64, 1961.

Niswander, K. R. Effect of diazepam on mepiridine requirements of patients during labor. Obstet Gynec 34:62, 1969.

Nyirjesy, I., Hawks, B. L., Herbert, J. E., Hopwood, H. G., and Falls, H. C. Hazards of the use of paracervical block anesthesia in obstetrics. Amer J Obstet Gynec 87:231, 1963.

Parmley, R. T., and Adriani, J. Saddle block anesthesia with Nupercaine in obstetrics. Amer J Obstet Gynec 52:636, 1946.

Phillips, O. C., Nelson, A. T., Lyons, W. B., Graff, T. D., Harris, L. C., and Frazier, T. M. Spinal anesthesia for vaginal delivery. A review of 2016 cases using xylocaine. Obstet Gynec 13:437, 1959.

Pitkin, G. P. Conduction Anesthesia, 2nd ed. Philadelphia, Lippincott, 1953.

Pittinger, C. B., and Morris, L. E. Placental transmission of d-tubocurarine chloride from maternal to fetal circulation in dogs. Anesthesiology 14:238, 1953.

Rodgers, C. D., Wickard, C. P., and McCaskill, M. R. Labor and delivery without terminal anesthesia. A report on the use of chlorpromazine. Obstet Gynec 17:92, 1961.

Roman-Vega, D. A., and Adriani, J. Spinal for cesarean section. New Orleans M & S J 20:449, 1950.

Rosefsky, J. B., and Petersiel, M. E. Perinatal deaths associated with mepivacaine paracervical-block anesthesia in labor. New Eng J Med 278:530, 1968.

Rovenstein, E. A., Adriana, J., and Studdiford, W. E. Gas changes in maternal and fetal blood during cyclopropane obstetric anesthesia. California and West Med 53:59, 1940.

Schultz, J. H., and Luthe, W. Autogenic Training. New York, Grune & Stratton, 1959.

Schumann, W. R. Demerol (S-140) and scopolamine in labor. A study of 1,000 cases. Amer J Obstet Gynec 47:93, 1944.

Sheridan, C. A., and Robson, J. G. Fluothane in obstetrical anaesthesia. Canad Anaesth Soc J 4:365, 1959.

Shnider, S. M., Asling, J. H., Margolis, A. J., Way, E. L., and Wilkinson, G. R. High fetal blood levels of mepivacaine and fetal bradycardia. New Eng J Med 279:947, 1968.

Smith, C. A. Effect of obstetrical anesthesia upon the oxygenation of maternal and fetal blood with particular reference to cyclopropane. Surg Gynec Obstet 69:584, 1939.

―――― and Barker, R. H. Ether in blood of the newborn infant; quantitative study. Amer J Obstet Gynec 43:763, 1942.

Spiegel, H. Current perspectives on hypnosis in obstetrics. New York J Med 63:2933, 1963.

Stenger, V., Andersen, T., Eitzman, D., and Prystowsky, H. Extradural anesthesia for cesarean section: Physiologic and biochemical observations. Obstet Gynec 25:802, 1965.

―――― Andersen, T. W., Eitzman, D. V., Blechner, J. N., and Prystowsky, H. Cyclopropane anesthesia. Physiologic and biochemical effects in human pregnancy. Amer J Obstet Gynec 96:201, 1966.

―――― Blechner, J. N., Andersen, T. W., Eitzman, D. V., Cestaric, E., and Prystowsky, H. Observations on pentothal, nitrous oxide, and succinylcholine anesthesia at cesarean section. Amer J Obstet Gynec 99:690, 1967.

Tafeen, C. H., Freedman, H. L., and Harris, H. A system of continuous paracervical block anesthesia. Amer J Obstet Gynec 94:854, 1966.

―――― Freedman, H. L., and Harris, H. Combined continuous paracervical and continuous pudendal nerve block anesthesia in labor. Amer J Obstet Gynec 100:55, 1968.

Usubiaga, J. E., LaIuppa, M., Moya, F., Wikinski, J. A., and Velazco, R. Passage of procaine hydrochloride and para-aminobenzoic acid across the human placenta. Amer J Obstet Gynec 100:918, 1968.

Van Liere, E. J., Bell, W. E., Mazzocco, T. R., and Northup, D. W. Mechanism of action of nitrous oxide, ether, and chloroform on the uterus. Amer J Obstet Gynec 90:811, 1964.

Vasicka, A., and Kretchmer, H. Effect of conduction and inhalation anesthesia on uterine contractions. Experimental study of the influence of anesthesia on intra-amniotic pressures. Amer J Obstet Gynec 82:600, 1961.

―――― Kretchmer, H., and Lawas, F. Cerebrospinal fluid pressures during labor. Amer J Obstet Gynec 84:206, 1962.

Ward, R. J., Bonica, J. J., Freund, F. G., Akamatsu, T., Danziger, F., and Englesson, S. Epidural and subarachnoid anesthesia. JAMA 191:275, 1965.

Waters, R. M. Chloroform. A Study after 100 Years. Madison, University of Wisconsin Press, 1951.

Wilds, P. L. Transvaginal pudendal-nerve block. An improved anatomic approach. Obstet Gynec 8:385, 1956.

Wolff, H. G., Hardy, J. D., and Goodell, H. Measurement of effect on pain threshold of acetylsalicylic acid. J Clin Invest 20:63, 1941.

18

THE PUERPERIUM

The puerperium is the period of a few weeks that starts immediately after delivery and is completed when the reproductive tract has returned to the normal nonpregnant condition. Although the changes occurring during this period are physiologic, in few, if any, other circumstances are there such marked and rapid catabolic events in the absence of disease.

ANATOMIC CHANGES IN THE PUERPERIUM

Involution of the Uterus. Immediately after expulsion of the placenta, the apex of the contracted corpus of the uterus is about midway between the umbilicus and symphysis, or slightly higher. It consists of a mass of tissue containing a flattened cavity with anterior and posterior walls in close apposition, each measuring 4 to 5 cm in thickness. Because its vessels are compressed by the contracted myometrium the puerperal uterus on section appears anemic, as contrasted with the purplish pregnant organ. During the next two days the uterus remains approximately the same size, and then atrophies so rapidly that by the tenth day it has descended into the cavity of the true pelvis and can no longer be felt above the symphysis. It regains its usual nonpregnant size after five or six weeks. The rapidity of the process is remarkable; the freshly delivered uterus weighs about 1,000 g; one week later it weighs 500 g, decreasing at the end of the second week to 300 g; and at the end of the puerperium it weighs less than 100 g. This rapid decrease in size is called *involution.* It was formerly believed that the myometrial cells underwent fatty degeneration during involution and that a large number of them completely disappeared. It is now known that the total number of muscle cells does not decrease greatly, but the individual cells decrease markedly in size. The mechanism by which the individual muscle cell divests itself of excess cytoplasm, including contractile protein, remains to be elucidated. The involution of the connective tissue framework occurs equally rapidly (Woessner).

Since the separation of the placenta and its membranes occurs in the spongy layer of the decidua, a portion of the decidua remains in the uterus. It presents striking variations in thickness, an irregular jagged appearance, and marked infiltration with blood, especially at the placental site.

465

Within two or three days after labor the portion of decidua remaining in the uterus becomes differentiated into two layers. The superficial layer becomes necrotic, whereas the layer adjacent to the myometrium does not. The former is cast off in the lochia, and the latter, which contains the fundi of the uterine glands, is the source of new endometrium. The epithelium arises from proliferation of the endometrial glandular remnants and the stroma from the interglandular connective tissue. The process of regeneration is rapid except at the placental site.

Elsewhere the free surface becomes covered by epithelium within a week or ten days, and the entire endometrium is restored by the end of the third week. Sharman, in an extensive histologic study of postpartum uteri, found that the endometrium in 626 biopsies was proliferative in 473 (147 in lactating women) and secretory in 153 (18 in lactating women). The earliest presumptive evidence of ovulation was the secretory endometrial pattern obtained on the forty-fourth day; in 7 other nonlactating women there were also secretory endometrial specimens in the seventh week. Fully restored endometrium was seen in all specimens examined histologically from the sixteenth day onward. The endometrium was normal except for occasional hyalinized decidual remnants and leukocytes. The so-called endometritis in the reparative days of the puerperium is but part of the normal process of repair of tissues and is not pathologic.

Involution of the Placental Site.   According to Williams, extrusion of the placental site takes up to six weeks. This process is of great clinical importance, for when it is defective *late puerperal* hemorrhage ensues.

Within a short time after delivery the placental site is reduced to an irregular, nodular, elevated area about the size of the palm of the hand. It rapidly decreases in size, measuring 3 to 4 cm in diameter at the end of the second week and only 1 to 2 cm at the completion of the puerperium. Very soon after the termination of labor the placental site consists of many thrombosed vascular sinusoids (Fig. 1). These thrombosed vessels undergo typical organization of the thrombus with invasion by fibroblasts, and eventual recanalization of some of the vessels with much smaller lumens. If involution of the placental site comprised only these events, each pregnancy would leave a fibrous scar in the endometrium, thus eventually limiting the number of future pregnancies. In his classic investigations Williams explained involution of the placental site as follows:

It is not effected by absorption in situ, but rather by a process of exfoliation which is in great part brought about by the undermining of the placental site by the growth of endometrial tissue. This is effected partly by extension and down growth of endometrium from the margins of the placental site and partly by the development of endometrial tissue from the glands and stroma left in the depths of the decidua basalis after the separation of the placenta. . . . Such a process of exfoliation should be regarded as very conservative, and as a wise provision on the part of nature; otherwise great difficulty might be experienced in getting rid of the obliterated arteries and organized thrombi which, if they remained in situ, would soon convert a considerable part of the mucosa into a mass of scar tissue with the result that after a few pregnancies it would no longer be possible for it to go through its usual cycle of changes, and the reproductive career would come to an untimely end.

Anderson and Davis, on the basis of their recent studies of involution of the placental site, differ from Williams in one detail. They conclude that exfoliation of the placental site is brought about as the consequence of a necrotic slough of

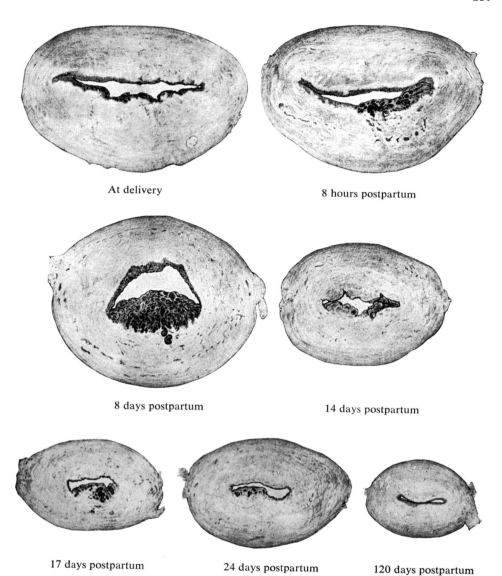

At delivery
8 hours postpartum

8 days postpartum
14 days postpartum

17 days postpartum
24 days postpartum
120 days postpartum

Fig. 1. Involution of the placental site. (From Williams. Amer J Obstet Gynec 22:664, 1931.)

infarcted superficial tissues followed by a reparative process not unlike that which takes place on any denuded epithelium-covered structure.

Changes in the Uterine Vessels. Since the pregnant uterus requires a much more abundant blood supply than does the nonpregnant organ, after delivery the lumens of its arteries must undergo a corresponding diminution in caliber. Formerly a compensatory endarteritis that disappeared in subsequent pregnancies was invoked as an explanation. Today, however, the prevailing belief is that the larger vessels are completely obliterated by hyaline changes and that new and smaller vessels develop in their place. The resorption of the hyaline is accomplished by processes similar to those observed in the ovaries, although the changes may persist for years, affording, under the microscope, a ready means of differentiating between the uteri of parous women and nulliparas.

Changes in the Cervix, Vagina, and Vaginal Outlet. Immediately after the completion of the third stage the cervix and lower uterine segment are collapsed, flabby structures. The margins that correspond to the external os are usually marked by depressions indicating lacerations. The cervical opening contracts slowly. For the few days immediately after labor it readily admits two fingers, but by the end of the first week it has become so narrow as to render difficult the introduction of one finger.

At the completion of involution, the external os does not resume its pregravid appearance completely. It remains somewhat wider, and lateral depressions at the site of lacerations remain as permanent changes that characterize the parous cervix.

The vagina and vaginal outlet in the first part of the puerperium form a capacious smooth-walled passage that gradually diminishes in size but rarely returns to the nulliparous condition. The rugae begin to reappear about the third week. The hymen is represented by several small tags of tissue, which during cicatrization are converted into the myrtiform caruncles characteristic of parous women.

Changes in the Peritoneum and Abdominal Wall. For the first few days after labor the peritoneum covering the lower part of the uterus forms folds, which soon disappear. The broad and round ligaments are much more lax than in the nonpregnant condition, and they require considerable time to recover from the stretching and loosening to which they have been subjected.

As a result of the rupture of the elastic fibers of the skin and the prolonged distention caused by the enlarged pregnant uterus, the abdominal walls remain soft and flabby for a while. The return to normal of these structures requires at least six weeks. Except for silvery striae, the abdominal wall resumes its normal appearance, but when the muscles are atonic, it may remain lax. There may be a marked separation, or *diastasis of the rectus muscles;* in that condition part of the abdominal wall is formed simply by peritoneum, thinned-out fascia, subcutaneous fat, and skin.

Changes in the Urinary Tract. Cystoscopic examination soon after delivery shows not only edema and hyperemia of the bladder wall but frequently submucous extravasation of blood. In addition, the puerperal bladder has an increased capacity and a relative insensitivity to intravesical fluid pressure. As a result, overdistention, incomplete emptying, and residual urine must be watched for closely. The paralyzing effect of anesthesia, especially conduction anesthesia, and the temporarily disturbed neural function of the bladder are undoubtedly contributory factors. Residual urine and bacteriuria in a traumatized bladder create optimal conditions for the development of urinary tract infection. After delivery the dilated ureters and renal pelves return to normal within four weeks. The stretching and dilatation do not continue long enough to cause permanent changes in the ureters unless infection has supervened.

Anatomy of the Breasts and Lactation. Each breast is made up of from 15 to 24 lobes, which are arranged more or less radially and separated from one another by a varying amount of fat. Each lobe consists of several lobules, which in turn are made up of large numbers of acini. The acini have a single layer of epithelium beneath which is a small amount of connective tissue richly supplied with capillaries. Every lobule is provided with a small duct, which joins others to form a single larger canal for each lobe. These so-called *lactiferous ducts* make their way to the nipple and open separately upon its surface, where they may be distinguished as minute isolated orifices. The acinar epithelium forms the various constituents of the milk (Figs. 2 and 3).

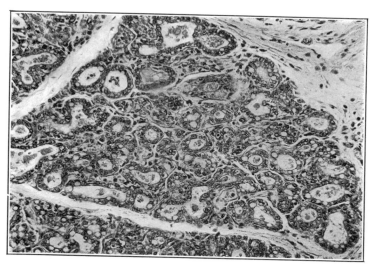

Fig. 2. Section of breast in late pregnancy. The lobules are large and the acinar cells contain fat droplets. (From Bell. Textbook of Pathology. Lea & Febiger.)

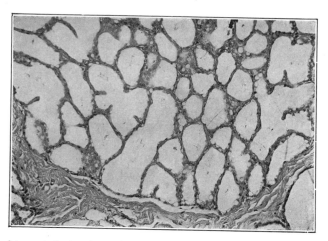

Fig. 3. Section of breast during lactation. The acini are distended and the cells are filled with fat. (From Bell. Textbook of Pathology. Lea & Febiger.)

The condition of the breasts during pregnancy is maintained for approximately the first two days after labor. At this time they do not contain milk, but a small amount of colostrum can be expressed from the nipples. Compared with the mature milk that is ultimately secreted by the breasts, colostrum contains more protein, much of which is globulin, and more minerals, but less sugar and fat. Colostrum, nevertheless, contains rather large fat globules in so-called *colostrum corpuscles,* which are thought by some to be epithelial cells that have undergone fatty degeneration and by others to be mononuclear phagocytes containing considerable fat. The secretion of colostrum persists for about a week, after which time gradual conversion to mature milk occurs. Antibodies are readily demonstrable in colostrum; IgA may offer protection against enteric infection.

Since mammary development and formation of milk in women rarely lend themselves to the experimental approach, knowledge of the physiology of the breast in pregnancy and the puerperium is limited. The alveolar cells, after completion of growth, begin to secrete about the middle of pregnancy. Progesterone, estrogen, and chorionic somatomammotropin produced by the placenta during pregnancy stimulate mammary growth. Estrogen promotes development of the ductal system, and progesterone, the alveolar system. Chorionic somatomammotropin, which has lactogenic properties, has been called "human placental lactogen." With the delivery of the placenta there is an abrupt decrease in the levels of estrogen, progesterone, and chorionic somatomammotropin. The withdrawal of these hormones coupled with the release of prolactin from the pituitary serves to initiate lactation during the early puerperium. The intensity and the duration of lactation in otherwise normal circumstances are controlled in large part by the stimulus of nursing. The precise humoral and neural mechanisms involved are complex.

The neurohypophysis secretes oxytocin, which stimulates the expression of milk from a lactating breast by causing contraction of myoepithelial cells in the alveoli and the small milk ducts. This mechanism has been utilized to assay oxytocin activity in biologic fluids (Ch. 6, p. 419). This ejection, or "letting" down, of milk is a reflex initiated especially by suckling, which stimulates the neurohypophysis to liberate oxytocin. The reflex in cows may be initiated by the sounds or actions associated with milking, such as the banging of milk pails in the dairy barn, and in women by the cry of their infants. The reflex may be inhibited by fright or stress. Successful lactation in cases of diabetes insipidus suggests that an intact posterior pituitary is not absolutely necessary for lactation in women. Prolactin activity, however, is essential; for example, women with extensive pituitary necrosis, as in Sheehan's disease, do not lactate (Ch. 33, p. 955).

Milk. On the second to fourth day after labor the breasts become larger, firmer, and more painful, indicating the onset of lacteal secretion. On pressure a small amount of bluish milk can be expressed from the nipples. Coincidentally the patient may experience lassitude and headache. At the same time she may have throbbing pains in the breasts and axillae. There is seldom any elevation of temperature. It was formerly believed that the establishment of the flow of milk could cause marked constitutional disturbances, including so-called *milk fever.* A rise of temperature, however, at this time is nearly always indicative of infection.

Nursing. The ideal food for the newborn child is the milk of the mother. In most instances, even though the supply of milk at first appears insufficient, it becomes adequate if suckling is continued. Nursing also exerts a beneficial effect upon the involution of the uterus, since repeated stimulation of the nipples through release of oxytocin from the neurohypophysis leads to stimulation of the myometrium.

Most drugs given to the mother are secreted in the milk. The list includes antibiotics, sulfonamides, most alkaloids, salicylates, bromides, quinine, alcohol, and several of the cathartics that are absorbed from the mother's intestinal tract. Unless large doses are administered or therapy is continued for a long period of time, the content of drugs in the milk in itself is generally not harmful to the infant. Recent concern has been expressed over the content of the pesticide DDT in both human and bovine milk.

Complications involving the breast are discussed in Chapter 35 (p. 993).

CLINICAL ASPECTS OF THE PUERPERIUM

Postpartum Chill. It was formerly common for the patient to have more or less violent chills shortly after the completion of the third stage of labor. Presumably because of better care during labor, these chills are rarely seen today.

Temperature. Occasionally the mother's temperature may become slightly elevated toward the end of a difficult labor, but rarely above 100.4°F (38°C); it most often falls to normal within 24 hours and does not rise again. A higher temperature during labor usually indicates intrapartum infection. Because *slight* rises of temperature occur frequently during the puerperium without apparent cause, it is customary to designate as normal all puerperas in whom the temperature remains below 100.4°F (38°C). For the purpose of ascertaining the frequency of puerperal morbidity, a puerperium is defined as febrile when the temperature exceeds 100.4°F (38°C) in any *two* 24-hour periods, excluding only the first 24 hours postpartum. This definition of maternal morbidity is of value only when the temperature is accurately recorded every four hours throughout the day and evening. In most instances recording the mother's temperature can be omitted during the night so that she can enjoy an otherwise uninterrupted sleep.

Breast engorgement on the third or fourth day of the puerperium was once thought to be accompanied by a rise in temperature. This so-called milk fever was regarded as normal. Although no such entity is recognized today, on rare occasions perhaps, extreme vascular and lymphatic engorgement may cause a sharp peak of fever for a few hours; it never lasts longer than 12 hours at the most, however. In general, any rise of temperature in the puerperium suggests an infection of the genitourinary tract.

Pulse. During the puerperium the pulse may be somewhat slower than at other times, averaging between 60 and 70. In nervous women, however, and in those who have had difficult labors or have lost considerable blood, a more rapid rate is not infrequent. In certain patients, however, a day or two after birth of the child the pulse becomes unusually slow, sometimes falling to 50 or 40, or even lower. Ordinarily the phenomenon is transient, the pulse attaining its normal rate by the end of the first week or 10 days. The slow pulse is usually regarded as a favorable prognostic sign, whereas tachycardia suggests disease. The slow pulse may result from a reduction in cardiac output without a concomitant reduction in stroke volume; the decrease in cardiac output, therefore, is accomplished by a fall in rate, which, in turn, may be related to the marked fall in blood flow through the placental site and relative hypervolemia.

Afterpains. In primiparas the puerperal uterus tends to remain tonically contracted unless blood clots, fragments of placenta, or other foreign bodies are retained in its cavity, causing active contractions in an effort to expel them. In multiparas, the uterus often contracts and relaxes at intervals, the contractions giving rise to painful sensations that are known as "afterpains" and that occasionally are sufficiently severe to require an analgesic. In some patients they may last for days. They are particularly noticeable when the child is put to the breast, presumably because of the release of oxytocin. Ordinarily, however, they decrease in intensity and become quite mild after the 48 hours immediately following delivery.

Lochia.   During the first part of the puerperium there is normally a variable amount of vaginal discharge, the lochia. For the first few days after delivery it consists of blood-stained fluid, *lochia rubra;* after three or four days it becomes paler, *lochia serosa;* and after the tenth day, because of a marked admixture with leukocytes, it assumes a whitish or yellowish white color, *lochia alba.* It has a peculiar fleshy odor suggesting fresh blood. Foul-smelling lochia indicates infection.

Adams and Flowers measured the lochia of 120 women during the first five and a half days after delivery. During this period the lochial weight in nursing and nonnursing women averaged 251 and 277 g, respectively. Similar patients also received 0.2 mg of methylergonovine maleate (Methergine) orally every four hours for the first three days after delivery. There was no appreciable difference in the amount of lochia between the women who received methylergonovine maleate and those who did not; the morbidity rates during the puerperium were the same, and the height of the fundus was identical in both the treated and untreated groups. The only real observed difference related to the patient's discomfort. Those who received the drug suffered much more from uterine cramping. These investigators concluded that the routine use of such medication is unwarranted. Newton and Bradford have similarly concluded that after the immediate period following delivery the routine administration of intramuscular oxytocin to normal women is of no value in decreasing blood loss or hastening involution of the uterus.

In many instances a reddish color in the lochia is maintained for a longer period; when it persists for more than two weeks, however, it indicates the retention of small portions of the placenta or imperfect involution of the placental site. Microscopically, the lochia during the first few days consists of red blood corpuscles, leukocytes, epithelial cells, shreds of degenerated decidua, and bacteria. Microorganisms can always be demonstrated in the vaginal lochia and are present in most cases when the discharge has been obtained from the uterine cavity. In uterine cultures carried out in normal afebrile puerperas three days postpartum, Douglas and Rhees obtained sterile specimens from only one fifth. The pathogen most frequently found was the anaerobic streptococcus, which was demonstrated in one half of the cultures. Similar results have been obtained at the Johns Hopkins Hospital by Guilbeau, Schaub, and Andrews, who obtained uterine cultures from normal afebrile puerperas from 36 to 72 hours postpartum; sterile cultures were obtained in only 6 per cent of the cases. The anaerobic streptococcus was present in 81 per cent. The coliform bacteria, various anaerobic gram-negative bacilli, staphyloccocci, and clostridia are also encountered occasionally.

Urine.   One of the most striking phenomena of the puerperium is the diuresis that regularly occurs between the second and fifth days. Normal pregnancy is associated with an increase in extracellular water of 2 to 3 liters; the puerperal diuresis supposedly represents a reversal of this process. In preeclampsia both retention of fluid and puerperal diuresis may be greatly increased (Ch. 26, p. 713).

Occasionally substantial amounts of sugar may be found in the urine during the first weeks of the puerperium. The sugar is lactose, which fortunately is non-reducing in test systems using glucose oxidase.

Acetone is markedly increased in the urine immediately after labor. It is greatest after difficult and prolonged labor, but disappears within the next three days.

Blood. A rather marked leukocytosis occurs during and after labor, the leukocyte count sometimes reaching levels as high as 30,000 per mm^3 (Ch. 8, p. 255). The increase is made up predominantly of granulocytes. There is a relative lymphopenia and an absolute eosinopenia.

During the first few days after delivery the hemoglobin, hematocrit, and red blood cell count may vary considerably. In general, however, if they fall much below the level present just before or during early labor, the patient has lost a considerable amount of blood. By one week after delivery the blood volume has returned to near the usual nonpregnant level.

The pregnancy-induced changes in blood coagulation factors persist for variable periods of time after delivery. The elevation of plasma fibrinogen is maintained at least through the first week of the puerperium. As a consequence, the elevated sedimentation rate normally found during much of pregnancy remains high during the early part of the puerperium.

Loss of Weight. In addition to the loss of about 12 pounds as the consequence of evacuation of the contents of the uterus, there is generally further loss of body weight during the puerperium of about 5 pounds. This weight loss is accounted for by fluid lost chiefly through urination and by sweating, which at times may be profuse even though the woman is afebrile. Chesley and co-workers have demonstrated a decrease in the sucrose and sodium spaces of about 2 liters, or nearly 5 pounds, during the first week after delivery.

CARE OF THE PATIENT DURING THE PUERPERIUM

Attention Immediately After Labor. After delivery of the placenta the uterus should be hard and round with its upper margin below the umbilicus. As long as it remains in this condition there is no danger of postpartum hemorrhage from uterine atony. To guard against such an occurrence the uterus should be gently palpated through the abdominal wall immediately after the conclusion of the third stage and the maneuver repeated at frequent intervals. If its size and consistency remain unaltered it should be left alone; but if any relaxation is detected, the uterus should be gently massaged through the abdominal walls until it remains contracted; at the same time an oxytocic agent should be administered.

Even in normal cases, the physician should remain in constant attendance for at least one hour after completion of the third stage. If at the end of that period the uterus remains satisfactorily contracted, he may safely leave. If the uterus is still relaxed, contractions should be stimulated by appropriate measures and the behavior of the organ carefully observed until the physician is sure that all danger of hemorrhage has passed. Occasionally a wait of several hours is required. Blood may accumulate within the uterus without external evidence of bleeding. This condition may be detected early by the frequent palpation of the fundus at regular intervals during the first few hours postpartum.

Care of the Vulva.   Shortly after completion of the third stage of labor and perineal repair, the drapings and soiled linen beneath the patient are removed, provided there is no excessive bleeding or other reason to keep the patient in the lithotomy position. The external genitalia and buttocks are then bathed with soap and water or a mild antiseptic solution. A sterile vulvar pad is then applied over the genitalia, held in place by a T-bandage, and replaced by a clean pad whenever necessary. The number of pads required in 24 hours varies according to the amount of lochial discharge and affords a means of estimating its quantity. After each bowel movement and before any local treatment or examination the external genitalia should be cleansed.

Binder.   An abdominal binder is unnecessary, although it was formerly believed to aid involution and help restore the patient's figure. It is now the consensus that it has no effect on involution. If, however, the abdomen is unusually flabby or pendulous or if the patient feels more comfortable with the binder, it may be applied for the first week of the puerperium. In these circumstances an ordinary girdle is often more satisfactory than the usual abdominal binder.

Afterpains.   Afterpains occur less frequently in primiparas than in multiparas. After the delivery of a multiparous patient it is often necessary to prescribe codeine or aspirin at intervals during the first few days of the puerperium if the pains are severe. Not infrequently the uterine contractions are accentuated during nursing, giving rise to an increase in symptoms at this time.

Early Ambulation.   Important changes have taken place in the management of the puerperium in the direction of early ambulation. It is now the general custom to allow normal patients out of bed within the first 24 hours postpartum. The many advantages of early ambulation are confirmed by numerous well-controlled studies. Patients state that they feel better and stronger after early ambulation. Bladder complications and constipation are less frequent. Early ambulation has reduced materially the frequency of thrombosis and pulmonary embolism during the puerperium.

Diet.   It was formerly customary to restrict the diet of the puerperal woman, but at present a liberal diet is recommended. If at the end of one hour after delivery there are no complications that are likely to necessitate another anesthetic, she should be given something to drink and, if hungry, something to eat. During the puerperium the appetite is usually normal, and the diet should be well-balanced and attractive. The intake of fluids should be neither restricted nor markedly increased. The diet of the lactating mother, compared with that consumed during pregnancy, should be increased somewhat, especially in calories and protein, as recommended by the Food and Nutrition Board of the National Research Council (Ch. 12, Table 1). If the mother does not breast-feed the infant her dietary requirements are the same as for a normal nonpregnant woman.

Urination.   Every effort should be made to induce patients to void within four hours after delivery. They should void at least 100 ml normally. If within the first eight hours after delivery the patient does not void 100 ml at any one time, she should be catheterized. If there is any suspicion that the bladder is distended, catheterization may be required earlier. Routine catheterization should be continued every eight hours unless the patient is able to void 100 ml or more at a time, and only then may it be discontinued. Patients who are receiving or have recently received intravenous fluids are very likely to develop a full bladder. They should be watched especially in this regard and treated accordingly. Moreover, patients who have had analgesia in labor and especially those who had conduction anesthesia for delivery may not be aware that the bladder is full and should be observed with particular care.

Bowels.   In view of the sluggishness of the bowels in the puerperium a mild cathartic should be administered on the evening of the second day, unless a bowel movement has previously occurred spontaneously. If the bowels have not moved by the morning of the third day, an enema may be employed. With early ambulation, constipation has become less of a problem in the puerperium.

Care of the Nipples.   The nipples require little attention in the puerperium other than cleanliness and attention to fissures. Since dried milk is likely to accumulate and irritate the nipples, cleansing of the areolae with water and soap before each nursing is desirable. Sore nipples are a frequent complaint. They are best treated with tincture of benzoin or one of the commercial compounds. Occasionally it is necessary to resort to a nipple shield for 24 hours.

Reappearance of Menstruation.   If the woman does not nurse her child, the menstrual flow will probably return within six to eight weeks after labor. The flow ordinarily does not appear so long as the child is nursed, however. The greatest possible variations are observed in this respect, for in lactating women the first period may occur as early as the second, or as late as the eighteenth, month after delivery; the most common time, however, is during the third to fourth month.

Sharman noted that at three months after childbirth menstrual function had returned in 91 per cent of the nonlactating primiparas, whereas only one third of the lactating primiparas had menstruated. In lactating multiparas, however, there is a greater tendency for menstruation to reestablish itself within three months. The bleeding may occur in an ovulatory or an anovulatory cycle. Sharman, by means of histologic dating of the endometrium, identified ovulation as early as 42 days after delivery.

In a study of normal lactating women who were amenorrheic, Udesky found that almost all had failed to ovulate. In women who continue to menstruate during lactation, the suppression of ovulation is much less complete. In the lactating women who were menstruating, Udesky observed an incidence of ovulation of 28 per cent after three or more periods.

Although it is often stated that amenorrhea during the period of lactation results from lack of ovarian stimulation by the pituitary gland, the pituitary-ovarian interrelation during this period is not well understood. Keettel and Bradbury noted very low pituitary gonadotropic activity, as anticipated, in the urine of some lactating women with amenorrhea. Much more frequently, however, they detected normal or even elevated amounts of gonadotropin in the urine, indicating that the absent or very limited estrogenic effect on the vaginal epithelium, as well as the amenorrhea and anovulation, resulted from the failure of the ovaries to respond to the gonadotropin. In this group of patients the ovaries must have been temporarily refractory to the stimulus of the gonadotropin.

Because of the absence of ovulation in a high percentage of cases, lactation confers a substantial degree of infertility, especially as long as it is associated with amenorrhea. Among 500 pregnancies studied by Gioiosa, pregnancy occurred during lactation in 9 per cent. In the great majority, the pregnancy occurred during the last few months of breast-feeding, or when weaning was taking place.

Time of Discharge.   In careful studies of early hospital discharge Hellman and associates, as well as Theobald, found no harm to either mother or babies released from the hospital within 72 hours postpartum. Puerperal women are usually up and about shortly after the birth of their children and consequently see no reason for further hospitalization. Moreover, the increase in the prevalence of antibiotic-resistant organisms militates against keeping well babies and well mothers in institutions. Finally, the cost of prolonged hospitalization has for many families become prohibitive.

Follow-up Examination.   The normal patient, who is having no difficulties during the puerperium, should return for examination three to not later than six weeks postpartum. At this time her general physical condition should be checked, her blood pressure measured, her urine examined for protein, the condition of her abdominal walls noted, her breasts inspected, and a thorough pelvic examination carried out. Abnormalities such as cervicitis can be treated at this time and arrangements made for further treatment or examinations when indicated. A very important obligation of the physician, at the time of the postpartum examination is to counsel the woman in family planning technics, discussed in Chapter 39.

Rᴇꜰᴇʀᴇɴᴄᴇꜱ

Adams, H., and Flowers, C. E.   Oral oxytocic drugs in the puerperium. Obstet Gynec 15:280, 1960.

Anderson, W. R., and Davis, J.   Placental site involution. Amer J Obstet Gynec 102:23, 1968.

Chesley, L. C., Valenti, C., and Uichanco, L.   Alterations in body fluid compartments and exchangeable sodium in early puerperium. Amer J Obstet Gynec 77:1054, 1959.

Douglas, R. G., and Rhees, H. S.   Bacteriological findings in the uterus during labor and the early puerperium. Amer J Obstet Gynec 27:203, 1934.

Eastman, N. J., and Lee, S. W.   Puerperal creatinuria. Chin Med J 46:143, 1932.

Gioiosa, R.   Incidence of pregnancy during lactation in 500 cases. Amer J Obstet Gynec 70:162, 1955.

Guilbeau, J. A., Schaub, I., and Andrews, M. C.   Penicillin treatment in the obstetrical patient. A study of its effect on the bacterial flora of the postpartum uterus. Amer J Obstet Gynec 58:101, 1949.

Hellman, L. M., Kohl, S. G., and Palmer, J.   Early hospital discharge in obstetrics. Lancet 1:227, 1962.

Keettel, W. C., and Bradbury, J. T.   Endocrine studies of lactation amenorrhea. Amer J Obstet Gynec 82:995, 1961.

Newton, M., and Bradford, W. M.   Postpartal blood loss. Obstet Gynec 17:229, 1961.

Sharman, A.   Menstruation after childbirth. J Obstet Gynaec Brit Emp 58:440, 1951.

———— Postpartum regeneration of the human endometrium. J Anat 87:1, 1953.

———— Ovulation in the post-partum period. Excerpta Medica International Congress Series, No. 133, p. 158, 1966.

Theobald, G. W.   Home on the second day: The Bradford experiment. Brit Med J 2:1364, 1959.

Udesky, I. C.   Ovulation in lactating women. Amer J Obstet Gynec 59:843, 1950.

Williams, J. W.   Regeneration of the uterine mucosa after delivery with especial reference to the placental site. Amer J Obstet Gynec 22:664, 1931.

Woessner, J. F.   Postpartum involution of the uterus connective tissue framework. Ob/Gyn Digest, p. 14, July, 1968.

19

THE NEWBORN

The First Breath. Considerable resistance must be overcome in the first expansion of the lung. The stiffness of the lung, the resistance of small airways to the passage of air, and the surface tension that tends to keep the moist linings of the distal air passages in apposition all contribute to this resistance. Both air spaces and surface active material must be present for ventilation to be effective. The functional capability of the lung is enhanced by a complex of phospholipids, particularly dipalmitoyl phosphatidyl choline, that line the terminal air spaces in normal lungs and decrease surface tension (Clements; Brumley and colleagues).

Initiation of Respiration. Normally the newborn infant begins to cry almost immediately after birth, indicating the establishment of active respiration, which is accompanied by important alterations in circulatory function. The mode of production of the first breath has been difficult to elucidate because many mechanisms involved occur simultaneously. Tactile, biochemical, thermal, and circulatory stimuli all play an important role. Various noteworthy explanations are as follows.

Physical Stimulation. The handling of the infant during delivery and its contact with air and with various relatively rough surfaces are believed to provoke respiration through stimuli reaching the respiratory center from the skin. Vigorous abdominal palpation, the application of forceps to the infant's head, and attempts at version and extraction do not, however, initiate breathing in the fetus with the placental circulation intact. James concluded that although strong tactile stimulation of the fetal lamb produces gasping, rhythmic respirations are not maintained. Occlusion of the umbilical cord precipitates a rise in blood pressure and is considered by some to be important in initiating respiration. Breathing can occur, however, with an intact umbilical circulation.

Compression of Fetal Thorax Incident to Delivery. The almost conical compression of the thorax during the second stage suggests, in the expansion that inevitably follows delivery of the shoulders, a possible explanation for the first inspiratory movement. Babies born by cesarean section, however, usually cry satisfactorily and sometimes just as quickly as babies born vaginally. The compression of the thorax incident to vaginal delivery may, nevertheless, be an auxiliary factor in the initiation of respiration.

Accumulation of Carbon Dioxide. Since mechanical theories fail to furnish a rational explanation of the onset of respiration, biochemical interpretations seem logical, particularly in view of the known chemical factors that influence respiration in the adult, such as the effects of increased tension of carbon dioxide in the blood. During the interval between the interruption of placental gaseous exchange and the establishment of pulmonary respiration, the level of carbon dioxide rises rapidly in the infant's blood while the pH falls. Studies of the ventilatory response of newborn infants to increased amounts of carbon dioxide in the inspired air show that infants increase their ventilation as pCO_2 rises (Avery and associates).

Deprivation of Oxygen. In Barcroft's opinion, based on animal experimentation, lack of oxygen is the cause of the onset of respiration at birth. He comments, "We are faced with the remarkable paradox that the dying (that is, anoxemic) gasp of the fetus is the earnest of life to the individual."

Both experimental work and observations of human beings at high altitudes, however, have shown that profound lack of oxygen produces apnea. If minor degrees of hypoxia produce the first respiration, certain observations become difficult to explain. For example, there is no relation between the concentration of oxygen in the blood at birth and the onset of respiration except possibly that infants with high levels of oxygen breathe more readily, whereas those with extremely low levels are often apneic. In response to hypoxia and hypercapnia in utero and increased muscular activity at term, respiratory activity is initiated with the inflow and egress of large volumes of air. Harned and associates, studying the partly delivered ewe, found that respiratory activity was not observed with either low oxygen tension or high carbon dioxide tension alone. Rhythmic breathing was soon induced, however, by the administration of a mixture of 5 per cent oxygen, 10 per cent carbon dioxide, and 85 per cent nitrogen to the mother. Blood samples obtained from catheters implanted into fetal vessels of experimental animals for prolonged periods of time without interruption of the pregnancy have revealed that arterial O_2 tension is low by adult standards. Nevertheless, a fall in pO_2 and pH accompanied by a rise in pCO_2 produces gasping in utero as well as after birth. If, however, the pO_2 drops and the pH is held stable, the fetus does not gasp.

Temperature. The effects of thermal stimuli have been recognized for many years, but only recently have they been quantitatively investigated. Adamsons and colleagues have shown that the newborn infant loses about 600 calories per minute. The fetal lamb delivered by cesarean section begins to gasp when cool; when the temperature is raised gasping diminishes.

Intrauterine Respiration. Snyder and Rosenfeld, chiefly on the basis of their experiments with rabbits, regard the onset of postnatal respiratory activity not as an event initiated abruptly at birth, but rather as a continuation of respiratory movements discernible during intrauterine life, as discussed in Chapter 7.

Becker and associates and Carter and colleagues, however, have noted in their extensive studies of rats and guinea pigs that in the absence of hypoxia there is no spontaneous respiratory activity and that following intraamniotic injection, neither a radiopaque contrast material nor a dye appeared in the fetal lungs unless intrauterine hypoxia had been induced.

It is quite unlikely that the diaphragm and thoracic muscles that are involved in respiration remain totally inactive during all of intrauterine life. It seems doubtful, however, that the fetus engages in regular forceful contractions of these muscles of sufficient magnitude to provide for the movement of large volumes of fluid into and out of the respiratory tract.

Windle seriously questions the concept of intrauterine respiration and its bearing on the onset of respiration at birth. His experiments, contrary to those of Snyder and Rosenfeld, indicate that experimental hypoxia induces aspiration by some but not all fetuses. Difficult labor with consequent fetal asphyxia, moreover, often leads to aspiration of meconium-tinged amniotic fluid, which has long been regarded as a cause of neonatal death. This moot question is still incompletely answered.

Immediate Care.   Immediately after birth, while the infant is still being held head down, it is thought to be beneficial to aspirate the excess mucus from the mouth and pharynx. A soft rubber ear syringe inserted with great care is quite suitable for the purpose. Once the cord has been divided, the infant should be placed in a heated crib or in a resuscitator such as the Kreiselman unit, which allows lowering of the child's head and provides oxygen, necessary equipment for suction, and adequate thermal regulation. During this period the obstetrician first evaluates the condition of the baby.

In the period immediately after birth the infant undergoes a characteristic series of reactions similar to those of an adult recovering from anesthesia. During the first few minutes, or first period of reactivity, the infant exhibits respiratory rales, flaring of the alae nasi, grunting, and substernal and subcostal retractions. Tachycardia and a fall in body temperature and alerting exploratory movements are usually present. Following this initial phase the infant enters a relatively quiescent period during which heart rate and respiratory rate decrease. Frequently the infant sleeps. A second period of reactivity follows the unresponsive interval, characterized by cardiac and respiratory irregularity. This sequence appears to occur generally, but is prolonged in depressed premature or compromised infants.

Evaluation of the Infant.   The result of the initial evaluation determines the need for and type of resuscitation. Attention to the condition of the mother and the clinical course of labor and to the fetal heart tones often provides an indication of the condition of the infant at birth. Cyanosis of the scalp and face during delivery of the infant indicates a functioning circulation; pallor is a poor sign. As the infant is held by the feet the obstetrician looks for gross malformations and observes the general muscular tone. After the first breath, the color of the infant's skin changes from dusky to ruddy, indicating adequate circulation and respiratory exchange. Immediate urination and erection of the infant's penis are good signs.

At this point the obstetrician records certain objective data, such as the time of first breath and cry. Most normal infants take the first breath within a few seconds of birth and cry within a half a minute. Prolongations of these intervals beyond one and two minutes, respectively, indicate difficulty. Gentle slapping of the heels or massage of the back may initiate breathing, but traumatic methods, such as "tubbing," "jackknifing," and dilatation of the sphincters, must be condemned as wasteful of valuable time and frequently severely injurious. A useful

Table 1. Apgar Scoring System

Sign	0	1	2
Heart rate	Absent	Slow (below 100)	Over 100
Respiratory effort	Absent	Slow, irregular	Good, crying
Muscle tone	Flaccid	Some flexion of extremities	Active motion
Reflex irritability	No response	Cry	Vigorous cry
Color	Blue, pale	Body pink, extremities blue	Completely pink

aid in the evaluation of the infant is the Apgar Scoring System (Table 1). A score of 3 or less indicates a severely jeopardized baby; the higher the score, up to a maximum of 10, the better is the condition of the infant. Most infants are in excellent condition, as indicated by Apgar scores of 7 to 10, and require no aid other than simple nasopharyngeal suction. The one-minute Apgar score determines the need for immediate resuscitation. The Apgar score at five minutes after birth has a direct relation to infant mortality and morbidity (Drage and Berendes).

Resuscitation.   Although resuscitation is required for only a small percentage of newborns, it is a lifesaving procedure, the success of which depends upon trained, efficient personnel and excellent equipment. Gentleness and deliberation are the hallmarks of the intelligent and well-trained physician at this period.

Each delivery room must be individually equipped for resuscitation, and the apparatus should be checked before each delivery. The equipment should include an apparatus for intermittent administration of oxygen under controlled pressure and suction (Fig. 1). Required items include a work table, with equipment for administration of oxygen and suction, on which the infant may be placed, a means of warming the infant, and a "resuscitation tray" (Fig. 2). The cardinal points of resuscitation are as follows.

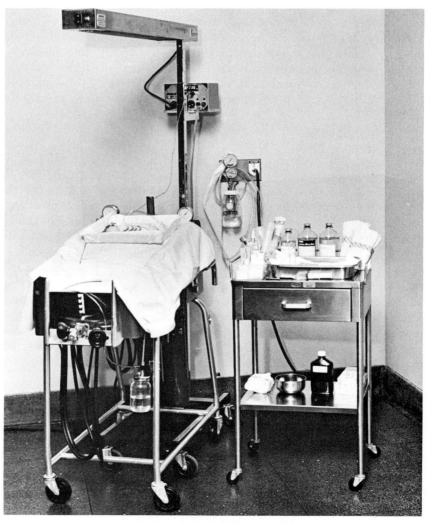

Fig. 1. Kreiselman infant resuscitator.

Proper temperature and humidity must be maintained. Babies who are in a state of vascular collapse should receive treatment for shock.

Adequate drainage of the upper respiratory tract must be provided. The baby's head should be declined about 30 degrees to favor drainage of fluids from the trachea. Gentle nasal and postpharyngeal suction is indicated (Fig. 3). Mucus

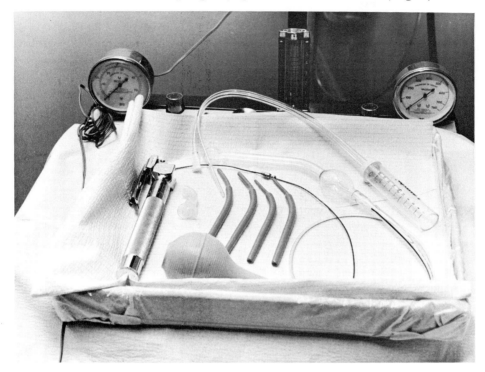

Fig. 2. Resuscitation tray.

must be removed through a catheter, by either oral suction or an electric aspirator. Suction from an electric aspirator should not be so great that it causes bleeding. Intratracheal aspiration is not without hazard, since it predisposes to laryngeal edema. It should therefore be reserved for certain cases of apnea secondary to obstruction. Intratracheal intubation should be performed under direct vision through the laryngoscope.

Oxygen must be administered. The lungs may be expanded by intermittent positive pressure in cases of primary apnea not caused by obstruction. Positive pressure oxygen should not be administered to infants with retraction, unequal expansion of the chest, or shallow and irregular respiration. Mouth-to-mouth insufflation should be avoided if equipment is available to give controlled pressure. In any case, great care should be exercised to keep the pressure below the alveolar bursting point. Smith and Chisholm believe that positive pressures of air between 20 and 30 cm of water are required to expand the human lung at birth and that the newborn infant, in struggling for a breath, can produce inflating pressures in excess of 40 cm of water. Day and co-workers advocate higher pressures at shorter intervals, simulating an infant's initial inspiratory gasp. A pressure of 40 cm is required when the interval is 0.15 second.

Most apneic infants respond to simple positive pressure. If, however, there

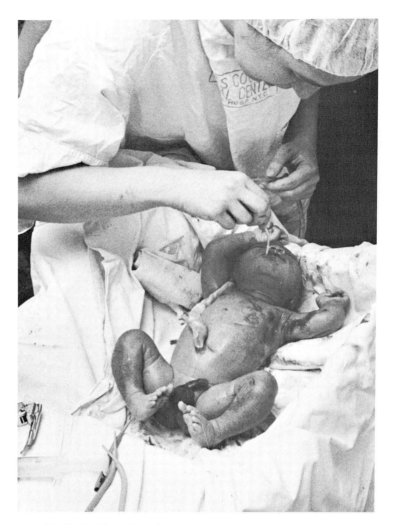

Fig. 3. Position of newborn during aspiration of the pharynx.

is no effort at voluntary respiration and the fetal heartbeat continues to slow with diminishing muscular tone, intubation is indicated.

Technic of Intubation. Direct endotracheal intubation, when necessary, must be instituted immediately. The decision must be made and carried out by an experienced person, regardless of the cause of the depression. When not clearly indicated, intubation leads to more trauma than benefit.

The necessary equipment includes a soft rubber catheter, a DeLee glass trap or suction machine, a pencil-battery laryngoscope handle with a "premature" blade, and Cole endotracheal tubes (Nos. 10, 12, 14) with a malleable but firm stylet (Fig. 2).

The infant is placed supine with its head toward the operator on a suitable work table. A small rolled towel is placed beneath the scapulae, bringing the level of the nasopharynx below that of the body. The towel raises the chest and increases the extension of the head, thereby facilitating visual intubation. The nasopharynx is gently cleaned of all vernix and blood. With the operator's right hand grasping the infant's right mandible and hyperextending the head, the right index finger is inserted into the mouth, pressing the tongue anteriorly. The laryngoscope is held in the left hand, and the blade is inserted into the mouth in the midline. It is then gently placed in the left corner, pressing the tongue to the same side. The tip of the blade is elevated and the larynx visualized. With the glottal orifice in view, the Cole endotracheal tube is inserted at the right corner of the mouth and passed beyond the vocal cords. The neck of the tube is held firmly and the laryngoscope is removed. The stylet is removed and mouth-to-tube resuscitation is instituted. Simultaneous ausculation of the chest enables the physician to ascertain the degree of aeration, the position of the tube with respect to the carina, and the presence of foreign matter beyond the tip of the tube. If the tube is in place, the child almost always gasps after the first or second insufflation. In addition, the heart rate increases if adequate oxygen is being delivered and the upper third of the chest rises. If the stomach expands, however, the esophagus has been intubated, and the position of the tube must be corrected. Endotracheal suction may be accomplished through a No. 10 or larger tube. An oxygen tube should be placed in the operator's mouth to increase the content of oxygen. Resuscitation is continued until spontaneous respirations are established and the color and muscular tone are good. Extubation is performed gently by simple withdrawal.

If the stimuli from these procedures have not initiated spontaneous breathing, the pH of the infant's blood should be corrected through an umbilical vessel. The umbilical cord should be cut to a length of 1 cm to permit intubation of an umbilical vessel with a No. 5 or 8 feeding tube. Care is required to prevent excessive bleeding from the cord, a common complication in apneic infants when the tie is removed. Air and blood clots must not be allowed to enter the circulation. Three mEq/kg of 7.5 per cent solution of sodium bicarbonate are given slowly. An assistant should maintain artificial respiration while the pH is being corrected. If the heart rate falls below 80 beats/min., the bicarbonate solution may not be distributed by the failing circulatory system. The heart rate may be improved by external cardiac massage. Epinephrine is ineffective before correction of the pH deficit. The initial dose may be carefully given in amounts not to exceed 0.1 ml of a 1:1,000 aqueous solution. The solution may be diluted before administration to increase the volume and to facilitate administration. If necessary, the dose can be titrated.

A special committee on infant mortality of the Medical Society of the County of New York gives the following instructions concerning resuscitation of the newborn:

If there is no audible heartbeat immediately upon birth, the initial resuscitative steps should be the same as those employed for infants born with respiratory depression. The airway is cleared, the infant is intubated, and ventilation is begun. If the heart has not begun to beat after ventilation, external cardiac massage is initiated. Two fingers are placed over the heart to the left of the lower sternal border. The chest wall is then firmly depressed one half to three quarters of an inch, 100 to 120 times a minute. Aortic pressures at least 80 per cent of normal may thus be achieved. Ventilation and external cardiac massage should be performed in sequence, with three massages after each insufflation to approximate the desirable cardiac and respiratory rates. Ventilation must be maintained, but massage should be stopped briefly every thirty seconds to detect a spontaneous heartbeat. Apparatus for intubation should always be available. If it is not, mouth-to-mouth insufflation, although not so effective, may be used. The infant's mouth must be cleared of all obstruction and the head must be hyperextended. Massage should be discontinued as soon as a rhythmical heartbeat can be readily heard, and resumed only if the heart stops again. Electrocardiographic monitoring of the heartbeat should be instituted promptly. Ventilation should be discontinued when the infant begins effective spontaneous breathing. Properly performed, cardiopulmonary resuscitation causes no damage to the liver capsule, ribs, or other organs. The resuscitated infant should, however, always be examined before transfer to the nursery. In some resuscitated infants, convulsions have been observed between 12 and 24 hours of age. These convulsions may be associated with recovery of the central nervous system from the asphyxial insult rather than with irreparable damage to the central nervous system. Convulsions may be controlled with barbiturates or other anticonvulsant drugs.

Most apneic infants require only the mildest form of resuscitation—namely, suction to clear the passages and oxygen under mild pressure. The great danger is overzealous treatment, especially unnecessarily frequent use of potentially traumatic intubation.

Nalorphine (Nalline) (0.2 mg) can be given intravenously into the umbilical vein to counter the narcotic effect of morphine or meperidine (Demerol) when either has been given to the mother in large amounts within four hours preceding delivery.

Gastric lavage is of little or no value.

After resuscitation, the infant should be placed in an incubator that maintains body temperature, humidity, and a concentration of oxygen that prevents cyanosis, usually 40 per cent or less.

The best management of neonatal apnea is its prevention. Adherence to the following obstetric principles leads to reduction in its frequency:

1. *Combat hypoxia.* Analgesia and anesthesia that allow adequate oxygenation of maternal blood should be employed.

2. *Avoid trauma.* Difficult vaginal operations that traumatize the fetal respiratory centers must be eliminated.

High-Risk Infant.   The majority of deaths of infants within the neonatal period can be predicted by maternal obstetric and perinatal factors. These infants are termed high-risk infants. Within the classification of high-risk infants are three prime categories:

1. Compromised newborns—namely, infants who have had one of the following: meconium-stained amniotic fluid, an Apgar score of 5 or below, a history of fetal distress, or birth by emergency cesarean section or breech presentation.

2. Maternal instability—namely, infants who are born of diabetic mothers, or infants who are born of mothers who have had vaginal bleeding in the last trimester, infants born of Rh-negative, sensitized mothers, infants whose mothers have had premature rupture of the membranes for 12 hours or more before delivery, and infants of mothers who are addicted to heroin, or other opiates.

3. Physically compromised newborns; infants who have grown too fast or too slowly or not long enough in utero—namely, infants of low birth weight, infants of excessive birth weight, postmature infants, or infants with life-threatening multiple congenital anomalies. As a group these infants are at high risk of dying in the neonatal period. It is, therefore, imperative that these newborns be placed in an area of especially close observation where their recovery from the birth process can be monitored carefully. A physician trained to recognize deviations from the normal should examine these high-risk infants shortly after birth, if delivery room attendance is not possible. Facilities must be provided to monitor blood gases, cardiac and respiratory status, and hematologic and thermal sta-

bility. The aim here is to prevent further compromise, correct deviations, and support the infant through this period of major adjustment.

Identification.   Proper identification of each infant is of prime importance. A foolproof system must be operative at all hours. It should prevent separation of infant from its mother until identification is complete, and it should provide a record easily recognized by the mother, such as an identification band or row of beads that spell the infant's name. It is crucial, furthermore, that a permanent record, such as footprints, be kept on file at the hospital (Fig. 4).

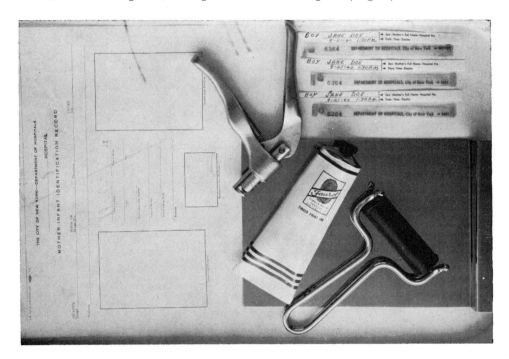

Fig. 4. Materials necessary for footprinting and Identa-bands.

Although the value of footprints in babies' identification has been occasionally questioned, the experience at Kings County Hospital in the past 20 years has shown that they may be of inestimable value. The definitive ridges on the palms, fingers, and feet of human beings begin to form several months before birth and remain throughout life. Most hospitals today use footprints rather than fingerprints or palmprints in identifying infants because the ridges in the feet are more pronounced and it is easier to obtain prints from them in newborn infants. The field of *dermatoglyphics* is making increasing use of footprints and fingerprints in the study of associated congenital anomalies and subtler hereditary disorders.

Temperature.   The temperature of the infant drops rapidly immediately after birth. If the naked newborn is left exposed in the usual air-conditioned delivery room, chilling so produced increases oxygen requirements. Consequently the infant should be cared for in a warm crib. During the first few days of life the temperature is unstable, responding to slight stimuli with considerable fluctuations above or below the normal level.

The Umbilical Cord.   Loss of water from Wharton's jelly leads to mummification of the cord shortly after birth. Within 24 hours it loses it characteristic bluish white, moist appearance and soon becomes dry and almost black (Fig. 5). Gradually the line of demarcation appears just beyond the skin of the abdomen, and in a few days the stump sloughs, leaving a small granulating wound, which after healing forms the umbilicus.

Separation usually takes place within the first two weeks after birth, most

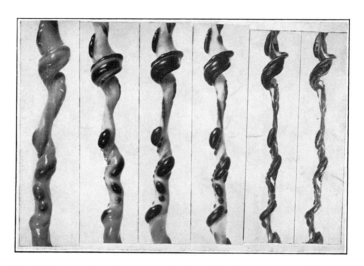

Fig. 5. Desiccation of a segment of umbilical cord exposed to air.

frequently around the tenth day, but occasionally only after several weeks. In the very rare instances in which the stump is still adherent at the end of the puerperium, it may become necessary to clip it off with a pair of scissors.

Formerly the care of the cord was considered trivial. Total neglect of asepsis in management of the cord, however, frequently resulted in an infection transmitted through the umbilical vessels and death of the infant from so-called puerperal fever or from tetanus.

Even today serious umbilical infections are occasionally encountered, usually, but not always, indicating gross lack of care. The offending organisms often are *Staphylococcus aureaus, E. coli,* or *Pseudomonas aeruginosa.* Since the umbilical stump in such cases frequently presents no outward sign of infection, the diagnosis cannot be made with certainty except by autopsy. Whenever infants die within three weeks after birth without an obvious cause, such an infection should be suspected. Examination of the intraabdominal portion of the umbilical vessels at autopsy sometimes reveals purulent thrombi, in which pyogenic microorganisms can be demonstrated. Strict aseptic precautions should, therefore, be observed in the immediate care of the cord. We believe that the cords dry more quickly and separate more readily when exposed to the air, and we therefore do not recommend umbilical dressings.

Care of the Eyes.   Because of the frequent infection of the eyes of the newborn during passage through the vagina of a mother with gonorrhea, Credé in 1884 introduced the practice of instilling into each eye immediately after birth one drop of a *1 per cent* solution of silver nitrate, which was later washed out with saline. This procedure has led to a marked decrease in the frequency of gonorrheal ophthalmia and resulting blindness. Some form of prophylaxis is a mandatory routine immediately after ligation of the cord. If silver nitrate is used, the following technic is recommended.

As a preliminary precaution the region about each eye should be irrigated with sterile water applied to the nasal side of the eye and allowed to run off from the opposite side. The lower lid should then be drawn down and the silver solution dropped into the lower cul-de-sac, whence in the course of two minutes it diffuses over the entire conjunctiva. After two minutes the lids are held apart and the conjunctival sac is freely flushed with warm normal salt solution by means of a rubber eye syringe, accomplishing the double purpose of washing out the excess of silver nitrate and forming an insoluble compound with any fraction that is retained.

The silver nitrate produces a discernible chemical conjunctivitis in over half the cases, manifested by redness, edema, or discharge. These signs of irritation are transient, however. Permanent damage to the infant's eyes does not result from prophylactic use of silver nitrate *in the correct concentration*.

Since penicillin is highly effective in eradicating gonococci, it serves as a preferable alternate to silver nitrate in prophylaxis of ophthalmia neonatorum. For many years at the Johns Hopkins Hospital and the Kings County Hospital penicillin ointment in the strength of 100,000 units per gram has been placed in the eyes of all newborn babies. A separate small tube is used for each infant. Our conclusions, based on experience with over 150,000 babies, are as follows:

1. Since no known case of gonorrheal ophthalmia has developed in this large number of cases, the efficacy of penicillin for this purpose, given locally as an ointment, cannot be questioned. It is, in fact, a more effective prophylactic agent than silver nitrate. Even when gonorrheal ophthalmia develops, it is cured by penicillin within a few hours, whereas silver nitrate has long since been abandoned for that purpose.

2. The incidence of chemical irritation with penicillin ointment (between 16 and 20 per cent) is much less than with silver nitrate and the irritation is generally milder.

3. Penicillin sensitivity, although rare, may occur. In summary, there are advantages and disadvantages to each technic. The most grave objection to silver nitrate, unless wax ampules are used, is the possibility of error in its preparation—for example, the use of a 10 per cent rather than a 1 per cent solution. Such mistakes have resulted in the blinding of babies. At the present time, the use of a silver preparation is still mandatory by statute in a number of states, but the general tendency among enlightened public health officials is to eliminate such restrictive legislation.

4. Tetracycline ointment containing the antibiotic in a concentration of 1 per cent has afforded effective prophylaxis in approximately 60,000 neonates cared for at Parkland Memorial Hospital. Tetracycline rather than penicillin was chosen on the basis that the rare risk of inducing drug sensitivity might be further lessened.

Care of the Skin.   In most clinics not all the vernix caseosa is removed, but the excess, as well as blood and meconium, is wiped off. The vernix caseosa is readily absorbed by the baby's skin and disappears entirely within 24 hours. Infants that are small for gestational age have less vernix caseosa. It is unwise to wash a newborn infant until its temperature has stabilized. Infants who require resuscitative measures should be patted dry during the procedure to minimize heat loss caused by evaporation. Handling of the baby should be minimized, and cuddling by nursing personnel must be entirely avoided.

Stools and Urine.   For the first few days after birth the contents of the colon are composed of soft, brownish green meconium, which comprises desquamated epithelial cells from the intestinal tract, a few epidermal cells, and lanugo hairs swallowed with the amniotic fluid. Its peculiar color results from bile pigments.

During intrauterine life and for a few hours after birth the intestinal contents are sterile, but bacteria soon gain access to them. The passage of meconium and urine in the minutes immediately after birth or during the next few hours indicates patency of the gastrointestinal and urinary tracts. Ninety per cent of the newborn infants pass meconium within the first 24 hours; most of the rest do so within 36 hours. Voiding may not occur until the second or third day of life. Failure of the infant to eliminate meconium or urine after these times suggests congenital defects such as imperforate anus or a urethral valve.

After the third or fourth day, with the establishment of feeding, the meconium disappears and is replaced by light yellow homogeneous feces with a characteristic odor. For the first few days the stools are unformed, but after a short time they assume their characteristic cylindric shape. The bowels usually move twice daily, but a single large stool is normal also.

Icterus Neonatorum.   About one third of all babies, between the second and fifth day of life, develop the so-called physiologic jaundice of the newborn. There is a hyperbilirubinemia at birth of 1 to 2 mg per 100 ml of serum. It increases during the next few days, but there is wide individual variation, as shown in Figure 6. Between the third and fourth day the median figure for bilirubin reaches

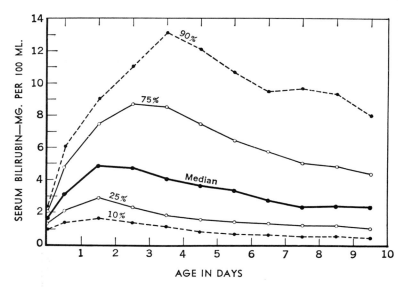

Fig. 6. Course of serum bilirubin during the first 10 days of life. The range between 75 per cent and 25 per cent includes 50 per cent of all observations; the range between 90 per cent and 10 per cent includes 80 per cent of all observations. (From Davidson, Merritt, and Weech. Amer J Dis Child 61:958, 1941.)

4 to 5 mg per 100 ml of serum, the concentration at which jaundice usually becomes noticeable. Most of the bilirubin is free, or unconjugated. The cause of this hyperbilirubinemia is presumably immaturity of the hepatic cells, resulting in very slight conjugation of bilirubin with glucuronic acid and reduced excretion of the conjugate in the bile. In premature infants jaundice is more common and usually more severe and prolonged than in term infants, because of greater

hepatic enzymatic immaturity. Infants that are small for gestational age, however, metabolize bilirubin in a manner similar to mature infants.

Initial Loss of Weight.   Because the child receives little nutriment for the first three or four days of life and at the same time produces considerable urine, feces, and sweat, it progressively loses weight until the flow of maternal milk or other feeding is established. The total loss is usually about 7 per cent of the birth weight. Premature infants lose relatively more weight and regain their birth weight more slowly than do term infants. Infants that are small for gestational age, however, regain their initial weight more quickly than do premature infants.

If the child is nourished properly, the birth weight is usually regained by the end of the tenth day, after which it normally increases steadily at the rate of about 25 g a day for the first few months, doubling by the time the child is five months of age, and trebling by the end of the first year.

Frequency of Feeding.   Despite the small quantity of colostrum available and its somewhat limited nutritive properties, it is advisable, because of the stimulating effect of nursing on mother and child, to commence regular nursing about 12 hours postpartum. Most mature infants thrive best when fed at intervals of four hours on a definite schedule, which is best arranged with reference to the daily bath. If the bath is given a little before 10:00 A.M., the first feeding would come at 6:00 A.M., with the evening feeding at the parents' bedtime, and only one during the night. With this arrangement six feedings will be given each day. They can frequently be reduced to five, since many children can be trained to sleep the entire night without awakening. Premature or frail infants not infrequently require feedings at shorter intervals; in most instances a three-hour interval is satisfactory. As soon as conditions permit, the four-hour interval should be commenced. "Demand feeding" is discussed in standard pediatric textbooks.

Duration of Feeding.   The proper length of each feeding depends on several factors, such as the quantity of milk, the readiness with which it can be obtained from the breast, and the avidity with which the child nurses. It is generally advisable to allow the child to remain at the breast for 10 minutes at first; 4 to 5 minutes are sufficient for some children, however, and 15 to 20 minutes are required by others. It is satisfactory for the baby to nurse for 5 minutes at each breast for the first four days, or until the mother has a supply of milk. After the fourth day the baby nurses up to 10 minutes on each breast. A child receiving proper nourishment should not spit up its food, should increase steadily in weight, and should have normal yellow homogeneous stools.

In the hospital the child should be weighed daily, but not at home, since minor variations in the weight curve may be the cause of great concern to the untrained mother. After the first few months the increase is more gradual.

Rooming-In.   Rooming-in involves keeping the infant in a crib at the mother's bedside rather than in the nursery. It is an outgrowth in part of early ambulation, which permits the mother to take care of the baby herself. It stems in part also from the modern trend to make all phases of childbearing as "natural" as possible and to foster proper mother-child relationships at an early date. By the end of 24 hours the mother is generally out of bed and thereafter with rooming-in may conduct practically all the routine care of herself and the infant. An advantage of this program is increased ability of the mother, when she arrives at home, to assume full care of the baby.

Circumcision of the healthy newborn male provides several advantages. Speert reported only one death attributable to circumcision in a huge number of such procedures, estimated at well over half a million. In the same period of time there were well over 200 deaths from carcinoma of the penis, a disease virtually abolished by circumcision of the newborn. Provided there is no defect in coagulation, there is no medical contraindication to the procedure in the healthy mature infant.

Circumcision formerly was generally performed on about the seventh day of life. With earlier discharge of mothers from the hospital, however, there has been a justifiable trend to earlier circumcision of the newborn.

Within the past few years a flurry of reports critical of routine circumcision has appeared. The adverse comments range from psychologic trauma to hypesthesia of the glans. These subjective allegations are at best difficult to prove. Objectively, the infrequent minor operative complications may be minimized by attention to surgical technic. Proper use of the Yellen (Gomco) clamp (Fig. 7) or the Plastibell provides an additional safeguard against accidents.

Because of the marked reduction in incidence of penile infection and the virtual elimination of penile cancer by adequate circumcision of the newborn, the procedure is recommended by the majority of American obstetricians.

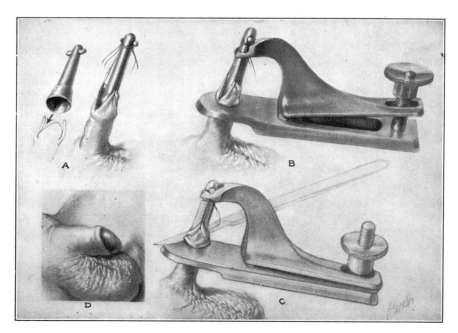

Fig. 7. Technic of circumcision with Yellen clamp. After cleansing area and stripping back prepuce, the cone of the Yellen clamp is placed over the glans and the prepuce put on a stretch with sutures (A). The prepuce is then drawn through the beveled hole of platform (B). Screwing down clamp crushes prepuce, producing hemostasis. Three to five minutes of such pressure are necessary to prevent subsequent bleeding. The excess of the prepuce is then cut away (C) and the clamp removed (D).

References

Adamsons, K., Gandy, G. M., and James, L. S. Influence of thermal factors upon oxygen consumption of the newborn human infant. J Pediat 66:495, 1965.

Apgar, V., Holaday, D. A., James, L. S., Weisbrot, I. M., and Berrien, C. Evaluation of the newborn infant: Second report. JAMA 168:1985, 1958.

Avery, M. E., Chernick, V., Duntton, R. E., and Permutt, S. Ventilatory response to inspired carbon dioxide in infants and adults. J Appl Physiol 18:895, 1963.

Barcroft, J., and Barron, D. H. The genesis of respiratory movements in the fetus of the sheep. J Physiol 88:56, 1936.

—— Elliott, R. H. E., Flexner, L. B., Hall, F. G., Herkel, W., McCarthy, E. F., McClurkin, T., and Talaat, M. Conditions of fetal respiration in the goat. J Physiol 83:192, 1934.

—— Kramer, K., and Millikan, G. A. The oxygen in the carotid blood at birth. J Physiol 94:571, 1939.

Becker, R. F., King, J. E., Marsh, R. H., and Wyrick, A. D. Intrauterine respiration in the rat fetus. I. Direct observations—Comparison with the guinea pig. Amer J Obstet Gynec 90:236, 1964.

Brumley, G. W., Hodson, W. A., and Avery, M. E. Lung phospholipid and surface tension correlation in infants with and without hyaline membrane disease and in adults. Pediatrics 40:13, 1967.

Carter, W. A., Becker, R. F., King, J. E., and Barry, W. F. Intrauterine respiration in the rat fetus. II. Analysis of roentgenological techniques. Amer J Obstet Gynec 90:247, 1964.

Clements, J. H. Surface phenomena in relation to pulmonary function. Physiologist 5:11, 1962.

Credé, C.S.F. Die Verhütung der Augenentzündung der Neugeborenen. Berlin, Hirschwald, 1884.

Davidson, L. T., Merritt, K. R., and Weech, A. A. Hyperbilirubinemia in the newborn. Amer J Dis Child 61:958, 1941.

Day, R., Goodfellow, A. M., Apgar, V., and Beck, G. J. Pressure-time relations in safe correction of atelectasis in animal lungs. Pediatrics 10:593, 1952.

Desmond, M. M., Rudolph, A. J., and Phitaksphraiwan, P. The transitional care nursery. Pediat Clin N Amer 13:655, 1966.

Drage, J. S., and Berendes, H. Apgar scores and outcome of the newborn. Pediat Clin N Amer 13:640, 1966.

Harned, H. S., Rowshan, G., MacKinney, L. G., and Sugioka, K. Relationships of pO_2, and pH to onset of breathing of term lamb as studied by flow-through cuvette electrode assembly. Pediatrics 33:672, 1964.

James, L. S. Onset of breathing and resuscitation. Pediat Clin N Amer 13:621, 1966.

King, J. E., and Becker, R. F. Intrauterine respiration in the rat fetus. 3. Aspiration and swallowing of Calcodur blue dye. Amer J Obstet Gynec 90:257, 1964.

Ploss, H. H., Bartels, M., and Bartels, P. Women: an historical, gynecological and anthropological compendium. St. Louis, C. V. Mosby Co., 1936.

Snyder, F. F., and Rosenfeld, M. Intrauterine respiratory movements of the human fetus. JAMA 108:1946, 1937.

—— and Rosenfeld, M. Direct observation of intrauterine respiratory movements of the fetus and the role of carbon dioxide and oxygen in their regulation. Amer J Physiol 119:153, 1937.

Special Committee on Infant Mortality of the Medical Society of New York. Resuscitation of the Newborn, Abramson, S., Chairman. Philadelphia, Smith, Kline and French, 1963.

Speert, H. Circumcision of the newborn. Obstet Gynec 2:164, 1953.

Steele, A. G., and Windle, W. F. Some correlations between respiratory movements and blood gases in cat fetuses. J Physiol 94:531, 1939.

Windle, W. F. Physiology and anatomy of the respiratory system in the fetus and newborn infant. J Pediat 19:437, 1941.

—— Monnier, M., and Steele, A. G. Fetal respiratory movements in the cat. Physiol Zool 11:425, 1938.

20

ABORTION AND PREMATURE LABOR

Abortion is the termination of a pregnancy at any time before the fetus has attained a stage of viability. Interpretations of the word "viability" have varied between fetal weights of 400 g (about 20 weeks of gestation) and 1,000 g (about 28 weeks of gestation). Since an infant reported by Monro that was said to weigh only 397 g survived, on the basis of this single precedent, an infant weighing 400 g or more may be regarded as capable of living. Although our smallest surviving infant weighed 540 g at birth, survival even at 700 or 800 g is unusual. Attainment of a weight of 1,000 g is therefore widely used as the criterion of viability. Infants below this weight have little chance of survival, whereas those over 1,000 g have a substantial chance, which increases greatly with each 100 g increment. Expert neonatal care, furthermore, has permitted survival of increasingly small infants.

An *abortion* is here defined as the termination of pregnancy at any time when the fetus weighs less than 500 g. Infants weighing between 500 and 999 g are defined as *immature,* although in many clinics they are included among the abortions.

Premature infants are born after the stage of viability but before their chances of survival approximate those of a term infant. By consensus premature infants weigh up to 2,500 g, or 5.5 pounds. The lower limit of prematurity depends on the definition of abortion, although a weight below 1,000 g is still frequently used. Recently infants born at or near term that weigh less than 2,500 g have been classified as small for date or dysmature. The subclassification is of clinical importance (see Ch. 37, p. 1026).

Since the term "abortion" suggests to the layman a criminal interruption of pregnancy, the word "miscarriage" is often employed in speaking to patients or their families, although it has no place in medical parlance.

Abortion may be classified as spontaneous and induced. *Spontaneous abortion* is the termination of conception before viability through natural causes, without mechanical or medicinal intervention. *Induced abortion* may be therapeutic or criminal. *Therapeutic abortion* is the artificial termination of pregnancy because of a physical or mental disorder that would make continuation of gestation undesirable. *Criminal abortion* is the termination of pregnancy without medicolegal justification. Variations in the clinical course of abortion lead to several possible outcomes. In a *complete abortion* all the products of conception are expelled. In an *incomplete abortion* some of the products of conception are passed, but some (usually part of the placenta and membranes) remain in the uterus. In a *missed abortion* the fetus dies, but the products of conception are retained within the uterus for two months or longer. In *habitual abortion* the accident occurs in a number of successive pregnancies, usually specified as three.

Sᴘᴏɴᴛᴀɴᴇᴏᴜs Aʙᴏʀᴛɪᴏɴ

Incidence.   The incidence of spontaneous abortion is usually quoted as 10 per cent of all pregnancies (United Nations; Tietze). This figure, derived by dividing the number of abortions in any series by the total number of births, may be termed the abortion ratio. Such data have at least two areas of instability: (1) failure to include early abortions and (2) the inclusion of induced abortions. In an attempt to reduce these sources of error, early investigators used large series of private patients. The unreliability of patients' histories and of public records of abortion, however, frustrates even the most careful efforts to uncover basic facts.

Studies now suggest that the estimate of 10 per cent may be too low and that at least 15 per cent of all pregnancies between the fourth and twentieth weeks of gestation may terminate in spontaneous abortion. These studies include

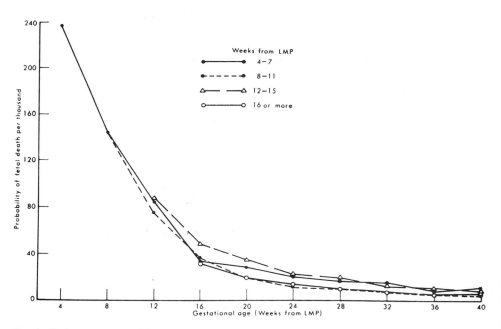

Fig. 1. Estimated probability of eventual fetal death per 1,000 pregnancies for women still pregnant at specified gestational age, for subcohorts of pregnancies first reported 4–7, 8–11, 12–15, and 16 weeks or more from last menstrual period, Kauai Pregnancy Study, 1953–56. (From French and Bierman. Public Health Rep 77:835, 1962.)

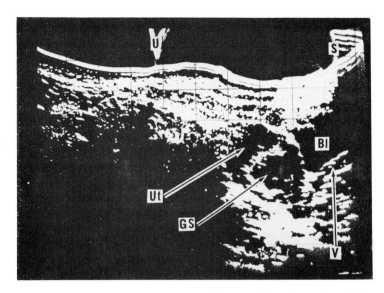

Fig. 2. Sonogram of a blighted ovum at 12 weeks (menstrual age). Longitudinal scan at mid-line. Bl, bladder; S, symphysis pubis; U, umbilicus; Ut, uterus; GS, gestational sac; V, va-. gina. Scanning was done about 10 hours before spontaneous abortion. The uterus is smaller than expected. The gestational sac is implanted low in the uterus and its outline is not clear. (From Hellman et al. Amer J Obstet Gynec 103:789-800, 1969.)

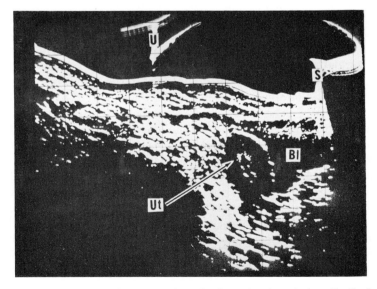

Fig. 3. Sonogram of an abnormal ovum at 6 weeks (menstrual age). Longitudinal scan at 3 cm to the right of the midline. Bl, bladder; S, symphysis pubis; U, umbilicus; Ut, uterus. Scanning was done 2 days before the patient began to bleed and pass necrotic decidua. (From Hellman et al. Amer J Obstet Gynec 103:789-800, 1969.)

both anterospective surveys (Tietze; Erhardt; Warburton and Fraser) and life table analyses (French and Bierman; Shapiro, Jones, and Densen). Tietze analyzed a carefully selected sample of the Kinsey data, whereas Erhardt derived his information from records of a large group of private obstetricians in New York City. Warburton studied the detailed family histories available through the Department of Medical Genetics at the Montreal General Children's Hospital. The figures of these three investigators are 14, 18, and 15 per cent, respectively.

Another current approach is the construction of life tables to give the expectancy of loss at any week of gestation. This method is advantageous because of the possibility that any study, retrospective or anterospective, underreports abortion in the first eight weeks of pregnancy. As pointed out by Hertig and Livingstone, the rate of loss is very high before the fourth week. Abortion at this time is rarely reported, however, because it is perceived by the patient as delayed menstruation or may not be recognized at all. Theoretically, these early high rates of loss should decrease rapidly with time, as shown in the life table graphs (Figure 1). Such calculations yield abortion rates about 20 per cent for the first 20 weeks of pregnancy. These higher estimates receive support from the recent findings of Donald's group in Glasgow and those of Hellman and co-workers, who by ultrasonic technics have independently described a surprisingly high incidence of early abnormal gestations (Figs. 2 and 3).

Etiology.   In the early months of pregnancy spontaneous expulsion of the ovum is nearly always preceded by death of the fetus. For this reason etiologic considerations of early abortion involve ascertaining the cause of fetal death. In the later months, on the contrary, the fetus is frequently born alive, and other explanations for its expulsion must be invoked. Fetal death may be caused by abnormalities in the ovum itself or in the generative tract, or by systemic disease of the mother and, occasionally, of the father.

Abnormal Development.   The most common cause of the fetal death is an abnormality of development that is incompatible with life. The investigations of Mall, Streeter, and Hertig reveal this etiologic factor in a large percentage of early abortions. In an analysis of 1,000 spontaneous abortions, Hertig noted pathologic ("blighted") ova (Figs. 4 and 5) in 48.9 per cent, embryos with localized anomalies in 3.2 per cent, and placental abnormalities in 9.6 per cent of his material. Significantly, he observed hydatidiform degeneration of the villi in 63 per cent of abnormal ova. The incidence of abnormal ova among spontaneous abortions decreases markedly from the first to the fourth month of gestation. The cause of such abnormalities in human beings is still unknown, but reasoning from experimental teratology, it seems probable that there are two main groups of factors: abnormalities in the earliest stages of segmentation of the ovum and changes in its environment. In the case of pathologic fetuses, Hertig found the average time of expulsion to be 10.2 weeks' menstrual age. In general, the embryo had been dead for an average of about 6 weeks before the abortion was completed.

In the absence of more precise knowledge, abnormalities in the early stages of segmentation are attributed to defective germ plasm from the mother, the father, or both. In many such cases the embryo is lacking or is represented by a formless mass of tissue, whereas the fetal membranes appear normal. In such circumstances it seems that the defect involves the cells forming the inner cell mass but not the trophoblast. In other cases, the trophoblast also may be involved. Grosser thought that whenever the entire periphery of a chorionic

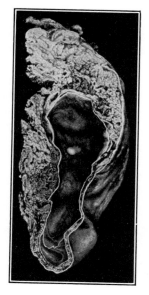

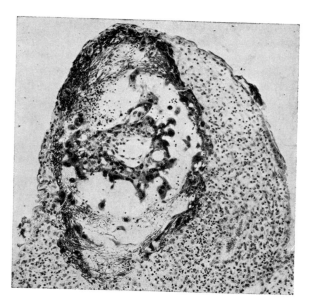

Fig. 4. Abortion result-
ing from defective germ
plasm. Note degenerated
embryo in center.

Fig. 5. Abnormal ovum. A cross section of a defective
ovum showing an empty chorionic sac embedded within
a polypoid mass of endometrium. (From Hertig and
Rock. Amer J Obstet Gynec 47:149, 1944.)

vesicle measuring less than 5 cm in diameter was not thickly covered with villi,
there was a primary trophoblastic defect; consequently, normal development
could not occur. In an attempt to differentiate between the cases with and without blighted ova, Rutherford, by means of decidual biopsy, studied 100 cases of
bleeding during the first four months of pregnancy and found that a diagnosis
could be made on such criteria as difference in staining reaction, vascular thrombosis, and infiltration of erythrocytes and leukocytes into the stroma.

The most conclusive evidence in favor of defective germ plasm is afforded
by the occurrence of double-ovum twins in which one vesicle contains a normal
and the other a rudimentary embryo. In such cases the abnormality cannot easily
be attributed to a defect in implantation, since both ova are presumably implanted in a similar decidua. In most cases, however, the evidence is inferential,
based upon the condition of the embryo, contrasted with that of the remainder
of the conceptus. Streeter thus concluded that defective germ plasm was the
essential cause of 81 of the 104 abortions reported by Huntington.

Failures of fertilization and of normal development of fertilized ova occur in all
mammals. In animals that produce multiple young, the extent of these anomalies may be
assessed by counting the numbers of embryos or young in a litter and comparing them
with the number of corpora lutea in both ovaries of the mother. The discrepancy is
termed "ovum loss." In a second method of study, ova may be recovered from the fallopian tubes and microscopically examined to ascertain the numbers of normal segmenting
eggs, unfertilized eggs, and abnormal fertilized eggs. By the first method, Corner found
a 24 per cent loss of ova in the sow, and by the second method Hartman found a 35
per cent loss in the opossum. In polytocous mammals the failure of some ova to become
fertilized and of others to develop is in large part a defect in germ plasm.

Only within the past decade has detailed information about the genetic basis of abortion become available. As a result of improved technics of tissue culture and cytogenetics, the chromosomes of human abortuses have been studied and the results applied in support of the classic Mall-Meyer hypothesis of defective germ plasm and the theories of Hertig and his co-workers that hold blighted ova to be primary etiologic factors in abortion.

There are considerable differences among the reported percentages of chromosomal anomalies in spontaneous abortion. On the one hand, for example, Thiede and Salm reported polyploidy, autosomal trisomy, and aberrations of sex chromosomes in almost 60 per cent of their cases (Fig. 6). On the other hand,

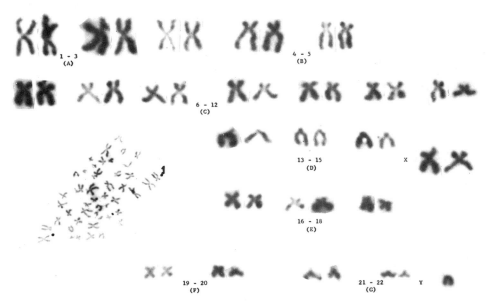

Fig. 6. Abnormal karyotype from a spontaneous abortion: 47,XXY. The extra chromosome, an X sex chromosome, characterizes the Klinefelter syndrome. (Courtesy of Dr. C. Valenti.)

in a careful study of 227 unselected spontaneous abortions, Carr found chromosomal abnormalities in only 22 per cent. The discrepancy apparently reflects the material studied. Singh and Carr reported chromosomal abnormalities in only 6 per cent of anatomically normal embryos, but in 48 per cent of abnormal specimens.

Although data on abortions induced for nonmedical reasons are not numerous, Sasaki and co-workers report an incidence of chromosomal anomalies of 2.8 per cent in a sizable series. Chromosomal anomalies, furthermore, may exhibit both a seasonal variation and a correlation with socioeconomic factors, according to Robinson and Puck.

Discrepancies were found in the primary sex ratios also, although according to Stevenson, the majority of anatomic studies and sex chromatin analyses showed an excess of males. In their study of spontaneous abortion Tricomi, Serr, and Solish noted a male to female ratio of 160 to 100, but Carr's investigations showed an excess of females. Szontagh, Jakobovits, and Mehes found a ratio of 122 male to 100 female in material from therapeutic abortions, whereas Makino and co-workers recorded a ratio approximating unity in similar material. These discrepancies may reflect differences in methods of investigation or possibly the failure to correct for the XO specimens.

These cytogenetic studies call attention to the prevalence of trisomy and polyploidy in spontaneous abortion and suggest that autosomal trisomy, previously associated with advanced maternal age, occurs in the fetuses of younger women also and may represent a genic predisposition to nondisjunction. Whereas previous cytogenetic studies were concerned with the neonate, investigations of malformations incompatible with intrauterine survival are now in progress. The earliest stages of development are particularly important from this point of view, since the earlier in pregnancy an abortion occurs, the more striking are the associated chromosomal anomalies likely to be. Problems such as the true primary sex ratio and the early major genetic anomalies will require cytogenetic study of the crucial but largely inaccessible zygote before implantation. At present, only the grossest chromosomal defects can be recognized: the absence of an entire chromosome, a major translocation, or the reduplication of an autosome (as in Down's syndrome) or a Y chromosome (as in Klinefelter's syndrome). The study of biochemical chromosomal defects has barely begun, and the electron microscope has not produced much valuable information in this area of reproductive wastage.

A suboptimal uterine environment, through its effects on implantation and early fetal nutrition, would be expected to cause defects in the conceptus. The delicate hormonal control of tubal and uterine peristalsis, the multiple endocrine factors associated with formation of the decidua, and the cellular relation of trophoblast and endometrium, must all be integrated to achieve implantation. It is perhaps remarkable that successful implantation occurs as often as it does. Immediately after implantation, furthermore, the trophoblast must obtain nutrition from the decidua and later tap maternal blood vessels, prior to the development of the villous circulation. If any of these mechanisms fails, survival of the ovum is jeopardized and abortion may occur.

Many factors affect both the intrauterine environment and the embryo. Some are well recognized, such as radiation, viruses, and chemicals. Because they can also produce congenital malformations, these factors are called *teratogens* (p. 1066). If they exert their effect at a particular time and at a particular concentration, however, they may produce abortion, either by direct action on the embryo or by alteration of its chromosomal constitution. It is therefore often difficult to assign the cause of abortion to either heredity or environment alone.

Abnormalities of the Placenta. Later in pregnancy, probably from the twentieth week on, certain abnormalities of the placenta may cause abortion, although more commonly they lead to premature labor. Endarteritis, not related to syphilis, may develop in the villi and interfere sufficiently with placental transfer to cause fetal death. Large infarcts may destroy so much placental tissue that the organ will no longer be adequate to meet fetal needs. Abnormalities such as placenta previa, premature separation, and velamentous insertion of the cord may cause circulatory disturbances leading to fetal death, although these accidents characteristically occur later in pregnancy and are not generally considered to be associated with early abortion.

Maternal Disease. ACUTE INFECTIONS. Severe acute infections, notably pneumonia, typhoid fever, and pyelonephritis, occasionally lead to abortion, although they are more likely to bring about premature labor. Malaria may cause abortion because of the high fever in the unprotected woman or rarely because of placental involvement or even placental transmission of the parasites (Lawson and Stewart). Toxins from the mother or specific bacterial invasion may injure the fetus or cause its death and expulsion. Toxic states of the mother, moreover, may initiate labor even when the fetus appears unaffected, especially in severe pneumonia, typhoid fever, and pyelonephritis. Anemia is probably a negligible cause of abortion in the developed countries of the world, but according to Lawson and Stewart, it is a common cause of abortion and premature labor in developing countries where the hemoglobin values may be extremely low. Poisoning with heavy metals or illuminating gas also occasionally produces abortion.

CʜʀOɴɪᴄ ɪɴꜰᴇᴄᴛɪᴏɴꜱ. Many chronic infections have been suspected of causing abortion. In particular, *Brucella abortus,* well known as a cause of chronic abortion in cattle, has been implicated. Many investigators, particularly Spink, have studied this organism and concluded that it has no significance in human abortion. According to some reports, *Listeria monocytogenes* (Rappaport and co-workers) and *Toxoplasma* (Ruffolo, Wilson, and Weed) may be etiologic agents, although they appear to be less important in this country than in other parts of the world.

CʜʀOɴɪᴄ ᴡᴀꜱᴛɪɴɢ ᴅɪꜱᴇᴀꜱᴇꜱ. In early pregnancy diseases such as tuberculosis or carcinomatosis rarely cause abortion; the patient often dies undelivered. In later pregnancy premature labor is not uncommonly associated with these conditions. Pregnancy-induced hypertension is almost never associated with abortion, but does lead to premature labor.

ꜱʏᴘʜɪʟɪꜱ. This disease was formerly considered to be a common cause of abortion. The spirochete does not cross the placental barrier until after the twentieth week, however. Since several weeks of syphilitic fetal infection are required to cause the death or expulsion of the fetus, it is now accepted that syphilis rarely, if ever, causes abortion.

ᴇɴᴅᴏᴄʀɪɴᴇ ᴅᴇꜰᴇᴄᴛꜱ. Abortion is often attributed, perhaps without adequate reason, to deficient secretion of progesterone by the corpus luteum or trophoblast. Since progesterone maintains the decidua, its relative deficiency would theoretically interfere with nutrition of the conceptus and thus contribute to its death. Other endocrine organs, especially the thyroid, may also be involved in some cases of abortion. This theoretical endocrine basis for habitual abortion is discussed on page 511.

ʟᴀᴘᴀʀᴏᴛᴏᴍʏ. The trauma of laparotomy may occasionally provoke abortion. Generalized peritonitis is especially likely to lead to abortion. The nearer the site of surgery is to the pelvic organs, the more likely is abortion to occur. Ovarian cysts and pedunculated myomas may, however, be removed during pregnancy without interfering with the gestation as a rule. Postoperative sedation and the administration of progesterone for the first week or ten days after operation are often prescribed to diminish the probability of abortion, although the efficacy of these drugs remains questionable.

ᴀʙɴᴏʀᴍᴀʟɪᴛɪᴇꜱ ᴏꜰ ᴛʜᴇ ʀᴇᴘʀᴏᴅᴜᴄᴛɪᴠᴇ ᴏʀɢᴀɴꜱ. Local abnormalities and diseases the generative tract are only infrequent causes of abortion. Adnexal inflammation, tumors of the uterus, and endocervicitis may result in sterility; however, they rarely if ever cause abortion.

Uncomplicated displacements of the uterus should not cause abortion. Incarceration, however, is usually accompanied by abortion unless the uterus is freed from the pelvis.

Even large, multiple myomas of the uterus do not necessarily cause abortion. The location of the myoma is more important in this regard than the size of the tumor. Submucous tumors are the most likely variety to cause abortion. The best way to judge the behavior of a myoma in pregnancy is to allow a clinical test.

Important lesions of the generative tract with regard to the causes of abortion are the congenitally short cervix and the cervix that has been shortened by surgical amputation, an operation to be avoided whenever possible during the childbearing years. Long cervical tears that are not properly repaired at the time of delivery or that heal poorly may also cause a late abortion. The "incompetent cervix" is discussed further on page 516.

PSYCHIC AND PHYSICAL TRAUMA. Both physicians and laymen often seek a simple explanation for commonplace medical phenomena. In the case of abortion, they may relate the accident to a fright or perhaps to a recent fall or blow. Multiple examples of trauma that failed to interrupt the pregnancy are forgotten. Only the particular event apparently related temporally to the abortion is remembered. An important argument against the role of trauma in causing spontaneous abortion is based on the factor of time. Most spontaneous abortions occur after fetal death. If trauma were the cause it would not be the recent incident but an event that happened six weeks before the abortion, as a rule. That the traumatic factor is probably overemphasized is borne out by Hertig and Sheldon's analysis of 1,000 cases of abortion, in only one of which they could definitely ascribe the cause to external trauma and psychic shock.

In rare instances, however, both physical and emotional trauma may cause abortion. The inciting mechanism in such cases is probably not death of the fetus but interference with the uterine circulation to the extent that placental separation occurs. Bleeding and abortion should therefore follow the initiating trauma by a short period of time. The products of conception, both fetus and placenta, should show no congenital abnormalities or signs of death antedating the trauma. The burden of proof, furthermore, is always on him who claims trauma to be the inciting cause of the abortion. In our hospitals, with very busy accident services, several abortions meeting these criteria have occurred after severe trauma. In the case of psychic trauma, proof is much more difficult to obtain. If this event is suspected, it is even more important that the criteria of proper time sequence and normal products of conception be rigidly observed.

Pathology. The most frequent lesion in spontaneous abortion is hemorrhage into the decidua basalis, followed by necrotic changes in the tissues adjacent to the bleeding. An inflammatory reaction may supervene. Because of the hemorrhage and necrosis, the ovum becomes detached in part or whole, acting as a foreign body in the uterus and eventually initiating contractions, which result in its expulsion. Until recently it was generally accepted that the decidual hemorrhage was primary and the death of the embryo secondary. McCombs and Craig, however, have shown that decidual hemorrhage is a common finding in normal early pregnancies. A typical early specimen consists of thickened, opaque, blood-infiltrated membranes with a thicker area at one point representing the placenta.

The expelled intact ovum is fluid-filled, and its walls seem rather lax and under little internal pressure. When the membranes are opened, clear fluid is found with a small macerated fetus depressed against a pleated, grayish amnion.

Under a dissecting microscope, the villi often appear thick and distended with fluid, the ends of the villous branches resembling little sausage-shaped sacs. In some the saclike termination seems about to drop off, since its base, where it arises from the villous stem, is often constricted. Such fluid-filled villi are undergoing hydatid degeneration, which probably follows the death of the fetus and is caused by the imbibition of tissue fluid.

On microscopic examination about 30 per cent of the placentas from spontaneous abortions show hydropic changes in the villi. These lesions, which have long been recognized, have been reinvestigated by Gray and his group and by Eckman and Carrow.

Before the tenth week, the ovum is likely to be expelled as an intact sac, often with the decidual cast of the uterus adherent to it. Before that time the anchoring villi of the chorion are not yet attached securely to the decidua, and complete separation of the loosely attached ovum is therefore easy. Between the tenth and twelfth weeks, however, the chorion undergoes striking development. Its anchoring villi establish firm connection with the decidua, leading to retention of chorionic elements in many of these later abortions.

Among the atypical forms of abortus is the *blighted or dropsical ovum,* a small sac with a relatively large volume of fluid and a fetus that is absent or represented by a small amorphous mass.

Blood or carneous mole (Fig. 7) is an ovum that is surrounded by a capsule of clotted blood. The capsule is of varying thickness, with degenerated chorionic villi scattered through it. The small, fluid-containing cavity within it appears compressed and distorted by the thick walls of old blood. This specimen is asso-

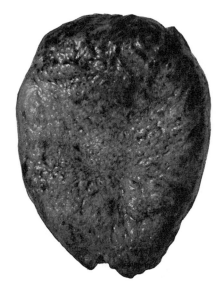

Fig. 7. Blood mole of a complete abortion.

ciated with an abortion that occurs rather slowly, allowing the blood collecting between the decidua and chorion to coagulate and form layers.

Tuberous mole, ovum tuberculosum, and tuberous subchorial hematoma of the decidua are three names applied to the same lesion (Fig. 8). The characteris-

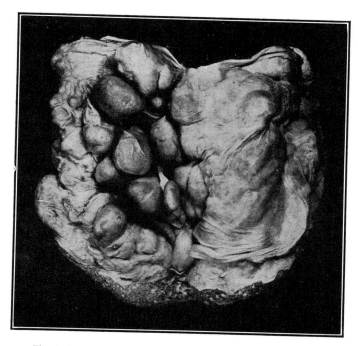

Fig. 8. Tuberous subchorial hematoma. (After H. Dumler.)

tic feature is a grossly nodular amnion, resulting from its elevation by localized hematomas of varying size between the amnion and the chorionic membrane.

Dissolution of the dead fetus is possible only in the early weeks of pregnancy. In abortions occurring after the fetus has attained considerable size, several outcomes are possible. First, the amniotic fluid may be absorbed when the fetus becomes compressed upon itself and desiccated to form a *fetus compressus.* At the same time the placental circulation is abolished, degeneration results, and the whole structure takes on a dry, whitish appearance. Occasionally the fetus becomes so dry and compressed that it resembles parchment. This process is called *mummification.* This outcome is rarely observed in ordinary abortion, although it is relatively frequent in twin pregnancy, particularly when one fetus has died at an early period and the other has gone on to full development. The dead twin becomes a *fetus papyraceus.*

In other cases the retained fetus may undergo *maceration.* In such circumstances the bones of the skull collapse, the abdomen becomes distended with a blood-stained fluid, and the entire fetus takes on a dull reddish color. At the same time the skin softens and peels off at the slightest touch, leaving behind the corium. The internal organs degenerate, becoming friable and losing their capacity for taking up the usual histologic stains.

PATHOLOGIC CLASSIFICATION OF ABORTUSES. Only about one half of all abortuses show embryologic malformations. The standard classification of these so-called pathologic ova (often called the "Carnegie Classification") is that of Mall (Mall and Meyer). This classification, modified by Hertig, is as follows:

Group I. Villi Only. This material contains only chorionic villi, whether normal or abnormal. Obviously this group is for convenience only, since it merely classifies the material submitted, which may or may not adequately represent the relation between maternal and ovular tissues. This group, therefore, includes curettings from cases of incomplete abortions.

Group II. Empty Chorionic Vesicle. This type of specimen when intact, as it often is, represents the most severely diseased type of ovum with which the pathologist has to deal. There is no derivative of the inner cell mass. If the chorion is ruptured, there may be reasonable doubt about the essential pathologic nature of the ovum; that is, the normal embryo with its surrounding amnion may have been lost during the abortion. If trauma has produced such an artifact in an otherwise normal ovum, however, there is usually evidence of the torn stump of a normal umbilical cord with its radiating vessels.

Group III. Chorion Containing Empty Amnion. This type of ovum is only slightly less pathologic than those of Group II. There is no evidence of an embryo, although the amnion is present. Members of this group are likewise valid if intact, as they often are. If ruptured, however, erstwhile normal ova with the embryos missing can usually be detected and differentiated from true Group III specimens.

Group IV. Chorion and Amnion Containing Nodular Embryo. This type is truly pathologic, for the embryonic mass consists merely of a disorganized group of cells. Artifacts in this group consist of the macerated remains of an otherwise normal umbilical cord within either a ruptured or an intact amnion.

Group V. Chorion and Amnion Containing Cylindric Embryo. If the cephalic end of the embryo can be recognized, even though it does not possess any other features of an embryo, such a specimen is valid for this group. It is quite rare, however.

Group VI. Chorion and Amnion Containing Stunted Embryo. It is possible to recognize the embryonic form, although it is much smaller than it should be for the menstrual age of the specimen. In addition, one or more portions of the embryo are atrophic, deformed, or degenerated. These embryos are usually not macerated. This is a valid group whether the chorion and amnion are ruptured or not, since the embryo has to be recognized before the specimen may be placed in this category.

The vast majority of these pathologic ova fall into Groups II, III, and IV. Hertig's modification consisted of eliminating Mall's Group VII, which comprises macerated embryos. This group contains embryos that are essentially normal anatomically.

Clinical Aspects. The clinical aspects of spontaneous abortion are most conveniently discussed under four subgroups: threatened, inevitable, incomplete, and missed.

Threatened Abortion. A *threatened abortion* is presumed to occur when any bloody vaginal discharge or frank vaginal bleeding appears during the first half of pregnancy. A threatened abortion may or may not be accompanied by mild cramps resembling those of a menstrual period or by backache. This interpretation of threatened abortion makes it an extremely commonplace occurrence, since one out of five pregnant women have vaginal spotting or actual bleeding during the early months of gestation. Of those who bleed, one half actually abort. There is reason to believe, however, that many patients who bleed in the first trimester are not threatening to abort. Some early bleeding may be physiologic, analogous to the placental sign described by Hartman in the rhesus monkey. In these animals there is always at least microscopic bleeding. The blood seems to make its way from ruptured paraplacental blood vessels and eroded uterine epithelium into the uterine cavity. Bleeding begins most commonly 17 days after conception, or about 29 days after the pregnant monkey's last menses. In many of Hartman's animals this bleeding could be observed grossly for several days. Microscopic evidence lasted on the average for 23 days. In the woman, furthermore, inflammatory lesions of the external os are likely to bleed in early pregnancy, especially postcoitum. Polyps presenting at the external os as well as decidual reactions of the cervix tend to bleed in early gestation. It is almost impossible to differentiate clinically some of these causes of bleeding in pregnancy from true instances of threatened abortion. For this reason most physicians term all bleeding in early pregnancy threatened abortion. As a result any treatment of so-called threatened abortion achieves a great likelihood of success. Most women who actually threaten to abort probably progress into the next stage of the process no matter what is done. If, however, the bleeding is attributable to some of the benign causes mentioned, it is likely to disappear, regardless of treatment.

The bleeding of threatened abortion is frequently slight, but it may persist for many days or even weeks. Sometimes it is fresh and therefore red, the color varying with the amount of mucus admixed. At other times, when the discharge consists of old blood, the color is dark brown. Lower abdominal cramps and persistent backache usually do not accompany bleeding from other causes.

Inevitable Abortion. *Inevitable abortion* is signalized by rupture of the membranes in the presence of cervical dilatation. Under these conditions, abortion is certain to occur. Very rarely a gush of fluid occurs during the first half of pregnancy without serious consequence. Such an event may be explained in several ways: the membranes may seal over the defect; fluid may collect between the amnion and chorion, with subsequent rupture of the chorion, the amnion remaining intact; and finally, incontinence of urine may be confused with the rupture of the membranes, in late or early pregnancy. The fate of the ruptured amnion is discussed in an experimental study by Wynn, Sever, and Hellman.

Incomplete Abortion. The fetus and placenta are likely to be passed together before the tenth week and separately thereafter. Even if the fetus and placenta appear to be expelled as an intact conceptus, some of the placenta may tear loose and remain adherent to the uterus. When the placenta, in whole or in part, is retained, bleeding ensues sooner or later, to produce the main, and often the only, sign of *incomplete abortion.* Bleeding is invariable in this condition; it is often profuse and may occasionally be massive to the point of profound shock. Such hemorrhage is explained on the basis of bleeding into the spongy layer of the decidua basalis, one of the earliest events in every abortion. As a result, separation of the ovum from the decidua occurs with opening of the underlying venous sinuses. As the process of abortion continues, the uterine contractions, together with the expulsion of the fetus and amniotic fluid, produce further separation. If the placenta separates completely, the muscle fibers clamp down on the blood vessels lying in their interstices and stop blood loss. If, however, placental tissue is partly attached and partly separated, the splintlike action of the attached portion of placenta interferes with myometrial contraction in the immediate vicinity. The vessels in the denuded segment of the placental site, deprived of the constriction by muscle fibers, bleed profusely.

This general principle that a partially separated placenta causes bleeding is one of the most important in all obstetrics. With a completely attached placenta, bleeding from the placental site is obviously impossible. With a completely detached placenta, hemorrhage from the placental site is usually controlled effectively by myometrial contraction. A partially separated placenta, however, always provokes bleeding and is a common cause of obstetric hemorrhage. In fact, it is the mechanism that explains blood loss in four of the most important hemorrhagic complications of pregnancy: third-stage hemorrhage, abruptio placentae, placenta previa, and incomplete abortion.

Missed Abortion. A *missed abortion* is the retention of the products of conception for *two months* or more after the death of the fetus. In the typical instance, the first few months of pregnancy are completely normal, with amenorrhea, nausea and vomiting, breast changes, and growth of the uterus. Upon death of the ovum there may or may not be vaginal bleeding or even transient symptoms denoting a threatened abortion. The uterus then seems to remain stationary in size and the mammary changes regress. The patient is likely to lose a few pounds in weight. Careful palpation and measurement of the uterus reveal that it has not only ceased to enlarge but is growing smaller, as a result of absorption of amniotic fluid and maceration of the fetus. Most patients have no symptoms during this period except persistent amenorrhea. Some, however, complain of lassitude, depression, and a bad taste in the mouth. If the missed abortion terminates spontaneously, as most do, the process of expulsion is quite the same as in any ordinary abortion. The product, if retained several weeks after fetal death, is a shriveled sac containing a greatly macerated embryo. If retained for months or years, it appears to be a mass of old tissue and blood, sometimes with areas of dense calcification.

Occasionally after prolonged retention of the dead products of conception, serious coagulation defects develop. At these times the patient may note troublesome bleeding from the nose or gums or from sites of slight trauma. The pathogenesis and treatment of this condition are discussed in detail on page 509.

The most accurate observations of this condition are those of Streeter, who reported a series of 437 cases of retention of the dead fetus. By comparing the size of the fetus, and thus its actual period of growth, with the menstrual age, he was able to point out the probable discrepancy in time between the death of the fetus and its birth. He found it to be about six weeks on the average, although it was usually somewhat shorter in the early stages of pregnancy and likely to be longer in advanced gestation.

ETIOLOGY OF MISSED ABORTION. The reasons why some abortions do not terminate within a few weeks after death of the fetus are not clear. One explanation depends on the role of progesterone. If the fetus and the placenta die simultaneously or if fetal death is closely followed by that of the placenta, abortion follows quite promptly. If, however, the placenta remains alive, continued production of progesterone will occur. According to one school of thought, the result will be prolonged retention of the products of conception (Bengtsson). The use of the more potent progestational compounds to treat threatened abortion may lead to missed abortion. For example, Piver and colleagues treated 57 women for threatened abortion with Depo-Provera (injectable medroxyprogesterone acetate); more than one third of them retained the dead fetus for more than eight weeks.

Treatment. *Threatened Abortion.* Threatened abortions will be divided into those with vaginal bleeding and no pain, and those with vaginal bleeding accompanied by pain.

VAGINAL BLEEDING WITHOUT PAIN, IN EARLY PREGNANCY. A patient should be instructed to notify her physician immediately whenever vaginal bleeding occurs during pregnancy. In early pregnancy, the utmost medical acumen is required to ascertain whether the bleeding is inconsequential or whether it presages abortion.

In either event, the problem should be discussed frankly with the patient. She should be reassured and an attempt should be made to allay her fears. Although there is no good evidence that any treatment changes the course of threatened abortion, most obstetricians have found it wise to restrict the patient's activity and to give mild sedation in the form of barbiturates. Prolonged bed rest is rarely indicated. Coitus should be interdicted for at least two weeks after the cessation of bleeding.

If the bleeding persists, it is wise to explain to the patient that she may abort and that further restriction of her activity is simply postponing the inevitable for perhaps a few days. The patient should, however, be examined at this time and the cervix viewed with a speculum, for bleeding may be caused by an abnormality unrelated to the pregnancy, such as a cervical polyp or carcinoma. Punch biopsy of the cervix or removal of a polyp will not ordinarily interfere with the progress of the pregnancy.

If, however, the bleeding stops promptly, the patient may resume her usual activities with reasonable assurance that her pregnancy will be normal. Rarely such bleeding is the first indication of serious blood dyscrasias, such as thrombocytopenic purpura or leukemia.

VAGINAL BLEEDING WITH PAIN, IN EARLY PREGNANCY. Usually, the vaginal bleeding begins first and the pain follows a few hours or several days later. The pain may be anterior and clearly rhythmic, simulating mild labor; it may be a persistent low backache, associated with a feeling of pelvic pressure; or it may be a dull, midline, suprasymphysial discomfort, often accompanied by urinary frequency and tenderness over the uterus. Whichever form the pain takes, the prognosis for continuation of the pregnancy is poor. Some threatened abortions with pain cease, however, resulting in a normal pregnancy. It may therefore be reasonable to try to save the pregnancy, since no harm can be done except prolonging the unpleasant process by several hours or days.

The patient should be thoroughly examined, for there is always the possibility that the cervix is already dilated and that abortion is inevitable, or that there is a serious complication such as extrauterine pregnancy or torsion of an unsuspected ovarian cyst. She may be kept at home in bed with mild sedation and codeine to relieve pain, but in general, if the symptoms are severe, she is more effectively treated in the hospital for a few days.

Many obstetricians treat threatened abortion with progesterone intramuscularly in daily doses of 10 to 20 mg or with a wide variety of progestins. As pointed out by Jacobson, among others, some of the progestins, particularly those structurally related to testosterone, may be virilizing to the fetus. Of greater importance is the unresolved controversy regarding the effectiveness of progestational agents in preventing abortion. The recent evidence of a high incidence of chromosomal defects in aborted fetuses lends support to a course of therapeutic nihilism in the case of threatened abortion. This policy is justified by controlled studies such as those of Fuchs and Stakemann on inhibition of labor and those of Shearman and Garrett on habitual abortion. These investigators could find no beneficial effect of steroids. Even in a group of habitual aborters who excreted low levels of pregnanediol, Goldzieher in a well-controlled study could not demonstrate a beneficial effect of exogenous progestational agents.

Occasionally, notwithstanding appropriate treatment and rest in bed, slight hemorrhage may persist for weeks. It then becomes essential to decide whether there is any possibility of continuation of the pregnancy. If two consecutive chorionic gonadtropin analyses of blood or urine are negative, it can be assumed that the outlook is hopeless. Positive findings, however, indicate simply that there is still living trophoblast, but they do not indicate whether the fetus is alive or dead. The problem cannot be settled at once; a delay of several weeks and repeated bimanual examinations are required. If at the end of this period the uterus has not increased in size, or has even become smaller, it is usually safe to conclude that the fetus is dead. An increase in uterine size probably indicates that the fetus is still alive. As soon as fetal death is definite, the uterus should be emptied. Sonographic examination may be helpful in ascertaining the normality of the products of conception. At the present time, however, except in a few clinics with vast experience, this procedure must be considered experimental.

If abortion appears imminent, it is wise to hospitalize the patient at once. As soon as she arrives, her blood should be grouped and matched for possible transfusion. If bleeding and pain persist unabated for six hours, it is probably best to face the reality of abortion and encourage its completion by injection of 0.5 ml of oxytocin intramuscularly every half hour, for six doses, or by use of the drug intravenously in concentrations of 10 to 20 units per liter of 5 per cent glucose in saline. Since oxytocin is likely to increase the pain, the injections should be preceded by the administration of an analgesic. All tissue passed should be kept and carefully studied to see whether the abortion is complete and to ascertain whether the abortion is related to defective germ plasm or another factor that has caused the uterus to empty itself of a normal ovum. Unless all of the fetus and placenta are identified the patient should be taken to the operating room for a sharp or suction curettage under anesthesia. Intravenous thiopental sodium (Pentothal) is an excellent form of anesthesia for such a short procedure in which anesthesia and not complete muscular relaxation is the prime requisite. Temporization is permissible if the patient is febrile, but with effective antibiotic therapy, completion of abortion promptly by curettage has become an acceptable and safe practice.

Inevitable Abortion. If in early pregnancy the sudden discharge of fluid, suggesting rupture of the membranes, occurs before any pain or bleeding, the patient is put to bed and observed. If after 48 hours there is no further fluid and no bleeding or pain, the patient may get up and after 48 hours more continue her usual activities.

If, however, the gush of fluid is followed by bleeding and pain, or if it occurs after pain and bleeding have already begun, abortion is inevitable. The patient should be hospitalized, her blood matched for transfusion, and oxytocin administered, as described. If oxytocin is ineffective, curettage should be performed promptly.

Incomplete Abortion. A patient with an incomplete abortion should be hospitalized, her blood matched for transfusion, and the retained tissue removed promptly. Since oxytocin is seldom effective in these patients, surgical completion of the abortion usually should be performed without delay. In many patients the retained placental tissue simply lies loose in the cervical canal and can be lifted from an exposed external os with ovum forceps. If not, ordinary curettage is performed. In an incomplete abortion it is often unnecessary to dilate the cervix before curettage. The suction technic is an acceptable alternative to sharp curettage for evacuation of the uterus. The technic of completion of an incomplete abortion is described on page 1089.

Although the prompt evacuation of the uterus in incomplete abortion has produced excellent results in our hands and in those of many colleagues, some believe that it is safer to delay curettage in the febrile patient until the fever has subsided or until the operation is forced by hemorrhage.

Hemorrhage from incomplete abortion is occasionally severe and shocking, but rarely fatal. Apparently, when the blood pressure drops to a critically low level, the bleeding from the uterus stops temporarily. Such patients will do best if blood is transfused before and during curettage.

Missed Abortion. Because of the mechanical difficulties involved in terminating by dilatation and curettage a missed abortion in which the fetus did not die until late in the first trimester or later, and because of the attendant high rate of infection, the treatment formerly was expectant. This method of management, although eventually successful, was emotionally trying for the patient and her relatives and was sometimes accompanied by some coagulation defect.

In the presence of certain fetal death, Loudon, Liggins, and others have advised emptying the uterus by administration of gradually increasing concentrations of intravenous oxytocin. We have found these technics quite satisfactory. Liggins begins the infusion with 10 units of synthetic oxytocin in 500 ml of 5 per cent dextrose in water running at the usual rate of 10 to 20 drops per minute. The concentration is increased by 20 units per hour until painful contractions ensue, and the infusion is allowed to run for 8 to 10 hours. If abortion has not occurred, the infusion is discontinued overnight and restarted the following day at a slightly lower concentration than the highest value last employed. As emphasized by Whalley and Pritchard and others, care must be taken to avoid water intoxication resulting from the antidiuretic effect of oxytocin and the electrolyte-free water given intravenously with this technic.

When fetal death occurs, and if the uterine fundus is easily palpable through the abdominal wall, abortion may be brought about by injecting hypertonic dextrose or saline into the uterine cavity. For details of this method of therapy see Chapter 39, page 1093.

HABITUAL ABORTION

Definition. Habitual abortion has been defined by various criteria of number and sequence, but probably the most generally accepted definition today refers to three or more consecutive spontaneous abortions.

In an attempt to give mathematical validity to this definition, Malpas and Eastman used three assumptions to construct a model that would indicate the percentage of women who could be expected to abort after any given number of previous abortions. The assumptions were (1) that the spontaneous abortion rate was known and constant regardless of parity; (2) that the patients who abort fall into two groups, those that are accidental and those that are recurrent; and (3) that the recurrent factors operate with an unvarying consistency. As indicated in Table 1, there was a clear distinction between women who had had two and those who had had three abortions.

Despite these statistical maneuvers the question remains whether there is in fact a clinical syndrome of habitual abortion or whether the results merely reflect

Table 1. Prediction of the Behavior of Women in Successive
Pregnancies in Respect to Repeated Abortion

Per Cent Will Abort

Previous Abortion	Malpas	Eastman	Warburton and Fraser
0	17.0	10.0	12.3
1	21.6	13.2	23.7
2	38.0	36.9	26.2
3	73.0	83.6	25.9

the laws of chance. Both laboratory and clinical experience supports the later proposition. A problem may well arise from attempts to group a variety of conditions of diverse cause under a single heading.

The Malpas-Eastman approach to this problem has been challenged on the basis of the assumptions and clinical observations. A much more precise attack on the problem, using detailed clinical histories, has been attempted by Warburton and Fraser, whose data are also shown in Table 1. Although Warburton and Fraser's expectancy clearly demonstrates two distinct populations—one with a lower rate when the pregnancy follows no previous abortions, and the other with a higher rate when there has been a previous abortion—this change takes place after the first abortion and does not vary significantly regardless of the number of subsequent abortions. Unfortunately, these data, particularly those of Malpas and Eastman, have been used as controls for a vast number of clinical experiments testing various therapeutic agents in the treatment of habitual abortion. Such an approach does not appear valid, however.

Etiology.   Although the multiplicity of mechanical and physiologic factors involved in the success of a normal term pregnancy suggests that the lesions and causes of repeated abortions must be manifold, the etiologic factors can nevertheless be divided into two main classes: (1) defective germ cells and (2) faulty maternal environment.

Defective Germ Cells. Either the spermatozoa or the ova are usually so defective that a pathologic conceptus results from every fertilization and is aborted. Although Mall and Meyer found a high incidence of anatomic defects in incidental spontaneous abortions, and Hertig found 48.9 per cent pathologic ova among a thousand abortuses, these data by themselves do not indicate that the embryos were conceived from defective ova or sperm. In other words, the germ plasm may not be defective genetically, although the data are often used to support this concept. Geneticists find that the probability of a lethal gene that will repeat in man is extremely low. It is therefore equally probable in repeated abortion that the defective product of conception has been produced by faulty maternal environment. For many years it has been contended that if a sperm can fertilize an ovum, it is normal and can therefore play no part in the production of a pathologic conceptus. More recent evidence, however, indicates that a sperm may in fact be sufficiently normal to fertilize an ovum but still lack the potential of contributing to a normally developed embryo (Roszkowski and Stroka; Joël). Joël believes also that hyporspermia may cause repeated abortion. Delfs and Jones noted this occurrence as a sole etiologic factor in abortion in a series of 74 patients with recurrent abortions. Joël, reporting 114 patients with habitual abortion, found 20 instances in which abnormal sperm were judged to be the etiologic factor in abortion. Six of these women had had normal pregnancies with their first husbands and abortions with their second husbands. Another woman had repeated abortions; her husband had been married to a woman with repeated abortions previously. A donor artificial insemination was performed, and the patient delivered a normal child.

Faulty Maternal Environment. It is known that 50 to 80 per cent of all abortuses are pathologic, often lacking an embryo. Whether they are usually caused by a primary defect in the germ cell or by faulty maternal environment remains to be ascertained, but it is possible that many, rather than a few, habitual abortions are caused by defective environment. Some of the possible causes of these maternal defects are as follows:

1. THYROID DYSFUNCTION. Litzenberg was one of the first clinicians to recognize the importance of the thyroid in reproduction. Several investigators have shown an elevation of the protein-bound iodine (PBI) and the butanol-extractable iodine (BEI) during pregnancy (Benson and co-workers). There are rather large variations, especially early in pregnancy, and the exact significance of low levels is unknown. Although hyperthyroidism in untreated patients may cause abortion, it is seldom the cause of repeated abortion.

2. OTHER HORMONAL ABNORMALITIES. As recently as a few years ago it was suggested that abnormal levels of one or more hormones might forecast an abortion or might even serve as therapeutic guides. Such reasoning held sway for more than a decade. Today, however, it is believed that although the values may be low or may fail to rise, the levels of chorionic gonadotropin, chorionic somatomammotropin, pregnanediol, estriol, and hormone secreted by the thyroid are not of great clinical value in predicting the outcome of a particular pregnancy or in determining therapy. Changes in the levels of these hormones usually fail to occur until after irreversible damage to the fetoplacental unit. This subject has recently been reviewed in detail by Klopper.

Because chorionic gonadotropin is a trophoblastic hormone, its level might be expected to indicate placental function. Brody and Carlström reported that patients with threatened abortion whose levels of HCG are low inevitably abort, whereas pregnancy usually continues in those whose levels are normal. The studies of Nesbitt and co-workers, of Hughes and colleagues, and of Watson suggest that chorionic gonadotropin values are of little prognostic significance in habitual abortion (p. 175).

Estriol excretion reflects primarily fetal function (p. 177). Estriol is theoretically, therefore, a more reliable index of possible abortion than is either HCG or pregnanediol, according to Klopper and Macnaughton. The average estriol excretion differentiates patients who will abort from those who will not earlier than does pregnanediol. Particularly after the ninth week of gestation, estriol excretion appears to have prognostic value. There is no proof, however, that estriol deficiency is causative or that estrogen has therapeutic value.

3. NUTRITIONAL FACTORS. Warkany has reviewed the literature showing that in women there is a definite relation between maternal diet and fetal development. The evidence suggests that during periods of prolonged famine there is a decreased birth rate, a lowering of babies' birth weights, and a higher rate of fetal malformation. The abortion rate in women is more difficult to assess, but

when these same defects occur in animals the resorption rates are increased; the assumption is that the abortion rate is also increased in women. In addition to general caloric deprivation, several vitamin deficiencies have been incriminated as etiologically important in abortion. Thiersch has reported fetal malformations and abortions from folic acid deficiencies. Since the growth effects of estrogen are inhibited in the absence of folic acid, this relative deprivation of estrogen is assumed to be the cause of the abortions. An association between folic acid deficiency and abortion is uncertain, however. Martin and co-workers and Hibbard report a higher frequency of abortion in women with folic acid deficiencies. Streiff and Little, however, in studies at the Boston City Hospital could not confirm this association. Jones and associates found that approximately 25 per cent of the women studied in their series showed a lowered level of alpha tocopherol in the serum. Since it was usually associated with other nutritional defects, however, they were inclined to regard the lowered vitamin E level as an index of general nutritional deficiency.

At this time it appears most likely that severe general malnutrition predisposes to increased likelihood of abortion. There is no conclusive evidence, however, that dietary deficiency of any one nutrient is an important cause of abortion.

4. ANATOMIC UTERINE DEFECTS. As demonstrated by Jones and Jones, the diagnosis of a double uterus in a woman with repeated abortions is not sufficient to prove that it is the etiologic factor. Only if all other possible factors can be excluded should it be so considered. In the small series studied at the Johns Hopkins Hospital, it appeared that about one of every four women with a double uterus would have serious reproductive problems. That 75 per cent of women with a double uterus have no serious problem emphasizes the necessity for making certain that the anomaly was indeed the causative factor. A review of the literature discloses abortion rates from 23 to 53 per cent. All of these figures are substantially higher than the incidence rate of 0.5 per cent of all pregnancies that result in habitual abortion or even the 10 to 15 per cent usually quoted as the rate of incidence of abortion in the general population, but they do not approach 100 per cent. In the study of Delfs and Jones, 4 per cent of the patients were found to have some degree of incomplete fusion of the uterus. This figure is significantly below that of 20 per cent reported by Sanchez or 32 per cent by Palmer, and possibly represents differences in population groups. The diagnosis of a double uterus can be made by roentgenologic examination, by manual exploration of the uterus at the time of delivery, and occasionally by dilatation and curettage in the nonpregnant patient. Palpation of the uterus is seriously misleading, and even inspection of the uterus at laparotomy may be inconclusive. *Myomas* can be regarded as the etiologic factor in abortion only if the rest of the clinical investigation is negative and the hysterogram demonstrates a true deformity of the cavity.

5. THE INCOMPETENT CERVIX. The term "incompetent cervix" has been applied to a rather discrete obstetric entity characterized by painless, bloodless dilatation of the cervix in the second trimester of pregnancy, followed by rupture of the membranes and subsequent expulsion of a fetus that is so immature that it almost always succumbs. This same sequence of events tends to repeat itself in each pregnancy, so that the presumptive diagnosis can usually be made if a woman gives a history of rupture of the membranes at midpregnancy in successive gestations with loss of the fetus.

Although the cause of cervical incompetence is obscure, previous trauma to the cervix, especially in the course of a dilatation and curettage or cauterization, appears to be a factor in many cases. In other instances, congenital, developmental, or endocrine factors may play a role. That it is rare in primigravidas who have had no cervical operations points strongly to trauma as the common cause.

The cervical dilatation characteristic of this condition rarely takes place before the sixteenth week, since before that time the products of conception are not sufficiently large to efface and dilate the cervix in the absence of painful uterine contractions. Abortion from incompetence of the cervix is an entirely different entity from spontaneous abortion in the first trimester, since it results from different factors, presents a different clinical picture, and requires different management. Whereas spontaneous abortion in the first trimester is an extremely common complication of pregnancy, incompetence of the cervix is relatively rare. Barter and others have observed only 19 cases of this disorder in some 35,000 pregnancies, and Danforth only 7 in 6,000.

6. SYPHILIS. Although never a cause of abortion before the fourth month, syphilis was formerly a common cause of late abortion or premature delivery and still has this potential if untreated.

7. HYPERTENSIVE VASCULAR DISEASE. Late abortions, fetal death, and premature delivery, sometimes as the result of abruptio placentae, are rather common accompaniments of this condition, particularly if there is associated glomerulonephritis or nephrosclerosis.

8. INCOMPATIBLE BLOOD GROUPS. Although Rh incompatibility may cause stillbirth from erythroblastosis, it very infrequently leads to late abortion. Evidence is accumulating, however, to suggest that ABO-incompatible blood groups may play some etiologic role in habitual abortion. Levine, in 1943, was the first to emphasize that spontaneous abortion appeared to be associated with an increased frequency of ABO incompatibility in the parents. Although some subsequent studies have failed to confirm this observation, the collective evidence of the majority of published reports, particularly the more recent, shows a slight but definite increase in the number of spontaneous abortions in marriages in which there was incompatibility among the ABO blood groups of the partners.

An alternative statistical approach, in which the frequency of abortions and fetal deaths in each ABO mating group is recorded, has also shown an increased frequency of abortions in ABO-incompatible matings. Matsunaga and Itoh, in their Japanese data, found that 15.3 per cent of all pregnancies terminated in abortions in incompatible matings, in contrast to 10.3 per cent in the compatible group. This result is significant at the 0.001 level. A study of American couples by Reed and Kelly also showed an increased number of abortions among ABO-incompatible matings, but the difference was not statistically significant.

9. PSYCHIATRIC. In a review of personality factors associated with habitual abortion, Tupper and Weil found that there were two types: the basically immature and the independent frustrated woman. Results suggest that supportive therapy is as effective as anything else in preventing loss.

Clinical Investigation. The most successful treatment of repeated abortion is accomplished before conception, since the disclosure of the factors involved can frequently be made only in the nonpregnant patient. Thus, treatment before conception for the correction of some factors is necessary for a successful outcome, as emphasized by Delfs and Jones, by Hughes, Lloyd, and Ledergerber, by Asplund, and by Levine and co-workers. A general outline for the investigation of etiologic factors in habitual abortion is given in Table 2.

Table 2. Outline for Clinical Investigation of Patients with Repeated Abortion

A. History
B. Physical examination
C. Diagnostic procedures: preconceptional
    1. X-ray examinations
        (a) Chest
        (b) Hysterosalpingogram
    2. Hematology
        (a) Hgb, WBC, differential
        (b) Blood type of patient and husband
        (c) Sedimentation rate
    3. Serologic test for syphilis
    4. Blood chemistry
        (a) Protein-bound serum iodine, or other specific indices of thyroid metabolism
        (b) Glucose tolerance test
    5. Special tests
        (a) Basal temperature chart
        (b) Endometrial biopsy, performed in luteal phase
    6. Serum progesterone assay, performed in luteal phase
D. Diagnostic procedures: postconceptional
    1. Serologic antibody titers if ABO blood type incompatibilities are suspected
    2. Protein-bound serum iodine, if thyroid dysfunction is suspected
    3. Quantitative serum chorionic gonadotropin (at least two values)
    4. Urinary pregnanediol at onset of pregnancy

Germ Plasm Defects. There is, of course, no known treatment for defective germ plasm, either sperm or ovum. The only recourse is to advise a good schedule of diet, exercise, and rest, with limitations of alcohol, tobacco, and drugs. Excessive fatigue, insufficient sleep, nervousness, and tension caused by overwork or social activities should be corrected.

Thyroid Dysfunction. Thyroid replacement may be indicated if the protein-bound iodine is below 4 μg/100 ml before pregnancy or below 6 μg/100 ml in the first trimester. Although most of these patients never develop definite symptoms or signs or myxedema, this is justifiable therapy for patients with a history of abortion, since there is evidence that reproductive difficulty may be one of the most sensitive indicators of thyroid deficiency in the adult and may be manifest long before other clinical signs. Dosage of thyroid should be adjusted to the patient's needs, but large amounts are rarely required. It should be continued throughout pregnancy with increase or reduction in dosage, depending on the protein-bound iodine values.

Steroid and Protein Hormonal Deficiencies. As indicated on page 511 the lowered values of these hormones cannot be taken as evidence that the apparent deficiency is in fact an etiologic factor in the abortion. Despite reports to the contrary, therefore, there is no scientific reason to expect any benefit from substitution therapy (Goldzieher; Shearman and Garrett).

Nutritional Deficiencies. The weight and nutritional status of patients should be carefully evaluated. Women who are obese should reduce before conception, and those who are underweight should be instructed in proper diet, rest, and hygiene. All patients with reproductive difficulties benefit from diets adequate in protein, vitamins, and calories.

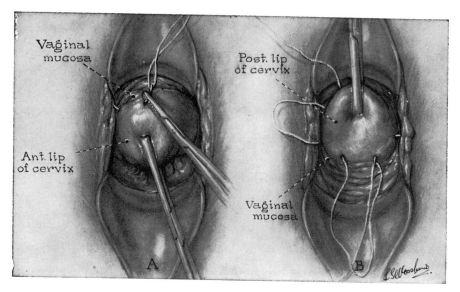

Fig. 9. The McDonald operation for repair of incompetent cervix. A, the purse-string suture of braided silk is started at the junction of the rugose vaginal mucosa and the smooth cervix. B, it is continued with two bites posteriorly; they should be placed deeply, because if the ligature subsequently pulls out, it does so posteriorly.

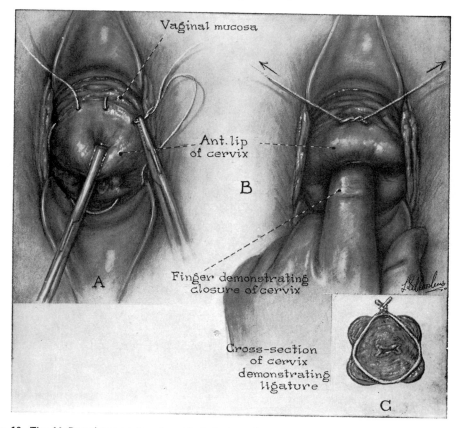

Fig. 10. The McDonald operation (cont.). A, laying of purse-string suture concluded. B, tying of ligature by assistant sufficiently tightly to admit just the tip of the operator's finger. C, anatomic result of operation.

Uterine Anomalies. In case of a double uterus in which the anomaly shown is considered to be the etiologic factor for the repeated abortions, a unification operation is justifiable. The rate of successful pregnancies following this operation is significant. Myomectomy, when indicated, should be performed.

Incompetent Cervix. With other causes of habitual abortion in midpregnancy ruled out, the treatment of the incompetent cervix is surgical. It consists in essence of reinforcing the weak cervix by some kind of purse-string suture. It is best performed between the fourteenth and eighteenth weeks and certainly before a dilatation of 4 cm is reached, if possible.

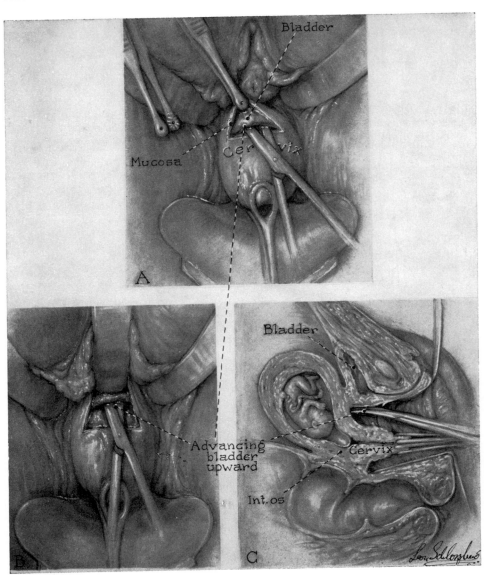

Fig. 11. Shirodkar-Barter operation for repair of incompetent cervix. A, after transverse incision of vaginal mucosa, the bladder is displaced upward by dissection with scissors. B and C, the bladder has been dissected upward to a level just above the internal os.

Two main types of operation are in current use for the patient already pregnant. One is a very simple procedure, as recommended by McDonald and illustrated in Figures 9 and 10. The other is the Shirodkar operation. Its modification by Barter and his colleagues is illustrated in Figures 11, 12, 13, and 14. In an analysis of 206 operations for cervical incompetence reported in the literature in which one or the other of these technics was used, Neser found a success rate of 67 per cent. As experience grows, success rates approaching 80 per cent are being achieved with both the McDonald and the Shirodkar technics, as amply demonstrated by the figures of Barter and of Gans, as well as by our own personal experience. In the event that the operation fails and signs of imminent abortion

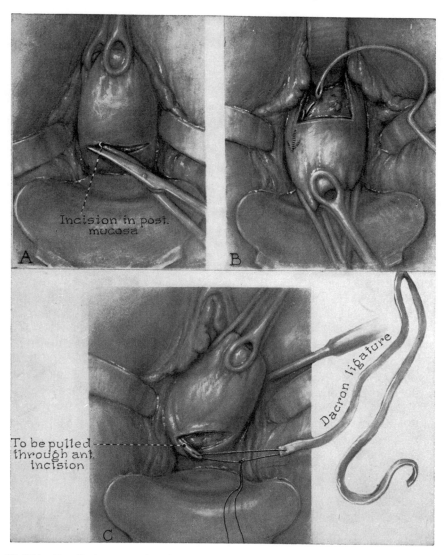

Fig. 12. Shirodkar-Barter operation (cont.). A, incision in posterior mucosa at a level corresponding to that of anterior incision. B, aneurysm needle is about to be passed through anterior incision, under the vaginal mucosa, and out through the posterior incision. C, a Dacron ligature is attached to the needle.

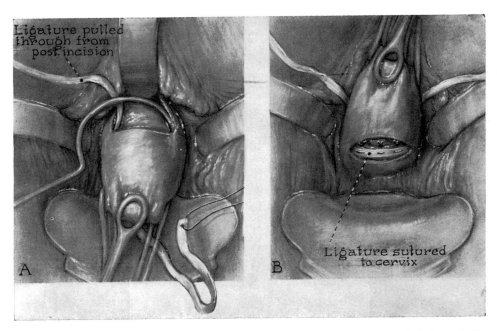

Fig. 13. Shirodkar-Barter operation (cont.). A, the ligature having been pulled through the incisions on the patient's right, the same procedure is carried out on the left side. B, the Dacron ligature is anchored to the posterior cervix by a silk suture to prevent its slipping over the posterior lip of the cervix.

develop, it is urgent that the suture be released at once, since failure to do so promptly may result in grave sequelae. In successful cases following the McDonald procedure, the suture must be removed at the thirty-eighth or thirty-ninth week to allow labor to progress. After the Shirodkar operation, the suture may be left in place and a cesarean section performed near term (a plan designed to prevent the necessity of repeating the procedure in subsequent pregnancies), or it may be released and vaginal delivery permitted, according to circumstances.

For the patient with a typical history of repeated abortions caused by an incompetent cervix, Lash and Lash have devised an operation that is performed when the patient is not pregnant. The mucosa is dissected from the anterior lip of the cervix, and an elliptical incision is made in the anterior lip between the internal and external os. A small amount of tissue is removed and the defect closed with interrupted sutures.

Blood Incompatibilities. To date, there is no treatment for blood incompatibilities. The only advice to a patient who wants to bear her own child may be therapeutic insemination using a donor with a compatible blood group.

Congenital Malformations of the Uterus (Double Uterus). Repairs of this defect by the technics described by Strassmann and by Jones and Jones lead to a successful pregnancy rate of around 85 per cent.

Prognosis. Except when there are definitely correctable surgical defects, one must guard against overoptimism. Overstreet states that whatever treatment is used, the apparent cure rate after three abortions will range between 70 and 80 per cent. In other words, the loss rate will be higher, but not much higher, than that anticipated for pregnancies in general.

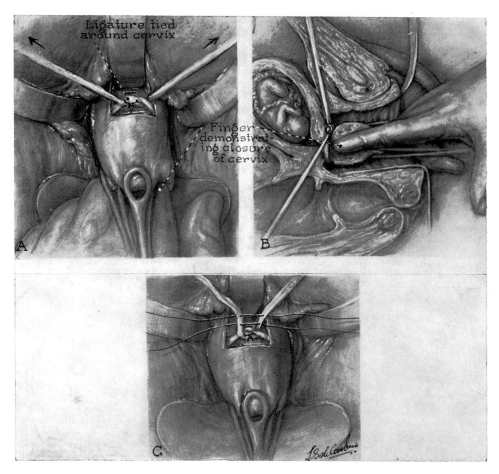

Fig. 14. Shirodkar-Barter operation (cont.). A, after tying the ligature anteriorly, it is anchored by a silk suture. B, testing size of internal os, which should admit just the fingertip. C, reinforcing ligature before cutting.

There is no evidence that the patient who has had habitual abortions will, when she finally carries her pregnancy to term, deliver an abnormal child.

INDUCED ABORTION

Therapeutic Abortion. This subject is discussed in Chapter 39.

Illegal Abortion. The incidence of illegal abortion is for obvious reasons unknown, but most observers believe that it is appallingly high. Some idea of the magnitude of the problem may be gleaned from the fact that in the recent past nearly half the maternal deaths in New York City were related to abortion. Former publications on the subject estimated the rate of illegal abortion in the United States to be in the range of 10 to 12 per cent. Currently, these figures are believed to be too low. An educated guess places the rate at not less than 15 per cent nor more than 25 per cent of the live births. In some Central American countries, the incidence approaches 50 per cent. There are no data to indicate the impact of recent changes in abortion laws on these estimates.

Consequences and Complications of Abortion

Serious complications of abortion are usually, but not always, associated with illegal abortion. Severe hemorrhage, sepsis, acute renal failure, and bacterial shock have all been found occasionally in spontaneous abortion also.

The most serious consequence of abortion is death. The incidence of abortion as obtained from death certificates is undoubtedly too low, since many abortions are hidden under the headings of hemorrhage or infection. At Kings County Hospital, for example, abortion accounted for one third of all the maternal deaths—a rate of 1.3 deaths per 1,000 abortions.

In New York City, before the recent repeal of the abortion law, Gold and his colleagues showed that the death rate from illegal abortion has risen from 1.6 to 3.1 per 10,000 live births in the past 20 years. It is a common fallacy, particularly in lay publications, to exaggerate the number of maternal deaths attributable to abortion each year. For example, Pilpel and Norwick state that "illegal (out-of-hospital) abortions account for as many as 8,000 maternal deaths each year." Although the exact number is unknown, in 1967 there was a total of only 50,683 deaths of women, aged 15 to 44, and only 987 maternal deaths. The often quoted high figure is therefore obviously impossible. The National Center for Health Statistics records 160 abortion deaths in 1967.

Febrility. Whereas elevation of temperature may, and usually does, accompany the serious complications of abortion, there is frequently fever just before and during the passage of the products of conception in noninduced abortion. For example, in 4,957 abortions the incidence of febrility was 27 per cent.* In this group serious complications occurred in 12.2 per cent, whereas the same complications were recorded in 7 per cent of the afebrile group.

The serious complications of abortion are related to infection and hemorrhage. For purpose of classification, acute renal failure and bacterial shock are placed in separate categories because these complications are highly lethal (Table 3). There is, in addition, a host of serious miscellaneous complications related to anesthesia, transfusions, and noxious agents used to induce abortion.

Table 3. Serious Complications of Abortion

	Per Cent Incidence
Infection (temperature of 101°F for 24 hours or more)	3.7
Hemorrhage (two or more transfusions needed)	0.8
Acute renal failure	0.1
Bacterial shock	0.1
Other, miscellaneous*	0.9

* Four perforations included.

Infection. Abortal infection is most often caused by enteric organisms, especially bacteria of the coli-aerogenes group. Second most common is the anaerobic streptococcus. Less common today are hemolytic streptococci, staphylococci, and

* Statistics in this section are from computed data of the Kings County Hospital unless otherwise specified. The term "febrility" indicates any elevation of temperature of 100.4°F or above.

clostridia. Infection is most commonly confined to the uterus in the form of endometritis. Parametritis, peritonitis (localized and general), and even septicemia are by no means rare. In the course of treating nearly 300 cases of septic abortion at Parkland Memorial Hospital during 1966 and 1967, a positive blood culture was found in one fourth. The organisms identified are listed in Table 4.

Table 4. **Bacteria Present in 76 Cases of Septic Abortion with Positive Blood Cultures**

Organisms Cultured	Frequency Per Cent
Anaerobic	63
Peptostreptococcus (anaerobic streptococcus)	41
Bacteroides	9
Both	9
Cl. perfringens	4
Aerobic	37
E. coli	14
Pseudomonas	9
β-hemolytic streptococcus	4
Enterococcus	3
Combination	7

From Smith, Southern, and Lehman. Obstet Gynec 35:704, 1970.

In our experience, infection is best treated by prompt evacuation of the products of conception. Although mild infections can be treated successfully with broad-spectrum antibiotics in usual dosage, any serious infection should be attacked with great vigor from the very start. We have found that penicillin in intravenous doses of 20 to 30 million units per day combined with either 1 g of streptomycin or 2 g of tetracycline yields excellent results.

When infection becomes chronic, with the formation of a pelvic abscess, a long and debilitating illness can be expected. In general, if drainage of these abscesses can be accomplished vaginally, it is the treatment of choice. Although a few patients will require abdominal operation with removal of the abscess along with the uterus, tubes, and ovaries, nothing is to be gained by abdominal removal of the indurated adnexa before the formation of an abscess.

Hemorrhage. In hospital practice, fatal hemorrhage from abortion is extremely rare. In Kings County Hospital, with nearly 40,000 abortions in the past 20 years, there has been but one death from this cause. Although patients are often admitted with extreme degrees of blood loss, the bleeding usually stops when the blood pressure drops to shock level. Treatment is support through transfusion and evacuation of the uterus.

Bacterial Endotoxic Shock. Bacteremia, caused usually by *E. coli* but also by other gram-negative bacteria, sometimes results in severe and often fatal shock. The endotoxin is contained in the cell wall of the offending organism. The phospholipid causes its toxicity and the polysaccharide its antigenicity. Such shock, fortunately rare, is seen most often in connection with induced abortion, although it may occur as a result of infection in the genital or urinary tracts at any time during pregnancy or the puerperium. It is not peculiar to obstetrics, but is seen in a wide variety of postoperative infections, especially in urology. Endotoxic shock complicates between 0.1 and 0.2 per cent of abortions, and the mortality rate may range from 50 to 70 per cent, depending on the severity of the process and the degree of renal involvement.

This rare but highly lethal complication of abortion has received current attention of investigators and clinicians alike. Bacterial endotoxic shock is characterized by shock in a febrile patient who does not respond readily to intravenous fluid including blood transfusion. Most shock associated with abortion is transient and usually alleviated by simple infusion. Bacterial shock, however, is not, and if intravenous therapy is long continued despite lack of response, the patient can drown while still hypotensive. The pathogenesis of endotoxic shock is still not clearly understood. Selective vasospasm has been suggested as the basic etiologic mechanism by Fine and co-workers, as well as by Lillehei and MacLean.

This theory postulates a release of catecholamines, stimulated by the endotoxin. In the final phase, tissue hypoxia results in vasodilatation. Good and Thomas, as well as McKay and Shapiro, believe, on the basis of human autopsies and animal studies, that disseminated intravascular coagulation is a basic mechanism. These different responses to the toxin have resulted in widely divergent courses of treatment. An outline of therapy that has proved relatively successful in our institutions is as follows:

Diagnosis and Treatment of Bacterial Endotoxic Shock

1. *Suspicion.* Blood pressure and urinary flow should be closely monitored. Bacterial shock should be strongly suspected in any case of infected abortion whenever there is any evidence of hypotension or oliguria.
2. *Recognition.* If hypotension and oliguria are not improved by rapid administration of a liter of electrolyte-containing fluid, such as lactated Ringer's solution, the shock is most likely caused by bacterial products.
3. *Treatment*
   a. Control of Infection
      (1) After obtaining cultures from blood and urine as well as from the cervix (anaerobic and aerobic), intensive broad-spectrum antibiotic therapy is begun. The kinds of organisms usually found in the blood are listed in Table 4. A combination of penicillin, tetracycline, and kanamycin or gentamycin has proved effective.
      (2) Once antibiotic therapy has been started and the patient's condition is somewhat stable, the infected products of conception are removed by curettage. Hysterectomy is seldom indicated unless the uterus has been lacerated or perforated by the abortionist's manipulations. Since bacterial shock can develop several hours after evacuating the infected products, careful monitoring must continue after curettage.
   b. Treatment of Shock. The primary goal is to establish adequate perfusion of vital organs. The adequacy of the circulation may be ascertained by continuously monitoring urinary flow using an indwelling catheter connected to a graduated cylinder. The commercially available Urinometer is quite satisfactory for this purpose.
      (1) *Fluid therapy.* Whole blood is given in amounts that maintain the hematocrit at or above 30. Electrolyte-containing fluids, such as lactated Ringer's solution, are given at a rate that maintains urinary flow at more than 0.5 ml, and preferably about 1.0 ml, per minute and the systolic blood pressure at 80 mm Hg or slightly higher. Sodium bicarbonate solution is of value in combating acidosis. *Central venous*

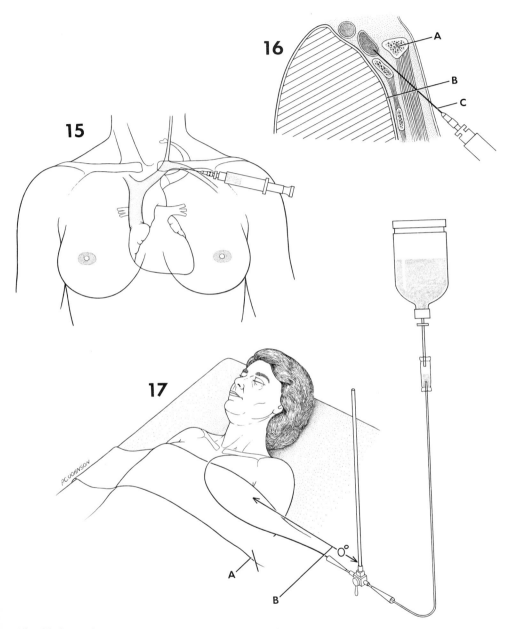

Fig. 15. Central venous pressure. Surface anatomy is shown in relation to the subclavian vein. (From Nelson. Atlas of Radical Pelvic Surgery. 1969. Courtesy of Appleton-Century-Crofts.)
Fig. 16. The anatomic relations of the subclavian vein are illustrated. Note the clavicle (A) overlying the vein, and the pleura (B) underlying it. C, needle in subclavian vein. (From Nelson. Atlas of Radical Pelvic Surgery. 1969. Courtesy of Appleton-Century-Crofts.)
Fig. 17. The catheter (A) in the subclavian vein is connected to a three-way stopcock. Remaining connections of the stopcock are with the manometer and an intravenous bottle. B, zero on manometer is lined up with midaxillary line. (From Nelson. Atlas of Radical Pelvic Surgery. 1969. Courtesy of Appleton-Century-Crofts.)

(right atrial) *pressure* is monitored continuously, as described by Wilson and colleagues (Figs. 15, 16, and 17). If central venous pressure rises beyond normal, intravenous fluids must be sharply restricted.

(2) *Adrenocortical steroids.* If control of the infection by antibiotics and curettage and the infusion of blood and aqueous fluids do not result in prompt improvement, large doses of corticosteroids are indicated. Lillehei and associates have recommended 10 g of Solu-Cortef or its equivalent rapidly administered intravenously. We have used 0.5 g of Solu-Medrol in this way. Steroid therapy need not be continued beyond the acute phase and it can be stopped abruptly.

(3) *Pressor agents.* These agents are not so popular as they were a decade ago. We have been impressed, however, by their occasional value in appropriate doses, especially metaraminol (Aramine). In response to infusion of metaraminol, a rise in blood pressure is frequently seen, accompanied by increase in urinary output, indicating improved perfusion. The drug has an additional powerful inotropic effect. It does not cause serious local necrosis, as does levarterenol bitartrate (Levophed). As little as 10 mg of metaraminol per liter may be effective, but as much as 500 mg per liter has been used without any deleterious effects. It may be necessary to decrease the dose of this drug gradually over the course of several days.

(4) *Vasodilating agents.* Drugs such as isoproterenol have been recommended to relieve vasoconstriction (Du Toit). Their role in cases of septic abortion with endotoxic shock is still questionable, however.

(5) *Heparin.* The concept that intravascular coagulation occludes the microcirculation in endotoxic shock has led to the recommendation that heparin be used in these circumstances (Phillips, Skrodelis, and Quigley). To date, however, no adequate clinical trial has been reported.

At Parkland Memorial Hospital during 1966 and 1967 there were nearly 300 cases of septic abortion with 3 deaths. In 2 there was some evidence before death of disturbances in the coagulation mechanism. At autopsy, material thought to be fibrin and platelets was found in the smaller blood vessels of vital organs. As yet there is no proof that heparin can prevent this complication. More important, the morbidity and mortality from heparin therapy in large numbers of women are unknown. Moreover, in other instances of septic abortion with gross disruption of the coagulation mechanism (including hypofibrinogenemia, thrombocytopenia, and accumulation of fibrin breakdown products, as indicated by a prolonged thrombin time), hemorrhage and sepsis were controlled by blood transfusions, fibrinogen, prompt curettage, and broad-spectrum antibiotics. Marked reduction in bleeding from the uterus, nose, and needle holes was noted immediately after injecting 4 g of fibrinogen, without evidence of deleterious vascular obstruction from the injected material (Pritchard). In similar instances, fibrinogen has been withheld and the hemorrhage treated with whole blood only. The majority of our patients so treated have recovered.

Acute Renal Failure. Persistent renal failure in abortion probably stems from the combined effects of infection. More rarely it can arise from toxic compounds employed to produce abortion, such as soap or Lysol. Abortion caused renal failure in 59 per cent of 70 pregnant women sufficiently ill to require some form of

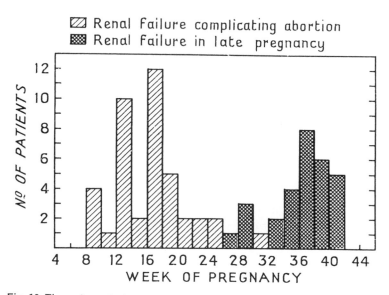

Fig. 18. Time of onset of renal failure. (From Smith et al. Lancet 8:351, 1965.)

dialysis according to Smith and co-workers (Fig. 18). Whereas very severe forms of bacterial endotoxic shock are frequently associated with renal damage, the milder forms rarely lead to overt renal failure. Most important is the early recognition of this very serious complication. It is therefore advisable to follow carefully for the first 24 hours the urinary output of all patients with abortion. The word "serious" is used advisedly in connection with acute renal failure in abortion, for the maternal mortality before the extensive use of dialysis exceeded 75

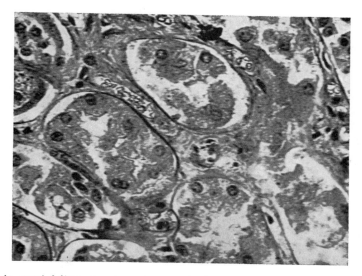

Fig. 19. Acute renal failure showing edema and disruption of the basement membrane of the renal tubules.

per cent (Knapp and Hellman). With modern therapy, Smith and his colleagues have reduced this figure to 27 per cent.

As Oliver, McDowell, and Tracy clearly stated, the fundamental lesion in some cases is not in the epithelial cells of the tubules but in the basement membrane (Fig. 19). Once the basement membrane is destroyed, the epithelium cannot regenerate to form a functioning nephron. In about 50 per cent of cases, however, no microscopic lesion is evident. Recovery depends on the proportion of tubules that are temporarily damaged to those that sustain permanent damage to the basement membrane.

Treatment is directed toward careful maintenance of fluid and electrolyte balance. Homeostasis is achieved by restriction of fluids, regulation of electrolytes, and dialysis. We agree with the plan of treatment recommended by Smith and co-workers as follows:

1. Rigid restriction of fluids and electrolytes.
2. Active cooperation with a renal dialysis unit.
3. Early use of peritoneal dialysis—*as soon as renal failure becomes manifest and before the advent of uremia.*
4. Hemodialysis if peritoneal dialysis is unsuccessful.

In experienced hands few if any of these patients will die of strictly renal causes. The great killer in abortion with or without renal failure is infection. Proper use of antibiotics is therefore crucial.

Perforation.   Accidental perforation of the uterus during dilatation or curettage is not unusual. As a rule, the accident is easy to recognize, the instrument passing without hindrance farther than it could have had uterine perforation not occurred. Observation may be sufficient if the hole in the uterus is small, as it well may be if produced by a sound or dilator. Such small defects may heal readily without complication.

A perforation made during the course of an illegally induced abortion is quite a different problem. In these patients, the rent may be large, involving a vascular portion of the uterus or even bowel or bladder. Such perforations may be obvious on admittance of the patient, who may present evidence of severe bleeding into the peritoneal cavity or generalized peritonitis. They may, however, be obscured by pelvic peritonitis or missed because neither serious bleeding nor infection is yet obvious. In face of a known induced abortion, radiologic examination of the patient in the standing position should always be performed. The films will usually show air beneath the diaphragm if there is a perforation, and sometimes even a foreign body in the peritoneal cavity (Figs. 20 and 21). In the likely event of uterine perforation in these circumstances, laparotomy should always be performed. At operation not only is it necessary to repair the rent in the uterus, but the bowel must be thoroughly searched for possible injury as well.

PREMATURE LABOR

As pointed out in Chapter 1, premature birth is by far the most common cause of neonatal mortality and morbidity, accounting for one half of all such deaths and a high percentage of neurologic, intellectual, and emotional deficits (Drillien). The incidence of premature labor, based on the 2,500 g criterion, varies with the race and economic status of the population. In the United States

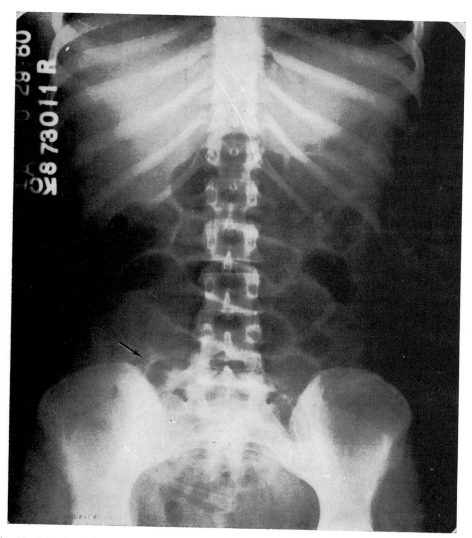

Fig. 20. Catheter lying free in the peritoneal cavity after uterine perforation during a criminal abortion.

the incidence of prematurity in the nonwhite population in 1958 was 12.9 per cent, as contrasted with 6.8 per cent for the white. The role of economic factors in the causation of premature labor has been most convincingly demonstrated by Baird, who has shown that in Aberdeen, Scotland, the incidence of prematurity is about two times greater among wives of unskilled workers than among those in the professional and managerial classes. This variability is further emphasized by comparing the figures from Hartford, Connecticut, the University of California, and the Kings County Hospital, where the race and economic status of the populations show considerable variation (Table 5). These factors influence the incidence of prematurity, but not the perinatal mortality rate for the premature infants. In Hartford the population is largely white. The University of California has a mixed population in regard to race and economic status. In contrast, the patients in the Kings County Hospital are indigent and mainly black.

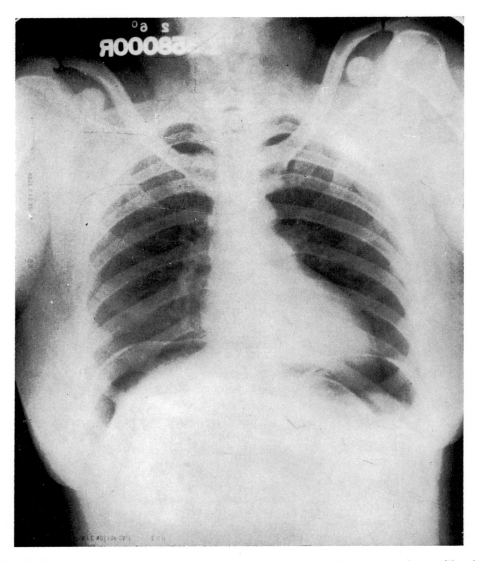

Fig. 21. Air under both domes of the diaphragm after perforation of the uterus after an illegal abortion.

In only about 40 per cent of patients can the cause of the premature delivery be demonstrated. On the basis of our experience, the maternal diseases that most frequently initiate the onset of premature labor are chronic hypertensive vascular disease, abruptio placentae, placenta previa, and, formerly, untreated syphilis. In other patients certain diseases, especially preeclampsia, demand termination of pregnancy prior to maturity of the fetus to safeguard the mother's life or health. If cases of multiple pregnancy and congenital abnormalities are added to these two groups, the total number of cases of premature labor in which the causative

Table 5. Incidence of Prematurity°

Hospital	Total No. of Births	Per Cent Incidence	Per Cent Perinatal Mortality in Prematures
Hartford	22,133	6.69	16.42
University of California	8,572	9.74	14.97
Kings County	27,416	14.18	15.05

° *Infants 1,000 g to 2,499 g.*
All data are for the period from January 1, 1961, to December 31, 1964.

factor can be demonstrated is less than 40 per cent. Although this percentage must be regarded as an approximation only, there is general agreement that a large proportion of premature labors, about one half, are without explanation. The search for the cause has been hindered by the use of weight alone as the index of prematurity. Etiologic factors in true prematurity and in growth retardation are mostly unknown. Infants that are small at or near term are obviously different from and have prognoses different from those of true premature infants (Ch. 37, p. 1026). Future studies must be discriminate between these two groups.

In a thoughtful review of the association between smoking and prematurity, Goldstein and co-workers indicate that both retrospective and anterospective studies show a positive correlation. Increasingly convincing evidence indicates that maternal smoking during pregnancy is associated with decreased birth weight and an increased incidence of prematurity, as defined by birth weight alone (U.S. Public Health Service Review Supplement, 1969). These conclusions are supported by investigations in many areas of the world (Russell in England; Terris and Gold in the United States; Kizer in Venezuela; and many others). Russell's studies suggest an association between smoking during pregnancy and abortion and perinatal loss, but an etiologic relation remains to be proved. The mechanism by which smoking affects pregnancy is unknown.

The hypothesis that nutrition plays a significant etiologic role in prematurity is attractive, but Thomson searched the available data in vain for proof. Very recently Pritchard and co-workers reported the frequency of prematurity, that is, low birth weight, among women with folate deficiency so severe as to cause overt megaloblastic anemia to be not greater than in the general obstetric population at Parkland Memorial Hospital. Eastman and Jackson have reopened the question of nutrition by showing that a small weight gain during pregnancy, especially in light women, tends to be associated with an increased incidence of prematurity.

In view of the profound effect of prematurity on reproductive efficiency, it is suprising that so little new etiologic information has been provided. Two etiologic correlations have recently been stressed: small cardiac volume and asymptomatic bacteriuria. Hedberg and Radberg investigated the former but were unable to show that either maternal weight or heart volume was of practical value in the prediction of prematurity.

The association between prematurity and asymptomatic bacteriuria was first suggested by Kass. Although his subsequent publications have stimulated a great many studies, such as those of Sleigh and colleagues, Whalley and co-workers, and Gold, there is no evident substantiation of the relation. Whereas Kass' figure of a

7 per cent incidence of bacteriuria in pregnancy and his positive correlation of bacteriuria and subsequent pyelonephritis have been confirmed repeatedly, the positive correlation of asymptomatic bacteriuria per se and prematurity remains to be proved. Current concepts of etiology and prognosis of prematurity have been reviewed by Abramowicz and Kass.

About one third of premature labors follow spontaneous rupture of the membranes. In isolated cases, the fluid stops leaking or pregnancy may progress to term despite the loss of fluid. In the majority of cases, however, labor supervenes in hours or days. Prolonged rupture of membranes leads to intrauterine infection in a high percentage of cases. Whereas maternal infection may be controlled with antibiotics, these drugs will not protect the fetus when given either prophylactically or after the onset of fever and other signs of infection (Lebherz and co-workers). The only safeguard for the baby is delivery and treatment after birth; even cesarean section may occasionally be required. Here the nicest judgment is necessary, for the odds in favor of survival of the infant out of the uterus must be carefully weighed against the degree of prematurity. It is probably unwise to perform a cesarean section to prevent infection of the fetus if the estimated fetal weight is less than approximately 1,800 g.

Bishop and Woutersz have produced evidence that premature labor may be arrested in some cases by the administration of isoxsuprine hydrochloride, and Fuchs has claimed success with intravenous alcohol. These therapeutic efforts are interesting and merit further trial. No greater error can be made than the administration of narcotizing or sedative drugs in an effort to stop labor. It is not only futile, as a rule, but also deleterious to the baby.

Management of Premature Labor.   Analgesic agents that cross the placenta should be administered with caution to patients in premature labor. Delivery is preferably performed under epidural, caudal, spinal, or infiltration anesthesia, with the aid of an adequate episiotomy. Inhalation of nitrous oxide with a substantial mixture of oxygen offers little risk to the infant.

The ideal procedure for the actual delivery of a premature infant, especially a small one, in our opinion is as follows. When the head is on the perineum and the vulvar ring is just beginning to distend, an episiotomy is made, followed by gentle fundal pressure. This method of delivery usually suffices, but with larger premature infants gentle forceps extraction may be advisable. The cord should be clamped immediately, because the livers of these infants cannot excrete bilirubin formed by the excess blood received by the infant if clamping is delayed until pulsations cease. Many pediatricians have reported significantly higher bilirubin levels in premature infants who were subjected to late cord clamping. After delivery the main immediate desiderata for the infant are a clear airway, oxygen, warmth, and a minimum of handling. (For further discussion of the premature infant, see Ch. 37.)

References

Abramowicz, M., and Kass, E. H.   The pathogenesis and prognosis of prematurity. New Eng J Med 275:878, 938, 1001, 1053, 1966 (four parts).

Asplund, J.   Factors concerned in the causation of habitual abortion, in La Prophylaxie en Gynécologie et Obstétrique. Geneva, Georg et Cie, 1954, p. 710.

Baird, D.   Environmental and obstetrical factors in prematurity, with special reference to experiences in Aberdeen. Bull WHO 26:291, 1962.

Barter, R. H., Dusbabek, J. A., Riva, H. L., and Parks, J. Surgical closure of incompetent cervix during pregnancy. Amer J Obstet Gynec 75:511, 1958.

Bengtsson, L. Ph. Missed abortion: The aetiology, endocrinology and treatment. Lancet 1:339, 1962.

Benson, R. C., Pickering, D. E., Kontaxis, N. E., and Fischer, D. A. Thyroid function in pregnancy. Obstet Gynec 14:11, 1959 (51 references cited).

Bishop, E. H., and Woutersz, T. B. Arrest of premature labor. JAMA 178:812, 1961.

Brody, S., and Carlström, G. Human chorionic gonadotropin in abnormal pregnancy. Serum and urinary findings using various immunoassay techniques. Acta Obstet Gynec Scand 44:32, 1965.

Carr, D. H. Chromosome anomalies as a cause of spontaneous abortions. Amer J Obstet Gynec 97:283, 1967.

Corner, G. W. Embryonic pathology in mammals, with observations upon intra-uterine mortality in the pig. Amer J Anat 31:523, 1923.

Danforth, D. N. Symposium: The incompetent cervix. Bull Sloane Hosp Wom 8:99, 1962.

Delfs, E., and Jones, G. E. S. Some aspects of habitual abortion. Southern Med J 41:809, 1948.

Donald, I. Diagnostic ultrasonic echo sounding in obstetrics and gynaecology. Trans Coll Phys Surg Gynaec So Africa 11:61, 1967.

Drillien, C. M. The Growth and Development of the Prematurely Born Infant. Baltimore, The Williams and Wilkins, 1964.

Du Toit, H. J., Du Plessis, J.M.E., Dommisse, J., Rorke, M. J., Theron, M. S., and De Villiers, V. P. Treatment of endotoxic shock with isoprenaline. Lancet 2:143, 1966.

Eastman, N. J. Habitual abortion, in Meigs, J. V., and Sturgis, S. H. (ed.) Progress in Gynecology. New York, Grune & Stratton, 1946, Vol. 1, p. 262.

——— Prematurity from the viewpoint of the obstetrician. Amer Pract 1:343, 1947.

——— Editorial Comment. Obstet Gynec Survey 21:740, 1966.

——— and Jackson, E. Weight relationships in pregnancy: The bearing of maternal weight gain and pre-pregnancy weight on birth weight in full term pregnancies. Obstet Gynec Survey 23:1003, 1968.

Eckman, T. R., and Carrow, L. Placental lesions in spontaneous abortion. Amer J Obstet Gynec 84:222, 1962.

Erhardt, C. L. Pregnancy losses in New York City, 1960. Amer J Public Health 53:1337, 1963.

Fine, J., Frank, E. D., Raven, H. A., Rutenberg, S. H., and Schweinberg, F. B. The bacterial factor in traumatic shock. New Eng J Med 260:214, 1959.

French, F. E., and Bierman, J. M. Probabilities of fetal mortality. Public Health Rep 77:835, 1962.

Fuchs, F., and Stakemann, G. Treatment of threatened premature labor with large doses of progesterone. Amer J Obstet Gynec 79:172, 1960.

——— Fuchs, A-R., Poblete, J. F., and Risk, A. Effect of alcohol on threatened premature labor. Amer J Obstet Gynec 99:627, 1967.

Gans, B., Eckerling, B., and Goldman, J. A. Cervical incompetence as an etiological factor in habitual abortion. Proc Staff Meet Beilinson Hosp 10:112, 1961.

Gold, E. M., Erhardt, C. L., and Jacobziner, H. Therapeutic abortions in New York City: A 20-year review. Amer J Public Health 55:964, 1965.

——— A symptomatic bacteriuria in pregnancy. Obstet Gynec 27:206, 1966.

Goldstein, H., Goldberg, I. D., Frazier, T. M., and Davis, G. E. Cigarette smoking and prematurity. (Rev.) Public Health Rep 79:553, 1964.

Goldzieher, J. W. Double-blind trial of a progestin in habitual abortion. JAMA 188:651, 1964.

Good, R. A., and Thomas, L. Studies on the generalized Shwartzman reaction; IV. Prevention of the local and generalized Shwartzman reactions with heparin. J Exp Med 97:871, 1953.

Gray, J. D., Tupper, C., and Rowse, J. A. The problem of spontaneous abortion. VII. Prematurity and spontaneous abortion. Amer J Obstet Gynec 78:325, 1959.

Grosser, O. (Trophoblastic growth and human non-villous eggs.) Z Mikr Anat Forsch 5:197, 1926.

Hartman, C. G. The interruption of pregnancy by ovariectomy in the aplacental opossum: A study in the physiology of implantation. Amer J Physiol 71:436, 1925.

——— Uterine bleeding as an early sign of pregnancy in the monkey (*Macaca rhesus*), together with observations on fertile period of menstrual cycle. Bull Hopkins Hosp 44:155, 1929.

——— Studies in the reproduction of the monkey. Contrib Embryol 23:1, 1932.

The Health Consequences of Smoking. 1969 Supplement, A Public Health Service Review: 1967. U.S. Department of Health, Education and Welfare, Washington, D.C.

Hedberg, E., and Radberg, C. Maternal heart volume and prematurity. Acta Obstet Gynec Scand 41:48, 1962.

Hellman, L. M., Kobayashi, M., Fillisti, L., and Lavenhar, M. Growth and development of the human fetus prior to the twentieth week of gestation. Amer J Obstet Gynec 103:789, 1969.

Hertig, A. T., and Livingstone, R. G. Medical Progress: Spontaneous threatened and habitual abortion; its pathogenesis and treatment. New Eng J Med 230:797, 1944.

———— and Rock, J. On the development of the early human ovum, with special reference to the trophoblast of the previllous stages; a description of 7 normal and 5 pathologic human ova. Amer J Obstet Gynec 47:149, 1944.

———— Rock, J., Adams, E. C., and Menkin, M. C. Thirty-four fertilized human ova, good, bad, and indifferent, recovered from 210 women of known fertility. A study of biologic wastage in early human pregnancy. Pediatrics 23:202, 1959.

———— and Sheldon, W. H. Minimal criteria required to prove prima facie case of traumatic abortion or miscarriage. An analysis of 1,000 spontaneous abortions. Ann Surg 117:596, 1943.

Hibbard, B. M. The role of folic acid in pregnancy. With particular reference to anaemia, abruption and abortion. J Obstet Gynaec Brit Comm 71:529, 1964.

Hughes, E. C., Lloyd, C. W., and Ledergerber, C. P. The role of preconceptional study and treatment in abortion and premature labor, in La Prophylaxie en Gynécologie et Obstétrique, Geneva, Georg et Cie, 1954, p. 715.

Hughes, H. E., Loraine, J. A., Bell, E. T., and Layton, R. Cytological observations, cervical mucus "ferning" and hormone assays in early pregnancy. Amer J Obstet Gynec 90:1297, 1964.

Huntington, J. L. A review of the pathology of 104 consecutive miscarriages in private obstetric practice. Amer J Obstet Gynec 17:32, 1929.

Jacobson, B. D. Hazards of norethindrone therapy during pregnancy. Amer J Obstet Gynec 84:962, 1962.

Joël, C. A. The etiology of habitual abortion with consideration of the male factors. Gynaecologia 154:257, 1962; also Obstet Gynec Survey 18:624, 1963.

Jones, G. E., Delfs, E., and Stran, H. M. The effect of alpha-tocopherol administration on pregnanediol excretion. J Clin Endocr 9:743, 1949.

Jones, H. W., and Jones, G. E. S. Double uterus as an etiological factor in repeated abortion: indications for surgical repair. Amer J Obstet Gynec 65:325, 1953.

Kass, E. H. Pyelonephritis and bacteriuria, a major problem in preventive medicine. Ann Intern Med 56:46, 1962.

Kinsey, A. C., Pomeroy, W. B., Martin, C. E., and Gebhard, P. H. Sexual Behavior in the Human Female. Philadelphia, W. B. Saunders Co., 1953.

Kizer, S. Influencia del habito de fumar sobre el embarazo, parto y recien nacido. Rev Obstet Ginec Venez 27:595, 1967.

Klopper, A., and Macnaughton, M. Hormones in recurrent abortion. J Obstet Gynaec Brit Comm 72:1022, 1965.

———— The assessment of feto-placental function by hormone assay. Amer J Obstet Gynec 107:807, 1970.

Knapp, R. C., and Hellman, L. M. Acute renal failure in pregnancy. Amer J Obstet Gynec 78:570, 1959.

Lash, A. F., and Lash, S. R. Habitual abortion: the incompetent internal os of the cervix. Amer J Obstet Gynec 59:68, 1950.

Lawson, J. B., and Stewart, D. B. Obstetrics and Gynaecology in the Tropics and Developing Countries. London, Edward Arnold, Ltd., 1967.

Lebherz, T. B., Hellman, L. P., Madding, R., Anctil, A., and Arje, S. L. Double-blind study of premature rupture of the membranes. A report of 1,896 cases. Amer J Obstet Gynec 87:218, 1963.

Levine, P. Serological factors as possible causes in spontaneous abortions. J Hered 34:71, 1943.

Levine, W., Aaron, J. B., and Gitman, L. Preconception studies in repeated fetal loss, in La Prophylaxie en Gynécologie et Obstétrique. Geneva, Georg et Cie, 1954, p. 724.

Liggins, G. C. The treatment of missed abortion by high dosage syntocinon intravenous infusion. J Obstet Gynaec Brit Comm 69:277, 1962.

Lillehei, R. C., and Maclean, L. D. The intestinal factor in irreversible endotoxin shock. Ann Surg 148:513, 1958.

Loudon, J. D. O. The use of high concentration of oxytocin I. V. drips in the management of missed abortion. J Obstet Gynaec Brit Emp 66:277, 1959.

Makino, S., Kikuchi, Y., Sasaki, M. S., Sasaki, M., and Yoshida, M. A further survey of chromosomes in the Japanese. Chromosoma 13:148, 1962.

Mall, F. P., and Meyer, A. W. Studies on abortuses: a survey of pathologic ova in the Carnegie Embryological Collection, Carnegie Inst. of Wash., 1921, Vol. 12, #56, Pub. No. 275.

Malpas, P. A study of abortion sequences. J Obstet Gynaec Brit Emp 45:932, 1938.

Martin, R. H., Harper, T. A., and Kelso, W. Serum-folic-acid in recurrent abortions. Lancet 1:670, 1965.

Matsunaga, E., and Itoh, S. Blood groups and fertility in a Japanese population, with special reference to intrauterine selection due to maternal-fetal incompatibility. Ann Hum Genet 22:111, 1958.

McCombs, H. L., and Craig, J. M. Decidual necrosis in normal pregnancy. Obstet Gynec 24:436, 1964.

McDonald, I. A. Incompetent cervix as a cause of recurrent abortion. J Obstet Gynaec Brit Comm 70:105, 1963.

McKay, D. G., and Shapiro, S. S. Alterations in the blood coagulation system induced by bacterial endotoxin. I. In vitro (Generalized Shwartzman Reaction). J Exp Med 107:353, 1958.

Monro, J. S. Premature infant weighing less than one pound at birth who survived and developed normally. Canad Med Ass J 40:69, 1939.

National Center for Health Statistics. Vital Statistics of the United States, Vol. 2, Mortality, 1967.

Nesbitt, R. E. L., Aubry, R. H., Goldberg, E. M., and Jacobs, R. D. Correlated hormone excretion patterns and cytohormone variations in normal and complicated pregnancies: Influence of administration of ovarian steroids or placebo in relation to outcome of pregnancy. Amer J Obstet Gynec 93:702, 1965.

Neser, F. N. Cervical incompetence and second trimester abortions. S Afr Med J 2:722, 1959.

Oliver, J., McDowell, M., and Tracy, A. The pathogenesis of acute renal failure associated with traumatic and toxic injury. Renal ischemia, nephrotoxic damage and the ischemuric episode. J Clin Invest 30:1307, 1951.

Overstreet, E. W. The newer progestins in threatened and habitual abortion. Pacif Med Surg 72:289, 1964.

Palmer, R. (Surgical treatment of recurring abortions due to double uterus). Bull Fed Soc Gynec et Obstet 14:107, 1962.

Phillips, L. L., Skrodelis, V., and Quigley, H. J. Intravascular coagulation and fibrinolysis in septic abortion. Obstet Gynec 30:350, 1967.

Pilpel, H. F., and Norwick, K. P. When should abortion be legal? Public Affairs Committee Inc., #429, New York, 1969.

Piver, M. S., Bolognese, R. J., and Feldman, J. D. Long-acting progesterone as a cause of missed abortion. Amer J Obstet Gynec 97:579, 1967.

Pritchard, J. A. A treatment of defibrination syndromes of pregnancy, in Ratnoff, O. D. (ed.), Modern Treatment of Acquired Hemorrhagic Disorders. New York, Hoeber Medical Division, Harper & Row, 1968, p. 401.

———— Scott, D. E., Whalley, P. J., and Haling, R. F. Infants of mothers with megaloblastic anemia due to folate deficiency. JAMA 211:1982, 1970.

Rappaport, F., Rubinovitz, M., Toaff, R., and Krochek, N. Genital Listeriosis as a cause of repeated abortion. Lancet 1:1273, 1960.

Reed, T. E., and Kelly, L. E. The completed reproductive performances of 161 couples selected before marriage and classified by ABO blood group. Ann Hum Genet 22:165, 1958.

Robinson, A., and Puck, T. T. Studies on chromosomal nondisjunction in man, II. Amer J Hum Genet 19:112, 1967.

Roszkowski, I., and Sroka, L. The effect of the male factor on abnormal pregnancy. Gynaecologia 154:321, 1962; also Obstet Gynec Survey 18:625, 1963.

Ruffolo, E. H., Wilson, R. B., and Weed, L. A. Listeria monocytogenes as a cause of pregnancy wastage. Obstet Gynec 19:533, 1962.

Russell, K. P., Maharry, J. S., and Stehly, J. W. Acute renal failure as an obstetric complication. JAMA 157:15, 1955.

Russell, C. S., Taylor, R., and Law, C. E. Smoking in pregnancy, maternal blood pressure, pregnancy outcome, baby weight and growth, and other related factors. A prospective study. Brit J Prev Soc Med 22:119, 1968.

Rutherford, R. N. The significance of bleeding in early pregnancy as evidenced by decidual biopsy. Surg Gynec Obstet 74:1139, 1942.

Sanchez Ibanez, J. M. (Hysterosalpingography in habitual abortion). Rev Esp Obstet Ginec 8:366, 1949.

Sasaki, M., Makino, S., Muramato, J., Ikeuchi, T., and Shumba, H. A chromosome survey of induced abortuses in a Japanese population. Chromosoma 20:267, 1967. Also see editorial comment, Obstet Gynec Survey 22:612, 1967.

Shapiro, S., Jones, E. W., and Densen, P. M. A life table of pregnancy terminations and correlates of fetal loss. Milbank Mem Fund Quart 40:7, 1962.

Shearman, R. P., and Garrett, W. J. Double-blind study of the effect of 17-hydroxyprogesterone caproate on abortion rate. Brit Med J 1:292, 1963.

Shirodkar, V. N. A new method of operative treatment for habitual abortions in the second trimester of pregnancy. Antiseptic 52:299, 1955.

Singh, R. P., and Carr, D. H. Anatomic findings in human abortions of known chromosomal constitution. Obstet Gynec 29:806, 1967.

Sleigh, J. D., Robertson, J. G., and Isdale, M. H. Asymptomatic bacteriuria in pregnancy. J Obstet Gynaec Brit Comm 71:74, 1964.

Smith, K., Browne, J. C., Shackman, R., and Wrong, O. M. Acute renal failure of obstetric origin: An analysis of 70 patients. Lancet 2:351, 1965.

Spink, W. W. The Nature of Brucellosis. Minneapolis, Univ. Minn. Press, 1956.

Stevenson, A. C. Sex chromatin and the sex ratio in man, in Moore, K. L. (ed.). The Sex Chromatin, Philadelphia, W. B. Saunders Co. 1966, p. 263.

Strassmann, P. F. (Operative treatment of double uterus). Zbl Gynaek 31:1322, 1907 (see also Obstet Gynec 10:701, 1957).

Streeter, G. L. Report on investigation, Department of Embryology, pathology, of the fetus. Contrib Embryol 30:15, 1931. (Printed by Carnegie Foundation, Washington, D.C.)

Streiff, R. R., and Little, A. B. Folic acid deficiency in pregnancy. New Eng J Med 276:776, 1967.

Szontagh, F. E., Jakobovits, A., and Mehes, C. Primary embryonal sex ratio in normal pregnancies determined by the nuclear chromatin. Nature 192:476, 1961.

Terris, M., and Gold, E. M. An epidemiologic study of prematurity. 1. Relation to smoking, heart volume, employment, and physique. Amer J Obstet Gynec 103:358, 1969.

Thiede, H. A., and Salm, S. B. Chromosome studies of human spontaneous abortions. Amer J Obstet Gynec 90:205, 1964.

Thiersch, J. B. Therapeutic abortions with a folic acid antagonist, 4-aminopteroylglutamic acid (4-amino PGA) administered by the oral route. Amer J Obstet Gynec 63:1298, 1952.

Thomson, A. M. Nutrition in pregnancy and lactation. WHO, Special Report of Expert Committee on Pregnancy and Lactation, 1964.

Tietze, C. Introduction to the Statistics of Abortion, in Engle, E. T. (ed.), Pregnancy Wastage. Springfield, Ill., Charles C Thomas, 1953, p. 135.

Tricomi, V., Serr, D., and Solish, G. The ratio of male to female embryos as determined by the sex chromatin. Amer J Obstet Gynec 79:504, 1960.

United Nations, Department of Social Affairs. Foetal, Infant and Early Childhood Mortality. I. The Statistics. New York, United Nations, 1954.

Warburton, D., and Fraser, F. C. Spontaneous abortion risks in man: Data from reproductive histories collected in a medical genetics unit. Amer J Hum Genet 16:1, 1964.

Warkany, J. Maternal nutrition during pregnancy and its relationship to reproductive failure, in La Prophylaxie en Gynécologie et Obstétrique. Geneva, Georg et Cie, 1954, p. 650.

Watson, D. Urinary chorionic gonadotrophin determination. Clin Chem 12:577, 1966.

Whalley, P. J., Martin, F. G., and Pritchard, J. A. Sickle cell trait and urinary tract infection during pregnancy. JAMA 189:903, 1964.

——— and Pritchard, J. A. Oxytocin and water intoxication. JAMA 186:601, 1963.

Winikoff, D., Dickinson, R. D., and Wade, G. Globulin-bound iodine levels in normal and abnormal pregnancy. J Obstet Gynaec Brit Emp 67:56, 1960.

Wynn, R. M., Sever, P. S., and Hellman, L. M. Morphologic studies of the ruptured amnion. Amer J Obstet Gynec 99:359, 1967.

21

ECTOPIC PREGNANCY

In a normal intrauterine pregnancy the blastocyst implants in the endometrium lining the uterine cavity. Implantation identified anywhere else is referred to as an ectopic pregnancy. Ectopic pregnancy is a broader term than extrauterine pregnancy, since it includes implantation in the interstitial portion of the oviduct and cervical pregnancy, as well as tubal, ovarian, and abdominal gestation. Although more than 95 per cent of ectopic pregnancies involve the fallopian tube, tubal pregnancy is not synonymous with, but rather a very common type of, ectopic gestation.

Incidence.   Among indigent and semiindigent, predominantly nonwhite populations, about one ectopic pregnancy is treated for every 100 to 150 infants delivered. At Parkland Memorial Hospital during the years 1966 through 1969 the ratio was almost exactly one ectopic pregnancy treated for every 150 infants delivered. Among populations of socioeconomically more fortunate, predominantly white private patients, ectopic pregnancy is perhaps only one half to one third as common. This difference is but one of several that implicate previous gonococcal salpingitis in the genesis of many cases of ectopic pregnancy. The increase in the frequency of ectopic pregnancy relates chronologically to the use of effective antimicrobial agents to treat gonococcal salpingitis. Such therapy may maintain a degree of fertility in women with tubal infection who formerly would have become sterile because of complete tubal occlusion. At the same time, however, enough damage may have occurred before arrest of the infection with antibiotics to initiate the formation of adhesions between mucosal folds or to impair tubal peristalsis.

The changing pattern in reproduction, as well as an increase in the prevalence of gonorrhea (Ch. 27, p. 800), may increase further the frequency of ectopic pregnancy, especially if its incidence is expressed relative to the number of births in a hospital or a community. Many fertile women without conditions predisposing to tubal gestation are currently limiting the number of their pregnancies. Moreover, although intrauterine contraceptive devices effectively prevent most intrauterine pregnancies, they do not appear to affect the occurrence of ectopic gestations (Tietze).

Etiology.   The following conditions have been implicated in the cause of ectopic pregnancy:

> A. *Conditions that prevent or retard the passage of the fertilized ovum into the uterine cavity.*

1. Endosalpingitis, which causes agglutination of the arborescent folds of the tubal mucosa with narrowing of the lumen or the formation of blind pockets.
2. Developmental abnormalities of the tube, especially diverticula, accessory ostia, and hypoplasia.
3. Peritubal adhesions subsequent to postabortal or puerperal infection or appendicitis, which cause kinking of the tube and narrowing of the lumen.
4. Tumors pressing against or otherwise distorting the tube.
5. Previous operations on the tube either to restore patency or occasionally in an attempt to disrupt continuity (tubal ligation or resection).
6. External migration of the ovum. By retarding the transport of the fertilized ovum into the uterine cavity, external migration theoretically enhances the development of invasive properties of the blastocyst while still within the tube. This is probably not an important factor in human ectopic gestation.
7. Menstrual reflux. Delayed fertilization of the ovum with menstrual bleeding at the usual time theoretically could either prevent the ovum from entering the uterus or flush it back into the tube. Little direct support for this concept is available.

B. *Increase in the receptivity of the tubal mucosa to the fertilized ovum.*
   1. Ectopic endometrial elements in the tubal mucosa.

Although endosalpingitis is generally recognized as the single most important cause predisposing to tubal pregnancy, there is a divergence of opinion as to what proportion of cases can be attributed to it. The point is well illustrated in Table 1 where, regardless of whether the information concerning the previous occurrence of the salpingitis was obtained from history, gross examination of the tubes at operation, or their microscopic appearance, tubal infection varied from

Table 1. The Prevalence of Salpingitis as a Cause of Ectopic Pregnancy
(A Review of the American and English Literature by Bone and Greene)

Source:	History	Gross Examination of Tubes	Microscopic Examination of Tubes
	0.5%–82.4%	8%–50%	19%–95%

a negligible causative factor to one of predominant importance.

Variability of the historical data is understandable. That the gross findings vary widely can also be explained, for the narrowing and mechanical obstruction of the tubes by the chronic inflammatory changes and the kinking caused by peritubal adhesions could be modified or even entirely abolished by the gestation itself. Endosalpingitis causes a denudation of tubal epithelium as well as other changes associated with acute inflammation. As healing takes place, adhesions form glandlike spaces and blind pouches that could trap the fertilized ovum. Thus, follicular salpingitis is the most important histopathologic criterion for the diagnosis of previous salpingitis. The extent to which this finding is confused with the subacute and acute inflammatory changes present in all tubal pregnancies may cause the wide variations in the association of ectopic pregnancy and salpingitis cited by Bone and Greene in a study of the American and English literature (Table 1). They carefully examined their own material and concluded that 38 per cent of patients with ectopic pregnancy showed residual evidence of previous tubal infection.

Osiakina-Rojdestvenskaia studied the tubes from 100 cases of tubal gestation using a histologic technic that permitted examination of all the potential obstacles to progress of the ovum and all the changes throughout the entire length of the tube. The author lists the etiologic factors in this series as follows: defective tubal development of post-embryonic origin, 21 cases; adhesions between the tubal folds caused by insufficient differentiation of the tubal mucosa, 21 cases; adenomyosis, 19 cases; inflammation, 14 cases; and tumors, 3 cases. Seventy-eight of the 100 cases, therefore, were the result of mechanical obstacles in the tube. Ten additional cases are explained on the basis of external migration of the ovum, with the result that the ovum had time to develop its capacity to implant before reaching the uterus. Of the 14 cases attributed to inflammatory changes in the tube, 6 were caused by perisalpingitis. In such cases the author found, in addition to adhesions that caused kinking of the tube, numerous scars in the muscular tissue that doubtless interfered with motor activity. Partial obliteration of the tubal lumen secondary to inflammatory processes was encountered in only 3 cases. Although the author concludes that the most important factor in the causation of ectopic pregnancy is defective postembryonic development of the tube, if the 21 cases of adhesions between the tubal folds are taken to be postinflammatory rather than congenital, as is likely, the figure for inflammatory changes associated with ectopic pregnancy is 35 per cent, a close agreement with Bone and Greene.

Although many observers have reported areas of endometriosis in fallopian tubes, it is an uncommon finding, particularly among indigent black patients, in whom tubal pregnancy is most prevalent. Although an occasional ovum might implant on such an area, endometriosis should be considered a rare cause of ectopic pregnancy, Bone and Greene having found it in only 2 of their 121 cases. A decidual reaction in the fallopian tube, furthermore, is the common response of

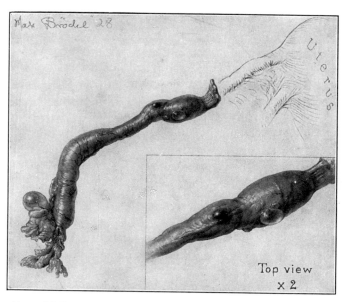

Fig. 1. Cross section of fallopian tube containing ectopic pregnancy. (From Cullen. J Missouri M A, p. 459, Oct. 1928.)

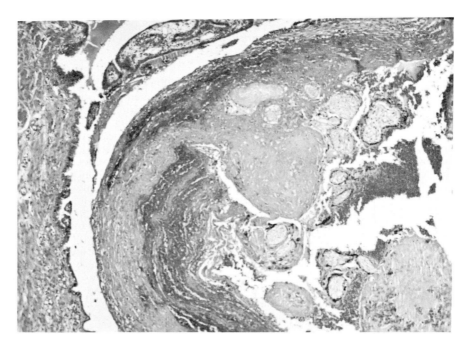

Fig. 2. Ectopic pregnancy, showing placental villi growing into wall of oviduct. (Courtesy of Dr. Ralph M. Wynn.)

that müllerian derivative to the implanting egg and not an indication of endometriosis. Finally, the significance of external migration of the human ovum is in doubt; the phenomenon should be considered mainly as a theoretical possibility in the cause of tubal pregnancy in women with anatomically normal pelvic organs.

Anatomic Considerations.   The fertilized ovum may develop in any portion of the tube, giving rise to ampullar, isthmic, and interstitial pregnancies (Figs. 1 and 2). In rare instances it may be implanted on the fimbriated extremity and occasionally even on the fimbria ovarica. From these primary types certain secondary forms occasionally develop: tuboabdominal, tuboovarian, and broad ligament. The ampulla is the most frequent site of implantation and the isthmus the next most common. Interstitial pregnancy is uncommon, occurring in only about 1 per cent of all tubal gestations.

  Mode of Implantation of the Ovum.   The ovum may implant in columnar or intercolumnar fashion. In the former, which is very rare, the ovum becomes attached to the tip or side of one of the folds of the mucosa; in the second, implantation occurs in a depression between two mucosal folds. In neither situation does the ovum remain on the surface, but at once burrows through the epithelium and comes to lie in the tissue just beneath it. At its periphery is a capsule of rapidly proliferating trophoblast, which invades and erodes the subjacent connective tissues and muscle of the tube. At the same time maternal blood vessels are opened, and the blood pours out into spaces of varying size lying within the trophoblast or between it and the adjacent tissue.

  In the usual intercolumnar implantation, since the tube lacks a submucosa and a well-developed decidua, as soon as the ovum penetrates the epithelium it comes to lie in the muscular wall. The ovum is separated from the lumen by a layer of tissue of varying thickness, the capsular or pseudocapsular membrane. In the rare columnar mode of implantation the ovum lies in the interior of a fold of mucosa and, except at its base, is surrounded on all sides by tubal epithelium with but slight room for initial expansion.

The subsequent course of the pregnancy depends in great part upon the portion of the tube in which implantation has occurred. In ampullary pregnancy, the growing ovum pushes the capsular membrane forward into the tubal lumen, which is occasionally compressed to form a mere crescentic slit. Later, if the course of the pregnancy is not interrupted, the capsular membrane may fuse with the neighboring mucosa, obliterating the lumen of the tube in the immediate vicinity of the ovum.

When implantation occurs in the isthmus, however, particularly in the portion immediately adjoining the uterus, the small size of the lumen precludes the possibility of such expansion. As a consequence the ovum distends the tubal wall eccentrically; the lumen may eventually separate completely, surrounded by placental villi and other fetal tissues, with the result that intraperitoneal rupture frequently occurs before the patient is even aware that she is pregnant.

Decidua. The tube does not normally form an extensive decidua, but decidual cells can usually be recognized and distinguished from trophoblast. The former are commonly found in discrete patches in the tips of some of the folds of the mucosa in the neighborhood of the ovum, or occasionally scattered among the fetal tissues at the placental site, but a continuous membrane analogous to the decidua in uterine pregnancy is much less commonly seen.

The comparatively scant decidual reaction is of both scientific interest and practical importance, since it seems to offer a satisfactory explanation for the invasion and destruction of the tubal wall by the trophoblast. In uterine pregnancy such invasion is noted only in the rare condition of placenta accreta, which is believed also to result from defective development of the decidua (Ch. 33, p. 962).

Decidua Capsularis. Because of the scant decidual reaction, the formation of a structure identical with the decidua capsularis of uterine pregnancy is unlikely. In all intact early tubal pregnancies, however, the ovum is separated from the lumen of the tube by a layer of connective and muscular tissue that may contain a few isolated decidual cells. As the pregnancy advances, this membrane is invaded by fetal cells; it then undergoes fibrinoid degeneration and, if rupture does not occur, eventually fuses with the mucosa of the opposite side of the tube.

Placenta. Since the early stages of development of the placenta are identical in tubal and uterine pregnancies, the different outcomes in the two reflect the differences in the sites of implantation, particularly the variations in decidual reaction. The tubal wall in contact with the ovum offers but slight resistance to invasion by the trophoblast, which soon burrows through it, opening up maternal vessels. There is often direct penetration through the peritoneal surface or through the capsular membrane, giving rise to intraperitoneal rupture and tubal abortion, respectively. In some instances, however, early rupture results from the sudden opening of a large vessel and disruption of the weakened tubal walls from the increased pressure. The microscopic structure of the fetal portion of the placenta is identical with that of normal uterine pregnancy of equivalent duration.

Structure of the Fetal Sac.   In tubal pregnancy there is a marked increase in the vascularity of the affected tube; the larger arteries and veins are greatly hypertrophied, whereas the smaller vessels, especially in the neighborhood of the placental site, are engorged.

Microscopic sections through the sac in the early months show definite hypertrophy of the muscle cells but no apparent increase in their number. Except at the placental site, the tubal wall is considerably thickened and its cells are spread apart by edema. At a still more advanced period, the muscular constituents of the gestational sac appear to diminish in number. At term almost its entire thickness is made up of connective tissue with sparse cells and only an occasional muscle fiber. Even though the muscularis of the tube occasionally undergoes marked hypertrophy, it lacks the enormous capacity of the uterus in that regard.

In many advanced cases the exterior of the tube shows evidence of peritonitis; a considerable portion of the thickness of the fetal sac is often the result of peritoneal adhesions. Occasionally, discrete patches of decidual tissue are found in the connective tissue cells of such adhesions. As shown by Mall, the embryo in ectopic pregnancy is often absent or stunted, a finding that is at least partially explained on the basis of the invariably deficient environment.

Uterine Changes.   The uterus undergoes some of the changes associated with normal pregnancy, such as softening of the lower segment and increase in size; the degree to which the endometrium is converted to decidua is variable. Although the finding of uterine decidua without trophoblast suggests ectopic pregnancy, it is by no means a positive indication. In 1954, Arias-Stella described in the endometrial glands and epithelium changes that he thought were caused by chorionic gonadotropin. The epithelial cells are enlarged and their nuclei are hypertrophic, hyperchromatic, lobular, and irregularly shaped. There is a loss of polarity, and the abnormal nuclei tend to occupy the luminal portion of the cells. The cytoplasm may be vacuolated and foamy, and occasional mitoses may be found. These endometrial changes are collectively referred to as the Arias-Stella phenomenon. Skulj found decidual changes in 55 of 124 patients with tubal pregnancy. Of the remaining 69, the Arias-Stella phenomenon confirmed the diagnosis in 29, yielding a diagnostic accuracy based on these two pathologic changes of 67 per cent.

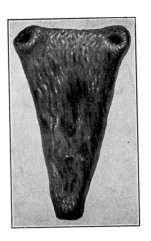

Fig. 3. Decidual cast of uterus in extrauterine pregnancy.

Soon after the death of the fetus, the decidua degenerates and is usually shed in small pieces, but occasionally it is cast off intact, as a *decidual cast* of the uterine cavity (Fig. 3). The absence of decidual tissue, however, does not exclude an ectopic pregnancy, for it is present in less than 20 per cent of cases.

The external bleeding seen in many cases of tubal pregnancy is uterine in origin and associated with degeneration and sloughing of the uterine decidua.

Termination of Tubal Pregnancy. *Tubal Abortion.* A common termination of tubal pregnancy is separation of the products of conception from the endosalpinx and extrusion of the abortus through the fimbriated end of the tube (Fig. 4). It occurs, as a rule, between the sixth and twelfth weeks. The frequency of tubal abortion depends in great part upon the site of implantation of the ovum. In ampullary pregnancy it is the rule, whereas intraperitoneal rupture is the usual outcome in isthmic pregnancy.

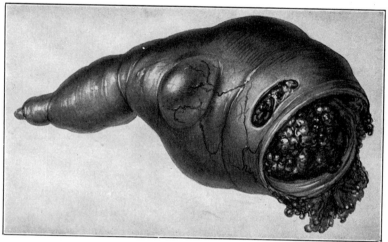

Fig. 4. Tubal abortion, ovum extruding through fimbriated extremity. (From Kelly. Operative Gynecology, 2nd ed., Vol. II. D. Appleton and Company, 1906.)

With regard to hemorrhage, tubal abortion does not differ from intraperitoneal rupture except that in the former bleeding occurs into the lumen of the tube, whereas in the latter it takes place directly into the peritoneal cavity. The immediate consequence of the hemorrhage is the loosening of the connection between the ovum and the tubal wall, the ovum completely or partially separating from its site of implantation. If separation is complete, the entire ovum is extruded into the lumen of the tube and is gradually forced by the effused blood toward the fimbriated end, through which it may be extruded into the peritoneal cavity. At that point hemorrhage may cease.

In incomplete tubal abortion, when the hemorrhage is moderate, the ovum may become infiltrated with blood and converted into a structure analogous to the blood mole observed in uterine abortion. Slight bleeding usually persists as long as the mole remains in the tube, and the blood slowly trickles from the fimbriated extremity into the rectouterine cul-de-sac, where it may become encapsulated, forming a *hematocele*. If the fimbriated extremity is occluded, the tube may gradually become distended by blood, forming a *hematosalpinx*.

After incomplete tubal abortion, pieces of the placenta or membranes may remain attached to the tubal wall and, after becoming surrounded by fibrin, give rise to a placental polyp, just as may occur after an incomplete uterine abortion.

Rupture into the Peritoneal Cavity. Many of the cases of tubal pregnancy end within the first 12 weeks by intraperitoneal rupture, which usually occurs spontaneously but occasionally is the result of external force. As a rule, whenever tubal rupture occurs in the first few weeks, the pregnancy is situated in the isthmus a short distance from the cornu of the uterus (Figs. 5 and 6). When the ovum is implanted in the interstitial portion of the tube, however, rupture usually does not occur until later.

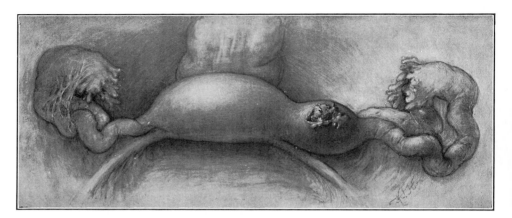

Fig. 5. Tubal pregnancy, isthmic portion, with rupture.

The prime factor in the causation of rupture is the intramural embedding of the ovum and the consequent invasion of the tubal wall by trophoblast with erosion of the muscular layer. Its immediate direct cause may be the trauma associated with coitus or a vaginal examination, although in the great majority of cases it occurs spontaneously. In the latter event, rupture results either from direct perforation by the growing villi or from the weakened tubal wall's yielding to a sudden increase of pressure following the opening up of a large vessel or the clogging of venous channels by the chorionic villi.

Occasionally, when the fimbriated end of the tube is occluded, secondary rupture may occur after a primary abortion. In such circumstances the weakened tubal wall yields to the pressure of the blood that has poured into its lumen and can find no other means of escape.

Rupture usually occurs in the neighborhood of the placental site either into the peritoneal cavity or between the folds of the broad ligaments, depending upon the original site of the ovum. These two outcomes differ so greatly that it is necessary to consider them separately.

In intraperitoneal rupture the entire ovum may be extruded from the tube, but if the rent is small, profuse hemorrhage may occur without its escape. In either event commonly the patient immediately shows signs of collapse. If the patient is not operated upon and does not die from hemorrhage, the fate of the fetus will depend on the damage it has sustained and the duration of the gestation. If an early conceptus is expelled into the peritoneal cavity, some believe that it can re-implant almost anywhere, establish adequate circulation, and survive and grow.

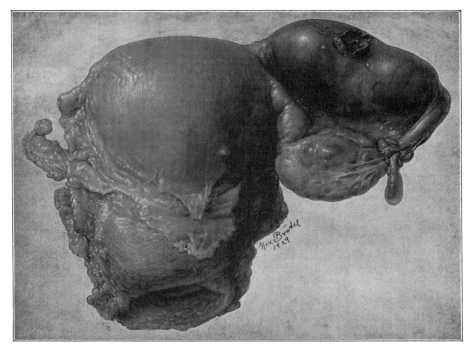

Fig. 6. Ruptured tubal pregnancy. Death from hemorrhage immediately after admittance to hospital. Left adnexa had been removed because of tubal pregnancy several years previously.

This outcome is unlikely, since the ovum is in all probability extensively damaged during the transition. The products of conception, if small, may be resorbed or, if larger, may remain in the cul-de-sac for years as an encapsulated mass or even become calcified to form a *lithopedion.*

If only the fetus escapes at the time of rupture, however, the effect upon the pregnancy will vary according to the extent of the injury sustained by the placenta. If it is much damaged, death of the fetus and termination of the pregnancy are inevitable, but if the greater portion of the placenta still retains its attachment to the tube, further development is possible. The fetus may then survive to term, giving rise to a *secondary abdominal pregnancy.* In such cases the tube may close down upon the placenta and form a sac in which it remains during the rest of the pregnancy; or while a portion of the placenta remains attached to the tubal wall, its growing periphery extends beyond it and establishes connections with the surrounding pelvic organs. In such circumstances the placenta may be attached partly to the uterus, pelvic floor, rectum, or even the intestines.

When the fetus escapes from the tube after rupture, it is nearly always surrounded by its membranes. Many authorities believe that further growth of the fetus is impossible unless it is enclosed within the amnion. Several cases, however, have been reported in which a term fetus lay perfectly free in the peritoneal cavity, with its residual membranes confined to the tubal sac.

Rupture into the Broad Ligament. In a small number of cases, especially when the original implantation of the ovum is toward the mesosalpinx, rupture may occur at the portion of the tube uncovered by peritoneum, so that the contents of the gestational sac are extruded into a space formed by the separation of the folds of the broad ligament. Generally this is the most favorable variety of rupture. It may terminate either in the death of the ovum and the formation of a *broad ligament hematoma* or in the further development of the pregnancy.

The outcome depends largely upon the degree of completeness with which the placenta has separated. If it remains attached to the interior of the tube, it is generally displaced upward as pregnancy advances and comes to lie above the fetus. When it is situated near the point of rupture, however, it gradually extends down between the folds of the broad ligament, implanted partly upon the interior of the tube and partly upon the pelvic connective tissue. In either event, the fetal sac lies entirely outside the peritoneal cavity; as it increases in size the peritoneum is gradually dissected off the pelvic and abdominal walls. This condition is designated an intraligamentous or *broad ligament pregnancy* (Fig. 7).

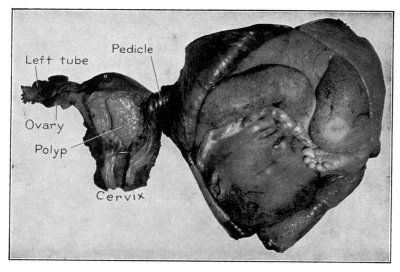

Fig. 7. Broad ligament pregnancy at term. The sac has been opened to expose the fetus, thus hiding most of proximal and all of distal end of elongated right tube, which almost completely encircles the sac. In the region of the isthmus the tube cannot be traced for some distance as it merges with the wall of the sac. It is probably at this site that early rupture occurred. The torn distal end of the tube has been carried laterally by the growing fetus. In the photograph the right ovary and ruptured vessels are hidden on the undersurface of the sac near the cervix. (Courtesy of Dr. Thomas J. Sims.)

Redgwick, Rumbolz, and Nace reported an intraligamentous pregnancy of 28 weeks' size with a macerated stillborn fetus and placenta on the undersurface of the anterior leaf of the right broad ligament. In an extensive review of the literature, these authors discovered 82 similar reported cases. Occasionally the broad ligament sac ruptures at a later period, and the fetus is extruded into the peritoneal cavity while the placenta retains its original position, forming a secondary abdominal pregnancy.

The so-called *tubouterine pregnancy* results from the gradual extension into the uterine cavity of an ovum that originally implanted in the interstitial portion of the tube. *Tuboabdominal pregnancy*, however, is derived from a tubal pregnancy in which the ovum, originally implanted in the neighborhood of the fimbriated extremity, gradually extends into the peritoneal cavity. In such circumstances the portion of the fetal sac projecting into the peritoneal cavity forms adhesions with the surrounding organs. As a result, removal of the sac is much more difficult. Neither of these conditions is common and neither requires separate classification. Both are merely pregnancies developing in unusual portions of the tubes.

The term *tuboovarian pregnancy* is employed when the fetal sac is composed partly of tubal and partly of ovarian tissue. Such cases arise from the development of an ovum in a tuboovarian cyst or in a tube, the fimbriated extremity of which was adherent to the ovary at the time of fertilization.

Signs and Symptoms. Before tubal rupture or abortion the manifestations of a tubal pregnancy are not characteristic; commonly the patient either believes she is normally pregnant or does not suspect that she is pregnant. Hence, the symptoms and signs of tubal pregnancy usually refer to the clinical picture encountered with rupture or abortion.

In the so-called classic, or textbook, case of ruptured tubal pregnancy, normal menstruation is replaced by slight vaginal bleeding, which is usually referred to as "spotting." Suddenly the woman is stricken with severe lower abdominal pain, frequently described as sharp, stabbing, or tearing in character. Vasomotor disturbances develop, ranging from vertigo to actual fainting, and the patient appears pale. Abdominal palpation discloses tenderness, and vaginal examination, especially motion of the cervix, causes exquisite pain. The posterior fornix of the vagina may bulge because of blood in the cul-de-sac, or a tender, boggy mass may be felt to one side of the uterus. The patient may or may not be hypotensive while lying supine; when she is placed in a sitting position, however, hypovolemia may be sufficiently intense to cause hypotension.

In cases of tubal pregnancy that present the aforementioned clinical picture there can be no question of the diagnosis, but ideally the diagnosis should be made earlier. Even though the symptoms and signs of ectopic pregnancy often range from indefinite to bizarre before rupture or abortion, increasing numbers of women are seeking medical care before the classic clinical picture develops. The physician must make every reasonable effort to diagnose the condition before the catastrophic events occur, but the task is seldom simple.

Pain. Pain may be unilateral or generalized over the lower abdomen. It may be lancinating or cramplike. In the presence of gross rupture and hemoperitoneum, pain radiating to the region of the shoulders and the side of the neck is a fairly common complaint.

It has been generally assumed that the abdominal pain, often excruciating, associated with rupture of an ectopic pregnancy is caused by the escape of blood into the peritoneal cavity. Since there may be considerable pain in instances in which there is little hemorrhage, it is obvious that blood is not the sole cause of the pain. There is no question, however, that the introduction of a relatively large amount of blood into the peritoneal cavity can lead to peritoneal irritation and varying degrees of discomfort. Pritchard and Adams noted that the instillation of 500 ml, or somewhat more, of citrated whole blood into the peritoneal cavity more often than not caused abdominal tenderness, moderate intestinal distention, and especially pain in the top of the shoulder and the side of the neck. The pain in the neck and shoulder is caused by diaphragmatic irritation. The volume of blood, shed as a result of tubal rupture or abortion, required to cause this pain must be sizable for a significant amount to reach the diaphragm. This fact probably accounts for the differences between the observations of Pritchard and Adams and those of Mengert and associates, who noted that the intraperitoneal infusion of up to 300 ml of blood in adult women produced only a feeling of fullness.

Amenorrhea. Hospital records indicate that a history of amenorrhea is not obtained in a quarter or more of the cases. One reason is that the patient mistakes the pathologic bleeding that frequently occurs in tubal pregnancy for a true menstrual period and so gives an erroneous date for the last period. This important source of diagnostic error can be eliminated in many cases by a more carefully obtained history. It is extremely important that the character of the last period be investigated in detail in respect to time of onset, duration, and amount, and it is advisable to ask whether it impressed the patient as abnormal in any way. Although the reason for the absence of true amenorrhea in certain cases of ectopic pregnancy may be obscure, the important fact is that no history of amenorrhea was obtained in a quarter to a half of the recorded cases. The absence of a missed menstrual period, therefore, by no means rules out tubal pregnancy.

Vaginal Spotting or Bleeding. The incidence of vaginal bleeding not considered to be normal menses is about the same as that of amenorrhea, namely, about 75 per cent. As long as the ovum remains intact, uterine bleeding is usually absent, but with the disturbance or death of the ovum, much of the endocrine support of the decidua is removed and the uterine mucosa bleeds. The bleeding is usually scanty, dark brown, and either intermittent or continuous. Although profuse vaginal bleeding suggests an incomplete intrauterine abortion rather than an ectopic gestation, it nevertheless occurs in about 5 per cent of tubal gestations.

Syncope and Hypovolemic Shock. The pallid, shocked patient, classically associated with ruptured tubal pregnancy, is seen in only the minority of cases. Fainting and weakness are not so common as usually supposed, being seen in fewer than one third of Marchetti's cases. Kohl and his colleagues found the classic signs of amenorrhea, bleeding, pain, and fainting in only one fifth of the black and one third of the white patients.

Vaginal Tenderness. By far the most common physical finding in ruptured tubal pregnancy is exquisite tenderness on vaginal examination, especially on *motion of the cervix.* It is demonstrable in over three quarters of the cases, but occasionally may be absent. Abdominal tenderness occurs in about the same proportion of cases.

Pelvic Mass. Several studies indicate that a pelvic mass is palpable in about only one half of the cases. The mass varies in size, consistency, and position, ranging as a rule between 5 and 15 cm in diameter, and is often soft and elastic. With extensive infiltration of the tubal wall with blood, however, it may be firm. It is rarely anterior to the uterus, but almost always either posterior or lateral.

Uterine Changes. Because of the action of placental hormones, the uterus grows during the first three months of a tubal gestation to nearly the same size as in an intrauterine pregnancy. Its consistency too is similar as long as the fetus is alive. The uterus may be pushed to one side or the other by the ectopic mass. In broad ligament pregnancies or when the broad ligament is filled with blood, the uterus may be greatly displaced, with the cervix high up behind the symphysis pubis. Uterine casts are passed by a small minority of patients, possibly 5 or 10 per cent.

Blood Pressure and Pulse.   As might be expected, the blood pressure usually falls in proportion to the extent and especially the rate of the intraabdominal hemorrhage. The initial response to hemorrhage, however, is occasionally the same as that encountered during the controlled phlebotomy of blood donation—namely, a slight rise in blood pressure. In these generally healthy young women, therefore, only if bleeding continues at a rapid rate and hypovolemia becomes fairly intense does the blood pressure fall and the pulse rate rise appreciably.

There are two simple means of detecting significant hypovolemia before the development of overt hypovolemic shock: (1) The blood pressure and pulse rate are compared with the patient in the sitting and supine positions. A distinct decrease in blood pressure and rise in pulse rate in the sitting position are indicative of a sizable loss of circulatory volume. (2) Urinary flow is closely monitored. Hypovolemia almost always causes oliguria before overt hypotension develops.

Anemia.   After hemorrhage the depleted blood volume is restored to normal by gradual hemodilution over the course of a day or two. Even after a substantial hemorrhage, therefore, the hemoglobin level or hematocrit may show only a slight immediately apparent reduction. For the first few hours after an acute hemorrhage the hemoglobin or hematocrit may be an unreliable index of the amount of blood lost. Because of progressive hemodilution, however, a decrease in hemoglobin concentration or hematocrit while the patient is under observation is a more valuable index of blood loss than is the initial reading, a most important practical point. Of course, in cases in which a pelvic hematocele has been gradually forming over a period of a week or more, there may be an extremely low hemoglobin concentration or hematocrit.

Temperature.   After acute hemorrhage the temperature may be normal or even low. Temperatures between 100°F and 101°F, perhaps related to hemoperitoneum, are noted in about one patient in three, but higher temperatures are rare in the absence of infection. Fever is important in distinguishing ruptured tubal pregnancy from acute salpingitis, in which the temperature is commonly above 101°F. In the Kings County Hospital only 1 per cent of all patients with ectopic pregnancies had a temperature above 101.5°F on admittance to the hospital.

Leukocyte Count.   The leukocyte count varies considerably in ruptured ectopic pregnancy. In about half the cases it is normal, but in the remainder varying leukocytosis up to 30,000 may be encountered. The white blood cell count, though of little aid in differential diagnosis, may be helpful in indicating the type of bleeding that has occurred. As a rule, in cases of old rupture or slow leakage the count is likely to be normal, whereas after sudden massive hemorrhage it usually exceeds 15,000.

Cullen's Sign.   A blue discoloration of the periumbilical skin may result from intraperitoneal hemorrhage. This rare sign may occasionally be discerned in thin women or in patients with an umbilical hernia.

The "Chronic Ruptured Ectopic."   In many cases of ruptured tubal pregnancy there is gradual disintegration of the tubal wall followed by a very slow leakage of blood into the tubal lumen, the peritoneal cavity, or both. Signs of active hemorrhage are absent, and even the mild symptoms may subside; but gradually the trickling blood collects in the pelvis, more or less walled off by adhesions, and a pelvic hematocele results. In some cases the hematocele is eventually absorbed, and the patient recovers without operation. In others it may rupture into the peritoneal cavity, producing a picture of hypovolemic shock, or it may become infected and form an abscess. Most commonly, however, the hematocele causes continued pain, and the physician is finally consulted weeks or even months after the original rupture. These cases present the most atypical manifestations. Since there are various gradations between the acute and chronic ruptures, it is understandable that tubal pregnancy may be associated with a wide and often confusing variety of clinical features.

Diagnosis.   Prompt diagnosis in ruptured tubal pregnancy is most important. Indeed, it is failure to make the correct diagnosis promptly that accounts for almost all deaths in this condition. Unfortunately, however, there is no other disorder in the field of obstetrics and gynecology that presents so many diagnostic pitfalls. For example, if many reports of ectopic pregnancy are surveyed, the preoperative diagnosis of ruptured tubal pregnancy is shown at operation to be wrong in about 15 to 20 per cent of cases.

The conditions most frequently confused with tubal pregnancy are (1) acute or chronic salpingitis, (2) threatened or incomplete abortion of an intrauterine pregnancy, (3) rupture of a corpus luteum or follicular cyst with intraperitoneal bleeding, (4) torsion of an ovarian cyst, and (5) appendicitis. The disease most commonly mistaken for ruptured tubal pregnancy is salpingitis, in which there is often a history of similar attacks and usually no missed period. In salpingitis there may be a history of metrorrhagia, but abnormal bleeding is not nearly so common as the spotting characteristic of tubal gestation. Pain and tenderness are more likely to be bilateral in pelvic inflammatory disease. A pelvic mass in tubal pregnancy, if palpable, is unilateral, whereas in salpingitis both fornices are likely to be equally resistant and tender. The temperature in acute salpingitis usually exceeds 101°F. A positive hormonal test for pregnancy is not uncommon in recently ruptured tubal pregnancies, but a negative test may be obtained in either condition and hence is of no diagnostic value.

In threatened or incomplete abortion of an intrauterine pregnancy, the vaginal bleeding is usually more profuse and the blood more likely to be bright red. Shock, when present, is usually in proportion to the extent of vaginal hemorrhage, but in tubal pregnancy shock is almost always far in excess of what might be expected from vaginal blood loss. The pain in uterine abortion is milder and located low in the midline of the abdomen, whereas in tubal pregnancy it is unilateral or generalized. In uterine abortions, the unilateral mass often found in tubal pregnancy is absent, the uterus may grow larger and softer, and the cervix may be more patulous. If products of conception are found in the vagina or at the external cervical os, the diagnosis of abortion is obvious, but it should be remember that combined extrauterine and intrauterine pregnancies may occur, albeit rarely. Conversely, decidual tissue without chorionic villi, or even an intact decidual cast, does not necessarily indicate ectopic pregnancy. The marked histologic variations in the endometrium in cases of ectopic pregnancy are such that endometrial biopsy provides an often unreliable diagnostic criterion. Romney, Hertig, and Reid, for example, reported that only 19 per cent of endometria associated with ectopic gestation show a decidual reaction.

In both torsion of an ovarian cyst and appendicitis, the signs and symptoms of pregnancy, including amenorrhea, are usually lacking and there is rarely a history of vaginal bleeding. The mass formed by a twisted ovarian cyst is more nearly discrete, whereas that of a tubal pregnancy is usually less well defined. In appendicitis there is no mass on vaginal examination, and pain on motion of the cervix is much less severe than in ruptured tubal pregnancy; the pain with appendicitis, furthermore, is often localized higher, over McBurney's point. If either appendicitis or a twisted ovarian cyst is mistaken for a tubal pregnancy, the error is not costly, since all three require prompt operation. Rupture of a follicle cyst or corpus luteum with bleeding into the peritoneal cavity may be extremely difficult, if not impossible, to distinguish clinically from a ruptured tubal gestation.

Because of the difficulties in diagnosis of ruptured tubal pregnancy, a variety of diagnostic aids have been utilized. Pregnancy tests have been used as an aid in the diagnosis of ectopic pregnancy, but because a substantial titer of chorionic gonadotropin is required for a positive test, a negative result does not necessarily indicate the absence of an ectopic pregnancy. Although Hall and Todd found that nearly 90 per cent of cases in their series of ectopic pregnancies had positive pregnancy tests, and thus regard the procedure as exceedingly valuable, our experience has been different. Various methods of entering the cul-de-sac for the purpose of demonstrating free blood have been employed—namely, culdocentesis, colpotomy, and culdoscopy.

Culdocentesis is the simplest technic for identifying hemoperitoneum, since it can be performed in the office, clinic, or emergency room. Fluid from the peritoneal cavity, of course, must be obtained for culdocentesis to be of aid. Usually a long 18-gauge needle can be inserted through the posterior fornix into the cul-de-sac, whence fluid can be aspirated. Absence of fluid can be interpreted only as unsatisfactory entry into the cul-de-sac. Fluid that looks like blood and does not clot is compatible with the diagnosis of hemoperitoneum resulting from tubal pregnancy (Beller, Maki, and Epstein). If the blood subsequently clots, it almost certainly was obtained from an adjacent perforated blood vessel rather than from the cul-de-sac. In the presence of very active bleeding from the tube, however, the aspirated blood may not yet have had time to clot. With bleeding of such intensity, however, culdocentesis is rarely necessary for diagnosing an intraabdominal catastrophe, which demands prompt replacement of fluids, including whole blood, and surgical intervention. Lucas and Hassim point out that culdocentesis is of greatest value for diagnosing ectopic pregnancy in populations in which anemia and pelvic infection are common. Armstrong and his colleagues, after reviewing 481 cases of ectopic pregnancy, conclude that needle puncture (culdocentesis) and particularly posterior *colpotomy* are invaluable diagnostic aids. Since the condition most frequently mistaken for ectopic pregnancy is pelvic inflammatory disease, which may bind intestines and other structures in the cul-de-sac, the blind introduction of a sharp instrument into the posterior fornix may be dangerous. Although these methods have many advocates, there are few data concerning their accuracy. That they are far from 100 per cent accurate, however, is attested by Hall and Todd, who cite 94 such procedures with 5 false negative, 2 false positive, and 4 inconclusive tests, a diagnostic error of nearly 12 per cent.

Laparoscopy has recently been reintroduced as a means of improving the accuracy of diagnosis of diseases of the pelvis, including ectopic pregnancy. Refined optic and electronic systems have overcome some of the objections that arose in the course of previous attempts to utilize transabdominal intraperitoneal lighted probes for visualization of organs. Nonetheless, successful laparoscopy demands fairly refined equipment, an experienced operator, an operating room, and surgical anesthesia (Fear; Cohen; Neuwirth). At this time, at least, laparoscopy does not appear to offer many advantages over the appropriate use of culdocentesis, colpotomy, and laparotomy. In our experience there is remarkably little morbidity associated with surgery limited to a carefully made and repaired suprapubic midline incision. At the same time diagnosis is often enhanced appreciably by direct visualization and palpation of the pelvic organs. If any doubt remains, laparotomy should be performed, since an unnecessary operation is far less tragic than a death from indecision or delay.

Sonography has been applied to the problem of diagnosis of tubal pregnancy (Kobayashi and colleagues). Identification of products of conception in the fallopian tube by this means is most often difficult, but if they are in the uterus they can usually be detected quite early in pregnancy (Ch. 9, p. 279). When an embryo is identified in the uterus the likelihood of an ectopic pregnancy becomes remote. Experience in sonographic diagnosis of tubal pregnancy is still quite limited, however.

The clinical diagnosis of ectopic pregnancy is subject to both false positive and false negative errors. About 15 to 20 per cent of patients operated upon with a diagnosis of ectopic pregnancy will have some other lesion; conversely, a small percentage of all ectopic pregnancies will be found in patients subjected to laparotomy with a different preoperative diagnosis.

Halpin recently reviewed the problems associated with the diagnosis of ectopic pregnancy encountered at Sloane Hospital for Women. Although culdocentesis, sequential hematocrits, pregnancy tests, and laparoscopy were helpful in making the diagnosis, no single reliable differential feature could be constantly elicited. Instead, careful investigation followed by exercise of good clinical judgment was essential for achieving the correct diagnosis. Undoubtedly, the diagnosis is most likely to be correctly made if the physician remains constantly alert to the possibility that abdominal pain in any woman during her reproductive years may represent tubal pregnancy and if he is diligent in obtaining an accurate history.

Prognosis.   The mortality of ectopic pregnancy for the nation as a whole has fallen. Reports covering a total of 2,478 cases (Sandmire, Malkasian, Torpin, Schiffer, Kostic, Riva) include 3 deaths, or 1 in 826 ectopic pregnancies. At Parkland Memorial Hospital in recent years mortality from ectopic pregnancy has not been greater than that from repeated cesarean section. This reduction from the 2 or 3 per cent figure of 25 years ago is the result of earlier diagnosis and the more liberal use of adequate transfusion. The mortality rate could be reduced still further by more rapid recognition of the acute emergency and by elimination of delay in hospitalization, operation, and transfusion of blood.

Subsequent Pregnancies.   Since the tubal lesions that predispose to ectopic pregnancy are commonly bilateral, a substantial number of women are sterile after one ectopic gestation or develop another extrauterine pregnancy in the remaining tube. About one half of all women operated upon for ectopic pregnancy fail to conceive subsequently; the sterility rate is even higher when the first pregnancy is ectopic. The rate of recurrence among subsequent pregnancies is estimated to be between 10 and 20 per cent. In some instances the surgical procedure to be done should be influenced by this high rate of recurrence. The woman with a reasonable number of children often would benefit from a procedure that provides protection against future ectopic pregnancies as well as cure of the current problem. If hypovolemic shock is absent, if anesthesia is satisfactory, and if technical surgical problems do not arise, hysterectomy may be indicated. Otherwise, the extent of the procedure could be scaled down to salpingectomy and partial resection of the opposite tube. Obviously these procedures must be discussed with the patient and her husband and permission obtained before operation.

Treatment. The usual treatment of tubal pregnancy is salpingectomy with or without ipsilateral oophorectomy. Simultaneous blood transfusion is, of course, a necessity if either hypovolemia or overt anemia is present. The response of most patients to the operation is dramatic, the blood pressure rising immediately after the major vessels are clamped.

The removal of the ovary on the affected side is sometimes necessitated by its involvement in the process, but elective oophorectomy is often performed. Jeffcoate advises removal of the ovary along with the tube to prevent future ectopic pregnancies that might result from external migration of the ovum. Ipsilateral oophorectomy at the time of salpingectomy has been suggested as a means of improving fertility on the basis that ovulation would always occur from an ovary immediately adjacent to a fallopian tube (Douglas and associates). Removal of a normal ovary is hardly justified by either theoretical possibility. Most gynecologists leave the ovary when possible and preserve its maximal blood supply, to prevent the formation of cysts, by clamping the vessels in the mesosalpinx close to the tube. In removing the tube, it is advisable to excise as a wedge the outer half of the interstitial portion of the fallopian tube (so-called cornual resection) and thereby minimize the rare recurrence of pregnancy in the tubal stump, as reported by Fulsher and others. Penetration into the cavity of the uterus is to be avoided, however, lest the defect so created lead to uterine rupture in a subsequent pregnancy.

In the face of serious blood loss, retransfusion of blood collected in the abdomen has been advocated. Although this procedure is effective in an emergency, it is not advised as a routine because of the danger of reaction. Some workers, however, have recommended that if such blood is left in the abdomen, it will be of benefit to the patient. Pritchard and Adams have shown by means of tagged red cells that absorption of erythrocytes from the adult peritoneal cavity is much too slow to be of significant help.

A series of reports deals with a more conservative surgical approach in an effort to preserve the affected tube and the fertility of the patient. By squeezing out or otherwise removing the products of conception from the tube and performing plastic procedures, the tube may occasionally be safely retained. Although no author recommends attempts at preservation of all tubes, there is a wide variation in the reported incidence of conservative procedures. Stromme, McKelvey, and Adkins cite a figure of 21 per cent, as compared with 17 per cent in the large series of Jarvinen and the perhaps optimistic 46 per cent of Rosenblum, Dowling, and Barnes. Although some of the reports are enthusiastic, it is doubtful that nonexcisional surgery will lower substantially the prevalent incidence of sterility or the possibility of future recurrence. Treatment should, nevertheless, be individualized.

Interstitial Pregnancy (Figs. 8 and 9). When the fertilized ovum implants in the segment of the tube that penetrates the uterine wall, an especially grave form of tubal gestation, *interstitial pregnancy*, results. It accounts for about 1 per cent of all tubal gestations. Bobrow and Bell, however, found this variety only 6 times in over 900 ectopic pregnancies at the Harlem Hospital. As the incidence of

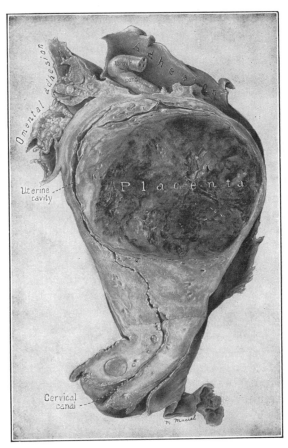

Fig. 8. Interstitial pregnancy. Note placenta in posterior wall of uterus and umbilical cord protruding through fundus. Rupture had occurred at the fourth month, and fetus remained alive in the abdominal cavity until shortly before the death of the patient at the eighth month.

ectopic pregnancy rises, there may be a relative decrease in the proportion of unusual varieties. Because of the site of implantation, no tubal mass is palpable, but rather an asymmetric uterus that is difficult to differentiate from an early intrauterine pregnancy. Hence, the early diagnosis is even more frequently overlooked than in other types of tubal implantation. Because of the greater distensibility of the myometrium compared with the tubal wall, rupture is likely to occur somewhat later, between the end of the second and the end of the fourth month. Because of the abundant blood supply from branches of both uterine and ovarian arteries immediately adjacent to the implantation site, the hemorrhage that attends the rupture may be fatal within an hour. In fact, most tubal pregnancies in which death occurs before the patient can be brought to the hospital fall into this group. Felmus and Pedowitz, however, reported only one death in their series of 45 cases. Because of the large uterine defect, hysterectomy is often required.

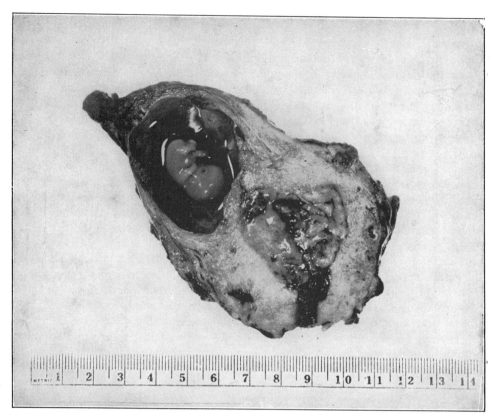

Fig. 9. Interstitial pregnancy with fetus in situ. Note thick decidua in empty uterus.

Combined and Multiple Pregnancies. In rare instances tubal pregnancy may be complicated by a coexisting intrauterine gestation, a condition designated as *combined pregnancy.* Combined pregnancy is very often quite difficult to diagnose. Typically laparotomy is performed because of a ruptured tubal pregnancy; at the same time the uterus also is noted to be congested, softened, and somewhat enlarged. Although these features suggest intrauterine pregnancy, they are commonly induced by a tubal pregnancy alone. This subject has been extensively reviewed by Vasicka and Grable and by Winer, Bergman, and Fields, who collected 466 cases from the world's literature. The incidence is estimated to be about 1 in 30,000 births.

Twin tubal pregnancy has been reported with both embryos in the same tube and with one in each tube, at the same stage of development. Arey considered the subject in detail and concluded that single-ovum twins form a far greater proportion of tubal than of uterine pregnancies. He postulated that difficulties in implantation retard the growth of the ovum with the result that two embryonic areas develop rather than one. Stewart, in an exhaustive search of the literature on bilateral ectopic gestation, brought the total number of reported cases to 212. Simultaneous pregnancy in both tubes is the rarest form of double-ovum twin pregnancy and one of the rarest anomalies of tubal gestation.

Frequency.   In the strict sense, abdominal pregnancy includes only gestations free in the peritoneal cavity rather than between the leaves of the broad ligament or in a greatly dilated fallopian tube. Beacham and his colleagues at Charity Hospital in New Orleans cite an incidence of 1 in 3,372 births, a figure that is in close agreement with that of Crawford and Ward. The incidence of abdominal pregnancy in most hospitals, however, is not nearly so high. The ability of patients to obtain care early in pregnancy, and the degree of suspicion of ectopic pregnancy exercised by those caring for them, are important determinants of the frequency with which advanced abdominal pregnancy will develop, since almost all cases are secondary to early rupture or abortion of a tubal pregnancy into the peritoneal cavity. Typically the trophoblast, after penetrating the wall of the oviduct, maintains its tubal attachment and gradually encroaches upon the neighboring peritoneum. Meanwhile the fetus, usually but not always surrounded by amnion, continues to grow within the peritoneal cavity. In such circumstances the placenta is found in the general region of the tube, no longer grossly identifiable as such, and over the posterior aspect of the broad ligament and uterus. In much rarer instances, the implanted ovum appears to have escaped from the tube after rupture to reimplant elsewhere in the peritoneal cavity.

Primary implantation of the ovum on the peritoneum is so rare that many authors have doubted its existence, as indicated in Cavanagh's extensive review. Conclusive proof of a primary abdominal pregnancy, however, was provided by Studdiford's well-documented case, which fulfills the following criteria upon which proof of such a pregnancy must rest: (1) normal tubes and ovaries with no evidence of recent or remote injury; (2) absence of any evidence of uteroplacental fistula; and (3) presence of a pregnancy related exclusively to the peritoneal surface and young enough to eliminate the possibility of secondary implantation following primary nidation in the tube.

E. L. King directed attention to a very rare cause of abdominal pregnancy—postoperative separation of the uterine wound of a previous cesarean section. In three of his four reported cases, the ovum had implanted upon the omentum plugging the uterine defect, whereas the fourth had become attached to the abdominal wall. He believes that in each case the fertilized ovum, escaping through the defect in the uterine wall, implanted as a primary abdominal pregnancy.

Since early rupture of a tubal pregnancy is the usual cause of abdominal pregnancy, a history suggestive of the accident can be obtained in the majority of cases. A history of early spotting, irregular bleeding, or pain can be elicited quite often. Gestation is likely to be uncomfortable because of peritoneal irritation. Nausea, vomiting, flatulence, constipation, diarrhea, and abdominal pain may each be found in varying degrees. Multiparas may state that the pregnancy does not "feel right." Late in pregnancy fetal movements may be very painful. Near term the empty uterus frequently goes into spurious labor.

The condition of the fetus in abdominal pregnancy is exceedingly precarious and the great majority succumb. A review of the world's literature by Ware cited a perinatal loss of 75.6 per cent; even that figure is probably falsely low because of the tendency to report cases with happy results. Beacham is probably more nearly correct in reporting a loss in his own series of about 95 per cent. Some authors, moreover, report an incidence of congenital malformations in the infants as high as 50 per cent, though others disagree. If the fetus dies after reaching a size too large to be resorbed, it must undergo suppuration, mummification, calcification, or formation of adipocere. Pyogenic bacteria may gain access to a gestational sac, particularly when it is adherent to the intestines, and cause suppuration of its contents. Eventually the abscess ruptures at the point of least resistance, and if the patient does not die from septicemia, fetal parts may be extruded through the abdominal wall or more commonly into the intestines or bladder. Mummification and the formation of a lithopedion occasionally ensue, and the calcified product of conception may be carried for years without producing symptoms until it causes dystocia in a subsequent pregnancy or symptoms from pressure. There are numerous instances in which a period of 20 to 30 years elapsed before removal of a lithopedion at operation or autopsy. Much more rarely the fetus is converted into a yellowish, greasy mass to which the term "adipocere" is applied. The various bizarre terminations of abdominal pregnancy are well discussed, with illustrative cases, by G. King.

Diagnosis.   As previously indicated, the history often gives the first clue in these cases. Frequently there is bleeding or spotting and perhaps pain early in pregnancy. The patient is usually uncomfortable, with more than the usual gastrointestinal symptoms, and aware that the fetus is carried unusually high and that the fetal movements are uncommonly painful.

On abdominal palpation, the abnormal position of the fetus, often a transverse lie, can frequently be confirmed. Ease of palpation of the fetal parts, however, is not a reliable sign, since they sometimes feel exceedingly close to the examining fingers in normal intrauterine pregnancies and especially so in thin multiparous women. Braxton Hicks contractions are absent, of course, and gentle massage of the pregnancy products through the abdominal wall does not stimulate the mass to become more firm, as it often does with intrauterine pregnancy. The cervix is usually displaced (Fig. 10), depending in part on the position of the fetus, and may dilate as much as 2 cm in spurious labor, but effacement does not occur. The uterus may be outlined in a few cases, and palpation of the fornices may occasionally reveal small parts or the fetal head clearly outside the uterus.

In their extensive paper on advanced extrauterine pregnancy, Dixon and Stewart stressed the diagnostic value of a maternal vascular souffle, distinctly louder than a normal uterine souffle, which is heard over a small area of the abdomen just medial to the iliac spine on the side on which the placenta is located. The souffle comes from the dilated and hypertrophied ovarian vessels that supply the abnormally situated placenta. Although not present if the fetus is dead, it is said to be a fairly constant sign of abdominal pregnancy with a living fetus.

Cross and his collaborators have emphasized that the oxytocin test is the single most valuable aid in the early diagnosis of abdominal pregnancy. One unit of oxytocin is given intramuscularly while the abdominal mass is carefully palpated. With an intrauterine pregnancy, contractions can be easily felt beginning about three minutes after the injection. A positive test—that is, a palpable contraction of the uterus surrounding the products of conception—does not invariably follow even though the pregnancy is intrauterine. Therefore the test is of value only if such a contraction is clearly identified.

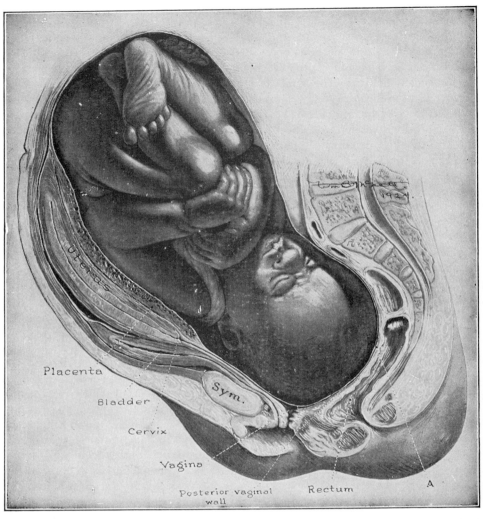

Fig. 10. Extrauterine pregnancy at term. Uterus and bladder have been displaced upward out of pelvis by development of fetal head. Its growth has stretched out the septum between vagina and pouch of Douglas to resemble the fetal membrane. (From Rowland. Surg Gynec Obstet 42:50, 1926.)

X-ray examination often reveals the fetus in a transverse or oblique lie with an unusual attitude and location. The mother's intestinal gas patterns may appear to be intermingled with the fetal parts. A lateral view may be particularly helpful by showing fetal parts overlying the maternal vertebrae.

A strong suspicion of abdominal pregnancy may be confirmed by x-ray examination with a probe or radiopaque material in the uterus. The fetus is then clearly shown to lie outside the uterine cavity, but such technics are not safe initial diagnostic procedures.

Treatment.   The operation for abdominal pregnancy frequently precipitates violent hemorrhage. Without massive blood transfusion the outlook for many such patients is hopeless. Hence, it is mandatory that at least 2,000 ml of compatible blood be immediately available in the operating room, and more in the blood bank. Preoperatively two intravenous infusion systems, each capable of delivering large volumes of fluid at a rapid rate, should be made operational. At the same time, systems for measuring central venous pressure and urine flow should be established to monitor the adequacy of the circulation. Whenever time allows, the bowel should be prepared using both mechanical cleansing and antimicrobial agents.

The massive hemorrhage that often occurs in the course of operations for abdominal pregnancy is related to the lack of constriction of the hypertrophied open vessels of the placental site after placental separation. It has therefore been recommended that operation be deferred until the fetus is dead in anticipation of diminished vascularity of the placental site. We believe, however, that regardless of the infant, procrastination may be dangerous and undesirable, since partial separation of the placenta with hemorrhage occasionally occurs spontaneously in the interval of waiting. Moreover, even though the fetus may have been dead several weeks, bleeding may still be torrential. For these reasons we believe that operation is indicated as soon as the diagnosis is established.

Another important consideration is the management of the placenta. Since its removal in abdominal pregnancy always carries the risk of hemorrhage, one should make certain that the vessels supplying the placenta can be ligated before

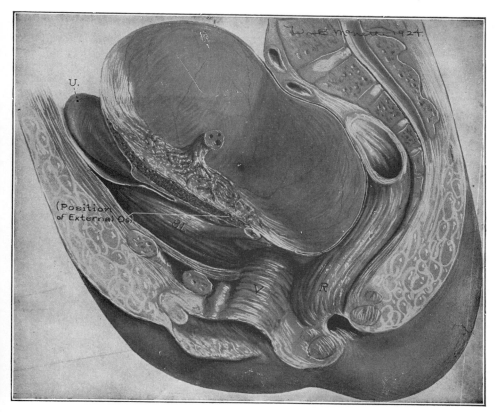

Fig. 11. Anatomic relations immediately after delivery of live child by laparotomy. Drawing shows how development of the head prevented downgrowth of the placenta, which was attached chiefly to the posterior surface of the broad ligaments and uterus. The latter was removed with the placental mass. (From Rowland. Surg Gynec Obstet 42:50, 1926.)

attempting removal of the organ (Fig. 11). In rare instances, partial separation may occur spontaneously or in the course of the operation. It is most likely to result from manipulation in attempting to locate the exact attachment of the placenta. Since in such cases the most massive hemorrhage can occur, it is, for the most part, best to avoid unnecessary exploration of the surrounding organs; the infant should be simply delivered, the cord severed close to the placenta, and the abdomen closed without drainage.

Unfortunately, the placenta, if left in the abdominal cavity, not infrequently causes complications in the form of infection, abscesses, adhesions, intestinal obstruction, and wound dehiscence. Although these complications are troublesome and usually lead to subsequent laparotomy, they are much less grave than the hemorrhage that sometimes results from placental removal.

Ware reports that when the placenta remains in situ, the test for chorionic gonadotropin may stay positive for as long as 35 days. Siegler and his colleagues have followed two such patients with quantitative urinary gonadotropin assays. The tests remained positive for 28 and 30 days, respectively, after the removal of the fetus.

Prognosis. The perinatal loss is so large that efforts at fetal salvage are almost fruitless. Ware quoted a maternal mortality of 14.5 per cent in 249 cases collected from the world's literature from 1935 to 1948. As expected, with improvement in operative technic and especially with extended use of transfusion, Beacham's maternal mortality rate for a later period was considerably lower. Even his 6 per cent figure, however, is high, indicating that abdominal pregnancy is still one of the most formidable of obstetric complications.

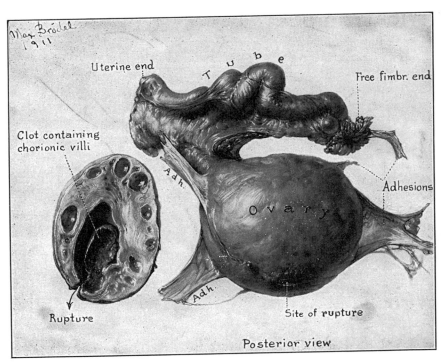

Fig. 12. E. K. Cullen's specimen of ovarian pregnancy. The four criteria of Spiegelberg are clearly illustrated.

OVARIAN PREGNANCY

Until 1878 there were no definite criteria by which specimens of suspected ovarian pregnancy could be classified. As a result, far too many ectopic pregnancies were incorrectly called ovarian. In that year, however, Spiegelberg formulated his criteria for the diagnosis of ovarian pregnancy. He required (1) that the tube on the affected side be intact; (2) that the fetal sac occupy the position of the ovary; (3) that it be connected to the uterus by the ovarian ligament; and (4) that definite ovarian tissue be found in its wall (Fig. 12). Bobrow and Winkelstein collected 154 cases from the literature that satisfied the four criteria of Spiegelberg and added one of their own. Modawi in 1962 reported a case of the exceedingly rare twin ovarian pregnancy. Even some of Spiegelberg's original cases are now subject to question, and the small number of authentic cases since 1878 attests the extreme rarity of true ovarian pregnancy.

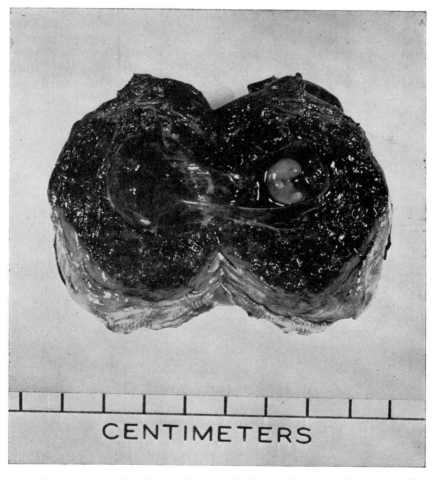

Fig. 13. Ovarian pregnancy showing the fetal sac implanted in the ovarian stroma. (Courtesy of Dr. Alexander H. Rosenthal.)

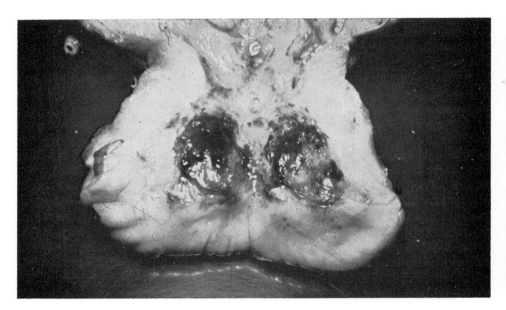

Fig. 14. Fetal sac implanted in the cervix.

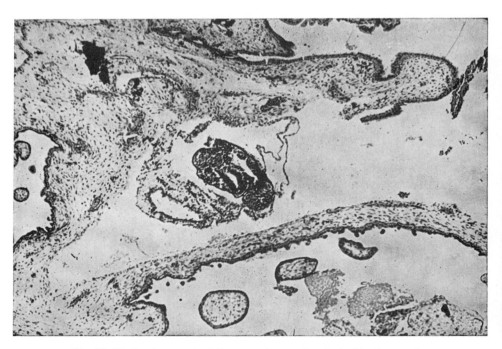

Fig. 15. Photomicrograph of three-week ovum implanted in the cervix.

In a considerable number of the recorded cases the pregnancy went to term, and in several instances lithopedia developed. Although the ovary can accommodate itself more readily than the tube to the expanding pregnancy, rupture at an early period is the usual termination. The product of conception may degenerate early without rupture and give rise to a tumor of varying size, consisting of a capsule of ovarian tissue enclosing a mass of blood, placental tissue, and possibly membranes. In ovarian pregnancy the absence of a distinct decidua leads to direct invasion of the ovarian stroma by the trophoblast (Fig. 13). A review of the subject is found in the paper of Baden and Heins.

CERVICAL PREGNANCY

Cervical pregnancy is a rare form of ectopic gestation in which the ovum implants in the cervical mucosa. In 1959, Paalman and McElin collected 52 cases from the literature and added 5 of their own. Several more cases have been added during the past 10 years.

As the endocervix is readily eroded by the trophoblast, the egg soon becomes anchored in the fibrous cervical wall, as illustrated by the three-week ovum, shown in Figures 14 and 15.

Usually, painless bleeding appearing shortly after nidation is the first sign. As pregnancy progresses, a distended thin-walled cervix with the external os partially dilated is found. Above the cervical mass, a slightly enlarged uterine fundus may be palpated.

Cervical pregnancy rarely goes beyond the twentieth week of gestation and is usually terminated surgically because of bleeding. Since attempts at removal of the placenta vaginally may result in profuse hemorrhage and even death of the patient, there should be little hesitation in performing hysterectomy to control the bleeding. Only in nulliparas very anxious to maintain fertility should so-called conservative vaginal procedures be attempted.

REFERENCES

Anderson, G. W. The racial incidence and mortality of ectopic pregnancy. Amer J Obstet Gynec 61:312, 1951.

Arey, L. B. The cause of tubal pregnancy and tubal twinning. Amer J Obstet Gynec 5:163, 1923.

Arias-Stella, J. Atypical endometrial changes associated with the presence of chorionic tissue. Arch Path 58:112, 1954.

Armstrong, J. T., Wills, S. H., Moore, J., and Lauden, A. E. Ectopic pregnancy. A review of 481 cases. Amer J Obstet Gynec 77:364, 1959.

Baden, W. F., and Heins, O. H. Ovarian pregnancy. Case report with discussion of controversial issues in the literature. Amer J Obstet Gynec 64:353, 1952.

Beacham, W. D., Hernquist, W. C., Beacham, D. W., and Webster, H. D. Abdominal pregnancy at Charity Hospital in New Orleans. Amer J Obstet Gynec 84:1257, 1962 (184 references cited).

Beller, F. K., Maki, M., and Epstein, M. D. Incoagulability of intraperitoneal blood. Amer J Obstet Gynec 102:1121, 1968.

Bobrow, M. L., and Bell, H. G. Ectopic pregnancy: A 16-year survey of 905 cases. Obstet Gynec 20:500, 1962.

———— and Winkelstein, L. B.   Intrafollicular ovarian pregnancy. Amer J Surg 91:991, 1956.

Bone, N. L., and Greene, R. R.   Histologic study of uterine tubes with tubal pregnancy. Amer J Obstet Gynec 82:1166, 1961 (50 references cited).

Cavanagh, D.   Primary peritoneal pregnancy. Rationalization or established entity? Omental transference as an alternative explanation. Amer J Obstet Gynec 76:523, 1958.

Cohen, M. R.   Culdoscopy vs. peritoneoscopy. Obstet Gynec 31:310, 1968.

Crawford, J. D., and Ward, J. V.   Advanced abdominal pregnancy. Obstet Gynec 10:549, 1957.

Cross, J. B., Lester, W. M., and McCain, J. R.   The diagnosis and management of abdominal pregnancy with a review of 19 cases. Amer J Obstet Gynec 62:303, 1951.

Cullen, T. S.   Bluish discoloration of the umbilicus as a diagnostic sign where ruptured extra-uterine pregnancy exists, in Contributions to Medical and Biological Research (Osler volume). 1919, Vol. 1, p. 420.

Dixon, H. G., and Stewart, D. B.   Advanced extrauterine pregnancy. Brit Med J 2:1103, 1960.

Douglas, E. S., Shingleton, H. M., and Crist, T.   Surgical management of tubal pregnancy: Effect on subsequent fertility. South Med J 62:954, 1969.

Fear, R. E.   Laparoscopy: A valuable aid in gynecologic diagnosis. Obstet Gynec 31:297, 1968.

Felmus, L. B., and Pedowitz, P.   Interstitial pregnancy: survey of 45 cases. Amer J Obstet Gynec 66:1271, 1953.

Fulsher, R.   Tubal pregnancy following homolateral salpingectomy. Amer J Obstet Gynec 78:355, 1959.

Funck-Brentano, P.   La Grossesse Extra-utérine. Paris, Masson et Cie, 1961.

Hall, R. E., and Todd, W. D.   The suspected ectopic pregnancy. A review of 500 cases. Amer J Obstet Gynec 81:1220, 1961.

Halpin, T. F.   Ectopic pregnancy: The problem of diagnosis. Amer J Obstet Gynec 106:227, 1970.

Hellman, L. M., Kobayashi, M., Fillisti, L., and Lavenhar, M.   The growth and development of the human fetus prior to the twentieth week of gestation. Amer J Obstet Gynec 103:789, 1969.

Jarvinen, P. A.   Value of conservative surgery in treatment of tubal pregnancy. Int J Fertil 6:269, 1961.

Jeffcoate, T.N.A.   Principles of Gynaecology, 3rd ed. New York, Appleton-Century-Crofts, 1967.

King, E. L.   Postoperative separation of the cesarean section wound, with subsequent abdominal pregnancy. Amer J Obstet Gynec 24:421, 1932.

King, G.   Advanced extrauterine pregnancy. Amer J Obstet Gynec 67:712, 1954.

Kobayashi, M., Hellman, L. M., and Fillisti, L.   Ultrasound—An aid in the diagnosis of ectopic pregnancy. Amer J Obstet Gynec 103:1131, 1969.

Kohl, S. G., Tricomi, V., and Siegler, A. M.   Ectopic pregnancy. New York J Med 56:850, 1956.

Kostic, P.   (Cause of extrauterine pregnancy: Analysis of clinical material of gynecologic hospital of the city of Belgrade). C R Soc Franc Gynéc 31:45, 1961.

Lucas, C., and Hassim, A. M.   Place of culdocentesis in the diagnosis of ectopic pregnancy. Brit Med J 1:200, 1970.

Malkasian, G. D., Hunter, J. S., and Re Mine, W. H.   Pregnancy in the tubal interstitium and tubal remnants. Amer J Obstet Gynec 77:1301, 1959.

Mall, F. P.   On the fate of the human embryo in ectopic pregnancy. Contrib Embryol 1:1, 1915.

Marchetti, A. A., Kuder, K., and Kuder, A.   A clinical evaluation of ectopic pregnancy. Amer J Obstet Gynec 52:544, 1946.

Mengert, W. F., Cobb, S. W., and Brown, W. W.   Introduction of blood into the peritoneal cavity. JAMA 147:34, 1951.

Modawi, O.   Primary twin ovarian pregnancy with ovarian endometriosis. J Obstet Gynaec Brit Comm 69:655, 1962.

Neuwirth, R. S.   Recent experience with diagnostic and surgical laparoscopy. Amer J Obstet Gynec 106:119, 1970.

Osiakina-Rojdestvenskaia, A. J.   The etiology of extrauterine pregnancy. Surg Obstet Gynec 67:308, 1938.

Overbeck, L. (The functional regeneration of the uterine mucosa in ectopic pregnancy). Z Geburtsh Gynaek 158 (Supplement), 1962.

Paalman, R. J., and McElin, T. W. Cervical pregnancy. A review of the literature and presentation of cases. Amer J Obstet Gynec 77:1261, 1959.

Pritchard, J. A., and Adams, R. H. The fate of blood in the peritoneal cavity. Surg Obstet Gynec 105:621, 1957.

Redgwick, J. P., Rumbolz, W. L., and Nace, F. M. Advanced intraligamentary pregnancy, review and case report. Western J Surg 58:424, 1950.

Riva, H. L., Kammeraad, L. A., and Andreson, P. S. Ectopic pregnancy: Report of 132 cases and comments on the role of the culdoscope in diagnosis. Obstet Gynec 20:189, 1962.

Romney, S. L., Hertig, A. T., and Reid, D. E. The endometria associated with ectopic pregnancy. Surg Obstet Gynec 91:605, 1950.

Rosenblum, J. M., Dowling, R. W., and Barnes, A. C. Treatment of tubal pregnancy. Amer J Obstet Gynec 80:274, 1960.

Sandmire, H. F., and Randall, J. H. Ectopic pregnancy: Review of 182 cases. Obstet Gynec 14:227, 1959.

Schiffer, M. A review of 268 ectopic pregnancies. Amer J Obstet Gynec 86:264, 1963.

Siegler, A., Zeichner, S., Rubenstein, I., Wallace, E. Z., and Carter, A. C. Endocrine studies in two instances of term abdominal pregnancy. Amer J Obstet Gynec 78:369, 1959.

Skulj, V. Significance of tubal pregnancy in the reproductive life of women. Amer J Obstet Gynec 80:278, 1960.

——— Bunarević, A., Dražančić, A., and Stoiljković, C. The Arias-Stella phenomenon in the diagnosis of ectopic pregnancy. Amer J Obstet Gynec 87:499, 1963.

Spiegelberg, O. (Casuistry in ovarian pregnancy). Arch Gynaek 13:73, 1878.

Stewart, H. L. Bilateral ectopic pregnancy. Western J Surg 58:648, 1950.

Stromme, W. B., McKelvey, J. L., and Adkins, C. D. Conservative surgery for ectopic pregnancy. Obstet Gynec 19:294, 1962.

Studdiford, W. E. Primary peritoneal pregnancy. Amer J Obstet Gynec 44:487, 1942.

——— Cervical pregnancy. Amer J Obstet Gynec 49:169, 1945.

Tietze, C. Progress report on intra-uterine devices, Proceedings of the Fifth World Congress on Fertility and Sterility, Stockholm, June 16-22, 1966. Excerpta Medica International Congress Series No. 133.

Torpin, R., Coleman, J., Seifi, M., and Arshadi, S. Ectopic pregnancy in Shiraz, Iran. Study of 10 year record (154 cases). Amer J Obstet Gynec 82:456, 1961.

Vasicka, A. I., and Grable, E. E. Simultaneous, extrauterine, and intrauterine pregnancies progressing to viability. A review of the literature and a report of two cases. Obstet Gynec Survey 11:603, 1956.

Ware, H. H. Observations on thirteen cases of late extrauterine pregnancy. Amer J Obstet Gynec 55:561, 1948.

Winer, A. E., Bergman, W. D., and Fields, C. Combined intra- and extrauterine pregnancy. Amer J Obstet Gynec 74:170, 1957.

22

DISEASES AND ABNORMALTIES OF THE PLACENTA AND FETAL MEMBRANES

Hydatidiform Mole, Invasive Mole, and Choriocarcinoma

Definitions.   *Hydatidiform mole* is a developmental anomaly of the placenta that is often regarded as a benign neoplasm. It is the commonest lesion anteceding *choriocarcinoma*, formerly called *chorionepithelioma*, which is a true malignant tumor of the trophoblast, characterized by a tendency to rapid and widespread metastasis. *Invasive mole* (*chorioadenoma destruens*) usually involves the myometrium and sometimes adjacent tissues, but metastasizes less frequently and less extensively than choriocarcinoma. From the viewpoint of spread, therefore, invasive mole falls between the other two lesions.

Although hydatidiform mole is uncommon and both choriocarcinoma and invasive mole are rare, their unusual biologic activity and the likelihood of their cure by chemotherapy have stimulated interest in them greater than their incidence alone would indicate. The frequently bizarre clinical behavior of the growths, the pathologic variations between benign moles and extremely malignant choriocarcinomas, and the relation of both to the normally invasive trophoblast, all raise many interesting and incompletely answered questions.

For a detailed account of these and other lesions of the placenta, the reader is referred to the scholarly volume by Benirschke and Driscoll.

HYDATIDIFORM MOLE

Pathology.   Some or all of the chorionic villi are converted into a mass of clear vesicles. Usually no embryo is present, though in occasional cases a mole arises in part of the placenta in association with a normal fetus. The vesicles vary in size from less than a millimeter to more than a centimeter in diameter and hang in grapelike clusters from thin pedicles (Fig. 1). The mass may grow large enough to fill the uterus to the size occupied by a six or seven months' normal pregnancy.

The microscopic structure is characterized by (1) hydropic degeneration and swelling of the villous stroma; (2) absence or scantiness of blood vessels; and (3) proliferation of the chorionic epithelium to a varying degree. Although both layers of the trophoblast usually undergo proliferation, the process may be limited mainly to the syncytium (Fig. 2). In a small minority of cases there may be little

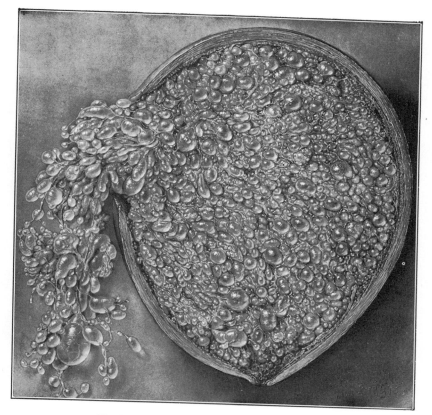

Fig. 1. Uterus containing a hydatidiform mole.

or no demonstrable proliferation. The stroma of the villi becomes hydropic and degenerates, with very few stromal cells and rare blood vessels to be seen. Most of the vesicles consist of such stroma surrounded by a very thin layer of trophoblast. In other moles the trophoblast may be moderately or markedly anaplastic or hyperplastic (Fig. 3). In rare instances, a small fetus may be present in addition to the hydatidiform mole, the condition called partial hydatidiform mole. In such cases, certain villi are not involved in the hydatidiform process and are sufficiently vascularized to sustain embryonic and fetal life for a variable period of time.

That hydatidiform mole was formerly considered primarily a degenerative rather than a neoplastic lesion is indicated by such terms as myxomatous and cystic degenerations of the chorion. In his classic study of 1895, Marchand demonstrated that trophoblastic proliferation is an essential feature, a viewpoint held by most current investigators. The mole may be considered a pathologic pregnancy, with the primary defect a blighted ovum.

Difference of opinion remains as to when hydatid change in the villi represents a true mole and when it is merely a degenerative reaction that resembles mole in its early stage. Hertig and Edmonds found that two thirds of the pathologic ova in their study showed early hydatid degeneration. They thought that many hydatid moles originated thus from defectively vascularized villi and that

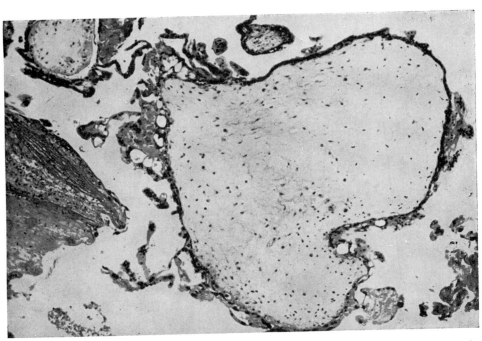

Fig. 2. Example of hydatidiform mole showing slight to moderate trophoblastic hyperplasia, confined to the syncytium and considered as probably benign. (From Smalbraak. Trophoblastic Growths. Elsevier Publishing Co.)

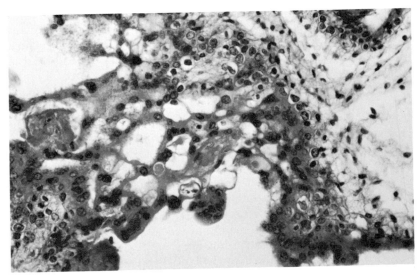

Fig. 3. Hydatidiform mole, showing moderate hyperplasia of trophoblast. (Courtesy of Dr. Ralph M. Wynn.)

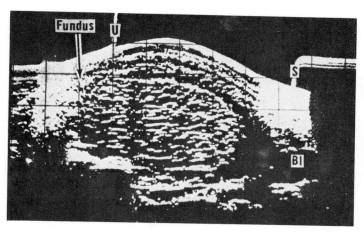

Fig. 4. Sonogram of hydatidiform mole, longitudinal scan at the midline. Bl, bladder; S, symphysis pubis; U, umbilicus; Fundus, fundus uteri.

if examined early enough at least a fetal sac could always be found. Support for this "transition theory" of the origin of hydatid mole is provided by Donald and by Hellman, who have demonstrated such structures in their ultrasonic examinations of patients with early moles (Fig. 4).

Carr noted that hydropic change, hydatidiform degeneration, and true moles all have pathologic and cytogenetic features in common. Triploidy was the commonest form of polyploidy noted in this group of lesions. In benign hydatidiform moles and invasive moles, the sex chromatin pattern was female in 29 out of 30 cases, according to Tominaga and Page. Baggish and co-workers also found that the sex chromatin pattern was predominantly female in their series of 90 hydatidiform moles; they reasoned, furthermore, that the findings could not be explained on the basis of polyploidy.

Attempts to relate the histologic structure of hydatidiform moles to their potential malignant tendencies with precision have been generally disappointing. Novak and Seah, for example, were unable to establish such a relation in 120 cases of hydatidiform mole or in the molar tissue submitted to them in 26 cases of choriocarcinoma following hydatidiform mole. The molar tissue from many patients that eventually developed choriocarcinoma showed only very slightly trophoblastic proliferation, whereas many of their patients with hydatidiform mole that had pronounced trophoblastic proliferation subsequently pursued a benign course after only a dilatation and curettage.

Wynn and Davies examined the hydatidiform mole with the electron microscope and found ultrastructural features resembling, in great detail, those of early normal trophoblast. The hyperplastic epithelium surrounding the vesicles showed ultrastructural evidence of intense metabolic activity, whereas the trophoblast covering the villi encased in fibrin, and thus excluded from maternal nourishment, exhibited varying degrees of degeneration.

In many cases of hydatidiform mole the ovaries show multiple lutein cysts (Fig. 5), which may vary from microscopic size to 10 cm or more in diameter.

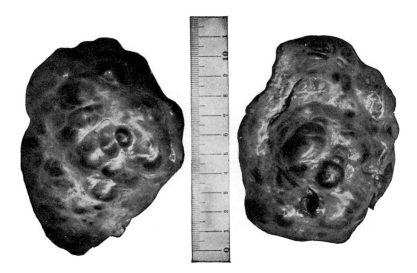

Fig. 5. Bilateral lutein cysts, associated with hydatidiform mole.

The surfaces of the cysts are smooth, often yellowish, and lined with lutein cells. The incidence of such cysts in association with mole is reported to be from 25 per cent to as high as 60 per cent. The variation in figures reflects the diagnostic criteria. Novak has emphasized that most of the ovaries lacking gross cysts show microscopic cystic change and luteal hyperreaction often involving both thecal and granulosal elements.

Lutein cysts of the ovaries are thought to result from overstimulation of lutein elements by large amounts of chorionic gonadtropin secreted by the proliferating trophoblast. That such extensive ovarian changes are not ordinarily seen in normal pregnancy may be explained by the fact that very high levels of gonadotropin are not maintained for long periods of time. In general, extensive cystic change is usually associated with the larger hydatidiform moles and a long period of stimulation.

Girouard, Barclay, and Collins collected 15 cases of typical theca lutein cysts without hydatid mole or choriocarcinoma during pregnancy and added 2 of their own. They are especially interesting because 11 were associated with placental hypertrophy, 6 with fetal hydrops, and 5 with multiple pregnancies. The remainder were from normal pregnancies. Oophorectomy should not be performed because of theca lutein cysts alone. After delivery of the mole, the cysts regress and eventually disappear.

Incidence. Hydatidiform mole occurs once in about 2,000 pregnancies in the United States and Europe but is much more frequent in parts of Asia and the South Pacific. King reports an incidence of hydatidiform mole of 1 in 530 pregnancies in Hong Kong over a 20-year period and 1 case of choriocarcinoma in 3,708 pregnancies. The data of Wei and Ouyang show that trophoblastic disease is particularly prevalent in Taiwan, where the incidence of hydatidiform mole is 1 in 125 pregnancies. Marquez-Monter and co-workers, furthermore, reported a surprisingly high incidence of 1 in 200 in the General Hospital of Mexico. The

Mexican study and data from the Philippines suggest that the high incidence in those countries is in some way related to poor social and economic status. In about 1 in 12,000 pregnancies hydatidiform mole and a fetus may coexist.

Recurrence of hydatid mole is uncommon but is seen in about 2 per cent of cases (Chesley and co-workers; Chun and associates; Acosta-Sison). Subsequent fecundity and childbearing are usually normal. According to Yen and MacMahon the chance of recurrence of a hydatidiform mole is 40 times as high as the incidence in the general population.

Age has an important bearing on the incidence of hydatidiform mole, as indicated by the relatively high frequency among pregnancies at the very beginning and, particularly, toward the end of the childbearing period. Age shows its most pronounced effect in woman older than 45, when the relative frequency of the lesion is more than ten times greater than at ages 20 to 40. There are numerous authenticated cases of hydatidiform mole in women 54 and 55 years old, whereas normal pregnancy at such advanced ages is practically unknown.

Clinical History.   In the early stages of development of the mole there are no characteristics distinguishing it from normal pregnancy. If early abortion does not occur, the growing uterus often enlarges more rapidly than usual, its size exceeding that expected from the supposed duration of gestation in about one half the cases; in the remainder the uterus is of average size or smaller. Uterine bleeding, the outstanding sign, may vary from spotting to profuse hemorrhage. It may appear just before abortion, but more often it occurs intermittently for weeks or even months. As a consequence of the bleeding, anemia is quite common. In some cases, however, the anemia is out of proportion to the amount of blood shed. In these instances usually there is rapidly developing and marked hypervolemia, which accounts to a considerable extent for the anemia (Pritchard). Occasionally hydatid vesicles are passed. Sooner or later the mole is aborted or removed by operation. Spontaneous expulsion is most likely to occur around the fourth month and is rarely delayed beyond the seventh month. In 72 cases of hydatidiform mole cited by Smalbraak, the average duration of the pregnancy was 18 weeks.

Uterine infection is common with hydatidiform mole, since there may be a period of threatening abortion with a patulous cervix, bleeding, and a large mass of poorly vascularized tissue in the uterus. Hyperemesis is more frequent and likely to be more severe and protracted in cases of hydatidiform mole than in normal pregnancy. Of special importance is the frequent association of severe preeclampsia and eclampsia with molar pregnancies. Since preeclampsia-eclampsia may arise early in the second trimester of molar gestations, and since in normal pregnancy the syndrome is hardly ever seen at so early a date, the development of severe preeclampsia or eclampsia before the twenty-fourth week of gestation should suggest hydatidiform mole. The syndrome is particularly likely to occur in moles in which uterine growth has been extremely rapid or in large tumors. Although seldom mentioned in the literature, pain is sometimes a conspicuous symptom, especially in association with rapid uterine growth.

Diagnosis.   Hydatidiform mole is often diagnosed only upon expulsion of the specimen. Since bleeding is the usual sign, the initial diagnosis is commonly simple threatened abortion. Occasionally vesicles may be passed, making the diagnosis clear. In a patient with persistent bleeding, a uterus larger than the expected size arouses the suspicion of mole. The possibilities of error in menstrual data, a pregnant uterus enlarged by myomas, hydramnios, and multiple pregnancy must also be considered. If pregnancy is advanced, palpation of fetal parts, perception of fetal movements or heart tones, and roentgenographic visualization of a fetal skeleton may be useful. Positive evidence is reliable; negative findings may be misleading.

Three diagnostic technics of relatively recent origin provide greater precision in the diagnosis of hydatidiform mole. Hendrickse and associates and Garcia and co-workers have demonstrated by properly timed arteriograms that the pregnant uterus shows early bilateral filling of the uterine veins only in the presence of mole or choriocarcinoma, presumably on the basis of arteriovenous shunts

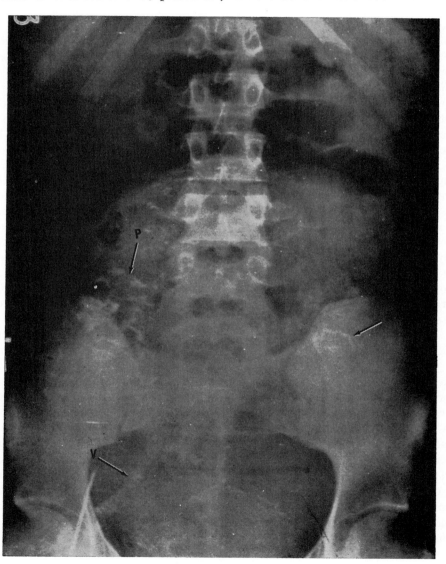

Fig. 6. Arteriogram in a case of hydatidiform mole. Arterial (A), placental (P), and venous (V) filling are simultaneously demonstrated in this roentgenogram. (Courtesy of Dr. James H. Nelson.)

(Fig. 6). Transabdominal intrauterine instillation of a radiopaque substance such as Hypaque produces a quite characteristic roentgenogram in cases of hydatidiform mole (Torres and Pelegrina; Zarou and associates). There is some risk of abortion from hypertonic contrast material. The greatest diagnostic accuracy may be obtained from the characteristic ultrasonogram of hydatidiform mole (Fig. 4). The safety and precision of sonography make it the technic of choice whenever it is available. According to Gottesfeld and co-workers, there were no false-positive diagnoses of hydatidiform mole by ultrasonography in their series. Tests for chorionic gonadotropin may be very useful if certain criteria are met: (1) a reliable quantitative method of assay must be used; and (2) there must be a correlation with clinical data and appreciation of the considerable variation in gonadotropin secretion in normal pregnancy (Ch. 6, p. 173).

Assays performed on serum are subject to fewer variables than are measurements of urinary gonadotropin. The assay involving weight of the immature rat's uterus has been most reliable. Recently a variety of immunoassays including radioimmunoassay have been popular. The result should be compared with the serum gonadotropin level for normal pregnancy at the stage in question. If it is far above the normal range for that stage of pregnancy, a presumptive diagnosis of mole may be made. It is clear from the gonadotropin curve for normal pregnancy that no *single* value can be established as the borderline between normal and abnormal pregnancy. Very high values in the first two or three months mean little, since they are encountered frequently in normal pregnancy, especially with multiple fetuses; hence the biologic test is not helpful in diagnosing the early cases of mole. Beyond 100 days after the last menstrual period, however, there is in normal pregnancy a rapid decline in gonadotropin; persistently high or rising levels after that time are therefore strong evidence of abnormal growth of trophoblast. If the slightest doubt demains, one or more repeated assays at intervals of a week should be performed in an attempt to observe the trend.

In summary, the diagnostic features of hydatidiform mole are (1) enlargement of the uterus out of proportion to the duration of pregnancy (in about one half of the cases); (2) continuous or intermittent bloody discharge, beginning about the twelfth week of pregnancy, usually not profuse, and often brownish rather than reddish; (3) absence of fetal parts on palpation or radiologic examination, even though the uterus may be enlarged to the level of the umbilicus or higher; (4) typical early venous shadows on the arteriogram; (5) characteristic ultrasonographic patterns; (6) signs and symptoms of preeclampsia, such as albuminuria, hypertension, or edema, earlier in pregnancy than usually found; and (7) a high chorionic gonadotropin level in the serum (or less dependably in the urine) 100 days or more after the last menstrual period. In differential diagnosis great care must be taken to rule out multiple pregnancy, which may simulate hydatidiform mole in several respects. Not a few normal twin pregnancies have been inadvertently interrupted because of the mistaken diagnosis of hydatidiform mole.

Prognosis. The immediate mortality from hydatidiform mole was formerly as high as 10 per cent, chiefly as a result of hemorrhage, infection, and uterine perforation. In a collective review of 576 cases, Mathieu found an immediate mortality of only 1.4 per cent, a figure that should be reduced practically to zero by the use of blood transfusion and antibiotics. Attempts to deliver large moles per vaginam, however, sometimes lead to uncontrollable and fatal hemorrhage.

The incidence of transformation of hydatidiform mole to frank choriocarcinoma is variously reported as from 2 to 8 per cent, but the figure rises sharply in older women. Years may sometimes intervene between the occurrence of a hydatidiform mole and the development of choriocarcinoma. In some of these cases the choriocarcinoma may have stemmed from a recent but unrecognized early abortion rather than from the previous hydatidiform mole. Nevertheless, cases in which an unrecognized pregnancy could be ruled out because an intervening hysterectomy had been performed leave no doubt that chorionic cells may lie dormant for long periods before manifesting malignancy. For instance, Natsume and Takada have reported a case in which choriocarcinoma developed nine years after a supravaginal hysterectomy for chorioadenoma destruens (invasive mole).

The subsequent course of 181 patients followed by Hertig and Sheldon (Table 1) shows that only a very small percentage of cases developed a true ma-

Table 1. **Subsequent Course of 181 Patients with Hydatid Mole**

	Per Cent
1. Initial spontaneous cure	73.5
2. Chorionepithelioma in situ*	3.5
3. Syncytial endometritis†	4.5
4. Chorioadenoma destruens	16.0
5. Choriocarcinoma	2.5
Total	100.0

* Chorionepithelioma in situ: *a term introduced by Hertig and Sheldon to describe a small, discrete mass of superficially invasive, apparently malignant trophoblast without villi found in uterine curettings in association with pregnancy, usually of molar type.*

† Syncytial endometritis: *a term that most pathologists agree refers to an accentuation of the morphologic features of the placental site. Endometrium and myometrium are infiltrated by trophoblastic cells with varying degrees of inflammation, but the lesion is clinically benign (Hertig and Mansell).*

lignant tumor, although over a quarter did not initially have an entirely benign course. A sizable proportion, however, will regress spontaneously or be cured by relatively simple procedures, such as a dilatation and curettage. It is precisely this spectrum of lesions, ranging from completely benign to highly malignant, with a rather unpredictable intermediate group, that has produced dilemmas in diagnosis unmatched by any other tumor.

Treatment.   The treatment of hydatidiform mole has two phases, the immediate abortion or evacuation of the mole and the later follow-up for detection of malignant change. In the majority of cases, abortion of the mole is imminent or in progress when diagnosis is made, and treatment is directed at completion of the abortion. Oxytocic stimulation may be useful. If bleeding is profuse, evacuation of the uterus by ovum forceps and completion by sharp or suction curettage may be necessary but must be done with great caution, since the uterus may be very soft and easily perforated. Since hemorrhage may be severe, ample blood for transfusion should be available. If intervention is not forced by hemorrhage, spontaneous completion may be awaited, with curettage deferred for several days, when beginning involution has rendered the uterus firmer. Unless the mole is passed spontaneously, it is far safer to complete evacuation of the uterus by abdominal hysterectomy or by suction curettage than to attempt sharp curettage, especially if the uterus is larger than 12 to 14 weeks' gestational size. Whether the mole is passed spontaneously or delivered by hysterotomy, it is important to curette the uterus. In hysterotomy, curettage is performed at the same time. These curettings give a much better indication of the invasiveness of the tumor than does the aborted mole itself.

Hysterectomy is a logical procedure in women of 40 or over, regardless of parity, and in women with three or more children, regardless of age, because of the frequency with which choriocarcinoma ensues in these age and parity groups. Although hysterectomy reduces greatly the likelihood of this sequel, it does not eliminate it entirely. In 69 cases of hydatidiform mole, reported by Chun and her associates, in which initial hysterectomy was done because of advanced age or parity, 2 patients developed choriocarcinoma two and a half and three years later, an incidence of 2.8 per cent. In contrast, in 166 cases treated by evacuation of the molar tissue with conservation of the uterus, 14 subsequently developed choriocarcinoma, a frequency of 8.4 per cent. In any event, hysterectomy does not eliminate the necessity for careful follow-up.

How long pregnancy should be interdicted after a mole is an unanswered question. Reid recommends one year; Donald more conservatively suggests an interval of two years. Hertig believes that there is insufficient basis for answering the question; the crux of the problem, in his opinion, is the likelihood of the pregnancy's interference with the diagnosis of a recurrent mole (personal communication). We have compromised on the following rule of thumb: if the chorionic gonadotropin titer remains negative for six months, and if recurrent ovulation is indicated by regular normal menstruation, biphasic temperature curves, and ovulatory vaginal smears, pregnancy can be safely undertaken.

Follow-up Procedures.   If these extremely important procedures are not carefully followed, a small but definite number of these patients will die of choriocarcinoma.

Whereas the serum chorionic gonadotropin becomes negative within a week after normal pregnancy, such is not the usual case with hydatid mole. In a very carefully studied series of patients, Delfs followed the levels of the serum chorionic gonadotropin after the delivery of a hydatid mole. Her data show that the chorionic gonadotropin titer falls in a parabola-shaped curve over a considerable period of time (Fig. 7). About one half of the patients will have negative tests at the beginning of the third week, and three quarters at the end of 40 days. From this time onward, the slope of the curve is gradual, with the result that concern may develop regarding the possibility of malignant change in the retained trophoblast. Delfs has clearly shown that many of these patients will subsequently develop negative tests, the longest recorded interval being 18 months. Although spontaneous disappearance of retained trophoblast is well known, the effectiveness of chemotherapeutic agents in the treatment of choriocarcinoma has led many authors to suggest the early use of these drugs in patients with retained molar trophoblast to preclude the development of subsequent choriocarcinoma and to hasten the disappearance of the retained trophoblast. Most chemotherapeutic agents, such as methotrexate, are highly toxic and potentially lethal; therefore the risk of chemotherapy must be carefully weighed against the chances of spontaneous regression.

The prime objective of follow-up is detection, at the earliest possible moment, of any change in behavior of the presumably benign mole in the direction of malignancy. Although microscopic examination of the original mole may provide prognostic criteria applicable in a general way to a series of patients, it

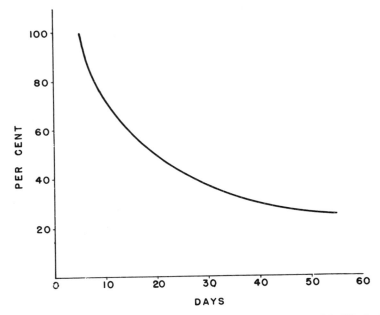

Fig. 7. Persistence of chorionic gonadotropin after hydatidiform mole. (Modified after Delfs. Obstet Gynec 9:1, 1957.)

furnishes little information for the individual specific case. It is therefore necessary to rely on the chorionic gonadotropin values to detect residual or proliferative
trophoblastic tissue. For this purpose the test must be sufficiently sensitive and
specific to detect levels of chorionic gonadotropin at least as low as 500 international units per liter. A dependable test should be employed at the time of passage
of the mole and biweekly for the next two months. Thereafter, the test should be
performed monthly for a full year unless, as previously indicated, a new pregnancy is permitted. An initial roentgenogram of the chest should be obtained
during the first examination of the patient to serve as a baseline should future
roentgenologic studies become necessary.

If chorionic gonadotropin persists after 30 days, a dilatation and curettage
should be performed, particularly if the *titers are rising*. If in such a case the curettings reveal malignant trophoblast, chemotherapy is indicated. Rising titers by
themselves, in the absence of pregnancy, are an indication for chemotherapy. If,
however, the levels of chorionic gonadotropin are rapidly falling and the curettings reveal either benign trophoblast or none at all, the patient may be followed
further.

A rising titer or the onset of vaginal bleeding necessitates a change in this
regimen. If maintenance of childbearing is not an important consideration or if
there is indication of impending perforation of the uterus by the tumor, hysterectomy will probably be adequate treatment. The chorionic gonadotropin levels
should be carefully followed, nevertheless, for such patients may already have
metastases to the lungs and elsewhere. If the uterus is to be preserved, a course

of chemotherapy should be instituted. Methotrexate, as discussed later, is usually the drug of choice.

Brewer and co-workers believe that measurement of levels of chorionic gonadotropin 60 days after termination of a molar pregnancy can be of great aid in detecting patients who have developed an invasive mole or a choriocarcinoma. By a combination of hormonal assays, clinical examination, and curettage to rule out retained molar tissue within the uterus, patients who need chemotherapy can be selected. Brewer and his group prefer this selective method of treatment to routine prophylaxis with powerful drugs such as methotrexate.

Human placental lactogen, more accurately termed human chorionic somato-mammotropin, may be of aid in distinguishing normal pregnancy from chorionic tumors. A high level of chorionic gonadotropin together with a low level of chorionic somatomammotropin after the early months of pregnancy should suggest chorionic neoplasia.

Saxena and co-workers found that the level of chorionic somatomammotropin in trophoblastic tumors was well below the range in early normal pregnancy of less than 10 weeks' duration. In molar pregnancy the values were 10 to 100 times lower than those expected in normal pregnancy of corresponding duration. In patients with trophoblastic tumors under treatment, the chorionic somatomammotropin in serum falls to undetectable levels before the fall in chorionic gonadotropin suggests complete remission. Relapse may be indicated by a subsequent rise in chorionic gonadotropin without a concomitant elevation in chorionic somatomammotropin. Yen and co-workers also have found radioimmunoassays of both hormones to be sensitive indices for monitoring patients who have delivered hydatidiform moles. Chorionic somatomammotropin may disappear promptly after evacuation of localized disease and may remain undetectable despite an active metastatic focus.

INVASIVE MOLE

Invasive mole occupies an intermediate position, between the benign hydatidiform mole and the highly malignant choriocarcinoma. It has also been called malignant hydatidiform mole, penetrative mole, and destructive mole. Although the term chorioadenoma destruens is firmly entrenched, it is histopathologically a misnomer, created in analogy with choriocarcinoma. The incidence of the condition, like that of choriocarcinoma, is very low.

The distinguishing features of invasive mole, as listed by Novak and Seah, are (1) excessive trophoblastic overgrowth and (2) extensive penetration of the trophoblastic elements, including whole villi, into the depths of the myometrium, sometimes involving the peritoneum or the adjacent parametrium or vaginal vault (Fig. 8). Such moles are thus locally invasive, though they generally lack the pronounced tendency to widespread metastasis that characterizes choriocarcinoma. As contrasted with the typically benign hydatidiform mole, invasive mole microscopically usually shows large fields of trophoblast. Even histologically entirely benign appearing moles with very little trophoblastic hyperplasia may, however, show the extreme invasiveness, the other feature of this lesion. Novak and Seah lay great stress on the fact that invasive mole, in contrast to choriocarcinoma, has a well-preserved villous pattern. They emphasize repeatedly that even a few villi should militate against the diagnosis of choriocarcinoma. In this connection, Tow

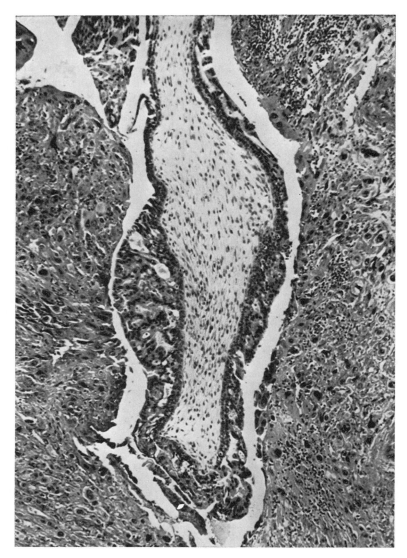

Fig. 8. Invasive hydatidiform mole (chorioadenoma destruens), showing molar villus with hyperplastic trophoblast penetrating deeply into myometrium. (Courtesy of Dr. Ralph M. Wynn.)

has suggested new histopathologic terms that deemphasize the importance of the villous pattern or its absence. According to him, chorioadenoma destruens may best be designated *villous choriocarcinoma*, and choriocarcinoma referred to specifically as *avillous choriocarcinoma*.

In an ultrastructural study of invasive mole, Wynn and Harris found relatively well preserved trophoblast deep within the myometrium. Relatively little fibrinoid was deposited around contiguous fetal and maternal cells, suggesting less reaction of uterine tissues to trophoblast in this lesion. (Fig. 9). The endometrial epithelium exhibited the Arias-Stella phenomenon (Ch. 21), which ultrastructurally appeared to represent cellular hyperactivity rather than involution (Fig. 10).

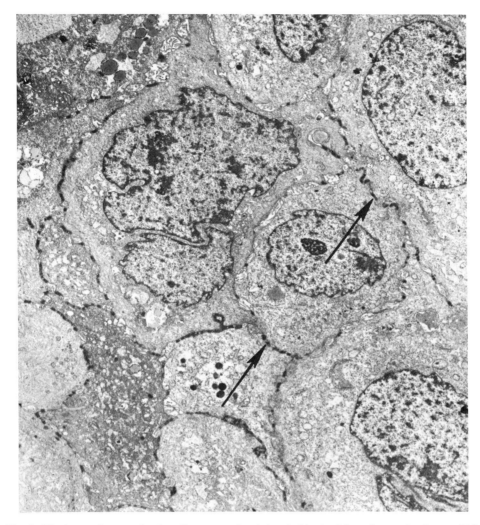

Fig. 9. Electron micrograph of well-preserved cytotrophoblast of invasive mole deep within myometrium. Arrows indicate desmosomes. (Courtesy of Dr. Ralph M. Wynn.)

Okudaira and Strauss have examined both the hydatidiform mole and chorioadenoma destruens with the electron microscope. In the invasive mole only, they found what they considered to be viruslike particles in the cytoplasm. This interesting suggestion remains to be confirmed.

In some cases invasive mole cannot be diagnosed until after hysterectomy, but in others it can frequently be recognized presumptively or at least suspected by the occurrence of intraabdominal hemorrhage or by the findings on palpation of parametrial invasion or the demonstration of vaginal extension. The treatment is often hysterectomy, because invasive moles may occasionally cause death through uterine perforation and massive intraabdominal hemorrhage and also because metastasis occurs in a certain minority of cases. Chemotherapy in the

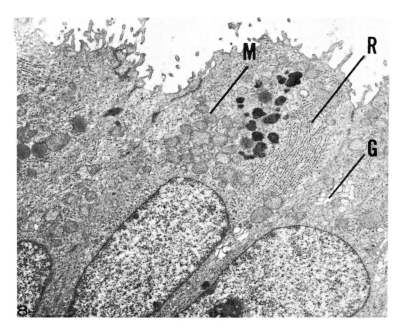

Fig. 10. Arias-Stella reaction in endometrial epithelium of patient with invasive mole shown in Figure 9. Electron micrograph shows Golgi complex (G), endoplasmic reticulum (R), and mitochondrion (M). (Courtesy of Dr. Ralph M. Wynn.)

treatment of this lesion is still insufficiently evaluated, but methotrexate without hysterectomy has brought about a complete remission in some cases.

CHORIOCARCINOMA

Frequency.   Since choriocarcinoma occurs only once in many thousands of pregnancies, estimates of incidence based on small series of cases are not significant. The tumor is confined to the reproductive period and, except for rare cases arising in teratomas, always follows pregnancy. Approximately 40 per cent of cases occur after hydatidiform mole, 40 per cent after abortions, and 20 per cent after term pregnancies. Choriocarcinoma may result from ectopic as well as intrauterine pregnancy. Very rarely it may coexist with the pregnancy, as shown by Brewer and Gerbie, but in most cases it develops immediately afterward. Occasionally it remains apparently dormant for amazingly long periods before undergoing active growth. Many such reported cases, however, may actually result from a subsequent pregnancy with early unrecognized abortion in the interim.

Etiology.   Iliya and co-workers have considered several etiologic factors in choriocarcinoma: low socioeconomic status, advanced maternal age, and poor nutrition. They appear to stress consanguinity, however. In parts of the Orient where choriocarcinoma is prevalent, consanguineous matings are also most common. The implication of these findings is that the high incidence of choriocarcinoma is related to a remarkable degree of compatibility between tissues of mother and fetus.

Pathology.   This extremely malignant tumor arises from the trophoblast. It may be considered a carcinoma of the chorionic epithelium, although in its growth and metastasis it often behaves like a sarcoma. The factors involved in malignant transformation of the chorion are unknown. In choriocarcinoma the tendencies of normal trophoblast to invasive growth and erosion of blood vessels are greatly exaggerated. The characteristic gross picture is that of a rapidly growing mass invading both uterine muscle and blood vessels with areas of hemorrhage and necrosis. The tumor is dark red or purple and ragged or friable. If it involves the endometrium, bleeding, sloughing, and infection of the surface usually occur early. Masses of tissue buried in the myometrium may extend outward, appearing on the uterus as dark, irregular nodules that eventually penetrate the peritoneum.

Microscopically, columns and sheets of trophoblast penetrate the muscle and blood vessels, sometimes in plexiform arrangement and at other times in complete disorganization, interspersed with clotted blood (Figs. 11 and 12). The most

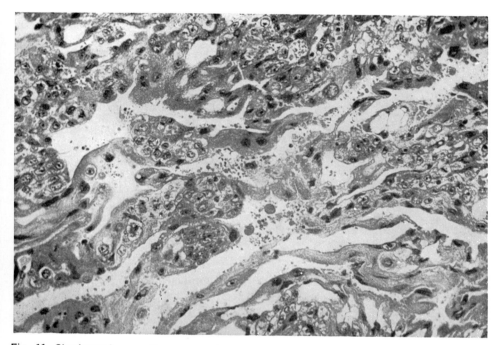

Fig. 11. Choriocarcinoma. Numerous mitoses can be seen in Langhans cells, mainly surrounded by syncytium, broad bands of which also border the tissue spaces. (From Smalbraak. Trophoblastic Growths. Elsevier Publishing Co.)

important diagnostic feature of choriocarcinoma is absence of a villous pattern. Only one of Novak and Seah's 74 cases showed any evidence of villi. Both Langhans cells and syncytial elements are involved, although one or the other may predominate. Cellular anaplasia exists in varying and often marked degrees, but is less valuable as a criterion of malignancy in trophoblastic than in other tumors. The difficulty of cytologic evaluation is one of the factors leading to error in the diagnosis of choriocarcinoma from uterine curettings, in which the general growth pattern may not be evident. Cells of normal trophoblast at the placental site have often been erroneously diagnosed as choriocarcinoma. In an interesting study of early choriocarcinoma in otherwise normal placentas, Brewer and Gerbie found the tumor to arise from normal villi. They regard the spontaneous degeneration of formed villi at the primary site to be characteristic of choriocarcinoma.

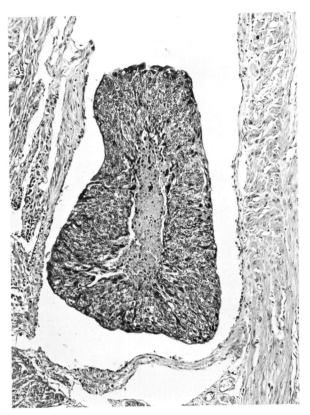

Fig. 12. Choriocarcinoma, showing plug of malignant trophoblast deeply invading myometrium. (Courtesy of Dr. Ralph M. Wynn.)

According to Brewer and Gerbie, the earliest stages of choriocarcinoma lack three of the histopathologic criteria usually associated with the lesion: absence of villi, hemorrhage into surrounding tissue, and necrosis of maternal tissue.

In their electron microscopic study of transplanted human choriocarcinoma, Wynn and Davies provided an ultrastructural explanation for the intense metabolic activity of the tumor. In addition to typical cellular and syncytial trophoblast, there is a spectrum of cells with fine structural features ranging from those of primitive cytotrophoblast to those of the mature, fully differentiated syncytium (Figs. 13 and 14). The growth of the choriocarcinoma in the hamster's cheek pouch provides a convenient method for study of the tumors.

Metastases often occur very early and they are generally blood-borne because of the affinity of trophoblast for blood vessels. The most common site is the lungs (over 75 per cent); the second most common is the vagina (about 50 per cent). The vulva, kidneys, liver, ovaries, and brain also show metastases in many cases. Lutein cysts occur in over one third of the cases. Mercer has reported a remarkable case of choriocarcinoma in mother and child.

Studies of the biologic activity of these unusual tumors have been hampered

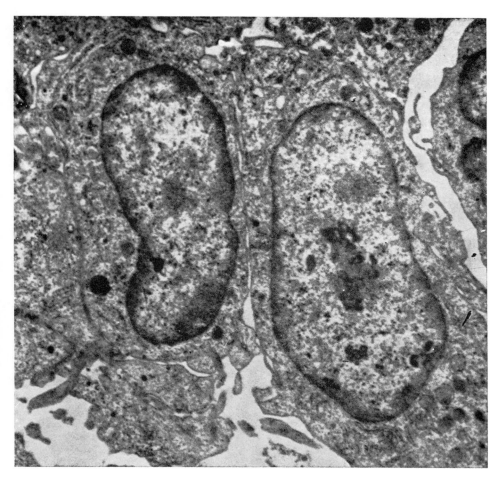

Fig. 13. Electron micrograph of cytotrophoblast of human choriocarcinoma. Note high nucleocytoplasmic ratio and poorly differentiated cytoplasm. Plasma membranes are prominent. Intracytoplasmic organelles other than ribosomes are scant. (Courtesy of Dr. Ralph M. Wynn.)

by the absence of spontaneous choriocarcinomas in experimental animals. With the discovery by Martin-Padilla and Benirschke of an apparent choriocarcinoma in the hemochorial villous placenta of the armadillo, means may now be available for studying the natural history of these extraordinary neoplasms.

Clinical History.   Choriocarcinoma may follow hydatid mole, abortion, or normal pregnancy. Except with moles, there is usually no evidence of malignancy immediately after the pregnancy. The most common, though not constant, sign is irregular bleeding after the immediate puerperium in association with subinvolution. The bleeding may be continuous or intermittent, with sudden and sometimes massive hemorrhages. Perforation of the uterus by the growth may cause intraperitoneal hemorrhage. Extension into the parametrium may cause pain and fixation suggestive of inflammatory disease. Secondary infection commonly accompanies the process.

     In many cases the first indication of the condition may be the metastatic lesions. Vaginal or vulvar tumors may be found. The patient may complain of cough

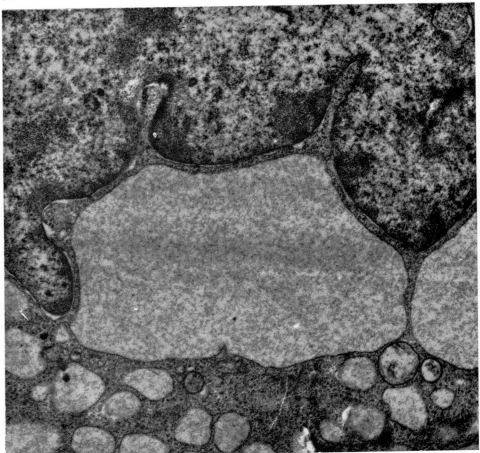

Fig. 14. Electron micrograph of syncytiotrophoblast of human choriocarcinoma. Note unevenly dense multilobular nuclei. Within cytoplasm are widely dilated cisternae of endoplasmic reticulum and dense accumulations of ribosomes. (Courtesy of Dr. Ralph M. Wynn.)

and bloody sputum arising from pulmonary metastases. In a few cases it has been impossible to find choriocarcinoma in the uterus or pelvis, the original lesion having disappeared, leaving only distant metastases growing actively.

Perforation of the uterine wall by choriocarcinoma with free and sometimes massive bleeding into the peritoneal cavity is probably a more common complication of this invasive neoplasm than is generally realized. Acosta-Sison and Espaniola encountered 8 instances of this accident in 32 cases of choriocarcinoma, or in 1 out of 4. The clinical course in these accidents may closely resemble that of ruptured tubal pregnancy. Since acute symptoms may appear almost immediately after pelvic examination, great care must be exercised in suspected cases.

If unmodified by treatment, the course of choriocarcinoma is rapidly progressive, death occurring usually within a few months to one year in the majority of cases. The most common cause of death is hemorrhage in various locations. Hou and Pang list the order of frequency as cerebral, vaginal, gastrointestinal, and abdominal, on the basis of autopsies performed on 28 patients.

Diagnosis.   Recognition of the possibility of the lesion is the most important factor in diagnosis. All cases of hydatidiform mole should be under suspicion and followed as described. Any case of unusual bleeding after term pregnancy or abortion should be investigated by curettage and measurements of chorionic gonadotropin.

Absolute reliance cannot be placed on curettings. Great experience and caution are required in making a positive diagnosis of choriocarcinoma from curettings unless the pattern is that of obvious malignancy, for normal trophoblast often penetrates deeply into the uterine wall at the placental site, thus simulating neoplastic invasion. Conversely, malignant tissue may be buried within the myometrium, inaccessible to the curette.

Chorionic gonadotropin normally disappears from the serum and urine a few days after normal pregnancy or uncomplicated complete abortion. Therefore, persistent or rising titers of gonadotropin after about a week are indicative of trophoblastic neoplasia. Correlation with clinical data is required to rule out a new intrauterine pregnancy. Assays should, of course, be repeated and checked before resorting to radical therapy. A positive gonadotropin assay, furthermore, confirms the diagnosis of distant lesions, such as pulmonary metastases.

Treatment.   Current treatment of choriocarcinoma is radically different from, and more successful than, that of the past. Formerly the only hope for cure was very early hysterectomy. In fact, Novak and Seah reported a one-year survival rate without evidence of recurrence in only 13 of their 74 cases. Since the advent of chemotherapy, the only reported series of patients treated surgically is that of Manahan, who achieved a five-year survival by hysterectomy alone in 10 out of 11 patients whose disease was confined to the uterus. Most other investigators consider the therapy of choice to be methotrexate (4-amino-N^{10}-methylpteroylglutamic acid), an antimetabolite that prevents the conversion of folic acid to folinic acid (citrovorum factor), which is essential to the synthesis of nucleic acids, as required in mitosis. Whereas all cells are affected by the drug, embryonic tissues, by virtue of their rapid cellular division and growth, are particularly sensitive. The usual dosage is 0.4 mg of methotrexate per kilogram per day parenterally or by mouth in courses of five days and repeated at least once unless toxicity supervenes. In Hertz's series of 87 patients treated initially with methotrexate, only 2 failed to show substantial regression of the tumor, and 45, or over half the total, experienced complete and sustained remission. Twenty-three of the patients with incomplete remission after repeated courses of methotrexate were then treated with actinomycin D; of the 23, 12 had subsequent complete remission, and the remainder showed varying responses of lesser degree. In Hertz's series about two out of every three of the patients appeared to be cured by the combined use of two chemotherapeutic agents. Actinomycin D is sometimes employed initially, as in patients with impaired hepatic function. It is given intravenously in doses ranging from 7 to 11 micrograms per kilogram per day for five days. The average patient requires more than one cause of treatment, usually at intervals of five days. Bagshawe has utilized a combination of methotrexate and 6-mercaptopurine in a series of 23 patients. Each course of therapy consisted of 75 to 125 mg of methotrexate and 300 to 3,000 mg of 6-mercaptopurine. As a result of the high toxicity of these drugs, 3 of Bagshawe's patients died of sepsis during hematopoietic depression, and 6 patients in Hertz's early series died as a result of therapy. The satisfactory and often amazing results of the drugs in otherwise hopeless cases, however, justify the risk in their use.

Although chemotherapy is the principal weapon against choriocarcinoma today, the role of surgical treatment has not been entirely eliminated. Lewis and co-workers, for example, point out the necessity for what they term "adjuvant surgery" in the occasional patient who does not respond to drugs. Tow and Cheng also believe that surgical treatment has a place in selected patients whose tumors are confined to the uterus. They agree, however, that chemotherapy is often decisive in management of metastatic choriocarcinoma.

In the past, cerebral metastases proved uniformly fatal. High voltage irradiation coupled with methotrexate and other chemotherapeutic agents has been shown to eradicate such lesions on occasion (Lewis, personal communication).

OTHER TUMORS OF THE PLACENTA

Angioma of the Placenta. Various tumors of the placenta ranging widely in size have been described. Most investigators agree that almost all have the same origin, and because of the resemblance of their components to the blood vessels and stroma of the chorionic villus, the term *chorangioma* or *chorioangioma* is the most appropriate designation. None of the theories regarding their mode of origin is entirely satisfactory, but it is most likely that groups of blood vessels and stroma originating in the chorionic mesenchyme proliferate and grow without relation to the normally developing chorionic villi.

Within the past few years several extensive studies of placental hemangiomas have appeared in print. These recent papers indicate that the incidence of this lesion is much greater than previously reported. Fox cites a figure of 1 in 100, and Wentworth 1 in 77.

The tumors are most likely hamartomas of primitive chorionic mesenchyme. The small growths are essentially asymptomatic, but the larger tumors may be associated with hydramnios or antepartum hemorrhage. Fetal death and malformations are uncommon complications, although there may be a positive correlation with low birth weight. According to Asadourian and Taylor, 27 of the 34 infants born in association with hemangioma of the placenta were girls.

Metastatic Tumors of the Placenta. Metastases of malignant tumors to the placenta are rare. Only 17 cases from the world's literature were collected in the reviews of Horner and of Freedman and MacMahon. Malignant melanoma is the most common, making up nearly one third of the reported cases, but any tumor with hematogenous spread is theoretically a source of potential placental metastases.

Cysts of the Placenta. Cystic structures are frequently observed upon the fetal surface and occasionally in the depths of the placenta. Small cysts a few millimeters in diameter were noted in 56 per cent of the placentas studied by Kermauner. Larger lesions, occasionally up to 8 to 10 cm in diameter, are much less common (Fig. 15).

Such cysts are derived from the chorionic membrane, as shown by the fact that the amnion can be readily stripped from them. Their contents are usually clear and transparent, but sometimes are bloody or grumous. The walls are lined in part by a dull whitish membrane, which occasionally reveals fibrinoid degeneration.

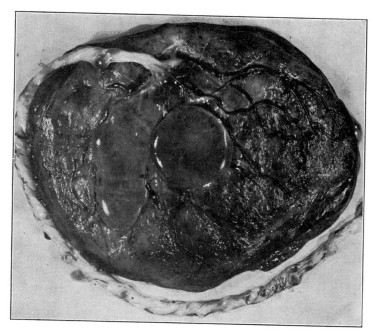

Fig. 15. Chorionic cyst of placenta.

Histologically the lining membrane consists of one or more layers of relatively large epithelial cells with round vesicular nuclei, in various stages of degeneration. Part of the wall may appear acellular after the trophoblastic elements, which presumably give rise to the cysts, have been obliterated by fibrinoid degeneration.

The cysts in the depths of the placenta rarely exceed 1 cm in diameter. They commonly occupy the center of an area of degeneration. Because their contents may be grumous, they were previously mistaken for abscesses.

Cysts arising either on the fetal surface or in the depths of the placenta are mainly of pathologic interest, since they exert little or no effect on the course of pregnancy or labor.

OTHER ABNORMALITIES OF THE PLACENTA

Abnormalities in Size, Shape, and Weight.   The normal placenta is a flattened, roundish, or discoid organ, which averages from 15 to 20 cm in diameter and from 1.5 to 3 cm in thickness. It weighs much more than the embryo very early in pregnancy, but the ratio gradually changes. At term it is generally only one sixth the weight of the fetus or less (Table 1, Ch. 6).

Rarely, when it develops in the vicinity of the internal os, the placenta assumes the form of an incomplete annulus.

The normal term placenta without cord and membranes, weighs on the average about 500 g. In certain diseases such as syphilis, the placenta may weigh one fourth, one third, or even one half as much as the fetus. The largest placentas are usually encountered in cases of erythroblastosis. In one such case, the fetus and placenta weighed 1,140 and 1,200 g, respectively, and in another the placenta weighed over 2,000 g.

Multiple Placentas in Single Pregnancies. Occasionally in a single pregnancy the placenta is divided into several parts that may be entirely separate or closely united. The conditions are thought to be related to abnormalities in the blood supply to the decidua.

In rare instances the placenta may be oblong with an aperture of varying size somewhere near its center (*placenta fenestrata*). Most frequently the organ is divided into two lobes. When the division is incomplete and the vessels extend from one lobe to the other before uniting to form the umbilical cord, the condition is termed *placenta dimidiata* or *bipartita*. If the two lobes are entirely separated, and the vessels remain distinct, not uniting until just before entering the cord, the condition is designated *placenta duplex*. Occasionally the organ may comprise three distinct lobes (*placenta triplex*). In very rare instances it may consist of as many as seven small lobes (*placenta septuplex*).

Placenta Succenturiata. An important and not infrequent anomaly is the so-called *placenta succenturiata*, in which one or more small accessory lobes are developed in the membrane at a distance from the periphery of the main placenta, to which they ordinarily have vascular connections; occasionally, however, the connections are lacking, and *placentae spuriae* result.

Placenta succenturiata is of considerable clinical importance because the accessory lobules are sometimes retained in the uterus after expulsion of the main placenta and may give rise to serious hemorrhage. If on examination of the placenta roundish defects are noted a short distance from the placental margin, retention of a succenturiate lobe should be suspected. The suspicion is confirmed if vessels extend from the placenta to the margins of the tear. In such cases, even if there is no hemorrhage at the moment, the retained lobe should be manually removed.

Placenta Membranacea. In rare instances the decidua capsularis is so abundantly supplied with blood that the chorion laeve in contact with it fails to undergo atrophy. In such circumstances the entire periphery of the ovum is covered by functioning villi, and the placenta develops as a thin membranous structure occupying the entire periphery of the chorion (*placenta membranacea*). This abnormality does not interfere with nutrition of the ovum but occasionally gives rise to serious hemorrhage during the third stage of labor, since the attenuated placenta does not readily separate from its area of attachment. Manual removal is sometimes very difficult in such cases.

Hertig and Sheldon, in an analysis of 1,000 spontaneous abortions, found a placental factor in 96 cases, 2 of which were examples of placenta membranacea. Finn reported 2 cases with constant vaginal bleeding sufficient to necessitate cesarean section at the twenty-sixth and twenty-third weeks, respectively. Bleeding often resembles that seen in central placenta previa, beginning in the second trimester and gradually increasing in severity to necessitate interruption of the pregnancy by hysterectomy or cesarean section.

Circumvallate Placenta. In certain cases the fetal surface of the placenta presents a central depression surrounded by a thickened, whitish ring, which is situated at a varying distance from the margin of the organ (Fig. 16).

Complete and incomplete rings are found in complete and incomplete circumvallate placentas, respectively. When the ring coincides with the placental

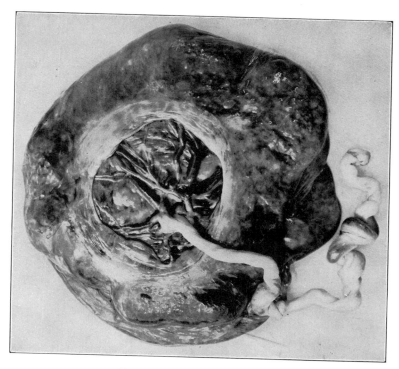

Fig. 16. Placenta circumvallata.

margin, the condition is sometimes described as a *placenta marginata*. Both circumvallate and circummarginate (marginate) placentas are varieties of *extrachorial* placentas. Within the ring the fetal surface presents the usual appearance, gives attachment to the umbilical cord, and shows the usual large vessels, which instead of coursing over the entire fetal surface terminate abruptly at the margin of the ring. In a circumvallate placenta the ring is composed of a double fold of amnion and chorion with degenerated decidua and fibrin in between. In a marginate placenta, the chorion and amnion are raised at the margin by interposed decidua and fibrin, without folding of the membranes. These relations are illustrated in Figure 17.

There has been a lengthy controversy concerning the morphogenesis of circumvallate and marginate placentas. Benirschke's review describes the two major theories of origin. One school holds that the original chorionic plate is too small in relation to the decidual plate, and the other attributes the condition to repetitive late marginal bleeding. Neither of these theories, however, explains the many varieties of this placental abnormality. The first theory cannot account for the absence of extrachorial placentas in very early pregnancy, and the hemorrhagic theory fails to explain the relative frequency of placenta marginata in twins. Benirschke believes that several factors may produce these same lesions in the placenta.

Scott cited an incidence of 18 per cent, whereas Pinkerton reported only 2.5 per cent for placenta circumvallate. The divergence probably reflects the varia-

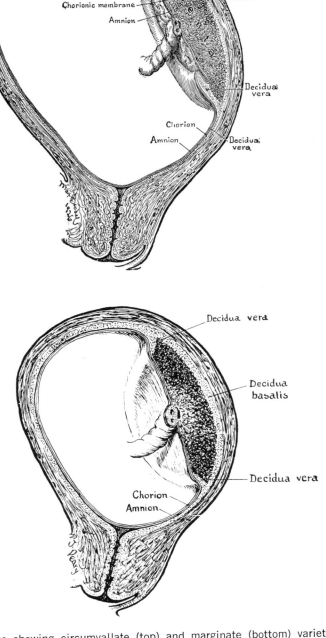

Fig. 17. Diagrams showing circumvallate (top) and marginate (bottom) varieties of extra-chorial placentas. (Bottom drawing modified after M. Brödel.)

tions in diagnostic criteria and the inclusion of incomplete varieties of the lesion in some reports but not in others. Various writers hold the condition responsible for a wide range of clinical manifestations. Both Scott and Pinkerton found a high incidence of hemorrhage into the decidua at the margin of the placenta, which inevitably leads to antepartum bleeding. In Scott's series, late antepartum hemorrhage, sometimes difficult to differentiate from that associated with placenta previa, occurred in 7 per cent of cases, in contrast to 3 per cent in a normal control group.

Current reports of circumvallate placentation continue to reflect differences in incidence and clinical significance. Wilson and Paalman, for example, cite a figure of 1 per cent as the incidence and state that bleeding is a common complication. They indicate, furthermore, a significant increase in fetal loss. Wentworth, however, cites figures of 6.5 per cent and 25.5 per cent for the incidences of circumvallate and circummarginate placentas, respectively. He indicates that these lesions have essentially no clinical significance, with no increase in associated antepartum hemorrhage, prematurity, or hydrorrhea.

Placenta Previa.   Once in several hundred cases the placenta, instead of being located upon the anterior or posterior wall of the corpus, is developed in the lower uterine segment in such a manner as to overlap more or less completely the internal os. Since this condition, known as *placenta previa,* is unavoidably associated with hemorrhage during the first stage of labor and is a most serious complication, it is dealt with separately in Chapter 23.

Placental Polyp.   Occasionally parts of a normal placenta or a succenturiate lobe may be retained after delivery. They may form polyps consisting of villi in varying stages of degeneration and covered by regenerated endometrium (Fig. 18). The clinical sequelae are often subinvolution of the uterus and late postpartum hemorrhage (Ch. 35).

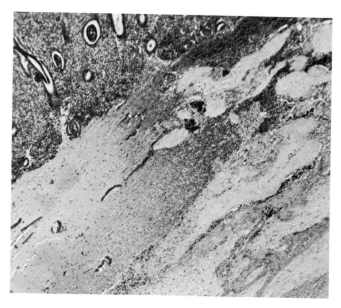

Fig. 18. Placental polyp, covered by regenerated endometrium. The bulk of this lesion consists of degenerating chorionic villi. (Courtesy of Dr. Ralph M. Wynn.)

Swan and Woodruff, in one of the few recent studies of placental polyps, state that menstrual irregularity and abdominal pain were found in one half and one third of patients with the lesion, respectively. They attach significance to the long-term viability of the apparently well-preserved chorionic tissue in many of these polyps.

Infarcts. The most common lesions of the placenta, though of diverse origin, are collectively referred to as "placental infarcts," Overclassification of these lesions has led to unnecessary confusion, which seems to increase with each attempt at further classification. In simplest terms, degenerative lesions of the placenta have two etiologic factors in common: changes associated with aging of the trophoblast, and vascular changes in the uteroplacental circulation and their sequelae. The lesions are easy to explain on the basis of the fundamental fact that nutrition of the placental villi is derived essentially from the maternal rather than the fetal circulation. The principal histopathologic features include fibrinoid degeneration of the trophoblast, calcification, and ischemic infarction, which is associated with occlusion of spiral arterioles.

In a lucid description of placental vascular anatomy, Wigglesworth provides a basis for classifying lesions. According to him, growth of the fetal lobules occurs preferentially around the entries of spiral arteries. Infarcts and placental hematomas have a lobular distribution. Thrombi occur in either arterial or venous regions of the intervillous space, but deposition of perivillous fibrin is predominantly a venous lesion.

The normal degeneration of the syncytium is increased and appears prematurely in preeclampsia-eclampsia. The process ultimately results in disappearance of the trophoblast, leaving only a thin hyalinized membrane covering the villus. Fibrinoid degeneration of the decidual vascular walls is also increased in preeclampsia. The vascular changes in the decidua may explain the greater incidence of placental infarcts and intervillous thromboses in preeclampsia as well as the diffuse changes in the syncytium.

Basically *ischemic necrosis of the villi* results from deposition of fibrin on their surfaces; a similar process may result from large areas of fibrin deposited in the intervillous space or from sudden coagulation of a large quantity of blood leading to intervillous thrombosis. A primarily degenerative lesion of the syncytium, which leads to clotting of maternal blood in contact with the exposed subepithelial tissues of the villi, may result in *hemovillous degeneration.* Moreover, vascular lesions of the decidua and primary syncytial degeneration may occur together in varying proportions to produce a host of mixed lesions.

About the edge of nearly every term placenta there is a more or less dense yellowish white fibrous ring representing a zone of degeneration, which is usually termed a "marginal infarct." It may be quite superficial in places but occasionally it extends a centimeter or two into the substance of the placenta. Underneath the chorionic plate, there are nearly always similar lesions, of more or less pyramidal shape, ranging from 0.2 cm to 2 or even 3 cm across the base, and extending downward with their apices in the intervillous space (subchorionic infarcts). Not infrequently similar lesions are noted about the intercotyledonary septa, in which case the broadest portion rests upon the maternal surface and the apex points toward the chorionic plate. Occasionally these lesions may meet and form a column of cartilagelike material extending from the maternal to the fetal surfaces. Less frequently, round or oval islands of similar tissue occupy the central portions of the placenta. Collectively these degenerative processes have been termed "white infacts" by many writers. Since the term may include many similar white lesions of varied origin, it is pathogenetically meaningless and should be discarded. By and large, the lesions represent *fibrinoid degeneration* of trophoblastic elements. In early placentas, they may be identified as islands or knots of trophoblast, located principally on the maternal side of the chorionic plate and over the decidua, particularly in the vicinity of septa and at the margins of the placenta. Later they may fuse to form large pale-staining masses and involve the tips of growing villi (Figs. 19 and 20).

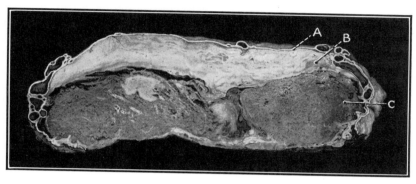

Fig. 19. Degeneration of the placenta. A, amnion and chorionic membrane; B, fibrinoid degeneration localized beneath the chorionic plate; C, unchanged placental tissue. (In this instance the infarct was unusually extensive, leading to the death of the fetus.)

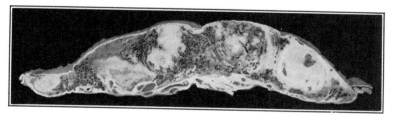

Fig. 20. Degeneration of the placenta. Generalized fibrinoid deposition with little normal tissue remaining.

Minute subchorionic and marginal areas of degeneration are present in every placenta. These lesions are of clinical significance only when they are large and abundant, in which case they may, by mechanical means, interfere with the function of a sufficiently large portion of the placenta to hamper seriously the nutrition of the fetus and on occasion cause its death.

Although the placenta is by no means a dying organ at term (Ch. 6, p. 148), there are morphologic indications of aging. A different type of lesion is formed as a result of the senescence of the syncytium. During the latter half of pregnancy syncytial degeneration begins and syncytial knots are formed; at the same time the villous stroma usually undergoes hyalinization. The syncytium may then break away or float off, exposing the connective tissue directly to maternal blood. As a result, clotting occurs; extensive propagation of the clot may result in the incorporation of other villi. Grossly such an area resembles closely an ordinary blood clot, but if not seen until it has become thoroughly organized, it reveals on section a firm, white island of tissue that looks like fibrinoid degeneration.

Pathologic Conditions Resulting from Accidents to the Maternal Vessels.   The arteries and veins of the decidua basalis, because of their extraordinarily thin walls composed of endothelium and a scant layer of connective tissue, not infrequently suffer damage, usually in the form of a tear or rupture, which is followed by extravasation of blood into the decidua, forming a retroplacental hematoma. Small hematomas detach only a small area of the placenta from the uterine wall and thus do little harm to the fetus. On examination of the maternal surface of the placenta, they may not infrequently be recognized as depressed areas, which sometimes contain a mass of clotted blood. The disruption of the blood supply may lead to extensive degeneration of the placenta. When the hematoma is larger, its accumulation in the decidua basalis causes greater detachment of the placenta, or *abruptio placentae,* a very important process discussed in detail in Chapter 23.

Clinical Significance of Degenerative Changes in the Placenta.   In general, "infarcts" of the placenta, caused either by local deposition of fibrin or by the more acute process of intervillous thrombosis, have little clinical significance, probably because of the large margin of safety in most placental functions. When these degenerative changes exceed those that normally accompany aging of the placenta, the efficiency of the organ may be greatly reduced. In certain maternal diseases, notably severe chronic hypertension, the reduction in placental function may be sufficient, on occasion, to cause fetal death.

Villous vessels may show endarteritic thickening and obliteration in association with fetal death. When the placental villi are excluded from their supply of maternal blood by fibrin deposits, hematomas, or direct blockage of the decidual circulation, they necessarily become infarcted and die. Histologically the compromised villi are characterized by fibrosis, obliteration of fetal vessels, and gradual disappearance of the syncytium. In other villi, however, there may be similar degenerative changes in the stroma, unassociated with necrosis of the epithelium or disturbances of the maternal circulation. Gruenwald refers to them as "avascular villi" and notes that the placentas in which they are common are often small and associated with retardation of intrauterine growth, but not prematurity.

Hypertrophic Lesions of the Chorionic Villi.   Striking enlargement of the chorionic villi is seen commonly in association with erythroblastosis of the hydropic variety (Ch. 37, Fig. 9). It has also been described in diabetes and occasionally in severe fetal disease, as, for example, in the case of congestive heart failure described by Gottschalk and Abramson. Hypertrophy of the villi, though seen most commonly and most strikingly in erythroblastosis, is by no means pathognomonic of that disease.

Despite the prime role of the placental villi as the means of nutrition and excretion of the fetus, relatively little new or basic information regarding their pathologic changes is available. The problem may be explained in part by the vast surface that the organ presents for microscopic examination and in part by the crude technics employed. The most serious shortcomings may result, however, from inadequate study of the pathologic placenta or from no examination whatsoever. The definitive work by Benirschke and Driscoll will undoubtedly serve to correct this neglect of an important field of study.

Inflammation of the Placenta.   Under the term "placentitis" were formerly described changes that are now recognized as various forms of degeneration. Moreover, small placental cysts with grumous contents were formerly thought to be abscesses. Although the frequency of acute inflammation of the placenta was greatly exaggerated formerly, the lesion is still occasionally encountered. The inflammation is usually not primary in the placenta, but secondary to extension of a similar process in the decidua, usually caused by pyogenic bacteria.

In cases of prolonged labor or rupture of the membranes, pyogenic bacteria may invade the fetal surface of the placenta and, after gaining access to the chorionic vessels, give rise to general infection of the fetus.

Frequently, histologic examination of placental tissue shows the decidua basalis and the inferior surface of the chorionic plate and the adjacent intervillous space to be infiltrated with polymorphonuclear leukocytes.

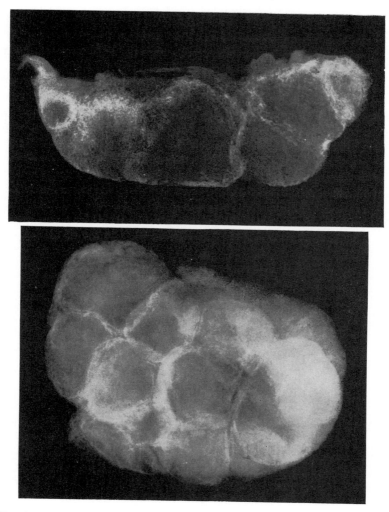

Fig. 21. Roentgenograms of the human placenta at term showing subchorionic and septal calcification. (Courtesy of Professor J. S. Scott.)

Tuberculosis of the Placenta.   Formation of tubercles in the fetal portion of the placenta is extremely infrequent. Whitman and Greene in 1922 collected 44 cases from the literature. Schaefer in 1939 reported that in 150 consecutive placentas of tuberculous women he was able to find only one with tuberculous lesions and acid-fast bacilli.

Calcification of the Placenta.   Small calcareous nodules or plaques are frequently observed upon the maternal surface of the placenta and are occasionally so abundant that the organ feels like coarse sandpaper. In view of the widespread degenerative changes in the placenta, calcification is not surprising. In fact, the conditions for deposition of calcium in the aging placenta are almost ideal. Moderate degrees of calcification may be detected in at least half of all placentas examined roentgenologically. An extensive deposition of calcium is shown in Figure 21. Tindall and Scott, in a study of 3,025 pregnancies, concluded that calcification in the placenta is a normal physiologic process.

ABNORMALITIES OF THE UMBILICAL CORD

Variations in Insertion.   The umbilical cord is usually inserted eccentrically on the fetal surface of the placenta between the center and periphery. A central insertion is less common; in a still smaller number of cases the junction is marginal, as in the *battledore placenta* (Fig. 22). In a series of 2,000 placentas the

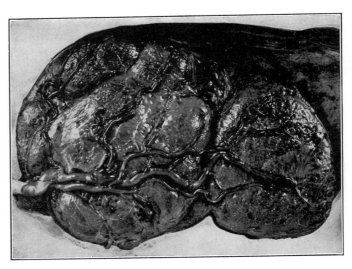

Fig. 22. Marginal insertion of cord, battledore placenta, and succenturiate lobe.

insertion was eccentric in 73 per cent, central in 18 per cent, and marginal in 7 per cent. Although these variations are without clinical significance, the so-called *velamentous insertion of the cord* is of considerable practical importance. In that condition the vessels of the cord separate at a distance from the placental margin, which they reach surrounded only by a fold of amnion. This mode of insertion was noted in a little over 1 per cent of our cases and in 1 per cent of those studied by Earn. Kobak and Cohen state that such insertions are nine times more frequent

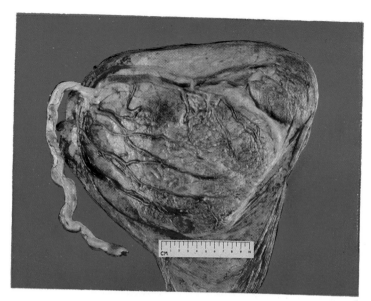

Fig. 23. Velamentous insertion of cord.

in twins and almost the rule in triplets (Fig. 23). Benirschke has noted a much higher incidence (7 per cent) of velamentous insertion in twins.

These variations of insertion may be determined at the time of implantation. The body stalk, which later becomes the umbilical cord, attaches the inner cell mass to the chorionic shell (Fig. 21, Ch. 5). Since the human egg implants with the inner cell mass down toward the endometrium, the placenta and body stalk are adjacent. According to one theory, minor degrees of rotation give rise to the usual eccentric location of the cord. The more marked the rotation of the egg, the farther the umbilical cord will be from the center of the placenta. In that way progressive rotation produces marginal and velamentous insertions. The theory goes on to explain that when the egg implants with the inner cell mass 180 degrees from the endometrium, the umbilical cord and placenta come to lie at opposite poles, and all the fetal vessels will be located in the membranes. When some of the fetal vessels cross the region of the internal os and present ahead of the infant, the condition is termed *vasa previa* (Fig. 24). Whenever fetal vessels are covered only by membranes, as in velamentous insertion and vasa previa, there is potential danger to the infant, for rupture of the membranes may also rupture a fetal vessel (Fig. 25) and lead to exsanguination of the infant.

Variations in Length of Cord. Normally the umbilical cord averages about 55 cm in length with a usual range of about 30 to 100 cm, though it may present marked variations from 0.5 to 198 cm. In rare instances it may be so short that the abdomen of the fetus is in contact with the placenta; in such circumstances a congenital umbilical hernia is usually found. The cord must be sufficiently long to reach from its placental insertion to the vulva, in order to allow normal delivery. In high and low locations of the placenta, the length must be about 35 and 20 cm, respectively. Excessively long cords may become twisted about the fetus and thus be relatively too short. The umbilical cord may therefore be relatively or abso-

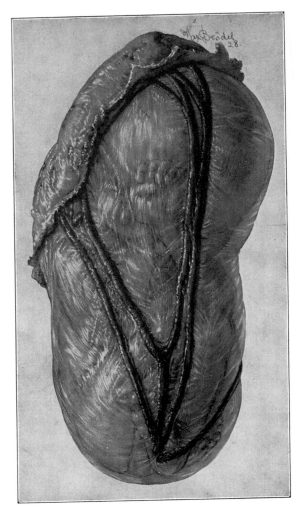

Fig. 24. Vasa previa with breech presentation. Note that cord arises from lowermost portion of fetal membranes.

lutely short. It is uncommon for the cord to be so short as to cause difficulties, but in rare instances short cords have been implicated in the causation of abruptio placentae, rupture of the cord, umbilical hernia, and even inversion of the uterus. **Knots of the Cord.** False knots, which result from kinking of the vessels to accommodate to the length of the cord, should be distinguished from true knots, which result from active movements of the fetus. In some 17,000 deliveries in The Collaborative Project on Cerebral Palsy, Spellacy and co-workers found an incidence of true knots of the umbilical cord of 1.1 per cent with a perinatal loss of 6.1 per cent.

Loops of the Cord. The cord frequently becomes coiled around portions of the fetus, usually the neck. In 1,000 consecutive deliveries studied by Kan and Eastman, the incidence of coiling of the umbilical cord around the fetal neck was as follows: one loop, 20.6 per cent; two loops, 2.5 per cent; and three loops, 0.2 per cent. Coiling of the cord around the fetal neck is sometimes alleged to be a

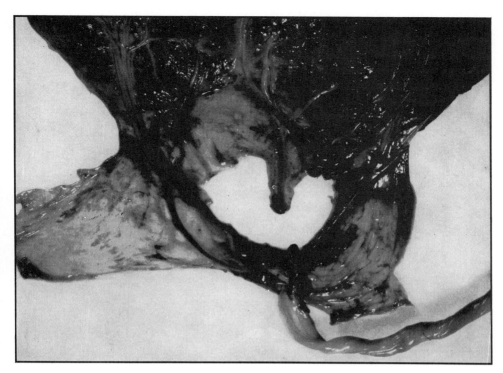

Fig. 25. Rupture of fetal vessel in a case of vasa previa and velamentous insertion of the cord.

cause of fetal death, but in the series of Kan and Eastman, no ill effects on the fetus could be attributed directly to the loops of cord. Coiling of the cord around the neck, therefore, should be considered an uncommon cause of fetal death. It is clear that the lethal role assigned to it has been exaggerated. The longer the cord, the greater, of course, is the likelihood of coiling. When there are as many as three loops, the cord is usually in excess of 70 cm in length.

In monoamnionic twinning, a significant fraction of the high perinatal mortality is attributed to entwining of the umbilical cords, which according to Salerno occurs in 71 per cent of cases.

Torsion of the Cord.   As a result of fetal movements the cord may become twisted. Occasionally the torsion is so marked that the fetal circulation is compromised. The extreme degrees of torsion occur only after the death of the fetus. In rare instances the cord may separate, though only after fetal death early in pregnancy.

Inflammation of the Cord.   Dominguez, Segal, and O'Sullivan found leukocytic infiltration of the umbilical cord in about one quarter of 986 single births. Although not all such infiltration represents true infection, inflammation is more likely when the umbilical cord is involved than when the findings are limited to the chorionic plate. Extensive inflammation of the cord with obliteration of the fetal vessels may be found after fetal death.

Varices of the Cord.   In rare instances varices of the cord may rupture as the result of undue pressure. Cases have been reported in which the death of the fetus was attributable to such an accident.

Tumors of the Cord.   Tumors involving the cord are rarely seen. Hematomas occasionally result from the rupture of a varix with subsequent effusion of blood into the cord (Fig. 26). Dippel found hematomas of the cord once in every 5,505

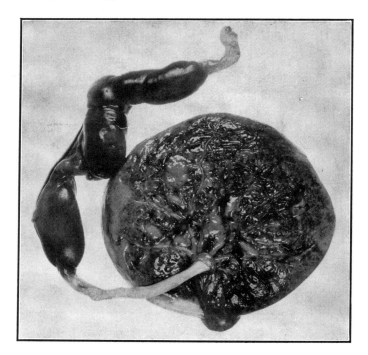

Fig. 26. Hematoma of the umbilical cord.

deliveries at or near term and stated that the hemorrhage usually results from rupture of the umbilical vein. He observed that about one half the fetuses with hematomas of the cord are stillborn. Myxomas and myxosarcomas have also been described.

Benirschke and Dodds described a large myxomatous degeneration of a marginally inserted cord, which contained a small angioma. One umbilical artery was atrophic. The anomaly is considered to be a manifestation of disturbed vascularization of the placenta.

Cysts occasionally occur along the course of the cord and are designated true and false, according to their origin. The former are always quite small and may be derived from remnants of the umbilical vesicle or of the allantois; the latter, which may attain considerable size, result from liquefaction of Wharton's jelly.

Edema of the Cord.   This condition rarely occurs by itself but is frequently associated with edema of the fetus. It is very common in macerated fetuses.

Absence of One Umbilical Artery.   Although formerly regarded as rare, the absence of one umbilical artery, according to Benirschke, may characterize about 1 per cent of all cords in singletons and up to 6 per cent of the cords of at least one twin. He states, futhermore, that at least 15 to 20 per cent of all infants with one umbilical artery have associated congenital anomalies.

A single umbilical artery was the most frequently detected malformation among over 12,000 infants in the study by Ainsworth and Davies. It occurred in

0.94 per cent of all children. Malformations, which occurred in one third of these children, were frequently multiple and severe. Esophageal atresia and imperforate anus with or without fistulas to the respective adjacent structures were the most common lesions. The incidence of the single umbilical artery was about equal in both sexes, but male infants had a higher number of associated malformations.

DISORDERS OF THE AMNION AND AMNIOTIC FLUID

HYDRAMNIOS

Hydramnios, sometimes called *polyhydramnios,* is an excessive quantity of liquor amnii. The normal volume of amniotic fluid near term is about 1,000 ml. In general, more than 2,000 ml may be considered excessive. In rare cases the uterus may contain an enormous quantity of fluid, with reports of at least 15 liters on record. In most cases the increase in amniotic fluid is gradual, in the condition commonly termed *chronic hydramnios.* When the fluid increases very suddenly, the uterus may become immensely distended within a few days; that condition is called *acute hydramnios.* The fluid in hydramnios is usually similar in appearance and composition to the amniotic fluid in normal conditions.

Incidence. Minor degrees of hydramnios, 2 to 3 liters, are common, but the more marked grades are not frequent. Because of the difficulty of complete collection of the amniotic fluid, the diagnosis is usually based on clinical impression only. In borderline cases the frequency of the diagnosis varies with the individual observer. For this reason the published data on incidence vary widely, from 1 in 62 deliveries, to 1 in 754. Murray, in one of the largest series ever collected, reported 846 cases in 128,042 deliveries, or 0.7 per cent, in the data from the Obstetrical Statistical Cooperative. Figures of 0.76 per cent, 0.3 per cent, and 0.2 per cent are quoted in the smaller series of cases collected by Lampé, Nagy, and Baszo; Moya and associates; and Buckingham and associates, respectively. Hydramnios sufficient to cause clinical symptoms (generally in excess of 3,000 ml of amniotic fluid) is less frequent; it probably occurs about once in a thousand pregnancies. Acute hydramnios is also rare, occurring 13 times in 46,805 births (0.03 per cent) in the cases reviewed by Buckingham, and 4 times in 49,793 (0.008 per cent) births in the cases studied by Mueller.

The incidence of hydramnios associated with fetal malformations, especially those of the central nervous system and gastrointestinal tract, is extremely high. For example, hydramnios accompanies nearly half the cases of anencephalus and nearly all cases of atresia of the esophagus (Scott and Wilson). Of the 178 cases of hydramnios in our clinic, 31, or 17.4 per cent, occurred in association with fetal deformities. In severe hydramnios, the percentage is much higher. In our 57 cases in which the volume of fluid exceeded 3,000 ml, 15, or more than one quarter, were accompanied by fetal malformations. The incidence of congenital anomalies in Mueller's cases of hydramnios was 29 per cent, and in Murray's series 22 per cent.

Excessive amniotic fluid is also common in twin pregnancies. Multiple gestation complicated 22 of Mueller's 178 cases of hydramnios, or 12.5 per cent. In Guttmacher's study of 573 twin pregnancies, hydramnios was diagnosed in 40, an incidence of 7 per cent. Most investigators have observed that hydramnios is more frequent in monozygotic than in dizygotic twinning. Of the 31 cases of hydramnios studied by Guttmacher in which the relations of the membranes gave a definite indication of the nature of the twinning, 7, or less than a quarter, were single ovum and 24, or more than three quarters, were double ovum; these figures represent the approximate proportion of single- to double-ovum pregnancies in the whole series. The incidence of hydramnios is also especially high in the hydropic variety of erythroblastosis and in pregnancies complicated by diabetes.

Etiology.   Very little is known about the underlying mechanism of hydramnios. Although the source of the amniotic fluid is assumed to be the amniotic epithelium, no histologic changes in the amnion or chemical changes in the amniotic fluid in cases of hydramnios have been found. In cases of anencephalus and spina bifida, increased transudation of fluid from the exposed meninges into the amniotic cavity is commonly believed to be an etiologic factor. Since the fetus normally swallows amniotic fluid, it has been assumed that this mechanism is one of the ways by which the volume of the fluid is controlled. The theory gains validity by the almost constant presence of hydramnios when swallowing is inhibited as, for example, in cases of atresia of the esophagus. Nichols and Schrepfer, however, indicated that fetal swallowing was by no means the only mechanism for preventing hydramnios. Moreover, both Pritchard and Abramovich have measured quantitatively amniotic fluid swallowing and found in some instances of gross hydramnios considerable volumes of fluid being swallowed.

Another explanation of the frequency of hydramnios in anencephalus is based on the theory that the increased fluid results from excessive urinary excretion brought about by stimulation of cerebrospinal centers that have been deprived of their protective coverings, as in piqûre experiments. On the contrary, fetal defects leading to anuria are almost equally frequent in cases of oligohydramnios. In hydramnios associated with monozygotic twin pregnancy the hypothesis has been advanced that one fetus usurps the greater part of the circulation common to both twins and develops cardiac hypertrophy, which in turn results in increased urine. Our own data, however, indicate that hydramnios is not more frequent with monozygotic than with dizygotic twins.

Hutchinson and colleagues have suggested that the interchange of water in normal pregnancy is relatively great. According to their studies, it averages 3,600 ml per hour between mother and fetus, whereas the amounts of water transferred between mother and amniotic fluid and between fetus and amniotic fluid are, by comparison, small. When the average figure of 3,600 ml per hour is compared with data in hydramnios, it is evident that hydramnios is associated with a profound reduction in the interchange of water between mother and fetus. On the basis of these studies, moreover, the *net* amount of water transferred from fetus to amniotic fluid in hydramnios is much greater than in normal pregnancy. In hydramnios, therefore, the role of the fetus in the interchange of water between mother and amniotic fluid is seriously deranged, an observation in line with the fact that congenital malformations predispose to hydramnios.

The weight of the placenta tends to be high in hydramnios. Our own observations indicate that the placenta weighed more than 800 g in 40 per cent and more than 900 g in 22 per cent of the cases. The figures are even more striking in view of the high rate of prematurity associated with hydramnios. Although the enlarged placenta theoretically may contribute to the increase in amniotic fluid, it is more likely that placental hypertrophy is a compensatory mechanism brought into play by failure of fetal homeostasis resulting from maternal diseases such as diabetes or fetal abnormalities, such as erythroblastosis or congenital malformations.

Symptoms.   The symptoms accompanying hydramnios arise from purely mechanical causes and result chiefly from the pressure exerted by the overdistended uterus upon adjacent organs. The effects on respiratory functions may be striking. When distention is excessive, the patient may suffer from severe dyspnea and cyanosis; in extreme cases she may be able to breathe only in the upright position. Edema is common, especially of the lower extremities, the vulva, and the abdominal wall. As the result of overstretching of the myometrium, generalized pain in the uterus itself is not uncommon; in our experience, it is a more frequent and distressing symptom than respiratory difficulty. When the accumulation of fluid takes place gradually, the patient may tolerate the excessive abdominal distention with relatively little discomfort. In acute hydramnios, however, the distention may lead to disturbances sufficiently serious to threaten the life of the patient. Acute hydramnios tends to occur earlier in pregnancy than does the chronic form, often as early as the fourth or fifth month, and it rapidly expands the uterus to enormous size. Pain may be intense and the dyspnea so severe that the patient is unable to lie flat. Edema of the abdomen, vulva, and thighs, together with nausea and vomiting, may present an alarming picture. As a rule, acute hydramnios leads to labor before the twenty-eighth week, or the symptoms become so severe that intervention is mandatory.

In the majority of cases of hydramnios, the amniotic fluid pressure is not higher than in normal pregnancy. It is usually so low as to necessitate negative pressure to withdraw the fluid during paracentesis. Caldeyro-Barcia and coworkers point out, however, that the pressure of the amniotic fluid may be elevated in certain cases characterized by high uterine contractility, especially in women who go to term despite the hydramnios.

Diagnosis.   Usually, uterine enlargement in association with difficulty in palpating fetal small parts and in hearing fetal heart tones, and ease of ballottement of the fetus, are the main diagnostic signs of hydramnios. In severe cases the uterine wall may be so tense and tender that it is impossible to palpate any part of the fetus (Fig. 27). Such findings call for immediate roentgenologic examination of the abdomen to rule out fetal abnormalities or multiple pregnancy. The differentiation between hydramnios, ascites, and a large ovarian cyst can usually be made without difficulty from the roentgenogram, since of the three, only hydramnios is always associated with pregnancy.

Prognosis.   The outlook for the infant in major degrees of hydramnios is notoriously poor. Even though the roentgenogram shows an apparently normal fetus, the prognosis must be guarded. The incidence of fetal malformations, many of which are incompatible with life, is at least 20 per cent. There is a further increase in perinatal mortality from prematurity, since the frequency of premature births in association with hydramnios is more than twice the overall rate. Prolapse of the umbilical cord, erythroblastosis, and the difficulties encountered by the infants of diabetic mothers add still further to the death rate. As the result of these factors, the total perinatal loss in hydramnios exceeds 50 per cent. Mueller's perinatal death rate at The New York Lying-In Hospital was 51 per cent, and that in the Johns Hopkins series was 48.3 per cent. In our cases in which the volume of fluid exceeded 3,000 ml, however, the mortality rate rose to 68.1 per cent. In general, the more severe the hydramnios, the higher is the perinatal mortality. In a review of the world's literature by Moya and associates, covering 1,745 cases of hydramnios, the perinatal mortality was 48.7 per cent. Jacoby and

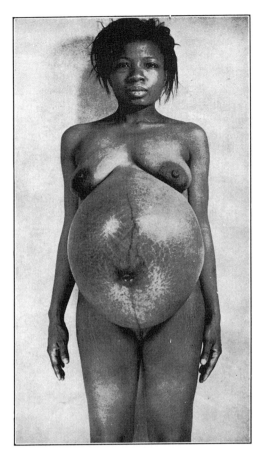

Fig. 27. Advanced degree of hydramnios; 5,500 ml of amniotic fluid were measured at delivery.

Charles concluded that the only conditions commonly associated with hydramnios were maternal diabetes and major fetal congenital anomalies.

The hazards imposed by hydramnios on the mother are rare but significant. They can usually be combated without serious threat to her life. The most frequent maternal complications are abruptio placentae, uterine dysfunction, and postpartum hemorrhage. Premature separation of the placenta sometimes follows escape of massive quantities of liquor amnii, presumably because of the decrease in area of uterine wall beneath the placenta. The last two complications are the result of the uterine atony consequent upon overdistention. Abnormal presentations are more common and operative interference is more frequently required.

Treatment.   Minor degrees of hydramnios rarely require treatment. Even moderate degrees of the complication, including cases in which there is some discomfort, can usually be managed without intervention until labor starts or until the membranes rupture spontaneously. If there is any dyspnea, abdominal pain, or edema of the abdominal wall, or if ambulation is difficult, hospitalization becomes necessary. There is no satisfactory treatment for symptomatic hydramnios other than removal of the excessive amniotic fluid. Bed rest with sedation may make the situation endurable, but it rarely has any effect on the accumulation of fluid. Diuretics and restriction of water and salt are likewise ineffective. If the discomfort becomes acute as a result of the growing uterine mass, amniocentesis may be performed either through the cervix (usually well dilated in such cases) or by abdominal paracentesis. The disadvantages inherent in rupture of the membranes through the cervix are the possibilities of prolapse of the cord, abruptio placentae, and uterine dysfunction. Very slow release of the fluid helps to obviate these dangers but is very difficult to accomplish through the cervical canal, since even a small nick in the membranes is usually quickly converted into a large rent. Neither prolapse of the cord nor abruptio placentae is a frequent complication of this method, however. The dangers of abdominal aminocentesis are largely theoretical, consisting in injury to adherent bowel or puncture of a fetal vessel. The former can be prevented by avoiding paracentesis in patients with previous uterine operations. If the abdominal tap is performed slowly, an anterior placenta will be recognized by the appearance of blood from the intervillous space before the chorionic plate has been punctured and a fetal vessel damaged.

For paracentesis, a 17-gauge, 3-inch needle is passed through the abdominal and uterine walls after a small amount of local anesthetic has been injected. Once amniotic fluid has been obtained, it can be withdrawn slowly with a syringe, or the needle can be replaced by a small polyethylene catheter passed through it and left within the amniotic cavity. As stressed by Barry, it is most important to withdraw the fluid slowly at a maximal rate of 500 ml per hour. In the average case of hydramnios, the procedure should take several hours.

To remove amniotic fluid from women with hydramnios who are not obese we have been using a commercially available plastic catheter that tightly covers a 2-inch, 18-gauge needle (Angiocath). The catheter is inserted into the amniotic sac, the needle is withdrawn, and an intravenous infusion set is connected to the catheter hub. The opposite end of the tubing is dropped into a graduated cylinder placed on the floor, and the rate of flow of amniotic fluid is controlled with the screw clamp so that about 500 ml per hour are withdrawn. After about 1,500 ml have escaped, the uterus usually has decreased in size sufficiently so that the plastic catheter has pulled out of the amniotic sac and the flow stops. Using strict aseptic technic this procedure can be repeated as often as necessary to make the woman comfortable.

The chief purpose of amniocentesis is relief of the patient's distress, and to that end it is eminently successful. Often, however, it initiates labor quite promptly, even though only a part of the fluid is removed; hence, relief of the patient's distress will seldom enable her to continue with the pregnancy. Especially in cases of anencephalus in which the uterus may be refractory to such stimulation, labor may not ensue. In such circumstances, it may be necessary to repeat the paracentesis weekly to keep the patient comfortable or to stimulate the uterus by some other means. Amniocentesis may also be helpful in avoiding the uterine dysfunction that often accompanies labor in the presence of hydramnios.

OLIGOHYDRAMNIOS

In rare instances the volume of amniotic fluid may fall far below the normal limits and occasionally be reduced to only a few ml of viscid fluid. The causation of this condition is not completely understood, but one association is with fetal renal agenesis.

When oligohydramnios occurs early in pregnancy it is attended by serious consequences to the fetus, since adhesions between the amnion and parts of the fetus may cause serious deformities including amputation. When occurring later, its effect upon the fetus is less marked. Subjected to pressure from all sides, the fetus assumes a peculiar appearance, and minor deformities, such as clubfoot, are frequently observed. In some cases of oligohydramnios the skin of the fetus is markedly thickened and it appears dry and leathery.

OTHER DISEASES OF THE AMNION

Inflammation of the Amnion. Since amnionitis is a manifestation of an intra-uterine infection, it is frequently associated with prolonged rupture of the membranes and long labors. When mononuclear and polymorphonuclear leukocytes infiltrate the chorion, the resulting lesion is properly designated *chorioamnionitis.* Inflammatory cells in the chorion do not necessarily indicate bacterial infection, for they generally appear there as early as five or six hours after rupture of the membranes.

Cysts of the Amnion. Small cysts lined by typical amniotic epithelium are occasionally formed. The common variety results from fusion of amniotic folds, with subsequent retention of fluid.

Amnion Nodosum. These nodules in the amnion are sometimes called *squamous metaplasia* of the amnion or amniotic caruncles. They occur most commonly in the amnion in contact with the chorionic plate but they may also be seen elsewhere. They usually appear near the insertion of the cord as multiple, rounded or oval, opaque elevations that vary from less than 1 to 5 or 6 mm in diameter. Microscopically, they consist of typical stratified squamous epithelium. The lowest layer is more cuboidal and continuous with the normal amniotic epithelium, whereas the upper layers become increasingly flattened and pale-staining toward the surface. They may become calcified and are common enough to be found as isolated nodules in about 60 per cent of placentas. Thompson has pointed out that these nodules occur in greater concentration in association with oligohydramnios and renal agenesis.

Bartman and Driscoll reported an association between amnion nodosum and multiple congenital abnormalities, including cystic hypoplastic kidneys. On the basis of ultrastructural studies, they point out the difficulty of deciding whether amnion nodosum arises from a primarily diseased amnion or from the incorporation of fetal ectodermal derivatives.

References

Abramovich, D. R. Fetal factors influencing the volume and composition of liquor amnii. J Obstet Gynaec Brit Comm 77:865, 1970.

Acosta-Sison, H. Diseases of the chorion: hydatidiform mole, syncytioma and choriocarcinoma, in J. P. Greenhill, Obstetrics, 13th ed. Philadelphia and London, W. B. Saunders, 1965. Ch. 53.

———— and Espaniola, N. A. Clinicopathologic study from 32 cases of chorio-epithelioma. Amer J Obstet Gynec 42:878, 1941.

Ainsworth, P., and Davies, P. A. The single umbilical artery: a five-year survey. Develop Med Child Neurol 11:297, 1969.

Asadourian, L. A., and Taylor, H. B.   Clinical significance of placental hemangiomas. Obstet Gynec 31:551, 1968.

Baggish, M. S., Woodruff, J. D., Tow, S. H., and Jones, H. W., Jr.   Sex chromatin pattern in hydatidiform mole. Amer J Obstet Gynec 102:362, 1968.

Bagshawe, K. D.   Trophoblastic tumors. Chemotherapy and developments. Brit Med J 2:1303, 1963.

Barry, A. P.   Hydramnios. Obstet Gynec 11:667, 1958.

Bartman, J., and Driscoll, S. G.   Amnion nodosum and hypoplastic cystic kidneys. Obstet Gynec 32:700, 1968.

Benirschke, K.   A review of the pathologic anatomy of the human placenta. Amer J Obstet Gynec 84:1595, 1962.

―――― Discussion of developmental anomalies of the placenta and membranes, in Wynn, R. M. (ed.), First Conference on Fetal Homeostasis, New York, New York Acad Sci, 1965, pp. 217–246.

―――― and Dodds, J. P.   Angiomyxoma of the umbilical cord with atrophy of an umbilical artery. Obstet Gynec 30:99, 1967.

―――― and Driscoll, S. G.   The Pathology of the Human Placenta. New York, Springer-Verlag, 1967.

Brewer, J. I., and Gerbie, A. B.   Early development of choriocarcinoma. Amer J Obstet Gynec 94:692, 1966.

―――― Torok, E. E., Webster, A., and Dolkart, R. E.   Hydatidiform mole: a follow-up regimen for identification of invasive mole and choriocarcinoma and for selection of patients for treatment. Amer J Obstet Gynec 101:557, 1968.

Buckingham, J. C., McElin, T. W., Bowers, V. M., and McVay, J.   A clinical study of hydramnios. Obstet Gynec 15:652, 1960.

Caldeyro-Barcia, R., Pose, S. V., and Alvarez, H.   Uterine contractility in polyhydramnios and the effects of withdrawal of the excess of amniotic fluid. Amer J Obstet Gynec 73:1238, 1957.

Carr, D. H.   Cytogenetics and the pathology of hydatidiform degeneration. Obstet Gynec 33:333, 1969.

Chesley, L. C., Cosgrove, S. A., and Preece, J.   Hydatid mole with special reference to recurrence and associated eclampsia. Amer J Obstet Gynec 52:311, 1946.

Chun, D., Braga, C., Chow, C., and Lok, L.   Clinical observations on some aspects of hydatidiform moles. J Obstet Gynaec Brit Comm 71:180, 1964.

―――― Braga, C., Chow, C., and Lok, L.   Treatment of hydatidiform mole. J Obstet Gynaec Brit Comm 71:185, 1964.

Delfs, E.   Quantitative chorionic gonadotrophin. Prognostic value in hydatidiform mole and chorionepithelioma. Obstet Gynec 9:1, 1957.

Dippel, A. L.   Hematomas of the umbilical cord. Surg Gynec Obstet 70:51, 1940.

Dominguez, R., Segal, A. J., and O'Sullivan, J. A.   Leukocytic infiltration of the umbilical cord. Manifestation of fetal hypoxia due to reduction of blood flow in the cord. JAMA 173:346, 1960.

Donald, I.   Ultrasonic echo sounding in obstetrical and gynecological diagnosis. Amer J Obstet Gynec 93:935, 1965.

―――― Practical Obstetric Problems, 4th ed. London, Lloyd-Luke, 1969.

Earn, A. A.   The effect of congenital abnormalities of the umbilical cord and placenta on the newborn and mother. A survey of 5675 consecutive deliveries. J Obstet Gynaec Brit Emp 58:456, 1951.

Finn, J. L.   Placenta membranacea. Obstet Gynec 3:438, 1954.

Fox, H.   Vascular tumors of the placenta. Obstet Gynec Survey 22:697, 1967.

Freedman, W. L., and MacMahon, F. J.   Placental metastasis. Review of the literature and report of a case of metastatic melanoma. Obstet Gynec 16:550, 1960.

Garcia, N. A., Nelson, J. H., Bernstine, R. L., Huston, J. W., and Gartenlaub. C.   Findings on retrograde femoral arteriography in choriocarcinoma. Amer J Obstet Gynec 81:706, 1961.

Girouard, D. P., Barclay, D. L., and Collins, C. G.   Hyperreactio luteinalis. A review of the literature and report of two cases. Obstet Gynec 23:513, 1964.

Gottesfeld, K. R., Taylor, E. S., Thompson, H. E., and Holmes, J. H.   Diagnosis of hydatidiform mole by ultrasound. Obstet Gynec 30:163, 1967.

Gottschalk, W., and Abramson, D.   Placental edema and fetal hydrops. A case of congenital cystic and adenomatoid malformation of the lung. Obstet Gynec 10:626, 1957.

Gruenwald, P.   Abnormalities of placental vascularity in relation to intrauterine deprivation and retardation of fetal growth. New York J Med 61:1508, 1961.

Guttmacher, A. F.   An analysis of 573 cases of twin pregnancy. II. The hazards of pregnancy itself. Amer J Obstet Gynec 38:277, 1939.

Hellman, L. M.   Sonographic measurement of fetal growth, in Wynn, R. M. (ed.), Fetal Homeostasis. New York, Appleton-Century-Crofts, 1969, Vol. 4, p. 185.

Hendrickse, J. P. de, Cockshott, W. P., Evans, K. T. E., and Barton, C. J.   Pelvic angiography in the diagnosis of malignant trophoblastic disease. New Eng J Med 271:859, 1964.

Hertig, A. T., and Edmonds, H. W.   Genesis of hydatidiform mole. Arch Path 30:260, 1940.

———— and Mansell, H.   Tumors of the Female Sex Organs, Part I. Hydatidiform Mole and Choriocarcinoma. Washington, D.C. Armed Forces Institute of Pathology, 1957.

———— and Sheldon, W. H.   Minimal criteria required to prove prima facie case of traumatic abortion or miscarriage. Ann Surg 117:596, 1943.

———— and Sheldon, W. H.   Hydatidiform mole—a pathologico-clinical correlation of 200 cases. Amer J Obstet Gynec 53:1, 1947.

Hertz, R., Bergenstal, D. M., Lipsett, M. B., Price, E. B., and Hilbish, T. F.   Chemotherapy of choriocarcinoma and related trophoblastic tumors in women. JAMA 168:845, 1958.

———— Ross, G. T., and Lipsett, M. B.   Chemotherapy in women with trophoblastic disease. Choriocarcinoma, chorioadenoma destruens, and complicated hydatid mole. Ann NY Acad Sci 114:881, 1964.

Horner, E. N.   Placental metastases. Case report: maternal deaths from ovarian cancer. Obstet Gynec 15:566, 1960.

Hou, P. C., and Pang, S. C.   Chorionepithelioma: an analytic study of 28 necropsied cases, with special reference to the possibility of spontaneous retrogression. J Path Bact 72:95, 1956.

Hutchinson, D. L., Gray, M. J., Plentl, A. A., Alvarez, H., Caldeyro-Barcia, R., Kaplan, B., and Lind, J.   The role of the fetus in the water exchange of the amniotic fluid of normal and hydramniotic patients. J Clin Invest 38:971, 1959.

Iliya, F. A., Williamson, S., and Azar, H. A.   Choriocarcinoma in the Near East. Consanguinity as a possible etiologic factor. Cancer 20:144, 1967.

Jacoby, H. E., and Charles, D.   Clinical conditions associated with hydramnios. Amer J Obstet Gynec 94:910, 1966.

Kan, P. S., and Eastman, N. J.   Coiling of the umbilical cord around the foetal neck. J Obstet Gynaec Brit Emp 64:227, 1957.

Kermauner, F.   (Studies of the development of cysts and infarcts of the human placenta). Z Heilk 1:273, 1900.

King, G.   Hydatidiform mole and chorionepithelioma—the problem of the borderline case. Proc Roy Soc Med 49:381, 1956.

Kobak, A. J., and Cohen, M. R.   Velamentous insertion of cord with spontaneous rupture of vasa previa in twin pregnancy. Amer J Obstet Gynec 38:1063, 1939.

Lampé, L., Nagy, T., and Baszo, J.   (Clinical importance of hydramnios: Study of the University Women's Clinic in Debrecen during a 27-year period, 1932–58). Zbl Gynaek 82:1387, 1960.

Lewis, J., Jr., Ketcham, A. S., and Hertz, R.   Surgical intervention during chemotherapy of gestational trophoblastic neoplasms. Cancer 19:1517, 1966.

Manahan, C. P., Manuel-Limson, G., and Abad, R.   Experience with choriocarcinoma in the Philippines. Ann NY Acad Sci 114:875, 1964.

Marchand, F.   (On the structure of hydatidiform mole). Z Geburtsh Gynaek 32:405, 1895.

————   (On the malignant chorionepithelioma, in connection with method of treatment of 2 new cases). Z Geburtsh Gynaek 39:173, 1898.

Marin-Padilla, M., and Benirschke, K.   Thalidomide induced alterations in the blastocyst and placenta of the armadillo, Dasypus novemcinctus mexicanus, including a choriocarcinoma. Amer J Path 43:999, 1963.

Marquez-Monter, H., Alfaro de la Vega, G., Robles, M., and Bolio-Cicero, A.   Epidemiology and pathology of hydatidiform mole in the General Hospital of Mexico. Amer J Obstet Gynec 85:856, 1963.

Mathieu, A.   Hydatidiform mole and chorio-epithelioma: collective review of literature for years 1935, 1936 and 1937. Int Abstr Surg 68:52, 181, 1939.

Mercer, R. D., Lammert, A. C., Anderson, R., and Hazard, J. B.   Choriocarcinoma in mother and child. JAMA 166:482, 1958.

Moya, F., Apgar, V., James, L. S., and Berrein, C. Hydramnios and congenital anomalies: Study of series of 74 patients. JAMA 173:1552, 1960.

Mueller, P. F. Acute hydramnios. Amer J Obstet Gynec 56:1069, 1948.

Murray, S. R. Hydramnios. A study of 846 cases. Amer J Obstet Gynec 88:65, 1964.

Natsume, M., and Takada, J. Choriocarcinoma. An unusual case recurring nine years after subtotal hysterectomy and followed by spontaneous regression of pulmonary metastases. Amer J Obstet Gynec 82:654, 1961.

Nichols, J., and Schrepfer, R. Polyhydramnios in anencephaly. JAMA 197:549, 1966.

Novak, E. Hydatidiform mole and chorionepithelioma. Amer J Surg 76:352, 1948.

———— Pathological aspects of hydatidiform mole and choriocarcinoma. Amer J Obstet Gynec 59:1355, 1950.

———— and Seah, C. S. Choriocarcinoma of the uterus. Amer J Obstet Gynec 67:933, 1954.

———— and Seah, C. S. Benign trophoblastic lesions in Mathieu Chorion-epithelioma Registry. Amer J Obstet Gynec 68:376, 1954.

Okudaira, Y., and Strauss, L. Ultrastructure of molar trophoblast. Observations on hydatidiform mole and chorioadenoma destruens. Obstet Gynec 30:172, 1967.

Pinkerton, J. H. M. Placenta circumvallata; its aetiology and clinical significance. J Obstet Gynaec Brit Emp 63:743, 1956.

Pritchard, J. A. Blood volume changes in pregnancy and the puerperium. IV. Anemia associated with hydatidiform mole. Amer J Obstet Gynec 91:621, 1965.

———— Fetal swallowing and amniotic fluid volume. Obstet Gynec 28:606, 1966.

Reid, D. E. A Textbook of Obstetrics. Philadelphia and London, W. B. Saunders, 1962, p. 270.

Salerno, L. J. Monoamniotic twinning. Obstet Gynec 14:205, 1959.

Saxena, B. N., Emerson, K., Jr., and Selenkow, H. A. Serum placental lactogen (HPL) levels as an index of placental function. New Eng J Med 281:225, 1969.

———— Goldstein, D. P., Emerson, K., Jr., and Selenkow, H. A. Serum placental lactogen levels in patients with molar pregnancy and trophoblastic tumors. Amer J Obstet Gynec 102:115, 1968.

Schaefer, G. Tuberculosis of the placenta. Quart Bull Sea View Hosp 4:457, 1939.

Scott, J. S. Placenta extrachorialis (placenta marginata and placenta circumvallata). J Obstet Gynaec Brit Emp 67:904, 1960 (51 references cited).

———— and Wilson, J. K. Hydramnios as an early sign of oesophageal atresia. Lancet 2:569, 1957.

Smalbraak, J. Trophoblastic Growths—A Clinical, Hormonal and Histopathologic Study of Hydatidiform Mole and Chorionepithelioma. Haarlem, The Netherlands, Elsevier Publishing Co., 1957.

Spellacy, W. N., Gravem, H., and Fisch, R. O. The umbilical cord complications of true knots, nuchal coils and cords around the body. Amer J Obstet Gynec 94:1136, 1966.

Swan, R. W., and Woodruff, J. D. Retained products of conception. Histologic viability of placental polyps. Obstet Gynec 34:506, 1969.

Thompson, V. M. Amnion nodosum. J Obstet Gynaec Brit Comm 67:611, 1960.

Tindall, V. R., and Scott, J. S. Placental calcification. A study of 3025 singleton and multiple pregnancies. J Obstet Gynaec Brit Comm 72:356, 1965.

Tominaga, T., and Page, E. W. Sex chromatin of trophoblastic tumors. Amer J Obstet Gynec 96:305, 1966.

Torres, A. H., and Pelegrina, I. A. Transabdominal intrauterine contrast medium injection. Amer J Obstet Gynec 94:936, 1966.

Tow, W. S. H. The classification of malignant growths of the chorion. J Obstet Gynaec Brit Comm 73:1000, 1966.

———— and Cheng, W. C. Recent trends in treatment of choriocarcinoma. Brit Med J 1:521, 1967.

Wei, P-Y., and Ouyang, P-C. Trophoblastic diseases in Taiwan. Amer J Obstet Gynec 85:844, 1963.

Wentworth, P. The incidence and significance of haemangioma of the placenta. J Obstet Gynaec Brit Comm 72:81, 1965.

———— Circumvallate and circummarginate placentas: their incidence and clinical significance. Amer J Obstet Gynec 102:44, 1968.

Whitman, R. C., and Greene, L. W. A case of disseminated miliary tuberculosis in a stillborn foetus. Arch Int Med 29:261, 1922.

Wigglesworth, J. S.   Vascular anatomy of the human placenta and its significance for placental pathology. J Obstet Gynaec Brit Comm 76:979, 1969.

Wilson, D., and Paalman, R. J.   Clinical significance of circumvallate placenta. Obstet Gynec 29:774, 1967.

Wynn, R. M., and Davies, J.   Ultrastructure of transplanted choriocarcinoma and its endocrine implications. Amer J Obstet Gynec 88:618, 1964.

———— and Davies, J.   Ultrastructure of hydatidiform mole: correlative electron microscopic and functional aspects. Amer J Obstet Gynec 90:293, 1964.

———— and Harris, J. R.   Ultrastructure of trophoblast and endometrium in invasive hydatidiform mole. Amer J Obstet Gynec 99:1125, 1967.

Yen, S., and MacMahon, B.   Epidemiologic features of trophoblastic disease. Amer J Obstet Gynec 101:126, 1968.

———— Pearson, O. H., and Rankin, J. S.   Radioimmunoassay of serum chorionic gonadotropin and placental lactogen in trophoblastic disease. Obstet Gynec 32:86, 1968.

Zarou, D. M., Imbleau, Y., and Zarou, G. S.   The radiographic diagnosis of molar pregnancy. Obstet Gynec 35:89, 1970.

23

PLACENTA PREVIA AND ABRUPTIO PLACENTAE

In the three preceding chapters the most frequent causes of bleeding in the first half of pregnancy were discussed—namely, abortion, ectopic pregnancy, and (a less common cause) hydatidiform mole. In the present chapter, placenta previa and abruptio placentae, the two most common causes of hemorrhage in the second half of pregnancy, will be reviewed.

Hemorrhage in the last half of pregnancy occurs in about 3 per cent of all births. Its seriousness is attested not only by the obvious maternal risk but by the associated high perinatal loss (Table 1).

Table 1. Prevalence and Perinatal Loss in Antepartum Hemorrhage

Etiology	Kings County Hospital, 1961–1967		Obstetrical Statistical Cooperative, 1965–1968	
	Prevalence %	Perinatal Loss %	Prevalence %	Perinatal Loss %
Placenta previa	0.5	23.8	0.5	17.6
Abruptio placentae	2.4	40.3	1.4	30.8
Other	0.3	24.3	0.8	14.7
Total	3.2	36.6	2.7	23.7

From Obstetrical Statistical Cooperative.

PLACENTA PREVIA

In placenta previa, the placenta, instead of being located high up in the uterus, is located low in the uterus, either overlying or reaching to the vicinity of the internal os. Three degrees of the abnormality are recognized:

Total Placenta Previa. The internal os is totally covered by placenta.

Partial Placenta Previa. The internal os is partially covered by placenta.

Low-Lying Placenta. The region of the internal os is encroached upon by the placenta, so that the placental edge can be palpated by the examining finger introduced through the cervix, but the placenta does not extend beyond the margin of the os. A variety of this abnormality in which the edge of the placenta involves the margin of the internal os to a considerable extent, without extending beyond it, is sometimes called *marginal placenta previa.*

The degrees of placenta previa are represented in Figures 1 and 2. It is clear that the degree of placenta previa will depend in large measure on the

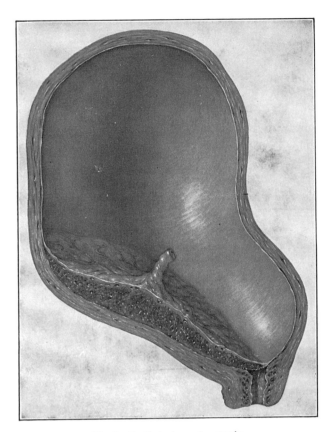

Fig. 1. Partial placenta previa.

cervical dilatation at the time of examination. For example, a low-lying placenta at 2 cm dilatation may become a partial placenta previa at 8 cm because the dilating cervix has uncovered placenta. Conversely, a placenta previa that appears to be total at 3 cm dilatation may become partial at full dilatation because the cervix dilates beyond the edge of the placenta. Since extensive exploration of the region of the internal os in placenta previa is one of the most dangerous undertakings in obstetrics, it is impractical to attempt to ascertain with any precision these changing relations between the edge of the placenta and the internal os as the cervix dilates. The diagnosis of the degree of the placenta previa is therefore based on the conditions at the first examination after the complication has been recognized.

In both the total and partial varieties, a certain degree of separation of the placenta is an inevitable consequence of the formation of the lower uterine segment and the dilatation of the cervix. It is always associated with disruption of blood vessels, which cannot constrict until after the uterus has been emptied. Rigby appropriately termed the resulting hemorrhage *unavoidable*.

Frequency.   Placenta previa is a serious but fairly uncommon complication, occurring once in about 200 deliveries. The contradictory statistics on the incidence of the various degrees of placenta previa reflect the lack of precision in their

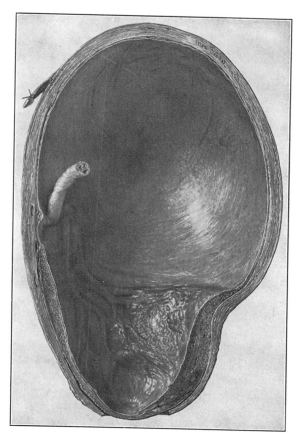

Fig. 2. Total placenta previa and velamentous insertion of cord. Note the cuplike form of the placenta and its varying thickness.

definitions. In 304 cases of this complication studied at the Johns Hopkins Hospital by Gutierrez-Yepes and Eastman, the total type was found in 23 per cent, the partial in 29 per cent, and low-lying in 48 per cent. At Kings County Hospital, the partial and total varieties occur with about equal frequency (Pedowitz).

Etiology.   Little is known about the cause of placenta previa. Multiparity and advancing age, however, appear to favor its occurrence.

The abnormality is about half as frequent in primigravidas as in multiparas, as shown in Tables 2 and 3. These data were derived from over 100,000 deliveries, in which 483 cases of placenta previa occurred in the Obstetrical Statistical Co-

Table 2. **The Relation of Placenta Previa to Age**

	Rate per 1,000 Births	
Age	*Primigravidas*	*Multiparas*
15–24	1.9	2.7
25–34	4.2	5.6
35+	7.0	10.4
Total rate	2.6	5.6

Table 3. The Relation of Placenta Previa to Parity

Parity	Rate per 1,000 Births
0	2.6
1–3	5.1
4–6	7.8
7–9	8.2
Total rate	4.7

operative during 1961 and 1962. Although placenta previa is supposed to be rare in primigravidas, our data show that at least 20 per cent of all cases occur in women who have had no previous pregnancies. In addition, our figures indicate that whereas age and parity both play a role in the cause of the condition, age may be more significant. Women over the age of 35 are about three and a half times more likely to have placenta previa than those under 25, regardless of parity. The same order of increase holds true when women of high parity are compared with primigravidas. When parity is excluded, by considering primigravidas alone, the increase of placenta previa with age is nevertheless still striking. Records demonstrated an increase in incidence with age in each parity group, but no increase with parity if age was held constant. In other words, age rather than parity appears to be the most important predisposing factor.

The chance that a patient with placenta previa has had the abnormality before is about 3 per cent. Although multiple occurrences of placenta previa are extremely rare, Fitzpatrick and Rivett each report a patient in whom placenta previa recurred in five successive pregnancies, and Gilliatt and MacCarthy each record the disorder four times in the same patient.

Estimation of the chance of recurrence of placenta previa with a succeeding pregnancy is more important. Pertinent data are scant and incomplete. Of Radtke's 80 patients with placenta previa, only 45 carried subsequent pregnancies to viability and 2 had a subsequent placenta previa. Similarly, of Penrose's 72 patients, 36 carried pregnancies to viability, with 3 instances of the condition. In other words, the chances of having a subsequent placenta previa if pregnancy is carried to viability is about 6 out of 100, or 12 times the general incidence.

One of the most important factors in the development of placenta previa is said to be defective vascularization of the decidua, the possible result of inflammatory or atrophic changes. Scarring of the endometrium may be increased by age or repeated pregnancies in rapid succession. When the blood supply to the placenta is limited, the placenta may compensate by spreading over a larger area of the uterus. In so doing its lower portion occasionally approaches the region of the internal os, completely or partially overlapping it. This view seems plausible, since the placenta in this abnormality is located over a greater area of the uterus than usual and is often considerably thinner. A similar situation occurs with the large placenta of erythroblastosis.

Rarely, placenta previa is associated with simple *placenta accreta* or one of its more advanced forms, *placenta increta* or *percreta* (p. 963). Such abnormally firm attachment of the placenta should be expected because of the poorly developed decidua in the lower uterine segment. Although placenta accreta is a rarity, it probably occurs more frequently in association with placenta previa than has previously been suspected. Millar and, more recently, Malkasian have cited an aggregate of 72 reported cases.

In most exceptional circumstances a part of the placenta develops on the upper portion of the cervix, forming an ectopic cervical pregnancy, discussed on page 561.

Signs and Symptoms. The most characteristic event in placenta previa is painless hemorrhage, which usually does not appear until after the seventh month of pregnancy. Many abortions, however, probably result from abnormal locations of the placenta. Ultrasonic investigations of early pregnancies that eventually abort disclose an unexpectedly large number of low-lying embryos (Hellman and co-workers).

The hemorrhage frequently occurs without warning in a pregnant woman who was previously in perfect health. Occasionally it makes its first appearance while the patient is asleep. On awakening, she is surprised to find herself in a pool of blood. The initial bleeding is rarely, if ever, so profuse as to prove fatal. It usually ceases spontaneously, recurring when least expected. In other cases, the bleeding does not cease entirely. The continuous discharge of small quantities of bloodstained fluid eventually so weakens the patient that a fairly small additional acute hemorrhage may be sufficient to cause death. In a certain proportion of cases, particularly with merely low-lying placentas, the bleeding does not appear until the onset of labor, when it may vary from a slight, bloodstained discharge to a profuse hemorrhage.

The cause of the hemorrhage is readily understood in terms of the changes that take place in the later weeks of pregnancy and at the time of labor. When the placenta is located over the internal os, the formation of the lower uterine segment and the dilatation of the internal os inevitably result in tearing of placental attachments, followed by hemorrhage from the uterine vessels. The bleeding is augmented by the inability of the stretched myometrial fibers of the lower uterine segment to compress the torn vessels, as occurs when the normally located placenta separates during the third stage of labor.

Since the placenta previa occupies the lower portion of the uterine cavity, it may interfere with the accommodations of the fetal head. As a consequence, abnormal presentations are unusually frequent. Schmitz, O'Dea, and Isaacs, for example, found shoulder presentations in 9 per cent of their cases, breech presentations in 16 per cent, and vertex presentations in only 70 per cent.

As the result of abnormal adherence or an excessively large area of attachment, the process of placental separation is sometimes impeded, and then hemorrhage frequently occurs after the birth of the child and, exceptionally, continues even after the manual removal of the placenta. In other instances hemorrhage may result from the overstretched lower segment, which commonly contracts poorly and is, therefore, unable to compress the vessels traversing its walls. In many cases, however, bleeding results from lacerations in the friable cervix and lower uterine segment.

Clinical Diagnosis. In patients with uterine hemorrhage during the last third of pregnancy, placenta previa or abruptio placentae should always be suspected. The possibility of the placenta previa should not be dismissed until careful examination has proved its absence, in which case the diagnosis of abruptio placentae should be made. Unfortunately, the diagnosis cannot be made clinically unless a finger is passed through the cervix and the placenta is palpated. **This**

procedure is never permissible unless the patient is in an operating room with all preparations for a cesarean section, for even the gentlest examination of this sort can cause torrential hemorrhage. Furthermore, such an examination is unwise unless delivery in the near future is contemplated, for the trauma may cause bleeding of such a degree that immediate delivery becomes necessary. It is unfortunate when an examination that could have been postponed for several weeks forces delivery of an infant too immature to survive. On the basis of these considerations, patients may be divided into two main groups: (1) those in whom the infant is premature and there is no pressing need for delivery; and (2) those in whom the fetus is within three weeks of term and estimated to weigh in excess of 2,500 g, or in whom labor is in progress, or in whom hemorrhage is so severe as to necessitate evacuation of the uterus despite the small size of the fetus. In the former group, the definitive diagnosis attainable only by pelvic examination can be postponed, but in the latter, the diagnosis must be clarified as soon as possible.

Malposition of the fetus (breech, transverse, or oblique lie) or a high head at term strengthens the suspicion of placenta previa. If all clinical and technical conditions have been satisfied, pelvic examination may be performed. The cervix should first be inspected and then palpated. In cases of placenta previa it is usually boggier and the canal is abnormally patulous, so that the examining finger can be passed with ease. The characteristic spongelike, slightly gritty placental mass interposed between the examining finger and the fetal head can be palpated with little difficulty and, with practice, can be distinguished from blood clot. The feel of placenta previa may be duplicated by placing a delivered placenta over a circle formed by the thumb and forefinger of the left hand. With his eyes shut, the examiner passes the gloved right forefinger through the circle, deriving an excellent impression of the palpatory findings in the real situation.

Technical Diagnostic Procedures.   Precise localization of the placenta in cases of suspected placenta previa is important only in certain circumstances. After the fetus has reached 2,500 g, or about three weeks before the expected date of confinement, the neonatal mortality rates are not greatly improved by further intrauterine development. In such cases, the cause of vaginal bleeding should be ascertained by pelvic examination. Additional diagnostic aids are purely academic, for if placenta previa is discovered, delivery could be accomplished forthwith. In the presence of severe hemorrhage the diagnosis must be made quickly by direct examination, so that the bleeding can be controlled by delivery. Only in patients with premature babies in whom delay in delivery is advisable is direct examination withheld. In such instances location of the placenta may be desirable information, but it does not alter management in all cases, for these patients must be carefully watched in any event. With proof that the placenta is normally located, the obstetrician may be more willing to discharge the patient from the hospital. Whether at home or hospitalized, however, all patients with bleeding are to be followed closely until delivery.

Ideally the diagnostic procedure should be accurate, simple, and harmless. It should, furthermore, differentiate between total and partial placenta previa (p. 963).

Ultrasonography is the simplest, most precise, and least hazardous method of placental localization yet developed. Unfortunately neither the equipment nor the technical experience is yet widely available.

Several radiologic technics can be used to localize the placenta. They include soft-tissue x-rays, intravenous injection of radioactive isotopes with localization of the placenta by noting the area of maximal counts, amniography using contrast material injected into the amniotic sac, and angiography. The most innocuous of these procedures, soft-tissue x-ray, is unfortunately the least accurate, giving a correct diagnosis in not more than 85 per cent of cases. In the remainder, the placenta cannot be visualized. The method often fails when most needed, as in hydramnios, multiple pregnancy, and obesity. Furthermore, diagnosis of posteriorly located placentas must be made by exclusion.

Isotopic procedures are safe and accurate, but they do not always differentiate between anteriorly and posteriorly located placentas or between the total and partial varieties. These methods have the added inconvenience of requiring a readily available isotope.

Angiography is accurate, but although we have had no accidents with this technic, it has the theoretical disadvantage of requiring injection into the maternal femoral artery and serial roentgenograms.

Studies on localization of the placenta by ultrasound were initiated by Gottesfeld and co-workers in Denver, who indicated a 97 per cent accuracy. These claims were supported by Donald's group in Glasgow, by Kohorn and co-workers, and later by our own studies in Brooklyn (Kobayashi and colleagues). The chorionic plate of the placenta is clearly visible on the sonogram as a more or less continuous white line. The intraplacental echoes produced by the blood and villi in the substance of the placenta are characteristic. The uterine wall and the region of the internal os are clearly defined (Fig. 3). Although the intraplacental echoes of a posteriorly located placenta are somewhat diminished, there is usually no difficulty in locating the structure. Often the degree to which the placenta covers the internal os can be ascertained. Ultrasonography locates the placenta with an accuracy of more than 95 per cent.

X-ray placentography can be extremely simple. Only one lateral 14- by 17-inch film is used. To achieve equal exposure of the front and back of the uterus, we cover the front half of one face of the cassette with black paper. Using a technic similar to that for the lateral lumbar spine, with fast film and cassettes, we obtain excellent pictures with properly graded exposure from front to rear (Fig. 4). The fetal and maternal gonadal dose with this technic is about 0.5 r. The placenta is well visualized in about 85 per cent of patients. Little is added by placing an opaque material in the bladder to measure the amount of separation between the bladder and the fetal head. Doing so, furthermore, requires an additional anteroposterior film.

Demonstration of placental location by this technic is based on visualization of an area of thickening of the structures between the fetal soft parts and the outside of the uterus. It is not possible to distinguish the placenta from the uterine wall because, except in instances of calcification, the radiopacity of these organs is similar and the shadows merge into one another. As shown by Moir, the subcutaneous tissues of the fetus produce a dark band demarcating the periphery of the fetal soft parts, as seen in Figure 4. By following this dark line and the anterior wall of the uterus, as illustrated in Figure 4, what appears to be a gradual thickening of the uterine wall in its upper third, believed to represent the placenta, can be seen. As shown by Brown and Dippel, the thickening of the uterine wall by the placenta is often better seen by viewing the film with a 200-watt frosted bulb in a gooseneck lamp with a shade.

Radioisotopes to locate the placenta were first used by Browne. About 50 microcuries of ^{24}Na in the form of 5 to 20 milliliters of isotonic saline were injected rapidly intravenously. After about 30 seconds, counts could be picked up from the abdomen using a scintillation counter. Localization of the placenta depends on the high count over

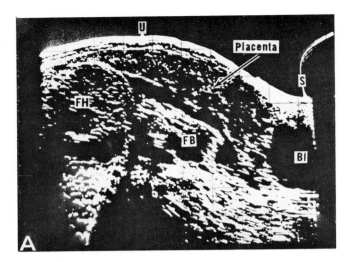

Fig. 3. A. Sonogram demonstrating anterior placenta previa (32 weeks). Bl, bladder; FB, fetal body; FH, fetal head; S, symphysis pubis; U, umbilicus. (From Kobayashi and colleagues. Amer J Obstet Gynec 106:279, 1970.)

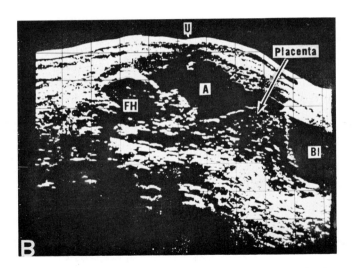

Fig. 3. B. Total posterior placenta previa (25 weeks). Bl, bladder; FH, fetal head; A, amniotic cavity; U, umbilicus.

the intervillous space caused by pooling of blood in that area. Weinberg and others and Hibbard have used radioiodinated serum albumin (RISA), both ^{131}I and [132]I, to localize the placenta. It is more satisfactory than radioactive sodium, for very little of the RISA traverses the placenta. Paul and colleagues have used ^{51}Cr similarly. Figure 5 shows how accurately the placenta can be mapped. Furthermore, de Rezende has pointed out that it gives 15 to 1,500 times less fetal radiation than x-ray diagnosis. The chief drawback is the difficulty in keeping the isotope always available. Accurate recording of the difference in counts from one area of the abdomen to another, moreover, requires considerable experience.

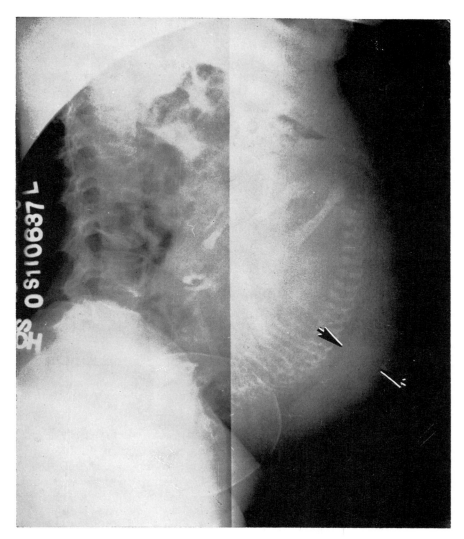

Fig. 4. Soft-tissue roentgenogram showing placenta on upper anterior surface of uterus.

Other isotopes such as ^{99}Tc-labeled serum albumin have been used. Several isotopic placentograms have utilized color scans to emphasize the pattern (Krohn and Jaffe; and also Adams).

If radiopaque material suitable for angiography is rapidly injected into the femoral artery and roentgenograms are taken rapidly thereafter, the spurts at the ends of the spiral arteries in the intervillous space (p. 163) will identify the placenta (Fig. 6). Solish, Masterson, and Hellman, as well as Fernström in Sweden and Hodge and others in this country, have all employed this technic to diagnose placenta previa. It is highly accurate, although somewhat time-consuming and complicated. For the several uses of femoral arteriography in obstetrics and gynecology, the comprehensive review by Nelson and his associates should be consulted.

The entire subject of radiologic localization of the placenta has been carefully reviewed by Weinberg. It seems that only the simplest and safest technics should be used routinely.

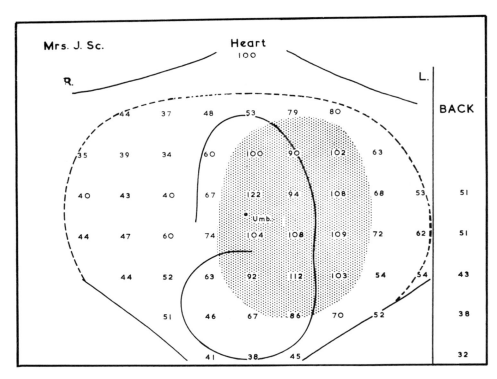

Fig. 5. Localization of the placenta with the use of R[132] ISA showing the very distinct elevation of the counts in the placental area. (From Hibbard and Herbert. Clin Sci 19:337, 1960.)

TREATMENT OF PLACENTA PREVIA

Every patient who bleeds in the latter half of pregnancy to an extent substantially greater than "show" should be sent to a hospital without either vaginal or rectal examination. This principle should be followed even though the hospital is 50 miles away. Any digital manipulation of the region of the cervix in placenta previa is likely to precipitate sudden, massive, and even fatal hemorrhage. It is therefore a firm rule that local examination should never be done in the home. Even in the hospital it must be carried out only in the operating room after all preparations have been made for surgical delivery and blood transfusion. It is both dangerous and unnecessary to resort to immediate action in all cases of placenta previa, since it is very rare for a woman with this complication to bleed to death from the initial hemorrhage, provided no vaginal or rectal examinations have been done. This principle has been emphasized by Johnson, who in his vast experience knew of no fatality from the initial bleeding of placenta previa, in the absence of digital manipulation of the cervix. Similarly, in a combined experience with placenta previa, which antedates transfusion and which comprises over 1,000 cases, there is no such death on record. In Macafee's extensive experience as well, a severe initial hemorrhage occurs only rarely with this complication.

Three facts form the basis for management of these patients: (1) the initial

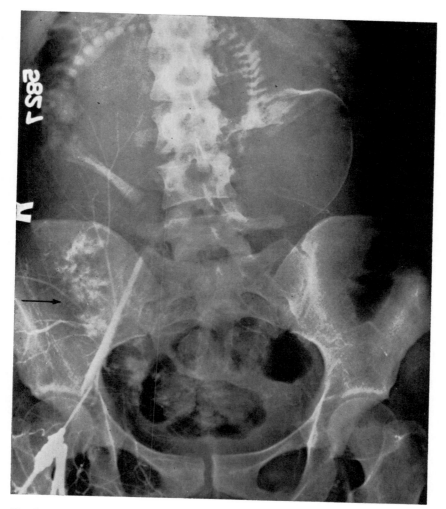

Fig. 6. Arteriogram showing low-lying placenta. (Courtesy of Dr. James H. Nelson.)

hemorrhage in placenta previa is rarely, if ever, fatal; (2) vaginal or rectal examination often precipitates severe hemorrhage; and (3) the major cause of perinatal loss in placenta previa is prematurity.

To recapitulate, vaginal or rectal examination should not be done in suspected cases of placenta previa except in an operating room, where all facilities are ready to combat massive hemorrhage. Vaginal packing is dangerous, since it may cause more bleeding and introduce infection and, moreover, is usually futile. After admittance of the patient to the hospital, there is ample time to arrange for blood transfusion, to prepare the operating room, and to plan the most judicious management of the case. In selected cases in which the fetus is premature, it is justifiable, with certain reservations, to postpone delivery until the infant has a better chance of survival. This *expectant treatment* of placenta previa will be discussed in more detail subsequently. Vaginal examination should be carried out with asepsis in an operating room prepared for cesarean section (*double setup*). It should be done only when expectant treatment is rendered unnecessary by closeness to term or impossible by labor or severe hemorrhage.

In placenta previa, as in other major hemorrhagic complications of obstetrics, blood transfusion is lifesaving and in many cases plays a larger role in the outcome than does the particular method used to combat bleeding. It should be the physician's first thought in every such case.

Methods Employed.   The procedures available for the treatment of placenta previa fall into two main categories: (1) vaginal methods, the rationale of which is to exert pressure against the placenta and placental site and thereby occlude the bleeding vessels; and (2) cesarean section, the rationale of which is twofold. First, through immediate delivery, it allows the uterus to contract and so stop the bleeding and second, it forestalls the possibility of cervical lacerations, a frequent complication of vaginal delivery in total and partial placenta previa.

Vaginal Methods.   There are four vaginal or "compression" methods, although only simple rupture of the membranes is now in general use. Willett's forceps, insertion of a bag, and Braxton Hicks version have all but disappeared from modern practice for a variety of reasons that will be mentioned.

1. Rupture of the membranes allows the head to drop down against the placenta and is often an efficacious procedure in multiparas with low-lying placentas. It has its greatest usefulness in multiparas with this least severe variety of placenta previa, which does not start to bleed until after onset of labor. After rupture of the membranes, fundal pressure should be exerted to force the head as tightly as possible against the placenta and lower uterine segment.

2. To put additional pressure on the placenta a T-shaped clamp (Willett's forceps) was formerly attached to the baby's scalp and a weight of one or two pounds applied to the clamp over a pulley. This procedure causes little more compression than simple rupture of the membranes and frequently inflicts severe damage to the fetal scalp. It has fallen into disuse except in rare instances of fetal death associated with minor degrees of placenta previa.

3. Before 1935, a 10 cm Voorhees bag filled with water and applied inside the cervix was frequently employed to compress the placenta. This procedure has been abandoned because the manipulations necessary to insert the bag frequently traumatize the friable and vascular lower segment. Additional disadvantages are the frequent failure of the bag to cause full dilatation, the danger of infection, and the high perinatal mortality associated with its use.

4. The Braxton Hicks procedure was not directed at immediate delivery. Its objective was rather the utilization of the fetal buttocks and thigh for tamponade of the placenta. It differed from conventional version and extraction in several important respects: two fingers and not the whole hand were inserted into the uterus to grasp the foot; Braxton Hicks version was done at 4 to 8 cm dilatation; and after a foot had been delivered no further effort at extraction was made, but simply enough traction exerted on the leg to control the bleeding. Only with complete dilatation was extraction effected. This procedure, too, has fallen into disrepute because of the difficulty of the operation, the high incidence of rupture of the friable lower uterine segment, and the almost inevitable death of the fetus.

Cesarean Section.   Cesarean section has now become the accepted method of delivery for the majority of patients with placenta previa, as borne out in many publications and hospital reports. For example, at the Kings County Hospital 67 per cent of patients with placenta previa are delivered by cesarean section, and 61 per cent of the patients in the Obstetrical Statistical Cooperative are so delivered. Nesbitt and associates cited a similar rate of about 65 per cent but believed that their results could be improved by raising the figure.

The rationale for performing cesarean section in placenta previa is twofold: (1) it decreases antepartum bleeding caused by the partially separated placenta by effecting immediate delivery and subsequent uterine contraction; and (2) it greatly reduces the likelihood of cervical and lower segment lacerations. Because of the extreme vascularity of the placental site, the cervix and lower uterine segment are so friable in placenta previa that they tear like wet blotting paper, especially in the total and partial varieties. In early reports, more than one third of the deaths from placenta previa were directly attributable to bleeding and lacerations of the cervix and lower uterine segment following vaginal manipulations and delivery. It is clear that cesarean section in placenta previa is performed primarily to safeguard the life of the mother.

Abdominal delivery yields an additional reward in better infant survival, but since about half of the infants are premature when bleeding occurs, cesarean section from the viewpoint of the infant must be evaluated with some reserve. In justifying cesarean section in the presence of a dead fetus, it is again necessary to understand that abdominal delivery is done primarily for the mother and that the delivery of a dead baby by vaginal methods also can cause lacerations. Cesarean section may therefore be the most judicious method of treatment even though the fetus has succumbed, especially in all cases of total placenta previa and in all total and partial varieties in primigravidas. In less severe varieties of placenta previa in a multipara, death of the fetus may justify attempts at vaginal delivery in certain circumstances, preferably by rupture of the membranes without further manipulation.

When the placenta lies far enough posteriorly that the anterior segment can be incised transversely, a low-segment cesarean section is to be preferred. If, however, the uterine incision must be carried through the placenta, bleeding, both maternal and fetal, can be severe, and extension of the incision to involve one or both uterine arteries can occur with surprising ease. With anterior placenta previa cannot be displaced from the region of the uterine incision, a vertical uterine incision may be safer. When placenta previa is complicated by degrees of placenta accreta that render control of bleeding from the placental bed difficult by conservative means, cesarean section and total hysterectomy is the procedure of choice.

Expectant Treatment. It was formerly taught that placenta previa demanded prompt delivery and that temporizing for any purpose was rarely, if ever, indicated. As the result of the important observations of Johnson, Macafee, and others, it is now clear that a policy of waiting is justifiable in certain cases in order to minimize the high neonatal mortality levied by prematurity in this complication. These authors based their contention on the fact that both the initial hemorrhage in placenta previa and subsequent hemorrhages are rarely, if ever, fatal in the absence of vaginal manipulation, provided the hemoglobin concentration is normal at the time of the hemorrhage. As already indicated, these general facts, which underlie the justification of the expectant treatment, are well documented. Since the sole purpose of expectant therapy is to allow small premature babies opportunity for longer intrauterine development, it does not apply to women who are near term or in whom the infant weighs clearly 2,500 g or more. If the fetus seems so small that the likelihood of its survival is poor and if labor has not begun, an expectant attitude may be adopted.

A speculum is gently inserted and inspection of the vagina and cervix carried out to eliminate the possibility of infrequent causes of bleeding, such as ruptured varices or cervical tumors, but the cervical canal should not be explored. No further vaginal examination should be done, for the risk of precipitating a potentially severe hemorrhage is so great that in this situation a definitive diagnosis is not desirable. If no sites of bleeding are seen, a presumptive diagnosis of placenta previa is made. This diagnosis may be confirmed by one of the methods described on page 614. As Pedowitz has pointed out, the perinatal mortality is higher and expectant treatment is less likely to succeed in cases of central placenta previa. These women should be kept under close observation, preferably in the hospital, although occasionally we may permit an intelligent, reliable patient to return home, with instructions to abstain from sexual intercourse, to permit no vaginal examination, and to return to the hospital at the first recurrence of bleeding. The mother's hemoglobin and hematocrit must be followed carefully. These data, rather than an alarming history derived from the patient's estimate of the amount of blood lost, must be the criteria for interruption of pregnancy before the fetus has clearly reached viability.

Delivery.   In selecting the best treatment for a given case of placenta previa, numerous factors must be given consideration. If there is any sign of infection, evidenced by fever or foul discharge, or a history of vaginal manipulations, the case falls into an especially dire category. Otherwise, the following factors and their significance must be reviewed: degree of placenta previa, parity, and extent of bleeding. In all cases of total placenta previa, regardless of other factors, cesarean section is the procedure of choice. In all primigravidas, both total and partial placenta previa are indications for abdominal delivery, regardless of other factors. If bleeding has been massive there is either a degree of placenta previa more advanced than examination may show or extreme vascularity of the cervix and lower uterine segment. Massive bleeding indicates the need for cesarean section, regardless of other factors. At the other extreme, multiparas who have low-lying placentas and are already in labor with 4 cm of cervical dilatation or more may be managed by rupture of the membranes. This least severe group will include a large proportion, perhaps one half, of any series. If a vaginal method of delivery is chosen, the simpler it is the better, since prolonged and complicated manipulations greatly increase the risk to both mother and child. If cesarean section is performed in anterior placenta previa, which cannot be avoided by low-segment technics, the classical operation is sometimes preferable to minimize the danger of both maternal and fetal hemorrhage.

If frank intrauterine infection complicates placenta previa, the outlook at once becomes grave, whether delivery is effected abdominally or vaginally. Intensive antimicrobial treatment should obviously be started at once and blood transfusions given to replace the amount lost. In all cases of total placenta previa and most cases of partial placenta previa, cesarean section is still the safest method of delivery, with reliance on the antimicrobials to combat infection. In patients of considerable parity, cesarean section and hysterectomy may be the operation of choice, but in multiparas with low-lying placentas and in some cases of partial placenta previa with minimal bleeding, the presence of outright uterine infection justifies the use of simple rupture of the membranes to ascertain whether this procedure will control bleeding. If it does, it is clearly the method of choice for delivery, but if it does not, cesarean section is the only reasonable alternative. Again, in all cases of placenta previa, liberal blood transfusions are frequently more decisive in lifesaving than is the type of local treatment employed.

Prognosis. A marked improvement in maternal mortality has been achieved, as can be seen in the reports of numerous large clinics. This trend began in 1927, when Bill advocated adequate transfusion and cesarean section in the treatment of placenta previa. At the Kings County Hospital we have had no deaths from placenta previa since 1950. Similarly, in the Obstetrical Statistical Cooperative, there were no maternal deaths during this period. With proper management and prompt hospitalization, the maternal death rate from placenta previa should approach zero. The prognosis is not nearly so good in developing countries, where the maternal death rate may exceed 15 per cent (Eastman).

Beginning in 1945, when Macafee and Johnson independently suggested expectant therapy, a similar trend has been evident in perinatal loss. Nesbitt's data taken from a very large sample in upstate New York indicate a current perinatal loss of between 15 and 20 per cent. Prematurity still poses a formidable problem, for only about one fourth of all patients with placenta previa can be treated expectantly. Half are already near term, and in half of the remainder delivery is forced by labor or profuse hemorrhage. Severe bleeding accounts for the nearly fourfold increase in perinatal loss in cases of total placenta previa.

ABRUPTIO PLACENTAE

Nomenclature. Whenever the normally located placenta undergoes separation from its uterine attachment between the twentieth week of prgnancy and the birth of the infant, the condition is known as *abruptio placentae*. Frequently employed synonyms are placental abruption, premature separation of the normally implanted placenta, ablatio placentae, and accidental hemorrhage. Detachment of the placenta before the twentieth week is a frequent cause of abortion. The reason for regarding placental separations early and late in pregnancy as different problems is that the clinical and pathologic features of the accidents at these two times are quite different. The earlier in pregnancy abruptio placentae occurs, the more it may resemble abortion and may frequently be treated as such. This accident in the middle trimester, however, may have serious consequences.

The term most descriptive of this complication is "premature separation of the normally implanted placenta." It is cumbersome, however, and hence the shorter phrases "abruptio placentae" and "placental abruption" have been employed. The Latin *abruptio placentae*, which means a rending asunder of the placenta, connotes a sudden accident, a clinical characteristic of most cases of this complication. *Ablatio placentae* means a carrying away of the placenta, analogous to *ablatio retinae;* this term is not extensively used. The term frequently employed in Great Britain for this complication is "accidental hemorrhage." The rationale for its use is that the condition is an "accident" in the sense of an event that takes place without expectation, in contrast to the "unavoidable" hemorrhage of placenta previa, in which bleeding is inevitable because of the anatomic relations. Since the term "accidental hemorrhage" may suggest an element of trauma, which is rarely a factor in these cases, it is sometimes misleading to students and is rarely employed in the United States.

Some of the bleeding of placental abruption usually insinuates itself between the membranes and uterus, escapes through the cervix, and appears externally,

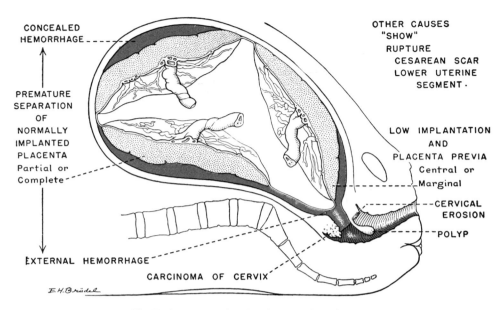

CONCEALED
HEMORRHAGE

OTHER CAUSES
"SHOW"
RUPTURE
CESAREAN SCAR
LOWER UTERINE
SEGMENT.

PREMATURE
SEPARATION
OF
NORMALLY
IMPLANTED
PLACENTA
Partial or
Complete

LOW IMPLANTATION
AND
PLACENTA PREVIA
Central or
Marginal

CERVICAL
EROSION

POLYP

EXTERNAL HEMORRHAGE

CARCINOMA OF CERVIX

E.H.Brödel

Fig. 7. Causes of bleeding in the third trimester.

causing an *external hemorrhage*. Less often, the blood does not escape externally but is retained between the detached placenta and the uterus, leading to *concealed hemorrhage* or *internal hemorrhage*. (Figs. 7 and 8). Abruptio placentae with concealed hemorrhage may be more catastrophic than placental abruption with external hemorrhage, and it carries with it much greater maternal hazards probably because the extent of the hemorrhage is not appreciated. Other important differences between abruptio placentae with external hemorrhage and with concealed hemorrhage are as follows: With external hemorrhage, detachment of the placenta is generally incomplete, whereas with concealed hemorrhage it is usually more extensive. Concealed hemorrhage, furthermore, is associated with hypertension in a substantial proportion of cases. This association is less common in cases with external bleeding. In about 80 per cent of cases of abruptio placentae the bleeding is predominantly external, but about 20 per cent is concealed.

Frequency.   The reported incidence ranges between 1 in 55 deliveries to 1 in 150, depending upon the diagnostic criteria.

All degrees of premature separation of the placenta may occur, from an area only a few millimeters in diameter to the entire placenta, with intermediate signs and symptoms. As a consequence, abruptio placentae is not a sharply defined condition. The placenta separating at its margin may disrupt the marginal sinus. Although such *marginal sinus ruptures* were formerly classified as separate clinical entities, it seems more likely that they represent merely slight degrees of placental separation at the margin with overt bleeding. This concept has been ably discussed by Wilkin and Picard. In this connection, it should be noted that of all cases of antepartum hemorrhage in the latter half of pregnancy, somewhat fewer than half can be ascribed positively to placenta previa and abruptio placentae. Of those remaining, a small number can be traced to lesions of the cervix, whereas bleeding in the rest is of uncertain origin. In all probability, much of

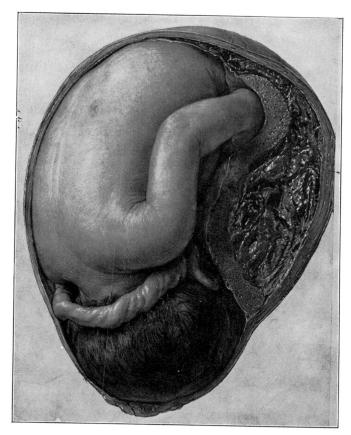

Fig. 8. Abruptio placentae with concealed hemorrhage.

this bleeding may result from minute marginal separations of the placenta, which are impossible to recognize with certainty either clinically or pathologically.

Because of the great variability in the clinical as well as in the pathologic manifestations of placental abruption, the classification of these cases is sometimes uncertain. In the main, the diagnosis of abruptio placentae is made only if, in addition to bleeding, there are definite clinical manifestations of the condition, such as abdominal pain, uterine tenderness or rigidity, and fetal distress or death, or if anatomic placental evidence is found in the form of clots and a depressed area on the maternal surface.

Etiology. The primary cause of abruptio placentae is unknown, but the following conditions have been evoked as etiologic factors: trauma, shortness of the umbilical cord, chronic hypertension, acute toxemia, pressure by the enlarged uterus on the inferior vena cava, and dietary deficiency. It was formerly held that a fall or blow to the abdomen might commonly cause the condition, but trauma is demonstrable in less than 5 per cent of cases. Sudden decompression of an overdistended uterus can cause placental separation. It cannot be demonstrated, however, that the average length of the umbilical cord is less than normal in abruptio placentae.

A relation between toxemia and abruptio placentae has long been postulated.

The frequency with which the two disorders are associated has been variously reported as from 25 to 60 per cent. Bartholomew and associates, for example, reported an association of 52.5 per cent; our previous data indicated 47 per cent, and Goethals recorded 24.2 per cent. Hibbard, however, reported that only 7.7 per cent of his patients had preeclampsia and 4.9 per cent chronic hypertension. Conversely, the incidence of abruptio placentae in patients suffering from preeclampsia was 1.6 per cent, and in patients with chronic hypertension 2.3 per cent. Similar data, expressing only a very slight association between toxemia and abruption of the placenta, have been presented by Hendelman and Fraser.

These figures agree with our own current findings. At the Kings County Hospital, if all degrees of abruption are considered, preeclampsia and chronic hypertension are present in 6.4 and 9.2 per cent of cases, respectively. However, if only those instances with more extensive separation are considered, hypertension is much more common. For example, at Parkland Memorial Hospital, 47 per cent of 192 cases of placental abruption so severe as to kill the fetus were complicated by hypertension (Pritchard). Placental abruption occurred in 6.5 per cent of cases of eclampsia (Pritchard and Stone).

There is, however, an association between parity and abruptio placentae. The disorder occurs three times as commonly in women of parity greater than five than in primigravidas. This association has been shown by Hibbard's data and by our own (Table 4). Unlike placenta previa, however, in abruptio placentae

Table 4. Relation of the Incidence of Abruptio Placentae to Parity

Parity	Incidence (Per Cent)
0	0.8
1–4	1.0
5+	2.3

After Hibbard. J Obstet Gynaec Brit Comm 69:282, 1962.

age itself, dissociated from parity, does not seem to play a significant etiologic role. Since age and chronic hypertension both increase with parity, there is a possible explanation for the higher incidence of abruptio placentae in patients with chronic hypertension. Nevertheless, we cannot conclude that either chronic hypertension or preeclampsia plays a significant etiologic role in abruptio placentae.

In 1915, Williams observed peculiar degenerative lesions in the intima of the smaller uterine arteries and suggested that the condition may be caused by a form of toxemia producing such vascular changes. McKelvey described lesions that he frequently observed in normal gestation in the arterioles of the upper part of the decidua basalis. He believed that in abruptio placentae there is an extension of these arteriolar changes that probably occur in all human placentas.

The pathologic changes in the spiral arterioles of the decidua compacta and spongiosa are discussed in detail in Chapter 6. Some support is lent to the etiologic role of vascular disease of the decidua basalis by the relation of abruptio placentae to age of the mother and the high recurrence rates in subsequent pregnancies. For patients who suffer severe placental abruption, Pritchard indicated a recurrence rate of this complication of 11 per cent, contrasted with a 0.2 per cent initial incidence rate, thus confirming the findings of Hibbard and Jeffcoate.

Although compression of the inferior vena cava has been shown to produce placental abruption in experimental animals, venous compression is virtually universal in supine gravidas (as mentioned on page 259), and it is, therefore, unlikely to be more than a very rare primary etiologic factor in human pregnancy. Stone and co-workers report two patients in the last trimester of pregnancy in whom the vena cava and both ovarian veins were ligated without producing abruptio placentae.

In a very small number of cases, direct trauma is the cause of separation. From the observations of Greig and on the basis of our own experience, it seems that trauma is an etiologic factor in about 1 per cent of cases.

Hibbard and others have suggested that folic acid deficiency may play an etiologic role. This hypothesis has been carefully examined by Menon and colleagues; by Rothman, by Kitay, as well as by Whalley and associates, and by Alperin and colleagues. All of these investigators can find no evidence to support it.

Pathology.   Abruptio placentae is initiated by hemorrhage into the decidua basalis, which sometimes appears to come from areas within the placenta itself and at other times from pathologic alterations in the smaller uterine vessels. The decidua then splits, so that a thin layer remains in contact with the maternal surface of the placenta, while a thicker layer adjoins the myometrium. Consequently, the process in its earliest stages consists in the development of a decidual hematoma that leads to separation, compression, and ultimate destruction of function of the portion of the placenta adjacent to it. In its early stage there may be no clinical symptoms. The condition is discovered only upon examination of the freshly delivered organ, which will present on its maternal surface a sharply circumscribed depression measuring a few centimeters in diameter and containing dark and partially disorganized clotted blood. In most instances the retroplacental hemorrhage is more profuse, so that the area of separation becomes more extensive and gradually reaches the margin of the placenta. Since the uterus is still distended by the products of conception, it is unable to contract and compress the torn vessels supplying the placental site; consequently, the escaping blood dissects the membranes from the uterine wall and eventually appears externally, although it may be retained within the uterus. Retention is likely to occur (1) when there is an effusion of blood behind the placenta, its margins still remaining adherent; (2) when the placenta is completely separated, while the membranes retain their attachment to the uterine wall; (3) when the blood gains access to the amniotic cavity after breaking through the membranes; and (4) when the head is so closely applied to the lower uterine segment that the blood cannot make its way past it. In the majority of such cases, however, the membranes are gradually dissected off the uterine wall, and part of the blood eventually escapes from the cervix.

Clinical Diagnosis.   The findings in a typical case of severe abruptio placentae are vaginal bleeding to a greater or lesser degree; a tightly contracted uterus of boardlike consistency; uterine tenderness, which may be general or localized; absence of the fetal heart sounds; and variable evidence of hypovolemia. The amniotic fluid may be blood-tinged. Many deviations from this typical picture occur, however. For example, unless more than half of the placenta has been separated, the fetal heart tones are usually audible. In concealed hemorrhage, of course, there is no vaginal bleeding, but uterine rigidity and tenderness are likely to be pronounced. Pain except on palpation is variable; it may be entirely absent or occasionally be excruciating. The most dependable sign of abruptio placentae is uterine rigidity. Even in mild cases, the uterus usually does not relax properly between contractions in labor.

It has long been held that the shock sometimes seen in abruptio placentae is out of proportion to the blood loss, even though a proper estimate is made of the original blood contained in the retroplacental hematoma. For example, in the case represented in Figure 9, the retroplacental hematoma weighed only 500 g, but the patient was in shock with a pulse rate of 140 on admittance to the hospital.

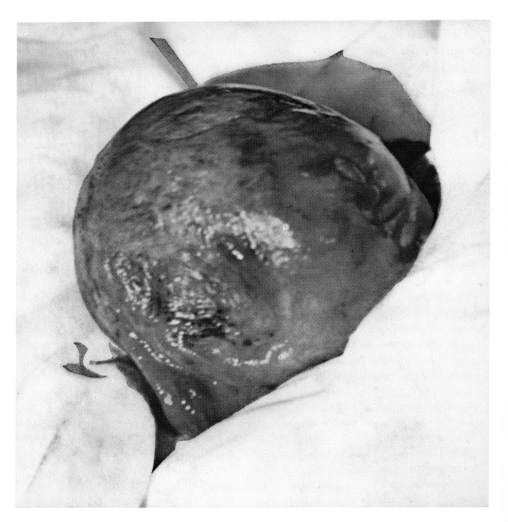

Fig. 9. Couvelaire uterus at cesarean section.

Weiner and associates express doubt about this old concept, pointing out that the volume of the clot is only 40 per cent of the amount of blood shed and that extravasation of blood into the broad ligament and retroperitoneum may reach substantial but unknown proportions. Pritchard and Brekken have studied the blood loss in 141 gravidas with severe abruptio placentae and fetal death. The blood loss often reached one half of the blood volume. In their experience blood pressure was often maintained in spite of hemorrhage of 2 liters or more. In these circumstances, oliguria caused by inadequate renal perfusion is frequently observed. Admittedly, the intravenous injection of large doses of thromboplastic material into experimental animals can cause profound shock, as shown by Schneider. In cases of abruptio placentae associated with fibrinogenopenia, furthermore, it is possible that shock may be aggravated, or even produced, by the passage of thromboplastic substances and thrombin into the maternal circulation. Despite these observations, however, the weight of evidence suggests that in most cases of abruptio placentae, the intensity of shock is not out of proportion to the maternal blood loss.

Although the severe case of abruptio placentae is usually marked by such classic signs and symptoms that the diagnosis is at once obvious, the milder and more common forms are difficult to distinguish clinically, and the diagnosis is often made by exclusion. Thus, in the face of persistent vaginal bleeding in the last trimester, it often becomes necessary to rule out placenta previa and other causes by inspection and direct transcervical palpation. Unfortunately, there are neither tests nor diagnostic methods to detect separation of the placenta, and the cause of the vaginal bleeding often remains obscure even after delivery.

Classic cases of abruptio placentae with pain, shock, and uterine rigidity occur infrequently in the middle trimester of pregnancy. These cases present the same complications and may even cause death. They must be treated according to the same general principles as those occurring at the more common period of gestation (Baker and Dewhurst).

Complications of Placental Abruption. The maternal, and to some extent the fetal, complications are time-related in the sense that their development and severity are dependent upon the duration as well as the magnitude of the separation. With extensive placental detachment (1) hemorrhage (which may be concealed or external), (2) intense *oliguria* indicative of *shock,* (3) *blood coagulation defects,* and (4) *severe fetal distress and death* can occur so rapidly that all of these complications are present at the time of admittance to the hospital. With lesser degrees of separation the rates at which these complications develop are somewhat slower, although the amount of placental separation can increase appreciably at any time.

The concept that some of the complications are time-related has a bearing on treatment, especially the need for supportive therapy and reasonably prompt delivery. Rupture of the membranes and the administration of oxytocin may retard the bleeding but will not stop it entirely. Similarly, steps to correct the coagulation defects might reduce bleeding somewhat. Uterine hemorrhage, however, can be effectively controlled only by delivery. Emptying the uterus will allow it to contract and retract sufficiently to constrict the severed blood vessels at the placental site.

The hemorrhage and the shock of placental abruption, of course, demand immediate treatment. Prompt restoration of an effective circulation by the intravenous administration of appropriate fluids, especially whole blood, is the first consideration and the sine qua non in the treatment of placental abruption.

Consumptive Coagulopathy. The commonest cause of blood-clotting defects in pregnancy is placental abruption, although they may occur also with amniotic fluid embolism, fetal death, sepsis, and postpartum hemorrhage. Hypofibrinogenemia occurs in about 10 per cent of patients with abruptio placentae, although it is probably much more common in the severe degrees of separation. Pritchard and Brekken noted severe hypofibrinogenemia (less than 100 mg per 100 ml) in 28 per cent of their 141 severe cases.

Dieckmann in 1936 called attention to hypofibrinogenemia associated with abruptio placentae. Since then there have been numerous reports of hypofibrino-genemia associated principally with abruptio placentae but also with amniotic fluid embolism (p. 950), fetal death (p. 1008), and severe postpartum hemorrhage. The significance of low fibrinogen levels must be interpreted in comparison with a normal plasma level in pregnant women at term of 450 mg per 100 ml, with a range of 300 to 700 per 100 ml. When levels of fibrinogen fall below 100 mg per 100 ml, the blood loses its ability to coagulate effectively. Uncontrollable hemorrhage may accompany this syndrome, particularly in cases of abdominal delivery.

The explanation of fibrinogenopenia suggested by Page and associates and championed by Schneider holds that in severe cases of abruptio placentae the retroplacental clot releases thromboplastin into the maternal circulation, producing intravascular coagulation with consumption of several coagulation factors, especially fibrinogen. Although this hypothesis is appealing because of its simplicity, confirmatory evidence, other than the depletion of fibrinogen and other coagulation factors, is lacking. The extent of intravascular clotting has been seriously questioned. If this were a phenomenon of prime importance, disseminated intravascular deposition of fibrin in fatal cases of abruptio placentae should not be so rarely described (Schneider). Sudden death, furthermore, similar to that following amniotic fluid embolism, should be more common. Nevertheless, the major mechanism in the genesis of the coagulation defects of abruptio placentae almost certainly is the induction of coagulation retroplacentally and especially intravascularly. As the result there is consumption of fibrinogen, platelets, factors V and VIII, and to a lesser degree prothrombin. Another consequence of importance is the induction of fibrinolytic activity, which lyses the microemboli of fibrin, thereby maintaining patency of the microcirculation. The degradation products of fibrin, in turn, can further alter the coagulation mechanism. These breakdown products are capable of slowing the rate of conversion of fibrinogen to fibrin clot by thrombin, qualitatively altering the fibrin threads that make up the clot, and impairing platelet function by inhibiting aggregation (Pritchard). Some of these changes in fibrinogen-fibrin conversion led Beller to propose the concept of dys-fibrinogenemia.

Fibrinolysis. Phillips believes that there is evidence to show that activation of the fibrinolytic system plays a role in coagulation defects associated with abruptio placentae. Although ϵ-aminocaproic acid therapy has been suggested to inhibit formation of plasmin (fibrinolysis), it should never be used unless there is unequivocal evidence of intense hyperplasminemia and other measures fail to control hemorrhage (Ratnoff). Hyperplasminemia is probably protective in the presence of intravascular coagulation.

Further discussions of fibrinogenopenia in abruptio placentae are found in the papers of Weiner, Reid, and Roby; Schneider; Page and associates; Jackson and co-workers; Pritchard; and Phillips and colleagues.

Uteroplacental Apoplexy (Couvelaire Uterus). In the severer forms of abruptio placentae, widespread extravasations of blood often take place into the uterine musculature and beneath the uterine serosa. Such effusions of blood are also seen occasionally beneath the tubal serosa, in the connective tissue of the broad ligaments, and in the substance of the ovaries. This hemorrhagic process, which often accompanies the more advanced degrees of abruptio placentae, was appropriately called "uteroplacental apoplexy" by Couvelaire, who first described it in 1912. The phenomenon, frequently called *Couvelaire uterus,* is an extreme form of uteroplacental apoplexy, in which the entire uterus may undergo a bluish, purplish, coppery discoloration, with the adnexa showing the same changes (Fig. 9). The blood that causes these alterations in color may also insinuate itself between the muscle fibers of the uterine wall, as shown in Figures 10 and 11.

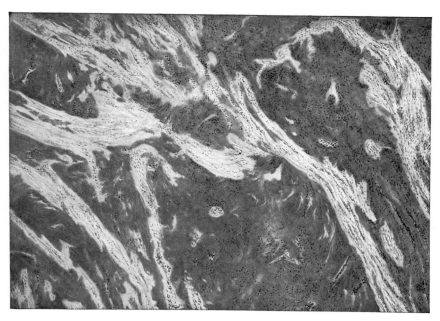

Fig. 10. Section through uterine wall from a case of abruptio placentae showing dissociation of the muscular fibers by hemorrhage. Light areas represent muscle; dark areas, effused blood.

These myometrial hematomas rarely interfere with uterine contractions sufficiently to produce postpartum hemorrhage.

It is impossible to give an accurate estimate of the incidence of Couvelaire uterus because the condition can only be demonstrated conclusively at cesarean section.

Acute Renal Failure. Acute renal failure that persists for any length of time is a rare occurrence in abruptio placentae and is probably seen only in the very severest forms. Many patients with placental abruption, however, show varying degrees of oliguria and a few show azotemia following delivery. At the Kings County Hospital, acute renal failure of a degree sufficient to merit treatment occurs in about 1 per cent of cases of abruptio placentae. Pritchard and Brekken found proteinuria in 48 per cent of their severe cases, but renal failure in only 4 per cent. Schreiner showed that about 25 per cent of patients with acute renal failure, in a dialysis unit emanated from the obstetric and gynecologic service. The data from Kings County Hospital are similar. Approximately 40 per cent of pa-

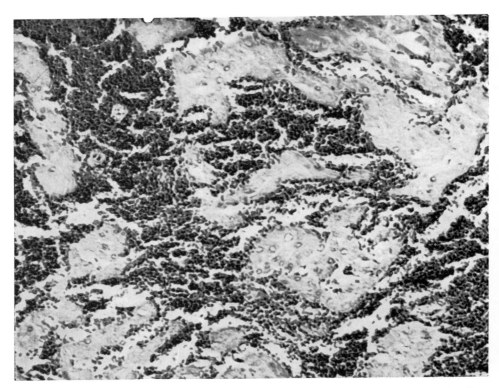

Fig. 11. Couvelaire uterus showing extrusion of blood between the uterine muscular bundles.

tients referred to our renal unit from the obstetric service have abruptio placentae. Complete cortical necrosis, however, is a rare complication of placental abruption.

The exact cause of the renal tubular damage associated with this condition is unknown. The major etiologic factor, however, is probably blood loss and severe intrarenal vasospasm. Carriere and co-workers showed that in dogs subjected to hemorrhagic hypotension, the renal medullary flow was well maintained for several hours after blood loss. The renal cortical flow, however, was diminished by trauma and mild hemorrhage even though the blood pressure remained normal. With further hemorrhage and prolonged shock there was marked shunting of the cortical blood flow to the medulla. The resulting cortical ischemia probably sometimes results in focal cortical necrosis. A similar mechanism is probably involved in human subjects with postoperative renal failure. There is no reason to believe that renal failure associated with abruptio placentae has a different cause.

These complications of placental abruption occur mainly with concealed hemorrhage. They are related to the intensity and the duration of the shock and hemorrhage. It is, therefore, evident that not only is restoration of adequate circulation by use of blood and electrolytes contained in aqueous fluid mandatory, but in severe cases with uncontrolled hemorrhage immediate delivery is necessary to prevent or ameliorate these complications. The low incidence of posttraumatic acute renal failure in the combat zone in Vietnam is further proof of the value of such prompt and vigorous treatment (Whelton and Donadio).

Treatment. The current treatment of placental abruption comprises (1) appropriate steps to make blood immediately available for multiple transfusions; (2) estimation of plasma fibrinogen by a simple, rapid technic, with repetition of the test approximately every hour until after delivery; (3) monitoring of urinary output; (4) monitoring of central venous pressure; (5) liberal use of intravenous fluids including blood transfusion; (6) administration of fibrinogen intravenously if the level in the plasma is critically reduced and there is excessive bleeding or a cesarean section is to be performed; (7) a program of obstetric management that includes delivery within about six hours of the onset of bleeding or symptoms; and (8) the general policy that no operative procedure (except artificial rupture of the membranes) be instituted until blood replacement has been initiated.

1. Blood for all patients must be typed and matched for possible transfusion promptly, although transfusion may not be needed in mild cases. If the case is even of moderate severity, 1,500 to 2,000 ml of blood should immediately be made available, because the process may progress, and in severe cases the total blood loss may exceed these amounts.

2. Since the more precise methods of measuring plasma fibrinogen consume time and demand full laboratory facilities, it is usually necessary to depend on some simple, rapid test to indicate whether the plasma fibrinogen has fallen to critical levels. The "clot observation test" of Weiner, Reid, and Roby meets these clinical needs. About 5 ml of blood are observed in a test tube for clotting. When fibrinogen concentration is reduced to a critical level, clotting may not occur at all. More frequently, however, clotting takes place, but when incubated at 37°C for one-half hour or so, the clot fragments and therefore appears to dissolve. This finding indicates a critically low level of fibrinogen. The test should be repeated about every hour until after delivery in all cases of abruptio placentae. For purposes of research a more precise quantitative test, such as that of Ratnoff and Menzie, should be employed.

3. Careful attention to the amount of urine excreted is essential to detect the earliest sign of renal failure. Barry and co-workers have suggested that acute renal failure can be prevented by reversing the oliguria with an infusion of mannitol. In severe cases of abruptio placentae, in which anuria or oliguria persists after sustained hydration, 20 g of hypertonic mannitol may be given intravenously during an interval of 5 to 10 minutes. Mannitol may be continued intermittently to maintain a urinary flow of 100 ml/hr.

It has been our experience that satisfactory results can be obtained if whole blood and lactated Ringer's solution are given in sufficient amounts to maintain the hematocrit above 30 per cent and the urinary output about 1.0 ml/min.

4. The central venous pressure furnishes an index of the status of cardiac return. If it exceeds 12 cm of water, it usually indicates overtransfusion, a common error in the treatment of shock. The insertion of a catheter into an antecubital vein is safer than the use of the subclavian vein in patients with a hemorrhagic diathesis (Wilson and colleagues).

5. Except in mild cases, blood transfusion is of transcendent importance. When shock and circulatory collapse are imminent, a venous cutdown should be performed to ensure uninterrupted parenteral therapy. In more advanced cases, simultaneous transfusion under pressure in both arms may be needed. This management demands the utmost in well-organized teamwork.

6. Ideally, 10 g of fibrinogen should be available at all times in every obstetric unit for cases of fibrinogenopenia. The amount of fibrinogen in blood

transfusions is usually less than 2 g per 1,000 ml. Although this amount is helpful in restoring fibrinogen levels, the quantity that can be so delivered is often insufficient in very severe cases. If plasma fibrinogen has been reduced to critical levels with clinical evidence of a clotting deficit, 4 g of fibrinogen dissolved in 10 per cent dextrose should be injected intravenously. Further administration may be gauged by the clot observation test. The danger of viral hepatitis is equivalent to, or greater than, that with the infusion of pooled plasma. This danger should not preclude the administration of fibrinogen; however, it should limit such therapy to cases of demonstrated need.

The use of heparin has been suggested on theoretical grounds to block active intravascular coagulation. Unfortunately, heparinization in the presence of a disrupted circulatory system as exists in abruptio placentae could lead to even more massive hemorrhage. Moreover, most evidence indicates that delivery is followed promptly by cessation of the consumptive coagulopathy.

7. Experience has shown that prolongation of the period of abruptio placentae is deleterious. The extent of the detachment may increase, the bleeding may increase, uteroplacental apoplexy may be aggravated, and the complications of hypofibrinogenemia and acute renal failure may supervene. For these reasons the injunction is to deliver the patient within about six hours. Rupture of the membranes therefore assumes a critical role in the management of abruptio placentae. This procedure should be carried out in all cases without obstetric contraindications, regardless of the condition of the cervix or level of the fetal head, as soon as possible after the diagnosis has been made. Intravenous oxytocin (10 units in 1,000 ml of 5 per cent lactated Ringers solution administered at the rate of 18 to 30 drops per minute) is an effective adjunct. If, however, the cervix is long and closed and the uterus is tetanically contracted, it is perhaps unreasonable to hope for vaginal delivery within a reasonable period of time. In such a case the abdominal route should be chosen.

8. Cesarean section becomes desirable in cases in which artificial rupture of the membranes and oxytocin do not bring on effective labor, so that delivery can be expected in approximately six hours. The time necessary to test the efficacy of the induction of labor should be utilized to replace the blood lost and combat the shock. In no circumstances should cesarean section be started until ample blood replacement is available and transfusion begun. It is a mistake to believe that the patient must be completely out of shock before beginning the operation, for in treating hemorrhage, of which abruption is in essence one form, the only effective method of therapy is control of the bleeding. This lesson has been demonstrated repeatedly in treating trauma and in managing ruptured tubal pregnancies, for example.

Rarely uteroplacental apoplexy may so interfere with uterine contraction that hysterectomy may be necessary; Couvelaire uterus in itself, however, is no indication for the operation.

Prognosis.   Although the maternal mortality of abruptio placentae was formerly very high, more intelligent methods of management have reduced it to 1 per cent or less, and many clinics can report series of several hundred cases without a maternal death. The maternal prognosis depends on the extent of placental detachment, total blood loss, degree of coagulation defects, extent of uteroplacental apoplexy, presence or absence of associated vascular disease, location of the hemorrhage (apparent or concealed), and finally the number of hours between the placental accident and treatment. Although it has been necessary to stress the importance of fibrinogenopenia and uteroplacental apoplexy in abruptio placentae, it must be understood that these grave complications occur in only a small minority of cases. In most cases, perhaps 80 to 95 per cent, the area of placental separation does not involve more than one or two cotyledons, and the maternal complications and mortality are negligible.

Since abruptio placentae is sometimes associated with acute or chronic hypertension, it has been customary to categorize cases of abruptio placentae as "toxic" or "nontoxic" and to regard the "toxic" cases as much more grave. When abruptio placentae is associated with acute or chronic hypertension, the hazards imposed by the two conditions are additive and the prognosis is inevitably worse. The severest examples of abruptio placentae, however, are sometimes seen in the absence of any previous hypertension. Proteinuria is usually evidence that some alteration of renal cortical blood flow has occurred; it does not necessarily indicate preexisting preeclampsia. Since proteinuria and oliguria may be signs of impending renal damage, they must be regarded quite seriously.

The mortality rate for the fetus in severe cases is almost 100 per cent. In mild or moderate cases the mortality rate depends primarily upon the stage of prematurity of the fetus at the time of the accident. The outlook for the fetus is further aggravated by any associated hypertensive disorder. Separation so extensive as to cause the loss of more than 2 liters of blood almost invariably results in fetal death. Because of these several factors the perinatal mortality is very high, ranging between 30 and 60 per cent, depending upon the criteria for diagnosis of abruptio placentae. Cesarean section may, however, reduce the perinatal mortality and morbidity in cases of placental abruption associated with fetal distress.

REFERENCES

Alperin, J. B., Haggard, M. E., and McGanity, W. J.   Folic acid, pregnancy, and abruptio placentae. Amer J Clin Nutr 22:1354, 1969.

Baker, J. L., and Dewhurst, C. J.   Accidental haemorrhage before the 28th week of pregnancy. J Obstet Gynaec Brit Comm 70:1063, 1963.

Barry, K. E., Brooks, M. H., and Hano, J. E.   Prevention of acute renal failure, in Renal Failure, Brest, H. N., and Moyer, J. G. (eds.). Philadelphia, J. B. Lippincott Co., 1967, p 259.

Bartholomew, R. A., Colvin, E. D., Grimes, W. H., and Fish, J. S.   Facts pertinent to a rational concept of abruptio placentae. Amer J Obstet Gynec 57:69, 1949.

Beller, F. K., Glas, P., and Roemer, H.   Fibrinogenolysis as a cause of obstetric hemorrhage. Amer J Obstet Gynec 82:620, 1961.

Bill, A. H.   The treatment of placenta previa by prophylactic blood transfusion and cesarean section. Amer J Obstet Gynec 14:523, 1927.

Brown, W. H., and Dippel, A. L.   The uses and limitations of soft tissue roentgenography in placenta previa and in certain other obstetrical conditions. Bull Johns Hopkins Hosp 66:90, 1940.

Browne, J. C. McC.   Localization of the placenta by means of radioactive sodium. Proc Roy Soc Med 44:715, 1951.

Carriere, S., Thorburn, G. D., O'Morchoe, C. C. C., and Barger, A. C.   Intrarenal distribution of blood flow in dogs during hemorrhagic hypotension. Circ Res 19:167, 1966.

Couvelaire, A.   (Two new observations on utero-placental apoplexy). Ann Gynec Obstet (Paris) 9:486, 1912.

de Rezende J., Nahoum, J. C., and Penna-Franca, E.   (Placental location by means of radioisotopes). Rev Ginec Obstet (Rio) 103:469, 1958.

Dieckmann, W. J.   Blood chemistry and renal function in abruptio placentae. Amer J Obstet Gynec 31:734, 1936.

Donald, I., and Abdullah, U. Placentography by sonar. J Obstet Gynaec Brit Comm 75:993, 1968.

Eastman, N. J. Editorial comments. Obstet Gynec Survey 20:506, 1965.

Fernström, L. Arteriography of uterine artery; its value in diagnosis of uterine fibromyoma, tubal pregnancy, adnexal tumor, and placental site localization in cases of intrauterine pregnancy. Acta Radiol, Suppl 122;3:55, 1955.

Fitzpatrick, E. H. The recurrence of placenta praevia in 5 consecutive pregnancies. Lancet 1:678, 1889.

Gilliatt, W. Placenta praevia in 4 successive pregnancies. Proc Roy Soc Med 17:3, 1923.

Goethals, T. R. Premature separation of the placenta; a statistical review. Amer J Obstet Gynec 15:627, 1928.

Gottesfeld, K. R., Thompson, H. E., Holmes, J. H., and Taylor, E. S. Ultrasonic placentography—a new method. Amer J Obstet Gynec 96:538, 1966.

Grieg, C. Observations on trauma as a cause of accidental hemorrhage. J Obstet Gynaec Brit Emp 58:817, 1951.

Gutierrez-Yepes, L., and Eastman, N. J. The management of placenta previa. Southern Med J 39:291, 1946.

Hendelman, M., and Fraser, W. D. A clinical analysis of abruptio placentae. Amer J Obstet Gynec 80:17, 1960.

Hibbard, B. M. Abruptio placentae, preeclampsia, and essential hypertension. J Obstet Gynaec Brit Comm 69:282, 1962.

———— The role of folic acid in pregnancy with particular reference to anaemia, abruption and abortion. J Obstet Gynaec Brit Comm 71:529, 1964.

———— and Herbert, R. J. D. Foetal radiation dose following administration of radioiodinated albumin. Clin Sci 19:337, 1960.

Hibbard, D. M., and Jeffcoate, T. N. A. Abruptio placentae. Obstet Gynec 27:155, 1966.

Hodge, K. E. Pelvic angiography; with particular reference to its value in intrauterine pregnancy after the fifth month of gestation. Amer J Roentgen 80:651, 1958.

Jackson, D. P., Hartmann, R. C., and Busby, T. Fibrinogenopenia complicating pregnancy. Obstet Gynec 5:223, 1955 (54 references cited).

Johnson, H. W. The conservative management of some varieties of placenta previa. Amer J Obstet Gynec 50:248, 1945.

Kitay, D. Z. Folic acid deficiency in pregnancy. Amer J Obstet Gynec 104:1067, 1969.

Kobayashi, M., Hellman, L. M., and Fillisti, L. Placental localization by ultrasound. Amer J Obstet Gynec 106:279, 1970.

Kohorn, E. I., Secker Walker, R. H., Morrison, J., and Campbell, S. Placental localization. A comparison between ultrasonic compound B scanning and radioisotope scanning. Amer J Obstet Gynec 103:868, 1969.

Krohn, L., Jaffe, H. L., and Adams, R. Radioisotope localization of the placenta by polaroid color scanning. Obstet Gynec 27:185, 1966.

Macafee, C. H. G. Placenta praevia. A study of 174 cases. J Obstet Gynaec Brit Emp 52:313, 1945.

———— Placenta praevia. Postgrad Med 38:254, 1962.

MacCarthy, T. Placenta praevia in 4 successive pregnancies. Brit Med J 1:95, 1928.

Malkasian, G. D., and Welch, J. S. Placenta previa percreta. Obstet Gynec 24:298, 1964.

Marais, W. D. Human decidual spiral arterial studies, Part VII. J Obstet Gynaec Brit Comm 70:777, 1963.

Martin, M. P., Bridgeforth, E., McGanity, W. J., and Darby, W. J. Vanderbilt cooperative study of maternal and infant nutrition. J Nutr 62:201, 1957.

McKelvey, J. L. Vascular lesions in the decidua basalis. Amer J Obstet Gynec 38:815, 1939.

Menon, M. K. K., Sengupta, M., and Kamaswamy, N. J Obstet Gynaec Brit Comm 73:49, 1966.

Millar, W. G. A clinical and pathological study of placenta accreta. J Obstet Gynaec Brit Emp 66:353, 1959.

Moir, C. Fallacies in soft tissue placentography. Amer J Obstet Gynec 47:198, 1944.

Nelson, J. H., Bernstein, R. L., Huston, J. W., Garcia, N. A., and Gartenlaub, C. Percutaneous retrograde femoral arteriography in obstetrics and gynecology. Obstet Gynec Survey 16:1, 1961.

Nesbitt, R. E. L., Yankauer, A., Schlesinger, E. R. and Allaway, N. C. Investigation of perinatal mortality rates associated with placenta previa in upstate New York, 1942–1958. New Eng J Med 267:381, 1962.

Page, E. W., Fulton, L. D., and Glendening, M. B. The cause of the blood coagulation defect following abruptio placentae. Amer J Obstet Gynec 61:1116, 1951.

Paintin, D. B. The epidemiology of ante-partum haemorrhage, a study of all births in a community. J Obstet Gynaec Brit Comm 69:614, 1962.

Paul, J. D., Gahres, E. E., Rhoads, J. C., and Dodek, S. M. Cr51 placenta localization and blood loss determinations in placenta previa accreta. Report of a case. Obstet Gynec 23:259, 1964.

Pedowitz, P. Placenta previa. An evaluation of expectant management and the factors responsible for fetal wastage. Amer J Obstet Gynec 93:16, 1965.

Penrose, L. S. Maternal age and parity in placenta praevia. J Obstet Gynaec Brit Emp 46:645, 1939.

Phillips, L. L., Skrodelis, V., and Taylor, H. C. Hemorrhage due to fibrinolysis in abruptio placentae. Amer J Obstet Gynec 84:1447, 1962.

Pritchard, J. A. Treatment of the defibrination syndromes of pregnancy, in Treatment of Hemorrhagic Disorders, Ratnoff, O. D. (ed.). New York, Hoeber Medical Division, Harper & Row, 1968.

———— Genesis of severe placental abruption. Amer J Obstet Gynec 108:22, 1970.

———— and Brekken, A. L. Clinical and laboratory studies on severe abruptio placentae. Amer J Obstet Gynec 97:681, 1967.

———— and Stone, S. R. Clinical and laboratory observations on eclampsia. Amer J Obstet Gynec 99:754, 1967.

Radtke, E. (On gynecological consequences of placenta previa). Zbl Gynaek 27:1521, 1903.

Ratnoff, O. D., and Menzie, C. A new method for the determination of fibrinogen in small samples of plasma. J Lab Clin Med 37:316, 1951.

———— Epsilon amniocaproic acid—A dangerous weapon. New Eng J Med 280:1124, 1969.

Record, R. G. Observations related to the aetiology of placenta praevia with special reference to influence of age and parity. Brit J Prev Soc Med 10:19, 1956.

Rigby, E. An essay on the uterine haemorrhage which precedes the delivery of the full-grown foetus, London, 1775.

Rivett, L. C., quoted by Dodd, B. J Obstet Gynaec Brit Emp 59:559, 1952.

Robertson, E. G., Millar, D. G., and Day, M. J. Placental localization by "colorscan" using iodine 132 labelled human serum albumin. J Obstet Gynaec Brit Comm 75:636, 1968.

Schmitz, H. E., O'Dea, N. J., and Isaacs, J. H. Placenta previa: A survey at the Lewis Memorial Hospital. Obstet Gynec 3:3, 1954.

Schneider, C. L. Coagulation defects in obstetric shock: meconium embolism and heparin; fibrin embolism and defibrination. Amer J Obstet Gynec 69:758, 1955 (60 references cited).

Schreiner, G. E. Causes of death in acute renal failure, in Acute Renal Failure, Shaldon S., and Cook, G. C. (eds.). Philadelphia, F. A. Davis Co., 1964, p. 107.

Solish, G. I., Masterson, J. G., and Hellman, L. M. Pelvic arteriography in obstetrics. Amer J Obstet Gynec 81:57, 1961.

Stone, S. R., Whalley, P. J., and Pritchard, J. A. Inferior vena cava and ovarian vein ligation during late pregnancy. Obstet Gynec 32:267, 1968.

Weinberg, A. Placentography: The radiological determination of the placental site. Obstet Gynec Survey 10:461, 1955.

———— Rizzi, J., McManus, R., and Rivera, J. Localization of the placental site by radioactive isotopes. Obstet Gynec 9:692, 1957.

Weiner, A. E., Reid, D. E., and Roby, C. C. Coagulation defects associated with premature separation of the normally implanted placenta. Amer J Obstet Gynec 60:379, 1950.

———— Reid, D. E., and Roby, C. C. Incoagulable blood in severe premature separation of the placenta: A method of management. Amer J Obstet Gynec 66:475, 1953.

Whalley, P. J., Scott, D. E., and Pritchard, J. A. Maternal folate deficiency and pregnancy wastage. I. Placental abruption. Amer J Obstet Gynec 105:670, 1969.

Whelton, A., and Donadio, J. V. Post-traumatic acute renal failure in Vietnam. Johns Hopkins Med J 124:95, 1969.

Wilkin, P., and Picard, C. (Does rupture of the marginal sinus exist? Anatomicoclinical study of vascular lesions of the marginal region of the human placenta). Bull Fed Gynec Obstet France 13:507, 1961.

Willett, J. A.   The treatment of placenta praevia by continuous weight traction—a report of seven cases. Proc Roy Soc Med 18:90, 1925.

Williams, J. W.   Premature separation of the normally implanted placenta. Surg Gynec Obstet 21:541, 1915.

Wilson, F., Nelson, J. H., and Moltz, A.   Methods and indications for central venous pressure monitoring. Amer J Obstet Gynec 101:137, 1968.

24

COMPLICATIONS CAUSED BY DISEASES AND ABNORMALITIES OF THE GENERATIVE TRACT

DISEASES OF THE VULVA, VAGINA, AND CERVIX

Varices.   Varicosities sometimes appear in the lower part of the vagina but are more common around the vulva, where they may attain considerable size and cause a sensation of weight and discomfort (Fig. 1). Vulvar varices may

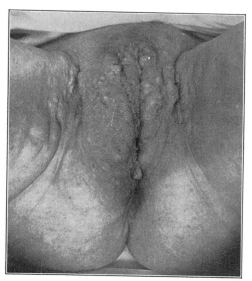

Fig. 1. Varicosities of vulva.

rupture during labor or cause increased bleeding during episiotomy, but the hemorrhage rarely leads to serious difficulties. In the case of vaginal varices, however, hemorrhage from rupture may be exceedingly profuse. Although both Solomons and Kimmel have shown that these varicosities can be injected safely and with excellent results during pregnancy, such a procedure is rarely necessary, for the discomfort can almost always be controlled by a perineal pad like that described by Nabatoff. In most instances, the varicosities disappear and become asymptomatic after delivery.

Inflammation of Bartholin's Glands.   Gonococci may gain access to Bartholin's glands and form abscesses. The labium majus on the side affected becomes swollen and painful, containing a collection of pus. Although the infection is usually gonococcal in origin, other bacteria may be secondary invaders. Aside from causing pain and discomfort, this complication may be the starting point of a puerperal infection. For these reasons drainage must be established whenever an abscess develops during pregnancy. The line of incision should be along the mucocutaneous junction between the vulva and vagina. After the contents have escaped, the cut edge of the abscess or cyst cavity is sutured to the overlying mucocutaneous margin using fine chromic catgut. A gauze wick is inserted to keep open the ostium so formed until granulation is complete.

The treatment of Bartholin's duct cysts, which are frequently the sequelae of abscesses, is best left until after delivery. They are usually small and therefore not the cause of dystocia. Occasionally a labial cyst is of sufficient size to cause trouble at delivery; in this case aspiration with syringe and small needle will suffice as a temporary measure. Definitive surgery, if necessary, should be postponed till later.

Condylomas (Condylomata).   Condylomata lata (Fig. 2) are small, flat, wartlike excrescences that are highly infectious. The *Treponema pallidum* of syphilis is usually present on dark field examination. Condylomata acuminata, however, are the result of neither syphilis nor gonorrhea. They are found with equal frequency in white and nonwhite women and have a high incidence in young primigravidas. Gorthey and Krembs believe that condylomata acuminata are often stimulated by the increased vaginal secretions associated with pregnancy. Rarely these lesions will regress during pregnancy. Infrequently, they attain enormous

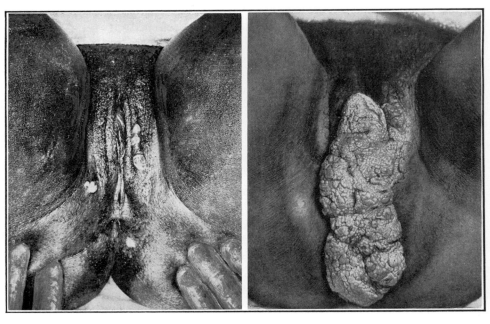

Fig. 2. Condylomata lata, annular lesions of secondary syphilis.

Fig. 3. Condylomata acuminata of vulva.

size (Fig. 3) and necessitate cesarean section. If the patient is seen several months before the end of pregnancy, the lesion can be removed by excision, fulguration, or painting with 25 per cent podophyllin. Gorthey and Krembs have reported one case in which treatment of an extensive lesion with podophyllin caused a severe systemic reaction and fetal death. We have had no bad results with small lesions.

Relaxation of the Vaginal Outlet.   Even in nulliparas the congestion incident to pregnancy frequently causes the anterior or posterior vaginal wall to protrude through the vulva as a redundant mass. In multiparas, particularly when the outlet is torn or relaxed, a distinct cystocele or rectocele may result. This condition is generally associated with dragging pains in the back and lower abdomen and may interfere with locomotion. It is not amenable to treatment during pregnancy, although the symptoms may be temporarily relieved by rest in bed.

Vaginitis.   This complication will be considered under the heading of gonorrhea and other infections (p. 802).

Vaginal Tumors.   Vaginal cysts, the most frequent of benign vaginal tumors, may be discovered during pregnancy or sometimes not until the time of labor. Such cysts, usually embryologic rests (Gartner's or müllerian), may be of sufficient size to cause serious dystocia. Treatment depends upon the size and location of the cyst as well as the time at which it is first recognized. Drainage or excision may be necessary. In other cases it may be more advisable to postpone treatment until after delivery and the puerperium. The treatment of vaginal cysts, as well as other vaginal tumors, is discussed on page 921.

Endocervicitis.   Gonorrheal and nonspecific infections of the cervical canal are frequently observed during pregnancy. The most prominent symptom is a profuse and persistent leukorrhea.

Papilloma of the Cervix.   Papillomas, as well as condylomata acuminata, are not quite so rare as suggested by Marsh's review, in which he was able to collect only 23 verified cases from the literature. Goforth and also Greene and Peckham have since added fairly large series. This lesion is frequently found in association with pregnancy. Grossly it is characterized by a wartlike area on the epithelial surface of the cervix, which may bleed quite easily. Microscopically it consists of an arborescent growth of connective tissue covered with normal-appearing epithelium. Occasionally there may be marked growth of the epithelium down into the wall of the cervix, and the cells may be disturbingly atypical. Such lesions are almost always benign, however, and are usually cured by local removal.

CARCINOMA OF THE CERVIX

The incidence of invasive carcinoma* of the cervix associated with pregnancy varies with race and environmental factors but shows an apparent increase as a result of the routine use of prenatal cervical smears. The lesion is reported to occur in from 1 in 450 to 1 in 6,000 pregnant women. The most recent reports, which give the highest incidence, no doubt reflect the improved case-finding. An additional factor contributing to the wide variation in reported incidence is the lack of uniform definition. In some reports only patients pregnant at the time of

---

* To avoid multiple repetitions of the adjective "invasive," the word "carcinoma" or "cancer" will be used hereafter to connote invasive neoplasm. The noninvasive variety will be designated by the term "carcinoma in situ" or "intraepithelial carcinoma."

diagnosis of cancer are included, whereas others comprise patients in whom the diagnosis of cancer is made up to one year postpartum.

Improvement in case-finding has lowered the average age from 36 to 32 years. Carcinoma of the cervix is uncommon in primigravidas; its highest incidence is in women who have given birth four or more times. In most cases the carcinoma probably antedates the pregnancy, but is first diagnosed at that time because of the requisite pelvic examination. Although a bloody, foul-smelling vaginal discharge is suggestive of the disease, most early cases are free of signs and symptoms and are detectable only by careful pelvic examination. Gross inspection of the cervix alone is no longer sufficient, but should be accompanied by a cervical cytologic smear in all patients regardless of age or parity. If the smears are abnormal, further diagnostic procedures should be carried out.

Although pregnancy was formerly thought to accelerate the growth of cervical carcinoma, more recent evidence does not support this concept. Progression of carcinoma in situ, furthermore, is probably not influenced by pregnancy (Johnson and co-authors). The age-specific and stage-specific cure rates are seemingly unaffected by whether the patient is pregnant or nonpregnant at the time of diagnosis (Waldrop and Palmer). The rate of growth appears to be an inherent characteristic of the neoplasm. The apparent acceleration of growth in some carcinomas during pregnancy may be related to the patient's age, which is often lower when carcinoma of the cervix is discovered in pregnant women. Way has shown that carcinoma of the cervix is often of a higher grade of malignancy in patients under 40 years of age.

Diagnosis.   Any persistent bleeding in pregnancy should suggest cervical carcinoma. Although in the vast majority of cases the hemorrhage is the result of threatened abortion, prolonged management of bleeding in pregnant women must not be based on that assumption without examination of the cervix. Failure to inspect the cervix and to obtain a Papanicolaou smear will cause occasional carcinomas to be overlooked.

When the cervix is exposed at the first prenatal visit, a Papanicolaou smear should be obtained routinely. It is also essential that a biopsy be taken of any suspicious lesions.

There is a divergence of opinion concerning diagnostic procedures and practice following the finding of a Class 3, 4, or 5[*] cervical smear in pregnancy. If there is no macroscopic lesion, some obstetricians believe a shallow cold-knife cone biopsy should be performed in all three situations. Others believe that a Class 3 smear, especially later in pregnancy, can be followed with punch biopsies and repeated smears; if malignant cells are present in the smear (Class 4 or 5), they hold that multiple punch biopsies are satisfactory. When these punch biopsies show carcinoma in situ, they then believe a cone biopsy should be performed in order to detect invasion. These diverse opinions are not likely to be reconciled, but all obstetricians insist that an accurate examination by a histo-

---

[*] Papanicolaou classification of vaginal smears:
   Class 1. Smear containing only normal cells.
   Class 2. Smear containing cells with atypical features, such as vacuolization, cytoplasmic granules, double nuclei, and nuclear enlargement, but not suggestive of malignant cells.
   Class 3. Smear containing cells with abnormal features suggestive, but not diagnostic, of malignant cells.
   Class 4. Smears containing malignant cells.
   Class 5. Smears containing malignant cells more bizarre than those in Class 4.

pathologist who is thoroughly familiar with the microscopic structure of the pregnant cervix is essential, to avoid confusing the normal gestational hyperplasia with carcinoma in situ. At Kings County Hospital, extensive experience with punch biopsy and conization of the cervix in pregnancy indicates that neither procedure when carefully performed leads to a greatly increased incidence of abortion.

Treatment. The treatment of carcinoma of the cervix in the pregnant woman is essentially the same as in the nonpregnant state. The underlying principle is the treatment of the disease, without regard to the pregnancy, except in the last trimester. Many clinics lean toward surgical treatment in Stage Ia (early stromal invasion or preclinical carcinoma). The choice of irradiation or surgical treatment in Stage Ib and Stage IIa depends on the medical condition of the patient and the training of the medical personnel. If the patient has a serious medical complication, such as organic heart disease, surgical treatment should not generally be employed. Where there are no medical complications either radiotherapy or surgical treatment, in well-trained hands, gives good results. If physicians with special training, in either radiotherapy or radical surgery, are not available, patients with cervical cancer should be sent elsewhere for treatment. In the first and second trimesters, radical hysterectomy with pelvic lymph node dissection can be carried out as soon as the diagnosis is confirmed. The prognosis is poorer after vaginal delivery if the pregnancy has progressed to the second trimester or beyond (Mikuta and co-workers). When irradiation is employed, it is better to perform hysterotomy before treatment if the pregnancy has progressed beyond the first trimester. In the first trimester, abortion usually follows the administration of 2,000 rads to the whole pelvis. The full dose of external radiation can then be completed. After involution of the uterus, radium is then given.

In the last trimester of pregnancy, a delay in treatment of a few weeks to assure adequate fetal development will not ordinarily aggravate the prognosis greatly. The infant should be delivered by cesarean section. If radical hysterectomy and pelvic lymph node dissection are to be performed, they can be carried out at the same time by properly trained gynecologists without greater difficulty than that encountered in the nonpregnant state. If irradiation is employed, external therapy can be started about ten days after cesarean section.

Prognosis. Kinch compared 75 pregnant patients with cancer of the cervix treated by irradiation with a control group of 402 nonpregnant patients of nearly the same age and stage of the disease similarly treated. The five-year survival rates for all stages were nearly identical, namely 44 and 45 per cent, respectively; those for Stage I were 64 and 68 per cent, respectively. Slightly higher survival rates were reported from the Radiumhemmet in Stockholm by Gustafsson and Kottmeier, who cite a rate for patients of all stages with a positive diagnosis during pregnancy of 52 per cent, and a five-year survival rate of 74 per cent for those with Stage I carcinoma.

The prognosis appears to be poorer if the diagnosis is made late in pregnancy. An explanation is difficult to find, but it may be related to delay and failure to diagnose the disease at the first prenatal visit.

Intraepithelial Carcinoma of the Cervix (Carcinoma In Situ). Intraepithelial carcinoma of the cervix, or carcinoma in situ, is a microscopic diagnosis, implying that the epithelial cells of the cervix manifest all the morphologic changes of cancer except stromal invasion. The International Classification of cervical cancer designates intraepithelial carcinoma as Stage 0.

The microscopic alterations in the cervical epithelium diagnostic of intraepithelial carcinoma are (1) loss of polarity of cells; (2) cellular pleomorphism; (3) alteration in nucleocytoplasmic ratio, with large, irreguar, and hyperchromatic nuclei containing numerous mitotic figures; (4) cellular changes ordinarily involving the full thickness of the epithelium; and (5) "basement membrane" that is relatively straight.

The normal changes in the epithelium lining the cervical canal during pregnancy have been described by Nesbitt and Hellman. According to Rosenthal and Hellman, the changes are caused by prolonged estrogenic stimulation, which they found to produce similar changes in the fetal cervix. Hyperplasia of the reserve or basal cells of the endocervix is often pronounced, and is occasionally so atypical that it may be mistaken for intraepithelial carcinoma by the inexperienced observer. Unlike carcinoma in situ, this estrogen-induced response is, of course, reversible. Carcinoma in situ, however, persists after pregnancy, as emphasized by Peckham and associates and later confirmed by Marsh and Fitzgerald and by Dean, Isbell, and Woodward. In an analysis of 28 women with preinvasive carcinoma of the cervix during pregnancy, Dean found that the lesion persisted in all cone biopsies performed six weeks to three months postpartum.

The increasing frequency with which intraepithelial carcinoma in pregnant women is being detected is illustrated by the following figures from Kings County Hospital:

1950–1959	1:2,000
1960–1964	1:1,074
1965–1969	1:455

Similar data are reported by others. Jones and co-workers found carcinoma in situ once in 328 pregnant women, and Shaffer and Merrill reported an incidence of 1 in 298. At Kings County Hospital one patient in three with a diagnosis of carcinoma in situ was pregnant or aborting (Hall, Boyce, and Nelson).

Carcinoma in situ associated with pregnancy is most common between the twenty-fifth and thirty-fifth years of life. The incidence is highest in women who have given birth several times. Once the diagnosis is made, pregnancy may be allowed to continue and vaginal delivery may be permitted without influencing the course of the disease. The two key points are accurate diagnosis and definitive therapy. The diagnosis must exclude invasive carcinoma, the treatment and prognosis of which are quite different. For accurate diagnosis, adequate tissue for histologic examination is essential. Multiple punch biopsies at least are required, but shallow conization is usually a much more satisfactory procedure in our experience. Mikuta, however, believes that conization should be avoided in the first trimester because of the danger of abortion. In some cases the smear may suggest invasive carcinoma. A visible lesion or indurated cervix requires punch biopsy, but a grossly normal cervix should be subjected to conization without delay.

According to Mussey and Decker, conization is not advisable during the last four weeks of pregnancy. If the cervical smear is suspicious or positive and if there is no obvious lesion for biopsy, it is wiser to delay conization until after delivery. If there is any possibility of invasive cancer, cesarean section is the wisest mode of delivery.

Transition of carcinoma in situ to invasive carcinoma often takes many years.

According to Petersen, who followed a large number of these patients, 4 per cent had invasive carcinoma after 1 year, 11 per cent after 3 years, and 33 per cent after 9 years. It is impossible to know how many years have already elapsed from the initiation of the lesion to the time of diagnosis. If the patient desires more children, particularly if she is nulliparous and under the age of 35, and if she is willing to submit to examination every few months, one or two more pregnancies may be permitted with reasonable safety. If, however, future childbearing is no longer desired, hysterectomy is the wisest course of action.

DEVELOPMENTAL ABNORMALITIES OF THE GENITAL TRACT

Incidence.   Developmental anomalies of the female genital tract are rare in obstetric practice, occurring in approximately 0.5 to 2 per cent of deliveries. Sheares found 134 congenital malformations in 29,726 patients, a ratio of 1:222. Zabriskie reported 92 malformations in 29,939 pregnant women, a ratio of 1:321. These figures doubtless represent underreporting, particularly of minor malformations. Since some of these anomalies contribute to serious fetal and maternal hazards, and since there has been recent revival of interest in plastic operations to correct these deformities, knowledge of the embryology of these defects and their obstetric significance is relevant.

Embryology and Significance.   Because fusion of the müllerian ducts to form a single reproductive tract in the human female takes place at three different levels at three different times, a variety of malformations may result. According to W. S. Jones, the three principal groups of deformities arising from three types of embryologic defects may be classified as follows:

    1. The most common is absent or faulty midline fusion of the müllerian ducts. If complete, it results in entirely separate uteri, cervices, and vaginas; if partial, the defect may arise at any of the three levels or in combinations of any two levels (Fig. 4).

    2. There may be unilateral maturation of the müllerian system with incom-

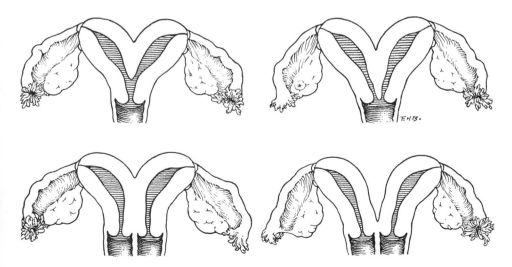

Fig. 4. Varying degrees of faulty midline fusion of müllerian ducts.

plete or absent development of the opposite side. The resulting defects are often associated with renal abnormalities on the affected side.

3. There may be defective canalization of the vagina resulting in a transverse septum or, in the most extreme form, absence of the vagina.

Various classifications of these anomalies have been proposed, but none is completely satisfactory. The terminology is often so complicated and replete with Latin words that the relative obstetric significance of the disorders is obscured. Both W. S. Jones and Semmens have proposed simpler classifications. The terminology used by Jones is outlined in Table 1.

Table 1. **Classification of Congenital Anomalies**

I. UTERUS (Four types of uterine fundi are recognized)
   1. *Single.* The normal symmetric uterus. In this category is included the saddle-shaped "arcuate" uterus, which some authors classify separately as the lowest grade of abnormality.
   2. *Septate.* Essentially normal on external examination, with little or no notching. Internally, a septum of varying thickness extends part or all of the way from fundus to cervix, dividing the uterine cavity into two more or less distinct compartments.
   3. *Bicornuate.* The Y-shaped forked uterus occurs in a wide range of varieties. Externally it may have only a shallow notch or a nubbin of rudimentary horn; or it may be cleft so deeply to the level of the cervix as to be called a "double uterus." The internal septum may be partial, or it may extend down to the cervix, dividing the interior into separate cavities. The distinguishing characteristic of this uterus, regardless of the extent of fundal notching, is the cervix. The term "bicornuate" should be limited to a forked uterus having a single or septate cervix, but never to one with a true double cervix.
   4. *Double.* This designation is reserved for complete failure of midline fusion, producing two small uteri each with its distinct cervix. This is the classical *uterus didelphys.* A comparable substandard miniature uterus results from maturation of a single müllerian tract. This small uterus derived from a single müllerian anlage may be referred to as a *hemiuterus.*

II. CERVIX (There are three types of cervices)
   1. *Single.* The normal cervix.
   2. *Septate.* A unit consisting of a single muscular ring partitioned by a septum that is either the downward continuation of a uterine septum or the upward extension of a vaginal septum.
   3. *Double.* Two distinct cervices. Both a septate and a true double cervix are frequently associated with vaginal septa, with the result that many septate cervices are erroneously classified as double. The diagnosis depends on careful visual and digital examination and is of great clinical importance. It is preferable to refer to the units of a true double cervix and to the cervix resulting from unilateral müllerian maturation as a *hemicervix.*

III. VAGINA (The vagina can be classified similarly)
   1. *Single.* The normal vagina.
   2. *Septate.* More or less complete *longitudinal septum.*
   3. *Double.* It is often difficult to distinguish the double from the completely septate vagina. The true double vagina includes a double introitus and resembles a double-barreled shotgun, with each passage terminating in a distinct, separate cervix.
      Transverse vaginal septa are of different developmental origin, resulting from faulty canalization of the united müllerian anlage.

   Modified from W. S. Jones.

The obstetric significance of these defects can be anticipated if a little thought is given to the function of each segment of the genital tract. The vagina rarely presents serious anomalies. The various septa are easily dilated, displaced, or surgically divided. The cervix, however, must undergo effacement and dilatation during labor. The septate cervix functions fairly well in these respects, but there is danger of septal rupture and consequent hemorrhage. The cervix that is derived from only one müllerian duct, as in the case of complete failure of fusion, may cause dystocia by its failure to dilate. The major difficulties arise from anomalies of the uterus, which not only must contract efficiently but must comprise a sufficient mass of tissue to permit enlargement during pregnancy adequate to accommodate a term-sized fetus in a proper longitudinal lie. The defects resulting from maturation of only one müllerian duct or from complete or almost complete lack of fusion often fail to allow for sufficient hypertrophy and thus give rise to a host of possible difficulties, including abortion, uterine rupture, uterine dysfunction, prematurity, pathologic lie, and abnormal placental adherence. Since lesser defects of fusion lead to proportionately less serious obstetric difficulties, patients with relatively common minor abnormalities such as arcuate or partially septate uteri may be expected to have relatively normal deliveries.

Diagnosis. Some malformations are discovered by simple inspection, and others by bimanual examination. They are occasionally noted first at delivery during manual removal of the placenta. Fundal notching, palpated abdominally in the third trimester, is indicative of a malformed uterus in 90 per cent of cases. Hysterography is important to ascertain the configuration of the uterine cavity (Figs. 5 and 6). Without radiologic examination or direct visualization of the

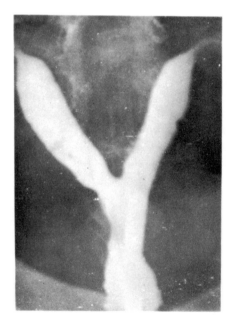

Fig. 5. Hysterogram of a bicornuate uterus. (Courtesy of Dr. Alvin Siegler.)

uterine surface, it is almost impossible to distinguish the septate from the bicornuate uterus (Siegler).

When a genital malformation is found, pyelography is indicated because of the frequent association of anomalies of the urinary tract. Woolf and Allen reported major renal involvement in 15 women who had asymmetric development of the müllerian ducts (unicornis, rudimentary horn, and didelphys with imperforate vagina). When there was uterine atresia on one side, ipsilateral urologic anomalies occurred in almost 100 per cent of cases. Renal agenesis was the most frequent malformation. Chromosomal studies may be relevant in these patients.

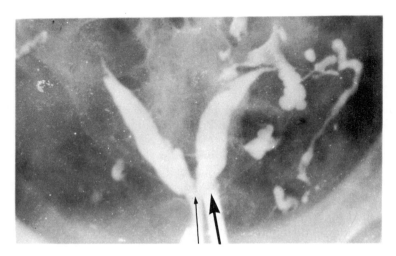

Fig. 6. Hysterogram of a uterus didelphys. (Courtesy of Dr. Alvin Siegler.)

Treatment.   Specific treatment is required in surprisingly few instances during labor. Vaginal septa can often be divided without causing serious hemorrhage. Even with more pronounced abnormalities, no special treatment is required if labor progresses normally. Abnormal presentations are generally treated in the same way as when they occur in normal uteri. If uterine inertia occurs, it is unwise to stimulate these defective uteri; cesarean section is the safe treatment. Unfortunately, however, the diagnosis is often unexpected. Rarely, pregnancy occurs simultaneously in both hemiuteri (Halbert and Longhead) or in a rudimentary horn. Rolen and colleagues have reviewed the histories of 70 pregnancies in rudimentary uterine horns. Although a few live births have been reported, the average duration of pregnancy before uterine rupture is only about 20 weeks. Intraperitoneal hemorrhage may be voluminous. Sometimes it is technically possible to remove only the damaged horn, in which case the larger horn may be preserved.

When a patient presents with a major uterine anomaly and a poor obstetric history with repeated abortions, plastic repair of the defect may be justified. Strassmann reviewed the results of 289 metroplasties. A fetal survival of 10 per cent before the operation contrasted with a figure of 86 per cent postoperatively.

Prognosis.   With minor uterine defects the prognosis is excellent. Most reports in the literature include only obvious major defects. In these situations also, except for uterine rupture, the prognosis for the mother is generally good. Cesarean section is, of course, more frequently required. It was employed by Semmens and by W. S. Jones in 15 and 29 per cent of their cases, respectively. The occurrence of prematurity is at least two or three times the normal rate, as shown in Table 2; consequently, the perinatal loss may range from 15 to 30 per cent. The abortion rate is also extremely high.

Sacculation of the Uterus.   This is a rare abnormality according to Eisenstein and Posner, who found fewer than 15 reported cases. It is essentially a pouch or sac in the uterine wall formed of very thin myometrium and often connected to the pregnant uterus by a relatively narrow neck (Fig. 7). Fetal parts often occupy the sac. Inasmuch as the abnormality appears most frequently in multigravidas,

Table 2. Abortion and Prematurity Associated with Congenital Malformations of the Uterus

(Total of Previous and Present Pregnancies)

	Abortion Rate (per cent)		Prematurity Rate (per cent)		Total No. of Pregnancies
	Series	Control	Series	Control	
Smith (1931)	23.15	14.5	29.4	12.7	81
Miller (1922)	28.3	—	10.4	—	67
Fenton and Singh (1952)	16.5	5.6	8.3	—	146
Baker et al. (1953)	18.9	—	20.0	—	127
MacGregor (1957)	45.0	—	22.0	—	42
Blair (1960)	48.0	—	—	—	147

From Blair, R. G. *J Obstet Gynaec Brit Emp* 67:36, 1960.

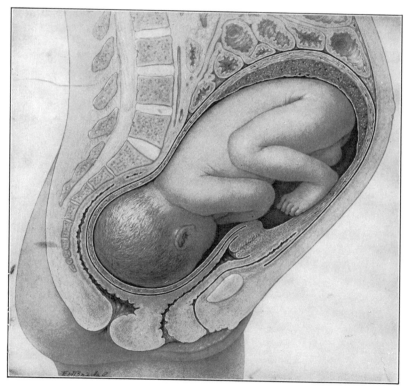

Fig. 7. Posterior sacculation of pregnant uterus.

the fundamental defect is thought to be a localized deficiency of uterine muscle, which gradually develops into a sac as a result of stretching incident to repeated pregnancies. Because fetal parts are often trapped in the sac and effective labor rarely supervenes, the diagnosis is most frequently made at cesarean section.

DISPLACEMENT OF THE UTERUS

Anteflexion. Exaggerated degrees of anteflexion are frequently observed in the early months of pregnancy, but are usually without significance. In the later months, particularly when the pelvis is markedly contracted or the abdominal walls are very lax, the uterus may fall forward; the sagging occasionally is so exaggerated that the fundus lies considerably below the lower margin of the symphysis pubis. Even in less striking instances of so-called *pendulous abdomen,* the patient may complain of various annoying symptoms, especially exhaustion on exertion and dragging pains in the back and lower abdomen. Amelioration of symptoms is frequently effected by wearing a properly fitted abdominal support.

Retrodisplacement of the Pregnant Uterus.   Retroflexion and retroversion of the uterus usually undergo spontaneous corrections during the third month of pregnancy. Posterior positions of the uterus are considered a normal variant of uterine position. They can no longer be regarded as factors predisposing to either abortion or the multitude of symptoms formerly attributed to them.

On very rare occasions the growing uterus is *incarcerated* in the hollow of the sacrum (Fig. 8). As the uterus grows, the cervix is pushed forward behind

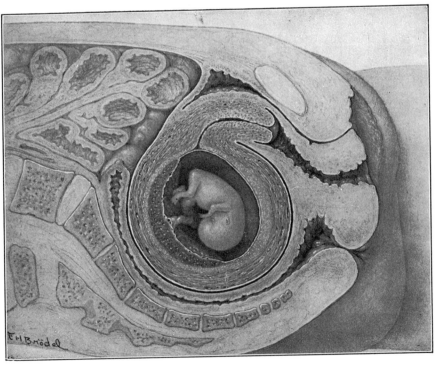

Fig. 8. Incarceration of retroflexed pregnant uterus.

the symphysis to impinge on the bladder neck. The patient is usually first seen complaining of abdominal discomfort and inability to void. As pressure from the full bladder increases, small amounts of urine are passed involuntarily, but the bladder can never empty itself entirely (*paradoxical incontinence*). After emptying the bladder by catheterization, the uterus can usually be easily pushed out of the pelvis when the patient is placed in the knee-chest position; anesthesia is rarely necessary. A retention catheter should be used until bladder tone returns.

Prolapse of the Pregnant Uterus. Impregnation in a totally prolapsed uterus is very rare because of the difficulty of successful coitus, but impregnation when the uterus is only partially prolapsed is comparatively frequent. In such cases the cervix (Fig. 9), and occasionally a portion of the corpus, may protrude to a vari-

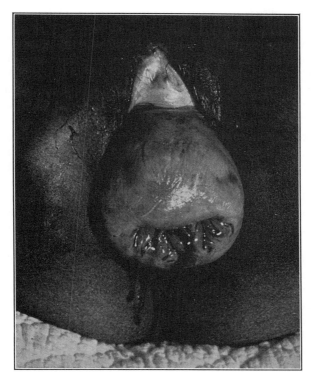

Fig. 9. Prolapse of cervix in pregnancy. Note extreme edema.

able extent from the vulva during the early months. As pregnancy progresses, however, the body of the uterus gradually rises in the pelvis, drawing the cervix up with it. As soon as the corpus has risen above the pelvic inlet, prolapse is, of course, no longer possible. If the uterus retains its abnormal position, symptoms of incarceration may appear during the third or fourth month, and abortion is the inevitable result. We have never seen pregnancy progress to term in the totally prolapsed uterus.

If there is a tendency toward prolapse during pregnancy, the uterus should be replaced and held in position with a suitable pessary. If, however, the pelvic floor is too relaxed to permit retention of the pessary, the patient should be kept recumbent as long as possible until after the fourth month. When the cervix reaches or slightly protrudes from the vulva, scrupulous hygiene is mandatory. Instances of fatal infection have been reported even without contamination by internal examination. If the uterus remains outside the vulva and cannot be replaced, it should be emptied of its contents.

When the vaginal outlet is markedly relaxed, the congested anterior or posterior vaginal walls sometimes prolapse during pregnancy, although the uterus may still retain its normal position. This condition may give rise to considerable discomfort and interfere with locomotion. It is not amenable to treatment until after delivery. During labor these structures may be forced down in front of the presenting part and interfere with its descent. In that event they should be carefully cleansed and pushed back over it.

In rare instances a true hernia may involve the vagina, and the resulting *enterocele* may form a mass of considerable size filled with loops of intestine. If the condition occurs during pregnancy, the protrusion should be replaced and the patient kept in the recumbent position. During labor the mass may interfere with the advance of the head. In such cases it should be pushed up or held as well out of the way as possible, to allow delivery of the head past it.

Torsion of the Pregnant Uterus.   Torsion of the pregnant uterus of sufficient degree to arrest the uterine circulation and produce an acute abdominal catastrophe is one of the rarest accidents of human gestation. Nesbitt and Corner reviewed this subject in 1956 and at that time collected 107 cases from the literature. Since then, Greening and Beck have added 5 more cases from North America alone. The rather frequent occurrence of this accident in cattle is of considerable importance, because it calls attention to one of the chief predisposing causes of the condition—namely, the bicornuate uterus. Whereas the normal human uterus is stayed on both sides by the round ligaments, which prevent undue rotation, such is not the case when pregnancy occurs in one horn of a bicornuate uterus. Congenital anomalies were present in 13 per cent of the collected cases, and myomas complicated torsion of the uterus in 30 per cent. In about 20 per cent of cases there are no visible etiologic factors. The pain and shock resemble those of abruptio placentae, but the vaginal bleeding in torsion of the uterus occurs rather late. Hysterectomy is the recommended treatment. The perinatal mortality exceeds 30 per cent.

Hypertrophy of the Cervix.   An abnormally elongated cervix seriously interferes with conception but, as a rule, does not complicate the course of pregnancy or labor. The canal usually becomes shorter preparatory to effacement and dilatation as term is approached. In one of our patients the vaginal portion of the cervix in the early months was 5 cm in length and the external os protruded from the vulva; later it underwent marked softening and reduction to normal dimensions, so that labor occurred spontaneously.

Acute Edema of the Cervix.   In very rare instances the cervix, particularly its anterior lip, may become so acutely edematous and enlarged during pregnancy that it protrudes from the vulva. This condition, if not associated with preexisting hypertrophy, may disappear on bed rest almost as suddenly as it developed.

Umbilical hernias are frequently noted during pregnancy but usually do not affect it. During the early months the uterus does not encroach upon the region of the hernial opening; later, when the fundus reaches the level of the umbilicus, it is usually too large to gain access to the hernial sac. When the abdomen is markedly pendulous, however, such an occurrence is possible. Much more common are cases in which the cicatrix of an abdominal incision yields as a consequence of the increased intraabdominal pressure of pregnancy and forms along the linea alba a hernial sac into which the pregnant uterus often makes it way, covered merely by a thin layer of skin, fascia, and peritoneum.

A similar condition is occasionally observed in women suffering from extensive *diastasis recti*. Ordinarily, such separation of the muscles of the abdominal wall has no effect upon pregnancy, although it may add markedly to the discomfort of the patient. Temporary relief is frequently obtained by maintaining the uterus in its normal position by a properly fitting binder. During labor, because of the loss of muscular tone in the abdominal walls, the second stage is likely to be prolonged, and the use of forceps often required.

MISCELLANEOUS CONDITIONS

Hydrorrhea Gravidarum.   Very rarely pregnant women may lose small amounts of clear fluid from the vagina throughout the greater part of pregnancy. Usually, only scant fluid is lost, but there are reports of the passage of more than 500 ml on several occasions. The cause of this condition is obscure. It has been said to arise from extramembranous pregnancy (Fig. 10), from hypertrophic changes in the decidua, or, as Paalman and others believe, from circumvallate placenta.

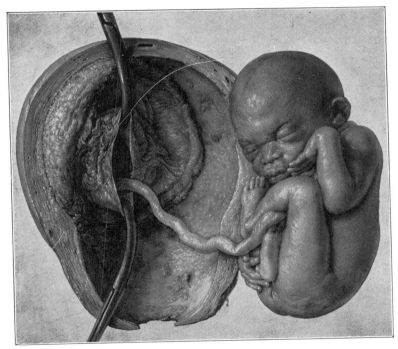

Fig. 10. Extramembranous pregnancy. Note collapsed fetal membranes held apart by clamps. (Drawing by Max Brödel, after Hofbauer.)

Previous Pelvic Inflammatory Disease.   When pregnancy occurs in women with previous pelvic inflammatory disease, considerable discomfort may result from the stretching of adhesions. Patients with extensive pelvic adhesions frequently have no symptoms during gestation; moreover, it is very unusual for such patients to have exacerbations of the inflammation at this time.

Pregnancy Complicated by Pelvic Tumors.   Pregnancy is occasionally complicated by ovarian or uterine tumors. Although, as a rule, they do not materially affect its course, they sometimes give rise to serious dystocia and will therefore be considered in detail in Chapter 31.

Because tumors of the ovary frequently cause dystocia, all disorders of the ovary will be discussed on page 928.

Endometriosis.   Since endometriosis is frequently associated with sterility, it is an uncommon complication of pregnancy. As emphasized in Scott's extensive study of the subject, however, patients suffering from endometriosis occasionally do become pregnant and, in the course of gestation, sometimes exhibit bizarre and vexing clinical pictures.

Rectovaginal endometriosis may present symptoms simulating threatening abortion. Ovarian endometriosis is perhaps less frequently seen, 7 cases having been published. Scott reported a very rare complication of ovarian endometriosis in pregnancy, rupture of an endometrial cyst, with clinical features suggesting acute appendicitis. We have seen an enlarging pelvic endometrioma that produced dystocia in labor. Many patients with unrecognized endometriosis doubtless go through pregnancy and labor without complications, however.

Of the 12 cases of adenomyosis associated with pregnancy that Scott was able to collect from the literature, 5 were complicated by uterine rupture, 3 by postpartum hemorrhage, and 2 by dystocia resulting from the adenomyoma.

REFERENCES

Blair, R. G.   Pregnancy associated with congenital malformations of the reproductive tract. J Obstet Gynaec Brit Emp 67:36, 1960.

Dean, R. E., Isbell, N. P., and Woodward, D. E.   Cervical carcinoma in situ in pregnancy. Obstet Gynec 20:633, 1962.

Eisenstein, M. I., and Posner, A. C.   Sacculation of the pregnant uterus at term. Review of the literature. Obstet Gynec 23:118, 1964.

Goforth, J. L.   Polyps and papillomas of the cervix uteri. Texas J Med 49:81, 1953.

Gorthey, R. L., and Krembs, M. A.   Vulvar condylomata acuminata complicating labor. Obstet Gynec 4:67, 1954.

Greene, R. R., and Peckham, B. M.   Squamous papillomas of the cervix. Amer J Obstet Gynec 67:883, 1954.

Greening, J. R., and Beck, R. P.   Torsion of the pregnant uterus. Report of a case. Obstet Gynec 21:421, 1963.

Gustafsson, D. C., and Kottmeier, H. L.   Carcinoma of the cervix associated with pregnancy. A study of the Radiumhemmet's series of invasive carcinoma during the period 1932–1956. Acta Obstet Gynec Scand 41:1, 1962.

Halbert, D. R., and Longhead, J. R.   Uterus didelphys: Two patients with pregnancy alternating in each hemiuterus with a review of pregnancy and uterus didelphys. J Reprod Med 1:571, 1968 (30 references cited).

Hall, J. E., Boyce, J. G., and Nelson, J. H.   Carcinoma in situ of the cervix uteri. Obstet Gynec 34:221, 1969.

Johnson, L. D., Hertig, A. T., Hinman, C. H., and Easterday, C. L.   Preinvasive cervical lesions in obstetrical patients. Obstet Gynec 16:133, 1960.

Jones, E. G., Schwinn, C. P., Bullock, W. K., Varga, A., Dunn, J. E., Friedmann, H., and Weir, J.   Cancer detection during pregnancy. Amer J Obstet Gynec 101:298, 1968.

Jones, W. N., and Osbund, R. Cancer of the cervix in pregnancy. Southern Med J 53:199, 1960.

Jones, W. S.   Obstetric significance of female genital anomalies. Obstet Gynec 10:113, 1957.

Kimmel, L.   Practical approach to the treatment of varicose veins in pregnancy. Bull Margaret Hague Maternity Hosp 5:72, 1952.

Kinch, R. A. H.   Factors affecting the prognosis of cancer of the cervix in pregnancy. Amer J Obstet Gynec 82:45, 1961.

Marsh, M. R.   Papilloma of the cervix. Amer J Obstet Gynec 64:281, 1952.

———— and Fitzgerald, P. J.   Carcinoma of the human uterine cervix in pregnancy. Cancer 9:1195, 1956.

Mikuta, J. J.   Invasive carcinoma of the cervix in pregnancy. Southern Med J 60:843, 1967.

——— Enterline, H. T., and Braun, T. E.   Carcinoma in situ of the cervix associated with pregnancy. JAMA 204:763, 1968.

Mussey, E., and Decker, D. G.   Intraepithelial carcinoma of the cervix in association with pregnancy. Amer J Obstet Gynec 97:30, 1967.

Nabatoff, R. A.   Vulval varicose veins during pregnancy. A new support for effective compression. JAMA 173:1932, 1960.

Nesbitt, R. E. L., and Corner, G. W.   Torsion of the human pregnant uterus. Obstet Gynec Survey 11:311, 1956.

——— and Hellman, L. M.   The histopathology and cytology of the cervix in pregnancy. Surg Gynec Obstet 94:10, 1952.

Paalman, R. J., and VanderVeer, C. G.   Circumvallate placenta. Amer J Obstet Gynec 65:491, 1953.

Peckham, B., Greene, R. R., Chung, J. T., Bayly, M. A., and Benaron, H. B. W.   Epithelial abnormalities of the cervix during pregnancy. Amer J Obstet Gynec 67:21, 1954.

Petersen, O.   Spontaneous course of cervical precancerous conditions. Amer J Obstet Gynec 72:1063, 1956.

Rolen, A. C., Choquette, A. J., and Semmens, J. P.   Rudimentary uterine horn: obstetric and gynecologic implications. Obstet Gynec 27:806, 1966.

Rosenthal, A., and Hellman, L. M.   The epithelial changes in the fetal cervix, including the role of the "reserve cell." Amer J Obstet Gynec 64:260, 1952.

Scott, R. B.   Endometriosis and pregnancy. Amer J Obstet Gynec 47:608, 1944.

Semmens, J. P.   Congenital anomalies of the female genital tract. Obstet Gynec 19:328, 1962 (260 references cited).

Shaffer, W. L., and Merrill, J. A.   Carcinoma of the cervix associated with pregnancy. Southern Med J 62:915, 1969.

Siegler, A. M.   Hysterosalpingography. New York, P. Hoeber, Harper & Row, 1967.

Solomons, E.   Treatment of varicose veins in pregnancy. Amer J Obstet Gynec, Suppl 61A:266, 1951.

Strassmann, E. O.   Fertility and unification of double uterus. Fertil Steril 17:165, 1966.

Waldrop, G. M., and Palmer, J. P.   Carcinoma of the cervix associated with pregnancy. Amer J. Obstet Gynec 86:202, 1963.

Way, S.   Malignant Disease of the Female Genital Tract. New York, The Blakiston Co., 1951.

Woolf, R. B., and Allen, W. M.   Concomitant malformations: Frequent simultaneous occurrence of congenital malformations of the reproductive and urinary tracts. Obstet Gynec 2:236, 1953.

Zabriskie, J. R.   Pregnancy and the malformed uterus. West J Surg 70:293, 1962.

25

MULTIPLE PREGNANCY

The number of young ordinarily resulting from a single pregnancy is an inherited characteristic that is fixed for each species. The average litter size of mammals is loosely related to several other characteristics. The number of young is, in general, inversely proportional to the adult size of the species: the larger the animal, the fewer her young. Animals with gestational periods exceeding 150 days rarely have multiple young. Species that have only two breasts usually give birth to one offspring during each gestation; those with many breasts have multiple young. Most animals with a simplex uterus have single young, whereas most animals with a bicornuate uterus usually have more than one. The life-span of the species is also related to the number of young, inasmuch as mammalian species that live longest usually produce the fewest offspring.

The anthropoids, including man, ordinarily give birth to single young.

Miraculous litter size has been imputed to man, the most extravagant recorded example remaining that of the Countess of Hagenau. Mauriceau discusses the events in his textbook of 1668: "But I esteem it either a miracle, or a fable, which is related in the history of the Lady Margaret, Countess of Holland, who in the year 1313 was brought to bed of 365 children at one and the same time." It is likely that some mathematically minded midwife counted each vesicle of a hydatid mole as an embryo.

Between fancy and fact is the story of the birth of seven children at one time, the famous septuplets of Hamelin, more famous for its thirteenth-century Pied Piper. A tablet erected at the supposed spot more than two centuries later purports to authenticate this birth. In part it reads: "It came about in the year 1600, as man reckons time, at 3 o'clock in the morning on the ninth of January, she was delivered of two small boys and five small girls. . . . All peacefully died by 12 o'clock of the twentieth of January."

Several valid births of sextuplets have been reported. A South African case in 1903 was investigated by two English medical officers. Their report contains a photograph of the children, five boys and one girl. Four placentas were involved. An earlier case published by Vassali is equally well established. The total weight of the six fetuses born on the hundred-and-fifteenth day of pregnancy was 1,739 g. The four boys and two girls had a single fused placenta.

The birth of the Dionne quintuplets in May, 1934, stimulated great interest in multiple births of this magnitude. MacArthur and Ford have summarized 45 cases from the world's literature from 1694 to 1936. Thirty-four were published in the past 100 years and 11 during the previous century and a half. Obviously a greater proportion of multiple births is being reported currently. The Dionne quintuplets, largely because of the early skillful medical care they received, shattered all previous records for both group and individual survival. Previously no single quintuplet had survived more than 50 days and no entire set more than 15 days.

Frequency of Multiple Births.   In a large population there is a mathematical relation between the frequencies of twins, triplets, and quadruplets. There is, furthermore, a consistent and significant variation in the frequency of multiple births among different racial stocks. A mathematical relation between the various orders of multiple births was first stated by Hellin, who wrote that twins occurred once in 89 births, triplets once in 89^2, and quadruplets once in 89^3. Zeleny, to take into account the variation in frequency between one racial stock and another, generalized Hellin's law: "If 1:N is the ratio of twin births to all births in a large population during any period, then the ratio of triplet births during the same period is very near $1:N^2$. . . . The expected number of quadruplets is $1:N^3$."

Guttmacher analyzed the occurrence of twins and triplets among 88,876,745 births reported by the U.S. National Office of Vital Statistics during the period of 1928 to 1957 inclusive. Twins occurred in 1.09 per cent (1:90.3) of all births; therefore, according to the Hellin-Zeleny hypothesis, triplets should have occurred in 0.0119 per cent (1:8,154). Actually triplets were recorded in 0.0105 per cent (1:9,800). On the basis of these data as well as the earlier findings of Strandskov and of Hamlett in smaller population samples, it appears that the hypothesis is more a biologic approximation than a law.

The marked variation in frequency of plural births among different racial stocks can be most clearly demonstrated by considering three racial groups: white, black, and yellow. Guttmacher found the mean frequency of twinning among 77 million white births in the United States to be 1.05 per cent (1:93.3), whereas among 11 million nonwhite births, well over 90 per cent of which were Negro, it was 1.35 per cent (1:73.3). The racial difference was even more striking for triplets. The proportion of triplets to single births among whites was 1:10,200 and among nonwhites 1:6,200. Hamlett demonstrated that this difference between whites and Negroes was racial rather than environmental or climatic, and found an equal difference between the two races in the northern and southern states. Twinning in Japan is about half as common as in the United States. We have exact data on the 10,427,779 Japanese births recorded between 1951 and 1955 inclusive. Twins occurred in 0.64 per cent (1:155) and triplets in 0.0056 per cent (1:17,710). Komai and Fukuoka explained the low incidence on the basis of a frequency of two-egg twin births in the Japanese of only one fourth to one third that in the Caucasians or Negroes, whereas one-egg twin births occur with the same frequency in all three races. All magnitudes of plural birth are most frequent among Negroes and least frequent among yellow races, with whites occupying an intermediate position.

Etiology.   Twin pregnancy may result from the fertilization of either two separate ova or a single ovum; the first gives rise to double-ovum (dizygotic, fraternal) twins and the second to single-ovum (monozygotic, identical) twins. In the former case the ova may be from the same ovary, or one may come from each ovary; in the latter case only a single ovum is involved.

Some marriages appear to have an inordinately high frequency of multiple births. Greulich reported the case of a 35-year-old mother who in nine births delivered six pairs of two-egg twins and three single children. In some instances there is no hereditary background, but in many there is a family history of plural gestation. Oettle states that there is no doubt about the influence of heredity on the tendency to polyzygotic births, but it remains quite uncertain whether heredity affects the frequency of monozygotic births.

White and Wyshak furnished a partial answer to the question of the role of heredity in a study of 4,000 records of the General Society of the Church of Jesus Christ of Latter-day Saints. They found that women who are dizygotic twins produce twins at the rate of 17.1 sets per 1,000 pregnancies, whereas the wives of male dizygotic twins produce multiple pregnancies at the rate of only 7.9 per 1,000. These data are consistent with the hypothesis that the genotype of the mother, but not that of the father, affects the frequency of twinning.

This frequency is affected not only by race and heredity but by age as well. The significant correlation between maternal age and frequency of twinning was known to the famous Scottish obstetrician J. Matthews Duncan, who in 1866 wrote: "From the earliest childbearing period till the age of 40 is reached, that is, till a period when fecundity has become extraordinarily diminished, the fertility of mothers in twins gradually increases." Waterhouse corroborated the observation in an anlysis of the total births in England and Wales for the 10-year period 1938–1948. He extended his study to include an analysis of the additive influence of parity. Table 1, reprinted from Waterhouse, is based on the number of twin births per 1,000 total births.

Table 1. The Effect of Maternal Age and Parity on Twinning Incidence

Age of Mother	Number of Previous Children										Total
	0	*1*	*2*	*3*	*4*	*5*	*6*	*7*	*8*	*9*	*Total*
Under 20	6.3	7.2	8.9								6.4
20–24	8.2	9.3	10.7	11.3	11.9						8.7
25–29	10.6	11.7	13.0	13.9	14.5	14.5	16.4	14.6			11.6
30–34	12.4	14.0	15.7	16.4	18.0	17.8	18.1	18.5	18.8	17.0	14.6
35–39	13.6	15.4	16.5	18.3	19.4	20.0	20.1	21.9	20.7	18.7	16.8
40–44	10.0	11.8	12.3	12.5	14.1	12.8	15.0	15.1	17.3	14.2	13.1
45–49	11.3	6.4	4.2	6.8	5.4	7.4	6.0	6.8	8.5	7.7	6.8
All ages	9.8	12.2	14.3	15.6	17.1	17.2	17.9	18.6	18.7	16.1	12.2

One must conclude from his data, which are in agreement with several earlier studies, that increasing maternal age and increasing parity exert separate and independent positive influences on the frequency of twinning.

The studies of Waterhouse, Strandskov, Guttmacher, and many others have shown that the frequency of single-ovum twinning is almost wholly independent of heredity, race, maternal age, and parity, whereas the incidence of double-ovum twinning is strongly influenced by all four factors.

Fraternal twins may be of the same or opposite sexes and do not necessarily resemble each other more than do other children of the same parents. Identical twins are necessarily of the same sex and resemble each other closely. Approximately 33 per cent of twins born in the United States are identical, as indicated by Strandskov and Edelen. Monozygotic twins account for 34 per cent of white twins and 29 per cent of nonwhite twins. The incidences of dizygotic twinning in nonwhites and whites were 1.01 per cent and 0.74 per cent, respectively, whereas the monozygotic frequency was 0.41 per cent and 0.39 per cent, respectively.

Double-ovum twins are in one sense not true twins, since they result from the maturation and fertilization of two ova during a single ovulatory cycle. Single-ovum twins, in any sense, are true twins. Newman writes, "Strictly speaking, twinning is twaining or two-ing—the division of an individual into two equivalent and more or less completely separate individuals." Their mode of production has given rise to a great deal of writing, to which American investigators have made important contributions. Biologic investigations have shown that single-ovum twinning occurs frequently in many species and can be produced experimentally in several varieties of fish. It is also fundamentally related to the production of monstrosities, normal twins representing the complete, and monstrosities an imperfect, form of the same process of reduplication.

Stockard has shown that retardation in growth of the egg at critical periods of development is the essential factor. He has demonstrated that it may be caused either by exposing the egg to cold or by diminishing its supply of oxygen. When exposed to such retarding influences just before gastrulation, the egg may die, or its development may be arrested or slowed for a time. As a result, when growth is resumed, two embryonic areas will develop instead of one. If they are far apart, two separate individuals will be formed, whereas if the two areas are in partial contact, double monsters with varying degrees of union will result. Stockard further showed that one can alter the degree of duplication by changing the time at which the retarding influences are brought into play, again illustrating the close relation between single-ovum twins and double monsters. In human beings one can identify gradations between typical identical twins and the well-known Siamese twins, and between double-headed or four-legged monsters, monsters by inclusion, and finally teratomas. The Stockard hypothesis receives further support from sonographic studies in our own laboratory and in that of Donald in Glasgow (personal communication). Women who eventually abort have a higher than expected frequency of double gestational sacs (Fig. 1).

The most striking example of monozygotic multiple pregnancy is afforded by the armadillo, which gives birth to four or more young at a time, always of the same sex and all enclosed within a common chorion. The details of the

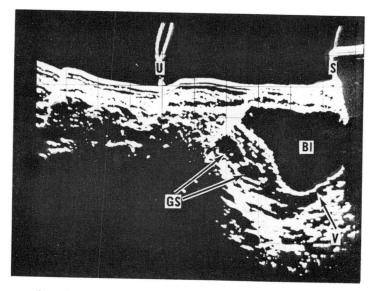

Fig. 1. Sonogram of an abnormal gestation. The uterus is small with apparently two gestational sacs. The growth rate was retarded and the patient eventually aborted. GS, gestational sac; Bl, bladder; S, symphysis pubis; U, umbilicus; V, vagina.

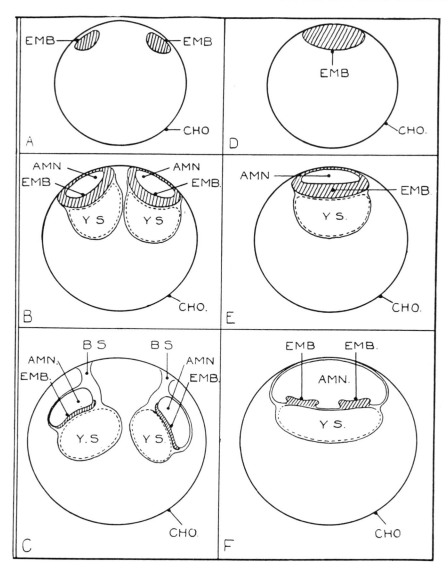

Duplication before formation of amniotic cavity.

Duplication after formation of amniotic cavity.

Fig. 2. Hypothetical diagrams of human monochorionic twins. (From Corner. Bull Hopkins Hosp 33:389, 1922.)

process have been exhaustively worked out by Newman and Patterson. An important feature is the prolonged period of delayed implantation with resulting retardation in growth and partial loss of polarity; when growth is then resumed, four embryonic areas develop instead of one. The biology of delayed implantation is presented in a modern symposium, edited by Enders.

Newman, in his two monographs *The Biology of Twins* and *The Physiology of Twinning*, states that single-ovum twins may be caused by (1) fission of the blastoderm, (2) double gastrulation, or (3) fission of the bilateral halves of a single embryonic axis. Corner does not discuss etiology but illustrates clearly the three processes by which a pair of monozygotic twins can be produced (Fig. 2): (1) separation of the early blastomeres, (2) duplication of the inner cell mass, and (3) duplication of the embryonic rudiment of the germ disc. In human beings single-ovum twinning does not necessarily represent an inherent attribute of the ovum; its cause may therefore be maternal environmental factors of which we are still ignorant.

Triplet pregnancy may be derived from one, two, or three ova. Single-ovum triplets are the least frequent, according to Sasse, who listed the ratios of frequency of the three varieties as 1:6:3. In the quintuplet pregnancy described by de Blécourt, three of the children shared a single placenta, and each of the other two had a separate placenta. The Dionne quintuplets, according to MacArthur, were derived from a single ovum. The Fisher quintuplets, born in 1963, had, according to Berbos, King, and Janusz, a placenta consisting of three main masses with a total weight of 1,800 g and a maximal diameter of 35 cm.

Since the introduction of agents to induce ovulation, largely the result of work by Gemzell in Sweden, the incidence of multiple births has increased. Fifty per cent of the first 100 women treated by Gemzell for anovulation with gonadotropins became pregnant. He reported 43 deliveries: 20 of a single infant, 14 of twins, and 9 of triplets or higher numbers. Since the birth of the Dionne quintuplets, Keast and Cooper have reported 3 additional sets who have survived the neonatal period. More recently Aiken has reported the birth of living sextuplets. The incidence of twinning in patients treated with clomiphene is reported by Kistner to be about 10 per cent, a figure lower than that induced by gonadotropins.

Sex of Children and Sex Ratio. In two thirds of twin deliveries only one sex is represented, and in one third of cases the twins are of opposite sex. In the 717,901 sets analyzed by Nichols, the children were both males in 234,497, both females in 219,312, and of opposite sex in 264,092 cases. The sex ratio of multiple births has been studied extensively (Strandskov, Edelen, and Siemens). The percentage of males in the human species decreases with increasing number of children per pregnancy. The sex ratio, or percentage of males, for 31 million United States single births was 51.59 per cent, whereas for three quarters of a million twins it was 50.85 per cent. The figure for triplets was 49.54 per cent and for quadruplets 46.48 per cent. Two explanations have been suggested. The differential mortality between the sexes of the fetus is well known, as it is for the infant during its delivery and for the child and adult during the postnatal period. Survival is always in favor of the female and against the male. The "population pressure" of a multiple pregnancy may possibly exaggerate the biologic tendency noted in single pregnancies. A second theory is that the female-producing egg has a greater tendency to divide into twins, triplets, or quadruplets. If so, the sex ratio of monozygotic pregnancies should be lower than that of dizygotic pregnancies, but an adequate analysis of the data has not been undertaken.

Anatomic Considerations: Relation of the Placentas and Membranes. The development of one child in either horn of a bicornuate uterus, or of one twin in the uterus and the other in a fallopian tube, affords indubitable evidence of their origin from two ova. In uterine twin pregnancy the examination of the placenta and fetal membranes frequently permits recognition of the mode of origin of the twins. When the fetuses are derived from a single ovum there is ordinarily a

single placenta from which two umbilical cords arise. When they develop from
two ova there are usually two separate placentas, although when originally inserted near each other their contiguous margins may fuse to form an apparently
single large placenta (Fig. 3).

In double-ovum twins, whether the placentas are separate or fused, there
are two chorions and two amnions, with each fetus enveloped in its two membranes. Single-ovum twins, as a rule, possess only a single chorion but two amnions. In rare instances a single amnion may be found. King and his associates
summarized the world's literature, collecting a total of 148 cases of monoamniotic

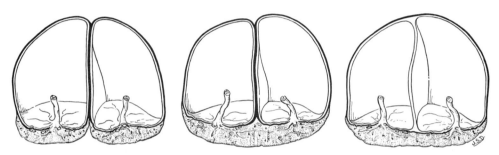

Fig. 3. Diagram showing relation of placenta and membranes in double and single twin
pregnancy. Left, double-ovum twins; middle, double-ovum twins, double membranes, single
placenta; right, single-ovum twins, one chorion, two amnions, and one placenta.

twins and adding five of their own. Since then, a number of isolated reports have
appeared. In 1963, Timmons and de Alvarez collected 62 cases from the American
literature. All of these reports emphasize the high perinatal loss associated with
knotting of the intertwining cords. Of the 124 babies in Timmons' series, in only
36 sets (72 babies) were both born alive. In another 6 sets, only 1 infant was born
alive, and in the remaining pairs both were stillborn. With 5 additional neonatal
deaths, the perinatal loss in this series was slightly over 41 per cent. There are
two etiologic suggestions: (1) the germ disc splits late, after formation of the
amnion; (2) the partition between the two amnions either is perforated or disappears early in pregnancy. Coulton and his colleagues postulate that late splitting
accounts for most monoamniotic twinning. Such division must occur between the
seventh and thirteenth day after fertilization, for later splitting gives rise to
conjoined twins. Despite the observation of a ridge on the chorionic surface of
the placenta in many monoamniotic pregnancies, it is doubtful that disappearance
of the amniotic septum accounts for more than a very small percentage of these
cases. Sinykin reported a monoamniotic triplet pregnancy with survival of all
three infants. The diagnosis may occasionally be made antenatally by the injection of a radiopaque dye to obtain an amniogram.

Siemens, Curtius, and others have questioned the possibility of ascertaining the
origin of twins from the relations between the placenta and its membranes; they lay
more stress upon the similarity or dissimilarity of the children particularly after infancy.

There is agreement that twins presenting two amnions with no chorion in the partition are from a single egg. If, however, there are two separate placentas, or one placenta with two amnions and two chorions in the partition, in some cases, the twins may still be monozygotic. If the fertilized ovum divides into two at a very early stage, each half may develop independently. Since there is not yet an embryo or a placenta, the separation is quite complete, with the result that two embryos (single-ovum but dichorionic twins), each with a distinct and separate placenta, are formed. If, however, separation occurs after differentiation into embryo and trophoblast, one placenta will form with a partition consisting of two amnions without intervening chorions.

The most frequently employed technic of ascertaining zygosity of twins is comparison of all blood factors, major and minor, which must show 100 per cent concordance. If such agreement is lacking, the twins must be from two eggs. A second technic is the comparison of handprints and footprints. These two methods together will establish zygosity in 96 per cent of cases. Robson and Harris have shown that human placentas may be classified into six distinct phenotypes according to the electrophoretic behavior of their alkaline phosphatases. Although concordance is not certain proof of monozygosity, discordance rules it out.

Several enzymes of the red blood cells can be differentiated into genetic types by starch gel electrophoresis. Identification of these isoenzymes provides further proof of zygosity.

Cameron and co-workers studied 1,424 pairs of twins in Ghent, Belgium, and Birmingham, England, employing blood groups and placental and red cell enzymes to ascertain the genotypes in 44 per cent of the cases where the sex of the infants was the same and the placentas were dichorionic. Approximately one quarter proved to be identical twins. Another highly reliable method employs reciprocal skin grafts. Only when the twins are from a single ovum will the graft behave like an autograft. The preliminary skin graft test was applied by Murray and his co-workers before they grafted a kidney from a healthy twin to his co-twin in renal failure. In their seven cases the skin grafts were observed for three weeks. In each instance they behaved like autografts, further justifying the subsequent renal transplantation.

Cameron and co-workers summarized their data on assessment of zygosity from the placenta in their study of 1,424 twin pairs as follows:

A. 22 per cent had monochorionic placentas and therefore presumably the twins were monozygotic.
B. 34 per cent of the twins were of opposite sexes and therefore dizygotic.
C. 44 per cent were of the same sex and the placentas were dichorionic.

The zygosity of this group was ascertained by the more refined technics previously described.

In summary, the anatomic relations of placenta and membranes will, in the majority of instances, indicate whether the twins are from the same or different eggs. In slightly less than half of the cases, however, a single ovum divides so early that the placental relations are precisely the same as those in a two-egg pregnancy. Benirschke and colleagues have reinterpreted the relations of the fetal membranes in multiple gestation in terms of the intersting hypothesis of "placental wandering," or *trophotropism.*

In triplet pregnancy the conditions are still more complicated. In the case of one egg, there may be a single large placenta with one chorion and three amnions, or with chorion as well as amnion in one or both of the partitions, depending upon the stage of division. In two-egg triplets, there may be a single large placenta resulting from fusion of the placenta of a single fetus with that of single-

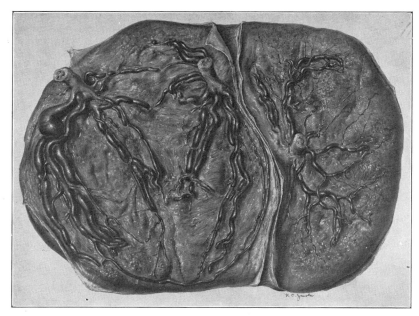

Fig. 4. Triplet pregnancy from two eggs. One child from the right side of the fused placenta, and single-ovum twins from the larger left side.

ovum twins, or the two placentas may remain separate (Fig. 4). In the case of three ova, there may be three separate placentas, each with its own chorion and amnion. Another possibility is two separate placentas, one single and the other fused, the latter a double-ovum twin placenta, as shown in Figure 5. A further anatomic result may be a huge single placenta, each embryo with its own chorion and amnion, as shown in Figure 6. In quadruplet and quintuplet pregnancies the conditions may be still more complicated.

In single-ovum twins especially, part of the placenta may have extensive anastomoses between the two vascular systems, resulting in mutual transfusion of the twins' blood. Theoretically, if during an early period the heart of one embryo is considerably stronger than that of the other, a gradually increasing area of the communicating portion of the placenta is taken over by the stronger twin, whose heart increases rapidly in size, while that of the weaker receives increasingly less blood and eventually atrophies. An explanation of the malformation known as acardius is thus provided. In extreme cases almost the entire placental circulation is appropriated by the normal embryo, while the malformed twin receives only enough blood to nourish its lower extremities; occasionally it is represented only by a shapeless mass of tissue, *acardius amorphus*. In its less severe form, a state resembling intrauterine parabiosis exists. In a review of the subject Naeye indicated that one twin receives most of the blood, becoming polycythemic with cardiomegaly. The other twin develops severe anemia and may require transfusions at birth, whereas the hypervolemic twin may require phlebotomy to prevent cardiac failure and hyperbilirubinemia. The hypervolemic twin may often

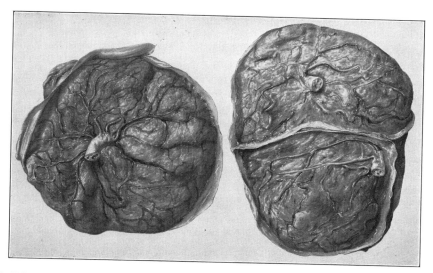

Fig. 5. Triplet pregnancy from three eggs. One child from the smaller placenta, and double-ovum twins from the larger fused organ.

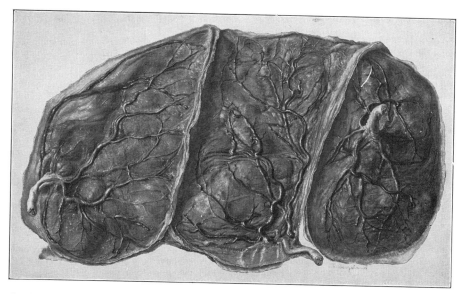

Fig 6. Fused three-egg placenta from a quadruplet pregnancy. One child from a single placenta not shown in the drawing, and three-egg triplets from the fused placenta.

have associated hydramnios, while very scant amniotic fluid may be found in relation to the other twin.

Infrequently in two-egg twins with a fused placenta a small area of vascular anastomosis is found, possibly accounting for certain cases of blood chimerism reported in adult twins. In such cases there is exchange of red and white blood cells in utero. Postnatally the twins have predominantly their own cells with a liberal admixture of blood cells of their co-twins. In the case reported by Booth, drumsticks were found in the nuclei of some of the polymorphonuclear leukocytes of the male twin. In another case the male twin's red cells were 86 per cent group A and 14 per cent group O, whereas the twin sister had 1 per cent group A and 99 per cent group O. The immunologic problems resulting from this chimerism are discussed by Benirschke and others in *Fetal Homeostasis* (Volume 4).

Ordinarily in twin pregnancies, whether derived from one or two ova, each child occupies roughly one half of the uterus, the long axis being directed vertically. Occasionally, however, they lie transversely with one fetus above the other. Twins are generally smaller and lighter than singletons, although their combined weight is usually greater than that of a single child. The smaller size may be considered normal, but in certain instances it may be explained by premature labor and birth of the twins several weeks before maturity, perhaps a result of the overdistention of the uterus.

It is not unusual for twins to differ considerably in size and weight. A remarkable difference is reported in a case of Sussi's, in which a living male weighing 3,110 g and measuring 48 cm was twin to a living female weighing 420 g and measuring 28 cm. In double-ovum twin pregnancy one fetus may die at an early stage of pregnancy and be expelled from the uterus soon afterward, whereas the other may achieve full maturity. More frequently, in both the single-ovum and double-ovum varieties of twinning, the dead fetus is retained until the end of pregnancy, compressed between the uterine wall and the membranes of the living child. This flattened and partially mummified twin is known as a *fetus papyraceus* or *fetus compressus* (Fig. 7).

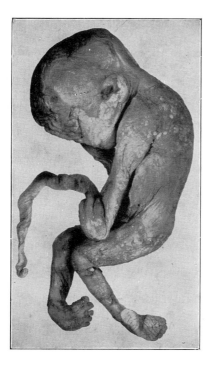

Fig. 7. Fetus papyraceus. Probably the result of a germinal defect; growth arrested in twentieth week. Twin pregnancy at term; other infant was normal. (Carnegie Collection No. 4159A.)

Superfecundation and Superfetation.

Superfecundation implies the fertilization of two ova within a short period, but not at the same coitus; in superfetation, several months, or an interval longer than an ovulatory cycle, intervene. Superfecundation is well recognized in lower animals and undoubtedly occurs in human beings, although it is impossible to ascertain its frequency. It is probable that in many cases twin ova are not fertilized at the same coitus, but the fact can be demonstrated only in exceptional circumstances. It is interesting that John Archer, the first physician to receive a medical degree in America, related in 1810 that a white woman, who had had intercourse with both a white and a colored man within a short period, was delivered of twins, one of which was white and the other mulatto. Since that time many instances of alleged superfecundation have been reported. In 1917 a most convincing case was recorded by Robertson in which a mare, covered by a horse and 10 minutes later by a jackass, gave birth to twins, one a horse and the other a mule.

The occurrence of superfetation has never been demonstrated, although it is theoretically possible until the uterine cavity is obliterated by the fusion of the decidua vera and capsularis. Superfetation requires, moreover, ovulation during the course of pregnancy, as yet unproved in women, though known to occur in the mare. Most authorities believe that the alleged cases of human superfetation result from either abortion of one twin or marked inequality of development. The arguments against the occurrence of superfetation were well reviewed by Meyer in 1919. Studdiford, in 1936, stated that he could find in the literature no proved case of human superfetation, but he presented complete histologic studies of two cases that superficially suggested superfetation. In each instance he was able to disprove the occurrence of superfetation. His explanation was ordinary twinning with the early death of one fetus and the continued growth of the twin, and he concluded that superfetation was most unlikely because of the inhibition of ovulation during pregnancy. A very interesting discussion of the legal aspects of superfetation appears in an editorial comment by Eastman.

Telegony implies that at the first conception the mother is affected by something that will be transmitted to later offspring, even though resulting from coitus with another mate. Some veterinarians hold that the breeding qualities of a prize mare or bitch inevitably suffer if she is ever covered by a male of inferior breed. Many physicians hold similar views, but qualified biologists contend that such opinions entirely lack foundation.

Conjoined Twins.

In this country united twins are commonly termed Siamese twins, after Chang and Eng Bunker, who were displayed all over the world for more than three decades by P. T. Barnum. Actually they were three-quarters Chinese and one-quarter Siamese. Double monsters have been known and recorded since antiquity. It was assumed until the nineteenth century that the phenomenon was caused by the intrauterine collision and fusion of two early twin embryos. It is now generally assumed that the cause is failure of the germ disc to split into two throughout its entirety. Most conjoined twins are *pygopagus* —that is, joined back to back with part of the buttocks, sacrum, rectum, and perineum in common. The females usually have a single vagina but separate uteri and cervices. Conjoined twins are of several other types, designated according to their shared structures. One of the common varieties is *omphalopagus*, a condition in which a portion of the abdominal wall is single. Conjoined twins of this form and of the *craniopagus* variety are the only types in which surgical separation has succeeded. Dystocia is rare in the birth of conjoined twins, since most of the union is of pliable soft tissue. If bone is shared, it is usually insufficiently ossified at the time of birth to prevent one twin from sliding ahead of the other in the birth canal, and the elastic bond is greatly stretched in the process. In one case of Siamese twins, the Blazek sisters, pregnancy occurred and delivery was uncomplicated.

Fertility of Twins.   There is an old canard that twins are less fertile than singletons. The misconception may result from the infertility of the female twin of a bull calf. In 95 per cent of such cases the female litter mate, termed a *freemartin,* has no uterus or ovaries and an infantile vagina, for in cattle twins of opposite sex the male gonadal hormone reaches the circulation of the female and inhibits the development of her whole generative tract. No such phenomenon occurs in the human being. As early as 1839, Duncan submitted the fertility of human twins to statistical analysis and found it not different from that of singletons.

Diagnosis.   The first indication of twins is sometimes afforded by the unusually large size of the uterus after the expulsion of the first child. Guttmacher, in his analysis of 573 cases of twin pregnancy, found that a correct diagnosis was made in only 50 per cent of the cases when both infants weighed less than 2,500 g, and in slightly more than 70 per cent when the larger twin was 2,500 g or more. Excessive size of the abdomen during pregnancy frequently leads to suspicion of twins, although the cause is usually some other condition. Because of relaxation of the abdominal wall and the resulting forward protrusion of the uterus after the birth of a first child, women pregnant for the second time sometimes think that they are carrying twins, although their suspicions are generally without foundation.

The diagnostic methods are abdominal palpation, ausculation, vaginal examination, roentgenography, and sonography. Sonograms obtained as early as the sixth or seventh week after the onset of the last menstrual period will sometimes reveal a double gestational sac. Sonograms of these patients should be repeated to detect the significant number of early double sacs that are abnormal and abort. If many small parts are palpated, twin pregnancy should always be suspected. Positive evidence is afforded by the palpation of two heads, two breeches, and two backs, or at least of one back and four fetal poles (Fig. 8). The detection of three fetal poles is not conclusive; in rare instances a myoma may be mistaken for the fetal head.

Auscultation frequently gives most valuable information. If two areas considerably removed from each other can be detected, in which the fetal heart tones can be heard, twins should be suspected. A positive diagnosis should not be made unless there is a difference of at least 10 beats per minute in the rate of the two hearts after counting the sounds simultaneously for at least a full minute. The diagnosis of multiple pregnancy by means of fetal electrocardiographic tracings has been reported by several authors.

In rare instances vaginal touch may reveal important findings. It is sometimes possible to distinguish a macerated head through the intact membranes. Occasionally a prolapsed and pulseless cord may be felt through the cervix, while auscultation gives positive evidence of a living child. Moreover, discovery of a

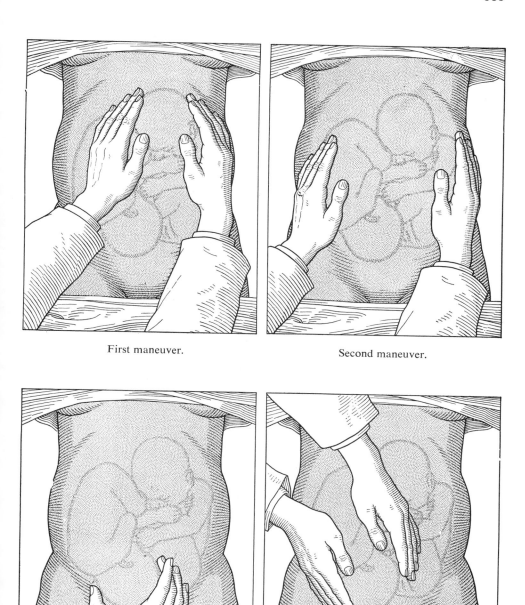

First maneuver.

Second maneuver.

Third maneuver.

Fourth maneuver.

Fig. 8. Palpation in twin pregnancy. Twin at left in ROA position; twin at right in LSP position.

small presenting part in the pelvis with the cervix obliterated and dilated 2 cm or more before the expected date of confinement, without evidence of labor, should arouse suspicion of multiple pregnancy. The diagnosis of a multiple pregnancy is frequently missed not so much because it is difficult, but because the examiner fails to keep the possibility in mind.

In doubtful cases, the use of x-ray usually leads to a positive diagnosis by detection of the skeletons of two fetuses. When two fetuses are suspected, roentgenograms or sonograms of the abdomen should be obtained (Figs. 9, 10, 11, and 12). Unless pregnancy is very early or hydramnios is marked, the additional fetus or fetuses are almost always visualized.

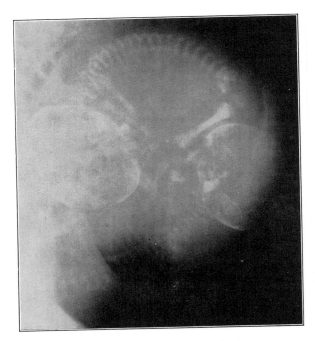

Fig. 9. Roentgenogram of twins in utero.

Clinical Course. Multiple pregnancy is frequently associated with hydramnios. Guttmacher was unable to ascertain the exact incidence of the complication, although it was diagnosed clinically in 7 per cent of the twin pregnancies in his series. Potter and Fuller report an incidence of hydramnios of slightly higher than 5 per cent. They found the complication associated with a significant increase in perinatal mortality, mainly because of the frequent occurrence of very premature labors.

Guttmacher, in an unpublished comparison of 1,200 multiple pregnancies with 80,000 singleton pregnancies, found hypertension in 20 per cent and 5 per cent, respectively. The increase was solely in preeclampsia and eclampsia; the incidence of chronic hypertensive disease was the same in both groups. One in three primigravidas with a multiple pregnancy and one in every eight multiparas had what appeared to be preeclampsia or eclampsia.

The distention of the uterus incidental to multiple pregnancy frequently leads

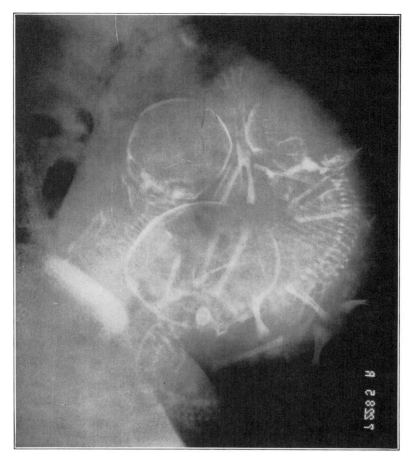

Fig. 10. Roentgenogram of triplets in utero. (Courtesy of Dr. Karl M. Wilson.)

to greater discomfort of the patient. Nausea and vomiting may be more frequent, although Guttmacher found no increased incidence of severe hyperemesis. Relaxation of the pelvic joints may possibly be more marked than in single gestations, resulting in greater difficulty of locomotion. If the multiple pregnancy is further complicated by hydramnios, interference with circulation and respiration may result, as indicated by marked dyspnea, extreme edema, or huge varicosities of the legs and vulva.

Guttmacher found that anemia was not only more frequent but also more pronounced in twin pregnancies. The increased tendency to premature labor has been noted by nearly all observers. Guttmacher and Kohl found the mean length of twin pregnancy to be 37.1 weeks and the median length 37.0 weeks.

MANAGEMENT OF MULTIPLE PREGNANCY

From the twentieth week on, physical examination may strongly suggest multiple pregnancy. If the diagnosis can be neither confirmed nor refuted, an x-ray film or sonogram of the abdomen should be obtained. If x-ray is employed

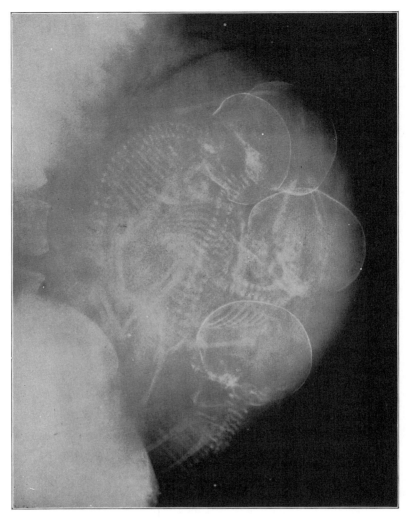

Fig. 11. Roentgenogram of quadruplets in utero. (Courtesy of Drs. J. C. Ullery, N. W. Vaux, and P. Bishop.)

it is wise to wait until after the twenty-eighth week. This precaution is unnecessary with sonography.

Conduct of a Multiple Pregnancy.   The two main complications associated with twinning—premature labor and increased frequency of preeclampsia-eclampsia—play dominant roles in management of pregnancy. When a diagnosis of twins is made, the pregnant woman must be advised to avoid physical strain by stopping work at 28 to 30 weeks' gestation instead of 6 to 8 weeks later, as usual. She also must give up travel, not only because it may predispose further to premature labor, but also because labor in a strange location may be hazardous as well as inconvenient. The patient should be advised to take long afternoon rests. Coitus probably should be eliminated during the last three months because of the possibility of a prematurely dilated cervix or the early onset of labor.

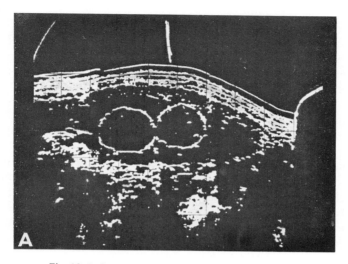

Fig. 12. A. Sonogram of a twin gestation (19 weeks).

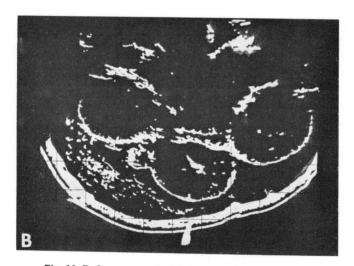

Fig. 12. B. Sonogram of a triplet gestation (31 weeks).

The obstetrician should make frequent careful vaginal or rectal examinations during the last three months to ascertain whether the cervix is effacing and beginning to dilate before the fetuses are mature. If so, in some instances labor may be postponed for several critical weeks by confining the patient to bed. Anderson and Bender report two small series of cases in which they confined mothers of twins to bed in the hospital from the thirtieth or thirty-second week until labor commenced. In both studies the incidence of prematurity was lessened. In our experience, hormones are of no value in delaying the onset of labor in either twin or single pregnancy.

As soon as the diagnosis of twins is made, the frequency of antepartum visits should be increased to detect incipient preeclampsia. If it appears the patient should be hospitalized promptly.

Maternal anemia is fairly common with multiple fetuses. Iron should be prescribed routinely, since the iron requirements for two fetuses together with the considerable increase in maternal blood volume normally total 1,000 mg or more. Supplemental folic acid may be of value.

The woman with a multiple pregnancy may be more comfortable if she wears a well-fitting maternity corset. Because of abdominal distention, her nights are particularly uncomfortable and a sedative may be required. The excessive abdominal pressure may make six small feedings preferable to three ordinary meals.

A patient with organic heart disease and a multiple pregnancy must be particularly careful to avoid all possible physical and emotional strain. We have seen one such patient decompensate at the thirty-fourth week of her twin gestation with what was thought to be a minimal rheumatic lesion. Since transfusions during labor or the early puerperium are more frequently and urgently needed in multiple pregnancies, it is essential that the blood group and Rh type of every such patient be known before labor begins. As soon as she enters the hospital in labor, blood should be matched and kept in reserve until it is definitely no longer needed.

Presentation.   In twins all possible combinations of position of the two fetuses are found. Either or both may present by the vertex, breech, or shoulder. The incidence of these combinations is approximately as follows:

Both vertex	31–47 per cent
Vertex and breech	34–40 per cent
Both breech	8–12 per cent
Longitudinal and shoulder	4–12 per cent
Both shoulder	0.3–10 per cent

In approximately 70 per cent of vertex-breech combinations, the first twin presents by the vertex. In about 90 per cent of the longitudinal-shoulder pairs, the longitudinal child is the first. Compound, face, and brow presentations are relatively common because of the small size of the fetuses and the frequent excess of amniotic fluid.

Labor. The conduct of labor in multiple pregnancy is an excellent test of the obstetrician's acumen, skill, judgment, and patience, for many complications, such as uterine dysfunction, abnormal presentations, prolapse of the cord, and postpartum hemorrhage, are significantly increased. Every statistical analysis demonstrates the twofold or threefold hazard of death that the woman faces with a plural delivery as compared with a single birth. To meet this challenge the obstetrician must be especially vigilant. He should manage the patient in a hospital where complications can be more effectively handled.

Induction of Labor.   Complications requiring the induction of labor are often better managed by cesarean section. In the occasional case of preeclampsia, however, or with a patient so ill from the overdistention of the abdomen that she has severe hyperemesis and respiratory distress and pain, induction of labor may be indicated. Ordinarily in multiple pregnancy artificial rupture of the membranes successfully initiates labor without the use of oxytocin. In a twin pregnancy near term, if the presenting part is fixed in the pelvis, the membranes may be ruptured before using oxytocin for either the induction or stimulation of labor, since release of the amniotic fluid diminishes the uterine distention and enhances the effectiveness of contractions. In our experience an intravenous oxytocin infusion for either induction or stimulation of labor, when properly administered with safeguards observed (p. 845), is not necessarily contraindicated because of multiple gestation alone.

Duration of Labor. There is a difference of opinion about the effects of multiple pregnancy on the length of labor. On the basis of a study of the literature and the statistical analysis of 418 births at the Johns Hopkins Hospital, Guttmacher came to the following conclusions. (1) Most twin labors are satisfactory. Because of the small size of the fetuses and the frequent effacement of the cervix before the onset of regular contractions, labor is usually shorter than with a single fetus. (2) There is a greater proportion of unsatisfactory desultory labors among plural pregnancies, frequently caused by hypotonic uterine dysfunction. (3) False labor is more common in multiple pregnancy. In confirmation of these findings Friedman and Sachtleben found the incidence of prolongation of one or more of the phases of labor with twins increased fourfold in nulliparas and twentyfold in multiparas.

Table 2. **Twin Gestation: Duration of Labor (Hours)**

	Primiparas	Multiparas
Mean	9.8 (14.5)*	6.0 (9.1)
Median	7.9 (11.3)	4.9 (6.6)

* *The numbers in parentheses refer to all deliveries.*
From the Obstetrical Statistical Cooperative

Table 2 indicates that the mean and median durations of labor are appreciably shorter in twin gestations than in single gestations, for both primiparas and multiparas. If the durations of all labors in twin gestations, regardless of parity,

Table 3. **Twin Gestation: Distribution of Patients by Duration of Labor**

Hours	No.	Per Cent
1–4	516	41.2
5–9	485	38.7
10–14	168	13.4
15 or more	83	6.7
Total	1,252	100.0

From the Obstetrical Statistical Cooperative

are tabulated (Table 3), it is evident that the huge majority will have been terminated in less than ten hours.

MANAGEMENT OF DELIVERY

In the ideal case, labor begins after the fetuses are mature. In such a situation the first stage is conducted as usual. If labor begins several weeks prematurely, however, or if the fetuses are judged to be very small at term, the amount of analgesic medication should be decreased as in the case of a single premature fetus.

A spontaneous delivery is especially desirable in twins because their birth is commonly followed by an increase in puerperal morbidity and blood loss. Furthermore, if the twins are small, a spontaneous delivery gives greater chance for fetal salvage. As soon as the first twin is delivered, the obstetrician ruptures the amniotic sac of the second twin. Then, by combined vaginal and abdominal manipulation, he attempts to bring the fetus into a longitudinal presentation, either vertex or breech. If he succeeds, pressure on the fundus, usually best administered by an assistant, will engage the presenting part and propel it downward through the birth canal, which has been so recently dilated. Such pressure is continued until either spontaneous delivery of the second twin eventuates or an easy forceps delivery or breech extraction is carried out. If it is impossible to manipulate the second fetus into a longitudinal position or if pressure does not engage it in the pelvis, version and extraction should then be carried out on the second twin. Delivery of the second twin should follow within a few minutes the birth of the first. Little and Friedman, in analyzing factors that influence the mortality of the second twin at the Sloane Hospital, caution against undue haste and undue delay. Optimal results were achieved when the interval between the first and second twins was between 5 and 15 minutes.

As soon as the first twin is delivered, its cord is doubly clamped and cut between the two clamps. It is particularly important that the placental end of the cord be thoroughly clamped, since it is possible for the undelivered twin to bleed to death through the leaking end of its twin's cord. It is usually undesirable and unnecessary to deliver the placenta of the first twin until after the birth of the second twin.

Immediately after the delivery of the second twin an oxytocic is given and the fundus is carefully observed to make sure that it is not being distended by an accumulation of blood. As soon as the placentas give evidence of separation they are expressed. Vigilant observation of the fundus for at least one hour after delivery of the placentas is particularly important, since uterine atony is a common complication after the delivery of twins. A prophylactic measure to prevent atony is the intravenous administration of 5 per cent dextrose in water during the delivery and, as soon as the placentas have been delivered, the addition of 20 to 30 units of oxytocin with maintenance of the oxytocin-dextrose infusion during the first hour. The uterus remains well contracted and hemorrhage resulting from atony is prevented.

Interval Between Infants.   Suprising intervals have been reported between the births of twins and triplets. Uthmöller records an interval of 4 days and 8 hours between the births of the first and second triplets, each weighing 4 pounds. In that case labor was reinitiated only after the obstetrician had ruptured the membranes of the second sac. Jahreiss gives the complete details of a twin birth in which there was an interval of 11 days and 7 hours. These two cases in no way establish a record. Williams and Cummings report twin births 56 days apart. The first delivery produced a living 3 pound 10¾ ounce male who weighed 6 pounds ½ ounce when his 5 pound 14¾ ounce vigorous brother was born almost two months later. The mother, as is frequently the case in women whose twins are born more than 72 hours apart, had a pregnancy in each horn of a double uterus. A double uterus is not always the explanation, however, for in the case reported by Drucker and colleagues, a patient with a normal uterus aborted one 375 g twin and then delivered the second twin live-born 65 days later.

Cesarean Section. In a study of 140 cesarean sections performed in twin pregnancies, Guttmacher and Kohl found the incidence of the operation to be 5.8 per cent. Sixty per cent were primary cesarean sections and 40 per cent repeated operations. The chief indication for primary sections was prolapse of the cord, particularly if the first fetus presented as a breech. Other important indications were toxemia, uterine dysfunction, and antepartum bleeding from placenta previa or abruption. Less frequent causes were shoulder presentation of the first fetus and intrapartum infection resulting from amnionitis. The frequency of premature rupture of the membranes is greatly increased in multiple pregnancy. Twins in themselves do not necessitate cesarean section. The indication is either a complication accompanying the multiple gestation or a complicated presentation, such as locking of the fetuses or twins in a uterus didelphys in which the emptied horn obstructs the birth of the undelivered fetus. Guttmacher and Kohl report 4 vaginal deliveries of twins following a previous low cervical cesarean section, and 56 cesarean sections repeated in patients pregnant with twins. After the 4 vaginal deliveries, the cavity of the uterus was explored digitally and found intact in all. Only 1 of the 56 repeated low cervical sections showed an incidental dehiscence, a frequency not greater than that in single pregnancies after low cervical sections. On this basis it is advised that the patient pregnant with twins after a low segment cesarean section be treated the same way as the patient with a single pregnancy, in regard to scheduling a repeated operation or allowing vaginal delivery. There were no maternal mortalities in the 140 cesarean sections in twin pregnancy, although the need for blood transfusions was double the incidence after cesarean sections for singletons. The choice of anesthetic for cesarean section is not affected by multiple pregnancy, although the prematurity of the infants must be a consideration. The low transverse incision of the uterus is usually adequate, but the low vertical type (Krönig) or classic incision may be better if the lower twin presents with a transverse lie. The 7.9 per cent perinatal loss could be materially reduced if the repeated cesarean sections in twin pregnancies were postponed at least until two weeks from term. It would probably be even safer for the infants to postpone operation until the onset of labor.

Collision. Collision, or the entrance of a pole of each fetus into the pelvis at the same time, is most likely when the fetuses are small or the pelvis is relatively large. The upward displacement of the presenting part of the less well engaged fetus usually solves the problem. A second and somewhat similar complication is locking (Fig. 13). In order for locking to occur, the first child must present by the breech and the second by the vertex. With descent of the breech the chin of the first child locks in the neck and chin of its cephalic twin. If unlocking cannot be achieved, either cesarean section or decapitation must be performed. The locking of twins is said to occur approximately once in 817 twin gestations (Cohen, Kohl, and Rosenthal). A report by Nissen summarizes the literature.

Anesthesia for Delivery. Because of the high incidence of prematurity it is probably wisest to deliver the first twin under local infiltration, pudendal block, and light nitrous oxide anesthesia. If operative measures are necessary in the delivery of the second twin, nitrous oxide or cyclopropane should be employed, unless version and extraction are necessary, in which case deep anesthesia, sufficient to relax the uterus, should be obtained before attempting the version. Version and extraction under conduction anesthesia are difficult and unwise except possibly in the hands of obstetricians highly experienced in these procedures.

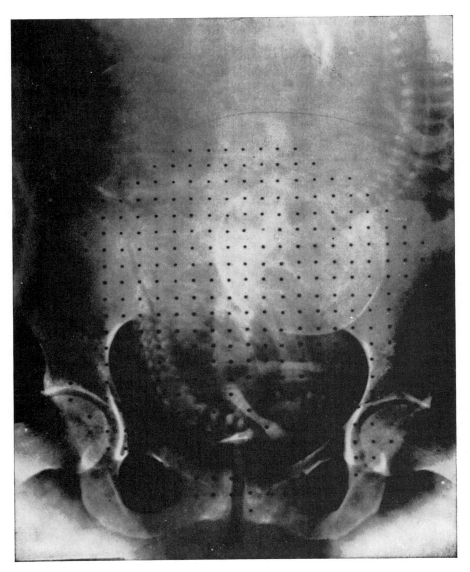

Fig. 13. Interlocked twins. (Courtesy of Dr. S. G. Kohl.)

Antepartum and Intrapartum Hemorrhage.   Placenta previa has been reported to be about twice as frequent in twin pregnancies as in singletons. Hawker and Allen report a 2.1 per cent incidence from the St. Louis City Hospital, Potter 1.2 per cent from the Chicago Lying-In Hospital, and Brown and Dixon 1.3 per cent, or double the expected incidence, from Hammersmith Hospital, London.

The increased incidence of placenta previa in multiple pregnancies is no doubt a result of the greater surface area of the uterus covered by the twin placentas. The course and treatment of placenta previa in multiple pregnancy do not differ from those in single pregnancy. Premature separation of the placenta probably is not more frequent before the birth of the first child than it is in single pregnancies; it is of the same origin in both cases. Premature separation of the placenta is not infrequent, however, between the births of the first and second twins. It may involve either the placenta of the twin already born or the second twin, or both. It results from the diminished area of attachment caused by the reduction in size of the uterus following expulsion of the first child. It causes external and concealed hemorrhage, with fetal distress if the placenta of the second twin is involved. Occasionally, one or both placentas are delivered before the birth of the second infant. The treatment of premature separation between a first and second twin is immediate vaginal delivery. Because of the greater incidence of velamentous insertion of the cord in multiple pregnancy, vasa previa are also more frequent than in single pregnancies. The diagnosis of rupture of the vessels depends on the simultaneous appearance of bleeding with either the spontaneous or artificial rupture of the membranes. Prompt delivery, when possible, is mandatory.

Prolapsed Cord. A multiple pregnancy often presents the ideal circumstances for prolapsed cord—namely, an excess of amniotic fluid and small fetuses. The incidence at the Johns Hopkins Hospital was 1.1 per cent, and in Brown and Dixon's series 1.3 per cent, or two to three times the expected rate. Treatment of the prolapse is not materially altered by a multiple gestation, but the prognosis is usually more favorable, since the infants are smaller and compression is ordinarily not so complete.

Constriction Ring. This complication may be encountered while performing a version on the second twin. In our experience, it bears no relation to protracted labor, but in each instance it followed the operative delivery of the first twin in a term pregnancy. The complication occurred in 0.9 per cent of the cases at the Johns Hopkins Hospital.

Postpartum Hemorrhage. The hazards of the third stage—postpartum hemorrhage, adherent placenta, and shock—are increased in plural pregnancy. The unusual frequency of these complications arises from the increased area of placental attachment and the abnormal uterine distention with resultant atony. Pritchard has measured blood loss associated with delivery of twins and found it to average very close to one liter, or twice that for the delivery of singletons. The importance of an intravenous infusion to which oxytocin may be readily added and of available crossmatched blood is obvious. Manual removal of the placenta is necessary twice as often after twins as after single births. The necessity is increased by operative twin deliveries and by an excessively long interval between the birth of the two infants. The increased incidence of shock after the delivery of twins has been stressed by several authors. It is therefore important in plural deliveries to minimize loss of blood, to eliminate traumatic procedures such as manual dilatation of the cervix whenever possible, and to provide for the adequate treatment of hypovolemia.

THE INFANT

Among the white patients at the Johns Hopkins Hospital the average viable single fetus weighed 3,350 g; among the black patients the average weighed 3,100 g. The average for viable white twins was 2,649 g, and 2,446 g for the black.

In other words, the average white singleton weighed about 700 g, or 1½ pounds, more than the average white twin at birth. Among the black patients the difference was slightly less, about 650 g. One important factor is the commonly abbreviated duration of twin pregnancies. In addition, as Stehle has proved in data collected from the University Clinic at Freiburg, the twin fetus weighs and measures less per unit time of intrauterine life than does the singleton. Stehle compared the weight and length of twins born during various weeks of pregnancy with tables of weights and lengths arranged in the same way for single fetuses. From the thirtieth to the fortieth weeks of gestation he found a mean difference of 536 g in weight and 2 cm in length between single fetuses and twins of equal intrauterine age. There is no adequate explanation of this discrepancy, but it seems probable that "placental insufficiency" is involved.

There is less relative difference in length than in weight between the single and twin fetus. The twin is thus thin at birth and viscerally more mature than its weight would indicate. It was formerly believed that a premature twin did as well after birth as a singleton 500 g heavier. Table 4 indicates, however, that the advantage is far less than 500 g.

Table 4. **Survival Rates for Single and Multiple Gestations (Born Alive)**

	Single		Multiple	
Birth Weight	No.	Per Cent Survival	No.	Per Cent Survival
401–1,000	196	4.1	112	8.9
1,001–1,500	253	52.2	174	60.3
1,501–2,000	599	81.6	392	91.8
2,001–2,500	2,312	96.2	799	97.6
Over 2,500	35,736	99.5	1,049	99.5
Total	39,096*	98.3	2,526*	91.0

* Obstetrical Statistical Cooperative, 1958.
S. G. Kohl

Guttmacher noted a steady rise in the weight of the average newborn twin with increasing parity. The rise was progressive up to the sixth pregnancy, after which no further increase in weight occurred. Of 684 twins analyzed, 21, or 3 per cent, exceeded 3,600 g at birth. The three largest weighed 4,060, 4,080, and 4,115 g. The heaviest pair in 346 sets totaled 7,680 g. These birth weights by no means establish a record. Holzapfel reported the delivery of a woman in her third pregnancy of twin boys weighing 4,670 g and 4,510 g, with survival of both infants. The placenta weighed 1,300 g, contributing, with about 3 liters of amniotic fluid, to 13.5 kg of intrauterine contents. According to several German authorities, there is a greater difference in weight and length between one-egg than between two-egg twins. The male twin is ordinarily larger than the female.

Occasionally one of a pair of discordant twins with a small placenta will show severe intrauterine growth retardation. According to Lubchenco and colleagues, the normal twin will behave as a singleton whereas the smaller will have smaller head measurements as well as lower weight. Sonographic technics may supply the correct intrauterine diagnosis in these cases.

Congenital malformations are more common in twins than in singly born children. Guttmacher and Kohl report an incidence of 7 per cent congenital malformations in twins, compared with an incidence of 4 per cent in a control series of singletons. Donnelly noted malformations in 3 per cent of singletons and 7.1 per cent of twins. It is believed that malformations are commoner in the one-egg than in the two-egg varieties. If one of a pair of monovular twins has an abnormality it is almost certain that the other twin will have a similar defect, on either the same side or on the opposite side, as in a mirror image. Some observers believe that two-egg twins never suffer from identical malformations and that both one-egg twins always exhibit the same malformation. The reported minor exceptions include cryptorchidism, congenital inguinal hernia, hydrocele, dislocation of the optic lens, and perhaps rare instances of clubfoot. All other congenital malformations appear in both identical twins.

PERINATAL AND MATERNAL MORTALITY

Perinatal Mortality.   Because of reproductive wastage, many breeders of horses and cattle consider it an undesirable trait when the stock is susceptible to multiple births. More of the mothers die, more pregnancies terminate in abortion, and a higher percentage of young succumbs. If human multiple births were viewed in that way, the same conclusion would be reached. All authorities agree that the total perinatal mortality in twins is two to three times that in single births. In her study at the Chicago Lying-In Hospital, Potter found an uncorrected mortality of 15.6 per cent in a series of twins. If the abortuses and fetuses weighing less than 1,000 g are excluded, the mortality is 8.2 per cent. If those of less than 1,500 g are excluded, it falls to 4.4 per cent. The latter figure is twice the total perinatal mortality of 2 per cent, for the same period, for all infants weighing more than 1,500 g. Guttmacher and Kohl report a total perinatal loss for all twin fetuses over 400 g of 13.3 per cent, and Donnelly, of 11.8 per cent. In almost all studies the ratio of stillbirths to neonatal deaths is 1:2. The predominant cause of the neonatal death is, of course, prematurity. The many complications of twin pregnancy, such as prolapsed cord, placenta previa, premature separation of the second placenta, contraction ring, and malformations, obviously contribute to the high mortality associated with multiple births. Nevertheless, all studies of the perinatal loss in multiple gestation point up the transcendent importance of prematurity. Several authors, especially in Great Britain, believe that bed rest, particularly before the thirty-sixth week, will materially reduce the perinatal loss by decreasing the incidence of very small babies. Although Jonas failed to confirm these findings, the relevant data of Robertson and of Ferguson, for example, are quite convincing.

Numerous reports from various parts of the world indicate an increased risk for the second twin (Bach and Kiffe, Germany; Spurway, Great Britain; and Ferguson, Canada). The reasons for this difference include the greater frequency of abnormal positions of the second twin, the increased likelihood of placental separation after delivery of the first twin, and the usually lighter weight of the second twin. Most authors stress the advantage of prompt delivery of the second twin.

Maternal Mortality.   In an earlier review of the literature, there were 29 maternal deaths in 2,595 cases of twin deliveries, a rate of 11.7 per 10,000. In three series, however, including those of Guttmacher and Kohl (1958), Brown and Dixon (1963), and Seski and Miller (1963), there were no deaths in 2,133 deliveries. The best way to protect the mother's life in a multiple pregnancy is through attentive antepartum care with the prompt recognition and treatment of preeclampsia, spontaneous delivery of the infants when possible, and immediate replacement of blood in excessive postpartum loss. Despite the many large series of multiple births without a maternal death, the potential hazards of antepartum and postpartum hemorrhage and of preeclampsia remain significantly higher in twin pregnancy.

REFERENCES

Aiken, R. A.   An account of the Birmingham "sextuplets."J Obstet Gynaec Brit Comm 76:684, 1969.

Anderson, W. J. R.   Stillbirth and neonatal mortality in twin pregnancy. J Obstet Gynaec Brit Emp 63:205, 1956.

Archer, J.   Observations showing that a white woman, by intercourse with a white man and a Negro, may conceive twins, one of which shall be white and the other a mulatto. Medical Repository, 3rd Hexade, 1:319, 1810.

Bach, H. G., and Kiffe, M.   (Twin births in the University Women's Clinic of Heidelberg from 1950 to 1959). Arch Gynaek 196:609, 1962.

Bender, S.   Twin pregnancy. J Obstet Gynaec Brit Emp 59:510, 1952.

Benirschke, K.   Discussion of blood chimerism, in Wynn, R. M. (ed.), Fetal Homeostasis, New York, Appleton-Century-Crofts, 1969, Vol. IV, p. 220.

———— Sullivan, M. M., and Marin-Padilla, M.   Size and number of umbilical vessels, a study of multiple pregnancy in man and the armadillo. Obstet Gynec 24:819, 1964.

Berbos, J. N., King, B. F., and Janusz, A.   Quintuple pregnancy. JAMA 188:813, 1964.

Booth, P. B., Plaut, G., James, J. D., Ikin, E. W., Moore, P., Sanger, R., and Race, R. R.   Blood chimerism in a pair of twins. Brit Med J 1:1456, 1957.

Brown, E. J., and Dixon, H. G.   Twin pregnancy. J Obstet Gynaec Brit Comm 70:251, 1963.

Cameron, A. H., Edwards, J. H., Derom, R., Thiery, M., and Boelaert, R.   The value of twin surveys in the study of malformations. Proceedings of the 6th World Congress on Fertility and Sterility, Tel Aviv, Israel, May, 1968. In press.

Cohen, M., Kohl, S. G., and Rosenthal, A. H.   Fetal interlocking complicating twin gestation. Amer J Obstet Gynec 91:407, 1965.

Corner, G. W.   The observed embryology of human single-ovum twins and other multiple births. Amer J Obstet Gynec 70:933, 1955.

Coulton, D., Hertig, A., and Long, W. N.   Monoamniotic twins. Amer J Obstet Gynec 54:119, 1947.

Curtius, F.   (Placental findings in twins and diagnosis of similarity). Arch Gynaek 140:361, 1930.

de Blécourt, J. J.   Fünflingsgeburten. Ein Fall von Fünflingsgeburt. Nebst einer Beschreibung des Präparats, und einer Casuistik und analytischer Uebersicht von 27 Fällen von Fünflingsgeburt, hrsg. von G. C. Nijhoff. Gröningen, J. B. Wolters, 1904, 74 pp.

Donnelly, M.   The influence of multiple births on perinatal loss. Amer J Obstet Gynec 72:998, 1956.

Drucker, P., Finkel, J., and Savel, L. E.   65-day interval between the birth of twins. Amer J Obstet Gynec 80:761, 1960.

Duncan, J. M.   Fecundity, Fertility, Sterility and Allied Topics. Edinburgh, A. & C. Black, 1866.

Eastman, N. J.   Editorial comment on sixty-five-day interval between the birth of twins. Obstet Gynec Survey 16:45, 1961.

Enders, A. C. (ed.). Delayed Implantation. Chicago, University of Chicago Press, 1963.

Ferguson, W. F.   Perinatal mortality in multiple gestations. A review of perinatal deaths from 1609 multiple gestations. Obstet Gynec 23:861, 1964.

Friedman, E. A., and Sachtleben, M. R.   The effect of uterine overdistension on labor. I. Multiple pregnancy. Obstet Gynec 23:164, 1964.

Gemzell, C. A.   The use of human gonadotropin in gynaecological disorders, in Kellar, R. J. (ed.), Modern Trends in Gynecology, London, Butterworth, 1963, p. 133.

References

683

———— Induction and control of ovulation, in Proceedings Part II: 2:709, 1965. Second International Congress of Endocrinology, London, 1964.

———— and Roos, P. Pregnancies following treatment with human gonadotropins with special reference to the problem of multiple births. Amer J Obstet Gynec 94:490, 1966.

Greulich, W. W. The birth of six pairs of fraternal twins to the same parents. A discussion of the possible significance of such cases in the light of some recent observations. JAMA 110: 559, 1938.

Guttmacher, A. F. An analysis of 521 cases of twin pregnancy. I. Differences in single and double ovum twinning. Amer J Obstet Gynec 34:76, 1937.

———— An analysis of 573 cases of twin pregnancy. II. The hazards of pregnancy itself. Amer J Obstet Gynec 38:277, 1939.

———— Clinical aspects of twin pregnancy. Med Clin N Amer 23:427, 1939.

———— The incidence of multiple births in man and some of the other uniparae. Obstet Gynec 2:22, 1953.

———— and Kohl, S. G. The fetus of multiple gestations. Obstet Gynec 12:528, 1958.

———— and Kohl, S. G. Cesarean section in twin pregnancy. Amer J Obstet Gynec 83:866, 1962.

Hamlett, G. W. Human twinning in the United States: Racial frequencies, sex ratios, and geographical variations. Genetics 20:250, 1935.

Hawker, W. D., and Allen, M. A study of 145 consecutive twin pregnancies. Amer J Obstet Gynec 57:996, 1949.

Hellin, D. Die Ursache der Multiparität der uniparen Tiere überhaupt und der Zwillingsschwangerschaft beim Menschen. München, Seitz und Schauer, 1895, 70 pp.

Holzapfel, K. (Very large twins). Monatschr Geburtsh u Gynäk 98:30, 1935.

Hytten, F. E. A strange case of Rosalie and Josefa Blazek. Zodiac. Journal of Aberdeen Medical Faculty 11:32, 1964.

Jahreiss, R. (Ten-day interval between birth of twins). Zbl Gynaek 46:1246, 1922.

Jonas, E. G. The value of prenatal bed-rest in multiple pregnancy. J Obstet Gynaec Brit Comm 70:461, 1963.

Keast, A. C., and Cooper, G. Z. The Tukutese quintuplets. S Afr J Obstet Gynaec 5:43, 1967.

King, J. A., Herring, J. S., Witt, E. D., and Blood, B. Monoamniotic twin pregnancy: Report of five new cases. Amer J Obstet Gynec 63:691, 1952.

Kistner, R. W. Induction of ovulation with clomiphène citrate (Clomid). S Afr J Obstet Gynaec 5:25, 1967.

Komai, T., and Fukuoka, G. Frequency of multiple births among the Japanese and related peoples. Amer J Phys Anthrop 21:433, 1936.

Little, W. A., and Friedman, E. A. The twin delivery factors influencing second twin mortality. Obstet Gynec Survey 13:611, 1958.

Lubchenco, L. O., Hansman, C., and Bäckström, L. Factors influencing fetal growth, in Jonxis, J. H. P., Visser, H. K. A., and Troelstra, J. A. (eds.), Aspects of Praematurity and Dysmaturity, Nutricia Symposium. Springfield, Ill., Charles C Thomas Co., 1968, p. 160 (149 articles).

MacArthur, J. Genetics of quintuplets: diagnosis of the Dionne quintuplets as a monozygotic set. J Hered 29:323, 1938.

———— and Ford, N. Collected Studies on the Dionne Quintuplets. Univ. Toronto Press, 1937.

Mauriceau, F. Traité des maladies des femmes grosses, Paris, 1668.

Meyer, A. W. The occurrence of superfetation. JAMA 72:769, 1919.

Murray, J. E., Merrell, J. P., and Harrison, J. H. Kidney transplantation between 7 pairs of identical twins. Ann Surg 148:343, 1958.

Naeye, R. L. Human intrauterine parabiotic syndrome and its complications. New Eng J Med 268:804, 1963.

Newman, H. H. The Physiology of Twinning. Chicago Press, 1923.

———— The Biology of Twins. Chicago Press, 1917.

———— Methods of diagnosing monozygotic and dizygotic twins. Biol Bull Boston 55:283, 1928.

———— and Patterson, J. T. The development of the nine-banded armadillo from the primitive streak stage to birth, etc. J Morphol 21:359, 1910.

Nichols, J. B. Statistics of births in the United States. Amer J Obstet Gynec 64:376, 1952.

Nissen, E. D. Twins: collision, impaction, compaction and interlocking. Obstet Gynec 11:514, 1958.

Oettle, A. G.   Paternal influence in polyzygotic births. J. Obstet Gynaec Brit Emp 60:775, 1953.

Potter, E. L., and Crunden, A. B.   Twin pregnancies in the service of the Chicago Lying-in Hospital. Amer J Obstet Gynec 42:870, 1941.

———— and Fuller, H.   Multiple pregnancies at the Chicago Lying-in Hospital, 1941–1947. Amer J Obstet Gynec 58:139, 1949.

Pritchard, J. A.   Changes in the blood volume during pregnancy and delivery. Anesthesiology 26:393, 1965.

Robertson, J. G.   Twin pregnancy. Influence of early admission on fetal survival. Obstet Gynec 23:854, 1964.

Robertson, W. R. B.   A mule and a horse as twins and the inheritance of twinning. Kansas Univ Sci Bull 10:293, 1917.

Robson, E. B., and Harris, H.   Genetics of the alkaline phosphatase polymorphism of the human placenta. Nature 207:1257, 1965.

Sasse, A.   (Contributions to the study of one-egg triplets). Acta Obstet Gynec Scand 4:79, 1925.

Seski, A. G., and Miller, L. A.   Plural pregnancies—the cause of plural problems. Obstet Gynec 21:227, 1963.

Siemens, H. W.   (The diagnosis of uniovular twins from obstetrical and dermatologic point of view). Arch Gynaek 126:623, 1925.

Sinykin, M. B.   Monoamniotic triplet pregnancy with triple survival. Obstet Gynec 12:78, 1958.

Spurway, J.   The fate and management of the second twin. Amer J Obstet Gynec 83:1377, 1962.

Stehle, F.   (Concerning the relations of size and duration of pregnancy in twins). Z Geburtsh Gynaek 119:159, 1939.

Stockard, C. B.   An experimental study of twins, "double monsters" and single deformities: Developmental rate and structural expression. Amer J Anat 28:115, 1921.

Strandskov, H. H.   Plural birth frequencies in the total, the "white" and the "colored" U.S. populations. Amer J Phys Anthrop 3:49, 1945.

———— and Edelen, E. W.   Monozygotic and dizygotic twin birth frequencies in the total white and colored U.S. population. Genetics 31:438, 1946.

———— Edelen, E. W., and Siemens, G. J.   Analysis of the sex ratios among single and plural births in the total "white" and "colored" U.S. populations. Amer J Phys Anthrop 4:491, 1946.

Studdiford, W. E.   Is superfetation possible in the human being? Amer J Obstet Gynec 31:845, 1936.

Sussi, L.   (A case of superfetation). Med Klin 31:1334, 1935.

Timmons, J. D., and de Alvarez, R. R.   Monoamniotic twin pregnancy. Amer J Obstet Gynec 86:875, 1963.

Uthmöller, A.   (Two sets of triplets). Zbl Gynaek 46:859, 1922.

Vassali, F.   Caso di gravidanza sesquigemellare. Gazz med Ital Lombardia 48:216-218, 1888. Cited in: A case of septuplets (Miscellany). Boston Medical & Surgical Journal 132:243, March 7, 1895.

Waterhouse, J. A. H.   Twinning in twin pedigrees. Brit J Soc Med 4:197, 1950.

White, C., and Wyshak, G.   Inheritance in human dizygotic twinning. New Eng J Med 271:1003, 1964.

Williams, B., and Cummings, G.   An unusual case of twins: Case report. J Obstet Gynaec Brit Emp 60:319, 1953.

Zeleny, C. L.   The relative numbers of twins and triplets. Science 53:262, 1921.

26

HYPERTENSIVE DISORDERS IN PREGNANCY

The hypertensive disorders in pregnancy are vascular derangements either antedating pregnancy or arising during gestation or the early puerperium. They are characterized by hypertension and are sometimes associated with proteinuria, edema, convulsions, coma, or other signs, alone or in various combinations. Because the disorders carry varying prognoses for mother and child, they should be differentiated. The hypertensive disorders are commonly called "toxemia of pregnancy," a term that is both illogical and ambiguous. No toxin has been found in the blood, and although the American Committee on Maternal Welfare defined the phrase as including both preeclampsia and chronic hypertension, many writers misuse it as a synonym for preeclampsia.

As described in Chapter 8, normal pregnancy is characterized by profound hemodynamic, metabolic, and hormonal changes and a substantial increase in body fluids. Whether preeclampsia represents an exaggeration of changes normally incident to pregnancy or depends upon some wholly new aberration is moot. The causes of preeclampsia, eclampsia, and essential hypertension are unknown, despite decades of intensive research, and they remain among the most important unsolved problems in obstetrics.

The hypertensive disorders in pregnancy are common complications of gestation, occurring in 6 or 7 per cent of all late pregnancies. They form one of the great triad of complications (hemorrhage, hypertension, and sepsis) responsible for most maternal deaths and they account for about one fifth of the maternal fatalities in the United States each year. As a cause of perinatal death they are even more important, for by a conservative estimate at least 25,000 stillbirths and neonatal deaths each year in this country are the result of the hypertensive disorders. Most neonatal deaths are caused by prematurity of the infant.

The huge toll taken by hypertension in pregnancy of maternal and infant lives is largely preventable. Good prenatal supervision, with the early detection of signs and symptoms of oncoming preeclampsia, and appropriate treatment will arrest many cases and sufficiently ameliorate others that the outcome for baby and mother is usually satisfactory.

CLASSIFICATION

Since the signs and symptoms of the various hypertensive disorders are non-specific, and since our knowledge about these syndromes is empiric and the prepregnancy status is unknown in most cases, accurate classification is very difficult. Although many schemes of classification have been proposed, that of the American Committee on Maternal Welfare is in widest use. It is now under revision by a committee of the American College of Obstetricians and Gynecologists and, independently, by a committee of German-speaking obstetricians. Neither revision has been completed. Tentatively, the German-speaking committee calls all of the disorders "Gestosis" or "EPH-Gestosis" and subdivides them as monosymptomatic, that is, with only one sign (E = edema, P = proteinuria, and H = hypertension), and polysymptomatic, that is, with two or more signs. As in the American classification they differentiate between signs antedating pregnancy and signs arising in pregnancy. The aggravation of antecedent signs or the addition of new signs during pregnancy is called superimposed Gestosis.

The tentative American revision divides the hypertensive disorders into (1) those arising in and peculiar to pregnancy, that is, preeclampsia and eclampsia; (2) chronic hypertension of whatever cause; (3) preeclampsia or eclampsia superimposed upon chronic hypertension; and (4) a new group, late, or transient, hypertension.

Preeclampsia and Eclampsia.   The acute or specific hypertensive disorder of pregnancy is peculiar to pregnant or puerperal women, although it occasionally occurs in other primates. Diagnosis is made on the basis of development of hypertension with proteinuria or edema, or both, after the twentieth week of gestation, although these signs may appear earlier with a hydatidiform mole. It is predominantly a disease of young nulliparas, and the diagnosis must be suspect in a multipara. In the nonconvulsive stage the disease is called *preeclampsia*; the added appearance of convulsions and coma makes the diagnosis *eclampsia*. Although the tentative decision of the committee permits the diagnosis of preeclampsia on the basis of hypertension and either proteinuria or edema, the diagnosis is shaky in the absence of proteinuria. The committee's justification is that proteinuria usually is a late sign and that some women with early, mild preeclampsia deliver before that sign appears.

Hypertension, for the diagnosis of preeclampsia, is defined as a rise of 30 mm Hg or more over the usual systolic blood pressure, an absolute systolic level of 140 or more, a rise of 15 mm Hg or more over the usual diastolic pressure, or an absolute diastolic level of 90 or more. The levels cited must be observed on at least two occasions six hours or more apart.

Proteinuria means urinary protein in concentrations greater than 0.3 g/L (1 or 2 plus) in a 24-hour collection or of 1 g/L or more in a random clean (midstream) or catheterized sample on two occasions at least six hours apart.

Edema is a generalized and excessive accumulation of fluid in the tissues. Pedal or pretibial edema is not significant in the diagnosis of preeclampsia. The sign is not specific, for Thomson and co-workers have noted generalized edema in 15 per cent of otherwise normal pregnant women. Generalized edema is often associated with a rapid gain in weight, of a kilogram or more per week, preceding detection of the edema.

Preeclampsia is classified as "severe" if any one of the following signs or symptoms occurs. If none is present the preeclampsia is classified as "mild":

1. Blood pressure of 160 mm Hg or more systolic, or 110 or more diastolic, on at least two occasions at least six hours apart, with the patient at bed rest

2. Proteinuria of 5 g or more in 24 hours (3 or 4 plus on qualitative examination)
3. Oliguria (400 ml or less per 24 hours)
4. Cerebral or visual disturbances
5. Pulmonary edema or cyanosis

Another sign of severity is epigastric pain.

The differentiation of mild and severe preeclampsia is not wholly desirable, except in retrospect, but the five criteria specified above are an improvement over the former differentiation on the basis of a blood pressure of 160/100. That widely employed dividing line between mild and severe preeclampsia can be dangerously misleading. The outlook in any given case cannot be so easily predicted. Blood pressure alone is not a dependable indication of severity, for a young girl with a pressure of 135/85 may develop convulsions, whereas many patients with pressures of 180/120 do not. The whole clinical picture—blood pressure, edema, facies, proteinuria, urinary output, age, ocular signs, and headache—must be evaluated in estimating prognosis. A clinical picture of such infinite variety cannot be classified accurately as mild or severe by any one or two criteria.

From the viewpoint of cause and anatomic, physiologic, and biochemical abnormalities, preeclampsia-eclampsia is a single entity. Clinically, eclampsia is distinguished from preeclampsia by the development of one or more convulsions. Fortunately, most patients suffering from preeclampsia never progress to convulsion. In some, the process is inherently mild and hence does not advance to the eclamptic stage. In others, suitable medication checks it. In a third group, the termination of pregnancy, either spontaneously or operatively, forestalls the development of convulsions, and the patient returns to normal shortly after delivery. Preeclampsia typically occurs in the last trimester of pregnancy, the incidence of the disease increasing as term approaches.

Chronic Hypertension of Whatever Cause. Chronic hypertension occurs in nonpregnant women and in men, but during pregnancy it often has a special significance. The differentiation of chronic hypertension from preeclampsia may be difficult in women first seen after the twentieth week of gestation, for few of them know what their blood pressures were before pregnancy. Patients with antecedent hypertension, moreover, frequently react to pregnancy with a fulminating vasculorenal syndrome that seems to be preeclampsia superimposed upon the underlying chronic disorder.

In the classification of the American Committee on Maternal Welfare, essential hypertension was singled out for inclusion as a "toxemia of pregnancy," in the mistaken belief that renal and other causes of hypertension could be recognized in most instances. In the tentative revision, all chronic hypertensions are included because probably all predispose to the development of superimposed preeclampsia, and all pose difficult problems of differential diagnosis.

The diagnosis of chronic hypertension is made on the history of hypertension (140/90 or higher) antedating pregnancy, or the discovery of hypertension before the twentieth week of pregnancy, with indefinite persistence after delivery. As in nonpregnant subjects, *essential hypertension* is a diagnosis made by exclusion of known causes of high blood pressure, such as primary renal disease.

Chronic hypertensive disease of whatever cause is a protean complex that may present a wide variety of clinical pictures depending upon the primary disease, the stage of the arteriolosclerosis, and the secondary effects on the heart, kidneys, and brain. Many patients manifest only hypertension with narrowing and tortuosity of the retinal vessels. In others, cardiac hypertrophy develops as a result of peripheral vascular resistance, and hypertensive cardiac failure may ensue. In some, the sclerosis affects the renal vessels. Combinations of secondary cardiac and secondary renal disease are often seen with all gradations of each. In still other patients, rupture of a cerebral vessel may occur. In advanced degrees of these disorders, therefore, chronic hypertensive cardiovascular disease or chronic hypertensive cardiovasculorenal disease may be a serious complication.

Chronic Hypertension with Superimposed Preeclampsia.   Patients with chronic hypertension often develop a syndrome called superimposed preeclampsia, the incidence of which depends upon the diagnostic criteria. The resultant clinical picture is characterized by an acute aggravation of the already existing hypertension (often to extreme levels), proteinuria, edema, and, not infrequently, acute retinal changes, such as hemorrhage, exudates, and edema. When preeclampsia develops in these chronic hypertensive patients it is likely to occur relatively early, sometimes between the twenty-fourth and thirtieth weeks, and it may progress to eclampsia.

The criteria for the diagnosis of chronic hypertension with superimposed preeclampsia are as follows: (1) evidence that the patient is suffering from chronic hypertension, and (2) evidence of the superimposition of an acute process, as demonstrated by an elevation of systolic pressure of 30 mm Hg or more, an elevation in diastolic pressure of 15 mm or more, and the development of a significant degree of proteinuria, usually with edema as well.

Transient Hypertension.   The tentatively revised classification adds a new category called "transient hypertension." The diagnosis is made when hypertension arises during pregnancy or within the first 24 hours postpartum in a previously normotensive woman, and disappears within 10 days after delivery. Generalized edema and proteinuria are absent. Some of these patients really have early mild preeclampsia and others have latent essential hypertension, but they do not satisfy the criteria for either diagnosis. Such findings are made in about one third of multiparous women whose first pregnancies were complicated by preeclampsia or eclampsia. In them, the condition has been called "recurrent toxemia of pregnancy."

"Recurrent toxemia" is regarded by some writers as another episode of preeclampsia (usually mild). Some consider it to be an entity, but Dieckmann, who appears to have been correct, wrote that it is a sign of latent essential hypertension or vasculorenal disease.

Necessarily, the classification is arbitrary. Preeclampsia on rare occasions appears before the twentieth week, and hypertensive disease may first become manifest after that time. Many believe that hypertensive disease predisposes to preeclampsia, but Dieckmann thought that the syndrome called superimposed preeclampsia represents an exacerbation of the hypertensive disease and is not preeclampsia. Finally, some believe that all of these subgroups merely form the spectrum of hypertensive disease colored by pregnancy.

An approximate idea of the relative incidences of the several types of hypertensive disorders, based upon the old classification, is shown in Table 1, which summarizes the ten-year observation of indigent patients at the Kings County

Table 1. **Hypertensive Disorders in Pregnancy at the Kings County Hospital**°

Type	Number of Cases	Incidence, Per Cent	Percentage of Total Hypertensive Disorders	Perinatal Mortality, Per Cent
Preeclampsia	1,229	1.94	33.0	5.7
Eclampsia	68	0.11	1.8	17.7
Chronic hypertensive disease	2,289	3.63	61.4	9.0
Preeclampsia superimposed upon chronic hypertension	122	0.19	3.2	24.6
Unclassified	21	0.03	0.6	4.8
Totals	3,729	5.9	100.0	8.5

° *Ten-year period, 1958–1967.*

Hospital. Many patients classified as having preeclampsia or, especially, chronic hypertensive disease would fall in the new category of "transient hypertension." The diagnosis of superimposed preeclampsia was made in only 5.1 per cent of the women thought to have chronic hypertension. That diagnosis was made only if the patient manifested both aggravated hypertension and sustained 3 or 4 plus proteinuria, which is a more stringent standard than that generally used. Many obstetricians make the diagnosis on the basis of a single sign: aggravated hypertension, any degree of proteinuria, or edema. The perinatal loss associated with superimposed preeclampsia obviously will vary with the diagnostic criteria. The high rate of loss (24.6 per cent) shown in Table 1 would be halved if the diagnosis were made more liberally, as would the perinatal loss of 9.0 per cent in uncomplicated hypertension. McCartney's study of renal biopsies indicates that the diagnosis is made too often and is usually wrong. Among his 152 multiparas with known chronic hypertension and apparent superimposition of preeclampsia, only 21, or 14 per cent, had the glomerular capillary endotheliosis that is said to be characteristic of preeclampsia.

The relative frequencies of preeclampsia and chronic hypertensive vascular disease vary widely from hospital to hospital, chiefly depending upon who makes the diagnoses. For instance, the relative frequency of preeclampsia ranged from 39 to 90 per cent among the eight hospitals listed in the first table of Dieckmann's monograph. This wide discrepancy is explained in part by the moot question of whether preeclampsia actually causes hypertensive vascular disease and in part by the varying proportions of black patients from hospital to hospital, since hypertensive disease is more prevalent in Negroes.

PREECLAMPSIA

Although the obstetric definition of hypertension is a blood pressure of 140/90 or higher, absolute figures are sometimes of less clinical significance than is the temporal trend of pressures, especially in young women. For instance, a rise from 105/70 to 135/85 does not fit the conventional definition of hypertension as used in nonpregnant subjects, but in a teen-age primigravida such an increase is alarming and may even be associated with convulsions.

Preeclampsia is overwhelmingly a disease of the first pregnancy. It may occur in later pregnancies, but when it does there is usually a predisposing factor such as antecedent hypertension, diabetes, or multiple pregnancy. In multiparas the diagnosis should always be suspect.

Clinical Course.   The earliest and most dependable warning sign of preeclampsia, in most cases, is acute hypertension, often heralded by an upward trend in the pressures at prior visits. The diastolic pressure is a more reliable prognostic sign than is the systolic, and any persisting diastolic pressure of 90 mm or more is abnormal. In the severer grades of preeclampsia the systolic pressure frequently reaches 180 mm and the diastolic 110, but systolic levels in excess of 200 mm are rarely seen. When the systolic blood pressure exceeds 200 it usually will be found that the underlying cause is chronic hypertensive disease with or without superimposed preeclampsia.

The next most important sign of preeclampsia is sudden and excessive weight

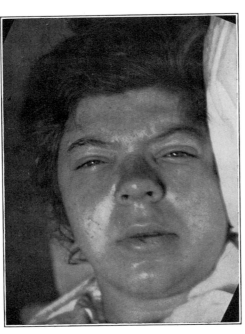

Fig. 1. Facies in fulminating preeclampsia. Note edema of eyelids, general puffiness of entire face, and coarseness of features of this 16-year-old girl.

gain. In many cases it is the first sign. Weight increments of about one pound a week may be regarded as normal, but when they reach two pounds in any given week, or as much as six pounds in a month, incipient preeclampsia is to be suspected. Sudden and excessive weight gain in gestation is attributable almost entirely to abnormal retention of fluid and is demonstrable, as a rule before visible signs of edema, such as swollen eyelids and puffiness of the fingers. In cases of fulminating preeclampsia, waterlogging may be extreme (Fig. 1), and in such patients increments of ten pounds or more in a week are not unusual. Especially characteristic of preeclampsia is the suddenness of the excessive weight gain rather than an increase distributed through gestation.

Proteinuria is a common finding in preeclampsia, but it varies greatly not only from case to case but also in the same patient from hour to hour. The fluctuations of proteinuria in preeclampsia, as well as in eclampsia, have been studied in detail by Chesley and his associates, who believe that the variability points to a functional (vasospastic) rather than an organic cause. In early preeclampsia, proteinuria may be entirely lacking or limited to a trace; in the severer grades, proteinuria is usually demonstrable and is often as much as 6 or 8 g per liter. Proteinuria usually develops later than the hypertension and weight gain and must therefore be regarded as a serious omen when superimposed on the two other findings. These three early and important signs of preeclampsia—hypertension, weight gain, and proteinuria—are changes of which the patient is usually totally unaware. By the time a preeclamptic patient has developed symptoms and signs that she herself can detect, such as headache, visual disturbances, puffiness of the eyelids and fingers, the disorder is usually advanced, and much ground has been lost. Hence, the transcendent importance of prenatal care in the early detection and early management of this complication becomes obvious.

Headache is rare in the milder cases but is increasingly frequent in the more severe grades. In patients who actually develop eclampsia, severe headache is a frequent forerunner of the first convulsion. It is most often frontal but may be occipital, and it is resistant to ordinary treatment. Epigastric pain is another late symptom in preeclampsia. It appears so late that it indicates imminent convulsions. It may be the result of stretching of the hepatic capsule by hemorrhage, although it is thought by some to be of central nervous origin.

Visual disturbances ranging from a slight blurring of vision to blindness frequently accompany preeclampsia. Although they are thought by some to be of central origin, they are more likely attributable to retinal arteriolar spasm, ischemia, edema, and in rare cases actual detachment.

Retinal Changes. The most common retinal findings in preeclampsia are spasm of the aterioles and, less frequently, edema. Pollak and Nettles observed retinal arteriolar spasm in 30 of 35 patients in whom the diagnosis of preeclampsia was confirmed by renal biopsy. On the basis of an extensive study, Hallum points out that the first change observed during preeclampsia is constriction of the arteriolar lumen. The constrictions may be localized; some are elongated and spindle-shaped, usually limited to the first half of the retinal arteriole, near the optic disc. The constrictions are seen more frequently in the nasal branches. In other patients the first change observed may be a generalized arteriolar constriction, changing the normal ratio of venous to arteriolar diameters (3 to 2) to 2 to 1. As the severity of the disease advances, the arterioles usually become more constricted until the ratio increases to 3 to 1, or more. As the retinal arterioles become progressively constricted in preeclampsia, there may be edema, which is ordinarily the first sign of retinal involvement. It usually makes its appearance at the upper and lower poles of the disc and progresses thence along the course of the retinal vessels. In the earlier stage of retinal edema the portion involved appears milky. On close examination with the very best focus of the ophthalmoscope, the retinal surface shows faint striations running in the direction of the layers of neural fibers. Retinal edema is illustrated in Figure 2. In rare instances retinal edema may progress to detachment of the retina, but in general the prognosis of such detachments is good, the retina reattaching, as a rule, within a few weeks after delivery. Hemorrhages and exudates are extremely rare in preeclampsia, usually indicating underlying chronic hypertensive vascular disease.

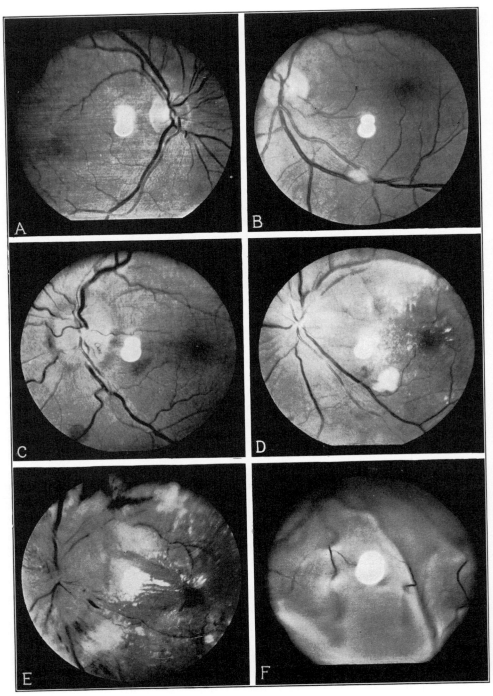

Fig. 2. The retinal changes in various types of toxemia. See description on opposite page. (Courtesy of Dr. A. J. Bedell.)

Finnerty has described a retinal sheen, probably attributable to edema, which he believes to be almost specific in pregnancy for preeclampsia. He stated that it is always found in this disorder and is often an early sign. Finnerty differentiates preeclampsia from hypertensive disease on this basis and accepts as preeclampsia only 14 per cent of the patients referred to him with that diagnosis by obstetricians.

Cause and Pathologic Anatomy. The cause of preeclampsia, whatever it may be, is doubtless identical with that of eclampsia and is discussed under the latter heading. What little is known about causation is, at the present writing, of theoretic importance only, for it has no bearing on the diagnosis, prognosis, and management of preeclampsia. Since patients rarely die in the preeclamptic stage of the process, few data are available on pathologic anatomy. It is assumed that organic alterations in preeclampsia are similar to those observed in eclampsia but of lesser degree. The morphologic changes seen in renal biopsy specimens are discussed on page 707. The physiologic and biochemical deviations of greatest importance in preeclampsia are generalized spasm of the smaller arterioles, retention of sodium and water, and possibly disseminated intravascular coagulation. Since most of the data are derived from eclamptic patients, these important underlying mechanisms are discussed in detail in connection with the physiologic and biochemical derangements of eclampsia (pp. 711 to 716).

Diagnosis. The clinical diagnosis of preeclampsia, made on the foregoing criteria, is frequently erroneous, for not only are cases of unrecognized renal disease included but cases of essential hypertension as well, in which the blood pressure had been in the normal range during midpregnancy. The difficulties of differential diagnosis are highlighted in a study by McCartney, who did renal biopsies in 62 primigravidas carefully selected for the clinical diagnosis of preeclampsia. Histologic study of the kidneys showed that 16 of these women had chronic renal disease, 3 had no lesion, and 43 had the glomerular capillary endotheliosis alleged to be specific for preeclampsia. Clinical preeclampsia appears to be a syndrome with any of several or even no underlying renal lesion. It probably includes (1) true preeclampsia, (2) latent hypertensive vascular disease brought to light by pregnancy, and (3) chronic hypertension of whatever cause, temporarily suppressed during midpregnancy.

Fig. 2 (cont.).

A, retinal vascular spasm, showing unequal caliber of inferior temporal arteriole near disc, as sometimes seen in preeclampsia.

B, early hypertensive retinitis. Cotton wool exudate forms the fluffy mass overlying the junction of the inferior temporal arteriole and vein.

C, papilledema with hypertension, showing rounded, elevated disc, distended veins, and unevenly contracted arterioles. Deep, dark, granular hemorrhages appear as black smudges.

D, advanced hypertensive retinitis (malignant nephrosclerosis). Terminal stage characterized by very marked constrictions in the inferior temporal arteriole, thick cotton wool spot, several hemorrhages, and an irregularly outlined macular star of exudate with widespread edema of the retina obscuring the disc.

E, terminal nephritis. Immense swelling of the disc with loss of outline. Striate and deep hemorrhages, massive exudates, macular star. Marked variation in the caliber of both veins and arterioles.

F, detachment of retina, showing the retinal folds forming ridges over which the vessels are clearly outlined. Usually transitory in eclampsia.

Carbon arc forms figure 8 image.

The complexities of diagnosis are further compounded when a woman is seen for the first time late in pregnancy with hypertension and with or without edema and proteinuria. In many such cases reliable diagnoses can only be made at follow-up examinations, months after delivery. In general, the following findings suggest chronic hypertensive vascular disease rather than preeclampsia: (1) a hypertensive disorder in a previous pregnancy; (2) multiparity; (3) retinal exudate and hemorrhage as well as narrowing, tortuosity, and sclerosis of the retinal arterioles; (4) cardiac enlargement; (5) absence of proteinuria and generalized edema; (6) systolic blood pressure over 200; and (7) age 30 years or more.

In view of the difficulties often encountered in differentiating preeclampsia from hypertensive disease, a number of tests have been suggested for the purpose. Chesley and Valenti used a battery of five such tests in patients in whom the clinical diagnosis seemed clear-cut and found no single test or combination of tests to be specific. The responses of the blood pressure to the cold pressor test and to intravenous tetraethylammonium chloride, a ganglionic blocking agent, were not significantly different in the two groups of patients. The response of the blood pressure to subcutaneous vasopressin was usually, but not always, greater in women with preeclampsia than in those with essential hypertension, however. In preeclampsia, the renal clearance of urate and the capacity for concentrating sodium in the urine after salt loading were significantly different from the findings in essential or chronic hypertension, but the tests still carried a diagnostic error of about 20 per cent. Aside from the clinical diagnoses, which may have been erroneous, the tests gave discordant results in that not all three of the seemingly significant tests indicated the same diagnosis in many of the patients. Other tests that have been used include urinary excretion of chorionic gonadotropin (often increased in preeclampsia), serum levels of betaglucuronidase, and degree of diuresis induced by water loading.

Immediate Prognosis.   The immediate prognosis for the mother depends almost entirely on whether eclampsia supervenes. In 2,418 cases of preeclampsia under surveillance at the Johns Hopkins Hospital between 1924 and 1943, 92 patients, or 3.8 per cent, developed eclampsia. As the result of improvements in antepartum care, the incidence has been lowered almost to zero. If eclampsia ensues, the prognosis immediately becomes grave, the death rate from eclampsia in this country approaching 5 per cent.

The perinatal mortality is increased in preeclampsia, as in the other hypertensive disorders, and it depends chiefly upon the time of onset and the severity of the disease. In the 1,229 cases of preeclampsia, shown in Table 1, the perinatal mortality was 5.7 per cent. Severe preeclampsia tends to appear earlier than the mild variety, often before the thirty-sixth week of gestation. Its associated perinatal death rate may approach 20 per cent. Much of the loss depends upon prematurity, either because of early spontaneous labor or because of therapeutic interruption necessitated by severe, progressive preeclampsia.

Treatment.   *Prophylaxis.*   Because women seldom notice the signs of incipient preeclampsia, the early detection of the disease demands close antepartum observation, especially in certain groups of patients known to be predisposed to preeclampsia. The major predisposing factors are (1) nulliparity, (2) a familial history of eclampsia or preeclampsia, (3) multiple fetuses, (4) diabetes, (5) chronic hypertension, (6) hydatidiform mole, and (7) fetal hydrops.

Rapid gain in weight, at any time after the twentieth week, or an upward trend in the diastolic blood pressure while still in the "normal" range are danger signals. Edema of the fingers frequently is an early sign, and may precede hypertension by several weeks. Hamlin and Hughes report that edema of the fingers had developed by the thirty-first week in almost every primigravida who six weeks later showed a rise in blood pressure. Dexter and Weiss, however, noted edema of the hands or face, or both, in 64 per cent of otherwise normal women during the last two months of pregnancy. Every patient should be examined by her obstetrician every week during the last month of pregnancy and every two weeks during the two previous months. At these visits, careful blood pressure readings, weighing of the patient, and urine analyses must be routine. Furthermore, all patients should be advised verbally and, preferably, also by means of suitable printed instructions to report between visits any of the well-known symptoms or signs of preeclampsia, such as persistent headaches, visual distrubances, and puffiness of the hands or face. The reporting of any such symptoms, of course, calls for an immediate examination to confirm or rule out preeclampsia.

Many obstetricians try to limit their patients' gain in weight to about 20 pounds, or even as little as 15 pounds, in the belief that preeclampsia can be prevented thereby. The total weight gained during pregnancy, however, probably has no relation to preeclampsia unless a large component of the gain is water. Stringent restriction of gain in weight, moreover, too often entails dietary restriction of protein, to the probable detriment of both mother and fetus. Experience seems to show that it is exceptional for patients with minimal intake of sodium to develop eclampsia (deSnoo), although rigid proof is lacking. Accordingly, restriction of sodium salts, including bicarbonate, is widely advised in all patients, especially during the last trimester, even though most of them can handle sodium perfectly well.

Saluretic drugs, such as chlorothiazide and its congeners, are grossly overused. In some obstetric practices, every patient is given a diuretic at some time during pregnancy. Although diuretics have been alleged to prevent the development of preeclampsia, the double-blind study of Kraus, Marchese, and Yen casts doubt on their real value. Their patients took either a placebo or 50 mg of hydrochlorothiazide daily during the last 16 weeks or more of gestation. The incidences of preeclampsia were identical (6.67 per cent) in 195 primigravidas who took the diuretic and in 210 primigravidas who took the placebo. Similarly, the development of hypertension was unaffected in 565 multiparas. The failure of saluretic drugs in the prevention of preeclampsia raises some doubt about the efficacy of dietary restriction of sodium.

The thiazide diuretics can induce serious depletion of both sodium and potassium. Minkowitz and associates have reported two fatal cases of depletion of electrolytes and hemorrhagic pancreatitis in preeclamptic women treated with chlorothiazide. Menzies and Prystowsky reported two more. Rodriguez and associates, moreover, have noted severe thrombocytopenia in some newborns whose mothers had received thiazide diuretics. If the drugs are to be used, they should be given for not more than five days. When the drug is discontinued, sodium retention usually occurs (rebound) and another short course of treatment may be started after several days. In general, the more severe the preeclampsia, the more resistant the edema is to diuretic agents. Gray has published an excellent review of the use and abuse of thiazides in pregnant women.

Whether preeclampsia can be prevented is uncertain and, to some extent, is a matter of semantics. Since the progression of early preeclampsia to diagnosable preeclampsia to severe preeclampsia to eclampsia can usually be arrested, prenatal care must be credited with much of the marked reduction in mortality from eclampsia. In New York City during 1920, there were 190 eclamptic deaths; in 1967 there were 3; and in 1968, there were none. Prenatal care with early detection and treatment of preeclampsia, however, is not the only factor that has been operating. Nearly a quarter of the indigent women delivering at the Kings County Hospital have had no prenatal care, and that probably is a fair reflection of the situation in depressed urban areas. Moreover, the incidence and severity of preeclampsia have fallen markedly in many areas of the nation, and eclampsia, when it does occur, seems to be milder than it formerly was.

Objectives of Treatment. If a case of preeclampsia is to be managed with complete success, a number of objectives must be attained, including (1) prevention of convulsions, (2) delivery of a surviving child, (3) delivery with minimal trauma, and (4) prevention of residual hypertension. The fourth of these objectives, which is controversial, is discussed on page 725; in our opinion, it is unnecessary to consider it in the management of preeclampsia.

In certain cases of preeclampsia, especially in patients near term, all four of these objectives may be served equally well by the same treatment, namely, prompt induction of labor. In other instances, however, the attainment of certain of these goals may so conflict with the realization of others as to make it virtually impossible to attain all four objectives. For instance, if a patient develops severe preeclampsia two or three months before her expected date of confinement, prompt termination of her pregnancy may seem indicated if the first and fourth objectives are to be realized, but this course may well result in the delivery of a grossly premature infant and consequent failure to attain the second objective. Again, when preeclampsia develops at such an early date, a long, closed cervix may make induction of labor hazardous. If in this case convulsions seem imminent, cesarean section may become almost mandatory. Although it may be impossible to attain all four of these objectives in every case, the extent to which we are able to do so is a rough gauge of our success in the management of this complication.

Foremost of these objectives is the prevention of eclampsia, because the development of convulsions in a patient with preeclampsia under observation is a grave catastrophe, representing grievous failure of antepartum care. In the 92 cases of eclampsia developing under observation at the Johns Hopkins Hospital (p. 694), 7 mothers and 20 infants died, yielding mortality rates of 7.6 and 21.7 per cent, respectively. By contrast, in the 2,326 cases of preeclampsia in which convulsions did not develop, only 4 mothers (0.2 per cent) and 158 infants (6.8 per cent) succumbed. Some of the more common causes of failure in the prevention of eclampsia in these 92 cases of preeclampsia were as follows: in 16 cases, failure to evaluate gravity of sudden weight gain; in 15 cases, failure to evaluate gravity of moderate deviations from normal (blood pressure, proteinuria, and edema) in young primigravidas; in 10 cases, failure to see patients every week during the last month; in 6 cases, failure to evaluate gravity of symptoms (headache, epigastric pain, and vomiting); in 3 cases, failure to evaluate gravity of moderate deviations from normal (blood pressure, proteinuria, edema) in twin pregnancy; and in 3 cases, failure to evaluate gravity of high diastolic pressure. These are all common potential sources of failure in the prevention of eclampsia and should be borne in mind in the management of every case of preeclampsia.

Ambulatory Treatment. An even more common cause of failure to forestall convulsions in the 92 cases of preeclampsia discussed here was tardiness in hospitalization, a lapse that was responsible for the outbreak of convulsions in 19 cases. Ambulatory treatment has no place in the management of preeclampsia as defined. Some patients, excluding young nulliparas whose systolic blood pressure does not exceed 135 mm and whose diastolic pressure does not exceed 85 mm and in whom edema and proteinuria are absent or minimal, may be managed tentatively at home pending the aggravation or abatement of signs and symptoms. The activities of such a patient should be confined to one floor. She should be instructed to add no salt to her food in the kitchen and none at the table. She should be given written instructions with a list of salt-containing foods to avoid, and she should be cautioned not to use baking soda for the relief of heartburn. Bed rest with the patient lying on her side throughout the greater part of the day should be encouraged. Such patients, moreover, should be examined twice a week rather than once and be instructed in detail about the reporting of symptoms. With minor elevations of blood pressure the response to this regimen is often immediate, but the patient must be cooperative and the obstetrician wary. If sodium restriction proves difficult for the patient, various salt substitutes are on the market (Rimmerman and Halpern). Many patients will not adhere to the low-salt diet. One of the best ways to check is to ask whether she likes the diet. If she says "yes," she is not on it.

Hospital Management. The indications for hospitalization in preeclampsia are (1) a systolic blood pressure of 140 mm or above or a diastolic of 90 mm or above, (2) significant proteinuria (1 plus or greater in a midstream catch or from catheterization), and (3) repeated weight gains of three pounds or more a week. In most cases the first and third of these indications will combine to emphasize the urgent desirability of hospitalization.

For an intelligent appraisal of the present severity of the case, a systematic method of study should be instituted upon admittance to the hospital: (1) a general physical examination and history, followed by daily search for the development of such signs and symptoms as headache, hyperreflexia, visual disturbances, and edema of the fingers and eyelids; (2) weight on admittance and every day thereafter; (3) blood pressure readings every four hours (except between midnight and morning unless the midnight pressure has risen); (4) record of daily fluid intake and urinary output; (5) daily quantitative analysis of the urine for protein and microscopic examination for casts; and (6) retinal examination on admittance and every second or third day thereafter, depending on findings. Blood chemical analyses in preeclampsia have yielded very little practical information, but if they can be readily obtained, the most informative measurements are uric acid and carbon dioxide content. Serial measurements of hematocrit are helpful in following hemoconcentration.

Complete bed rest is essential, and the patient should be instructed to lie on her side. The most important dietary specification is salt-poor food containing sodium equivalent to 3 g per day or less of sodium chloride. Ample proteins should be included in the diet in the form of lean meats, eggs, and one quart of milk daily. Brewer, in a flood of personal communications, believes that such a diet earlier in pregnancy will prevent preeclampsia. The fluid intake should be neither limited nor forced and is best set at 2,500 ml except in hot weather when 3,000 ml are permissible. In severe cases, with persistent oliguria, the fluid intake should be limited to reduce the danger of pulmonary edema. Even in milder cases small doses of a sedative drug are helpful—for example, 0.03 g of pheno-barbital four times daily, or twice that dose in cases of moderate severity. Oral magnesium sulfate and citrate of magnesia, widely used in the past, are inef-fective because they divert excreted water from the kidney to the bowel without an equivalent loss of sodium.

The further management of a case of preeclampsia will depend upon (1) its severity as demonstrated by the course in the hospital, (2) the condition of the cervix, and (3) other factors. Fortunately, most cases prove to be sufficiently mild and near enough to term that they can be managed conservatively until labor starts spontaneously or the cervix becomes suitable for induction. Com-plete abatement of all signs and symptoms, however, is uncommon until after delivery.

Occasionally preeclampsia is fulminating, as evidenced by blood pressure in excess of 160/110, massive edema, heavy proteinuria, and general nervousness, indicating that convulsions are imminent. Such severe preeclampsia demands immediate and intensive medicinal therapy for 12 to 24 hours. The prime ob-jectives are to forestall convulsions and to deliver a living infant. Some clinics use magnesium sulfate alone, but sedatives are widely employed in others. The doses of sedative drugs should be regulated to produce drowsiness or light sleep from which the patient can be easily awakened, but not coma. Sedation may well be initiated by a hypodermic injection of 15 mg of morphine sulfate fol-lowed by either paraldehyde per rectum or one of the barbiturates. There are two objections to paraldehyde. First, in the usual dosage it sedates the patient to the point that it may be difficult to differentiate the effect of the drug from the progression of the preeclampsia to coma; second, the rectal instillation may not be retained. Some of the barbiturates are subject to the objection that they increase cerebral vascular resistance and decrease cerebral oxygen consumption, abnormalities already present in severe preeclampsia (McCall). Effective doses of any of them, furthermore, depress the fetus.

If paraldehyde is employed, the dose should be about 10 ml for a woman weighing under 160 pounds, or 15 ml if she appears to weigh more, administered rectally in 30 ml of olive oil, with repetition every 6 to 10 hours, the interval depending on restlessness and blood pressure. Paraldehyde usually produces a fall in blood pressure, is dependable prophylaxis against convulsions, does not depend upon renal excretion for disposal, and has a wide margin of safety.

If the paraldehyde is expelled, one of the longer-acting barbiturates may be used—for example, phenobarbital sodium 0.1 g orally every 6 to 8 hours, or sodium amytal 0.2 g intramuscularly every 8 to 12 hours.

In fulminating preeclampsia, as well as in eclampsia, parenteral magnesium sulfate is a most valuable anticonvulsant agent, as attested by the experience of many clinics over many years. The magnesium sulfate may be given intramus-cularly or intravenously by single injections or continuous infusion. Its use will be discussed in detail on page 728. If labor is to be induced, magnesium sulfate injections should be started before the procedure is initiated.

In severe preeclampsia associated with oliguria (urinary output of less than

400 ml during 24 hours of observation), intravenous dextrose or mannitol may be indicated. In many clinics this treatment is routine in all severe cases for the purpose of increasing the urinary output. Over the years the trend has been toward the use of less concentrated solutions of dextrose. Fifty per cent solutions were formerly in vogue because they were supposed to produce an osmotic (artificial diabetic) diuresis, reduce intracranial pressure, and protect the liver by deposition of glycogen. The osmotic diuresis produced by the customary dose of 50 ml of 50 per cent dextrose is fleeting and almost negligible; the transitory reduction in intracranial pressure is followed by a rebound to even higher levels; moreover, the concentrated solutions cause sclerosis of the veins and conduce to thrombosis. Other concentrations used have been 30, 25, 20, 10, and 5 per cent. With the possible exception of the 20 per cent solution, the increase in urinary volume often falls short of the volume of fluid infused. Mannitol, a nonmetabolized alcohol derived from fructose, is an osmotic diuretic that finds its chief clinical use in the prophylaxis and early treatment of acute renal failure. When used in treating the oliguria of preeclampsia-eclampsia, the initial dose should be 12.5 g in 25 per cent solution given intravenously over about five minutes. If the urinary flow increases to more than 60 ml per hour, mannitol can then be given by continuous infusion, adjusted to produce a urinary flow of about 100 ml per hour. Not more than 200 g should be given in a day. Since there is a risk of overloading the circulation, the central venous pressure should be monitored if mannitol is to be infused for more than two hours. In general, persistent oliguria in preeclampsia is an indication for termination of pregnancy.

Termination of Pregnancy. The only specific treatment of preeclampsia is termination of the pregnancy. There are two main reasons why prompt delivery is desirable: prevention of convulsions and prevention of fetal death. Abruptio placentae, which poses additional hazards to mother and infant (Ch. 23, p. 634), is alleged by some workers to be an additional risk. Because the baby may be premature, however, the tendency is widespread to temporize in many of these cases in the hope that a few more weeks of intrauterine life will give the infant a better chance. In the milder varieties of preeclampsia such a policy is often justifiable, at least until the thirty-seventh week of gestation. In severe preeclampsia, however, as McLane has emphasized, waiting may be ill-advised, since preeclampsia itself may kill the fetus and, even in the lower weight brackets, the likelihood of survival in severe preeclampsia may be better outside than inside the uterus.

Assessment of fetal and placental function is of practical value when there is hesitation to deliver the fetus because of prematurity. Serial measurements of plasma or urinary estriol, plasma heat-stable alkaline phosphatase or cystine aminopeptidase, or placental lactogen (human chorionic somatomammotropin) may show abnormal values when the fetoplacental unit is compromised. Failure of the fetus to grow, as estimated clinically or by sonography, is another sign that he is in jeopardy. Analyses of the amniotic fluid for bilirubin, creatinine, and fetal sebaceous material may provide additional indices of fetal maturity.

The decision whether to terminate pregnancy in preeclampsia involves, on the one hand, allowing the pregnancy to continue with the hazards of convulsions and possible fetal death, and, on the other, termination of the pregnancy with the risks attendant upon operative interference and the possibility of a premature baby that succumbs. In a patient near term with a soft, open, and partially effaced cervix, even the mildest degrees of preeclampsia probably carry more risk to the mother and her infant than does induction of labor by simple rupture of the membranes or with oxytocin stimulation. If, however, the preeclampsia is mild but the cervix is firm and closed (indicating a reasonable likelihood of abdominal delivery if pregnancy is to be terminated), the hazard of cesarean section may be greater than that of allowing the pregnancy to continue for a few weeks under treatment, at the end of which time the cervix may be suitable for induction. If severe preeclampsia, as judged by the general condition of the patient, does not improve with medicinal therapy after one or two days, termination of pregnancy is usually advisable for both the mother and the infant. Labor may be induced by administration of oxytocin and rupture of the membranes. This procedure is often successful, even when the cervix appears unfavorable. If attempts at induction of labor are not successful after a short trial, cesarean section may be the procedure of choice (see p. 733).

The termination of pregnancy in preeclampsia should rarely be performed until after 12 to 24 hours of intensive treatment in the hospital. After this period of stabilization the patient will invariably be a much better operative risk for either procedure than she was on admittance. If cesarean section is to be done, general anesthesia with thiopental nitrous oxide, and a muscle relaxant has many advantages (p. 457). With local infiltration there is always danger of a convulsion. With subarachnoid or epidural block severe hypotension may occur (Ch. 18, p. 452).

ECLAMPSIA

Eclampsia is an acute disorder peculiar to pregnant and puerperal women, characterized by clonic and tonic convulsions during which there is a loss of consciousness followed by more or less prolonged coma. It may result in death. The word "eclampsia" is derived from the Greek term used by Hippocrates to designate a fever of sudden onset. The word means a flash or shining forth and is indicative of the fulminating character of the disease that has come to be generally known as eclampsia.

Incidence. Eclampsia is becoming rarer each year as more and more women receive better prenatal care. The incidence throughout the country is probably 1 in every 1,500 to 2,000 deliveries, but there are wide deviations from this figure in different localities and countries. In interpreting data on the incidence of eclampsia, three fundamental factors must be kept in mind: (1) the extent of antepartum care, (2) the proportion of nulliparas, and (3) the source of the statistics. Eclampsia is usually preventable and will therefore be less prevalent and cause fewer deaths in localities where most women seek antepartum care. Eclampsia occurs more often in nulliparas than in multiparas, in a ratio of about 3 to 1. Moreover, many of the multiparous eclamptics have underlying hypertensive disease, and some may really have hypertensive encephalopathy. Nearly all statistics, except for deaths, are derived from hospital experiences. In many areas of the world, and formerly in some of the United States, women plan for home deliveries and are transported scores of miles to a hospital because of a complication such as eclampsia. Hospital statistics in the northeastern metropolitan areas of the United States reflect fairly well the local incidence of the hypertensive disorders. In the past, those of the hospitals in the southeastern United States have not. The uncritical acceptance of data on incidence of eclampsia and eclamptic deaths has led to many publications proposing that the cause is a high-protein diet, a low-protein diet, a deficiency of one vitamin or another, unwholesome city life, mental stress, the weather, and innumerable other factors.

Depending on whether the disorder first appears before labor, during labor, or in the puerperium, it is designated as *antepartum, intrapartum,* or *postpartum* eclampsia, respectively. Roughly about one half of the cases develop antepartum, approximately one quarter intrapartum, and another quarter postpartum. Nearly all cases of postpartum eclampsia appear within 24 hours after delivery, and cases in which the first convulsion is observed more than 48 hours postpartum should be regarded with some skepticism. Nevertheless, in rare instances, cases are said to have begun as late as six days after delivery. Convulsions beginning more than one week after delivery may be confidently attributed to some other origin. Eclampsia occurs almost exclusively in the last third of pregnancy and becomes increasingly frequent as term is approached.

The disorder is noted four times more often in twin than in single pregnancies, and four or five times more frequently when the pregnancy is complicated by hydramnios, although the significant correlation may be with the cause of the hydramnios, for example, diabetes (Jeffcoate and Scott). Eclampsia may occur during the course of advanced extrauterine gestation. Pride and Rucker have reported a case occurring in a woman with an ovarian pregnancy.

The association of preeclampsia with hydatidiform mole has long been known. Page observed 30 women with moles and arbitrarily divided the cases into early stages (less than four months' amenorrhea, or a tumor below the level of the umbilicus), and late stages (from four to seven months' amenorrhea, or a tumor above the level of the umbilicus). Among the 16 early cases, there were no instances of preeclampsia. Three severe and 7 mild cases of preeclampsia were found among 14 women with hydatidiform moles of four to seven months' duration, an incidence of about three out of four. In a study of 57 consecutive cases of hydatidiform mole by Chesley, Cosgrove, and Preece, it was found that one of the patients developed eclampsia between the fourth and fifth months. The case was of extraordinary interest in that the patient had developed severe preeclampsia in a previous molar pregnancy but had manifested no evidence of hypertension in three intervening normal pregnancies without mole. These authors found in the literature 35 cases of probable or alleged eclampsia occurring in association with hydatidiform mole or with partial hydatidiform degeneration of the placenta. In practically all these cases eclampsia was said to have occurred extremely early—that is, between the third and sixth months. Lembrych found 14 additional cases in the more recent literature and added one of his own, the fiftieth.

There appears to be a familial tendency to preeclampsia. In a unique study of this question, Chesley, Annitto, and Cosgrove traced more than 96 per cent of the grown daughters of women who had had eclampsia at the Margaret Hague Maternity Hospital. Among the 187 who carried pregnancies to viability, the incidence of preeclampsia in the first pregnancy was 26 per cent; four of the daughters, or 1 in 47, had eclampsia. Adams and Finlayson, in a study of sisters, also found a strong familial factor. Humphries has studied the question from another angle. Since many parturients at the Johns Hopkins Hospital today were born there themselves, obstetric charts are available for mother and daughter pairs. The mothers of 100 hypertensive daughters had had an incidence of hypertension of 28 per cent. In contrast, the mothers of 200 normal daughters delivering in the same decade and selected at random had had an incidence of hypertension of only 13 per cent. (The term "hypertensive" here includes preeclampsia as well as the other hypertensive disorders.)

Clinical Course.   Almost without exception, the outbreak of convulsions is preceded by clinical preeclampsia. Isolated cases are occasionally cited in which an eclamptic convulsion is said to have occurred without warning in women who were apparently in good health. Usually such a patient had not been examined by her physician for some days or weeks previously, and she had neglected to report symptoms of preeclampsia. Occasionally a distinct aura precedes the onset, but it is usually lacking. Severe epigastric pain and a sensation of constriction of the thorax, frequent precursors of a seizure, are signs that should excite grave concern. Apprehension, excitability, and hyperreflexia often precede the convulsion. The hyperreflexia is so characteristic that testing of the reflexes at intervals should be part of the routine assessment of any patient with preeclampsia; convulsions may, however, occur in the absence of hyperreflexia.

The attack may come on at any time, sometimes while the patient is sleeping. If she is awake, the first sign of the impending convulsion is a fixed expression of the eyes and a tense turning of the head to one side. The pupils are usually dilated; less often they may be contracted. The convulsive movements begin about the mouth in the form of facial twitchings. This *stage of invasion* of the convulsion lasts only a few seconds.

The whole body then becomes rigid in a generalized muscular contraction. The face is distorted, the eyes protrude, the arms are flexed, the hands are clenched, and the legs are inverted. Since all the muscles of the body are now in a state of tonic contraction, this phase may be regarded as the *stage of contraction,* which lasts 15 to 20 seconds.

Suddenly the jaws begin to open and close violently, and forthwith the eyelids also. The other facial muscles and then all the muscles of the body alternately contract and relax in rapid succession. So forceful are the muscular movements that the patient may throw herself out of bed, and almost invariably, unless protected, the tongue is bitten by the violent action of the jaws. Foam, often blood-tinged, exudes from the mouth. The face is congested and purple, and the eyes are bloodshot. Few clinical pictures are so terrifying. This phase, in which the muscles alternately contract and relax, is called the *stage of convulsion,* which may last about a minute. Gradually the muscular movements become smaller and less frequent, and finally the patient lies motionless.

Throughout the seizure the diaphragm has been fixed, with respiration halted. For a few seconds the woman appears to be dying from respiratory arrest, but just when a fatal outcome seems almost inevitable, she takes a long, deep, stertorous inhalation, and breathing is resumed. Coma ensues. The patient will remember nothing of the convulsion or, in all probability, of events immediately before and afterward.

When the disorder appears in the latter part of labor or during the puerperium, only a single convulsion may be observed. More often, however, the first is the forerunner of other convulsions, which may vary in number from one or two in mild cases to 10 to 20 or even 100 or more in severe cases, the intervals between them becoming shorter in inverse proportion to the number. In rare instances they follow one another so rapidly that the patient appears to be in a prolonged, almost continuous convulsion.

The duration of the coma is quite variable. When the convulsions are infrequent, the patient usually recovers consciousness after each attack. In severe cases the coma persists from one convulsion to another, and death may result before the patient awakens. In rare instances a single convulsion may be followed by profound coma from which the patient never emerges, although, as a rule, death does not occur until after a frequent repetition of the convulsive attacks. The immediate cause of death is usually pulmonary edema, apoplexy, or acidosis, although if death is postponed for several days it may be attributable to aspiration pneumonia, marked hepatic degeneration, or acute renal failure.

Whereas the convulsions are by far the most striking clinical manifestation of eclampsia, rarely they are absent, with the patient dying in coma and presenting at autopsy the hepatic and renal lesions compatible with the disorder. For instance, Dieckmann and Wegner reported a case without convulsions in which the hepatic lesion was typical of eclampsia. Moreover, Reis and Bernick have reported a case, which they refer to as eclampsia, in which there occurred no convulsions, hypertension, or coma. It is probably clearer to limit the diagnosis of eclampsia to convulsive cases, regarding fatal nonconvulsive cases as exceedingly severe preeclampsia. Such a policy would bring more forcibly to our attention the fact that preeclampsia and eclampsia are one disorder with all gradations of pathologic changes and with a clinical picture that may show wide variations. In some cases the absence of convulsive attacks has led to an erroneous clinical diagnosis, the condition having been regarded as uremic coma, poisoning by phosphorus, fulminating bacterial infection, Weil's disease, or acute yellow atrophy of the liver.

In most but not all cases of eclampsia the arterial pressure is markedly augmented. Very rarely, little or no increase is observed above levels that are accepted as normal, and patients may occasionally go through the eclamptic attacks with a maximal systolic pressure of 140 mm or less. Such patients usually are young girls in whom the antecedent blood pressure had been of the order of 105 systolic and 60 diastolic. In them, an elevation to 135 systolic and 90 diastolic would represent hypertension. The pulse is usually full and bounding, but in very severe cases it is rapid but weak, and becomes weaker with each succeeding convulsion. The temperature rises to 101°F or above in a third or more of the cases. Temperatures of 103° and 104° are of very grave prognostic import. The cause of the fever is probably central.

Respiration in eclampsia is usually increased in rate and is stertorous. The rate may reach 50 or more per minute, exerting profound effects on the acid-base balance. Cyanosis may be observed in severe cases.

Proteinuria is almost always present and is frequently pronounced. The urinary protein excreted in eclampsia has an albumin to globulin ratio of 2 or 3 to 1, probably the direct result of increased glomerular capillary permeability. The output of urine is invariably diminished and occasionally is entirely suppressed. On microscopic examination various types of casts are found in great abundance, with the hyaline and granular varieties predominating. Epithelial casts also occur, as well as isolated renal cells, and blood is nearly always present. Hemoglobinuria may also be observed.

Edema is probably present in all eclamptic patients, but in 10 or 15 per cent it is occult and not demonstrable on superficial examination. Often it is massive, eclamptic patients occasionally gaining 70 or more pounds during gestation.

In antepartum eclampsia, labor begins as a rule after a short while and often progresses rapidly to completion, sometimes before the attendants are even aware that the patient is having contractions. If the attack occurs during labor, the contractions usually increase in frequency and severity, and the duration of labor is shortened. Improvement after delivery with subsidence of convulsions may be expected, provided proper treatment has been instituted. Not infrequently labor does not supervene, but the patient improves greatly, convulsions cease, the coma disappears, and the patient becomes completely oriented. This improved state may continue for several days or longer, a condition known as *intercurrent eclampsia*. It has been claimed that such patients may often return entirely to normal with complete subsidence of the hypertension and proteinuria, but that event has been extremely rare in our experience. Although convulsions and coma may entirely subside and the blood pressure and proteinuria may decrease to a certain extent, such patients usually continue to show substantial hypertension and demonstrable proteinuria. It is likely that they have merely returned to the preeclamptic state. It is not uncommon for such patients, after a few days of apparent improvement, to develop convulsions again. This second attack may be exceedingly severe, even fatal. Accordingly, one must be wary about these cases of so-called intercurrent eclampsia, for unless delivery occurs, return of convulsions is always a threat.

Improvement is most likely to be observed 12 to 14 hours after delivery, when the convulsions usually decrease in frequency and then subside entirely. The duration of coma before complete mental orientation varies from a few hours to several days. As the patient arouses from her coma, there often ensues a semiconscious, combative state that may last as long as a day. The first sign of improvement is usually an increase in urinary output. The proteinuria and edema ordinarily disappear within four or five days. The hypertension is likely to persist for seven to ten days, but in most cases the blood pressure returns to normal within two weeks after delivery.

In fatal cases pulmonary edema is common, especially during the terminal hours. It may be present also in patients who survive, but it is always a grave prognostic sign. Other signs of cardiac failure appear in the terminal stage of fatal eclampsia, especially cyanosis, a rising pulse rate, and a falling blood pressure. As the cardiovascular system fails, convulsions usually cease and may not occur at all during the last six or eight hours of life. In some cases of eclampsia, death occurs suddenly, synchronously with or shortly after a convulsion, as the result of massive cerebral hemorrhage.

In about every twentieth case, eclampsia is followed by an acute psychosis in which the patient may become violent (Sioli). The psychosis usually appears on the second or third day after delivery, or about the time that the patient is coming out of coma. It ordinarily lasts for one or two weeks. The prognosis in general is good except when the patient has a preexisting mental illness. In rare instances hemiplegia may result from a sublethal cerebral hemorrhage (Parks and Pearson).

In 1 or 2 per cent of cases, the patient finds herself blind as she begins to arouse from her coma. Most frequently the disturbed vision, sometimes preceding the attack, is caused by retinal edema, which usually disappears spontaneously. It is sometimes central in origin, caused by a disturbance in the optic nerve or in the visual centers in the occipital lobe; the most logical explanation is edema of these structures. The blindness may persist for a few hours or for several weeks. Usually, however, the vision returns to normal within a week and the prognosis for sight is good. Occasionally, hemorrhagic retinitis or detachment of the retina is observed. In an ophthalmologic study of 132 eclamptic patients, Schiötz found 7 cases of retinal detachment, in 2 of whom the detachment persisted for years. Clapp reported 6 cases of detachment, with complete recovery in all. Doggart stresses four points of distinction in retinal detachment in eclampsia: (1) rapidity of onset, (2) subretinal fluid, (3) no hemorrhage or exudate with extensive bilateral detachment, and (4) a generally good prognosis. The prognosis of ocular lesions accompanying eclampsia is surprisingly favorable. Most cases of incomplete detachment of the retina and many cases of complete detachment result in no permanent impairment of vision.

Pathologic Anatomy.   The most common alterations found in eclampsia are in the liver, kidneys, brain, lungs, and heart.

The characteristic *hepatic* lesion is hemorrhagic necrosis in the periphery of the lobules (Fig. 3). It may appear grossly as irregularly shaped reddish areas both beneath the capsule and on the cut surface, giving the liver a mottled appearance. The hemorrhages are most commonly found in the right lobe of the liver. The areas of hemorrhagic necrosis begin about a periportal space and are usually associated with extensive thrombosis in the smallest vessels in the periportal connective tissue. In the opinion of Sheehan the lesion is the result primarily of the escape of blood or plasma into the peripheral base of the hepatic cell cords. Thus the cords are pushed up in their connective tissue sleeves. At the base, the sleeves may be distended by fibrin masses, which then compress the blood sinuses. Secondary necrotic changes often appear in the few cells at the base of the cord. Diffuse lesions result from the dissection of the liver cords from their sleeves by plasma or whole blood. The artificial channels may erupt into the sinuses at almost any point, and an extravascular circulation may thus be established. Although fibrin is usually seen in the focal lesion, it is rare in the diffuse lesion.

Although the characteristic hepatic necrosis of eclampsia is periportal, the lesion may sometimes extend into the center of the hepatic lobule, as has been described by Acosta-Sison, Way, and others. As Dieckmann pointed out, it is barely possible that the central and midzonal necrosis is the result of relative starvation. The most characteristic feature of the hepatic lesion in eclampsia is its variability in extent and severity. Many cases have been reported with no hepatic necrosis whatsoever. In Acosta-Sison's series of cases the hepatic necrosis was so variable and bizarre in distribution that she was unable to confirm the view, then prevalent, that focal necrosis around the portal areas is the characteristic lesion of eclampsia. Bell, Theobald, and Davidson, furthermore, are all of the opinion that peripheral necrosis is not always the typical or frequent

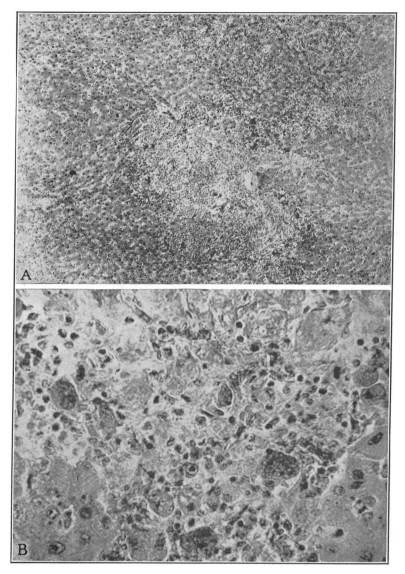

Fig. 3. Liver from eclampsia. A, section showing periportal necrosis. B, area of same section showing damage of hepatic cells.

hepatic lesion in this disorder. Moreover, nearly all observers agree that there is no correlation between the clinical severity of eclampsia and the extent of the hepatic lesion. It is therefore generally agreed that the hepatic lesions of eclampsia can be the result but certainly not the cause of the disorder.

Hepatic biopsies have been performed in five cases of eclampsia by Ingerslev and Teilum. The liver was apparently quite normal in two cases, but in two others it showed changes attributed to eclampsia. Their two patients with the severest hepatic changes survived.

In rare instances hemorrhage beneath the hepatic capsule may be so extensive as to cause rupture of the capsule with massive hemorrhage into the peritoneal cavity. Salzmann and Malkary have reported such a case of their own and have reviewed 21 other published cases of rupture of the hepatic capsule. Of the six women who survived, only one did not have hypertension; eclampsia or severe preeclampsia was present in nearly all of the fatal cases. Two or three additional cases are reported annually.

Renal lesions are usually found. Sheehan, who has studied a large number of cases brought to necropsy within an hour of death, writes that all of the glomeruli are enlarged by about 20 per cent, often pouting into the neck of the tubule. The capillary loops vary from a contraction to a twofold increase in diameter. The endothelial cells are swollen, and they deposit fibrils that share some of the staining reactions of collagen and have been mistaken for thickening and reduplication of the basement membrane. The changes are exaggerated in elderly primigravidas and multiparas who die of eclampsia. Sheehan's interpretations have been confirmed by electron microscopic studies of renal biopsies taken from patients with preeclampsia. Most (Farquhar; Mautner and associates; Pollak and Nettles; and others), but not all (Ishikawa), of the electron microscopic studies agree that the characteristic change is glomerular capillary endothelial swelling, which Spargo and associates called "glomerular capillary endotheliosis." Whether intercapillary cells are increased in number is controversial. Various changes in the basal lamina (basement membrane), the glomer-

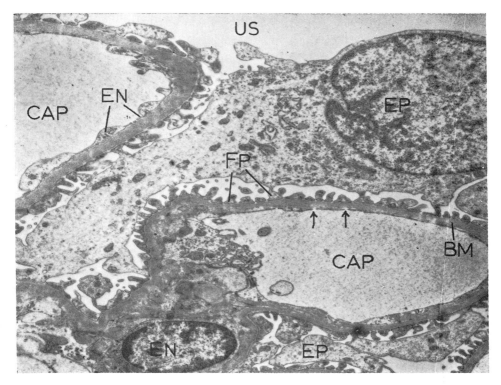

Fig. 4. Electron micrograph of renal glomerular capillaries in a biopsy from a normal subject. Abbreviations: BM, basement membrane; CAP, capillary lumen; EN, endothelium; EP, epithelium; FP, epithelial foot process; US, urinary space in Bowman's capsule. (From Hopper et al. Obstet Gynec 17:271, 1961.)

ular epithelial cells and their podocytic processes, and the mesangium have been affirmed and denied. The endothelial cells are so swollen as to block, partially or even completely, the capillary lumens. Homogeneous deposits of an electro-dense substance are found between the basal lamina and the endothelial cell and within the cells themselves (Figs. 4 and 5). Vassalli, Morris, and McCluskey, using immunofluorescent staining, have identified the material as fibrinogen or a fibrinogen derivative and regard its presence as characteristic of preeclampsia.

Faith and Trump, in comparing the renal lesions of preeclampsia with those of systemic lupus erythematosus and acute glomerulonephritis, noted several common features. In each disease there is a characteristic exaggeration of one or more changes, the differences involving chiefly the appearance and location of abnormal deposits in the glomerular wall. The morphologic alterations prob-ably result from the endothelial phagocytosis, transport, and deposition of ma-terial from the circulating plasma.

The renal changes almost always regress rapidly after delivery, as Sheehan wrote. Tubular lesions are also common in eclampsia, but what has been in-terpreted as degenerative change may represent only an accumulation within the cells of protein reabsorbed from the glomerular filtrate. The collecting tubules are often obstructed by casts, from derivatives of protein and hemoglobin. The hemoglobin casts may be associated with the typical damage resulting in oliguria. Altchek, Albright, and Sommers have reported a lesion in Henle's loop, the severity of which is positively correlated with the degree of hyperuricemia. They also confirmed the finding by McManus, Pollak and Nettles, and Fisher and co-workers of hyperplasia of the juxtaglomerular apparatus, with evidence of high activity.

The renal changes have been held out by some as pathognomonic of pre-eclampsia, always present in that disease and specific for it. The uncertainties of clinical diagnosis are so great, however, as to preclude acceptance of such a one-to-one relation, except as an act of faith. The morphologic findings of McCartney, in carefully selected cases of clinical preeclampsia, are described on page 692. The history of "pathognomonic" lesions in eclampsia engenders skepti-cism. One such lesion accepted in the past was the peripheral, hemorrhagic necrosis of the hepatic lobules, discussed on page 705.

In rare cases the major portion of the cortex of both kidneys undergoes complete necrosis, as the result of thrombosis of the intralobular arteries with extension from or into the glomerular capillaries. Infarction and necrosis ensue. The condition probably results from spasm of the renal arteries with resultant thrombosis and anemic infarcts. Although cortical necrosis of the kidney is known to have occurred in nonpregnant women and in men, many cases have been associated with pregnancy. In a group of 45 authentic and 16 questionable cases collected by Dieckmann from the literature, 9 were encountered during autopsies of eclamptic patients. The disease is characterized clinically by oliguria or anuria and rapidly developing azotemia.

The main postmortem lesions described in the *brain* in eclampsia are edema, hyperemia, focal anemia, thrombosis, and hemorrhage. Prutz noted edema in 42 per cent, hyperemia in 35 per cent, and hemorrhage in 13 per cent, while the brain was apparently normal in only 10 per cent of his cases. Schmorl, in 58 out of 65 autopsies, noted the presence of petechial hemorrhages and thrombi in the smaller cerebral vessels and regarded them as the cause of the small areas of

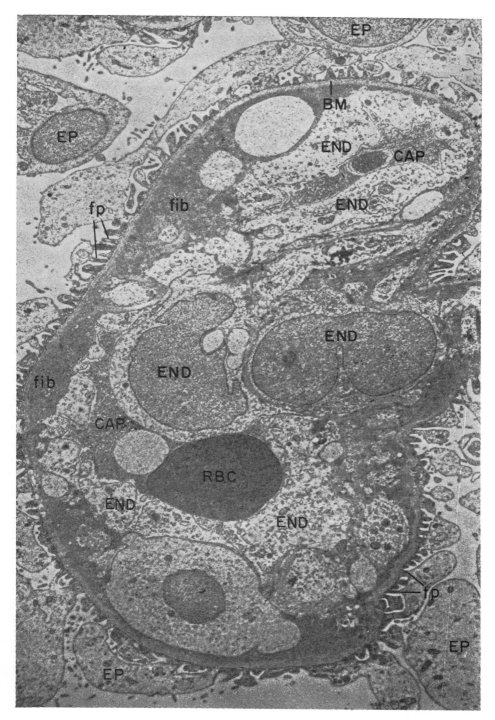

Fig. 5. Electron micrograph of a renal glomerular capillary in a biopsy from a patient with preeclampsia. Abbreviations: BM, basement membrane (normal); CAP, capillary lumen (severely reduced); END, endothelium (markedly swollen); EP, epithelium (normal); fib, "fibrinoid" (abnormal); fp, epithelial foot processes (normal); RBC, red blood cell. (From Farquhar. Review of normal and pathologic glomerular ultrastructure, in Proceedings Tenth Annual Conference on the Nephrotic Syndrome. National Kidney Disease Foundation, 1959.)

necrosis that are often observed. In Way's more recent study of 33 autopsies of eclamptic patients, cerebral hemorrhage was present in 3 cases, in 2 of which it was massive. These 2 cases also demonstrated cerebral arteritis and arteriolitis with necrosis of the vascular walls. Sheehan examined the brains of 48 eclamptic women within about an hour after their death. Hemorrhages, ranging from petechiae to gross bleeding, were found in 56 per cent of the cases. According to Sheehan, if the brain is examined within an hour after death, it is as firm as normal and there is no obvious edema. Cisternal pressures are normal, according to Spoljanskij and Juzhelevskiy. Govan ascertained the cause of death in 110 fatal cases of eclampsia and found that cerebral hemorrhage was responsible in 39. Forty-seven women died of cardiorespiratory failure; small hemorrhagic lesions were found in the brains of 85 per cent of them. Govan describes fibrinoid changes as a regular finding in the walls of the cerebral vessels. The lesions sometimes appear to have been present for some time, as judged from the surrounding leukocytic response and infiltration by pigmented macrophages. These findings suggest that the prodromal neurologic symptoms and the convulsions may be explained by the lesions.

In most cases of eclampsia the *heart* is involved to a greater or lesser extent. According to Schmorl, the changes usually consist in degenerative lesions of the myocardium. Disregarding cloudy swelling and fatty degeneration, which were very frequently present, he found hemorrhage and necrosis in the myocardium in 43 of 73 autopsies. Around the hemorrhages the muscle fibers undergo hyaline degeneration. Among Way's 33 cases, the heart was the site of hemorrhage in 12 patients. Four of them showed focal necrosis of the myocardium with slight cellular reaction. There were two cases of myocarditis, one characterized by the focal aggregation of polymorphonuclear leukocytes and the other by a diffuse scattering of round cells. Sheehan described subendocardial hemorrhages on the left side of the interventricular septum in about two thirds of the women who died within the first two days after the onset of convulsions.

The *lungs* show varying degrees of pulmonary edema, often extreme, while in about half the cases bronchopneumonia is demonstrable as the result of aspiration of infectious material during coma. On the same basis, a few cases of pulmonary abscess have been known to follow eclampsia.

Lesions in the *adrenal glands* are frequent, consisting essentially of necrosis and hemorrhage of varying degrees. Eleven, or one third, of Way's cases showed this pathologic change. Of these 11, 5 were classified as severe in that practically no functional adrenal cortical tissue remained. The other 6 showed involvement of approximately half of the cortical tissue. There were no cases with minimal lesions. In Way's opinion, adrenal insufficiency secondary to recent widespread injury may be a contributory factor in the terminal shocklike syndrome in eclampsia and in the death of certain patients. Sheehan, however, writes that the adrenal cortical necrosis is not more common in fatal eclampsia than in other deaths, and Govan found extensive adrenal hemorrhage in only 3 of 110 women dying of eclampsia.

Placental Changes.   The frequency of so-called *infarcts of the placenta* is increased somewhat in hypertensive cases over the 60 per cent incidence observed in the placentas of normal cases (p. 590). Tenney and Parker believe that the characteristic placental change is primarily a premature aging. As has been known for many years, the term placenta shows a certain amount of syncytial degeneration, involving 10 to 50 per cent of the small terminal villi. Tenney and Parker noted that in preeclampsia most of the villi are involved, and in severe preeclampsia and eclampsia all may be affected. After the trophoblast degenerates, the villi appear to be covered by only a thin irregular layer of hyaline material. They also observed a marked congestion of the villous blood vessels. In early stages of preeclampsia, as in other conditions in which placental dysfunction may occur, there may be an apparent hyperplasia of trophoblast. When preeclampsia accompanies multiple gestation and chorionic neoplasms, marked trophoblastic hyperplasia and degeneration may occur in the same placenta.

The Common Denominator in the Pathology of Eclampsia. Although pathologic changes in eclampsia are widespread and varied, factors common to all of them may be found in the intravascular coagulation and the abnormal behavior of the vascular tree, especially its terminal branches. The widespread deposition of fibrin, the thrombosis of the hepatic arteries with rupture and hemorrhage, the glomerular changes, and the hemorrhages in the brain, heart, and adrenal glands all attest this fact. Eclampsia is not a disease of the liver, the kidneys, or any single organ, but of all the smaller arterioles. Hertig believes that the essential lesion is an arteriolitis, probably initiated by widespread vasospasm.

Pathologic Physiology. As noted, vasospasm looms large in the mechanism of the whole disease process of preeclampsia. This concept, first advanced by Volhard, has been widely accepted. It is based upon direct observation of minute blood vessels in the nail beds, ocular fundi, and bulbar conjunctivae and has been surmised from histologic changes seen in the affected organs.

The vascular constriction accounts for the hypertension. It imposes a resistance to blood flow and may produce focal areas of hypoxia, although the total blood flow to various organs, except the uterus, liver, and kidney, seems to be normal except in severe, decompensated cases. Vasospasm probably has a noxious effect in interfering with circulation in the vasa vasorum, thus leading to damage of the vascular walls. These vascular changes, together with local hypoxia of the tissues, presumably cause the hemorrhage, the necrosis, and most of the other disturbances observed in the disease. Deposition of fibrinoid is widespread. In the kidney, at least, some of this material is believed to be derived from fibrinogen.

In women with preeclampsia, even in its incipient stages, there appears to be a sensitization of the arterioles to pressor hormones. Browne reported that preeclamptic women who had shown minimal rises in blood pressure in response to vasopressin during early pregnancy gave exaggerated hypertensive responses during preeclampsia. The sensitivity to vasopressin disappears after delivery. Raab and co-workers found a similar response to norepinephrine, as did Talledo, Chesley, and Zuspan with respect to both norepinephrine and angiotensin.

In preeclampsia, Hinselmann, and later several others, noted changes in the smaller vessels of the nail bed, comprising alterations in the size of the arterioles with evidence of spasm, which produced alternate regions of contraction and dilatation, together with elongation of the capillary loops and some degree of stasis. Similar changes have been found in a large number of eclamptic patients. Even more striking changes can be seen in the bulbar conjunctivae. Landesman, Douglas, and Holze describe marked arteriolar constriction, even to the point that capillary circulation is intermittently abolished.

Further evidence that vascular changes play an important role in preeclampsia and eclampsia is afforded by the constancy with which spasms of the retinal arterioles are met in these disorders. Mylius demonstrated that in association with rise of blood pressure the primary and most commonly observed lesions of the fundus were spasms and tonic constrictions of the retinal arterioles. In the opinion of Wagener and of Hallum, the first visible sign in the retina of a preeclamptic patient is a spastic contraction of the arterioles. This change, according to Wagener, may disappear entirely if there is an early and permanent fall in blood pressure, but at some later stage of the spastic process, permanent sclerotic changes occur in the walls of the arterioles. These lesions are apparently a response to ischemia of the vascular walls, a result of the continual compression of the vasa vasorum by the spastic contractions. Agarwal, Chawla, and Saxena have estimated the blood pressure in the retinal arterioles (or perhaps the ophthalmic artery) by ophthalmodynamometry and have concluded that the diastolic pressure increases early in the development of preeclampsia, before the pressure in the brachial artery rises. The greater the disproportionate rise in retinal pressure in preeclampsia and eclampsia, the graver is the prognosis.

Important as vascular constriction is in rationalizing the pathology of preeclampsia, it seems to be a secondary manifestation of the disease. Its morbid effects, however, cannot be denied nor can the value of empirical measures designed to ameliorate the vasospasm. The hypertension caused by vascular constriction also seems to compensate for it, with the result that the blood supply to many areas of the body is not significantly reduced. Munnell and Taylor measured the hepatic blood flow in a very few cases and found that it is not decreased in preeclampsia. Hoshino, however, found rather marked reductions in the hepatic blood flow. The renal blood flow is somewhat diminished, on the average, but the range is very wide (Chesley). McCall found normal cerebral blood flows in preeclampsia and eclampsia. Burt reported that the cutaneous blood flow of the hand is considerably increased and that the blood flow in the forearm, probably representative of the musculoskeletal system, is either normal or increased.

These measurements of blood flow cover nearly all of the circulation, except that of the uterus, without finding an organ (with the possible exception of the liver) in which vasospasm reduces the total blood supply significantly. Other arguments against the primacy of vasospasm in preeclampsia can be adduced. For instance, rapid weight gain, increases in thiocyanate-available water (Chesley), increased urinary excretion of gonadotropin, and decreased excretion of estrogens and pregnanediol (Smith and Smith) sometimes precede hypertension or any other recognized sign of vasospasm, sometimes even by weeks.

Clinically, the frequency of pulmonary edema and cyanosis in severe eclampsia suggests cardiac failure, and the autopsy findings indicate that cardiac damage is common in fatal cases. Stroganoff included digitalis in his famous treatment of eclampsia. Cardiologists today are divided on the question. Paul White described toxic myocarditis, cardiac failure, and pulmonary edema in association with eclampsia. Hamilton, however, wrote "Our present opinion is that uncomplicated preeclampsia or eclampsia causes neither heart failure nor significant acute myocarditis." Wallace and co-workers, in an electrocardiographic study of 12 women with preeclampsia, found significant changes in 6, with cardiac failure in 2. Szekely and Snaith made similar observations in 19 unselected cases and found 7 cases showing significant clinical or cardiographic changes, with left ventricular failure in 3.

Some of the physiologic changes of normal pregnancy, together with the deviations in preeclampsia, are summarized in Table 2. A few of the data are tentative and some qualifications must be specified. For instance, the measures

Table 2. **Physiologic Changes in Normal and Preeclamptic Pregnancies**

	Normal Nonpregnant Women	Last Weeks of Normal Pregnancy		Preeclampsia Compared with Normal in Last Weeks
		Mean Value	Absolute Change	
Plasma volume (ml)	1,900	3,030	+1,130 ml	Decreased
Red cell volume (ml)	1,360	1,790	+430	Decreased
Thiocyanate space (ml/kg)	230	300	+6.3 liter	Increased
Exchangeable sodium (mEq/kg)	39.4	39.4	+600 mEq	Increased
Total body water (ml/kg)	525	566	+8.5 liter	Increased
Capillary filtration (ml/100 g forearm/min)	0.111	0.160		Decreased
Cardiac output (L/min)	5.2	6.9†	+1.7 liter	Normal
Cerebral blood flow (ml/100 g/min)	54	54		Normal; decreased during coma
Hepatic blood flow (ml/min)*	1,830	1,790		Decreased
Cutaneous blood flow (ml/100 g hand/min)	1	13		Increased
Musculoskeletal blood flow (ml/100 g forearm/min)	4.56	8.73		Normal (?)
Renal blood flow (ml/min)*	940	1,300†		Decreased
Glomerular filtration (ml/min)*	120	180		Decreased
Diodrast T_m (mg/min)*	42	46		Normal
Uterine blood flow ml/min		600		Decreased
ml/100 g/min		10		Decreased

* *Corrected to body surface area of 1.73 sq m (Illogical in pregnancy unless based upon weight before pregnancy).*

† *There is a strong postural effect late in pregnancy. The alleged regression in cardiac output, renal blood flow, and glomerular filtration during the last weeks of pregnancy seems to depend upon impaired venous return to the heart. The bulky uterus occludes the vena cava when the woman lies supine (the position in which most measurements have been made) and occludes the common iliac veins when she sits or stands. The data shown are derived from observations made with the patients lying on their side.*

Note: *Some of the data are tentative and are based upon very few cases from a single publication.*

of Diodrast T_m (*maximal tubular excretory capacity*) are based upon only a few cases from one report.

Pathologic Biochemistry. The outstanding biochemical alteration in preeclampsia and eclampsia is retention of sodium and water beyond that found in normal pregnancy. It is not clear whether the edema of preeclampsia is merely an exaggeration of that in normal pregnancy or whether it is a wholly new aberration. The second possibility seems more probable. Retention of water and sodium is so inseparably connected that it is not possible to say whether the edema seen in preeclampsia represents a metabolic disorder affecting water or sodium primarily.

There is multiple evidence that sodium is retained in preeclampsia (Chesley). Measurements of the sodium space and total exchangeable sodium (Plentl and Gray) by means of radioactive sodium give direct evidence. The postpartum loss of weight, water, and sodium, furthermore, is greater in the preeclamptic patient than in the normal. Harding and Van Wyck gave several patients with preeclampsia intravenous injections of 300 ml of 6 per cent sodium chloride solution. The results were virtually disastrous. One patient who had received two such injections within 24 hours developed fulminating eclampsia with dramatic suddenness and had three typical convulsions; meanwhile the blood pressure had risen from 128/100 to 200/140, and the proteinuria had more than doubled. Harding and Van Wyck believed firmly that a high intake of salt ingested at a particular time during development of preeclampsia will produce proteinuria, increase the blood pressure, and even cause convulsions in a short period of time.

Zangemeister in 1903 observed that the urine is almost free of chlorides during eclampsia and that in all women with preeclampsia or eclampsia the contribution of chloride to total urinary osmolality is small before delivery and large during postpartum recovery. Several German investigators of that era confirmed the observation and described an impairment in the excretion of salt loads given to women with preeclampsia and eclampsia. Dieckmann and co-workers made extensive studies of salt tolerance, giving as much as 36 g of salt daily for many consecutive days. The normal patient in late pregnancy does not concentrate sodium in the urine so greatly as she does in the nonpregnant state, but excretes the load normally. Patients with hypertensive disease show no untoward effects of the high intake of salt although they do not concentrate it in the urine so well as do normals. Patients with the clinical diagnosis of preeclampsia differ in their response to high intake of salt. About 20 per cent of the mild cases are not affected adversely, as judged by response of the blood pressure or degree of proteinuria. They concentrate sodium to more than 144 mEq per liter in the urine, and were called "pseudopreeclamptic" by Dieckmann (compare McCartney's findings in renal biopsies, page 692, in which 26 per cent of primigravidas with clinical preeclampsia proved to have renal disease). The other 80 per cent often react to the salt with increased proteinuria, aggravated hypertension, progression of edema, the appearance or aggravation of symptoms, and even convulsions. The concentration of sodium in their urine was less than that in their plasma.

The mechanism of the sodium and water retention is unknown. Apparently it cannot be explained on the basis of the simple causes of edema, such as increased intracapillary pressure, decreased plasma oncotic pressure, or increased capillary permeability. Estrogens, which may play a role in the sodium and water retention of normal pregnancy, are decreased early in the development of preeclampsia. Aldosterone, a potent adrenal cortical hormone that promotes sodium retention, does not appear to be responsible. In preeclampsia both the urinary excretion and the adrenal secretory rate of that steroid are subnormal (Watanabe and co-workers). The spironolactone antagonists of aldosterone, moreover, have little effect in patients with preeclampsia, although they do enhance sodium excretion by normal pregnant women (Barnes and Buckingham). The role of the kidney still has not been assessed. Normally, excretion of sodium appears to depend upon a balance between glomerular filtration and tubular reabsorption. The tubular reabsorption of sodium is modified by steroidal hormones, most notably aldosterone, by renal vascular resistance, renal perfusion pressure and plasma oncotic pressure, and by an elusive additional factor that may be a hormone that depresses tubular reabsorption in response to expansion of the extracellular fluid volume.

In normal pregnancy there must be a substantial readjustment of tubular function to maintain glomerulotubular balance, for the rate of glomerular filtration is increased by an average of 50 per cent. Obviously tubular reabsorption of sodium must be augmented to a similar degree, for certainly the sodium balance does not become negative during pregnancy. Although the role of the "third factor" has not been assessed, the adrenal secretory rate of aldosterone is increased severalfold (Watanabe and co-workers), probably stimulated by angiotensin resulting from the increased plasma levels of renin, renin activity (Brown and co-workers), and renin substrate (Helmer and Judson).

Nearly every patient with preeclampsia has a marked reduction in glomerular filtration rate. Unless there were an offsetting depression in tubular reabsorption of sodium, sodium would be retained. Presumably tubular function does change, for during preeclampsia the adrenal secretory rate of aldosterone is diminished (Watanabe and co-workers), as is plasma renin (Brown and co-workers), but normal balance is not established, as indicated by abnormally great retention of sodium. Since it has not yet been shown that the rate of glomerular filtration falls at the very beginning of preeclampsia, it cannot be considered the primary mechanism.

Another important biochemical alteration in eclampsia is hemoconcentration, a change noted by Zangemeister, and studied and emphasized especially by Dieckmann. Table 10 in Dieckmann's exhaustive monograph, *The Toxemias of Pregnancy*, shows that during the two days before the eclamptic attack the serum proteins usually rise from about 5.7 g per 100 ml to about 6.7; meanwhile the hematocrit increases from 41 to 45 per cent on the average, while hemoglobin rises from 87 to 108 per cent. The hemoconcentration, which is seen in both severe preeclampsia and eclampsia, is associated with a decrease in plasma volume. Dieckmann has emphasized the association of clinical improvement in eclampsia with hemodilution, stressing that failure of the blood to undergo dilution with the usual treatment indicates that the eclampsia is very severe.

Eclampsia is seldom accompanied by any significant degree of nitrogenous retention, but an increased concentration of uric acid in the blood is typical. Although it was originally thought that the elevated uric acid seen in preeclampsia and eclampsia was the result of hepatic injury, and hence might be regarded as a valuable prognostic sign (Stander and Cadden), Chesley has shown that this phenomenon is related simply to a decreased ability of the kidney to excrete uric acid, as evidenced by a diminution in its clearance.

The bicarbonate content of the blood is usually reduced in eclampsia. It is not uncommon to find values below 13.5 millimoles per liter, but the reduction is transitory unless convulsions continue. Stander and co-workers demonstrated a definite increase in the hydrogen ion concentration of the blood in association with eclamptic convulsions. They concluded that the eclamptic patient usually overcomes the true acidosis by lowering the carbonic acid through deepened breathing; but when she is unable to overcome acidosis, death may result. The accumulation of lactic and other organic acids in the blood following the muscular activity during convulsion probably leads to acidosis. The organic acids are neutralized by sodium bicarbonate, thus reducing the CO_2 combining power. After convulsions cease, the organic acids are oxidized, releasing sodium to combine with water and carbon dioxide and thus restoring the alkali reserve.

Although many attempts have been made to establish a relation between the serum proteins, especially the alubumin-globulin ratio, and eclampsia, no correlation has been demonstrated, except some elevation in total serum proteins as the result of hemoconcentration. The slightly reduced albumin-globulin ratio may play an auxiliary role in the production of edema. The inorganic elements are within normal limits, except for a slightly increased phosphorus, resulting in an elevation of the ratio of phosphorus to calcium. The blood sugar is not greatly disturbed, except that occasionally hyperglycemia follows the eclamptic fit, perhaps because of the muscular activity. Blood thioneine, glutathione, and nucleotide nitrogen are within normal limits (Bonsnes and Stander). Lactate usually is not elevated in venous blood except after convulsions, but in severe cases of eclampsia the total organic acids are definitely increased. Handler reports that arterial blood levels of lactate are increased in preeclampsia, a finding that may relate to the depressed renal clearance of uric acid.

Cause.   So many ideas have been advanced concerning the cause of eclampsia that Zweifel called it "the disease of theories." Appropriately, he doubted the theories. In earlier editions of this book, it was suggested that any acceptable theory must explain: (1) the predisposing influence of nulliparity, multiple pregnancy, hydatidiform mole, and hydramnios; (2) its higher incidence in certain localities and among the indigent; (3) the increasing incidence as term approaches; (4) the rarity of repeated eclampsia; (5) the improvement that usually ensues after death of the fetus; (6) the hypertension, edema, proteinuria, convulsions, and coma; and (7) the characteristic hepatic and renal lesions. These criteria may now be revised slightly. Much of the geographic variation in the incidence of eclampsia depends upon the availability of prenatal care, although additional factors are probably involved. In Jersey City, eclampsia is more freqeunt in private than in clinic patients. Although many of the clinic patients are indigent, their antepartum care is better than that of many private cases. As for the alleged improvement following the death of the fetus, Dexter and Weiss found that in less than one third of cases did the improvement occur. Theirs is the only well-controlled study of the question, although they quote earlier investigators who had reached the same conclusion. The association of preeclampsia and eclampsia with hydramnios in the absence of other factors predisposing to preeclampsia is doubtful (Jeffcoate and Scott).

Everyone from allergist to zoologist has proposed hypotheses and suggested rational therapies based upon them, such as mastectomy, oophorectomy, renal decapsulation, trephination, alignment of the patient with the earth's magnetic field with her head pointing to the North Pole, and all sorts of medical regimens. Only a few of the many hypotheses will be discussed here.

1. RENAL FACTORS.   A century ago eclampsia was thought to be *uremia*. With the development of renal function tests, estimates of the severity of the supposedly causative renal disorder have been reduced progressively. The *glomerular* capillary endotheliosis (p. 707) probably is secondary to the trapping and transport of derivatives of fibrinogen (Vassalli and co-workers; Faith and Trump). The levels of *renin and renin activity* in

the plasma are lower than in normal pregnancy (Brown and co-workers), but the increased arteriolar reactivity to angiotensin (Talledo and co-workers) may offset that factor. Gordon and co-workers, in a prospective study, found that apparently normal women with high plasma renin activity in the second trimester were more likely to develop preeclampsia later.

Sophian has postulated a *uterorenal reflex*. Distention of the uterus, as in multiple pregnancy, for instance, elicits a diversion of the blood flow from the renal cortex to the medulla (Trueta shunt), thereby causing oliguria, retention of sodium, hypertension, and so on. Objection: there is no evidence that the Trueta shunt occurs in the human kidney, even in acute renal failure. Eclampsia, furthermore, is sometimes associated with extrauterine pregnancy, and hydramnios does not predispose to preeclampsia unless associated with factors that do, such as multiple pregnancy and diabetes.

Peters reported a high incidence (13 per cent) of urinary tract infection in patients with hypertensive disorders of pregnancy and a 27 per cent incidence of hypertension or edema in pregnant women with such infections. He therefore regarded infection of the urinary tract as an important cause of preeclampsia. Objection: the observations cannot be confirmed by other investigators.

2. BIOLOGIC REACTIONS. (a) *Incompatibility between maternal and fetal blood* has been suggested as a cause. Objection: incompatibility of maternal and fetal blood is just as frequent in normal as in eclamptic patients (Allen). Preeclampsia is common in cases of hydatidiform mole, where there is no fetal blood. The Rh factor is not involved, except in cases of fetal hydrops with large placentas.

(b) *Immune response.* The belief that the mother becomes sensitized to small quantities of fetal protein and later reacts to it has been advanced by many investigators (e.g., Jegorow). Objection: Preeclampsia and eclampsia seldom recur in later pregnancies. The renal lesion of preeclampsia is not associated with the deposition of complement or antigen-antibody complexes (Vassalli and McCluskey).

3. INCREASED ABDOMINAL PRESSURE. Paramore, Davis and Snook, and Wylie all have suggested that increased abdominal pressure reduces the blood flow to the placenta, kidneys, and liver, resulting in pathologic changes responsible for eclampsia. Objection: eclampsia occurs with special frequency in hydatidiform mole at periods when pressure of the uterus on surrounding organs is negligible (see theory of uterine ischemia).

4. FETAL METABOLIC PRODUCTS. Objection: preeclampsia occurs with especial frequency with hydatidiform moles in which there is no fetus.

5. PLACENTAL DECOMPOSITION PRODUCTS. Inasmuch as eclampsia sometimes occurs in the absence of a fetus (as with mole) and sometimes with ectopic pregnancy, attention has focused on the placenta as the cause of the disorder.

(a) *Placental endotoxins.* Countless placental extracts, autolysates, and press juices have been injected into laboratory animals with production of convulsions or hepatic lesions. Objection: the same results are elicited by extracts of other organs. Furthermore, Lichtenstein has demonstrated that the effects have been chiefly mechanical and that large quantities of such preparations can be injected with impunity, provided all suspended particles and thromboplastin have been previously removed by filtration. Subsequent writers have confirmed his observations, and there is no evidence that eclampsia can be produced by normal placental tissue.

(b) *Placental infarcts.* So-called infarcts of a diameter of 1 cm or more are present in about 60 per cent of all placentas (p. 590). Since all types of infarcts are somewhat more frequent and extensive in placentas associated with preeclampsia, Fehling originally suggested a relation between infarction and proteinuria of pregnancy. In modern times the main proponents of this theory have been Young in England and Bartholomew and Kracke in the United States. They laid particular emphasis on the red infarct as a causative factor and claimed to have produced eclampsia experimentally by injecting autolyzed infarcts. Objections: students of the placenta have been unable to discover any correlation between infarcts and preeclampsia and regard any increased incidence of infarction as the result rather than the cause of the disease. Dieckmann, moreover, cites the frequent occurrence of preeclampsia in patients with hydatidiform mole, in which typical placental infarcts do not occur.

6. UTEROPLACENTAL ISCHEMIA. The uterine ischemia theory of eclampsia has been proposed in various forms by Beker, by Dexter and Weiss, by Page, by Dieckmann, and by many others.

Several factors that predispose to preeclampsia might be associated with an impaired uterine supply of blood. With approach to term and in multiple gestation, overstretching of the uterine wall with a resulting increase in myometrial tension may offer increased resistance to the flow of blood. (Hydramnios, however, does not predispose the patient to preeclampsia unless it is associated with multiple pregnancy or other factors previously discussed.) Hydatidiform mole may result in an insufficient supply of blood because the vesicular placenta may grow more rapidly than does the normal placenta of the same age. In chronic hypertensive vascular disease, generalized sclerosis of the arterioles might well hinder the vasodilatation necessary for adequate blood supply to the uterus. The fact that 5 to 15 per cent of the patients with chronic hypertensive vascular disease develop preeclampsia fits well with this theory. In women with long-standing diabetes the uterine arteries are often calcified; such diabetics are especially likely to develop preeclampsia (White). There is also, however, an increased incidence of preeclampsia in early diabetes, as well as in early chronic hypertension, before such vascular changes are recognizable. The lower incidence of eclampsia in multiparas is explained on the ground that once the uterine vessels have undergone gestational hypertrophy, they might be expected to do so again without difficulty. Beker has shown that the arteries in the multiparous uterus, before as well as during pregnancy, are of distinctly larger caliber than in the primigravid uterus. Moreover, the greater tone of the abdominal walls in primigravidas might conceivably play a role in uterine ischemia. This hypothesis could thus be correlated with that of Paramore (p. 717). The aggravation of preeclampsia during labor, as well as the increased incidence of convulsions at that time, might be explained by the ischemic effect of the uterine contractions. With the inclusion of the thromboplastin concept (p. 719), the lesions may possibly be explained.

Although the role of the autonomic nervous system in vasomotor function is well known, the part it plays in the hypertension of preeclampsia, if any, is not established. The studies of Brust, Assali, and Ferris with ganglionic blockade indicate that the neurogenic factor is much less important than the humoral in preeclamptic hypertension.

The experimental production of uterine ischemia in pregnant animals has been frustrating, for if the blood supply is reduced too much, abortion occurs. When abortion does not occur, collateral circulation develops rapidly. Kumar, working with pregnant dogs, successively tied off the uterine and ovarian arteries in a three-stage operation over several days, thus leaving the pregnant uterus with only collateral circulation. The few animals that did not abort developed hypertension, proteinuria, or both, but no edema. Berger and Cavanagh induced hypertension in intact and nephrectomized pregnant rabbits by placing sutures through the placentas in such a way as to impede the blood flow. The blood pressure began to rise progressively, 5 to 10 minutes after the sutures were placed, and reached a maximum in 25 to 95 minutes; thereafter it either decreased or remained constant for an unspecified length of time. Blood from hypertensive animals had a pressor effect when transfused into nonpregnant rabbits. It would be of great interest to know how long hypertension would persist in the rabbits with placental ischemia and why it often began to regress within an hour or two. Hodari ligated the ovarian arteries and placed snugly fitting Teflon bands around the uterine arteries of nonpregnant dogs before breeding them. Some were sterile and some aborted after conception, but those that carried pregnancies developed progressive hypertension, proteinuria, and hypernatremia, all of which disappeared after delivery. The abnormalities were found at the first observation, during the first trimester of pregnancy, a time much earlier than that at which preeclampsia appears in women. The hypernatremia, moreover, has no counterpart in the human disorder. This interesting work has not been repeated.

Few relevant observations have been made in human subjects. Hertig, Zeek and Assali, and Dixon and Robertson have described in the subplacental decidual arteries of women with preeclampsia a marked atherosclerosis, which presumably impeded blood flow. Dixon and Robertson, however, regard the lesions as secondary to the hypertension. Assali and co-workers have estimated the uterine blood flow by the nitrous oxide method and found a reduction of about 40 per cent in four cases of preeclampsia.

Browne and Veall injected radioactive sodium into the maternal placental blood lake and from its rate of disappearance calculated that the placental blood flow is reduced by more than 50 per cent in preeclampsia. They found comparable reductions in pregnant women with uncomplicated hypertensive disease. These findings in preeclampsia are impressive because they seem to support the hypothesis, but the comparable reductions in patients with essential hypertension raise the possibility that the diminished blood flow may be secondary to local vasospasm and therefore an effect rather than a cause of preeclampsia. Valid answers to these questions may well be forthcoming in the future, but meanwhile the hypothesis, appealing though it may be, is still open to question.

7. DISORDERS OF BLOOD COAGULATION. Page suggested that the liberation of thromboplastin from the ischemic placenta plays an important role in the causation of eclampsia. Schneider killed mice by intravenous injections of human placental extracts and identified the lethal factor as thromboplastin. In these animals the liver appears to be the primary site of fibrin deposition and capillary thrombosis, just as in human eclampsia. Dieckmann produced similar lesions in dogs, although he called his injected material "tissue fibrinogen." The concept that thrombokinase (thromboplastin in the presence of calcium ions) may play a role in the production of certain eclamptic lesions was discussed by Hinselmann in his monograph and credited to Dienst, but the general hypothesis was advanced in the nineteenth century by Wooldridge (1888) and Schmorl (1893). Chargaff has shown that the placenta is the richest source of thromboplastin in the body. As the result of injury from ischemia and hypoxia, lysis of the syncytial trophoblast would be expected, followed by entry of thromboplastin into the maternal circulation, explaining the high incidence of "infarcts" in placentas and the generalized deposition of fibrinoid. Jäämeri, Koivuniemi, and Carpén, in sampling uterine venous blood at the time of cesarean section, found that patients with preeclampsia had about twenty times as much "deported" trophoblastic tissue as did normal subjects. Presumably the material is trapped in the pulmonary circulation, where it is degraded with the release of thromboplastin and many other substances into the systemic circulation, as Schmorl suggested three quarters of a century ago.

McKay has reviewed the evidence for disseminated intravascular coagulation as the major mechanism accounting for the lesions of eclampsia and has shown that there are certain disorders of the clotting mechanism in preeclampsia, as well. Although deposition of fibrin may be found in almost any placenta, it is increased in preeclampsia. The generalized deposition of fibrin and fibrinoid is discussed on page 711. McKay found increases in cryofibrinogen and adhesiveness of platelets in preeclampsia. Pritchard and co-workers reported decreases in the platelets, especially, and less frequently in prothrombin and fibrinogen of women with severe preeclampsia; the fibrinogen, however, is more often elevated than depressed. McKay contends that the lesions of preeclampsia and eclampsia may represent a generalized Shwartzman reaction to products of decidual or trophoblastic degeneration. He has produced many of the typical lesions in pregnant rats by feeding a diet deficient in tocopherol and containing oxidized cod liver oil. The sequence of events is partial blockade of the reticuloendothelial system, injury to the endothelium and trophoblast, agglutination of blood platelets on the vascular walls, and intravascular coagulation. The placenta appears to be essential and it is the first organ to show damage. Presumably, thromboplastin is released from both the platelets and the trophoblast. Douglas and Langford confirmed McKay's observations, but found no hypertension, proteinuria, or edema in experimental rats. Bonnar and co-workers have measured the circulating levels of decomposition products of fibrinogen in pregnant women and found normal values during normal pregnancies. In the two eclamptic women studied, however, they found high levels (25-fold increases), as they did in women with abruptio placentae. In association with the rise in decomposition products of fibrinogen, they found decreased levels of platelets, plasminogen (the enzyme that degrades fibrinogen and fibrin), and fibrinogen; the euglobulin lysis time was prolonged, indicating low levels of plasminogen activator. Pritchard and Mason have not identified increased levels of degradation products of fibrinogen or fibrin in the serum of women with eclampsia.

8. HORMONAL DISTURBANCES. *Hypothyroidism* has been suggested as a cause of preeclampsia (Colvin). Objection: the clinical picture does not suggest hypothyroidism,

the basal metabolic rate is not depressed significantly, and the protein concentration in edema fluid is very low. There is no valid evidence, moreover, that points to *hyperthyroidism* as a cause.

Hofbauer postulated that eclampsia is caused by *hyperfunction* of the *posterior lobe of the pituitary body,* and Hoffmann and Anselmino attempted to show that preeclampsia and eclampsia are dependent upon an increased amount of pituitary antidiuretic and vasopressor hormone (vasopressin). Several investigators have reported the presence of antidiuretic activity in the urine or blood of patients with preeclampsia. The validity of most of this work has been called into question by the demonstration by Krieger and co-workers that bacterial contamination of the preparations assayed is responsible for most of the antidiuresis induced in test animals. On that basis, they retracted their own previous conclusion that preeclamptic patients often excrete an antidiuretic substance. Paterson, however, has reported that vasopressin (identified as such) is increased in plasma and urine in rough proportion to the degree of preeclamptic edema. Objection: clinical syndromes associated with excessive secretion of vasopressin are not accompanied by edema; cases of preeclampsia have been reported in women with diabetes insipidus.

Excessive chorionic gonadotropin in the blood, urine, and placentas of patients with preeclampsia was first reported by Smith and Smith. The increase, however, is not demonstrable in all cases, bears no direct relation to the severity of the disease, and is associated also with stillbirth and premature delivery in the absence of preeclamptic signs. Others have confirmed the inconstancy and nonspecificity.

Smith and Smith found also a progressive *deficiency of progesterone and estrogen before and during preeclampsia.* They postulated premature senility of the placental syncytium and withdrawal of the steroidal hormones secondary to either an intrinsic metabolic abnormality or a decrease in blood supply to the placenta, or both. Smith and Smith have shown that decreased blood supply to the placenta results in a decrease in the secretion of estrogen and progesterone; they postulated a vicious cycle in which vascular and hormonal deficiencies potentiate each other.

9. DIETARY ALTERATIONS.   During World War I there was a startling reduction in the incidence of eclampsia in central Europe, with return to the prewar frequency thereafter. At that time the decrease was attributed to the shortage of meats and fats. It was therefore deduced that a diet rich in meat led to the development of preeclampsia and eclampsia. Much of the decrease in the occurrence of eclampsia during World War I, however, was the result of a great decrease in the percentage of primigravidas among childbearing women, although Hinselmann noted a reduction in eclampsia among primigravidas as well.

The geographic variation in the incidence of eclampsia, such as its high incidence in the southeastern states of this country, in the Philippines, and in China, has suggested the possibility of dietary deficiency of one kind or another as a cause. For instance, in the southeastern quadrant of the United States, where eclampsia has been notoriously common (and antepartum care uncommon), there occurs almost all of the pellagra in the nation. Siddall adduced evidence to show that in countries where pellagra is rare, eclampsia is also uncommon. More recently Hobson has positively correlated deficiency of nicotinic acid, or at least some deficiency of the B complex, with the incidence of eclampsia. Folic acid deficiency has been suggested, but Whalley and co-workers, using several of the biochemical and biologic criteria for folate deficiency, could find no evidence for that hypothesis.

On the basis of extensive experience with eclampsia in China, the Philippines, and the midsouth of the United States, Whitacre believes that the disease increases in proportion to indigency and *that dietary deficiency,* especially *in first-class proteins, vitamins, and essential minerals,* plays an important causative role. Burke has reported, on the basis of antepartum dietary ratings, that there was no preeclampsia among the women she studied whose diets were fair but that it occurred in 44 per cent of those with the poorest diets.

Davies surveyed the diets of pregnant women in Jerusalem, attempting to interview patients with suspected early preeclampsia and controls matched for country of origin, age, parity, expected month of delivery, year of immigration to Israel, and years of schooling. A final diagnosis of preeclampsia was made in 196; 16 were rejected for one reason or another, leaving 180 and their 360 controls. Dietitians ascertained the menus and amounts of food eaten for three days, quantities of individual foods purchased for the families, frequency tables for 66 items of food, consumption of salt and other condiments, and changes in dietary habits during pregnancy. In the patients with preeclampsia the dietary intake of calories, protein, fats, and sugar was somewhat lower than that of the control women. Further analysis of the data, however, indicated that the 66 preeclamptic women who had not changed their diets ate the same kinds and amounts of food as did the controls. The 114 women with preeclampsia who had changed their diets spontaneously did so because they were not feeling well. That is, the reduction in intake of food was the result rather than the cause of preeclampsia.

Although there are suggestions that dietary deficiencies may possibly predispose to eclampsia, this hypothesis must be regarded as far from proved. Eclampsia remains primarily a disease of primigravidas, but the fetal drain imposed by repeated pregnancies undoubtedly aggravates dietary deficiencies.

10. SOCIOECONOMIC FACTORS. Preeclampsia-eclampsia is now said to have its highest incidence among indigent women, but it has not always been the case. In the early years of the present century, eclampsia was thought to be most common in middle- and upper-class women. Indeed, that observation led to the ready acceptance of the hypothesis that the dietary restriction of protein (meat) accounted for the reduction in the incidence of eclampsia in Germany during World War I. The proponents of the hypothesis that dietary protein is related to eclampsia appear to have swung from "too much" to "too little."

Eastman analyzed the national maternal mortality from the hypertensive disorders in pregnancy, chiefly eclampsia, for the period 1961 through 1965. Nine of the ten states having the highest mortality rates were in the South, with an average of 13.2 per 100,000 live births, as compared with the national figure of 6.2. The mortality rates bore an inverse relation to the average income per capita. The southern states, of course, have a large proportion of black women, but a racial factor probably does not account for the high mortality. The District of Columbia has a higher average income per capita and a higher percentage of black births than any of the 50 states, but the incidence of fatal hypertensive disorders in pregnancy was only 5.2 per 100,000, or less than the national average.

Undoubtedly, mortality from eclampsia is increased in areas of poverty. Interpretation of the data is difficult, but a significant factor must be the availability, utilization, and quality of prenatal care, because eclampsia is usually preventable.

The most carefully controlled epidemiologic study of pregnancy has been made in Aberdeen, Scotland, where for many years the relevant data have been available for nearly all deliveries. Baird found that the incidences of preeclampsia did not differ significantly among the five social classes ranging from the professional and well-to-do (Class I) through the unskilled laborers (Class V), except for some slight increase in Class III (skilled manual occupations).

Preeclampsia-eclampsia is a disease of primigravidas. Among them the susceptibility is highest at each end of the age scale. The older primigravidas are increasingly likely to have chronic hypertension, which predisposes to the development of preeclampsia. Whatever the explanation, teen-age primigravidas are at high risk, and pregnancies among teen-agers have been increasing spectacularly. Through ignorance, and often shame because of an illegitimate pregnancy, many such girls do not seek prenatal care.

A common belief is that black women are more susceptible to preeclampsia-eclampsia than are white women. The incidence of eclamptic deaths among the blacks is greatly increased, but it appears to reflect their lack of prenatal care. At the Kings County Hospital, the incidences of preeclampsia have been identical at 2.0 per cent in black and white women during the years 1962 to 1967. The prevalence of chronic hypertension, however, has been almost three times greater in the blacks than in the whites. At the Margaret Hague Maternity Hospital, during the years 1931 through 1951, 8 per cent of the babies were delivered of black women, and 8 per cent of the patients with eclampsia were black.

Diagnosis. The recognition of eclampsia usually offers no difficulty. It might be confounded with acute poisoning from strychnine, phosphorus, or nitrobenzol, as in certain reported cases. Such instances, however, are extremely rare; and careful inquiry into the history of the patient should prevent error. Generally, one is much more likely to make a diagnosis of eclampsia too frequently than to overlook the disease, because epilepsy, encephalitis, meningitis, cerebral tumor, acute porphyria, ruptured cerebral aneurysm, acute yellow atrophy of the liver, and even hysteria may simulate it. Consequently such conditions should be borne in mind whenever convulsions or coma occur during pregnancy, labor, or the puerperium; and they must be excluded before a positive diagnosis is made. Until eclampsia can be ruled out, however, all pregnant patients with convulsions must be suspect and kept under close observation on the *obstetric* service of the hospital. It is unusual for eclampsia to develop after the first 24 hours postpartum, although a few seemingly authentic cases have been reported as late as the sixth day. Convulsions developing later than one week postpartum are probably never caused by eclampsia.

Prognosis. The prognosis is always serious, for eclampsia is one of the most dangerous conditions with which the obstetrician has to deal. The maternal mortality in eclampsia has fallen notably in the past three decades, and the disorder itself has become so infrequent in the United States that no large, contemporary series is available for analysis. Kyank and co-workers surveyed 1,013 patients treated in 72 German clinics, between 1957 and 1960, and 510 patients treated in 97 Hungarian clinics. The uncorrected maternal mortality in Germany was 5.3 per cent and in Hungary 3.7 per cent. Perinatal mortality has approached 45 per cent in the past, but was 19.9 per cent in Germany, 16.8 per cent in Hungary, and is 17.7 per cent in the Kings County Hospital. The reduction in perinatal mortality may depend, in part, upon the growing tendency to initiate efforts to effect delivery once the convulsions are controlled and the patient is responsive. In the German series, 45 per cent of the women with antepartum eclampsia were delivered by cesarean section, as were 63 per cent in Hungary and 64 per cent at Kings County Hospital. Whereas early delivery is effected in the mother's interest, it additionally decreases the chance of fetal death, which often outweighs the hazard of prematurity.

Although the bearing of parity on prognosis has been disputed, the consensus is that the outlook is worse in multiparas. If so, it is probably because many of them have underlying hypertensive vascular disease and hence are handicapped by preexisting pathologic changes in their vessels, heart, and kidneys. In this connection the age factor also plays a role. In general, the prognosis is much graver in women over 35. Naturally, the prognosis is more favorable for the patient seen immediately after the first convulsion than for neglected patients sent to the hospital only as the last resort. By the same token the outlook is better in women who have had good antepartum care.

In individual cases the most important prognostic sign is urinary output. Eclamptic patients who excrete urine at the rate of 800 ml or more per 24 hours (or 200 ml or more every 6 hours) may be regarded as having a favorable prognosis, whereas extreme degrees of oliguria indicate a grave outlook. Other bad prognostic signs, known as Eden's criteria, are (1) prolonged coma; (2) pulse rate above 120; (3) temperature 103°F or higher; (4) blood pressure above 200 mm; (5) more than 10 convulsions; (6) urinary protein of 10 g or more per liter; and (7) absence of edema. If none or only one of these signs was present, Eden classified the case as "mild"; if two or more were observed, he called it "severe." In 706 of his cases that could be so classified, the mortalities were 6.6 and 37.2 per cent in the mild and severe groups, respectively. Using the same criteria, Peckham, in an analysis of 129 cases of eclampsia observed at the Johns Hopkins Hospital between 1924 and 1933, found that the maternal mortality in the mild cases was slightly under 3 per cent and, in the severe, about 21 per cent. By amending these criteria slightly (omitting proteinuria and changing the blood pressure figure to 180 and the number of convulsions to 20), Peckham was able to demonstrate that the maternal death rate increases progressively with the number of signs. Although it is impossible to set any fixed standards by which the prognosis in eclampsia can be established with precision, the criteria of Eden are often helpful and at least permit the obstetrician to differentiate between very mild and very severe cases of the disorder. A graver prognostic sign than any of those mentioned by Eden is pulmonary edema. If pronounced, it is a forerunner of death in most cases. Apoplexy and paralysis are two other serious complications that usually end fatally.

In general, the maternal prognosis in eclampsia must always be guarded, since extremely severe cases sometimes survive, whereas patients with apparently mild disorders occasionally become severe and die. Some patients survive after a huge number of convulsions, Jardine and Kennedy, for example, have reported a recovery after 200. Despite these rare lucky outcomes, however, convulsions must be regarded as serious signs that must be prevented or, at least, promptly terminated.

Ultimate Prognosis. Because of the catastrophic implications of convulsions, patients who have suffered them (and especially their families) are often loath to consider subsequent pregnancies. Moreover, the literature in general presents a rather gloomy forecast for these women in later childbearing. The recurrence rates of hypertensive complications (not necessarily eclampsia) in some series run as high as 80.0 and 94.5 per cent (Browne and Dodds; Peters); the average for all recent reports is near 35 per cent. The actual outlook of posteclamptic women in subsequent pregnancies assumes great practical importance because most of them were primigravidas, many of whom had lost their babies.

Chesley, Cosgrove, and Annitto found that 189 women who had had eclampsia at the Margaret Hague Maternity Hospital have had 466 later pregnancies, with a fetal salvage rate of 76 per cent (Table 3). Much of the loss was in early abortion, whereas in pregnancies carrying to 28 weeks or more the salvage rate was 93 per cent. There were 83 later abortions (7 therapeutic), 21 stillbirths (16 with recurrent hypertension), and 4 neonatal deaths (2 with recurrent hypertension). Twenty-five per cent of the later pregnancies were complicated by hypertensive states, usually merely a mild hypertension. About 20 per cent of these women did have severe hypertensive complications, and 4 women had eclampsia for the second time.

The eight factors associated with an increased prevalence of hypertension as found at follow-up (p. 725) also bear upon the rate of recurrence of the hypertensive disorders, as shown in Table 4, which deals only with women who had eclampsia in the first pregnancy carried to 28 weeks or more. Many of the re-

Table 3. Outcome of 466 Pregnancies Subsequent to Eclampsia

Percentage Incidences

No. of Pregnancies per Patient Subsequent to Eclampsia	No. of Patients	Total Pregnancies Subsequent to Eclampsia	Hypertensive Disorder*		Abortion	Stillbirths*	Neonatal Deaths*	Abruptio Placentae*	Hypertension at 8 to 28 yrs after Eclampsia
			By Pregnancies	By Patients					
Primigravid Eclamptics									
1	53	53	30.6	30.6	7.6	2.0	2.0	4.1	32.1
2	43	86	19.7	30.8	17.5	9.9	1.4	2.8	18.6
3	28	84	18.2	37.0	21.4	3.0	0	1.5	32.1
4 or more	34	186	18.8	42.4	17.2	2.0	0.6	1.3	20.6
Totals	158	409	20.6	34.5	16.8	3.8	0.9	2.1	26.0
Multiparous Eclamptics									
1	19	19	35.7	35.7	26.3	7.1	0	0	68.4
2	5	10	62.5	60.0	20.0	25.0	0	0	40.0
3	2	6	50.0	50.0	33.3	50.0	0	25.0	50.0
4 or more	5	22	64.7	80.0	22.7	11.8	5.9	11.8	60.0
Totals	31	57	53.5	50.0	24.6	16.3	2.3	7.0	61.3
ALL CASES	189	466	24.3	36.8	17.8	5.2	1.0	2.6	31.8

* Incidences based upon pregnancies carrying past the twentieth week.

Table 4. Relation Between Adverse Prognostic Factors (p. 725) and the Recurrence Rate of Hypertension in Pregnancies Subsequent to Eclampsia in the First Pregnancy

Number of Adverse Factors	0	1	2	3	4 or more
Cases	26	24	26	23	28
Incidence of recurrent hypertension	8	18	27	52	68

currences represent nothing more than chronic hypertension. Some women do have normal blood pressures between pregnancies and at follow-up; but in general, pregnancies following eclampsia are an excellent screening test for latent hypertensive disease. Nearly all women who develop recurrences ultimately become hypertensive, whereas the prevalence of ultimate hypertension is extremely low in those whose later pregnancies are normal.

Chesley, Annitto, and Cosgrove have traced to 1966 all but two of the 270 women surviving eclampsia at the Margaret Hague Maternity Hospital in the period 1931 through 1951. White women who had eclampsia in the first pregnancy carried to 28 weeks or more have shown no increase over the expected number of remote deaths, and only 4 of 16 such deaths were related to cardiovascular-renal disease. In sharp contrast, white women who had eclampsia as multiparas, and all black women, have shown three times the expected number of deaths. At least 22 of the 28 deaths were related to cardiovascular-renal disease, because of the high prevalence of hypertensive disease antedating the eclamptic pregnancies.

Relation of Preeclampsia and Eclampsia to Chronic Hypertension. There appears to be a correlation between the duration and severity of a preeclamptic or eclamptic attack and the development of permanent hypertension. Whether preeclampsia actually *causes* ensuing chronic hypertension is a subject of debate, however. One point of view is that preeclampsia and eclampsia represent an acute vascular disorder in the form of muscle spasm, which, if allowed to continue for several weeks, results in a permanent structural injury to the vascular wall through hypoxia. This injury manifests itself by arteriolar fibrosis, consequent hypertension, and possible renal vascular damage. These findings lead to the suggestion that permanent hypertension might be prevented by delivery of patients within two or three weeks after onset of preeclampsia. For many years Chesley was of this school, but reappraisal of his data has forced him to a reversal of his conclusions. The problem has been confused by the mistaken diagnosis of preeclampsia, even in primigravidas, in women who really had renal disease or essential hypertension. Many studies have included a substantial proportion of multiparas, few of whom really had preeclampsia (p. 689). Furthermore, nearly 40 per cent of women with essential hypertension have significant drops in blood pressure during much of pregnancy. In many of them, normal pressures may be observed from early in gestation. Typically, the blood pressure rises again early in the third trimester, and some edema, with perhaps minimal proteinuria, may occur. Inasmuch as blood pressures before pregnancy are seldom known, the erroneous diagnosis of preeclampsia is likely to be made.

Many follow-up studies have been made of women thought to have had preeclampsia, and the frequency of chronic hypertension has ranged from 2 to more than 60 per cent, with 45 per cent as a fair average. The prevalence of such hypertension has been found to increase with (1) age of the patient in pregnancy or at follow-up; (2) higher blood pressures, in the "normal" range, as initially observed in pregnancy; (3) higher blood pressures during the supposedly acute episode; (4) earlier stage in pregnancy of the onset of hypertension; (5) longer duration of the hypertension (4 and 5 are obviously interrelated); (6) lesser degrees of proteinuria; (7) longer persistence of hypertension in the puerperium; and (8) greater obesity. (When the weight in pounds divided by the height in inches exceeds 2.2, the prevalence of chronic hypertension mounts rapidly.)

The recurrence of a hypertensive disorder in later pregnancy is related to these eight factors in the same way as is the prevalence of chronic hypertension found at follow-up examination. All, or nearly all, of these factors are stigmas of hypertensive disease, which often antedated the complicated pregnancy.

The long-term follow-up studies of Chesley, Annitto, and Cosgrove and of Bryans, who have reexamined women repeatedly for up to 44 years after eclampsia in the first pregnancy, indicate that the prevalence of hypertension is not increased over that in unselected women matched for age and race. Tillman accumulated a series of 377 women whose blood pressures were recorded before, during, and at intervals after pregnancy. He could find no indication that normal, preeclamptic, or hypertensive pregnancies had any effect on the blood pressure at follow-up examination and concluded that preeclampsia neither causes residual hypertension nor aggravates preexisting hypertension.

Treatment.   *Prophylaxis.*   Since eclampsia is preceded in most cases by premonitory signs and symptoms, its prophylaxis is in many ways more important than its cure and is identical with the treatment of preeclampsia. Indeed, a major aim in treating the preeclampsia is to prevent convulsions. The necessity of regular and frequent blood pressure measurements thus becomes clear, as well as the importance of detection of rapid gain of weight and of proteinuria, and the immediate institution of appropriate dietary and medical treatment as soon as the earliest signs and symptoms appear. By the employment of these precautionary measures and by prompt termination of pregnancy in those cases that do not improve or that become progressively worse under treatment, the frequency of eclampsia will be greatly diminished and many lives will be saved. Prophylaxis, while valuable, is not invariably successful. Since eclampsia is generally but not wholly preventable, it does not always indicate neglect on the part of the obstetrician.

General Rationale of Therapy.   It has been recognized for at least two centuries that eclampsia is caused by pregnancy and that the disease abates after delivery. Denman wrote in 1768 that nearly all of his colleagues advocated delivery as soon as possible because that was the only means of saving mother and child. He noted, however, that "the most eminent men of the present time" disagreed and awaited the onset of labor. The radicals dilated the cervix with instruments and delivered the baby forcibly. Although Dührssen (1890) is generally credited with the introduction of cervical incisions as a means of expediting delivery, Theobald notes that Velpeau used them nearly 60 years earlier. Cesarean section, despite its dangers in that era. also was employed.

The maternal mortality of about 30 per cent associated with forced delivery and cesarean section late in the nineteenth century led to more conservative medical therapy. During the first quarter of the twentieth century, obstetricians were divided into radicals and conservatives, with some following a "middle line." In the mid-1920's reviews of the literature and comparison of the maternal mortalities associated with radical and conservative managements indicated that the mortality was doubled by immediate cesarean section. Plass, for instance, tabulated 4,607 cases treated radically, with a maternal mortality of 21.7 per cent; the mortality in 5,976 cases managed conservatively was 11.1 per cent. Holland, in surveying the cesarean sections performed in Great Britain and Ireland, found that the mortality in eclampsia was 32 per cent. Eden, in analyzing the thousands of cases collected by the Eclampsia Committee of the British Congress of Obstetrics and Gynaecology in 1922, confirmed the disastrous results of radical therapy, as shown in Table 5. In the late 1920's the slogan became

Table 5. **Increase in Maternal Mortality in Eclampsia as a Result of Radical Methods of Delivery (Eden)**

	Mild Cases, Per Cent Mortality	Severe Cases, Per Cent Mortality
Natural delivery, assisted delivery, or induction of labor	5	34
Cesarean section	11	46
Accouchement forcé	18	63

"Treat the eclampsia medically and ignore the pregnancy," and an overly conservative attitude prevailed. Women with intercurrent eclampsia were carried for as long as several weeks, with a resultant soaring rate of stillbirths, occasional recurrence of convulsions, and preventable maternal mortality.

The treatment of eclampsia today is medical, with delivery delayed until the patient is free of convulsions, coma, and acidosis.

First Steps in Management. Morphine sulfate is the drug most often given at the patient's home to allay convulsions during transport to the hospital or in the admitting room of a hospital. The initial dose should be between 15 and 30 mg, depending on the size of the patient. The 15 mg dose may be administered intravenously. Repeated doses are not desirable because they reduce urinary output, increase intracranial pressure, and tend to cause acidosis through decreased pulmonary ventilation.

All eclamptic patients should be hospitalized and placed as soon as possible in a quiet room and kept on their sides. The patients may have their eyes shielded but the room should be light enough so that jaundice, cyanosis, and the earliest twitchings of an oncoming convulsion can be detected. If the patient is comatose, the foot of the bed should be elevated about four inches to expedite drainage of any bronchial or pharyngeal secretions. Constant expert nursing care is of paramount importance, and the patient should never be left alone for a second. In the throes of a convulsion she may strike her head against the bed or throw herself onto the floor, or she may bite her tongue violently. To prevent injury to the tongue, a piece of very heavy rubber tubing, a rolled towel, or a padded clothespin should be readily available for insertion between the jaws at the first sign of a convulsion. An eclamptic patient must not be given fluids by mouth lest she aspirate them and develop pneumonia. Meanwhile every effort should be made to keep the room quiet and to shield the patient's face from any bright light, because any form of stimulation may provoke a convulsion.

The physician now evaluates the patient's pulse rate, character of respiration, blood pressure, degree of coma, the presence or absence of cyanosis, reflexes, and the fetal heart tones. By this time, the initial dose of morphine should have given the patient some degree of protection against convulsions. Only then should more stimulating manipulations, such as catheterization or intramuscular or intravenous therapy, be considered. Continual irritation of the patient with needles and other disturbances may do more harm than good. The catheter should be left in place, secured to the patient's thigh with adhesive, and connected with a sterile plastic bag under the bed, so that urinary output may be estimated from hour to hour.

The treatment is based on three main objectives: (1) to provide sedation and thereby allay convulsions, (2) to combat vasospasm, and (3) to promote diuresis. A reliable guide to the need for sedation, in preeclampsia or eclampsia, is hyperreflexia. Dieckmann has found that failure of hemoconcentration to reverse itself is often associated with a fatal outcome. Forcing fluids in an effort to promote hemodilution, however, is usually futile and can be dangerous. Patients with severe preeclampsia or eclampsia should have serial measurements of the hematocrit (or red cell count or hemoglobin) performed as an index of the degree of hemoconcentration. The initial value is often meaningless, but repeated measurements, which will indicate whether the blood is becoming more concentrated or diluted, can provide a reliable prognostic sign.

MAGNESIUM SULFATE. The efficacy of magnesium sulfate as a depressant of the neuromuscular junction is well known. Its use in the treatment of eclampsia stemmed from its success in allaying the convulsions of tetanus, without other evidence of depression of the central nervous system. Blackfan and Hamilton observed that intravenous injections of magnesium sulfate have a favorable effect in lowering the blood pressure and increasing the urinary output in children suffering from hemorrhagic nephritis. These observations have been confirmed by numerous workers. Harbert and co-workers, moreover, have shown that magnesium sulfate increases the uterine blood flow of pregnant monkeys.

Toxic signs and symptoms induced by magnesium do not develop until its concentration in plasma reaches 10 to 12 mg per 100 ml (8.3 to 10 mEq/L). At or near this level the knee jerks disappear. At a level of between 12 and 15 mg per 100 ml, respirations are likely to cease; when the level reaches 15, cardiac arrest may occur. At the Johns Hopkins Hospital this drug has been used intramuscularly in a great number of patients with rather large total dosages (up to 110 g in three days). Following the intramuscular injection of magnesium sulfate there is a lag of 90 to 120 minutes before the plasma level of magnesium reaches a plateau. Pritchard, as well as Chesley and Tepper, therefore combines an intravenous dose of 3 or 4 g (in 10 per cent solution) with the first intramuscular injection of 10 g (in 50 per cent solution). The plasma magnesium reaches the desired level immediately, and a fairly good plateau is maintained for three to four hours. The level attained varies with the body weight of the patient and with renal function; it usually is between 4 and 6 mg per 100 ml. The initial dose is safe; subsequent doses of 5 g intramuscularly every four hours must not be given unless certain precautions are observed: (1) the knee jerks should be tested before each injection and the drug given only if they are active; (2) the respirations should be counted before each injection and the drug given only if they are 16 or more per minute; (3) each of the successive doses, after the initial one, should be contingent upon the patient's having excreted at least 100 ml of urine since the preceding dose, because the kidneys are the only route of its excretion; and (4) as a further precautionary measure, an intravenous calcium preparation (calcium gluconate, 1 g in 10 ml) should always be by the bedside, for it is an immediate antidote. If the patient has been given digitalis, calcium must be injected very slowly and cautiously.

The technic of administering magnesium is important. The injection is made in the upper outer gluteal quadrant, the skin having been prepared with ether, iodine, and alcohol as for a surgical operation. A 50 per cent solution of magnesium sulfate is employed, in which a 1 per cent concentration of procaine has been introduced in order to reduce discomfort from the injection. The initial dose is divided, with 10 ml given into each buttock. The needle is moved about while injecting the solution in order to obtain wider dispersion. After withdrawal of the needle the area is massaged with a dry, warm pack.

Intramuscular rather than intravenous administration of magnesium sulfate is preferred at Kings County and Parkland Memorial Hospitals, for example, in the belief that it is just as efficacious, is safer from the viewpoint of sudden respiratory depression, and, in restless patients, is easier to administer. One disadvantage of repeated injections is pygalgia. Dieckmann also preferred intramuscular administration of this drug, but used it in smaller doses. Several authorities, however, have had satisfactory results from the intravenous use of magnesium sulfate, either as intermittent injections or by continuous infusion, as currently administered at the University of Illinois Hospital. Lazard gave 20 ml of a 10 per cent solution intravenously and repeated the dose every hour until the convulsions were under control. Subsequent dosage was based on a recurrence of convulsions, elevation of blood pressure, and other signs. McNeile, using this regimen, reported that the maternal mortality in 259 cases of eclampsia was 13 per cent, as against 36 per cent before the use of magnesium sulfate. Dorsett and Dieckmann, using intramuscular injections, reported a mortality of 7 per cent in 186 cases of eclampsia. Stroganoff and Davidovitch used magnesium sulfate subcutaneously along with other measures in the treatment of 201 cases of eclampsia with a mortality rate of only 3 per cent. Pritchard and Stone use magnesium sulfate in the treatment of eclampsia, and except for Apresoline in selected cases with persistent and severe hypertension, they employ no other drug; they have reported 77 consecutive cases without a maternal death. Zuspan at the University of Chicago uses magnesium sulfate alone, giving a priming dose of 3 or 4 g intravenously followed by the constant infusion of 1 g per hour. Occasionally, magnesium sulfate does not stop the convulsions; intravenous sodium pentobarbital (0.2 to 0.3 g) or sodium amobarbital (0.25 to 0.5 g) will do so. The doses are smaller than would be necessary if magnesium sulfate were not used.

Lipsitz and English reported depression in newborn infants of 3 eclamptic and 3 severely preeclamptic women who had been treated with magnesium sulfate alone, and attributed the depression to fetal hypermagnesemia. Stone and Pritchard, however, could find no relation between the concentration of magnesium in cord blood and the Apgar score of 118 newborn infants whose mothers had been treated with magnesium sulfate. Since 1955, 80 infants were born to eclamptic mothers treated with magnesium sulfate before delivery. In every case in which fetal heart tones were heard when treatment was started, the infant was born alive and every infant weighing 1,800 g or more survived. In 1967 and 1968, 1,248 infants were born to mothers whose hypertension was treated with magnesium; the neonatal death rate was 1.9 per cent, as compared with 2.5 per cent in all live births.

BARBITURATES. Many barbiturates are available, differing mainly in their effective dose, speed and persistence of action, and untoward side reactions. Some of them depress cerebral consumption of oxygen, thus aggravating an abnormality already present in eclampsia. They are all capable of preventing or suppressing convulsions, but anticonvulsant doses inhibit or arrest uterine contractions. The barbiturates most commonly employed in eclampsia are perhaps sodium phenobarbital and sodium amobarbital. Phenobarbital may be given subcutaneously in a dose of 0.3 g, repeated in 12 hours. Dieckmann preferred sodium amobarbital subcutaneously. If convulsions prove very difficult to control, sodium amobarbital intravenously is a valuable agent in a dose between 0.25 and 0.5 g, with care taken to administer it slowly over a period of three or four minutes. When sodium phenobarbital or any other barbiturate is employed intravenously, however, the blood pressure must be carefully watched, since precipitous falls occasionally occur. Pentobarbital and other barbiturate derivatives have also been used to control convulsions in eclampsia and have proved generally satisfactory.

PARALDEHYDE. In the opinion of Douglass and Linn, paraldehyde in sufficient dosage without exception prevents convulsions, keeps the patient quiet, and lowers the blood pressure. The fall in pressure may not be pronounced and is never precipitous, but there is usually a drop of 30 to 40 mm Hg in the systolic and 10 to 20 mm Hg in the diastolic pressure with continuation of such levels for several hours. The initial rectal dose of paraldehyde recommended by Douglass and Linn is 40 ml in 20 or 25 ml of olive or mineral oil. In their 48 cases of eclampsia treated with paraldehyde, there was only one maternal death. In contrast, in a control series of 49 cases, comparable in every respect except the absence of paraldehyde, there were 7 maternal deaths. The profound sedative effect of the drug may lead the obstetrician to confuse sedation and coma.

INTRAVENOUS DEXTROSE. In many clinics, treatment with more or less concentrated dextrose is started after admittance, regardless of the urinary output. The use of dextrose or mannitol is discussed on page 699. In the presence of a rapid pulse (120 or over), cyanosis, pulmonary edema, or other evidence of cardiac failure, intravenous fluids must be administered cautiously.

In patients who have been in coma more than 12 hours, 5 or 10 per cent dextrose may be given to provide fluid and caloric needs, to prevent ketosis, and to provide added protection to the liver. An eclamptic or preeclamptic patient, however, can be given too much fluid. A number of eclamptic deaths have been caused by forcing intravenous fluid to the extent of 5,000 or 6,000 ml in 24 hours. As a rule, the amount given should be 1,000 ml plus an amount equivalent to the urinary volume. The total volume administered should not exceed 2,500 ml; in the face of persistent oliguria, the fluid volume should be restricted to 1,500 ml.

The individual therapeutic measures just discussed—morphine, magnesium sulfate, barbiturates, paraldehyde, and intravenous dextrose—are generally accepted procedures in eclampsia and have been widely employed. There are several other methods of treatment, however, that are reported to give satisfactory results in certain clinics.

VERATRUM VIRIDE. Toward the end of the nineteenth century and in the first decade or two of this century, veratrum was one of the most widely employed drugs in the treatment of eclampsia, but it was largely abandoned because of the grave and unpredictable fall in blood pressure often attending its administration. Its use has been revived by Bryant and Fleming, who reported a gross maternal mortality of 1.6 per cent in 253 cases in which veratrum or hydrazinophthalazine (Apresoline) was used, together with sedation, dextrose, magnesium sulfate, and the induction of labor. Actually, two of the four maternal deaths in their series occurred late in the puerperium and were caused by sepsis rather than eclampsia. The death rate from eclampsia itself was only 0.8 per cent, a superlatively good record. Irving has also reported favorably on the use of veratrum in eclampsia at the Boston Lying-In Hospital.

OTHER ANTIHYPERTENSIVE DRUGS. Assali and co-workers have been particularly active in the trial of antihypertensive drugs, not only in the treatment of acute pre-eclampsia-eclampsia, but also in assessing the hemodynamic effects of these preparations. In general, drugs that act by blockade of the autonomic nervous system or by adrenolysis have a negligible effect upon preeclamptic hypertension. The veratrum alkaloids, the rauwolfia alkaloids, and hydralazine (Apresoline) decrease peripheral (arteriolar) resistance with a consequent drop in blood pressure. Unlike such agents as spinal anesthesia, for instance, they do not decrease the venous tone significantly and therefore do not lead to pooling of the blood on the venous side of the circulation, do not decrease the venous return to the heart, and do not cause a fall in cardiac output. Hydralazine increases the cardiac output, renal blood flow, and cerebral blood flow and oxygen consumption, while decreasing the vascular resistance. The effect on uterine blood flow is uncertain. Johnson and Clayton found that this drug given intravenously accelerated the clearance of radioactive sodium from the myometrium in three cases of severe preeclampsia, suggesting that the blood flow was increased. Dixon and co-workers, however, found no improvement in the clearance of ^{24}Na from the placental blood lake. Ladner and co-workers, studying normal pregnant sheep, observed that the uterine blood flow decreased in proportion to the decrement in blood pressure.

Both Assali and McCall have recommended the combination of hydralazine with a veratrum preparation, although Assali has not used veratrum in the past decade. The reduced dose of each drug minimizes side effects. The combination appears to ameliorate the disturbance in hemodynamics seen in preeclampsia, and each drug cancels out deviations that the other alone would produce. Typically, the urinary output drops when the blood pressure falls in response to these drugs, but the drop is transitory, the output subsequently increasing. Dieckmann believed that the hypertension is "protective" or compensatory. For that reason attempts ordinarily should not be made to lower it drastically. Insofar as the hemodynamics have been studied, the treatment appears to remove the abnormality (vasospasm) for which the hypertension compensates. An eclamptic may continue to have convulsions even though the blood pressure has been kept at normal levels by these drugs. Obviously, the antihypertensive drugs are not specific treatment for preeclampsia but only counter empirically one of the abnormalities, albeit an important one.

The arguments in favor of such treatment are: (1) vasospasm is relieved; (2) relaxation of vasospasm may prevent vascular damage; (3) reduction of marked hypertension may prevent the rupture of damaged vessels in the brain and elsewhere; (4) reduction of peripheral resistance certainly will ease the strain acutely imposed upon the heart; (5) circulation to the kidney is improved. The place for such drugs seems to be in the treatment of severe hypertension. Patients with mild hypertension perhaps do not need such therapy. McCall concluded that it is of no value in patients with mild preeclampsia or uncomplicated hypertensive disease.

Assali's scheme of treatment is to give 30 to 40 mg of hydralazine intravenously, repeating the injection as often as necessary to keep the blood pressure 20 to 25 per cent below the level before treatment. The amount given should depend upon the response of the blood pressure. If the hypertension is refractory to this drug or if the side effects are troublesome, reserpine alone or in combination with veratrum is given intravenously. Veratrum alkaloids may be given by continuous infusion in 5 per cent dextrose at a rate determined by the response of the blood pressure. The two drugs may be combined for injection, using 10 mg of hydralazine (Apresoline) and 0.3 ml of cryptenamine (Unitensen). Headache induced by hydralazine is alleviated by barbiturates. In addition to the hypotensive drugs, Assali uses intramuscular magnesium sulfate, intravenous 5 per cent dextrose up to about 1,500 ml over the urinary output, diuretics, barbiturates, and, of course, bed rest and restriction of salt.

McCall gave a continuous infusion of 20 per cent dextrose containing 20 mg of hydralazine and 5 mg of cryptenamine in 500 ml. The infusion is started at 20 drops a minute, with frequent checks on the blood pressure. The infusion rate is then regulated to maintain the desired level of blood pressure.

Initial treatment is usually by intravenous administration of the drug chosen. After the blood pressure has been stabilized, the veratrum preparations may be given subcutaneously. Hydralazine or reserpine may be given orally. Reserpine causes depletion of the catecholamines and increases the hazards of anesthesia for the mother. It crosses the placenta and may depress the respiratory center of the fetus.

Another drug used extensively in the treatment of eclampsia, especially in the Far East, is chlorpromazine (Thorazine, Largactil). Although this agent has many actions, its depressant effect on the central nervous system and its antihypertensive properties are the rationale for its use in eclampsia. Menon, of Madras, India, has employed chlorpromazine in conjunction with meperidine (Demerol) and diethazine (Diparcol) in 402 cases of eclampsia, with a maternal mortality rate of 2.2 per cent—one of the lowest figures on record. Diethazine is characterized by its depressant action on the autonomic nervous system and has been used extensively in the treatment of Parkinson's disease. Menon gives 25 mg of chlorpromazine and 100 mg of meperidine in 20 ml of 5 per cent dextrose intravenously, and 50 mg of diethazine intramuscularly as initial doses. Meperidine (200 mg in a liter of 20 per cent dextrose) is then infused slowly; not more than a liter is given in 24 hours. Diethazine and chlorpromazine in 50 mg doses are alternately injected intramuscularly every 4 hours for 48 hours. If convulsions are not controlled within 10 hours, the membranes are ruptured if the cervix is favorable and the fetal head engaged; otherwise, cesarean section is done.

VENESECTION.   Historically, bloodletting has been a favorite therapeutic procedure in a wide range of circulatory disorders, including eclampsia. In view of the tendency to circulatory collapse and shock in eclampsia, venesection should be used with discrimination. The chief indication is pulmonary edema.

LUMBAR PUNCTURE.   The drainage of various quantities of spinal fluid has been used sporadically in the treatment of eclampsia since the beginning of the present century. It has not been beneficial (Spillman) and is of historic interest only.

CONDUCTION ANESTHESIA.   Continuous caudal or spinal anesthesia has been proposed for the treatment of eclampsia. Whitacre, Hingson, and Turner reported 74 cases of eclampsia treated by conduction anesthesia (with or without magnesium sulfate) with only 3 maternal deaths. The blood pressure was regularly reduced, convulsions were controlled, urinary excretion was augmented, and in many instances patients promptly came out of coma. The method should be attempted only by the expert anesthesiologist or by the obstetrician with special training and experience. As discussed on page 731, the effects of conduction anesthesia are unphysiologic.

ADJUVANT MEASURES.   For a number of years many clinics have had a policy of prophylactic digitalization of all eclamptic patients. Whether this measure is necessary as a routine procedure remains a moot question, but there is general agreement that digitalization is always indicated in the presence of pulmonary edema associated with evidence of circulatory collapse. Oxygen should be given to all patients who show the slightest evidence of cyanosis or in whom the respiratory rate exceeds 30 per minute. Oxygen should also be administered after each convulsion and continued until the respiration is normal. Many obstetricians believe that supplementary oxygen should be routine as long as convulsions and coma persist. In very severe cases in which convulsions follow one another in rapid succession, light anesthesia may be necessary to control them. In general, however, magnesium sulfate or one of the barbiturates is preferable.

The Question of Delivery.   The generally accepted management of antepartum eclampsia is to defer delivery until the patient has been free of convulsions and coma. Some women, of course, will go into labor spontaneously.

In many clinics an attempt is made to induce labor by administering oxytocin and rupturing the membranes when possible. These trials of induction often succeed even though the fetal head is high and the cervix appears unfavorable. If they are not successful, within a relatively short period of time, delivery should be accomplished by cesarean section.

The uterus of a patient with eclampsia is irritable, its spontaneous activity is increased, hypertonus is often present, and the sensitivity to oxytocin is increased (Caldeyro-Barcia; Cobo; Talledo and Zuspan). Zuspan and Talledo report the successful induction of labor in eclamptic women whose cervices were unfavorable. Of 18 such women, 12 went into labor with a single infusion of oxytocin, and 3 with the second infusion. The perinatal loss was nearly doubled in the group with unfavorable cervices, but the pregnancies were farther from term than in women with favorable cervices.

Cesarean section has certain advantages over induction of labor in women with severe preeclampsia and eclampsia. The eclamptic patient has been compared with a frog under the influence of strychnine: a slight stimulus will set off a convulsion and labor may do so. During labor the blood pressure characteristically increases. In about one quarter of all cases of eclampsia the first convulsion occurs during the few hours of labor. Additionally, the fetus is often compromised in severe preeclampsia and eclampsia, and there is some indication that the fetal salvage is better in deliveries by cesarean section.

Improved modern methods of anesthesia, better control of fluid, electrolyte, and acid-base balances, and the availability of blood and antibiotics have led a few obstetricians to retest the radical management of eclampsia, but their results were not good. Recently, however, Crichton and co-workers have advocated a modified radical approach. As quickly as possible they prepare the patient for delivery by correcting acidosis, reducing the blood pressure by intravenous hydralazine (Nepresol), and sedating with meperidine (Pethidine). In many cases medications were omitted and cesarean section under general anesthesia was performed at once. Among the 240 women delivered by cesarean section the maternal mortality was 4.2 per cent and the perinatal loss 35.4 per cent. Vaginal deliveries occurred in 106 women, 83 by forceps and 23 spontaneously before admittance; the maternal mortality was 4.8 and the perinatal loss 47 per cent.

Occasionally an obstetrician will perform cesarean section as a last resort in patients whose condition deteriorates under conservative therapy; such women usually are acidotic and are such poor risks that the operation may spell death.

For vaginal delivery moderate sedation with terminal local block anesthesia is satisfactory. For cesarean section, however, general anesthesia should be employed.

CHRONIC HYPERTENSION

A diagnosis of chronic hypertension is made in association with pregnancy whenever the evidence supports the chronicity of the disorder: (1) a well-authenticated history of elevated blood pressure (140 systolic or above and 90 diastolic or above) before the present pregnancy; and (2) the discovery of such hypertension prior to the twentieth week, that is, before the time in gestation when preeclampsia is likely to develop. The finding of hypertension before the twentieth week, is taken to mean that the pressure had been elevated prior to pregnancy and is high whether the patient is pregnant or not. As in preeclampsia, the hypertensive readings must be demonstrated on two occasions six or more hours apart.

In addition to instances of frank chronic hypertension, there are many cases in which successive pregnancies are associated with hypertension but in which the pressure is normal between pregnancies. Many authors, notably Dieckmann, regard these recurrent bouts as evidence of latent hypertensive vascular disease. Others have thought that they are repeated attacks of preeclampsia, and still others have regarded recurrent hypertension as a separate entity. The long-term follow-up studies of Chesley and co-workers support Dieckmann's view.

In the classification of the American Committee on Maternal Welfare, only essential hypertension was included as a "toxemia of pregnancy." In the tentative revision, hypertension of any cause is encompassed in the phrase "hypertensive disorders in pregnancy." There are many diseases and syndromes associated with hypertension that may be encountered in pregnant women. Sims has proposed the following classification, which is presented here with slight modifications:

I. Hypertensive disease
    A. Essential hypertension (hypertensive vascular disease)
        1. Mild; 2. Moderate; 3. Severe; 4. Accelerated (malignant)
    B. Renal vascular disease (renovascular hypertension)
    C. Coarctation of the aorta
    D. Primary aldosteronism
    E. Pheochromocytoma
II. Renal and urinary tract disease
    A. Glomerulonephritis
        1. Acute; 2. Chronic; 3. Nephrotic syndrome
        (may occur in several other diseases as well)
    B. Pyelonephritis
        1. Acute; 2. Chronic
    C. Lupus erythematosus
        1. With glomerulitis; 2. With glomerulonephritis
    D. Scleroderma with renal involvement
    E. Periarteritis nodosa with renal involvement
    F. Acute renal failure
        1. Acute renal insufficiency; 2. Cortical necrosis
    G. Polycystic disease
    H. Diabetic nephropathy

Essential hypertension is by far the most common of these diseases in pregnant women. Chronic glomerulonephritis may be more frequent than previously thought, for in his study of renal biopsies from women with "clinical preeclampsia," McCartney found it in 21 per cent of the primigravidas and in 6.6 per cent of the multiparas. Fisher and co-workers, however, did not confirm a high prevalence in their own patients; Janisch found the lesions of glomerulonephritis in 20 of 169 women with hypertensive disorders in pregnancy. Essential hypertension (hypertensive vascular disease) is discussed in this chapter. Other hypertensive disorders, which may occur independently of pregnancy, are discussed in Chapter 27.

In most cases of chronic hypertensive vascular disease, hypertension is the only demonstrable finding. A few patients, however, show secondary alterations that are often grave, in relation not only to pregnancy but also to life expectancy. They include hypertensive cardiac disease, arteriolosclerotic renal disease, and retinal hemorrhages and exudate. The blood pressure, moreover, may vary from levels scarcely above normal to extreme heights of 300 or more systolic and 160 or more diastolic. In other words, it is a disease in which all gradations of vascular lesions may be encountered with or without secondary changes in the heart, kidney, retina, and brain.

Hypertensive vascular disease in pregnancy is met most frequently in women in the older age group and in multiparas. In addition to age, obesity seems to be an important factor predisposing to chronic hypertension. More than 25 per cent of pregnant women weighing over 200 pounds show elevated blood pressures. Heredity also seems to play a role in the development of this condition. Frequently many members of one family show hypertension; upon questioning, the patient will often say that a sister or mother suffered from this disease.

Aside from persisting hypertension, signs and symptoms may be negligible or absent. Ranking next to hypertension among physical findings are retinal changes, which are demonstrable in more than 75 per cent of the more chronic or more severe cases. They comprise irregular tortuosity of the small vessels and variations in their caliber, visibility of the walls of the smaller macular arterioles, and arteriovenous compression. Retinal hemorrhages and exudates are often encountered in advanced stages of the disease, especially if there is renal involvement. Usually the patients feel well and are often annoyed by the discovery of the high blood pressure and by the examinations incident to its study. Except in advanced cases, headache is the only common symptom, and it too may be absent. The blood pressure often falls during the second trimester, but the decrement is usually temporary, since it is followed in most cases by a rise during the last trimester to levels somewhat above those observed early in pregnancy. Sometimes the babies of mothers with chronic hypertension are smaller than expected for their gestational ages, and they seem to grow in utero less rapidly than the average fetus. It is possible in some cases to correlate the small size of these babies with placental infarcts and consequent interference with fetal nutrition, but in many cases there is no unequivocal explanation for the phenomenon. The incidence of abruptio placentae is probably increased in chronic hypertensive women, although the association has been denied in some recent publications (Ch. 23, p. 625).

Superimposed Preeclampsia.   The most common hazard faced by pregnant women with chronic hypertensive vascular disease, or probably any form of hypertension, is the superimposition of preeclampsia. The frequency with which it occurs is hard to specify, for the incidence varies with the diagnostic criteria employed. If the diagnosis is made only on the basis of (1) a significant aggravation of the hypertension (rise of 30 mm Hg systolic and 15 mm Hg diastolic), (2) sustained three- or four-plus proteinuria, and (3) significant edema, then the incidence will be less than 10 per cent. If, however, the diagnosis is made on the appearance of any single sign and lesser proteinuria, then the incidence approaches 50 per cent. Preeclampsia superimposed on chronic hypertensive disease manifests itself by a more or less sudden rise in blood pressure and is almost always associated with the appearance of substantial proteinuria and edema. The picture is often explosive and is characterized by extreme hypertension (systolic of 280 to 300 and diastolic of 140 to 160), oliguria, and nitrogenous retention; the retina may show extensive hemorrhages and many old and new cotton-wool exudates. In somewhat less than 1 per cent of cases of chronic hypertensive vascular disease in pregnancy, actual eclampsia, at least convulsions and coma, is superimposed. Here, in its full-blown form, the resultant syndrome is very similar to hypertensive encephalopathy. With the superimposition of preeclampsia, the outlook for both the infant and the mother becomes more grave. About 20 per cent of the babies are lost, and the maternal mortality is of the order of 1 to 2 per cent.

The diagnosis of superimposed preeclampsia in a patient with antecedent renal disease, such as glomerulonephritis, must be uncertain unless confirmed by renal biopsy, for increases in hypertension, proteinuria, and edema might represent either preeclampsia or an exacerbation of the renal disease.

Prognosis.   Fully 85 per cent of women with chronic hypertensive vascular disease may be expected to go through pregnancy successfully without aggravation of the hypertension. In approximately 5 to 15 per cent, preeclampsia of varying degrees is superimposed. When preeclampsia develops in such patients it is likely to occur earlier than it does in normotensive women. In about 10 per cent of cases it appears toward the end of the second trimester. When it does, the outlook for the baby is extremely grave. If gestation is allowed to continue, fetal death is common; if delivery is effected, prematurity takes a large toll. To summarize, the total perinatal mortality for cases of preeclampsia superimposed on chronic hypertensive vascular disease is about 20 per cent.

Jones analyzed 203 pregnancies occurring in women with mild essential hypertension who were delivered at the Providence Lying-In Hospital between 1939 and 1948. In the uncomplicated hypertensive pregnancies, the perinatal mortality was 8.5 per cent, as against 21.9 per cent in pregnancies with superimposed preeclampsia.

In recent years the fetal salvage has been improved. Gate studied 71 women whose blood pressures were 150/100 or higher before the twentieth week of gestation. One therapeutic abortion, four stillbirths, and one neonatal death added up to a total perinatal loss of about 1 in 12. Gate attributed the high salvage to the frequent interruption of pregnancy before term; labor was induced in 26 women and cesarean section was done in 15.

Townsend personally cared for 109 women found to have blood pressures of 140/90 or higher before the twentieth week; 8 therapeutic abortions were done, and in the 101 pregnancies allowed to continue the perinatal loss was 8 per cent, giving a total fetal salvage of 85.3 per cent. Although he wrote that he could not single out any factor in his management as playing a major role in the reduction of perinatal mortality, it may be significant that he induced labor in 68 per cent of his cases.

At the Kings County Hospital it had been the practice to await the spontaneous onset of labor in most women with uncomplicated hypertensive disease. The results of that method of management showed that death of fetuses weighing more than 2,500 g accounts for one quarter of the total perinatal loss. The perinatal mortality in that weight group is 5.5 per cent, with stillbirths accounting for 60 per cent of the loss. It seems likely that the induction of labor at the thirty-seventh week, for example, would have forestalled some of the stillbirths. Most pregnant women with hypertensive disease are multiparas, and induction of labor would very likely be successful in many of them.

Dunlop analyzed the pregnancies of 1,226 hypertensive women seen in the Royal Infirmary of Edinburgh between 1955 and 1964. Abortion occurred in 44;

the perinatal loss in cases delivering after the twenty-eighth week was 4.25 per cent. Superimposed preeclampsia was diagnosed in 11.5 per cent; with that complication the perinatal loss was 15.1 per cent. Women with mild or moderate hypertension had a low incidence of abruptio placentae, but in women whose systolic pressures exceeded 180 mm Hg the incidence was 6.5 per cent. How many of Dunlop's patients had established chronic hypertension is not clear. His diagnosis was made on the basis of two or more blood pressure readings of 140/90 or higher after admittance to the hospital. He defined the group of mild hypertensives as those whose blood pressure "hovered around 140/90" and the moderate hypertensives as those with pressures "hovering around 160/90." Cases of preeclampsia were excluded.

Harley reported that in the Royal Maternity Hospital of Belfast the perinatal mortality was 15.1 per cent in a group of 563 hypertensive patients not treated with hypotensive drugs. Oral hydralazine, reserpine, protoveratrine, and methyl dopa, singly or in combinations, were used to control the blood pressure of 69 patients; in that group the perinatal loss was 19 per cent. In analyzing factors associated with perinatal loss, Harley found that mortality increased with higher initial diastolic pressures and with a history of previously unfruitful pregnancies. Factors of little or no significance were age, parity, systolic pressure, control of the pressure by hypotensive drugs, and proteinuria. Nearly all investigators have found the perinatal loss to rise with the appearance and degree of proteinuria, but the proteinuria may roughtly parallel the diastolic pressure.

In some hypertensive women careful observation indicates that the fetus is not growing normally. In such cases termination of the pregnancy should be considered in the light of possible placental insufficiency, especially if tests of placental function (p. 699) indicate deterioration.

With certain important exceptions, women with chronic hypertensive vascular disease can go through pregnancy without great hazard. The great threat is superimposed preeclampsia, but even in that complication, prompt termination of pregnancy will safeguard the patient's life as a rule. There is ordinarily no residual effect of pregnancy on the vascular disease, provided preeclampsia is not superimposed. If it is superimposed but cut short by appropriate treatment, the prognosis probably remains the same. There are, however, the following important exceptions to the relatively sanguine forecast:

1. Patients with cardiac enlargement or electrocardiographic changes face a grave outlook in pregnancy, for cardiac failure is the most common cause of death in hypertensive vascular disease. In Chesley's study of the 35 remote deaths following pregnancy in chronic hypertensive women, 9 were caused by cardiac failure. Aggravation of hypertension, as in the case of superimposition of preeclampsia, may impose acutely an intolerable burden on an impaired heart.

2. If renal function is markedly impaired, the life expectancy of the mother is poor regardless of pregnancy, but even moderate diminution in renal function augurs ill for the success of gestation. In a study by Chesley, among 82 patients who failed to concentrate urine to a specific gravity as high as 1.022 there were 36 perinatal deaths. Urea clearances were done in the patients who failed to concentrate to 1.022. There were 11 pregnancies in 11 patients in whom the clearances were less than 70 per cent. Nine of the babies were lost, a mortality rate of 81.8 per cent.

3. Patients with old retinal exudates or fresh hemorrhages will usually show

evidence of renal disease also or of superimposed preeclampsia; but whatever the cause, the presence of these advanced retinal changes is of such grave importance as to deserve special mention.

4. Patients with initial blood pressure of 200 systolic or above, or 120 diastolic or above, face a perinatal mortality rate in excess of 50 per cent and a higher incidence of maternal complications than do milder chronic hypertensives, although the risk of superimposed preeclampsia is not increased by higher initial blood pressure levels.

5. If in a previous pregnancy preeclampsia was superimposed on chronic hypertensive disease, the chances of repetition are so great as to render another pregnancy hazardous and often futile. Chesley notes a 71 per cent rate of recurrence of superimposed preeclampsia.

Management.   All pregnant women with chronic hypertensive vascular disease should be admitted to the hospital for evaluation of their blood pressure levels at rest, cardiac assay (including, if possible, roentgenographic study of cardiac size), investigations of urine and renal function, and a careful survey of the retina. Upon the basis of this evidence an impression is gained about the degree of the hypertension at rest, the presence or absence of secondary alterations in the heart, kidney, and retina, and the general hazard that pregnancy will possibly impose.

In patients who fall in the five categories just enumerated, pregnancy is a sufficient threat to the life of the mother and sufficiently futile from the standpoint of fetal survival that interruption of gestation, combined with tubal sterilization, is often the best management of the problem. As Cosgrove has said, "If there is any legitimate indication for therapeutic abortion it is in that type of case (fixed hypertension)." Therapeutic abortion was done in 11.5 per cent of the patients with chronic hypertension at the Johns Hopkins Hospital between 1935 and 1960. With a few exceptions, the operation was combined with tubal ligation. Since many of these patients were referred in advanced stages of the disease, the incidence of therapeutic abortion there is undoubtedly higher than in unselected chronic hypertensives. At the Kings County Hospital, therapeutic abortion was performed in only 5 of the women with hypertensive disorders in the period 1958 through 1967 (Table 1). One was a late abortion in an eclamptic patient. Thus, among 2,411 women with chronic hypertension, with or without renal disease, only 4, or 0.17 per cent, were aborted. A large proportion of our patients, however, are not seen until late in pregnancy. If any chronic, irreversible disease indicates therapeutic abortion it also calls for sterilization as a rule. Tubal ligation may be indicated also in selected patients with chronic hypertensive disease who have been allowed to complete their current pregnancies. In general, those with cardiac, renal, or advanced retinal changes would fall in this group, as might those who have had superimposed preeclampsia. At the Kings County Hospital, 94, or 3.9 per cent of the women with chronic hypertension were sterilized (Table 1).

The treatment of uncomplicated hypertensive disease itself in pregnancy is the same as in the nonpregnant person. Abundant rest with limitation of any strenuous activity, a salt-poor diet, curtailment of weight gain, and mild sedation are the main features of treatment. These patients should be seen at least every two weeks and warned especially about reporting headache, visual disturbances, scanty urine, and other signs of preeclampsia. Provided preeclampsia is not superimposed, the patients are carried to 37 weeks, at which time interruption of pregnancy should be considered. In many of them, however, puerperal tubal ligation is warranted.

Control of the blood pressure by antihypertensive drugs has been disappointing. The perinatal mortality has not been reduced (Landesman and co-workers; Harley), nor has the incidence of superimposed preeclampsia. Landesman and co-workers reported that the signs of developing preeclampsia are hidden by the use of antihypertensive drugs, but the disorder may appear later in fulminating form, often during labor.

If the patient has moderate to severe hypertension, her own interests probably are best served by reduction of her blood pressure. Internists treating nonpregnant hypertensive patients with antihypertensive drugs have reduced mortality from cardiac failure almost to the vanishing point. It was formerly the mode of death in about 70 per cent of hypertensive subjects. Treated hypertensive patients now die of other causes and presumably live longer. At the Kings County Hospital women with severe hypertension are seldom seen until late in pregnancy. If they are seen earlier and already are on antihypertensive drugs, we continue this treatment; if not, they may be started if the patient's diastolic pressure exceeds 120 mm Hg. Most women are not treated during pregnancy, but are referred to the Medical Clinic after delivery.

If unequivocal evidence of superimposed preeclampsia becomes manifest, hospitalization and intensive treatment of the preeclampsia are indicated. If, after 24 to 48 hours, the signs and symptoms of the acute disorder continue, interruption of pregnancy is usually desirable and sometimes imperative. This decision is often disturbing, since the infant is usually premature. The mother will unquestionably benefit by such interference, and the chances for the baby in these circumstances are usually better outside than inside the uterus at any time after the thirty-second week. In many such cases, cesarean section is the procedure of choice.

Several successful pregnancies have been reported following the Smithwick operation (lumbodorsal splanchnicectomy) for hypertension (Kellogg; Newell and Smithwick; Austin and Frymire). The operation has been largely supplanted by medical treatment, however.

REFERENCES

Acosta-Sison, H. Clinicopathologic study of eclampsia based upon 38 autopsied cases. Amer J Obstet Gynec 22:35, 1931.

Adams, E. M., and Finlayson, A. Familial aspects of pre-eclampsia and hypertension in pregnancy. Lancet 2:1375, 1961.

Agarwal, L. P., Chawla, S. R., and Saxena, R. P. Ophthalmodynamometry in toxemias of pregnancy. Amer J Obstet Gynec 74:521, 1957.

Allen, W. M. Interagglutination of maternal and fetal blood in the late toxemias of pregnancy. Bull Hopkins Hosp 38:217, 1926.

Altchek, A. Electron microscopy of renal biopsies in toxemia of pregnancy. JAMA 175:791, 1961.

——— Albright, N. L., and Sommers, S. C. The renal pathology of toxemia of pregnancy. Obstet Gynec 31:595, 1968.

Anselmino, K. J., and Hoffmann, F. (The similarity of the clinical symptoms of toxemic and eclamptic women to the activity of the hormone of the posterior lobe of the pituitary gland). Arch Gynaek 147:597, 1931.

Assali, N. S.   Hemodynamic effects of hypotensive drugs used in obstetrics. Obstet Gynec Survey 9:776, 1954.

———— Douglass, R. A., Baird, W. W., and Nicholson, D. B.   Measurement of uterine blood flow and uterine metabolism with the N₂O method in normotensive and toxemic pregnancies. Clin Res Proc 2:102, 1954.

Austin, B. R., and Frymire, L. J.   Pregnancy following the Smithwick operation for hypertension. Amer J Obstet Gynec 56:805, 1948.

Baird, D.   Combined Textbook of Obstetrics and Gynaecology for Students and Practitioners. Edinburgh and London, E. & S. Livingstone, Ltd., 1969, p. 631.

Barnes, A. C., and Buckingham, J. C.   Electrolyte balance studies with the antihormones. Amer J Obstet Gynec 76:955, 1958.

Bartholomew, R. A., and Kracke, R. R.   The probable role of the hypercholesteremia of pregnancy in producing vascular changes in the placenta, predisposing to placental infarction and eclampsia. Amer J Obstet Gynec 31:549, 1936.

Beker, J. C.   The effects of pregnancy on blood circulation in their relation to so-called toxemia. Amer J Obstet Gynec 18:368, 1929.

———— Aetiology of eclampsia. J. Obstet Gynaec Brit Emp 55:757, 1948.

Bell, J. W.   Postmortem findings in ten cases of toxemia of pregnancy. Amer J Obstet Gynec 12:792, 1926.

Berger, M., and Boucek, R. J.   Irreversible uterine and renal changes induced by placental ischemia (rabbit). Amer J Obstet Gynec 89:230, 1964.

———— and Cavanagh, D.   Toxemia of pregnancy; the hypertensive effect of acute experimental placental ischemia. Amer J Obstet Gynec 87:293, 1963.

Blackfan, K. D., and Hamilton, B.   Uremia in acute glomerular nephritis (the cause and treatment in children). Boston Med Surg J 193:617, 1925.

Bonnar, J., Davidson, J. F., Pidgeon, C. F., McNichol, G. P., and Douglas, A. S.   Fibrin degradation products in normal and abnormal pregnancy and parturition. Brit Med J 3:137, 1969.

Bonsnes, R. W., and Stander, H. J.   Blood nucleotides in pregnancy and in the toxemias of pregnancy. Amer J Obstet Gynec 45:827, 1943.

Brown, J. J., Davis, D. L., Doak, P. B., Lever, A. F., and Robertson, J. I. S.   Plasma-renin in normal pregnancy. Lancet 2:900, 1963.

———— Davies, D. L., Doak, P. B., Lever, A. F., Robertson, J. I. S., and Trust, P.   Plasma renin concentration in the hypertensive diseases of pregnancy. J Obstet Gynaec Brit Comm 73:410, 1966.

Browne, F. J.   Sensitization of the vascular system in pre-eclamptic toxaemia and eclampsia. J Obstet Gynaec Brit Emp 53:510, 1946.

———— and Dodds, G. H.   Remote prognosis of toxaemias of pregnancy based on follow-up study of 40 patients in 589 pregnancies for periods varying from 6 months to 12 years. J Obstet Gynaec Brit Emp 46:443, 1939.

Browne, J. C. M., and Veall, N.   The maternal placental blood flow in normotensive and hypertensive women. J. Obstet Gynaec Brit Emp 60:141, 1953.

Brust, A. A., Assali, N. S., and Ferris, E. B.   Evaluation of neurogenic and humoral factors in blood pressure maintenance in normal and toxemic pregnancy using tetra-ethyl-ammonium chloride. J Clin Invest 27:717, 1948.

Bryans, C. I.   The remote prognosis in toxemia of pregnancy. Clin Obstet Gynec 9:973, 1966.

Bryant, R. D., and Fleming, J. G.   Veratrum viride in the treatment of eclampsia. III.   Obstet Gynec 19:372, 1962.

Burke, B. S., Beal, V. A., Kirkwood, S. B., and Stuart, H. C.   Nutrition studies during pregnancy. Amer J Obstet Gynec 46:38, 1943.

Burt, C.   Forearm and hand blood flow in pregnancy, in Toxaemias of Pregnancy, Human and Veterinary. Philadelphia, Blakiston Co., 1950.

Caldeyro-Barcia, R.   Uterine contractility in obstetrics. In Extrait du Deuxième Congrès International de Gynécologie et d'Obstétrique de Montréal, Vol. 1, 1958, p. 65.

Chargaff, E.   The isolation of preparations of thromboplastic protein from human organs. J Biol Chem 161:389, 1945.

Chesley, L. C.   Certain laboratory findings and interpretations in eclampsia. Amer J Obstet Gynec 38:430, 1939.

———— The variability of proteinuria in the hypertensive complications of pregnancy. J Clin Invest 18:617, 1939.

———— Weight changes and water balance in normal and toxic pregnancy. Amer J Obstet Gynec 48:565, 1944.

———— Toxemia of pregnancy in relation to chronic hypertension. Western J Surg 64:284, 1956.

———— Sodium retention and pre-eclampsia. Amer J Obstet Gynec 95:127, 1966.

———— and Annitto, J. E.   Pregnancy in the patient with hypertensive disease. Amer J Obstet Gynec 53:372, 1947.

———— Annitto, J. E., and Cosgrove, R. A.   Prognostic significance of recurrent toxemia of pregnancy. Obstet Gynec 23:874, 1964.

———— Annitto, J. E., and Cosgrove, R. A.   The familial factor in toxemia of pregnancy. Obstet Gynec 32:303, 1968.

———— Annitto, J. E., and Cosgrove, R. A.   Long-term follow-up study of eclamptic women: fifth periodic report. Amer J Obstet Gynec 101:886, 1968.

———— Annitto, J. E., and Jarvis, D. G.   A study of the interaction of pregnancy and hypertensive disease. Amer J Obstet Gynec 53:851, 1947.

———— Connell, E. J., Chesley, E. R., Katz, J. D., and Glisson, C. S.   The diodrast clearance and renal blood flow in toxemias of pregnancy. J Clin Invest 19:219, 1940.

———— Cosgrove, R. A., and Annitto, J. E.   A follow-up study of eclamptic women: Fourth periodic report. Amer J Obstet Gynec 83:1360, 1962.

———— Cosgrove, S. A., and Preece, J.   Hydatidiform mole with special reference to recurrence and associated eclampsia. Amer J Obstet Gynec 52:311, 1946.

———— Markowitz, I., and Wetchler, B. B.   Proteinuria following momentary vascular constriction. J Clin Invest 18:51, 1939.

———— and Tepper, I.   Plasma levels of magnesium attained in magnesium sulfate therapy for preeclampsia and eclampsia. Surg Clin N Amer April 1957, p. 353.

———— and Valenti, C.   The evaluation of tests to differentiate pre-eclampsia from hypertensive disease. Amer J Obstet Gynec 75:1165, 1958.

———— and Williams, L. O.   Renal glomerular and tubular function in relation to the hyperuricemia of pre-eclampsia and eclampsia. Amer J Obstet Gynec 50:367, 1945.

Clapp, C. A.   Detachment of the retina in eclampsia and toxemia of pregnancy. Amer J Ophthal 2:473, 1919.

Cobo, E.   Uterine hypercontractility in toxemia of pregnancy. Amer J Obstet Gynec 90:505, 1964.

Colvin, E. D., Bartholomew, R. A., and Grimes, W. H.   A comparison of thyroid extract and iodine therapy in the prevention of toxemia of pregnancy. Amer J Obstet Gynec 43:183, 1942.

Crichton, D., Notelovitz, M., and Heller, I.   Less conservatism in the treatment of eclampsia. J Obstet Gynaec Brit Comm 75:1019, 1968.

Davidson, J.   Eclampsia and puerperal toxaemia: study of histological changes occurring in liver and kidneys. Edinburgh M J, April, 1931. Trans Edinburgh Obst Soc 1930–31, p. 24.

Davies, M.   The Jerusalem toxemia study.   III. Diet and toxemia in pregnancy. Working Group on Relation of Nutrition to the Toxemias of Pregnancy. National Research Council. November, 1968.

Davis, J. A., and Snook, L. O.   The "pressure theory" of eclampsia. Surg Gynec Obstet 73:336, 1941.

Denman, T.   Essays on the Puerperal Fever and on Puerperal Convulsions. London, J. Walter, 1768.

DeSnoo, K.   The prevention of eclampsia. Amer J Obstet Gynec 34:911, 1937.

Dexter, L., and Weiss, S.   Pre-eclamptic and Eclamptic Toxemia of Pregnancy. Boston, Little, Brown & Co., 1941.

Dieckmann, W. J.   The hepatic lesion in eclampsia. Amer J Obstet Gynec 17:454, 1929.

———— Further observations on the hepatic lesion in eclampsia. Amer J Obstet Gynec 18:757, 1929.

———— Blood and plasma volume changes in eclampsia. Amer J Obstet Gynec 32:927, 1936.

———— The geographic distribution and effect of climate on eclampsia, toxemia of pregnancy, hyperemesis gravidarum, and abruptio placentae. Amer J Obstet Gynec 36:623, 1938.

———— The Toxemias of Pregnancy, 2nd ed. St. Louis, C. V. Mosby Co., 1952.

———— and Brown, I.   Do eclampsia and pre-eclampsia cause permanent vascular renal pathology? Amer J Obstet Gynec 37:762, 1939.

———— Pottinger, R. E., and Rynkiewicz, L. M.   Etiology of pre-eclampsia-eclampsia.   IV. Sodium chloride test for the diagnosis of pre-eclampsia. Amer J Obstet Gynec 63:783, 1952.

———— and Wegner, C. R.   Eclampsia without convulsions or coma. Amer J Obstet Gynec 23:657, 1932.

Dill, L. V., Isenhour, C. E., Cadden, J. F., and Schaffer, N. K.   Glomerular filtration and renal blood flow in the toxemias of pregnancy. Amer J Obstet Gynec 43:32, 1942.

Dixon, H. G., Browne, J. C. M., and Davey, D. A.   Choriodecidual and myometrial blood flow. Lancet 2:369, 1963.

———— and Robertson, W. B.   Vascular changes in the placental bed. Path Microbiol (Basel) 24:622, 1961.

Doggart, J. H.   Eclamptic detachment of retina. Proc Roy Soc Med 29:753, 1936.

Dorsett, L., and Dieckmann, W. J.   Unpublished. Cited in Dieckmann, W. J., The Toxemias of Pregnancy, 2nd ed. St. Louis, C. V. Mosby Co., 1952, p. 519.

Douglas, B. H., and Langford, H. G.   Toxemia of pregnancy: production of lesions in the absence of signs. Amer J Obstet Gynec 95:534, 1966.

Douglass, L. H., and Linn, R. F.   Paraldehyde in obstetrics, with particular reference to its use in eclampsia. Amer J Obstet Gynec 43:844, 1942.

Dunlop, J. C. H.   Chronic hypertension and perinatal mortality. Proc Roy Soc Med 59:838, 1966.

Eastman, N. J.   The vascular factor in the toxemias of late pregnancy. Amer J Obstet Gynec 34:549, 1937.

————   The geographic distribution of toxemia of pregnancy in the United States. Working Group on Relation of Nutrition to the Toxemias of Pregnancy, National Research Council, November, 1968.

———— Bell, E. T., Dieckmann, W. J., Kellog, F. S., Mussey, R. D., Chesley, L. C., Peters, J. P., Page, E. W., Ross, R. A., Johnson, H. W., and Van Wyck, H. B.   Definition and Classification of Toxemias Brought Up-to-Date, American Committee on Maternal Welfare, Chicago, 1952.

———— and Steptoe, P. P.   The management of pre-eclampsia. Canad Med Ass J 52:562, 1945.

Eden, T. W.   Eclampsia: a commentary on the reports presented to the British Congress of Obstetrics and Gynaecology, June 29, 1922. J Obstet Gynaec Brit Emp 29:386, 1922.

Faith, G. C., and Trump, B. F.   The glomerular capillary wall in human kidney disease: acute glomerulonephritis, systemic lupus erythematosus, and preeclampsia-eclampsia. Lab Invest 15:1682, 1966.

Farquhar, M.   Review of normal and pathologic glomerular ultrastructure, in Proceedings of the Tenth Annual Conference on the Nephrotic Syndrome. New York, National Kidney Disease Foundation, 1959.

Fehling, H.   (On habitual fetal death associated with maternal renal disease). Arch Gynaek 27:300, 1886.

Finnerty, F. A.   Does vascular damage follow toxemia of pregnancy? JAMA 154:1075, 1954.

Fisher, E. R., Pardo, V., Paul, R., and Hayashi, T. T.   Ultrastructural studies in hypertension. IV. Toxemia of pregnancy. Amer J Path 55:901, 1969.

Gate, J. M.   Foetal mortality in essential hypertension. Lancet 1:901, 1960.

Gordon, R. D., Parsons, S., and Symonds, E. M.   A prospective study of plasma-renin activity in normal and toxaemic pregnancy. Lancet 1:347, 1969.

Govan, A. D. T.   The pathogenesis of eclamptic lesions. Path Microbiol (Basel) 24:561, 1961.

Gray, M. J.   Use and abuse of thiazides in pregnancy. Clin Obstet Gynec 11:568, 1968.

———— and Plentl, A. A.   The variations of the sodium space and the total exchangeable sodium during pregnancy. J Clin Invest 33:347, 1954.

Hallum, A. V.   Eye changes in hypertensive toxemia of pregnancy, a study of 300 cases. JAMA 106:1649, 1936.

Hamilton, B. E., and Thomson, K. J.   The Heart in Pregnancy and the Childbearing Age. Boston, Little, Brown & Co., 1941.

Hamlin, R. H. J.   The prevention of eclampsia and pre-eclampsia. Lancet 1:64, 1952.

Handler, J. S.   The role of lactic acid in the reduced excretion of uric acid in toxemia of pregnancy. J Clin Invest 39:1526, 1960.

Harbert, G. M., Cornell, G. W., and Thornton, W. N.   Effect of toxemia therapy on uterine dynamics. Amer J Obstet Gynec 105:94, 1969.

Harding, V. J., and Van Wyck, H. B.   Effects of hypertonic saline in the toxaemias of later pregnancy. Brit Med J 2:589, 1930.

Harley, J. M. G.   Pregnancy in the chronic hypertensive woman. Essential hypertension complicating pregnancy: factors affecting the foetal mortality. Proc Roy Soc Med 59:835, 1966.

Helmer, O. M., and Judson, W. E.   Influence of high renin substrate levels on renin-angiotensian system in pregnancy. Amer J Obstet Gynec 99:9, 1967.

Herrick, W. W., and Tillman, A. J. B.   Toxemia of pregnancy; its relation to cardiovascular and renal disease; clinical and necropsy observations with a long follow-up. Arch Intern Med 55:643, 1935.

Hertig, A. T.   Vascular pathology in the hypertensive albuminuric toxemias of pregnancy. Clinics 4:602, 1945.

Hinselmann, H.   Die Eklampsie. Bonn, F. Cohen, 1924.

Hobson, W.   A dietary and clinical survey of pregnant women with particular reference to toxaemia of pregnancy. J Hyg (Camb) 46:198, 1948.

Hodari, A. A.   Chronic uterine ischemia and reversible experimental "toxemia of pregnancy." Amer J Obstet Gynec 97:597, 1967.

Hofbauer, J.   (Toxemias of pregnancy). Z Geburtsh Gynaek 61:258, 1908.

———— (Clarification of the problem of eclampsia). Zbl Gynaek 45:1797, 1921.

Hoffmann, F., and Anselmino, K. J.   (Detection of the antidiuretic factor of the posterior pituitary and of a pressor substance in the blood in toxemia and eclampsia). Arch Gynaek 147:604, 1931.

Holland, E.   The results of a collective investigation into Caesarean sections performed in Great Britain and Ireland from the year 1911 to 1920 inclusive. J Obstet Gynaec Brit Emp 28:358, 1921.

Hoshino, H.   Hemodynamic studies on liver in toxemias of late pregnancy. J Jap Obstet Gynec Soc 6:42, 1959.

Hughes, T. D.   The importance of the relativity of blood pressure and other signs in the prevention of eclampsia. Med J Aust 2:871, 1951.

Humphries, J. O.   Occurrence of hypertensive toxemia of pregnancy in mother-daughter pairs. Bull Hopkins Hosp 107:271, 1960.

Ingerslev, M., and Teilum, G.   Biopsy studies of the liver in pregnancy. Acta Obstet Gynec Scand 25:339, 1946.

Irving, F. C.   The treatment of eclampsia and pre-eclampsia with veratrum viride and magnesium sulfate. Amer J Obstet Gynec 54:731, 1947.

Ishikawa, E.   The kidney in the toxemias of pregnancy. Path Microbiol (Basel) 24:576, 1961.

Jäämeri, K. E. U., Koivuniemi, A. P., and Carpén, E. O.   Occurrence of trophoblasts in the blood of toxaemic patients. Gynaecologia 160:315, 1965.

Janisch, H.   (Renal changes in pregnancy toxemia). Wien Klin Wschr 81:749, 1969.

Jardine, R., and Kennedy, A. M.   Three cases of symmetrical necrosis of the cortex of the kidney associated with puerperal eclampsia and suppression of urine. Trans Edinburgh Obstet Soc 38:158, 1912–1913.

Jeffcoate, T. N. A., and Scott, J. S.   Some observations on the placental factor in pregnancy toxemia. Amer J Obstet Gynec 77:475, 1959.

Jegorow, B.   (The principle of allergy and pregnancy). Zbl Gynaek 59:1455, 1935.

Johnson, T., and Clayton, C. G.   Diffusion of radioactive sodium in normotensive and pre-eclamptic pregnancies. Brit Med J 1:312, 1957.

Jones, W. S.   Essential hypertension with superimposed preeclampsia. Amer J Obstet Gynec 62:387, 1951.

Kellogg, F. S.   Toxemias of pregnancy. Clinics 4:585, 1945.

Kraus, G. W., Marchese, J. R., and Yen, S. S. C.   Prophylactic use of hydrochlorothiazide in pregnancy. JAMA 198:1150, 1966.

Krieger, V. I., Butler, H. M., and Kilvington, T. B.   Antidiuretic substance in the urine during pregnancy and its frequent association with bacterial growth. J Obstet Gynaec Brit Emp 58:5, 1951.

Kumar, D.   Chronic placental ischemia in relation to toxemias of pregnancy. Amer J Obstet Gynec 84:1323, 1962.

Kyank, H., Schubert, E., and Gyöngyössy, A.   Evaluation of cases of eclampsia treated between 1957 and 1960 at 72 German obstetric clinics. German Med Monthly 9:108, 1964.

Ladner, C. N., Weston, P. V., Brinkman, C. R., and Assali, N. S. Effects of hydralazine on uteroplacental and fetal circulations. Amer J Obstet Gynec 108:375, 1970.

Landesman, R., Douglas, R. G., and Holze, E. The bulbar conjunctival vascular bed in the toxemias of pregnancy. Amer J Obstet Gynec 68:170, 1954.

────── McLarn, W. D., Ollstein, R. N., and Mendelsohn, B. Reserpine in toxemia of pregnancy. Obstet Gynec 9:377, 1957.

Lazard, E. M. Analysis of 575 cases of eclamptic and preeclamptic toxemias treated by intravenous injections of magnesium sulphate. Amer J Obstet Gynec 26:647, 1933.

────── Irwin, J. C., and Vruwink, J. The intravenous magnesium sulphate treatment of eclampsia. Amer J Obstet Gynec 12:104, 1926.

Lembrych, S. (Severe toxemia [eclampsia] with hydatidiform mole). Zbl Gynaek 88:1622, 1966.

Lichtenstein, F. (Critical and experimental studies of the toxicity of the placenta, with a contribution in opposition to the placental theory of the etiology of eclampsia). Arch Gynaek 86:434, 1908.

Lipsitz, P. J., and English, I. C. Hypermagnesemia in the newborn infant. Pediatrics 40:856, 1967.

Mautner, W., Churg, J., Grishman, E., and Dachs, S. Preeclamptic nephropathy; an electron microscopic study. Lab Invest 11:518, 1962.

McCall, M. L. Continuing vasodilator infusion therapy. Utilization of a blend of 1-hydrazinophthalazine (Apresoline) and cryptenamine (Unitensin) in toxemia of pregnancy. Obstet Gynec 4:403, 1954.

────── and Taylor, H. W. Effects of barbiturate sedation on the brain in toxemia of pregnancy. JAMA 149:51, 1952.

McCartney, C. P. Pathological anatomy of acute hypertension of pregnancy. Circulation 30 (Suppl. 2):37, 1964.

McKay, D. G. Clinical significance of the pathology of toxemia of pregnancy. Circulation 30 (Suppl. 2):66, 1964.

────── Goldenberg, V., Kaunitz, H., and Csavossy, I. Experimental eclampsia. Arch Path 84:557, 1967.

McLane, C. M. Results in the treatment of severe pre-eclampsia. Med Rec Ann 42:669, 1948 (abstract in Obstet Gynec Survey 4:36, 1949).

────── and Kuder, K. Severe pre-eclampsia. Amer J Obstet Gynec 46:549, 1943.

McLennan, C. E. Antecubital and femoral venous pressure in normal and toxemic pregnancy. Amer J Obstet Gynec 45:568, 1943.

────── The rate of filtration through the capillary walls in pregnancy. Amer J Obstet Gynec 46:63, 1943.

McManus, J. F. A. Medical Diseases of the Kidney. Philadelphia, Lea & Febiger, 1950.

McNeile, L. G. Conservative treatment of the late toxemias of pregnancy, with special reference to intravenous use of magnesium sulphate. JAMA 103:548, 1934.

Menon, M. K. K. The evolution of the treatment of eclampsia. J Obstet Gynaec Brit Comm 68:417, 1961.

Menzher, D., and Prystowsky, H. Acute hemorrhagic pancreatitis during pregnancy and the puerperium associated with thiazide therapy. J Florida Med Ass 54:564, 1967.

Minkowitz, S., Soloway, H. B., Hall, J. E., and Yermakov, V. Fatal hemorrhagic pancreatitis following chlorothiazide administration in pregnancy. Obstet Gynec 24:337, 1964.

Munnell, E. W., and Taylor, H. C. Liver blood flow in pregnancy—hepatic vein catheterization. J Clin Invest 26:952, 1947.

Mylius, K. (Spastic and tetanic changes in retinal vessels in eclampsia). Berichte über der Versammlung der deutsch ophth Gesellsch 47:379, 1929.

Newell, J. L., and Smithwick, R. H. Pregnancy following lumbodorsal splanchnicectomy for essential and malignant hypertension. New Eng J Med 236:851, 1947.

Page, E. W. The effect of eclamptic blood upon the urinary output and blood pressure of human recipients. J Clin Invest 17:207, 1938.

────── The relation between hydatid moles, relative ischemia of the gravid uterus, and the placental origin of eclampsia. Amer J Obstet Gynec 37:291, 1939.

────── Placental dysfunction in eclamptogenic toxemias. Obstet Gynec Survey 3:615, 1948.

────── The Hypertensive Disorders of Pregnancy. Springfield, Ill., Charles C Thomas, 1953.

Paramore, R. H.   An introduction to the mechanistic conception of eclampsia. Lancet 2:914, 1928.

Parks, J., and Pearson, J. W.   Cerebral complications occurring in the toxemias of pregnancy. Amer J Obstet Gynec 45:774, 1943.

Paterson, M. L.   The role of the posterior pituitary antidiuretic hormone in toxaemia of pregnancy. J. Obstet Gynaec Brit 67: 883, 1960.

Peckham, C. H.   An analysis of 127 cases of eclampsia treated by the modified Stroganoff method. Amer J Obstet Gynec 29:27, 1935.

Peters, J. P.   The nature of the toxemias of pregnancy. JAMA 110:329, 1938.

Plass, E. D.   The conservative treatment of eclampsia. Med Herald Physiotherapist 46:153, 1927.

Plentl, A. A., and Gray, M. J.   Total body water, sodium space, and total exchangeable sodium in normal and toxemic pregnant women. Amer J Obstet Gynec 78:472, 1959.

Pollak, V. E., and Nettles, J. B.   The kidney in toxemia of pregnancy; a clinical and pathologic study based on renal biopsies. Medicine 39:469, 1960.

Pride, C. B., and Rucker, M. P.   Eclampsia and ovarian pregnancy. Amer J Obstet Gynec 44:575, 1942.

Pritchard, J. A.   Use of the magnesium ion in the management of eclamptogenic toxemias. Surg Gynec Obstet 100:131, 1955.

———— and Stone, S. R.   Clinical and laboratory observations on eclampsia. Amer J Obstet Gynec 99:754, 1967.

———— Weisman, R., Ratnoff, O. D., and Vosburgh, G. J.   Intravascular hemolysis, thrombocytopenia and other hematologic abnormalities associated with severe toxemia of pregnancy. New Eng J Med 250:89, 1954.

———— and Mason, R.   Unpublished observations.

Prutz, W.   (The anatomical state of the kidneys in puerperal eclampsia). Z Geburtsh Gynaek 23:1, 1892.

Raab, W., Schroeder, G., Wagner, R., and Gigee, W.   Vascular reactivity and electrolytes in normal and toxemic pregnancy. J Clin Endocr 16:1196, 1956.

Reis, R. A., and Bernick, E. A.   Eclampsia without convulsions, hypertension or coma. Amer J Obstet Gynec 48:257, 1944.

Rimmerman, A. B., and Halpern, A.   A comparative study of sodium-free salt substitutes. Amer Pract 2:168, 1951.

Rodriguez, S. U., Leikin, S. L., and Hiller, M. C.   Neonatal thrombocytopenia associated with antepartum administration of thiazide drugs. New Eng J Med 270:881, 1964.

Ross, R. A., Perlzweig, W. A., Taylor, H. M., McBryde, A., Yates, A., and Kondritzer, A. A.   A study of certain dietary factors of possible etiologic significance in toxemias of pregnancy. Amer J Obstet Gynec 35:426, 1938.

Salzmann, B., and Malkary, J.   Hepatic hemorrhage in pregnancy. Obstet Gynec 19:436, 1962.

Schiötz, I.   (Retinal detachment during pregnancy). Klin Mbl Augenheilk 62:234, 1919.

Schmorl, G.   Pathologisch-anatomische Untersuchungen ueber Puerperal-Eklampsie. Leipzig, F. C. W. Vogel, 1893.

———— (Studies of eclampsia). Arch Gynaek 65:504, 1902.

Schneider, C. L.   Thromboplastin complications of pregnancy. Bull Margaret Hague Mat Hosp 4:2, 1951.

Sheehan, H. L.   Pathological lesions in the hypertensive toxaemias of pregnancy, in Hammond, J., Browne, F. J., and Wolstenholme, G. E. W. (eds.), Toxaemias of Pregnancy, Human and Veterinary. Philadelphia, The Blakiston Co., 1950.

———— Causes of maternal death in toxemia. Clin Obstet Gynec 1:397, 1958.

Siddall, A. C.   Vitamin B₁ deficiency as an etiologic factor in pregnancy toxemias. Amer J Obstet Gynec 39:818, 1940.

Sims, E. A. H.   Pre-eclampsia and related complications of pregnancy. Amer J Obstet Gynec, 107:154, 1970.

Sioli, F.   (Eclamptic and post-eclamptic psychoses), in Hinselmann (ed.), Die Eklampsie, Bonn, 1924, p. 597.

Smith, G. V., and Smith, O. W.   Estrogen and progestin metabolism in pregnant women, with especial reference to pre-eclamptic toxemia and the effect of hormone administration. Amer J Obstet Gynec 39:405, 1940.

———— and Smith, O. W. The anterior pituitary-like hormone in late pregnancy toxemia. A summary of results since 1932. Amer J Obstet Gynec 38:618, 1939.

Sophian, J. Toxaemias of Pregnancy. London, Butterworth, 1953.

Spargo, B., McCartney, C. P., and Winemiller, R. Glomerular capillary endotheliosis in toxemia of pregnancy. Arch Path 68:593, 1959.

Spillman, R. Lumbar puncture in the treatment of eclampsia. Collective review. Amer J Obstet Gynec 4:568, 1922.

Spoljanskij, G., and Juzhelevskiy, A. S. (Cerebral pressure in eclampsia in relation to the cause of convulsions). Mschr Geburtsh Gynaek 96:190, 1934.

Stander, H. J., and Cadden, J. F. Blood chemistry in pre-eclampsia and eclampsia. Amer J Obstet Gynec 28:856, 1934.

———— Eastman, N. J., Harrison, E.P.H., and Cadden, J. F. The acid-base equilibrium of the blood in eclampsia. J Biol Chem 85:233, 1929.

Stone, S. R., and Pritchard, J. A. The effect of maternally-administered magnesium-sulfate on the neonate. Obstet Gynec 35:574, 1970.

Stroganoff, W. Results obtained in the treatment of eclampsia by the improved prophylactic method. Trans Edinburgh Obstet Soc, Edinburgh M J, 1928, p. 161.

———— (The management of eclampsia). Zbl Gynaek 25:1309, 1901.

———— and Davidovitch, O. Two hundred cases of eclampsia treated with magnesium sulphate. J Obstet Gynaec Brit Emp 44:289, 1937.

Szekely, P., and Snaith, L. The heart in toxaemia of pregnancy. Brit Heart J 9:128, 1947.

Talledo, O. E., Chesley, L. C., and Zuspan, F. P. Renin-angiotensin system in normal and toxemic pregnancies. III. Differential sensitivity to angiotensin II and norepinephrine in toxemia of pregnancy. Amer J Obstet Gynec 100:218, 1968.

———— and Zuspan, F. P. Spontaneous uterine contractility in eclampsia. Clin Obstet Gynec 9:910, 1966.

Tenney, B., and Parker, F. The placenta in toxemia of pregnancy. Amer J Obstet Gynec 39:1000, 1940.

Theobald, G. W. Hepatic lesions associated with eclampsia and those caused by raising intra-abdominal pressure. J Path Bact 35:843, 1932.

———— The Pregnancy Toxemias or the Encymonic Atelositeses. New York, Paul B. Hoeber, Inc., 1956.

Thomson, A. M., Hytten, F. E., and Billewicz, W. Z. The epidemiology of oedema during pregnancy. J Obstet Gynaec Brit Comm 74:1, 1967.

Tillman, A. J. B. The effect of normal and toxemic pregnancy on blood pressure. Amer J Obstet Gynec 70:589, 1955.

Townsend, L. High Blood Pressure and Pregnancy. New York, Cambridge University Press, 1959.

Vassalli, P., and McCluskey, R. T. The coagulation process and glomerular disease. Amer J Med 39:179, 1965.

———— Morris, R. H., and McCluskey, R. T. The pathogenic role of fibrin deposition in the glomerular lesions of toxemia of pregnancy. J Exp Med 118:467, 1963.

Vital Statistics of the United States 1965, Vol. II—Mortality, Part A, p. 1–40, Published 1967, U.S. Department of Health, Education and Welfare, Public Health Service, National Center for Health Statistics.

Volhard, F. Die doppelseitigen haematogenen Nierenerkrankungen. Berlin, Julius Springer, 1918.

Wagener, H. P. Arterioles of the retina in toxemia of pregnancy. JAMA 101:1380, 1933.

———— and Keith, N. M. Diffuse arteriolar disease with hypertension and the associated retinal lesions. Medicine 18:317, 1939.

Wallace, L., Katz, L. N., Langendorf, R., and Buxbaum, H. Electrocardiogram in toxemias of pregnancy. Arch Intern Med 77:405, 1946.

Watanabe, M. C., Meeker, C. I., Gray, M. J., Sims, E. A. H., and Solomon, S. Secretion rates of aldosterone in normal pregnancy. J Clin Invest 42:1619, 1963.

———— Meeker, C. I., Gray, M. J., Sims, E. A. H., and Solomon, S. Aldosterone secretion rates in abnormal pregnancy. J Clin Endocr 25:1665, 1965.

Way, G. T. C. Fatal eclampsia. A clinical and anatomic correlative study. Amer J Obstet Gynec 54:928, 1947.

References

Welsh, C. A., Wellen, I., Taylor, H. C., and Rosenthal, A. The filtration rate, effective renal blood flow, tubular excretory mass and phenol red clearance in normal pregnancy. J Clin Invest 21:57, 1942.

Whalley, P. J., Scott, D. E., and Pritchard, J. A. Maternal folate deficiency and pregnancy wastage. III. Pregnancy-induced hypertension. Obstet Gynec 36:29, 1970.

Whitacre, F. E., Hingson, R. A., and Turner, H. B. The treatment of eclampsia by means of regional nerve block. Southern Med J 41:920, 1948.

———— Loeb, W. M., and Chin, H. A contribution to the study of eclampsia. A consideration of 200 cases. JAMA 133:445, 1947.

White, P. Pregnancy complicating diabetes of more than twenty years' duration. Med Clin N Amer 31:395, 1947.

White, P. D. Heart Disease, 3rd ed. New York, The Macmillan Co., 1944.

Wooldridge, L. C. On haemorrhagic infarction of the liver. Trans Path Soc London 39:421, 1888.

Wylie, B. Toxemia of pregnancy and altered renal circulation. Amer J Obstet Gynec 66:254, 1953.

Young, J. The aetiology of eclampsia and albuminuria and their relation to accidental haemorrhage. J Obstet Gynaec Brit Emp 26:1, 1914.

———— Recurrent pregnancy toxaemia and its relation to placental damage. Trans Edinburgh Obst Soc, Edinburgh M J, p. 61, 1927.

Zangemeister, W. (Investigations of the properties of blood and urinary excretion during eclampsia). Z Geburtsh Gynaek 50:385, 1903.

Zeek, P. M., and Assali, N. S. Vascular changes in decidua associated with eclamptogenic toxemia of pregnancy. Amer J Clin Path 20:1099, 1950.

Zuspan, F. P. Treatment of severe preeclampsia and eclampsia. Clin Obstet Gynec 9:954, 1966.

———— and Talledo, E. Factors affecting delivery in eclampsia. The condition of the cervix and uterine activity. Amer J Obstet Gynec 100:672, 1968.

Zweifel, P. (Eclampsia), in Doederlein (ed.), Handbuch der Geburtshilfe. Weisbaden, J. F. Bergmann, 1916, p. 672.

27

MEDICAL AND SURGICAL ILLNESSES DURING PREGNANCY AND THE PUERPERIUM

For the great majority of systemic illnesses the physiologic and anatomic changes inherent in normal pregnancy not infrequently influence the symptoms, signs, and laboratory values to a considerable degree. As a consequence the physician who is not aware of these changes induced by normal pregnancy may not be able to recognize a disease or may diagnose incorrectly some other disease, to the jeopardy of the mother and her fetus. Throughout this chapter emphasis has been placed on the effects of any interaction between the disease and the pregnancy as well as the problems in diagnosis and treatment imposed by the gestational state.

Essentially all diseases that affect a woman when nonpregnant may be contracted during pregnancy. Moreover, the presence of the majority of diseases does not prevent conception. It is imperative that the physician appreciate the significance of the many variations that may occur when any of a great variety of diseases coincides with pregnancy. In practically all instances the following questions are pertinent to diagnosis, treatment, and prognosis:

1. Is pregnancy likely to make the disease more serious, and if so, how?
2. Does the disease jeopardize the pregnancy, and if so, how and to what degree?
3. Should the pregnancy be terminated because of either gross risk to the mother or likelihood of grave damage to the fetus?
4. Should the pregnancy be allowed to continue under a very carefully defined regimen of therapy?
5. If the disease exists before pregnancy, is pregnancy contraindicated, and if so, what steps should be taken to protect the woman from pregnancy?

INFECTIONS OF THE URINARY SYSTEM

The term "pyelitis of pregnancy," which has been widely used to describe infections of the urinary tract during pregnancy, should be discarded, for it implies that the infection is confined to the renal pelvis. Although occasionally a urinary infection may involve only the bladder and thus represent true cystitis,

infection of the renal calyces and pelvis is invariably accompanied by involvement of the renal parenchyma, a condition better described as pyelonephritis.
The term "pyelonephritis" is here used to designate a disease involving the renal
pelves, calyces, and parenchyma and resulting from the immediate or late effects of bacterial infection. Accordingly, the disease may be acute or chronic, or
both.

Cystitis.   Cystitis is inflammation of the bladder resulting almost always
from bacterial infection. Typically, it is characterized by dysuria, particularly
at the end of urination, as well as urgency and frequency. There are few associated systemic findings. The urine is usually free of protein, but there is an
abnormally large number of white blood cells, and bacteria may usually be
identified. Erythrocytes are commonly found in the urinary sediment, and occasionally even gross hematuria is seen. The term "cystitis" implies an infection
confined to the bladder without involvement of the upper urinary tract. Although
uncomplicated cystitis occurs, the upper urinary tract is often soon involved in
an ascending infection.

Acute Pyelonephritis.   Acute pyelonephritis is one of the most common medical complications of pregnancy. Not only is this disease an important cause of
maternal morbidity, but the acute disease may also play a significant role in the
natural history of chronic pyelonephritis. The reported incidence of acute pyelonephritis complicating pregnancy and the puerperium approximates 2 per cent,
with about an equal frequency antepartum and postpartum. The disease is often
bilateral, but when unilateral it is more frequently right-sided. It most often appears in the latter part of pregnancy, as shown in the series of 98 cases of antepartum pyelonephritis reported by McLane, in which 3 occurred in the first
trimester, 35 in the second, and 60 in the third.

The onset of signs and symptoms of the disease is usually rather abrupt. The
patient who has previously been well or has complained of slight bladder irritation or hematuria suddenly develops fever, shaking chills, and aching pain in one
or both lumbar regions. There may be anorexia, nausea, and vomiting. Physical
examination reveals a temperature usually greater than 100°F and tenderness to
palpation in the region of one or both kidneys. The urinary sediment contains
many leukocytes, frequently in clumps, and white blood cell casts. Examination
of the stained sediment reveals numerous bacteria, predominantly gram-negative
bacilli. *Escherichia coli* is the microorganism cultured from the urine of over 90
per cent of patients with this disease. Infrequently, culture of the blood may
also reveal the same organism.

Pain in one lumbar region and the characteristic urinary findings, as well as
fever and costovertebral tenderness, should make the diagnosis clear. The condition may be mistaken, however, for labor, appendicitis, placental abruption or
infarction of a myoma, and, in the puerperium, for uterine infection. Pyelonephritis with hypertension and proteinuria may occasionally be confused with preeclampsia.

Acute pyelonephritis is the direct result of bacterial infection, which may
extend upward from the bladder or through the blood vessels and lymphatics.
The weight of clinical evidence suggests that the ascending route of infection is
very much more common, with bacteria passing from the bladder to the kidney
via the ureter. The urine in the bladder is normally sterile, for bacteria are not
excreted by the kidney except in cases of active infection of the renal parenchyma.

During pregnancy the two major causes of active multiplication of bacteria within the bladder are recent instrumentation of the urinary tract and persistent asymptomatic bacteriuria.

Since bacteria are normally found in the outer portion of the urethra, single catheterization or the use of an indwelling catheter may introduce bacteria into the bladder, where the organisms encounter ideal conditions for multiplication, particularly during the puerperium. In nonpregnant women a single catheterization of the bladder is followed by significant bacteriuria in 2 to 4 per cent of patients, whereas a catheter that remains in the bladder for more than 72 hours results in bacteriuria in 100 per cent of cases. As shown by Brumfitt and associates, routine bladder catheterization before parturition initiates infection in approximately 9 per cent of puerperal women. It follows that the number of puerperal urinary infections can be reduced appreciably by avoiding routine catheterization of the bladder at the time of delivery. When catheterization is unavoidable, prophylactic administration of antibacterial agents for 3 to 5 days postpartum often will prevent these infections (Turck and Petersdorf). In addition, approximately 6 per cent of pregnant women already have bacteriuria at the time of the first prenatal visit; provided there has been no instrumentation of the urinary tract, acute pyelonephritis complicating pregnancy occurs chiefly among this group of women with preexisting bacteriuria. Approximately 25 per cent of women with asymptomatic bacteriuria subsequently develop a symptomatic infection of the urinary tract during the course of pregnancy.

Once bacteria gain entrance to the bladder, several factors predispose the pregnant woman to acute pyelonephritis. As a result of the hormonal changes, as well as the mechanical effect of the enlarging uterus and ovarian vein ligation, there is a gradual dilatation of the renal calyces, pelves, and ureters, accompanied by a decrease in tone and peristalsis (Bellina and associates). These changes lead to stasis, a factor known to increase the susceptibility to renal infection (Figs. 1 through 4). Moreover, the bladder in the early puerperium has an increased capacity and a decreased sensitivity to intravesical fluid tension compared with the nonpregnant state; as a result, overdistention, incomplete emptying, and residual urine are common. In addition, evacuation of the uterus is associated with stretching and trauma to the base of the bladder. Residual urine and a traumatized bladder provide an excellent environment for multiplication of bacteria.

Asymptomatic Bacteriuria.   The term "asymptomatic bacteriuria" is used to indicate actively multiplying bacteria within the urinary tract without symptoms of a urinary infection. The reported prevalence of bacteriuria during pregnancy varies from 2 to 7 per cent, depending on the parity, race, and socioeconomic status of the women surveyed. The highest incidence has been reported in Negro multiparas, and the lowest incidence has been found in white private patients. Bacteriuria is typically present at the time of the first prenatal visit; after an initial negative culture of the urine fewer than 1.5 per cent acquire a urinary infection in the subsequent months until delivery. The diagnosis of asymptomatic bacteriuria requires the demonstration of significant numbers of bacteria in the urine. In most instances this can be accomplished by culturing clean voided specimens of urine without resorting to catheterization. A clean voided specimen of urine containing more than 100,000 organisms per milliliter of urine is most often evidence of infection. Smaller numbers of bacteria usually represent contamination of the specimen during collection.

Several studies listed in Table 1 indicate that approximately 25 per cent of

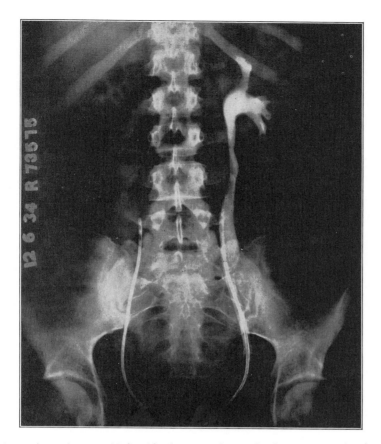

Fig. 1. Retrograde pyelogram obtained in the seventh month of pregnancy, showing moderate hydronephrosis and hydroureter. This degree of dilatation is not uncommon.

Table 1. **Symptomatic Infections of the Urinary Tract Following Asymptomatic Bacteriuria**

Author	No. of Patients with Asymptomatic Bacteriuria	Per Cent Who Developed Pyelonephritis
Grüneberg	86	23
Little	141	25
Norden	110	23
Savage	98	26
Whalley	179	26
Total	614	25

women with asymptomatic bacteriuria during pregnancy subsequently develop an acute symptomatic urinary infection during that pregnancy. Moreover, as depicted in Table 2, eradication of bacteriuria with antimicrobial agents has been shown to be effective in the prevention of these infections.

Bacteriuria has been thought by some investigators to cause premature labor and, in turn, increased neonatal morbidity and mortality. In an early study by Kass, the incidence of premature births, defined as a birth weight of 2,500 g or less, among 95 women with bacteriuria who received only placebos during preg-

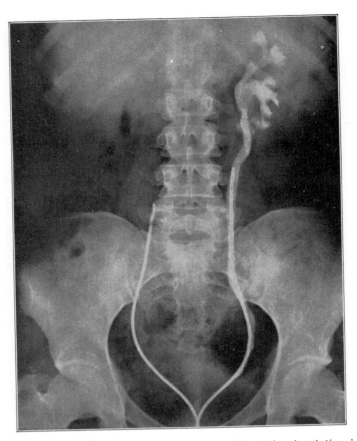

Fig. 2. Retrograde pyelogram, three weeks postpartum, illustrating involution in the ureter and renal pelvis. The pregnancy-induced marked hydronephrosis and hydroureter have returned almost to normal. This outcome may be expected unless infection produces edema fibrosis.

nancy was 27 per cent, whereas among 84 women with bacteriuria who were treated with antimicrobial agents, the rate was only 7 per cent. The corresponding rates of perinatal death were 14 and 0 per cent, respectively. On the basis of an extensive study in Australia, Kincaid-Smith and Bullen also reported a relatively high proportion of infants of low birth weight among untreated bacteriuric women, but these investigators were unable to reduce significantly this proportion with antimicrobial therapy (21.5 per cent compared with 17.3 per cent). They concluded that bacteriuria in pregnancy is commonly a manifestation of

Table 2. Effect of Antibacterial Therapy on the Subsequent Occurrence of Antepartum Pyelonephritis in Women with Asymptomatic Bacteriuria

Author	No of Patients	No Who Developed Pyelonephritis	Per Cent
Grüneberg	285	8	2.8
Kincaid-Smith	61	2	3.3
Little	124	4	3.2
Savage	93	1	1.1

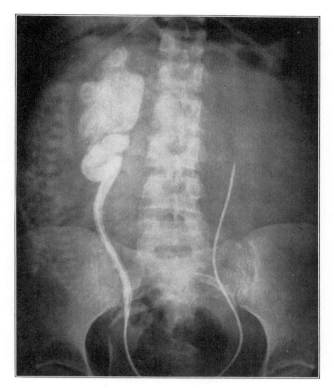

Fig. 3. Retrograde pyelogram obtained during the eighth month of pregnancy. This multiparous woman suffered from pyonephrosis as well as hydronephrosis of pregnancy. The renal pelvis and ureter had a capacity of 85 ml.

underlying chronic renal disease, which accounts for the higher incidence of low-birth-weight infants and perinatal loss. As demonstrated in Table 3, several other

Table 3. Incidences of Premature Deliveries in Women With and Without Bacteriuria During Pregnancy

Author	Bacteriuric		Nonbacteriuric	
	No of Patients	*Per Cent*	*No of Patients*	*Per Cent*
Little	141	9	4,735	8
Norden	114	15	109	13
Sleigh	100	7	100	7
Whalley	176	15	176	12
Wilson	230	11	6,216	10

investigators have been unable to corroborate this alleged relation between bacteriuria and low birth weight. Therefore, from the evidence currently available it must be concluded that although there may be a relation between bacteriuria and prematurity, bacteriuria is not a prominent factor in the genesis of low birth weight or prematurity, and eradication of bacteriuria would reduce the overall rate of prematurity very little.

Even though bacteriuria plays a prominent role in the cause of acute pyelonephritis during pregnancy, the majority of women with bacteriuria remain asymptomatic throughout pregnancy. Some of these women certainly have bac-

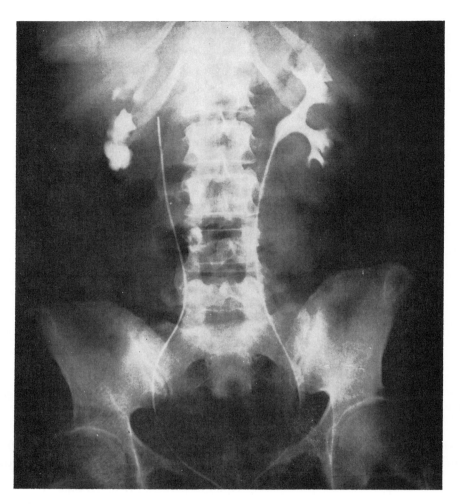

Fig. 4. Retrograde pyelogram obtained three months postpartum, showing marked destruction of the right calyceal system from long-standing asymptomatic infection. The patient, a multipara, had asymptomatic bacteriuria during pregnancy. There was no history of infection of the urinary tract. (Courtesy of Dr. P. J. Whalley.)

teriuria limited to the bladder without involvement of the kidney, but several studies clearly demonstrate that some of these women have potentially serious renal disease. Postpartum urologic investigation of patients shown to have bacteriuria during pregnancy indicates that, in many, bacteriuria persists after delivery. Moreover, in a significant number of these women there is pyelographic evidence of chronic infection, obstructive lesions, or congenital abnormalities of the urinary tract (Monzon and associates; Low and associates; Whalley and associates; Kincaid-Smith and Bullen).

At present it is difficult to identify the patients who will eventually develop serious renal disease. Accordingly, many authors now believe that it is advisable to screen routinely all obstetric patients to detect bacteriuria, and when positive cultures are obtained an attempt should then be made to eradicate the infection. Women who do not respond to treatment, who subsequently become reinfected, or who relapse should be thoroughly evaluated urologically after the puerperium.

Chronic Pyelonephritis.   In contrast to acute pyelonephritis, chronic pyelonephritis may be associated with few or no symptoms referable to the urinary tract. In advanced cases the major symptoms are those of renal insufficiency. There may or may not be a history of prior symptomatic infection of the urinary tract; in fact, in less than half of women with chronic pyelonephritis is there a history of preceding cystitis or acute pyelonephritis. The pathogenesis of this disease is therefore obscure. Two good reviews of the subject are those of Freedman and of Kleeman, Hewitt, and Guze. As in all chronic progressive renal diseases, the maternal and fetal prognosis in a particular case depends on the extent of renal destruction. Women with hypertension or renal insufficiency have a poor prognosis, whereas those with adequate renal function may go through pregnancy without complications. Regardless of the extent of renal destruction, chronic pyelonephritis complicated by pregnancy is associated with an increased risk of superimposed acute pyelonephritis, which, in turn, may lead to further deterioration of renal function; in that event, termination of pregnancy is justified.

Management of Infections of the Urinary Tract.   A variety of drugs are now available for the treatment of urinary infections. Ideally, the choice of a particular antimicrobial agent should be based upon studies of the sensitivity of the infecting microorganism. In practice, however, most bacteria causing urinary tract infections in pregnancy are sensitive to the short-acting sulfonamides, nitrofurantoin, and ampicillin. Since sensitivity is predictable, treatment can be initiated with one of these three agents and changed if necessary, when the laboratory results are available. Except for ampicillin, the broad-spectrum antibiotics used for treating urinary tract infections have certain disadvantages when used in pregnancy, as do the sulfonamides. However, these disadvantages do not preclude their use when treatment with one of them is essential.

Women with asymptomatic bacteriuria or symptoms confined to the lower urinary tract may be treated without being hospitalized, but in general it is better for pregnant women with systemic manifestations of acute pyelonephritis to be hospitalized during the initiation of treatment and until clinical improvement is observed. During the first few days of therapy, patients with acute pyelonephritis should be watched carefully to detect signs or symptoms suggesting bacterial shock. Although this serious complication is quite uncommon, its gravity demands early recognition and prompt therapy. Urinary output should therefore be recorded carefully and blood pressure measured frequently during the initial stage of therapy in all patients with acute pyelonephritis. The levels of urea nitrogen and creatinine in plasma should be ascertained early in the course of therapy. If there is no retention of nitrogen and the clinical course is satisfactory, further chemical studies of the blood are usually not required.

Antimicrobial agents used to treat infections of the urinary tract during pregnancy may, in certain circumstances, produce undesirable side effects, both maternal and fetal. Large doses of sulfonamides given to the mother late in pregnancy have been reported to cause kernicterus in the newborn infant, particularly the premature infant. These drugs cross the placenta and compete with bilirubin for binding by albumin. As a result there is an increase in unbound, unconjugated bilirubin. The sulfonamides, furthermore, may compete with bilirubin for glucuronyl transferase, which is required for conversion of free bilirubin to conjugated pigment (see Ch. 37, p. 1048). Nitrofurantoin (Furadantin) may lead to hemolytic anemia in patients whose erythrocytes are deficient in glucose-6-phosphate dehydrogenase, an inherited enzymatic deficiency that is fairly common among Negroes.

Tetracycline administered in the last trimester of pregnancy may cause discoloration of the deciduous teeth of the infant. Tetracycline, when used to treat pyelonephritis, may also produce a syndrome of azotemia, jaundice, and pancreatitis in pregnant women with impaired renal excretory function (Whalley, Adams, and Combes). Any woman who exhibits a rising plasma urea nitrogen concentration during the course of therapy must be assumed to have impaired renal function and consequently impaired excretion of the drug (Whalley and associates). Therefore, when the plasma urea nitrogen concentration is elevated, the dosage of tetracycline should be decreased or discontinued. Chloramphenicol may produce serious and even fatal blood dyscrasias, such as aplastic anemia and thrombocytopenia.

Streptomycin, kanamycin, and gentamicin may be both ototoxic and nephrotoxic. Streptomycin rapidly induces bacterial resistance. At the present writing gentamicin appears to be superior to streptomycin and kanamycin in the treatment of serious urinary infections caused by resistant organisms. The antibacterial spectrum of gentamicin is broader, and to date bacterial resistance appears less likely to develop.

The potential seriousness of urinary infections during pregnancy demands treatment with effective antimicrobial agents, but the physician must be aware of possible deleterious effects from their use. Should they occur, most often the drug should be promptly discontinued and appropriate measures instituted to combat complications.

Most urinary infections respond rapidly to adequate antimicrobial therapy. Clinical symptoms for the most part disappear during the first two days of therapy. Even though the symptoms promptly abate, therapy should be continued for at least 10 days. Cultures of urine usually become sterile within the first 24 hours if the microorganism is sensitive to the chosen drug. Since, however, the physiologic changes in the urinary tract are unaltered by treatment, a reinfection for the same reasons that caused the initial infection is always possible. If the subsequent culture of the urine is positive, additional therapy is indicated.

In long-standing chronic pyelonephritis nothing more than temporary relief is usually afforded by drugs. The major symptoms of infection can usually be controlled, but it may sometimes be necessary to terminate the pregnancy to prevent further irreversible damage to the kidneys. If after delivery evidence of the infection recurs another course or courses of therapy should be instituted.

The prognosis for patients with infections of the urinary tract in pregnancy is variable. Pyelonephritis during pregnancy must not be considered cured even though the symptoms subside completely and spontaneously, unless specific therapy has been given and the urine remains sterile on repeated examination. The untreated woman harbors infection for a variable time after delivery. Although the majority of patients who develop urinary infections during pregnancy may never have significant renal damage, at least some of these patients eventually develop serious renal disease. It is therefore imperative to treat adequately all infections of the urinary tract during pregnancy. The responsibilities of the physician are not discharged until he is certain that the urine is free from organisms after repeated cultures; absence of pyuria is not in itself adequate evidence of cure. Finally, all patients who develop an acute infection of the urinary tract prenatally should be examined by intravenous pyelography after the puerperium.

Renal Tuberculosis. Tuberculosis of the kidney is a serious, but rare, complication of pregnancy. Renal tuberculosis is believed by some to pursue a rapidly unfavorable course, particularly during the later months of pregnancy. The question of the advisability of allowing the pregnancy to continue in any case of proved renal tuberculosis is therefore raised. A decision regarding termination of pregnancy should be based upon the individual findings in each case, however.

Whether the patient who has undergone nephrectomy for tuberculosis should be allowed to become pregnant is another question. The consensus is that pregnancy should be interdicted for about two years until absence of involvement and good function of the remaining kidney have been demonstrated.

OTHER DISEASES OF THE URINARY SYSTEM

Urinary Calculi. Renal and ureteral lithiasis is an uncommon complication of pregnancy. Prather and Crabtree reported an incidence of 0.04 per cent for renal stones and 0.08 per cent for ureteral stones in 9,823 deliveries. In a more recent paper, Harris and Dunnihoo report a similar incidence for urinary calculi. The reason for this low incidence seems to be that renal lithiasis is distinctly a disease of middle age, whereas the vast majority of pregnancies occur before the age of 35. Since in many pregnant women there are some of the cardinal prerequisites for the formation of stones—namely, urinary stasis and infection—the incidence might be expected to be higher were it not for counteracting factors, one of which is undoubtedly the relatively short duration of pregnancy.

The calculi are much less likely to cause pain during pregnancy, presumably because of the reduced muscular tonus of the urinary tract; only a few cases of ureteral colic have been reported. The stones are usually discovered during roentgenography or ureteral catheterization in the study of the patient with infection of the urinary tract. Very rarely do they cause acute symptomatic obstruction. In all patients in whom urinary calculi are discovered during pregnancy the possibility of hyperparathyroidism should be considered.

Treatment depends on the symptoms and the duration of pregnancy. If the symptoms are acute, surgical removal is usually mandatory regardless of other considerations. Usually, however, a therapeutic choice is available. During the first five months of pregnancy surgical removal is frequently desirable. Operative procedures are not likely to affect adversely the gestation; more significantly, they may prevent serious damage to the urinary tract. Late in pregnancy it is sometimes wiser to continue palliation to term, if possible, reserving surgical procedure until after delivery. Therapy in each case, however, requires individualization. During the latter half of pregnancy the blood vessels to the kidney and ureter are tremendously enlarged, and proper exposure of the lower ureter without emptying the uterus is often impossible.

Acute Glomerulonephritis. Acute glomerulonephritis is characterized by the sudden appearance of hematuria, edema, and hypertension in a previously normal person. In addition, the syndrome may be complicated by hypertensive encephalopathy with convulsions, acute pulmonary edema, or acute renal failure with oliguria, azotemia, and uremia. The urine usually has a high specific gravity, and the urinary sediment contains erythrocytes and hyaline, granular, and red blood cell casts. Proteinuria is frequent. By far the most common cause of acute glomerulonephritis is infection with a nephritogenic strain of group A streptococcus.

Acute poststreptococcal glomerulonephritis rarely develops during pregnancy. In reviewing the literature, Nadler and co-workers were able to find reports of only 19 women with acute glomerulonephritis occurring between weeks 8 and 37 of pregnancy, and in only 3 of them was the diagnosis verified by biopsy.

The diagnosis of acute poststreptococcal glomerulonephritis during pregnancy is based upon the history of a streptococcal infection two weeks before the onset of the findings just described. Supporting evidence is provided by an elevated antistreptolysin titer. Acute nephritis appearing during the last trimester of pregnancy may sometimes be clinically indistinguishable from pregnancy-induced hypertension, that is, preeclampsia and eclampsia. Prolonged hematuria or persistence of hematuria after delivery suggests acute hemorrhagic nephritis.

In general the treatment of acute glomerulonephritis is the same in the pregnant as in the nonpregnant patient. Bed rest, restriction of sodium intake, drugs to lower an excessively elevated blood pressure, careful maintenance of fluid balance, and avoidance of hyperkalemia constitute sufficient therapy in most instances. In addition, an attempt should be made to eradicate the streptococcal infection with penicillin. There are insufficient data available to predict fetal or maternal prognosis. Some investigators have noted a high fetal loss from abortion, immaturity, or stillbirth; others have documented otherwise uneventful pregnancies. Since the clinical syndrome usually subsides within two weeks, a course of expectant observation is warranted. In particularly severe cases or when the disease persists longer than two weeks, interruption of the pregnancy may be advisable. In nonpregnant women the mortality rate is less than 5 per cent, death usually resulting from severe venous congestion or unrelenting renal failure. Some patients never completely recover, lapsing gradually into chronic glomerulonephritis. Patients with a history of acute hemorrhagic nephritis that has subsequently healed may undergo additional pregnancies without any appreciable increase in the incidence of complications, according to Felding's survey.

Chronic Glomerulonephritis.   Chronic glomerulonephritis is characterized by the progressive destruction of renal glomeruli, eventually producing the so-called contracted, or end-stage, kidney. In most cases the cause is unknown, although a few patients appear to develop the disease after a bout of acute glomerulonephritis that fails to heal.

The disease may present in one of four ways: (1) Some patients may remain asymptomatic for years, with persistent proteinuria or an abnormal urinary sediment, or both, as the only indications of disease; (2) the disease may first become manifest as the nephrotic syndrome; (3) the disease may present in an acute form quite similar to acute glomerulonephritis; or (4) renal failure may be the first manifestation. Regardless of the mode of onset, all patients with chronic glomerulonephritis eventually develop signs and symptoms of renal insufficiency and hypertensive cardiovascular disease.

The prognosis for the outcome of pregnancy in any given case is related to the level of renal function and the presence or absence of hypertension. Except for an increased risk of superimposed preeclampsia, those patients with relatively normal renal function and no hypertension may be carried successfully through pregnancy. Because of the likelihood of progression of the disease, however, the ultimate maternal prognosis is poor. Conversely, in patients with extreme hypertension or azotemia the outcome is poor, and therapeutic abortion often is advisable. Fetal salvage in the unfavorable group is relatively low; some are infertile and others may abort early in pregnancy (Mackay; Felding).

Because of the varying rates of renal destruction it is difficult to evaluate the influence of pregnancy on the progress of the disease. Pregnancy usually does not appear to accelerate appreciably deterioration in renal function. On the contrary, certain studies of renal function during pregnancy in patients with chronic glomerulonephritis indicate that in some cases the affected kidney shows the same pattern of response as does the normal kidney, with an increase in both glomerular filtration and renal plasma flow (Werkö and Bucht).

Nephrosis.   The nephrotic syndrome, or nephrosis, is a disorder of multiple causes, characterized by massive proteinuria (in excess of 5 g per day), hypoalbuminemia, and hypercholesteremia, usually with lipemia and edema. Diseases known to be associated with the nephrotic syndrome include chronic glomerulonephritis, lupus erythematosus, diabetes mellitus, amyloidosis, syphilis, and thrombosis of the renal vein. In addition, the syndrome may result from poisoning by heavy metals, therapy with anticonvulsant drugs, and allergies to poison ivy or bee and wasp venom.

When the nephrotic syndrome complicates pregnancy, the maternal and fetal prognosis and the treatment depend on the underlying cause of the disease and the extent of renal insufficiency. Whenever possible the specific cause should be ascertained and renal function assessed. In this regard percutaneous renal biopsy may be of value. Serial studies of renal function in two of our patients with the nephrotic syndrome associated with chronic glomerulonephritis revealed the usual augmentation of renal function that characterizes pregnancy; neither patient became hypertensive. A review of additional reported cases of nephrosis indicates that the majority of patients who are not hypertensive and do not have severe renal insufficiency may undergo a successful pregnancy, particularly since the advent of adrenocorticosteroid therapy (Marcus; Seftel and Schewitz; Studd and Blainey). In certain cases, however, in which there is evidence of renal insufficiency or moderate to severe hypertension, or both, the prognosis for mother and fetus is poorer, and interruption of the pregnancy is often indicated, particularly if renal function is deteriorating.

Polycystic Disease of the Kidney.   The decision to allow pregnancy to continue depends almost entirely on the degree of renal involvement. If the disease has not progressed to the stage of hypertension, proteinuria, and azotemia, the outlook for the pregnancy is good. With mild hypertension and normal renal function, pregnancy carries the same risk as in women with other forms of chronic hypertension. With azotemia, the chance of a successful pregnancy is slight and the risk to the mother and fetus considerable (Landesman and Scherr).

Pregnancy After Nephrectomy.   Large series of cases of women who became pregnant after unilateral nephrectomy have been reported by Matthews, by Prather and Crabtree, and by others. The predominant indications for the nephrectomies were tuberculosis in 55 per cent, pyonephrosis in 10 per cent, and calculi in 9 per cent.

Because the excretory capacity of the kidneys is much in excess of ordinary needs, and because the surviving kidney usually undergoes parenchymatous hypertrophy with increased excretory capacity, women with one normal kidney most often have no difficulty in pregnancy. If the remaining kidney is chronically infected, however, further damage may result from the stasis induced by pregnancy, with the likelihood of more intense infection. Accordingly, before advising a woman with one kidney about the risk of future pregnancy, a thorough functional evaluation of the remaining organ is essential. Should it be found impaired, further childbearing is inadvisable. Even asymptomatic women should be carefully monitored to make certain that the single kidney is functioning satisfactorily. If, however, the patient has chronic renal disease and is early in pregnancy, abortion should be promptly performed. Late in pregnancy, labor should be induced at the first sign of pregnancy-induced hypertension or infection of the urinary tract.

Acute Tubular Necrosis.   Acute tubular necrosis is the major cause of acute renal failure during pregnancy. This lesion is a result of ischemia related to either acute and severe blood loss, sudden intravascular hemolysis, severe sepsis, or a combination of these complications. The disease is therefore largely preventable by means of (1) prompt replacement of blood in instances of massive hemorrhage, as in abruptio placentae, placenta previa, rupture of the uterus, and postpartum uterine atony; (2) careful observation for early signs of bacterial shock in patients with septic abortion, amnionitis, or pyelonephritis; (3) early detection and prompt therapy of infections caused by *Clostridium perfringens* (*welchii*); and (4) meticulous care to prevent the administration of incompatible blood. The disease is not progressive; after healing takes place renal function usually returns to normal or near normal. Future pregnancies are therefore not necessarily contraindicated.

Cortical Necrosis of the Kidney.   Bilateral necrosis of the renal cortex is rare. Most of the reported cases in pregnant women have followed such complications as abruptio placentae, preeclampsia-eclampsia, or bacterial shock. The histologic lesion appears to result from thrombosis of segments of the renal vascular system. The lesions may be focal, patchy, confluent. or gross (Sheehan and Moore). Antecedent nephrosclerosis appears to increase the vulnerability of the kidney to this complication (Ober and associates). Clinically the disease follows the course of acute renal failure with oliguria or anuria, uremia, and generally death in 7 to 14 days. Differentiation from acute tubular necrosis during the early phase is possible only by renal biopsy. The prognosis depends on the extent of the necrosis, since recovery is a function of the amount of renal tissue spared; when the lesion is confluent the mortality rate approaches 100 per cent. The management of this condition is that of acute renal failure in general.

Postpartum Acute Renal Failure.   Both Wagoner and associates and Robson and associates describe what they believe to be a new syndrome of acute irreversible renal failure occurring within the first six weeks postpartum. Pregnancy and delivery appeared to have been normal in each of the seven cases; none of the known causes of renal failure was present. The pathologic changes identified by renal biopsy were glomerular necrosis, glomerular endothelial proliferation, and necrosis, thrombosis, and intimal thickening of the arterioles. No vascular abnormalities were demonstrated in the other visceral organs in the four cases in which autopsy was performed. Morphologic changes in the erythrocytes consistent with microangiopathic hemolytic anemia were present in the majority of cases. The cause of this syndrome is obscure; suggested factors in the pathogenesis included drug sensitivity (all seven patients had received an ergot preparation), consumptive coagulopathy, and a primary immunologic mechanism. Recently two puerperal women with idiopathic renal failure were referred to the Renal Unit of Parkland Memorial Hospital where deformed and fragmented red cells characteristic of microangiopathic hemolytic anemia and evidence of consumptive coagulopathy were identified, as well as severe azotemia. Therapy consisted of hemodialysis and prolonged heparinization. Initially renal function improved somewhat in both, although neither was cured.

Pregnancy After Renal Transplantation. Murray and associates in 1963 reported two successful pregnancies in a woman who had a kidney transplanted from her identical twin sister. Since that time there have been several reports of pregnancy in women who previously had received a kidney from immunologically nonidentical donors. Penn and co-workers report the largest experience. Of 10 pregnancies in 8 women, 6 resulted in live births, 2 in therapeutic abortion, and 2 were still pregnant at the time of the report. No significant changes in immunosuppression with azathioprine and prednisone were made during pregnancy except to give supplemental hydrocortisone at the time of delivery. No cesarean sections were performed. Three women developed hypertension severe enough to treat and 2 of the 3 demonstrated appreciable proteinuria. The deterioration of renal function noted in 3 women was reversed after termination of the pregnancy. Only 2 of the 5 surviving infants demonstrated an uncomplicated newborn course. One had pulmonary valvular stenosis, two demonstrated evidence of adrenocortical insufficiency plus lymphopenia, and one developed the respiratory distress syndrome. Caplan and co-workers report an instance of pregnancy after transplantation of a cadaver's kidney. Throughout much of the pregnancy the mother was plagued by several serious problems, including rejection reaction, aseptic necrosis of weight-bearing bones, lung abscesses with fungi, and severe anemia. After spontaneous labor a somewhat premature infant was delivered vaginally. The infant was relatively small for the duration of gestation but otherwise appeared normal, despite the azathioprine and prednisone. The mother did not improve and finally expired.

As pointed out by Penn and associates, there are special implications of parenthood by immunosuppressed individuals, male as well as female. Despite the formidable body of evidence in animals that azathioprine and prednisone can cause chromosomal aberrations and fetal malformation, there is enough clinical evidence to indicate that the risks of fetal malformation are not excessive.

ANEMIA AND OTHER DISEASES OF THE BLOOD

Definition of Anemia. The definition of anemia is complicated by the differences in the concentrations of hemoglobin between women and men, between women who are pregnant and those who are not, and between pregnant women who receive iron supplements and those who do not. On the basis of the observations summarized in Table 4 and for reasons that follow, it can be said that anemia exists in women if the hemoglobin is less than 12.0 g per 100 ml in the nonpregnant state, or is less than 10.0 g per 100 ml during pregnancy or the puerperium. Both early in pregnancy and near term, the hemoglobin level of healthy women, however, is usually 11.0 g per 100 ml or higher. During the

Table 4. Hemoglobin Concentration in Healthy Women with Proven Iron Stores

| | Mean | Hemoglobin (g per 100 ml) | | | Lowest |
		<12.0 (%)	<11.0 (%)	<10.0 (%)	
Nonpregnant	13.7	1	0	0	11.7
Midpregnancy	11.5	72	29	4	9.7
Late pregnancy	12.3	36	6	1	9.8

puerperium the hemoglobin concentration normally is not lower than before delivery. After delivery the hemoglobin level commonly fluctuates for a few days and then rises toward the nonpregnant level. The magnitude of the increase is to a considerable degree the resultant of the amount of hemoglobin added to the circulation during pregnancy and the amount shed during and after delivery.

Extensive hematologic measurements have been made in healthy women, none of whom were iron-deficient, since each had histochemically proven iron stores. Nor were any of them overtly deficient in metabolically active forms of folic acid, since marrow erythropoiesis was normoblastic (Scott, Pritchard, and co-workers). Pertinent observations are presented in Table 4. The hemoglobin concentration of 85 healthy iron-sufficient nonpregnant women averaged 13.7 g per 100 ml and ranged from 12.0 g to 15.0 g for ±2 standard deviations from the mean. In healthy iron-sufficient women who were 16 to 22 weeks pregnant, the mean hemoglobin was only 11.5 g per 100 ml, and in 3 of the 81 evaluated it was 9.7 or 9.8 g per 100 ml. The hemoglobin at or very near term averaged 12.3 g per 100 ml; in only 7 out of 95 was the hemoglobin less than 11.0 g per 100 ml with the lowest value 9.8 g per 100 ml.

The modest fall in hemoglobin levels observed during pregnancy in healthy women not deficient in iron or folate is caused by relatively greater expansion of the volume of plasma compared with the increase in hemoglobin mass and volume of red cells. The disproportion between the rates at which plasma and red cells are added to the maternal circulation normally is greatest during the second trimester. Later in pregnancy plasma expansion ceases while red cell production continues.

Frequency of Anemia.   Although anemia is somewhat more common among indigent patients, it is by no means restricted to them. The frequency of anemia during pregnancy varies considerably, depending primarily upon whether supplemental iron is taken during pregnancy. For example, at Parkland Memorial Hospital the hemoglobin levels at the time of delivery among women who took iron supplements averaged 12.4 g per 100 ml, whereas it was only 11.3 g per 100 ml among those who received no iron. Moreover, in none of the group receiving iron supplements was the hemoglobin less than 10.0 g per 100 ml, but it was below this level in 16 per cent of the group who received no supplements (Pritchard and Hunt).

Etiology of Anemia.   A classification based primarily on etiology and including most of the common causes of anemia in pregnant women is presented in Table 5. Although laboratory error as a cause of apparent anemia has not been included in this table, the results from clinical laboratories may sometimes be grossly inaccurate. A common source of error during pregnancy stems from the rapid sedimentation rate of erythrocytes, which is induced by the hyperfibrino-

Table 5. Causes of Anemia During Pregnancy

Acquired

    1. Iron-deficiency anemia
    2. Anemia caused by acute blood loss
    3. Anemia caused by infection
    4. Megaloblastic anemia
    5. Acquired hemolytic anemia
    6. Aplastic or hypoplastic anemia

Hereditary

    1. Thalassemia
    2. Sickle-cell anemia
    3. Sickle-cell–hemoglobin C disease
    4. Sickle-cell–thalessemia disease
    5. Homozygous hemoglobin C disease
    6. Other hemoglobinopathies
    7. Hereditary hemolytic anemia without hemoglobinopathy

genemia of pregnancy. If the specimen of blood is not thoroughly mixed immediately before pipetting the sample for the hemoglobin measurement or before filling the hemotocrit tube, the results will probably be grossly inaccurate.

The observed differences between the hemoglobin levels in pregnant and nonpregnant women, coupled with the well-recognized phenomenon of hypervolemia induced by normal pregnancy, have led to the use by some of the term *physiologic anemia*. This poor term for describing a normal process is a source of confusion and should be discarded.

A limited but practical hematologic evaluation may be rather easily and promptly carried out at the time of the patient's visit to the clinic or office. The equipment and reagents required are simple and inexpensive. A few milliliters of venous blood are anticoagulated with Versenate. A centrifuge for performing microhematocrit measurements and a hematocrit reading device are employed to detect anemia. The plasma in the hematocrit tube is examined for icterus, and the thickness of the buffy coat is noted. If icterus is observed, studies to detect hemolytic disease or hepatic dysfunction are initiated. For Negro patients a sickle-cell preparation is made using isotonic sodium metabisulfite; if positive, hemoglobin electrophoresis is usually indicated. Whenever the hematocrit approaches 30 or less, or when there is icterus, or when sickling is demonstrated, a blood smear with Wright's stain is used to evaluate the blood cells morphologically. These rather simple studies not only detect anemia but also provide important etiologic clues.

ACQUIRED ANEMIAS

The two most common causes of anemia during pregnancy and the puerperium are iron deficiency and acute blood loss. Not infrequently the two are intimately related, since excessive blood loss with its concomitant loss of hemoglobin iron in one pregnancy can be an important cause of iron-deficiency anemia in the next pregnancy.

Iron-Deficiency Anemia. As discussed in Chapter 8 (p. 252), the iron requirements of pregnancy are considerable, but the majority of women undoubtedly have small stores of iron (Scott and Pritchard; Hallberg and co-workers; DeLeeuw and associates; Pritchard and Scott). In a typical gestation with a single fetus the maternal need induced by pregnancy for iron averages close to 800 mg, of which nearly 300 mg go to the fetus and placenta whereas about 500 mg are used to expand the maternal hemoglobin mass. This amount of iron usually exceeds considerably the iron stores available for such purposes. Unless the difference between the amount of stored iron available to the mother and the iron requirements of normal pregnancy is made up by absorption of iron from the gastrointestinal tract during pregnancy, iron-deficiency anemia develops.

With the rather rapid expansion of the blood volume during the second trimester, the lack of iron often manifests itself by an appreciable drop in the maternal hemoglobin concentration. Although the rate of expansion of the blood volume is not so great in the third trimester, the need for iron remains high because augmentation of the maternal hemoglobin mass continues and even more iron is transported at this time across the placenta from mother to fetus. Since the amount of iron diverted to the fetus from an iron-deficient mother is not much less than the amount normally transferred, the newborn infant of even a severely anemic mother does not necessarily suffer from iron-deficiency anemia.

Classic morphologic evidence of iron-deficiency anemia—erythrocytic hypochromia and microcytosis—is much less likely to be as prominent in the pregnant woman as in the nonpregnant woman with the same hemoglobin concentration. Iron-deficiency anemia during pregnancy, with a hemoglobin concentration of 9 to 11 g per 100 ml, is usually not accompanied by obvious morphologic changes in the circulating erythrocytes. With this degree of anemia from iron deficiency the serum iron is lower than normal, and there is no stainable iron in the bone marrow. The serum iron-binding capacity is elevated but is in itself of little diagnostic value, since it is also elevated during normal pregnancy in the absence of iron deficiency. Moderate normoblastic hyperplasia of the bone marrow is also found to be similar to that in normal pregnancy.

The initial evaluation of a pregnant patient with moderate anemia should include measurements of hemoglobin and hematocrit, careful examination of a well-prepared smear of the peripheral blood, a sickle-cell preparation if the patient is Negro, and the measurement of the serum iron concentration. Examination of the bone marrow at this point is seldom done, although the demonstration of hemosiderin rules out iron deficiency. The diagnosis of iron deficiency in moderately anemic pregnant women is usually presumptive; it is based largely on the exclusion of other causes of anemia.

If the pregnant woman with iron-deficiency anemia of moderate degree receives adequate iron therapy, hematologic response can be detected first in a blood smear. New red blood cells, normal or slightly larger than normal in size and polychromatophilic or basophilic, soon appear in the peripheral blood. Examination of a blood smear is simpler than a reticulocyte count and is probably a more accurate index of response in the moderately anemic patient. The rate of increase of the concentration of hemoglobin or of the hematocrit varies considerably but is usually somewhat slower than in nonpregnant women. The reason is related largely to the differences in blood volumes. During the latter half of pregnancy the newly formed hemoglobin is added to the characteristically larger volume of blood. Since, furthermore, the blood volume commonly continues to expand during the period of therapy, the production of a given amount of hemoglobin by the pregnant woman may not result in a rapid increase in hemoglobin concentration. There is little evidence, however, that pregnancy itself depresses erythropoiesis to any degree.

In severe iron-deficiency anemia during pregnancy the red blood cells undergo the classic morphologic changes of hypochromia and microcytosis, and the diagnosis is usually easily made on examination of a well-prepared smear of the peripheral blood.

There has been some divergence of opinion regarding the best way to treat iron-deficiency anemia during pregnancy and the puerperium. The use of an effective parenteral iron medication guarantees that the mother receives the iron. Oral preparations are preferred, however, if the patient understands the importance of taking the medication regularly. If she will not or, much less likely, cannot take the oral doses of iron, parenteral therapy is the alternative. Whatever treatment is employed, the objectives are reasonably prompt correction of the anemia and eventual restitution of iron stores. Both of these objectives can be accomplished with adequate doses of oral iron compounds supplying a daily dose of about 200 mg of iron (Table 6). To replenish iron stores, oral therapy

Table 6. Iron Content of Commonly Used Ferrous Compounds

	Iron Content (per g)	Usual Size of Pill	No of Pills to Supply About 200 mg Iron
Ferrous sulfate	200 mg	0.3 g	3
Exsiccated ferrous sulfate (Feosol)	300 mg	0.2 g	3
Ferrous gluconate (Fergon)	110 mg	0.3 g	6
Ferrous fumarate (Ircon)	330 mg	0.2 g	3

should usually be continued for three to six months after the anemia is corrected (Pritchard and Mason). The major disadvantages of therapy with oral iron, therefore, are the possibility of failure of the woman to take the medication in adequate amounts and the danger of iron intoxication if young children should ingest large doses of the usually attractive tablets.

Whenever parenteral iron therapy is judged advisable during pregnancy, a satisfactory dose in most instances is one 5 ml ampule of iron-dextran providing 250 mg of iron for each 1.0 g per 100 ml deficit in maternal hemoglobin concentration. Accordingly, if the hemoglobin level is 8.0 g per 100 ml, the number of ampules to be injected is 13 minus 8, or 5 ampules. If the woman is unusually small, somewhat less iron-dextran is needed, and if quite large, the opposite is true. To provide sufficient iron for effective erythropoiesis, 250 mg of iron should be injected every 4 to 7 days. If after the first few injections of iron-dextran there is no evidence of hematologic response, it is important that the injections be stopped and the cause of the anemia reevaluated.

Folic acid may be given along with the iron as a safeguard against folate deficiency, although in our experience the response of pregnant women with iron-deficiency anemia treated with iron and folic acid is usually not better than when iron is given alone. There is no good evidence that the addition of cobalt, copper, molybdenum, or ascorbic acid to the iron tablet is advantageous. Ascorbic acid enhances iron absorption somewhat, so that less iron need be ingested to achieve a comparable level of absorption. The adverse effects of oral iron, however, relate primarily to the amount of iron absorbed rather than to the amount ingested (Hallberg and associates). Most often, iron preparations that contain significant amounts of iron but are completely free of adverse effects are very poorly absorbed and consequently ineffective.

Iron-dextran administered intravenously has been evaluated extensively, especially in other countries. Although the frequency and intensity of adverse systemic reactions appear to be not greater than when iron-dextran is given intramuscularly, the United States Food and Drug Administration has not yet approved iron-dextran for intravenous use.

Transfusions of whole blood or packed red cells are seldom indicated for the treatment of iron-deficiency anemia unless hypovolemia from blood loss coexists or an operative procedure must be performed on a severely anemic woman. Whereas hypovolemia is commonly a prominent feature of anemia caused by acute blood loss, very severe anemia from failure of production of red cells or their accelerated destruction may lead to some degree of cardiac insufficiency and pathologic hypervolemia. With acute blood loss and hypovolemia it is essential to restore an adequate blood volume as well as to provide hemoglobin for oxygen transport; therefore, transfusions of whole blood are usually indicated. In case of severe anemia with compromised cardiac function and pathologic hypervolemia, however, the administration of whole blood can lead to severe circulatory overloading, pulmonary edema, and death.

Exchange transfusion is an effective way to raise the hemoglobin concentration of severely anemic women without inducing or intensifying circulatory overloading (Fullerton and Turner). A measured small volume of venous blood is withdrawn and immediately an equal volume of packed red cells is injected; this sequence is repeated until the hemoglobin concentration is raised to a level adequate for supplying the oxygen needs of the mother and fetus. The use of a potent diuretic such as ethacrynic acid or preferably furosemide (Lasix) before transfusing packed red cells may be of value in reducing plasma volume and thereby allowing the intravascular compartment to accommodate the added red blood cells without causing circulatory overloading (Harrison).

Anemia Resulting from Acute Loss of Blood.   Anemia resulting from recent hemorrhage is more likely to be evident during the puerperium. Both abruptio placentae and placenta previa may be sources of serious blood loss and anemia. Earlier in pregnancy, anemia caused by acute loss of blood commonly results from abortion, tubal pregnancy with rupture or abortion, and hydatidiform mole.

Acute hemorrhage may have no immediate effect on the hemoglobin concentration even though the hemorrhage leads to hypovolemia so severe as to cause overt collapse. Severe hemorrhage demands immediate blood replacement in amounts that restore and maintain adequate perfusion of vital organs. Even though the amount of blood replaced commonly does not completely make up the deficit of hemoglobin created by the hemorrhage, in general, once dangerous hypovolemia has been overcome and hemostasis has been achieved, the residual anemia should be treated with iron. Certainly the moderately anemic woman who no longer faces the likelihood of further gross hemorrhage, who can ambulate, and who is not seriously febrile is better treated with iron than with more blood transfusions.

Anemia Associated with Inflammation.   A large variety of subacute and chronic infections may produce moderate and sometimes severe anemia, usually with normocytic or very slightly microcytic erythrocytes. The bone marrow is not markedly altered, but there may be hyperplasia of the leukocytic series that might be misinterpreted as a relative reduction in precursors of the red cells or slight erythrocytic hypoplasia. The serum iron concentration is decreased, and the serum iron-binding capacity, although lower than in normal pregnancy, is not necessarily much below the normal nonpregnant range. The anemia appears to result, at least in part, from alterations in reticuloendothelial function and iron metabolism (Freireich and associates). Iron released from the patient's senescent red blood cells is retained rather than returned to the plasma to be reutilized by the bone marrow for production of hemoglobin. The fate of iron administered in therapeutic doses is similar. The life-span of the erythrocyte, furthermore, is usually slightly shortened (Wintrobe). The anemia, therefore, results from decreased erythropoiesis coupled with slightly increased destruction.

Chronic renal disease, suppuration, granulomatous infections, malignancies, and rheumatoid arthritis may also cause anemia, presumably by these same mechanisms. At least some cases of so-called *refractory anemia of pregnancy* probably are the consequence of one of these diseases that has gone unrecognized. The anemia of infection, chronic renal disease, and malignancy is refractory in the sense that it is not corrected by treatment with iron, folic acid, vitamin B_{12}, or any other known hematinic agent. Nonetheless, prophylaxis with iron and folic acid usually is desirable to offset any deficiency induced by pregnancy.

Megaloblastic Anemia.   The prevalence of megaloblastic anemia during pregnancy varies considerably through the world. In the United States overt anemia with frankly megaloblastic erythropoiesis demonstrable in the bone marrow is an uncommon complication of pregnancy, but in other parts of the world it is much more frequent. In this country megaloblastic anemia beginning during pregnancy almost always results from folic acid deficiency. It is usually found in pregnant women who consume neither fresh vegetables, especially of the uncooked green leafy variety, nor foods with a high content of animal protein. Not infrequently patients with megaloblastic anemia develop troublesome nausea, vomiting, and anorexia during pregnancy. As the anemia increases, the anorexia often becomes more intense, thus aggravating the dietary deficiency.

Deficiency of metabolically active forms of folic acid induces many biochemical and hematologic changes. Some of these changes are listed in Table 7

Table 7. **The Sequence of Changes Induced by Dietary Deprivation of Folic Acid in a Normal Adult**

	Weeks After Starting Folate-Poor Diet
1. Low concentration of serum folate	3
2. Hypersegmentation of neutrophils	7
3. Increased urinary formiminoglutamic acid	14
4. Low folate in erythrocytes	16
5. Erythrocytic macrocytosis	18
6. Megaloblastic marrow	19
7. Anemia	19

Data from Herbert.

in the order that they have been observed to develop in experimentally induced folate deficiency in man. The sequence of changes resulting from folate deficiency, as recorded by Herbert, is probably unaltered by pregnancy. In the peripheral blood the earliest morphologic evidence of deficiency usually is hypersegmentation of some of the neutrophilic leukocytes. Five or more distinct lobes in some of the neutrophils during pregnancy suggest folic acid deficiency. As anemia develops, the newly formed erythrocytes are produced in reduced numbers and are macrocytic, even if there has been previous iron deficiency with microcytosis. With preexisting iron deficiency the more recently formed macrocytic erythrocytes would not be detected from the measurement of the mean corpuscular volume of the erythrocytes. Careful examination of a well-prepared smear of the peripheral blood, however, usually will reveal some macrocytes. As the anemia becomes more intense, an occasional nucleated erythrocyte appears in the peripheral blood. If smears of the buffy coat from peripheral blood are made in order to concentrate the nucleated red blood cells, several such cells with the distinct features of megaloblasts are usually demonstrable (Goodall; Pritchard). At the same time, examination of the bone marrow reveals megaloblastic erythropoiesis. As the maternal folate deficiency and, in turn, the anemia become severe, thrombocytopenia, leukopenia, or both may develop.

Herbert estimates that in the normal nonpregnant woman the daily folate requirements expressed as folic acid are in the range of 50 to 100 mcg per day. During pregnancy, however, the requirements for metabolically active forms of folic acid are considerably increased. The fetus and placenta extract folate from the maternal circulation so effectively that the fetus is not anemic even when the mother is severely anemic from folate deficiency. Cases have been recorded in which the newborn hemoglobin levels were 18.0 g or more per 100 ml, while the maternal values were as low as 3.6 g per 100 ml (Pritchard and co-workers).

The treatment of megaloblastic anemia induced by pregnancy should include folic acid, a well-balanced diet, and usually iron. As little as 1 mg of folic acid administered orally once a day produces a striking hematologic response. Within three to six days after the beginning of treatment the reticulocyte count is appreciably increased, and leukopenia and thrombocytopenia are promptly corrected. Sometimes the rate of increase in hemoglobin concentration or hematocrit is disappointing, especially when compared with the usual exuberant reticulocytosis that starts soon after therapy is begun. Severe megaloblastic anemia during pregnancy is accompanied frequently by a smaller blood volume than that of a normal pregnancy, but soon after folic acid therapy is started the blood volume usually increases considerably. Therefore, even though hemoglobin is being rapidly added to the circulation, the hemoglobin concentration does not precisely reflect the total amount of additional hemoglobin because of the simultaneous expansion of the blood volume (Lowenstein, Pick, and Philpott; Pritchard).

Women who develop megaloblastic anemia during pregnancy commonly are also deficient in iron, although the lack of effective erythropoiesis resulting from the folate deficiency usually produces a considerable elevation of the plasma iron. With the onset of effective erythropoiesis, however, the concentration of iron in the plasma falls precipitously. Iron may then become the limiting factor in production of hemoglobin.

Megaloblastic anemia not infrequently recurs in subsequent pregnancies, very likely because of repeated dietary inadequacies but also perhaps in part because of a peculiarity in the absorption or utilization of folic acid.

During the past decade a great deal of attention has been devoted to the frequency of maternal folate deficiency and megaloblastic anemia in pregnancy and the puerperium, the possible role of folate deficiency in various forms of reproductive failure, and the value of prophylactic administration of folic acid throughout pregnancy and perhaps the puerperium as well. The frequency with which maternal folate deficiency is detected will vary considerably, depending in large measure upon the intensity of the search and the criteria for diagnosis.

Markedly divergent views have been expressed concerning the value of the measurement of urinary formiminoglutamic acid (FIGLU) excretion after an oral load of histidine in the detection of folate deficiency during pregnancy. Hibbard and Hibbard, for instance, state that the FIGLU test provides a reliable index of defective folic acid metabolism. They report an excellent correlation between elevated FIGLU excretion and morphologic evidence of megaloblastic erythropoiesis in the marrow. Chanarin and associates, however, as well as Chisholm and Sharp, have found that in any individual case, at least, the estimation of FIGLU excretion during pregnancy is of little value in ascertaining the cause of anemia and is not a substitute for biopsy of the bone marrow. Although these several British workers do not agree about the validity of the FIGLU test as a specific measure of maternal folate deficiency, they all believe that in Great Britain some degree of folic acid deficiency is common among pregnant women.

Hibbard, Hibbard, and co-workers maintain that faulty folate metabolism is an important cause of placental abruption, abortion, and fetal malformation. They conclude that the dangers of folate deficiency to mother and fetus are so great that early prophylaxis, even before conception, is advisable in any woman at increased risk unless facilities for regular assessment of folate status are available. These investigators, and some others, claim a high frequency of folate deficiency in women who suffer any of several forms of pregnancy wastage and propose a causal relation. Other investigators find maternal folate deficiency to be no more common among women who experience some form of reproductive failure than in the general obstetric population. For example, in Dallas we find little difference in maternal plasma folate levels, neutrophil hypersegmentation, and pattern of marrow erythropoiesis in mothers with placental abruption, fetal malformation, or pregnancy-induced hypertension when compared with women whose pregnancies are not thus complicated (Whalley, Scott, and Pritchard). Moreover, to try to ascertain the effects of severe maternal folate deficiency on the products of conception, we have investigated the fate of 88 infants of women with folate deficiency so severe as to cause overt megaloblastic anemia. Perinatal mortality, fetal malformation, birth weight, and neonatal hemoglobin concentration were very similar to those of the general obstetric population cared for at the same institution. Consequently it appears very unlikely that intensive public health measures focused on providing folic acid supplementation to eradicate all suspicions of maternal folate deficiency would have a marked effect on reducing these various kinds of pregnancy wastage.

The actual folic acid requirements of pregnancy are not known, although 400 mcg per day of folic acid orally sometimes produces a hematologic remission in the severely anemic pregnant woman who is consuming a diet poor in folate, and 1,000 mcg per day is quite effective (Pritchard and co-workers). The studies of Hansen and Rybo in Sweden and of Chanarin and associates in England suggest that 100 mcg of folic acid daily probably is adequate for populations in which megaloblastic anemia is rarely found. If, however, the pregnant women are members of a population in which megaloblastic anemia develops rather commonly during pregnancy, this level of supplementation seems inadequate, according to the studies of Willoughby and Jewell.

Whether to administer folic acid routinely to all pregnant women still seems debatable. If, however, prenatal vitamin supplements are prescribed, folic acid should be included, since there is more evidence that the pregnant woman might suffer from a deficiency of that vitamin than of the several others that are almost always included.

Megaloblastic anemia caused by lack of vitamin B_{12} during pregnancy is quite rare. *Addisonian pernicious anemia,* in which there is failure to absorb vitamin B_{12} because of lack of intrinsic factor, is extremely uncommon in women of reproductive age; moreover, unless women with this disease are treated with vitamin B_{12}, infertility may be a complication (Ball and Giles). There is little reason for withholding folic acid during pregnancy simply out of fear of jeopardizing the neurologic integrity of women who might be pregnant and simultaneously have unrecognized, and therefore untreated, Addisonian pernicious anemia.

Acquired Hemolytic Anemia.   Women with an acquired hemolytic anemia and a positive direct Coombs test sometimes demonstrate marked acceleration of the rate of hemolysis during pregnancy. Prednisone and similar compounds seem to be nearly as effective as in the nonpregnant state. Associated thrombocytopenia may also be favorably affected by such steroid therapy. Pregnancy is not a contraindication to the use of the drugs, but since the underlying disease is usually chronic and progressive, repeated pregnancies are not advisable in women with acquired hemolytic anemia caused by autoimmune disease.

Drug-induced hemolytic anemia is occasionally encountered during pregnancy. Infrequently the hemolysis results from an antibody that, in the presence of a drug such as quinine, may cause lysis of red blood cells. Especially in Negro women the hemolysis may much more often be related to an inherited specific enzymatic defect of the erythrocytes, the deficiency of glucose-6-phosphate dehydrogenase (G-6-PD). The red blood cells of about 2 per cent of Negro women are markedly deficient in this enzyme. In such instances both X chromosomes are genetically deficient. The heterozygous state, with one deficient and one normal X chromosome, occurs in 10 to 15 per cent of Negro women and results in a moderate deficiency of the enzyme. Several oxidant drugs can induce hemolysis in susceptible women. Among the more common agents are antimalarials such as primaquine and quinine, several sulfonamides, nitrofurans including nitrofurantoin (Furadantin), analgesics, and antipyretics including phenacetin and aspirin. Infection or acidosis intensifies drug-induced hemolysis (Kellermeyer and co-workers).

Since young red blood cells contain more G-6-PD than do older erythrocytes, the anemia ultimately becomes stabilized. In the absence of depression of the bone marrow the anemia is rather promptly corrected after the drug is discontinued.

Intravascular hemolysis infrequently complicates eclampsia; the precise cause of the hemolysis is unknown. Baker and Brain suggest that the process of microangiopathic hemolytic anemia may be responsible for the hemolysis. The most fulminant acquired hemolytic anemia encountered during pregnancy is caused by the exotoxin of *Clostridium perfringens,* and this condition is often fatal.

Aplastic or Hypoplastic Anemia.   Although rarely encountered during pregnancy, aplastic anemia is a grave complication. The diagnosis is readily made when anemia, usually with thrombocytopenia and leukopenia, and markedly hypocellular bone marrow are demonstrated. None of the erythropoietic agents that produce remission of the other anemias is effective. Corticosteroids such as prednisone may be of some value, and large doses of testosterone or other androgenic steroids are occasionally effective in treating aplastic anemia, especially in children. The effects of large doses of testosterone or other potent androgens during pregnancy are unknown, but a female fetus would most likely develop the stigmata of androgen excess.

The two greatest risks to the woman with aplastic anemia during pregnancy are hemorrhage caused by thrombocytopenia and infection. Blood transfusion will combat, but not cure, aplastic anemia. A continuous search for infection should be made, and when it is found, specific antibiotic therapy should be started promptly.

When hypoplastic anemia antedates the pregnancy, marked improvement is unlikely after interrupting the pregnancy (Rovinsky). When the disease develops during pregnancy, termination of the pregnancy may sometimes result in remission (Danforth and co-workers; Fleming).

Delivery should be accomplished vaginally, if possible. If there are no large lacerations or incisions of the birth canal, and if the uterus is kept firmly contracted after delivery, intense thrombocytopenia or other defects of coagulation are not likely to cause fatal hemorrhage.

Whether pregnancy itself impairs erythropoiesis except through the induction of iron or folate deficiency is not clear. Certainly a few cases have been described of recurrent severe aplastic anemia during pregnancy with essentially a normal blood picture between pregnancies. Holly has described pregnant women with moderate to severe normochromic normocytic anemia and a reduction in the ratio of erythroid to myeloid precursors in the bone marrow. None of the hematinic agents tried was effective. He concluded that pregnancy caused bone marrow depression, which was relieved when the pregnancy was terminated. Further investigations are needed in which newer technics are used to measure quantitatively erythrocyte production and destruction.

HEREDITARY ANEMIAS

Hereditary anemias are much less common than the acquired forms. Nonetheless, certain of the hereditary anemias, especially the hemoglobinopathies, rather often lead to serious complications in both the mother and the fetus.

Thalassemia. Hypochromic microcytic anemia in obstetric patients is not always caused by iron deficiency. A slight to moderate reduction in hemoglobin concentration with hypochromia and microcytosis in families of Mediterranean stock has long been recognized as a distinct entity, usually designated thalassemia minor (Wintrobe). An inherited anemia with these features is occasionally found during pregnancy not only in white women without known Mediterranean ancestors but in Negro women as well.

The most prevalent and characteristic form of thalassemia is *beta thalassemia minor*, in which the synthesis of the beta chains of globin is impaired and the A_2 hemoglobin fraction is elevated to a range of about 4 per cent or more, as compared with a value of 3 per cent or less in the normal population. Pregnancy itself does not alter the percentage of A_2 hemoglobin. The hematologic abnormalities of thalassemia minor result from the combination of an abnormal autosomal gene from one parent and a normal allelic gene from the other. In the affected children neither the morphologically abnormal erythrocyte nor the elevated level of A_2 hemoglobin appears immediately after birth. *Beta thalassemia major*, or *Cooley's anemia*, a very severe anemia that is nearly always fatal during childhood, results from the homozygous condition. Rarely do these women live long enough to become pregnant.

Beta thalassemia minor has been detected in 10 per cent or more of the population in some areas of Italy (Wintrobe). Its frequency in the United States in white women without known Mediterranean ancestors and in Negro women is much lower. The anemia of thalassemia minor is probably caused by impaired erythropoiesis coupled with slightly accelerated destruction of some red blood cells. The hemoglobin concentration is typically 8 to 10 g per 100 ml late in the second trimester, with an increase to between 9 and 11 g per 100 ml near term, as compared with a hemoglobin level of 10 to 12 g per 100 ml in the nonpregnant state (Pritchard; Freedman). There is a significant augmentation of erythropoiesis in these patients during pregnancy, as in normal women.

There is no specific therapy for beta thalassemia minor during pregnancy. In general, the outcome of these patients and of the pregnancy is satisfactory. Blood transfusions are very seldom indicated except for hemorrhage. Iron and folic acid in prophylactic daily doses of about 30 mg and 1 mg, respectively, may be of value. Any disease that depresses the function of the bone marrow or increases destruction of erythrocytes naturally intensifies the anemia. Infections, therefore, should be promptly and adequately treated.

Alpha thalassemia, an abnormality characterized by impaired synthesis of the alpha chains of globin, is rare in this country but relatively common in southeast Asia. The homozygous state in the fetus is characterized by very high levels of hemoglobin Bart's and uniformly fatal erythroblastosis fetalis. Presumably both parents have the heterozygous form of alpha thalassemia, which typically causes only very slight hematologic changes (Lehmann and Huntsman).

Sickle-Cell Anemia.   The inheritance of the gene for the production of sickle, or S, hemoglobin from each parent results in sickle-cell anemia. In most communities approximately 1 out of every 12 Negroes has the sickle-cell trait, which results from inheritance of one gene for the production of S hemoglobin and one for normal hemoglobin A. The theoretical incidence of sickle-cell anemia among Negroes is one out of every 576 ($\frac{1}{12} \times \frac{1}{12} \times \frac{1}{4} = 1/576$), but the disease is not nearly so common in pregnant black women, perhaps only one fourth to one third of the theoretically calculated frequency. Undoubtedly there are many deaths from this disease during childhood or early adulthood, and the fertility of women with sickle-cell anemia is reduced.

Although usually made earlier, the diagnosis of sickle-cell anemia is occasionally first made during pregnancy. Pregnancy is a serious burden to the woman with the disease, for the anemia usually becomes more intense, the attacks of pain, or the so-called pain crises, usually become more frequent, and infections and pulmonary disease are more common. Fetal wastage is usually rather high. One half to one third of all known pregnancies in women with sickle-cell anemia terminate in abortion, stillbirth, or neonatal death (Curtis; Ricks; McCurdy; Pritchard).

In our experience, adequate care of patients with sickle-cell disease in pregnancy involves close observation with careful evaluation of all symptoms, physical findings, and laboratory studies. One rather common danger is that these patients may categorically be considered to be suffering from "sickle-cell crisis." As a result, ectopic pregnancy, placental abruption, pyelonephritis, and other serious obstetric problems that cause pain or anemia or both may be overlooked. The term "sickle-cell crisis," if used at all, is to be applied only after all other possible causes of pain or reduction in hemoglobin concentration have been excluded.

The value of blood transfusions in sickle-cell anemia is difficult to ascertain. The hazards of blood transfusions contraindicate their routine use in these patients. In our experience, in the absence of infection or nutritional deficiency, the hemoglobin concentration does not fall much below 7 g per 100 ml, a level at or above which pregnant women with sickle-cell anemia usually have no symptoms from the low level of hemoglobin. Since these women maintain their hemoglobin concentration by great augmentation of erythropoiesis to compensate for the markedly shortened life-span of the erythrocytes, any factor that impairs erythropoiesis or increases destruction of red cells results in aggravation of the anemia. The folic acid requirements during pregnancy complicated by sickle-cell anemia are considerable. Since the dietary intake of folic acid may be inadequate, especially during episodes of pain, supplementary folic acid is usually indicated.

Labor in the patient with sickle-cell disease should be managed essentially in the same way as for the patient with cardiac disease. The patient should be kept comfortable but not oversedated. In all cases compatible whole blood should be readily available. If a difficult vaginal delivery or cesarean section is contemplated, the hemoglobin concentration should be raised by giving carefully either packed red blood cells before delivery or whole blood during delivery. Continuous oxygen therapy, furthermore, should be instituted during times of increased oxygen need.

According to Hendrickse and Watson-Williams, acute sequestration of sickled red cells is common late in pregnancy, during labor and delivery, and in the early puerperium. Dangerous anemia rapidly appears and is accompanied by an increase in the size of the liver and of the spleen, unless the spleen has been previously destroyed by fibrosis. The acute sequestration is usually accompanied by intense bone pain and can be anticipated by frequently monitoring the hemoglobin concentration at the time of risk. Whenever the hemoglobin drops below 6.0 g per 100 ml or decreases at a rate of 2 g or more per 24 hours, Hendrickse and Watson-Williams recommend exchange transfusion with donor blood known to contain only hemoglobin A. The advantages derived from reducing the population of red cells containing S hemoglobin through exchange transfusion, however, must be weighed against the dangers, which include homologous serum hepatitis and other infections transmitted by donor blood, pathologic hemosiderosis, circulatory overloading, and maternal isoimmunization. Transfusion-induced isoimmunization may lead to erythroblastosis fetalis as well as intense donor blood incompatibility in the mother. We have encountered adult women with sickle-cell anemia who, because of previous transfusions, have reacted adversely to practically all available blood.

For some time we have administered transfusions of whole blood or of packed normal red cells only to replace excessive blood loss or to augment circulating red cell volume when anemia is very severe—that is, with a hemoglobin concentration of less than 7.0 g per 100 ml. Before delivery, however, at least a liter of appropriately crossmatched blood is available, and a well-anchored intravenous infusion system is established. Excessive blood loss is promptly replaced with normal whole blood. We have managed in this manner a considerable number of pregnancies complicated by sickle-cell anemia with no maternal deaths.

Hendrickse and Watson-Williams advocate heparin therapy in patients with sickle-cell anemia who develop severe bone pain during late pregnancy or the puerperium. The benefits derived from heparin administration, however, have not been firmly established. Dextran infusion was originally claimed to reduce bone pain and marrow infarction, but a well-controlled study subsequently failed to demonstrate any benefit (Barnes and co-workers).

Because of the chronic debility from sickle-cell anemia, the further complications caused by pregnancy, and the predictably shortened life-span of these patients, sterilization, or at least a very effective means of contraception, is indicated, even in women of low parity. Oral contraceptives in the form of estrogen-progestin combinations probably are contraindicated in women with sickle-cell anemia since red cell sequestration and vascular occlusion inherent in the disease might be intensified.

Sickle-Cell–Hemoglobin C Disease.   Although about 1 out of 12 American Negroes possesses the gene for production of hemoglobin S, only about 1 in 50 carries the gene for hemoglobin C. Therefore, the probability of this genetic combination in a Negro couple is about 1 in 600, and the probability of their child's inheriting the gene for hemoglobin S and an allelic gene for hemoglobin C is 1 in 4. As the consequence of these genetic frequencies, about 1 out of every 2,400 ($\frac{1}{12} \times \frac{1}{50} \times \frac{1}{4}$) pregnant black women can be expected to have sickle-cell–hemoglobin C disease, barring any significant mortality either before or during the years of reproductivity. We have found the disease to occur at this level of frequency among pregnant Negro women.

In nonpregnant women the morbidity and mortality from the sickle-cell–hemoglobin C disease are appreciably lower than those of sickle-cell anemia. During pregnancy and the puerperium, however, the morbidity and mortality are increased (Curtis; Fullerton and co-workers; Pritchard). Attacks of severe bone pain and episodes of "pneumonitis" are fairly common during these times. The "pneumonitis" appears to be related to embolization of necrotic bone marrow. In a fifteen-year anterospective study at Parkland Memorial Hospital, the maternal mortality for a large series of pregnancies in women with sickle-cell–hemoglobin C disease was close to 2 per cent, and one out of 6 pregnancies resulted in abortion, stillbirth, or neonatal death. The pregnancy wastage was greater than in the general population but was not so great as with sickle-cell anemia. These values for abortion and for perinatal loss are similar to those reported by McCurdy and by Anderson.

As in other pregnancies complicated by overt hemolytic anemia, the need for metabolically active forms of folic acid in women with sickle-cell–hemoglobin C disease is increased, especially when anorexia is present. Iron deficiency is less common than in the general population of pregnant women, but it occasionally occurs, especially if the mother has not received transfusions previously. Therefore supplementation with folic acid and in some instances with iron is of value. Whenever the hemoglobin concentration drops below 8.0 g per 100 ml, a thorough search for the cause or causes is essential. The guidelines for blood transfusion are similar to those in sickle-cell anemia.

Fullerton and co-workers in Africa urge that pregnant women with sickle-cell–hemoglobin C disease receive iron and folic acid routinely, exchange transfusions with blood containing only hemoglobin A whenever a sudden decrease in hemoglobin concentration develops, and heparinization for severe bone pain to try to prevent embolization of necrotic marrow. They estimate the "natural" maternal mortality rate for pregnancy complicated by sickle-cell–hemoglobin C disease in Africa to be 10 per cent. They believe that the application of these several measures combined with good general medical care, including antimalarial therapy, has been responsible for reducing their maternal mortality to 2.4 per cent.

The frequent morbidity and relatively high mortality during pregnancy and the puerperium in women with sickle-cell–hemoglobin C disease warrant limitation of family size.

Sickle-Cell–Thalassemia Disease.   The inheritance of the gene for hemoglobin S from one parent and the allelic gene for beta thalassemia from the other results in sickle-cell–beta-thalassemia disease. Our experience indicates that the maternal and perinatal mortality and morbidity of this disease are similar to those of sickle-cell–hemoglobin C disease. The recommendations for prenatal care, labor and delivery, and the restriction of future pregnancies are the same in sickle-cell–thalassemia, sickle-cell–hemoglobin C disease, and sickle-cell anemia.

Hemoglobin C and C-Thalassemia Diseases.   Pregnancy and homozygous hemoglobin C disease or hemoglobin C–thalassemia disease appear to be rather benign associations (Smith and Krevans; Pritchard). The anemia is usually mild but, if severe, may be related to folic acid deficiency or some other superimposed cause. Supplementation with folic acid and sometimes with iron is of value in pregnant women with any hemoglobinopathy.

Sickle-Cell and Hemoglobin C Traits.   The inheritance of the gene for the production of S (sickle) hemoglobin from one parent and for normal or A (normal adult) hemoglobin from the other results in sickle-cell trait. In this circumstance the amount of S hemoglobin produced is less than the amount of A hemoglobin and, on the average, makes up only about one third of the total hemoglobin. The prevalence of sickle-cell trait in Negroes varies throughout the country, averaging about 8 per cent. Hemoglobin C trait is found in approximately 2 per cent of the Negro population.

Erythrocytes in smears of blood from patients with sickle-cell trait usually appear normal unless the blood has previously been markedly depleted of oxygen to produce sickled forms. Target cells are prominent in blood from women with hemoglobin C trait.

A rather extensive study with matched controls of the effect of sickle-cell trait on pregnancy has been reported by Whalley and co-workers. Sickle-cell trait did not influence the frequency of abortion, perinatal mortality, prematurity, or preeclampsia-eclampsia. Infection of the urinary tract, however, was about twice as common in the group with sickle-cell trait. Further investigations revealed that almost 14 per cent of pregnant women with sickle-cell trait had asymptomatic bacteriuria, as compared with 6.4 per cent in pregnant black women whose red blood cells did not sickle. One third of the group with sickle trait and bacteriuria developed clinically evident pyelonephritis later in the antepartum period.

Blank and Freedman state that iron-deficiency anemia in women with sickle trait may be refractory to the usual methods of treatment, but our experience has been different. Moreover, in a survey carried out at Parkland Memorial Hospital, hemoglobin levels were as high during pregnancy in women with sickle trait as in Negro women whose red cells did not sickle.

Other Hereditary Hemolytic Anemias.   Hemolytic anemia resulting from the combination of the genes for S and D hemoglobins is a rare disease. In the one case that we have followed throughout two pregnancies, bone pain developed, the hemolysis became more intense, the anemia became worse, and overt megaloblastic erythropoiesis occurred.

Congenital hemolytic anemia with or without spherocytosis is rarely encountered during pregnancy. If erythropoiesis is not impaired, these women have no major difficulty during pregnancy. In the case of congenital spherocytic anemia, splenectomy before pregnancy results in considerable reduction in the intensity of the hemolysis and, in turn, the anemia. The newborn may have congenital spherocytosis and soon become anemic.

Genetic Counseling.   Identification of the more common hemoglobinopathies and their trait forms involves relatively simple laboratory procedures, and the genetic aspects of these diseases are straightforward. Therefore, genetic counseling can be readily provided. One out of every 4 children, on the average, will be afflicted with the disease whenever both parents have a trait form, as pointed out in the discussion of sickle-cell anemia and sickle-cell–hemoglobin C disease. If one parent has the hemoglobinopathy and the other only the trait form, one half of their children can be expected to inherit the hemoglobinopathy and the other half the trait form. If both parents have a hemoglobinopathy, so will all of their children.

OTHER HEMATOLOGIC DISORDERS

Polycythemia.   Polycythemia during pregnancy is usually related to hypoxia, most often resulting from congenital cardiac disease or a pulmonary disorder. If the polycythemia is severe, the probability of a successful outcome of the pregnancy is remote.

Polycythemia vera and pregnancy rarely coexist. Ruch and Klein have described a case in which the hematocrit in the nonpregnant state was as high as 63. During each of two pregnancies, however, the hematocrit ranged from a low of about 35 during the second trimester to about 44 at term. Fetal loss seems to be high in women with polycythemia vera.

Thrombocytopenic Purpura.   Thrombocytopenic purpura may be idiopathic or, more often, associated with aplastic anemia, acquired hemolytic anemia, eclampsia or severe preeclampsia, acquired hypofibrinogenemia related to placental abruption or similar hypofibrinogenemic states, lupus erythematosus, megaloblastic anemia caused by severe folate deficiency, drugs, infections, allergies, or radiation.

Idiopathic thrombocytopenic purpura is a rare complication of pregnancy. Peterson and Larson report a maternal mortality rate of 2 per cent and a perinatal mortality rate of 15 per cent. Investigations by Harrington and associates and by Stefanini, Chatterjea, and Adelson point toward a platelet autoagglutinin or isoagglutinin that causes idiopathic thrombocytopenia, but not all investigators find such an antibody in the majority of the cases of idiopathic thrombocytopenic purpura. Most often the transfer of an abnormal platelet agglutinin to the fetus is the cause of the so-called congenital thrombocytopenia in the newborn. Such passively acquired thrombocytopenia in the newborn is seldom a grave problem, but circumcision should be delayed until the platelet count is normal. Rarely has it been necessary to give the child a transfusion of blood or platelets.

A pregnant woman with idiopathic thrombocytopenic purpura should be under careful medical supervision. Prednisone and similar corticosteroids have produced somewhat inconsistent results; they are apparently of greatest value in correcting the abnormal capillary fragility, but their effect on the platelet count varies. During a period of uncontrollable bleeding, or when major surgery is to be performed, transient improvement in platelet function may sometimes be achieved by transfusing platelets carefully collected from compatible very fresh blood. Blood from donors with polycythemia vera or thrombocytosis yields the greatest number of platelets.

For women with thrombocytopenia, vaginal delivery without lacerations or large episiotomies is most desirable. Deep anesthesia should be avoided, and for several hours after delivery the myometrium should be kept firmly contracted. Cesarean section is likely to lead to serious hemorrhage.

Leukemia.   Of 100 cases of leukemia in pregnancy collected from the literature by Erf, the following distribution was noted: acute myeloid, 24; chronic myeloid, 63; acute lymphatic, 10; chronic lymphatic, 3. Erf observed that the survival of these 100 patients was the same as in nonpregnant leukemic patients. These data suggest that pregnancy exerts no effect on the course of leukemia. Shub, Black, and Speer, however, believe that pregnancy may transform chronic leukemia into the acute form; several observers, furthermore, have noted a tendency toward exacerbations in the puerperium. The most common effect of leukemia on pregnancy is premature labor, and in general the perinatal mortality is high. There is not a very effective treatment for this rapidly fatal disease; however, vincristine, 6-mercaptopurine, methotrexate, and prednisone have been administered during the second and third trimesters without any apparent bad effects in the fetus (Coopland and associates).

As pointed out by Harris, no case of transmission of leukemia to the fetus has been authenticated, but several cases of congenital leukemia in infants born of nonleukemic mothers have been recorded.

Hodgkin's Disease.   In the extensive study by Kasdon, no evidence was presented that pregnancy exerts any deleterious effect on Hodgkin's disease, nor is the incidence of obstetric complications increased by coincidental Hodgkin's disease. In about 10 per cent of the reported cases, however, the disease appears to be transmitted from the mother to the fetus across the placenta. If roentgen therapy is employed, adequate shielding of the fetus should be attempted.

DISEASES OF THE HEART

Heart disease is estimated to occur in approximately 1 per cent of pregnancies. Rheumatic heart disease formerly accounted for the great majority of the cases (Burwell and Metcalfe), but in recent years congenital heart disease has become relatively more prevalent. Prophylaxis with antimicrobial agents has reduced the cardiac complications of rheumatic fever, and better medical management, together with a number of newer surgical technics, has enabled more girls with congenital heart disease to live into the childbearing age. Cardiac disease from hypertension contributes only a few per cent of all cases of organic heart disease in pregnancy, whereas other varieties, such as coronary, thyroid, syphilitic, and kyphoscoliotic cardiac diseases, cor pulmonale, constrictive pericarditis, various forms of heart block, and isolated myocarditis are even less common.

Heart disease may be a very serious complication of pregnancy leading to maternal death, but as will be pointed out, in the great majority of instances it need not do so.

Diagnosis. As discussed at some length in Chapter 8 (p. 257), many of the physiologic changes of normal pregnancy tend to make the diagnosis of heart disease much more difficult than in the nonpregnant state. For example, in normal pregnancy systolic heart murmurs that are functional are quite common. Moreover, as the uterus enlarges and the diaphragm is elevated, the heart is elevated and rotated in such a way that the apex is moved laterally while the heart is somewhat closer to the anterior chest wall. Cardiac filling is increased, furthermore, accounting for the greater stroke volume during much of pregnancy. Respiratory effort in normal pregnancy is accentuated, at times suggesting dyspnea. Presumably this change is brought about in large part by a stimulatory effect of progesterone on the respiratory center. Edema, a further source of confusion, is prevalent in the lower extremities during the latter half of pregnancy. Therefore, systolic murmurs and edema, as well as changes that suggest cardiac enlargement and dyspnea, are commonplace in normal pregnancy. It becomes obvious that the physician must be quite careful not to diagnose heart disease during pregnancy when none exists, but not fail to detect and treat appropriately heart disease when it does exist.

Burwell and Metcalfe list the following criteria, any one of which confirms the diagnosis of heart disease in pregnancy: (1) a diastolic, presystolic, or continuous heart murmur; (2) unequivocal cardiac enlargement; (3) a loud harsh systolic murmur, especially if associated with a thrill; and (4) severe arrhythmia. Patients fulfilling none of these criteria rarely have heart disease. A history of rheumatic fever accompanied by the changes of normal pregnancy just summarized does not suffice for the diagnosis of valvular cardiac disease.

Prognosis. The likelihood of a favorable outcome for the mother with heart disease and her child-to-be depends upon (1) the functional capacity of her heart, (2) the likelihood of other complications that increase further the cardiac load during pregnancy and the puerperium, (3) the quality of medical care provided, and (4) the psychologic and socioeconomic capabilities of the patient, her family, and the community. The last item may assume great importance, since a favorable outcome for the pregnancy is often achieved even in instances of markedly impaired cardiac function if the mother, her family, and the community will accept the need for, and provide an environment suitable for, a very sedentary life. For some women these requirements may amount to hospitalization with complete bed rest throughout pregnancy and the puerperium.

The prognosis and recommended treatment of cardiac disease have been influenced inappropriately in some instances by certain physiologic measurements, the imprecise or incorrect interpretation of which led the authors to conclude that there was a peak maternal hemodynamic burden some weeks before term. Considerable emphasis has been placed, for example, on an apparent reduction in cardiac output after the twenty-eighth to thirty-third week of pregnancy (Ch. 8, p. 257). The misconception persists that cardiac decompensation would seldom occur after this time, a belief not well supported by clinical observations. The decrease in maternal blood volume during the last weeks of pregnancy reported by some has been similarly considered to bring about a decrease in cardiac work. Most reported measurements, however, fail to identify a decrease in blood volume of any appreciable magnitude during the last several weeks. It is important that the physician understand that cardiac failure may develop during the last few weeks of the antepartum period, during labor, or during the puerperium.

Classification of Patients. There is no clinically applicable test for accurately measuring the functional capacity of the heart. In general, the best index is provided by the classification of the New York Heart Association, which is based on the patient's history of past and present disability and is uninfluenced by the presence or absence of physical signs:

Class I. Patients with cardiac disease and *no limitation of physical activity*. Patients in this class do not have symptoms of cardiac insufficiency, nor do they experience anginal pain.

Class II. Patients with cardiac disease and *slight limitation of physical activity*. They are comfortable at rest, but if ordinary physical activity is undertaken, discomfort results in the form of excessive fatigue, palpitation, dyspnea, or anginal pain.

Class III. Patients with cardiac disease and *marked limitation of physical activity*. They are comfortable at rest, but less than ordinary activity causes discomfort in the form of excessive fatigue, palpitation, dyspnea, or anginal pain.

Class IV. Patients with cardiac disease and *inability to perform any physical activity without discomfort*. Symptoms of cardiac insufficiency or of the anginal syndrome may occur even at rest, and if any physical activity is undertaken, discomfort is increased.

Hamilton and Thomson have tabulated several complications, previous or current, that point toward an unfavorable outcome for the pregnancy: (1) history of previous heart failure exclusive of failure at the time of acute rheumatic carditis; (2) prior heart disease and recent active rheumatic fever; (3) atrial fibrillation; (4) hemoptysis; (5) overt enlargement of any of the cardiac chambers; (6) aortic stenosis; (7) cardiac disease causing cyanosis.

Treatment. The treatment of heart disease in pregnancy is dictated by the functional capacity of the heart. In all pregnant women, especially those with cardiac disease, excessive weight gain, abnormal retention of fluid, and anemia should be prevented. Increased bodily bulk increases the cardiac work, and anemia with its compensatory rise in cardiac output also predisposes to cardiac failure. The development of pregnancy-induced hypertension is particularly hazardous, for in this circumstance cardiac output can be maintained only by an increase in cardiac work commensurate with the increase in blood pressure. At the same time, hypotension is undesirable, especially in women with septal defects that allow shunting of blood.

Classes I and II. With rare exceptions, patients in Class I and most patients in Class II may be allowed to go through pregnancy. Throughout pregnancy and the puerperium special attention should be directed toward the prevention and the early recognition of heart failure. A specific routine that assures adequate rest should be outlined for each patient. The recommendations of Hamilton and Thomson are often pertinent: The patient must rest in bed 10 hours each night and in addition, must lie down for half an hour after each meal. Light housework and walking about on the level may be permitted, but climbing should be restricted. The patient should do no heavy housework or shopping. If possible, another woman should remain in the house throughout the pregnancy, not only to help with the housework but also to enable the pregnant woman to go to bed at once should any signs of a failing heart develop. In essence, the pregnant woman must learn to spare herself all unnecessary effort and must rest as much as possible. Not infrequently infection has proved to be an important factor in precipitating cardiac failure. Each woman should receive instructions to avoid contact with others who have respiratory infections, including the common cold, and to report to her physician at once if she develops any evidence of an infection.

The onset of congestive heart failure is often gradual and may be detected if attention is continually directed to certain particular signs. Hamilton and Thomson concur in the earlier observations of Mackenzie that the first warning sign of cardiac failure is likely to be persistent rales at the base of the lungs, frequently with a cough. To be significant the rales must still be audible after the patient has taken two or three deep breaths, for the rales that are sometimes heard in normal pregnant women disappear after one or two deep inspirations. A sudden diminution in the woman's ability to carry out her household duties, increasing dyspnea on exertion, attacks of smothering with cough, and hemoptysis are other signals warning of serious heart failure, as are progressive edema and tachycardia. Measurements appropriately made of the vital capacity at each visit are of value, for a sudden decrease may denote cardiac failure. Although the program outlined for the early detection of cardiac failure may seem scarcely applicable to patients in Class I or Class II, since they rarely, if ever, decompensate during pregnancy, the interests of the mother and the fetus dictate that all cases of cardiac disease in pregnancy be regarded as at risk of possible decompensation.

LABOR AND DELIVERY. Hospitalization for about a week before delivery of patients with cardiac disease is common practice. Delivery should be accomplished vaginally except in circumstances in which other obstetric complications require cesarean section. In spite of the physical effort inherent in labor and vaginal delivery, less morbidity and mortality have been recorded when delivery has been so accomplished.

Relief from pain and apprehension without undue depression of the infant or the mother is especially important during labor and delivery of women with cardiac disease. In the multiparous woman with a soft, effaced, somewhat dilated cervix, in whom little soft-tissue resistance is offered by the vagina and perineum, analgesics in moderate doses usually provide satisfactory pain relief. For women, especially nulliparas, in whom cervical dilatation, descent of the presenting part, and delivery will require greater force over a longer time, continuous conduction anesthesia—epidural or caudal—often proves valuable for reducing pain and apprehension. The major danger of conduction anesthesia is maternal hypotension. Hypotension may be rapidly fatal in patients with cardiac shunts, in whom flow may be reversed from the right to the left side of the heart or the aorta, thereby bypassing the lungs. The technics of continuous conduction anesthesia are detailed in Chapter 17.

For cesarean section the combination of thiopental, succinyl choline, and nitrous oxide with at least 30 per cent oxygen, with an endotracheal airway in place, has proved quite satisfactory. If spinal anesthesia is used for cesarean section, great care must be exercised to prevent hypotension.

During labor the patient should be kept in a semirecumbent position. Measurements of the pulse and respiratory rates should be made three to four times every hour during the first stage of labor, and every 10 minutes during the second stage. Increases in the pulse rate much above 100 per minute or in the respiratory rate above 28, particularly when associated with dyspnea, are signs of cardiac embarrassment that may progress to overt cardiac failure. With any evidence of cardiac embarrassment, intensive medical management must be instituted immediately. Only in the presence of the completely dilated cervix and an engaged presenting part may these changes be taken as indication for delivery. With the cervix only partially dilated and the mother showing evidence of cardiac embarrassment, there is no method of delivery that will not tend to precipitate rather than to forestall heart failure.

Immediate medical treatment calls for the use of morphine, oxygen, a digitalis preparation, and, at times, rotating tourniquets and diuretics. Morphine should be given intramuscularly in a dose of 10 to 15 mg. It will serve to allay apprehension, reduce the elevated respiratory rate, and perhaps reduce transiently, at least, the frequency and intensity of the uterine contractions. Oxygen is best given in the form of intermittent positive-pressure breathing to promote adequate oxygenation and to prevent or minimize pulmonary edema. Digitalis in the form of a rapidly acting glycoside such as deslanoside (Cedilanid D) should be given intravenously. The total dose of deslanoside for a patient who has not previously received a digitalis preparation is usually 1.2 to 1.6 mg. The initial dose should be 0.8 mg followed by 0.4 mg given once or twice at intervals of one to two hours. Care must be exercised to avoid toxicity in the patient who is depleted of potassium as the consequence of previous diuretic therapy. If pulmonary edema is developing, rotating tourniquets to the extremities may prove of value. In these circumstances the potent diuretic furosemide (Lasix) may be given intravenously in a dose of 40 to 80 mg.

Signs of cardiac embarrassment developing after complete dilatation of the cervix and engagement of the vertex are indications for prompt forceps delivery unless spontaneous birth is expected within a few minutes.

PUERPERIUM. Patients who have shown little or no evidence of cardiac distress during pregnancy, labor, or delivery sometimes collapse after delivery. Therefore, it is important that the same meticulous care provided during the antepartum and intrapartum periods be continued into the puerperium. Postpartum hemorrhage, puerperal infection, and puerperal thromboembolism are much more serious complications of pregnancy in the woman with heart disease. If there was no evidence of cardiac embarrassment during labor, delivery, and the early puerperium, nursing is usually not contraindicated. In general, if tubal sterilization is to be performed, it should be delayed for several days until it is obvious that the patient is afebrile, not anemic, and capable of limited exercise, at least, without symptoms. Patients who do not undergo tubal sterilization should be given detailed contraceptive advice, as should all puerperal women.

Class III. Women whose cardiac function is so diminished as to fall in Class III present difficult problems that demand expert medical judgment and care. The important question is whether they should become pregnant. The rational answer is no, but many women will risk much for a baby. They and their families must understand the risk and be willing and able to cooperate to the fullest extent. To avoid cardiac decompensation these women ideally should be kept in bed and observed very closely throughout all of the pregnancy until after delivery. The method of delivery is vaginal, as in Classes I and II, with cesarean section limited to strictly obstetric indications. A pregnant woman with a history of previous cardiac failure that was not associated with acute rheumatic carditis and the patient whose cardiac lesion causing the failure has not been corrected surgically are best managed as Class III patients regardless of their current functional classification.

Should frank cardiac failure develop during the course of pregnancy, without exception the woman must remain in bed in the hospital throughout the remainder of the pregnancy. With strict bed rest, digitalization, diuresis, and sodium restriction, the signs and symptoms of decompensation often disappear rapidly; but should the rule be broken and the patient be allowed to go home, she will very likely return to the hospital in severe or even fatal cardiac failure.

Even though the woman has recently been in failure or is in failure at the time of labor, vaginal delivery, in general, is far safer than cesarean section. Abundant evidence shows that these very sick women withstand major surgical procedures poorly and that heart disease itself is not an indication for cesarean section; on the contrary, is a contraindication.

As shown by the study of Bunim and Appel, about one third of Class III cardiac patients will decompensate during pregnancy, unless preventive measures are taken. When such a patient is seen in the first trimester, a question of therapeutic abortion inevitably arises. The desire of the patient for a child may be a determining factor, but Class III cardiac disease is an urgent indication for therapeutic abortion unless the patient can be hospitalized for the duration of the pregnancy.

The experience of Gorenberg and Chesley at the Margaret Hague Maternity Hospital led them to conclude that any patient with heart disease seen early in gestation can be carried through pregnancy successfully if she and her family are willing to abide by certain strict rules. Their recommended regimen includes bed rest in the hospital for the duration of pregnancy in any patient with Class III disease or with a history of cardiac failure. The application of this basic principle, together with good medical and obstetric care to well over 1,000 patients in the cardiac clinic, reduced the maternal death rate to not much more than that of the general obstetric population. The extreme importance of rigid adherence to their rules is clearly demonstrated by the fact that cardiac disease was the leading cause of maternal death at the hospital, but those who died were not patients attending their cardiac clinic.

Whereas it is well established that the woman with cardiac disease who receives appropriate care rarely dies during pregnancy or the puerperium, the possibility has been raised that pregnancy causes obscure deleterious effects that ultimately shorten her life-span. In other words, it is suggested that pregnancy in some way might accelerate the rate of deterioration of cardiac function. The comprehensive studies by Chesley of a large number of pregnant women observed over a long period do not demonstrate or even suggest that pregnancy has a deleterious remote effect on the course of rheumatic heart disease.

Hospitalization for many months for the woman who has other children, or who perhaps is unmarried and does not desire the pregnancy, is a great price, psychologic as well as financial, for her, her family, and in many instances the community to pay. Moreover, the life expectancy of the woman with serious cardiac disease is appreciably shortened. Sometimes, therefore, the child will be

motherless at a young age. Thus, even though therapeutic abortion is not mandatory to save the life of the mother when prolonged hospitalization and competent medical care can be provided, if these conditions are not available or are
not acceptable to the patient, therapeutic abortion and sterilization or at least
effective contraception are indicated. Therapeutic abortion demands the application of all of the safeguards discussed previously for safely accomplishing delivery, including correction of cardiac decompensation before the procedure.

Class IV. The treatment of women with Class IV heart disease is essentially that of cardiac failure in pregnancy, labor, and the puerperium. In the
presence of cardiac failure, delivery by any known method carries a high
maternal mortality. Accordingly, the treatment of heart failure in pregnancy is
primarily medical rather than obstetric. The prime objective is to correct the
decompensation, for only then will delivery be safe.

EFFECTS ON FETUS AND NEWBORN. In general, any disease complicated by
severe maternal hypoxia is likely to lead to abortion, premature delivery, and
intrauterine death. A relation of chronic hypoxia and the polycythemia it causes
to the outcome of pregnancy has been demonstrated in the studies of Hellegers
and Neill on women with cyanotic heart disease. When hypoxia was so intense
as to stimulate a rise in hematocrit above 65 per cent, all pregnancies ended in
abortion. Intrauterine growth retardation and prematurity were identified with
lesser degrees of hypoxia and polycythemia.

SURGICAL REPAIR. In recent years several operations have been performed
on the heart and the large vessels to try to improve cardiovascular function.
Schenker and Polishuk have analyzed the experiences of 182 women who conceived and delivered after *mitral valvotomy.* The procedure was performed on
30 patients during pregnancy with no deaths during or immediately after the
operation, although 3 died later in the antepartum period. Apparently good
clinical results after mitral valvotomy were not always followed by uncomplicated pregnancy and delivery. In fact, 10 of the 18 deaths after the operation
were attributed to the effects of pregnancy and delivery. In 42 per cent of all
patients who had their first delivery after the operation, various stages of congestive heart failure were encountered The puerperium was a particularly dangerous time. The reports of some others are more favorable.

In the past decade a number of women of reproductive age have received
a *cardiac valvar prosthesis* to replace a severely damaged mitral or aortic valve.
Continuous anticoagulant therapy is recommended by most authorities to prevent emboli. In the absence of pregnancy, agents such as Coumadin or Dicumarol are satisfactory, but these drugs cross the placenta and may cause hemorrhage and death in the fetus and newborn. Heparin is therefore the anticoagulant
of choice antepartum (Radnich and Jacobs). The pregnant woman can usually
be instructed to inject heparin deeply into the subcutaneous tissue. Just before
delivery the heparin is stopped; if delivery occurs while the anticoagulant is still
effective and extensive bleeding is encountered, protamine sulfate should be
given. Anticoagulant therapy with Coumadin, Dicumarol, or heparin may be
restarted the day after delivery, usually with no problems.

Laros and associates have recently presented their experiences in two instances of successful pregnancies in women with Starr-Edwards prosthetic mitral
valves and have summarized those reported by others. Some of the reported
complications are cardiac failure, thromboembolism, morbidity from anticoagu-

lant therapy, and premature labor. Even though cardiac function may be adequate, the difficulties associated with prolonged administration of heparin to prevent arterial embolization tend to preclude repeated pregnancies; therefore, in these women sterilization frequently has merit. Oral contraceptives containing estrogen and a progestin may be contraindicated, although MacDonald states that risk of thromboembolism is slight as long as the patients are receiving anticoagulants. Bemiller and associates report the successful outcome of pregnancy in a woman with an aortic valve prosthesis and congenital complete heart block.

Some patients with *patent ductus arteriosus* develop pulmonary hypertension and, particularly if the systemic blood pressure falls, may have a reversal of blood flow from the pulmonary artery to the aorta with consequent cyanosis. Sudden drops in blood pressure at delivery, as with conduction anesthesia or hemorrhage, may lead to fatal collapse. Therefore, hypotension should be avoided whenever possible and treated vigorously if it occurs. Burwell and Metcalfe suggest that the ductus should not be ligated during pregnancy. In our own limited experience, however, the operation has proved to be relatively simple, and cardiac function improves dramatically.

Various operations have been performed on women with *tetralogy of Fallot* with variable results. The hematocrit often provides an index of the success of the procedure. As pointed out previously, if the hematocrit is very high (greater than 65), abortion is the rule. With somewhat lesser degrees of polycythemia there is an increased incidence of abortion, premature delivery, and underweight infants. If signs of cardiac failure develop in early pregnancy and do not yield to medical treatment, therapeutic abortion is advisable.

Coarctation of the aorta is a relatively rare lesion. The collateral circulation arising above the level of the coarctation expands, often to a striking extent, to cause localized erosion of the margins of the ribs by the hypertrophied intercostal arteries. The typical findings on physical examination are hypertension in the upper extremities and normal to reduced arterial blood pressures in the lower extremities.

The major complications of coarctation of the aorta are congestive heart failure when there has been long-standing severe hypertension, bacterial endocarditis, and rupture of the aorta. The aortic ruptures are likely to occur late in pregnancy or early in the puerperium and are associated with changes in the media that are histologically similar to those characterizing Erdheim's idiopathic medial cystic necrosis. Congestive heart failure demands vigorous efforts to improve cardiac function and usually warrants interruption of the pregnancy. Bacterial endocarditis can be effectively treated by appropriate antibiotics. It has been recommended by some that resection of the coarctation be undertaken during pregnancy to protect against the possibility of dissecting aneurysm and rupture of the aorta. The operation, however, is not without significant risk, especially to the fetus, because all of the collaterals must be clamped for variable periods of time during the procedure, possibly leading to serious fetal hypoxia. Some authorities have recommended that the woman with coarctation of the aorta be delivered by cesarean section lest the transient elevation of arterial blood pressure that commonly accompanies labor lead to rupture of either the aorta or a coexisting cerebral aneurysm. The available evidence, however, suggests that cesarean section probably should be limited to obstetric indications.

Coronary thrombosis and *ischemic heart disease* are rare complications of pregnancy. The treatment is quite similar to that of the nonpregnant patient. If anticoagulants are given, the possibility of the toxic effects of Coumadin or Dicumarol on the fetus must be considered. The advisability of a woman's undertaking a pregnancy after a myocardial infarction is not clear. Since the underlying vascular disease is usually progressive, and since it not infrequently is associated with hypertension, pregnancy in general appears to be contra-indicated. There are, however, reported instances of uncomplicated pregnancies after myocardial infarction. Ginz has recently reported 3 cases of myocardial infarction during pregnancy and reviewed 36 others described previously.

Postpartum heart disease is an obscure form of cardiac failure that develops either very late in pregnancy or more often during the several weeks after delivery, unassociated with antecedent organic cardiac disease. If the patient survives the episode of cardiac decompensation, she usually makes a complete recovery. The disease has been reported to recur occasionally in a subsequent pregnancy. Some believe that it is a unique syndrome induced in some way by pregnancy and characterized by congestive heart failure with cardiomegaly, pulmonary congestion, and electrocardiographic evidence of nonspecific myocardial damage. It is far from clear, however, whether postpartum heart disease is a distinct clinical entity.

During pregnancy especially, severe degrees of kyphoscoliosis commonly cause serious cardiopulmonary problems, sometimes referred to as *kypho-scoliotic heart disease*. In these circumstances some regions of the lungs in the markedly deformed thoracic cage may be quite emphysematous, while others are atelectatic, with both lesions contributing to an inadequate ventilatory capacity. In these circumstances *cor pulmonale* is a frequent complication.

The increased oxygen demands and the cardiac work imposed by pregnancy and delivery must be taken into account in reaching a decision whether to allow the pregnancy to continue or to perform a therapeutic abortion. If pulmonary function studies indicate that the vital capacity is not reduced appreciably, the outcome most often is favorable. In women with more marked degrees of kyphoscoliosis and impaired pulmonary function, therapeutic abortion may be indicated.

Frequently the bony pelvis is so distorted that cesarean section is necessary. The supine position during delivery may result in serious hypotension. The commonly used analgesics such as meperidine should not be given in large doses, since respiratory depression is very poorly tolerated. During and after delivery meticulous care should be directed toward the prevention of further atelectasis, which could lead rapidly to severe hypoxia and death. Intermittent positive-pressure breathing using appropriate concentrations of oxygen with mucolytic agents is of value. Sterilization or effective contraception is usually indicated.

BACTERIAL ENDOCARDITIS. Since the advent of antibiotics bacterial endocarditis, acute or subacute, is rarely encountered during pregnancy and the puerperium. Treatment is the same as in the absence of pregnancy. The use of antibiotics prophylactically at the time of delivery of a woman with an underlying lesion of the endocardium of the valves or elsewhere is moot. Procaine penicillin G (1.2 million units) plus tetracycline (1 g) or ampicillin (2 g) given during labor or before cesarean section and daily for several days thereafter have been suggested for prophylaxis. All women who are treated for an infection during pregnancy and the puerperium and who have valvular heart lesions should have blood cultures for anaerobic as well as aerobic organisms before instituting antibiotic therapy.

DISEASES OF THE RESPIRATORY SYSTEM

Pregnancy induces a number of changes in the respiratory system. Enlargement of the uterus causes the diaphragm to rise, the transverse thoracic diameter to increase, the vertical chest diameter to decrease, and the residual volume of air in the lungs to be reduced. The respiratory rate increases somewhat, and in response to the modest hyperventilation the plasma carbon dioxide is lowered slightly. During the latter part of pregnancy the oxygen consumption is increased approximately 25 per cent above that of normal nonpregnant women.

Pneumonia. In general, pneumonitis causing an appreciable loss of ventilatory capacity is tolerated less well by women during pregnancy. This generalization seems to hold true irrespective of whether the cause of the pneumonia is bacterial, viral, or chemical. Moreover, as has been pointed out in the discussions of heart disease and of diabetes, hypoxia and acidosis are poorly tolerated by the fetus. Therefore, it is important to the pregnant woman and her fetus that pneumonia be diagnosed as soon as possible and that she be promptly hospitalized so that the disease can be treated.

Aspiration of gastric contents during anesthesia for delivery often results in severe chemical pneumonitis, primarily as the consequence of the necrotizing effects of hydrochloric acid (Mendelson). Even though the woman has been fasting for some time, gastric juice that may be strongly acid is likely to accumulate in the stomach. This relatively common anesthetic accident should be promptly recognized and immediately treated. When general anesthesia with endotracheal intubation is used, the times of greatest danger from aspiration are during insertion and removal of the endotracheal tube; not infrequently the gastric juices are observed to enter the pharynx and thence reach the trachea. The aspiration of gastric contents is not limited to anesthesia for delivery. Treatment of eclampsia with large doses of morphine or barbiturates, for example, has sometimes been followed by the aspiration of gastric contents.

The physical findings after aspiration vary, depending on the volume of the fluid and its acidity and on the extent of the dispersion of the fluid in the lungs. Bronchospasm is a common early finding, with rales developing soon thereafter. Roentgenographic findings may be variable. As soon as the accident is recognized or even strongly suspected, treatment should be initiated with adrenocorticosteroids. Methylprednisolone sodium succinate (Solu-Medrol) in a dose of about 250 mg rapidly injected intravenously or equivalent amounts of other corticosteroids are recommended to reduce the inflammatory reaction in the lungs. Somewhat smaller doses are then given at three-hour to four-hour intervals during the remainder of the day. The steroid therapy then can usually be stopped. Oxygen given by intermittent positive pressure is of value to overcome hypoxia and to try to inhibit pulmonary congestion. Broad-spectrum antibiotics are indicated to prevent secondary infection of the injured lungs. Serial roentgenograms of the chest and measurements of blood gases are of value in following the course of the disease. Results with the relatively recent use of large doses of steroids seem to be greatly improved over those obtained during the era in which bronchoscopy and saline flushing of the pulmonary airways were commonly used methods of treatment. The experiences with *aspiration pneumonitis* at Parkland Memorial Hospital have recently been reviewed by Bailey and Giesecke.

Varicella pneumonia is a very uncommon but very serious illness during pregnancy; several maternal deaths have been reported (Pickard; Mendelow and Lewis). Whether gamma globulin or convalescent sera are of any value is not clear.

Thromboembolism and Pulmonary Infarction.   It may be encountered during pregnancy, but they occur much more often during the puerperium. Diagnosis and treatment of these serious problems are discussed in Chapter 35 (p. 1001).

Asthma.   This is a rather common respiratory illness, which consequently is encountered relatively often in pregnant women. Pregnancy does not seem to exert any consistent predictable effect on bronchial asthma. In some pregnant women asthma appears to be less of a problem; in others, it is more of a problem; and in still others, it remains about the same as in the nonpregnant state. The great majority of women with asthma can be safely carried through pregnancy, labor, and delivery. Respiratory infections and sometimes emotional stress may intensify the asthmatic attacks. Most drugs that have proved effective before pregnancy may be continued during pregnancy with one major exception: The use of medications that contain iodide must be avoided, for iodide is transported across the placenta to the fetus and concentrated in the fetal thyroid. When the mother ingests large doses of iodide over a prolonged period of time, the large amount of iodide reaching the fetus may induce a large goiter. We have observed this sequence of events in a patient who ingested considerable amounts of a preparation containing ephedrine, phenobarbital, theophylline, calcium salicylate, and potassium iodide (Quadrinal). Carswell and associates have recently reported several instances of congenital goiter and hypothyroidism caused by the maternal ingestion of iodides.

When severe attacks of asthma cannot be relieved by other types of medication, cortisone or similar steroid compounds may be given. Although there is evidence that cortisone is teratogenic when given to pregnant rabbits, rats, and some other animals, there is no strong evidence that it is teratogenic in human pregnancy. For example, Williams has reported that of 33 infants whose mothers were receiving steroids for asthma at the onset of pregnancy, one had a serious anomaly. Asthma is not a contraindication to the use of most forms of analgesia and anesthesia for labor and delivery. Therapeutic abortion might be indicated in the uncommon patient who, as the consequence of long-standing asthma, has reduced cardiopulmonary function. Since asthma is a chronic disease that in the adult predictably will persist for many years after the pregnancy, sterilization may have merit for the woman who desires no more children.

Pulmonary Resection.   The effect of *pulmonary resection,* usually for bronchiectasis or tuberculosis, will depend upon the functional capacity of the remaining pulmonary tissue. In general, if function is equivalent to one normal lung and active pulmonary disease is not present, pregnancy is tolerated without undue risk to the mother and with a good likelihood of delivery of a healthy infant.

Tuberculosis.   In recent years the prognosis has improved remarkably for the woman with active pulmonary tuberculosis. Chemotherapy that has proved to be effective in the absence of pregnancy is also effective during pregnancy.

Fortunately, the drugs in common use do not appear to affect the fetus adversely.

The diagnosis of active tuberculosis may be difficult during pregnancy. The identification of *Mycobacterium tuberculosis* by culture or animal inoculation may take many weeks to months. Evaluation of the degree of activity of the pulmonary disease may require several serial roentgenograms over a considerable period of time. Moreover, as pregnancy advances and the diaphragm rises, the lungs undergo some degree of compression, which may mask the extent of the tuberculous lesion. In fact, this mechanical effect of pregnancy on the lung may conceal actual pulmonary cavitation. Therefore, treatment may have to be undertaken in the pregnant woman on less firm ground than if she were not pregnant. Treatment consists specifically of isoniazid, para-aminosalicylic acid, and streptomycin or dihydrostreptomycin. Supportive therapy consists of bed rest and good diet. In the absence of seriously impaired pulmonary function, analgesia and anesthesia for labor and delivery can usually be accomplished with any of the technics used for normal pregnancy. Therapeutic abortion is seldom indicated unless there is disseminated tuberculosis or severely compromised cardiopulmonary function. Sterilization is often warranted for women who desire no more children. Congenital tuberculosis is rare even when the mother has widespread disease. The newborn infant, however, is quite susceptible to tuberculosis. Therefore, the infant should be isolated immediately from the mother with active disease.

Pelvic tuberculosis usually causes intractable sterility. According to Schaefer, for example, only 31 term pregnancies have been reported in authenticated cases of genital tuberculosis. Other cases of pregnancy often terminate ectopically or in abortion and are frequently followed by activation of the pelvic infection. Kistner, Hertig, and Rock collected 42 cases of tubal pregnancy with pelvic tuberculosis. Although treatment is still controversial, the consensus favors a combination of chemotherapy and surgical extirpation of the pelvic organs. In certain younger women, however, more conservative therapy may be justified. Both Studdiford and Schaefer have reviewed the problems of pelvic tuberculosis in relation to pregnancy.

Sarcoidosis. This disease is rarely identified in pregnant women. The available evidence implies that sarcoidosis does not affect pregnancy adversely, and some authors suggest that pregnancy may actually be beneficial (Dines and Banner). Pregnancy is not a contraindication to the use of corticosteroids if they are needed. O'Leary noted that only women with extensive pulmonary involvement were at risk during pregnancy; the development of respiratory infection warrants hospitalization.

ENDOCRINE DISORDERS

Diabetes Mellitus. Before the advent of insulin in 1921 most women with diabetes were too ill to conceive. For example, in 1909 Williams, after thirteen years as Chief of the Obstetrical Service of the Johns Hopkins Hospital, with a large consulting practice in addition, had encountered only one case of pregnancy complicated by diabetes. The exact cause of the infertility in diabetic women during the preinsulin era is not clear, but amenorrhea was common, the incidence having been placed as high as 50 per cent. Of the infrequent cases in which pregnancy occurred, about a fourth of the mothers and about half of the fetuses and infants died.

Incidence. The lack of agreement about the minimal requirements for the diagnosis of diabetes makes it difficult to acquire satisfactory figures for its prevalence. There are approximately two million diagnosed cases, but quite likely an even larger number have not been diagnosed. The prevalence, but not necessarily the severity, of diabetes increases sharply with age. Its frequency in women aged 35 to 44, for example, is five times that of women aged 15 to 24. Diabetes is most likely to develop in women who are obese and who have a family history of diabetes. The probability of development of diabetes in people whose blood relatives have the disease is summarized in Table 8.

Table 8. **Probability of Diabetes within Families with Known Diabetes**

Relatives with Diabetes	Probability of Abnormal Glucose Metabolism (%)
Both parents	approaches 100
Identical twin	approaches 100
One parent and one sibling	approximately 50
One sibling or one parent	approximately 25

From Steinberg, Eugenics Quart 2:26, 1955.

Diagnosis. The patient who presents with high plasma glucose levels, glucosuria, ketonemia, and ketonuria is no problem in diagnosis. The woman at the opposite end of the spectrum, with only minimal metabolic derangement caused by diabetes, may be difficult to identify. The likelihood of impaired carbohydrate metabolism and related metabolic stigmata of diabetes is increased appreciably in women who have a strong familial history of diabetes, or have given birth to large infants, or demonstrate persistent glucosuria.

Reducing substances are commonly found in the urine of pregnant women, but their presence does not necessarily mean diabetes. Sometimes the material is lactose, but it should not be a source of needless concern if the urine is tested by a method that is specific for glucose. The commercially available testing substances, Tes-Tape and Clinistix, may be used to identify glucose in the urine while avoiding a positive reaction from lactose. Even when lactosuria is excluded, glycosuria caused by glucose is occasionally identified. Most often the glucosuria does not reflect hyperglycemia and impaired glucose tolerance, but rather the lowered renal threshold for glucose induced by normal pregnancy, as discussed in Chapter 8 (p. 250). Sutherland and associates have recently reported that the presence or absence of glucose in the second voided urine specimen during continuation of an overnight fast is of diagnostic importance. According to them there is a significant positive correlation between glucosuria detected in the second specimen, using the glucose oxidase test strip (Clinistix), and chemical diabetes. Nonetheless, the detection of glucosuria during pregnancy probably warrants a glucose tolerance test.

GLUCOSE TOLERANCE TEST. A true plasma sugar level above 130 mg per 100 ml, confirmed by repeated analyses of plasma obtained from the fasting patient on different days, is considered to be evidence of diabetes by most authorities. Measurement of the fasting plasma sugar level is not sufficient, however, for the diagnosis of milder degrees of diabetes, since some patients with a significantly decreased glucose tolerance have fasting plasma sugar levels within normal limits.

The oral glucose tolerance test measures the balance between the absorption of glucose from the intestinal tract, its uptake by tissues, and its excretion in the urine. In the absence of pregnancy the oral test is often preferred to the intravenous glucose tolerance test because of its greater sensitivity.

The intravenous test, however, is usually preferred for pregnant women because of the variability in gastric emptying time and glucose absorption induced by pregnancy. Typically the woman has been prepared by consuming a diet relatively high in carbohydrates for a few days before testing. A blood sample is drawn from the fasting patient, 50 ml of a 50 per cent glucose solution are injected intravenously in a period of about four minutes, and serial blood specimens are obtained. An important end point is the plasma sugar level two hours after the administration of the glucose. If the fasting sugar level is less than 100 mg per 100 ml and the level at two hours is not greater than the fasting level, it is unlikely that the patient has any significant degree of metabolic impairment.

A somewhat more complicated method of evaluation involves plotting the plasma glucose concentrations on semilogarithmic graph paper, with the ordinate expressing the concentration and the abscissa the time after injection. A line is drawn through the values, and the time for the glucose concentration to decrease 50 per cent is ascertained. The so-called K-value is then calculated ($K = 0.693 \div t_{1/2} \times 100$). The K-value, or the rate of utilization of glucose expressed as per cent per minute, in women with diabetes is lower than in normals.

Several investigators believe the intravenous test with the calculation of the K-value to be the most sensitive and reliable diagnostic test for diabetes in pregnancy, especially in predicting obstetric complications. They recommend that patients in whom diabetes is suspected be screened for glucose intolerance with a two-hour postprandial plasma glucose measurement and, then, if indicated, there be further evaluation early in the third trimester with an intravenous glucose tolerance test. Burt and Leake urge caution in employing an oral glucose tolerance test during pregnancy or the early puerperium for identification of the prediabetic woman or the patient susceptible to pregnancy wastage. These investigators point out that approximately 25 per cent of the patients tested showed abnormal plasma glucose levels by criteria employed in the nonpregnant state. Benjamin and Casper contend, however, that the main drawback of the intravenous glucose tolerance test is a false negative rate approaching 47 per cent, compared with 12 per cent with the oral test.

The confusion that persists results, in part at least, from the variation in criteria for diagnosing diabetes. The precise levels for diagnosing diabetes by any form of test of carbohydrate tolerance are far from settled, for many of the experts in the field of diabetes are unable to reach an agreement.

The *cortisone glucose tolerance test* and the *tolbutamide response test* are seldom used for identifying abnormalities in glucose tolerance in pregnant women.

Effect of Pregnancy on Diabetes. The diabetogenic properties of pregnancy are borne out by the fact that some women who have no evidence of diabetes when not pregnant develop, during pregnancy, abnormalities in glucose tolerance and, at times, clinically evident diabetes. Most often these changes are reversible. After delivery the evidence for diabetes usually disappears rapidly, and the ability of the mother to metabolize carbohydrate returns to that of the prepregnant state. As pointed out in Chapter 8 (p. 250), pregnancy induces an increase in the peripheral resistance to insulin. The action of insulin is antagonized during pregnancy by chorionic somatomammotropin and to lesser degrees by estrogens and progesterone. At the same time the rate of destruction of insulin is increased by a potent insulinase in the placenta.

During pregnancy the management of diabetes may be made more difficult by a variety of complications. Nausea and vomiting may lead, on the one hand, to insulin shock in women who are receiving insulin and, on the other, to insulin resistance if the starvation is severe enough to cause ketosis. Infection during pregnancy commonly results in insulin resistance and ketoacidosis unless the infection is promptly recognized and both the infection and the diabetes are effectively treated. The vigorous muscular exertion of labor accompanied by the ingestion of little or no carbohydrate may result in profound hypoglycemia unless the amount of insulin given is reduced appropriately or an intravenous infusion of glucose is provided. After delivery, insulin requirements usually, but not always, decrease at a rapid rate and to a considerable degree. Puerperal infection, however, may obtund this response or even increase the insulin requirements. Presumably the rapid decrease in insulin requirements that is usually seen in the absence of other complications stems from the removal of the placenta. The direct consequence is the exclusion of the placental insulinase as well as the rapid disappearance from the circulation of chorionic somatomammotropin, estrogens, and progesterone of placental origin.

It was previously thought that the fetus ameliorates maternal diabetes by producing insulin, which is transferred in significant amounts across the placenta to the mother. There is no good evidence, however, that the fetal pancreas is capable of providing insulin to the mother in amounts sufficient to ameliorate her disease to any appreciable degree or that the insulin is transferred across the placenta in physiologic amounts.

The pregnant woman, even in the absence of diabetes, appears much more likely to develop metabolic acidosis. Presumably chorionic somatomammotropin is responsible for this tendency by virtue of its carbohydrate-sparing and lipolytic actions. With diabetes the likelihood of severe metabolic acidosis is increased markedly.

Effects of Diabetes on Pregnancy. Diabetes is deleterious to pregnancy in a number of ways. The adverse maternal effects that are likely to be encountered include the following: (1) The likelihood of preeclampsia-eclampsia is increased about fourfold. A considerable increase is noted even in the absence of demonstrated preexisting vascular disease. (2) Infection occurs more often and is likely to be more severe in women with diabetes. (3) The fetus frequently is much larger (Fig. 5), and its size may lead to difficult delivery with injury to the birth canal. (4) The tendency of the fetus to succumb before the onset of spontaneous labor, as well as the possibility of dystocia, increases the frequency of cesarean section and the maternal risks that are imposed by this operation. (5) Postpartum hemorrhage after vaginal delivery is more common than in the general obstetric population. (6) Hydramnios is common, and at times the large volume of amniotic fluid coupled with fetal macrosomia may even cause cardiorespiratory symptoms in the mother.

Maternal diabetes adversely affects the fetus and newborn infant in a variety of ways: (1) The perinatal death rate is considerably elevated compared with that of the general population. For example, at the University of Iowa during the past three decades 14.9 per cent of infants weighing 1,000 g or more

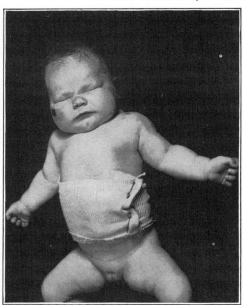

Fig. 5. Characteristic large baby of diabetic mother. Birth weight: 5,200 g.

were lost. Nine per cent were stillborn, and 6 per cent died during the neonatal period (Delaney and Ptacek). Moreover, the death rate in more recent years has not differed significantly from that of earlier years. Although the perinatal death rate is increased severalfold, abortion is not much more likely to occur than in the general obstetric population. (2) Morbidity is common in the newborn infant of a mother with diabetes. In some instances the morbidity is the direct result of birth injury as the consequence of fetal macrosomia with disproportion between the size of the infant and the maternal pelvis. In others it takes the form of severe respiratory distress. (3) Anomalies have been identified somewhat more often in the fetuses of women with diabetes. (4) The infant is likely to inherit diabetes, as pointed out in Table 8. (5) Maternal diabetes in some instances may lead to neurologic and psychologic deficits in the child. Churchill and co-workers have reported recently that children whose diabetic mothers developed ketosis during pregnancy have a somewhat lower intelligence quotient than do the offspring of diabetic women without acetonuria.

Except for the brain, all organs of the fetus are affected by macrosomia that commonly characterizes the fetus of the woman with diabetes (Fig. 5). The mechanisms responsible for the extra growth are not clear. One attractive possible explanation is that maternal hyperglycemia and, in turn, fetal hyperglycemia provide a stimulus for hyperinsulinism in the fetus, thereby facilitating the utilization of the extra glucose for growth. There is recent experimental evidence to support this concept. Hutchinson and associates have injected the antibiotic streptozotocin into the circulation of the pregnant monkey to destroy the beta cells of the islets of Langerhans. Maternal diabetes so produced was followed by fetal macrosomia. Cheek has injected streptozotocin into the circulation of the monkey fetus to destroy the capacity of the fetus to make insulin. Fetal size was reduced appreciably.

Some of the other changes wrought by diabetes mellitus in human pregnancy may be reproduced in experimental animals with alloxan-induced diabetes, even though the disease is extremely mild. Pregnant rats, for example, in which the only evidence of diabetes is an altered glucose tolerance curve, not only gave birth to oversized young four times more frequently than did nondiabetic rats, and the combined stillbirth and neonatal death rate was three times greater (Lazarow).

A fairly common finding at autopsy in the newborn infant of a diabetic mother is hypertrophy and hyperplasia of the islets of Langerhans. Although the changes are not specific, since they are also noted in erythroblastotic infants, they are sufficiently characteristic when found to suggest that the mother has diabetes or prediabetes. This information may be useful in subsequent pregnancies. It has been suggested that maternal hyperglycemia and, in turn, fetal hyperglycemia are responsible for the striking increase in the size, and sometimes the number, of islets, but this explanation does not account for the enlargement noted in infants of prediabetic women or in erythroblastotic infants.

Maternal Prognosis. In two large series of diabetic pregnancies reported from England by Oakley, the maternal mortality rates were 1.4 and 2.8 per cent, respectively. There were 3 maternal deaths in the course of the 357 pregnancies complicated by diabetes that were cared for at the University of Iowa (Delaney and Ptacek). Each of the 3 deaths was cardiac or vascular in origin—one caused by myocardial infarction, another by eclampsia, and the third by pulmonary embolism after cesarean section. It is apparent from these studies that, in general, good medical and obstetric care throughout all of the pregnancy and puerperium usually assures a favorable outcome for the mother. Today almost all maternal deaths from diabetes are the result of less than optimal care. The experiences of White at the Joslin Clinic certainly attest to the validity of this statement; 99.8 per cent of the diabetic mothers cared for by that group survived the pregnancy and the puerperium. Moreover, 90 per cent were alive 20 or more years after the first pregnancy. White concludes that the course of maternal diabetes need not be affected unfavorably by intercurrent pregnancies.

Fetal Prognosis. The prognosis for the fetus, although vastly better than in the preinsulin era, is still guarded. The lowest perinatal mortality rates reported are of the order of 10 per cent, and most are 15 per cent or even somewhat higher (White; Delaney and Ptacek; Horger and associates).

The prognosis for the fetus depends to a considerable degree, although not totally, upon the intensity of the diabetes, its duration, and the extent of pre-existing vascular and renal disease, as well as the development of complications of pregnancy. Delaney and Ptacek, for example, noted perinatal loss for infants weighing 1,000 g or more to be only 3.6 per cent when the mother had chemical diabetes (White's Class A, Table 9), whereas in those with overt diabetes, fetal loss ranged from 16 to 23 per cent.

Table 9. **A Classification of Diabetes**

Class	Definition
A	Chemical diabetes only
B	Diabetes of adult onset (after 20 years of age)
C	Diabetes of long duration (10 to 19 years)
D	Duration more than 20 years, or onset before age of 10, or vascular lesions, benign retinopathy, or calcified leg arteries
E	Calcification of iliac or uterine arteries
F	Diabetic nephropathy
R	Proliferating retinopathy

From White, P. Med Clin N Amer 49:1015, 1965.

Management. Our own experiences with a large obstetric clinic are comparable with those reported by others. If the mother does not obtain prenatal care, the fetal outcome most often is bad. With close observation in a clinic organized especially for obstetric complications, the outcome is improved remarkably.

The main objective in the management of diabetes throughout the pregnancy is continuous control of the disease. A select group of physicians skilled in the treatment of diabetes and in obstetrics ideally should assume primary responsibility for the medical and obstetric care throughout the pregnancy. From the moment of birth it is important that a physician expert in the care of the newborn, especially in the recognition and treatment of the problems of the newborn whose mother has diabetes, assume the responsibility for care of the infant. Similarly, an anesthesiologist especially cognizant of the problems of the diabetic mother and her fetus is a most desirable addition to the team providing care.

Effective counseling of the mother is an extremely important function of prenatal care. She must not only be seen often but also be instructed carefully how to recognize and deal with problems that arise in the interim. She must be encouraged to report immediately any of a variety of events to the physician who has primary responsibility for her care. For example, respiratory or urinary infection, rather common occurrences during pregnancy, can rapidly precipitate ketoacidosis that is very poorly tolerated by the fetus. The common complications of pregnancy—nausea and vomiting—may, if the mother does not eat appropriately, lead to the characteristic reaction of hyperinsulinism; but if more severe and prolonged, the starvation may lead to both serious acidosis and insulin resistance much sooner than if she were not pregnant.

The diabetic woman who is pregnant may have to be reeducated about the significance of glucosuria. Similar to the normal pregnant woman, she is likely to develop glucosuria as the consequence of the pregnancy-induced increase in glomerular filtration without increased tubular reabsorption. If she were to increase her insulin dosage to a level that avoids glucosuria, she would likely develop symptomatic hypoglycemia. Therefore, she must be instructed to note slight to moderate glucosuria but not to be especially concerned about it unless it is accompanied by acetonuria. Frank acetonuria usually means that the insulin dosage should be increased somewhat.

Preclinical (Chemical) Diabetes.   The most favorable category of diabetic pregnancies includes that group of mothers with only chemical evidence of diabetes (Class A diabetes, Table 9) who enroll in clinic early and attend faithfully and whose previous pregnancies terminated successfully in infants who survived. In general, in these circumstances pregnancies can be allowed to progress to term unless complications develop (Schwarz and associates). The detection of hypertension, generalized edema, or marked hydramnios, however, signals the likelihood of fetal demise unless delivery is soon accomplished.

Clinically Evident Diabetes.   Most patients in this broad category receive insulin or an oral hypoglycemic agent. Most often tolbutamide (Orinase) and the other oral hypoglycemic agents are not used during pregnancy, but instead insulin is given when indicated. Tolbutamide in large doses is teratogenic in some species, but there is no evidence that doses used clinically are teratogenic in women. Serious hypoglycemia has been observed, however, in the newborn of mothers treated with tolbutamide.

For many years White has administered an estrogen and a progestational agent to diabetic mothers throughout much of pregnancy. Compounds used in the past include the estrogen estradiol or stilbestrol and either progesterone or ethisterone. More recently White has prescribed a mixture of estradiol valerate and 17-hydroxyprogesterone caproate (Deluteval-2X). Although the fetal outcome has been good in patients treated in this way by White, comparable results have been obtained by others without administering these often expensive and, at times, troublesome drugs. Therefore, we agree with the majority who do not recommend their use.

In institutions that have achieved the best outcome, it has often been the practice to admit the woman to the hospital periodically for careful evaluation of her diabetic status. It is usually not practical for the patient to be hospitalized longer than a few days; but on occasion, control of the disease proves more difficult, and hospitalization is required for a longer period of time.

The time set for admitting the mother in preparation for delivery varies in different institutions. Most likely the perinatal death rate would be favorably influenced by admitting all mothers with diabetes to the hospital eight to ten weeks before term and providing very close medical and obstetric supervision throughout the remainder of the pregnancy. Driscoll and Gillespie recommend that all diabetic mothers be hospitalized a minimum of one week before the date selected for delivery. In accordance with the classification of White for maternal diabetes outlined in Table 9, they recommend the following: Patients in Class B are admitted not later than the end of the thirty-sixth week of gestation; a patient in Class C, not later than the end of the thirty-fifth week; in Class D, at the end of the thirty-fourth week; and in Class E or F, at the end of the thirty-second week. They urge that the mother be hospitalized for as long as necessary whenever a complication of the diabetes or of the pregnancy arises. They would recommend hospitalization for all diabetic patients for the last several weeks antepartum were it not for economic considerations.

Delivery. The ideal time for delivery is when the fetus is not only mature enough to survive but also mature enough not to suffer any subsequent physical or psychologic impairment. To achieve just the first goal—a liveborn infant that survives—has proved to be a difficult task. The approaches used have ranged from a fixed policy of delivery of all women with diabetes by cesarean section not later than the thirty-seventh week of gestation to individualization of the time of delivery, depending upon the presence or absence of a variety of complications as well as the outcome of previous pregnancies.

In general, the welfare of the fetus is best served when each case is individualized. In instances of clinically evident diabetes without other complications, with a favorable history of any previous pregnancies, and with a known duration of gestation, delivery should be carried out at about 38 weeks. If, however, the fetus of a previous gestation expired late in pregnancy without apparent cause, delivery usually should be planned for about the thirty-sixth week—if the duration of gestation is precisely known.

If overt chronic vascular or renal disease, preeclampsia, or marked hydramnios complicates the pregnancy, delivery is indicated at the thirty-fourth or thirty-fifth week.

The measurement of 24-hour urinary estriol excretion to monitor fetal well-being has received considerable attention in recent years (Ch. 6, p. 181). There is no doubt that unusually low excretion of estriol in urine most often, but not always, indicates that the fetus is in jeopardy (Greene and co-workers). It remains to be proved, however, that the widespread application of measurements of urinary estriol to identify such a fetus will reduce perinatal mortality significantly in diabetic pregnancies. To deliver a fetus in jeopardy of dying in utero, only to have him succumb from immaturity, accomplishes little, as emphasized by Barnes. Klopper points out that for this reason estriol assays are not of value much before the thirty-fourth week of gestation. Studies are in progress at several centers to evaluate the benefits that might be achieved from monitoring estriol excretion at close intervals during the latter half of the third trimester. The results will be of considerable interest.

In some clinics all women with diabetes are delivered by cesarean section. Our own preference is to attempt induction of labor when the following criteria are met: (1) Parity is not great. (2) The fetus is not excessively large nor is the pelvis contracted. (3) The cervix is soft, appreciably effaced, and somewhat dilated. (4) The presenting part is the vertex and is fixed in the pelvis.

Dilute oxytocin is slowly administered intravenously and the fetal heart rate is monitored toward the end and immediately after each contraction. Once regular, effective contractions are established and the cervix begins to dilate, the oxytocin infusion is either stopped or reduced to deliver the minimal amount that maintains labor. Fetal depression from oversedation is avoided and delivery is accomplished using pudendal block, perineal infiltration, and nitrous oxide-oxygen. Low spinal anesthesia is often the choice for nulliparas in whom low forceps and a more extensive episiotomy are commonly employed to effect delivery. If any of these criteria for induction of labor and vaginal delivery is not met, or if labor is not established promptly using oxytocin, cesarean section is employed. Either conduction anesthesia or general anesthesia with thiopental, succinyl choline, and nitrous oxide and oxygen are recommended for the operation.

It is important to reduce considerably the dose of long-acting insulin given on the day of delivery. Regular insulin should be utilized to meet most or all of the insulin needs of the patient at this time, since the insulin requirements may drop markedly after delivery. During and after either cesarean section or labor and delivery, the mothers should be adequately hydrated as well as supplied with glucose. As a rule, 3 liters of fluid—in the form of 2 liters of 5 per cent glucose in distilled water and 1 liter of 5 per cent glucose in normal saline or in lactated Ringer's solution—are indicated during the day of delivery. Plasma glucose levels should be checked frequently and regular insulin administered accordingly. The urine, or preferably the plasma, should be checked for ketones. The insulin requirements may fluctuate markedly during the first few days after delivery.

It is extremely important that the robust appearance of the newly delivered infant not lead to inappropriate care. Although the infant may appear mature on the basis of his size, functionally he may be quite premature and must be so treated.

Sterilization should be considered for multiparous women with diabetes, especially those with vascular or renal disease.

Diabetes Insipidus.   This condition is a rare complication of pregnancy. We have cared for only one case in the past 15 years, during which there were approximately 90,000 deliveries. While the patient took vasopressin for replacement therapy, the pregnancy progressed without serious complication. This experience is similar to those reported by others (Hendricks; Alexander and Downs; Chau and associates). In some instances there appears to have been an impairment of labor, possibly caused by lack of or reduced amounts of endogenous oxytocin. A patient recently described by Chau and associates lactated normally, with measured milk ejection pressures comparable to those of normal lactating women.

Adrenal Dysfunction. Before 1953 only 50 published cases of *Addison's disease* in pregnancy had been identified, suggesting that untreated adrenal hypofunction causes sterility. With the advent of cortisone and related compounds, pregnancy has become much more common in women with adrenocortical hypofunction. For example, during the past decade we have cared for four pregnancies in three women, two of whom had Addison's disease and one of whom had undergone *bilateral adrenalectomy* for Cushing's syndrome. The four infants, as well as the mothers, all survived, although one mother close to the time of delivery developed pyelonephritis, bacterial shock, and bleeding from a central placenta previa.

It is essential during pregnancy and the puerperium to observe the mother quite closely for evidence of either inadequate or excessive steroid replacement. Except at times of stress, replacement therapy need not be greater and sometimes may be less than in the nonpregnant state. There may be little or no need during pregnancy for compounds with potent mineralocorticoid action. During and after labor and delivery or a surgical procedure, the amount of steroid replacement would be increased appreciably to approximate the normal response at that time in women with intact adrenals. It is important that shock from causes other than adrenocortical insufficiency be promptly recognized and treated, especially that caused by blood loss or bacterial infection, as in the case described.

Pregnancy associated with *Cushing's syndrome* is rare, since anovulation is a typical feature of the illness, but seven such pregnancies are reported by Hunt and McConahey.

Although aldosterone is produced in large amounts during much of pregnancy, it is not essential for a successful outcome. A few cases of primary aldosteronism in association with pregnancy are reported. In view of the very high levels of aldosterone in normal pregnancies, it is not surprising that there may be amelioration of symptoms as well as electrolyte disturbances during pregnancy (Biglieri and Slaton).

Pheochromocytoma. Pheochromocytoma is a rare complication of pregnancy; both the maternal and the fetal mortalities have been extremely high (Bowen and associates; Fox and associates).

Porphyria. Acute idiopathic porphyria is a rare metabolic dysfunction caused by an inborn error of porphyrin metabolism. It may present a wide range of symptoms affecting the skin, gastrointestinal tract, pelvic organs, and nervous system. It is of special importance to obstetricians to understand that the symptoms may be greatly aggravated by barbiturates. The subject is discussed by O'Dwyer and reviewed by Tricomi and Baum.

Thyroid Disease. Pregnancy normally induces a number of changes in the thyroid, some of which might be erroneously interpreted as indicating disease.

The variations include modest diffuse enlargement of the gland, elevation of the level of circulating thyroxin and thyroid-binding proteins, increased thyroid uptake of radioiodide, and decreased binding in vitro of triiodothyronine by resin (Ch. 8, p. 267). Therefore it is very important, but at times difficult, to differentiate changes of normal pregnancy from actual disease.

Helpful signs for identifying *hyperthyroidism* during pregnancy are persistent tachycardia, including a high pulse rate while sleeping, and exophthalmos. The level of circulating thyroid hormone measured as thyroxin, protein-bound iodine, or butanol-extractable iodine is markedly elevated compared with normal values in the nonpregnant state. Most often the serum protein-bound iodine concentration, for example, is 12 mcg per 100 ml or higher. At the same time, in vitro tests fail to demonstrate the decreased uptake of triiodothyronine that is characteristic of normal pregnancy. Measurement of radioiodine uptake by the thyroid is contradindicated during pregnancy.

Treatment may be medical or surgical, or initially medical until such time as the mother is nearly euthyroid, and then surgical. Hyperthyroidism nearly always can be controlled by antithyroid drugs, so that the disease, if treated adequately, need not be a serious threat to the mother. Medical treatment, however, has the potential for causing severe fetal complications. Propylthiouracil and similar compounds readily cross the placenta and may induce fetal hypothyroidism and goiter. Therefore, it has been recommended commonly that the drug be given in doses that effectively suppress maternal thyroid activity while the mother receives thyroid hormone simultaneously to provide hormone to the fetus. It now seems doubtful that the hormone in the doses so administered crosses the placenta to the fetus in significant amounts; therefore, it serves only to increase the requirements for propylthiouracil. Consequently, a regimen employing propylthiouracil or compounds with similar actions without thyroid hormone is favored in our clinic. The dose of propylthiouracil should be increased until the woman appears to be only minimally toxic and the level of thyroid hormone in the blood is reduced to the upper normal range for pregnancy. In case of very severe hyperthyroidism, treatment with adrenocorticosteroids or chlorpromazine is not contraindicated by the pregnancy.

Burrow and associates have carried out a long-term study of the intellectual and physical development, including thyroid function, of the children born to thyrotoxic mothers treated with propylthiouracil during pregnancy. Although the number of children studied was small, the data do not suggest that propylthiouracil therapy during pregnancy had an adverse effect on subsequent growth and development of the child. The prolonged administration of iodide to the mother along with propylthiouracil appears to increase appreciably the likelihood of gross goiter in the fetus. Therefore iodide should be used only preceding the time of thyroidectomy and not for long-term therapy.

Thyroidectomy may be carried out after the thyrotoxicosis has been brought under control. Opinions differ as to the wisdom of surgical treatment during the first trimester, a time when abortion is relatively common, or during the third trimester, when delivery may occur prematurely. From the beginning of the second until early in the third trimester, however, subtotal thyroidectomy often is the treatment of choice after achieving control medically (Talbert and associates).

Women with *Graves' disease*, even though they are no longer hyperthyroid, may give birth to infants with manifestations of thyrotoxicosis, including goiter and exophthalmos. Long-acting thyroid stimulator (LATS), a gamma globulin synthesized by the mother presumably as an autoimmune phenomenon, is transferred across the placenta to the fetus. Its activity persists for some time in the infant after birth.

Overt *hypothyroidism* is often associated with infertility, and in women who do become pregnant the likelihood of abortion seems to be increased considerably. In general, hypothyroidism can be diagnosed if the expected rise, during pregnancy, of the level of circulating thyroxin or hormonal iodine fails to take place. Measurement of serum cholesterol is of little value, since pregnancy induces an increase in the cholesterol concentration. The infant of a mother with severe hypothyroidism may be a cretin but is most often normal.

Simple colloid goiter if unassociated with hypothyroidism has no influence on pregnancy.

Parathyroid Diseases. *Hyperparathyroidism* rarely complicates pregnancy, even though the disease is more common in women and has a peak incidence before the menopause. Whalley has described four cases cared for at Parkland Memorial Hospital. One case with parathyroid storm characterized by hypercalcemia and convulsions was especially interesting. The convulsions together with chronic pyelonephritis and chronic hypertension might erroneously have been considered to be caused by eclampsia.

Tetany has been noted occasionally in the newborn infants of mothers with hyperparathyroidism. At times it has led to a search that identified a maternal parathyroid adenoma (Hartenstein and Gardner).

Hypoparathyroidism is equally uncommon in pregnancy. Treatment with dihydrotachysterol or large doses of vitamin D, together with calcium gluconate or calcium lactate and a diet low in phosphates, usually prevents symptomatic hypocalcemia (O'Leary and associates). The risk to the fetus from large doses of either dihydrotachysterol or vitamin D_2 is not established. Whether these compounds cause cardiovascular and other anomalies is not clear.

Obesity. Marked obesity is a hazard to the pregnant woman and her fetus. For example, Tracy and Miller, in the course of reviewing the pregnancies of 48 women whose weights averaged 284 pounds, noted that nearly two thirds developed some obstetric complication. One of the 5 mothers diagnosed as having diabetes expired. Over half of the 48 were considered hypertensive, and pyelonephritis developed in 5.

In our experience a large variety of serious complications of pregnancy is more likely to develop, including hypertension, diabetes, aspiration of gastric contents during anesthesia, wound complications, and thromboembolism. The most extreme case of obesity we have encountered during pregnancy was in a young multipara who early in the third trimester weighed 508 pounds although she was only 62 inches tall. In spite of a variety of complications 6 pregnancies have produced 8 living children.

Management of obesity during pregnancy is a challenge. A program of weight reduction utilizing a diet restricted in calories but providing all essential nutrients has commonly been recommended for obese pregnant women. If such a regimen is used, however, it is mandatory that the quality of the diet be monitored closely and that ketosis not be allowed to develop. Ketosis during pregnancy has been implicated in the genesis of impaired intelligence of the offspring (Ch. 12, p. 343).

Syphilis. During the past few years there has been a disturbing increase in the incidence of syphilis, leaving no doubt about the need for intensive control programs. An unusually critical time to detect and treat syphilis is during pregnancy—to protect the mother and her sexual partner from the numerous complications of syphilis and, especially important, to promptly treat the mother to prevent the extensive pathologic changes that characterize congenital syphilis (Ch. 37, p. 1053). The need for vigilant programs for detecting and treating syphilis in obstetric clinics is emphasized by the recent observations of Coblentz and associates, who report a sixfold increase in congenital syphilis at Los Angeles County–University of Southern California Medical Center. A decade ago the incidence of congenital syphilis at that institution was 2 cases per 10,000 births; now it is 12 per 10,000 births.

When infection is acquired during pregnancy, the primary lesion, or sometimes multiple lesions, involving the genital tract may be of such size or so located as to go unnoticed. In some instances, however, it may be somewhat larger than usual, presumably because of the increased vascularity of the genitalia. The lesions of secondary syphilis are often slight; they may be limited to the genitalia, where they appear usually as elevated areas, or condylomata lata, which occasionally cause ulceration of the vulva. Unfortunately, in many patients no history of a local sore or rash can be elicited. The first suggestion of the disease is the delivery of an infant that may be either stillborn or liveborn but severely afflicted with congenital syphilis. A suitable serologic screening test such as the Venereal Disease Research Laboratory (VDRL) slide test must be performed on blood obtained at the time of the first prenatal visit. This procedure is required by law in many states. Fortunately, serologic tests for syphilis will almost always be positive by four to six weeks after contracting the disease.

It is firmly established that adequate treatment of the mother before the eighteenth week of pregnancy prevents infection of the fetus, since the fetus rarely if ever becomes infected before that time; and because penicillin crosses the placenta, treatment of the mother practically always will also successfully treat the infected fetus. Hardy and associates, however, have recently reported an instance of congenital syphilis in which penicillin in acceptable doses given to the mother 10 days before delivery and to the newborn in massive doses for 17 days after birth failed to rid the infant of *Treponema pallidum*. The infant succumbed from widespread lues.

The Bureau of Disease Prevention and Environmental Control of the National Communicable Disease Center recommends, for people not allergic to penicillin, the use of either benzathine penicillin G (Bicillin) or procaine penicillin G (Crysticillin, Duracillin). For primary, secondary, or early latent syphilis a single treatment of 2.4 million units of benzathine penicillin G intramuscularly (one half of the dose in each buttock) or 4.8 million units of aqueous procaine penicillin G in 8 daily doses of 600,000 units intramuscularly should be used. For late syphilis these same drugs are recommended, but in total doses of 6 million to 9 million units given intramuscularly in divided doses.

If the mother is allergic to penicillin, several of the broad-spectrum anti-biotics are effective, including erythromycin and tetracycline. Erythromycin is usually preferred because of lower toxicity; the effective dose is 500 mg orally 4 times a day for 15 days for a total of 30 g.

The obstetrician is sometimes faced with the problem of the pregnant woman who is known to have been exposed to infectious syphilis but has no obvious stigmata of the disease. Occasionally in early syphilis neither local nor generalized lesions develop, or they are so slight as to escape notice. Although every effort, including physical examination, should be made to arrive at a diagnosis before administering treatment to someone known to have been exposed to infectious syphilis, it is fallacious to procrastinate until clinical or laboratory stigmata appear. Adequate treatment is 2.4 million units of benzathine penicillin G, intramuscularly, one half of the dose in each buttock.

The mother who has been treated successfully often remains susceptible to a subsequent syphilitic infection, as does her fetus. Therefore, it is very important during pregnancy to treat her sexual partner and to observe her closely for evidence of reinfection. When reinfection is detected, retreatment is necessary.

Gonorrhea.   In women infection caused by *Neisseria gonorrhoeae* may be limited to the lower genital tract, including the cervix, urethra and periurethral glands, and Bartholin's glands, or it may spread across the endometrium to involve the oviducts and the peritoneum. The organism enters the bloodstream to cause arthritis uncommonly and endocarditis rarely.

Acute gonococcal salpingitis is not a problem in pregnancy after the third month when the chorion laeve has fused with the decidua parietalis to obliterate the endometrial cavity between the cervix and oviduct. Rarely a fallopian tube previously damaged by infection with *Neisseria gonorrhoeae*, however, may become reinfected during pregnancy with other organisms that reach the oviduct through the bloodstream or lymphatics.

Bacteriologic evidence of gonorrheal infection, as well as increased resistance of the organism to penicillin, is currently noted with alarming frequency. There has been a steady increase in the incidence of gonorrhea in the United States for several years. In 1968, there were 431,280 cases recorded, but it has been estimated that the true figure for that year was over 1,500,000. The greatly increased prevalence of gonorrhea in recent years has not spared pregnant women; many obstetric clinics have noted gonococcal infections of the lower genitourinary tract quite commonly. Kraus and Yen, for example, in a study of all pregnant women near term attending a prenatal clinic in Cleveland found that cultures of cervical swabbings were positive for *Neisseria gonorrhoeae* in 5.7 per cent. Cave and associates have obtained almost identical results in obstetric patients studied in the clinic of a large voluntary hospital in Brooklyn.

The pregnant woman may have asymptomatic local infection involving, singly or in combination, the lower genital tract, the lower urinary tract, the vagina, and the rectum (Table 10). The infection may antedate the pregnancy; or the patient may have acquired the disease at the time of the insemination that resulted in pregnancy, in which case she is likely to develop symptomatic acute salpingitis; or she may have become infected locally after the uterine cavity had been obliterated by fusion of chorion and decidua, and a well-formed mucous plug had sealed the cervical canal. In any event either no treatment or inadequate treatment with persistence of the infection allows her to infect her sexual partner, to suffer gonococcal arthritis, to infect her infant at the time of delivery,

Table 10. Frequency of Cultures Positive for *Neisseria gonorrhoeae*

Site Cultured	First Visit (%)	Second Visit° (%)
Cervix	94	89
Vagina	78	82
Urethra	78	71
Rectum	49	57

° *No treatment during interval from previous culture.*
From Schmale, Martin, and Domescik. JAMA 210:312, 1969.

thereby causing gonorrheal ophthalmia (Ch. 19, p. 486), and to develop an ascending infection of the genital tract after delivery. Consequently, even asymptomatic disease during pregnancy should be identified and eradicated.

Unfortunately, positive identification of *Neisseria gonorrhoeae* has not been simple, because of difficulties associated with culturing the organism as well as the relative inaccuracy of examination of smears for intracellular gram-negative diplococci. Schmale and associates have recommended that specimens be taken for culture with a sterile cotton-tipped applicator, be immediately rolled onto Thayer-Martin medium, and be placed in a candle jar at room temperature. Subsequently all cultures from that day are taken to the laboratory for streak dilution and incubation. After overnight incubation in the candle jar, the cultures are examined; if typical colonies on the selective medium are oxidase-positive and show gram-negative diplococci on gram stain, they are judged to be presumptively positive for *Neisseria gonorrhoeae*. Identification is confirmed by sugar fermentation or by direct fluorescent antibody staining. Schmale and co-workers carefully remove the mucous plug and obtain the specimens for smear from the endocervix. They also obtain cultures from the urethra, vagina, and rectal crypts. As shown in Table 10, cultures from the cervix are most often positive. The observations of Schmale and associates indicate that, in spite of obtaining cultures from all four sites, 6 to 8 per cent of women infected with *Neisseria gonorrhoeae* will not be identified except by repeated cultures.

There is evidence of increased resistance of *Neisseria gonorrhoeae* especially in Southeast Asia (Johnson and associates), penicillin remains the treatment of choice in most instances. Procaine penicillin G suspension, 2.4 million units intramuscularly daily for 2 to 4 days, most often effectively eradicates infections of the lower genital tract. In a few instances, especially if there is rectal involvement, the dose may be inadequate and it should then be repeated. Ampicillin in a single oral dose of 3.5 g has been found to be effective by Johnson and associates. In case of infections other than those of the lower genitourinary tract—for example, gonococcal arthritis—penicillin therapy should be continued for at least 10 days.

If the woman is sensitive to penicillin, other antibiotics may be used. Erythromycin, 0.5 g orally 4 times a day for 5 to 10 days, or tetracycline, 0.25 g orally 4 times a day for a similar period of time, is usually effective in eradicating the infection. McLone and co-workers point out that tetracycline in a single dose of 1.5 g is an acceptable alternative to penicillin. Johnson and associates, however, have noted recently increasing resistance of *Neisseria gonorrhoeae* to tetracycline. Recently kanamycin (Kantrex) has been recommended for treatment of some cases of gonorrhea in women. Shapiro and Lentz report a cure rate of 91 per cent after a single treatment with 2 g of kanamycin intramuscularly, 1 g in each buttock. They emphasize that ototoxicity and nephrotoxicity are very unlikely unless kanamycin therapy is prolonged. Differing from penicillin, erythromycin, and tetracycline, kanamycin has no effect on *Treponema pallidum* and therefore does not alter the course of a syphilitic infection.

Other Venereal Diseases. Chancroid, granuloma inguinale, and lymphopathia venereum are uncommon. In the pregnant woman the lesions of *granuloma inguinale* tend to be multiple, large, quite foul-smelling ulcerations of the vulva, lower vagina, perineum, and cervix. The causative organism, *Donovania granulomatis,* at times disseminates to cause lesions remote from the lower genital tract, especially in bone. Diagnosis depends upon identification of Donovan bodies in large mononuclear cells in Giemsa-stained smears from the lesion. Tetracycline, 2 g per day in divided doses for 15 to 20 days, is usually effective, although at times a vulvar lesion may heal incompletely or with gross deformity, ultimately requiring vulvectomy.

The primary genital infection of *lymphopathia venereum* is transient and seldom recognized. Inguinal adenitis may follow and at times lead to suppuration. Ultimately the lymphatics of the lower genital tract and the perirectal tissues may be involved in sclerosis and fibrosis, which cause vulvar elephantiasis and especially severe rectal stricture. Sometimes attention is first drawn to the disease in pregnant women when rectal examination is attempted. The Frei test is usually positive, as is the complement-fixation test. Sulfadiazine has been the standard treatment of the early disease; tetracycline is of value for treating draining buboes.

A careful vaginal examination is of utmost importance in deciding upon the method of delivery. If there is widespread pelvic scarring, cesarean section is indicated. Marked perirectal fibrosis with cicatricial changes in the rectovaginal septum is usually indicative of an extensive process that requires abdominal delivery. The extent and intensity of these fibrotic changes rather than the size of the rectal stricture dictate cesarean section. As the data of Kaiser and King indicate, 9 out of 10 patients with lymphopathia venereum can be delivered safely by the vaginal route. It is crucial, however, to avoid difficult vaginal delivery, since most ruptures of the rectum reported in this complication have occurred in association with traumatic vaginal operations. Colostomy presents no special problems in abdominal or vaginal delivery. Although treatment with tetracyclines may arrest the infection of lymphopathia venereum and clear up secondary infections, they, of course, fail to influence preexisting fibrotic changes.

Chancroid is usually a self-limiting disease that produces a painful, nonindurated ulcer, or "soft chancre," in the lower genital tract and painful inguinal lymphadenopathy. The causative organism, *Hemophilus ducreyi,* is sensitive to sulfisoxazole (Gantrisin) and to tetracycline as well as other antibiotics.

DISEASES OF THE LIVER AND ALIMENTARY TRACT

Viral Hepatitis. Classification of viral hepatitis as either infectious or serum hepatitis on the basis of a history of parenteral administration of blood or some blood products is no longer tenable. It now appears quite certain that there are two viruses that cause hepatitis. Each is capable of inducing hepatitis after either ingestion or parenteral administration of infected material, and each causes hepatitis after a relatively well-defined period of incubation (Krugman and Giles).

Adams and Combes at Parkland Memorial Hospital noted one maternal death in 34 instances of viral hepatitis complicating pregnancy. Two women aborted and two infants that were delivered prematurely succumbed. These results are much more favorable than those reported by investigators in some developing countries. For example, D'Cruz and associates in Bombay, India, noted a mortality rate of 54 per cent among 143 hospitalized pregnant or puerperal women compared with 26 per cent in nonpregnant women. By American standards, the mortality rates are very high for both groups. The causes are probably malnutrition and the restriction of hospitalization to only the most seriously ill patients.

Our regimen for the treatment of hepatitis in pregnancy consists basically in hospitalization, bed rest, and a good diet. Fluids, electrolytes, and calories are provided intravenously if vomiting is a problem. Corticosteroids are used in severe cases.

It is important that the pregnant woman with hepatitis be diagnosed and so treated long before she becomes moribund. The physician must not ignore the possibility of hepatitis in any pregnant woman who complains of nausea and vomiting. Unfortunately, these symptoms are sometimes incorrectly ascribed to pregnancy itself rather than to hepatitis. As a result, supportive treatment may be ignored until the mother becomes gravely ill.

Australia antigen is a viruslike particle that quite likely is the infective agent in cases of so-called serum, or long incubation, hepatitis. More recently the detection of another antigen called epidemic-hepatitis-associated antigen has been reported by DelPrete and co-workers. This antigen is believed to be the infective agent that causes epidemic, or short incubation, hepatitis.

Neither London and associates nor Schweitzer and Spears were able to identify Australia antigen in cord blood even though the mothers' sera were positive. Subsequently the infants' sera became positive suggesting that the long incubation hepatitis associated antigen need not cross the placenta to infect the infant. Schweitzer and Spears also noted the antigen to be present in the infant for long periods without causing hepatitis. A great many more such studies are needed, of course, to ascertain further the ability of the infectious agents causing viral hepatitis to cross the placenta and reach the fetus. Viral hepatitis transmitted to the fetus from the mother has been described (Stokes and associates), although we have not identified this process in newborn infants at Parkland Memorial Hospital.

Acute Yellow Atrophy of the Liver.   This extremely rare complication of pregnancy occurs in two forms: (1) true acute yellow atrophy, a disease seen in pregnant as well as nonpregnant women and characterized by massive hepatocellular necrosis; and (2) "obstetric" acute yellow atrophy, a disease characterized by fatty infiltration of the hepatic cells without necrosis (Fig. 6).

The association of true acute yellow atrophy with infectious hepatitis was shown conclusively by Lucké. Similar cases were studied by Zondek and Bromberg in Israel in pregnant women during an epidemic of infectious hepatitis. The clinical picture includes profound prostration, mahogany jaundice, and coma.

The belief that there is a type of yellow atrophy peculiar to pregnancy has received strong support from the studies of Sheehan, as well as those of Ober and LeCompte and of Kahil and associates, who presented 2 new cases and 39 others collected from the literature up to 1964. This disease is often fatal, although rare cases with recovery have been reported. The characteristic pathologic change is infiltration of all the hepatic cells by fine fatty droplets, without the necrosis that

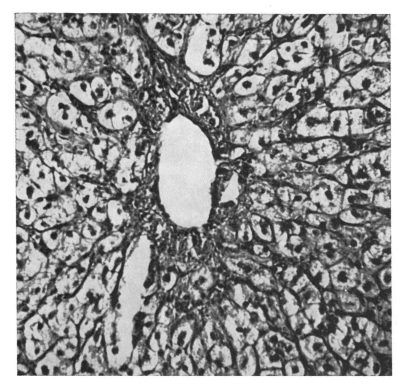

Fig. 6. Fatty metamorphosis of liver.

characterizes viral hepatitis. Although sporadic cases without obvious cause occur in pregnancy, indistinguishable cases resulting from toxicity of tetracycline have been reported in nonpregnant women by Schultz and associates, as well as by Schiffer, and in similarly treated pregnant women with pyelonephritis by Whalley, Adams, and Combes. Kunelis, Peters, and Edmondson also have discussed the relation of the fatty liver of pregnancy to therapy with tetracyclines.

Obstetric Hepatosis.   Described under a variety of names, including recurrent jaundice of pregnancy, idiopathic cholestasis of pregnancy, cholestatic hepatosis, and icterus gravidarum, this condition is characterized clinically by either icterus, pruritus, or both. The major lesion is intrahepatic cholestasis with centrolobular bile staining without inflammatory cells or proliferation of mesenchymal cells.

The modest hyperbilirubinemia results predominantly from conjugated pigment. Bromsulphalein excretion is impaired, and serum alkaline phosphatase may be elevated above the usual levels for pregnancy. Serum glutamic oxalacetic transaminase activity may be moderately elevated. These changes disappear after delivery but often recur in a subsequent pregnancy or when an oral contraceptive containing potent estrogen is employed (Kreek and associates).

Pruritus associated with obstetric hepatosis may be quite troublesome; cholestyramine has been reported to provide relief in most cases (Lutz and Margolis).

Cholelithiasis and Cholecystitis.   The greater frequency (twice or three times as high) of cholelithiasis in women than in men suggests a possible association with the increase in cholesterol in the blood during pregnancy. In a review of the literature, however, Robertson and Dochat conclude that pregnancy does not account significantly for the higher incidence of gallstones in women.

Acute attacks of gallbladder disease during pregnancy or the puerperium, in general, are managed the same way as in the nonpregnant woman. When surgery is thought to be indicated in the pregnant woman, procrastination should be avoided. Delay can only place the woman and her fetus in greater jeopardy. At times just drainage of the gallbladder is the procedure of choice. Recent surgery does not complicate labor unduly.

Cirrhosis of the Liver. Borhanmanesh and Haghighi, on the basis of their own observations, as well as a review of the experiences reported by others, conclude that pregnancy does not have a deleterious effect on cirrhosis. On the other hand, cirrhosis exerts an adverse effect on pregnancy; they noted a high rate of both stillbirths and prematurity.

Hyperemesis Gravidarum. Nausea and vomiting of moderate intensity are especially common complaints from the second to the fourth month of gestation (Ch. 12, p. 343). Fortunately, vomiting sufficiently pernicious to produce weight loss, dehydration, acidosis from starvation, alkalosis from loss of hydrochloric acid in vomitus, and hypokalemia has become quite rare.

Treatment of pernicious vomiting of pregnancy comprises correction of deficits of fluid and electrolytes and of acidosis or alkalosis by means of appropriate amounts of sodium, potassium, chloride, lactate or bicarbonate, glucose, and water, which should be administered parenterally until the vomiting has been controlled. Appropriate steps should be taken to detect other diseases—for example, gastroenteritis, cholecystitis, hepatitis, peptic ulcer, and pyelonephritis. Drugs such as dimenhydrinate (Dramamine) or chlorpromazine (Thorazine) administered parenterally may be of considerable value. In many instances social and psychologic factors contribute to the illness, as in the case of the young unwed mother who continues to live with her parents while they harass her because of her "sin." Therefore positive assistance with psychologic and social problems often proves quite beneficial. Rarely is it necessary to interrupt the pregnancy. Not infrequently the patient improves remarkably while hospitalized only to relapse after discharge. The subject of nausea and vomiting in pregnancy has been reviewed extensively by Fairweather.

Appendicitis. Gestation does not predispose to appendicitis, but because of the general prevalence of the disease, there is an incidence of about 1 in every 2,000 pregnancies, as shown in Black's extensive review (Table 11). Pregnancy

Table 11. **The Maternal Mortality from Acute Appendicitis in Pregnancy According to Time of Occurrence**

	Present Series	Literature	Total	Per Cent Incidence	Per Cent Mortality
First trimester	2	122	124	35.1	0
Second trimester	13	107	120	33.9	4.0
Third trimester	6	89	95	26.9	11.5
Labor	2	4	6	1.7	16.7
Puerperium	2	6	8	2.3	0
Total	25	328	353		

Modified from Black. Brit Med J. 1:1938, 1960.

often makes diagnosis more difficult. First, anorexia, nausea, and vomiting caused by pregnancy itself are fairly common. Second, as the uterus enlarges, the appendix commonly moves upward and outward toward the flank, so that pain and tenderness may not be prominent in the right lower quadrant. Third, some degree of leukocytosis is the rule during normal pregnancy. Fourth, during pregnancy especially, other diseases may be readily confused with appendicitis, such as pyelonephritis, renal colic caused by a stone or kinking of a ureter, placental abruption, and red, or carneous, degeneration of a myoma.

Appendicitis increases the likelihood of abortion or premature labor, especially if peritonitis develops. The fetal loss rate, therefore, in most series is about 15 per cent. As pointed out by Hoffman and Suzuki, the maternal mortality depends upon the duration of the infection and the period of gestation. As the appendix is pushed progressively higher by the growing uterus, walling off of the infection becomes increasingly unlikely and appendiceal rupture causes widespread peritonitis. Acute appendicitis in the last trimester, therefore carries a grave prognosis, as shown in Table 11, and in the work of King and Anderson. Although antibiotics have reduced the mortality from acute appendicitis in pregnancy, the disease remains one of the more serious complications of gestation.

The treatment, regardless of the stage of gestation, is immediate operation. Even though diagnostic errors sometimes lead to the removal of a normal appendix, it is better to operate unnecessarily than to postpone intervention until generalized peritonitis has developed. The mortality of appendicitis today in the obstetric patient is essentially that associated with surgical delay.

It is important that during the operation and period of recovery both hypoxia and hypotension be avoided. If they are avoided and generalized peritonitis does not develop, the prognosis is quite good. Seldom, if ever, is cesarean section indicated at the time of appendectomy. Aside from local soreness, a recent abdominal incision presents no problem during labor and vaginal delivery.

Peptic Ulcer. An active peptic ulcer is rare during pregnancy, and complications such as perforation or hemorrhage are even rarer (Honiotes and associates). Vasicka, Lin, and Bright, however, indicate that in a small proportion of cases, peptic ulcers become aggravated by pregnancy, and massive hemorrhage may occur.

Pancreatitis. Pancreatitis during pregnancy is rare. The principles of therapy, in general, are the same as for nonpregnant patients; treatment is medical rather than surgical. Two commonly used drugs—tetracycline and the thiazides—have been implicated in pancreatitis in pregnant women (Whalley and co-investigators; Minkowitz and associates). Montgomery and Miller have recently reviewed the published reports concerned with pancreatitis and pregnancy.

Intestinal Obstruction. This grave complication of pregnancy results most frequently from pressure of the growing uterus on intestinal adhesions resulting from previous abdominal operations. Of 10 cases reported by Bellingham, Mackey, and Winston, there was a history of previous abdominal operation in 9. As emphasized by these authors, as well as by Waters and McCall, the mortality rate tends to be very high, chiefly because of error in diagnosis, late diagnosis, reluctance to operate on a pregnant woman, and inadequate preparation for surgery. The large pregnant uterus, furthermore, lying anterior to the intestinal obstruction, may mask the abdominal signs, thus contributing greatly to the difficulty of diagnosis.

Kohn, Briele, and Douglass have reported a remarkable case in which the same patient was operated upon for *volvulus* four times, three of the operations having been performed in the course of two pregnancies. In a review of the literature, they collected 79 cases of volvulus in pregnancy. In a third of the cases reported by Harer and Harer, emptying the uterus by cesarean section was necessary to obtain proper exposure.

Carcinoma of the Bowel.   Carcinoma of the rectum and colon is a rare complication of pregnancy, 65 cases having been reported in a review of the literature by Waters and Fenimore.

Ulcerative Colitis.   In an analysis of one of the largest series of cases reported, Crohn and his associates found that colitis quiescent at the beginning of gestation is reactivated by pregnancy, usually in the first trimester, in about half the cases. If the colitis is already active at the time of conception, it is materially aggravated in three quarters of the cases. They emphasize also the excessive and prolonged severity of postpartum recurrences. Felsen and Wolarsky, in an analysis of the clinical course of 34 women with ulcerative colitis in 50 pregnancies, found that in one third of the pregnancies the colitis was somewhat aggravated in the first trimester but was definitely ameliorated in about one half. When this disease becomes worse in gestation, the etiologic factor may be psychogenic, rather than related to any intrinsic effect of pregnancy. The patient's fear that pregnancy will aggravate her disease, for example, may precipitate an exacerbation. Reassurance is therefore an important part of management.

Patients with *colostomies* usually go through pregnancy without difficulty. Intestinal obstruction caused by pressure of the enlarged uterus on the proximal loop of intestine concerned rarely occurs. Some of the problems that may be anticipated in this group of patients have been reviewed by Scudamore and associates.

Regional Enteritis.   Fielding and Cooke have recently reported their extensive experiences with pregnancies complicated by Crohn's disease. In those women who became pregnant there was no evidence that pregnancy exerted adverse effects on the course of the disease or increased the mortality rate. Moreover, abortion, prematurity, and stillbirth were not increased. Sterility was the main problem encountered.

Gingivitis.   Rarely the gums of pregnant women become inflamed and spongy, bleeding upon the slightest touch. In many cases the condition clears almost immediately after delivery. It is best treated by a combination of oral hygiene and a well-balanced diet. An *epulis*, a focal, highly vascular swelling of the gingiva, is an occasional complication (Ch. 8, Fig. 14).

OTHER VIRAL INFECTIONS

Various viruses have been recovered from the fetus, but only three—rubella virus, cytomegalovirus, and herpesvirus hominis—have proved to be teratogenic. Others that may reach the fetus include the viruses causing measles (rubeola) chickenpox (varicella), smallpox (variola), vaccinia, poliomyelitis, hepatitis, Western equine encephalitis, mumps, and the Coxsackie B group (Sever).

About 5 per cent of pregnancies are complicated by clinically apparent viral infections, according to the Collaborative Perinatal Research Study. Excluding the common cold, the most frequent viral infections are influenza, flulike disease, cold sore-herpesvirus infections, viral gastroenteritis, and viral infection of larynx, pharynx, and tonsils.

Rubella (German Measles).   Rubella, a disease of minor importance in the absence of pregnancy, has been directly responsible for inestimable perinatal loss and, perhaps even more important, serious malformations in the liveborn infant. The relation between maternal rubella and grave congenital malformations was first recognized by Gregg in 1941.

The diagnosis of rubella is at times quite difficult. Not only are the clinical features of other illnesses quite similar, but subclinical cases with viremia and the capability of infecting the embryo and fetus are not rare. Diagnosis of rubella, therefore, can be made with certainty only by isolation of the virus or by the more practical demonstration of a rising rubella antibody titer in the serum. Absence of rubella antibody detected by hemagglutination inhibition indicates lack of immunity. The presence of antibody denotes an immune response to rubella viremia that may have been acquired anywhere from a few weeks to many years earlier.

Various studies have shown that from 10 to nearly 20 per cent of adult women in the United States are susceptible to rubella (Skinner; Burroughs and Bollman; Bowes and co-workers). In the far western states as many as 50 to 75 per cent of women are susceptible (Sever). Of considerable importance, a poor correlation has been noted between the presence or absence of rubella antibody and a history of previous rubella infection.

The nonimmune person who acquires rubella viremia demonstrates peak antibody titers one to two weeks after the onset of the rash, or two to three weeks after the onset of viremia, since the viremia precedes clinically evident disease by about one week (Cooper and Krugman). The promptness of the antibody response, therefore, may complicate serodiagnosis unless serum is collected initially within a very few days after the onset of the rash. If, for example, the first specimen was obtained approximately ten days after the rash, detection of antibodies would fail to differentiate between two possibilities: one, that the very recent disease was actually rubella and, two, that it was not rubella, but the person was already immune to rubella. Since the primary antibody response to rubella virus is the production of a specific IgM antibody, it is possible sometimes to identify recent infection by treating the serum with a sulfhydryl reducing compound such as 2-mercaptoethanol, which inactivates IgM antibody. Failure of such treatment to reduce the hemagglutination-inhibition rubella antibody titer, however, does not always exclude recent infection (Cooper and associates). The detection of rubella antibody by hemagglutination inhibition with a negative complement-fixation test more precisely identifies previous rubella infection with immunity.

There is no known chemotherapeutic or antibiotic agent that will prevent viremia in nonimmune subjects exposed to rubella. The use of gamma globulin for this purpose remains controversial. Brody and co-workers, during a rubella outbreak in an isolated community, gave relatively large doses of gamma globulin to boys but not to girls at the time of, or even before, exposure. The attack rate, measured by seroconversion, among the boys was 44 per cent and among the girls 85 per cent. The group that received gamma globulin, therefore, was only partially protected. The data of Brody and associates also suggest that large doses of gamma globulin given at or before exposure to rubella may only minimize the clinical features of the disease. Viremia without clinically apparent disease can, of course, lead to fetal infection with disastrous consequences.

Even though effective vaccines for rubella are now available, there are problems inherent in immunizing the estimated two million or more women of child-bearing age who are susceptible. A lesser problem is the occurrence of arthralgia or arthritis after administration of some vaccines. Preliminary studies indicate, however, that of those currently available the Cendehill rubella vaccine is not so likely to cause troublesome arthralgia or arthritis in adult women (Halstead). The major problem is the hazard of congenital rubella infection caused by inadvertent vaccination of a woman either a short time before or during pregnancy. The evidence reported by Vaheri and associates strongly suggests that the intrauterine rubella infection can be produced by the vaccination. Rubella vaccination of women during the childbearing period, consequently, should be considered only for those women not at risk of pregnancy.

Strict adherence to the following program for immunizing women of childbearing age susceptible to rubella should prove satisfactory: (1) Identify susceptible women by means of the hemagglutination-inhibition antibody test. The majority of women will be immune to the rubella virus and can be so assured. (2) Non-immune women would be eligible for vaccination only if pregnancy can be avoided for a minimum of three months after vaccination. (3) On the basis of available evidence, abortion is probably indicated for women who are subsequently shown to have been in early pregnancy at the time of vaccination or who conceive during the next several weeks.

There will be failures in any program of contraception. Women least likely to become pregnant are those who have been delivered within the week before vaccination and those who take oral contraceptives in the approved way. Farquhar has reported the results of administration of the Cendehill strain of rubella virus vaccine to 115 rubella-susceptible women a few days after they had been delivered. Rubella antibody was detected subsequently by hemagglutination inhibition in 98 per cent. Troublesome side effects were very uncommon. Each vaccinated patient agreed in writing to adhere to a reliable method of birth control for a minimum of two months after vaccination. Horstmann and associates have made identical observations.

Mass vaccination programs in children are currently underway. A very important question concerning the value of such immunization programs has yet to be answered: Will the antibody titers persist at levels sufficient to maintain immunity or will they fall to leave the woman vaccinated as a child susceptible to rubella?

The numerous reports concerned with the frequency of major fetal developmental defects thought due to rubella are difficult to interpret because of the lack of precision inherent previously in the diagnosis of rubella. Forbes believes that the diagnosis of rubella may have been erroneous in as many as 50 per cent of the cases. The frequency of congenital malformations, therefore, is probably higher than some reports have indicated. Rubella during the first month of pregnancy probably causes serious defects in up to 50 per cent of the embryos and perhaps even more if those that abort spontaneously are considered. During the second month the rate appears to be halved to about 25 per cent, and during the third month approximately halved again to about 15 per cent. The incidence of embryopathy identified in 200 reported cases of rubella at various weeks of pregnancy is shown in Figure 7.

It is now evident that many infants who are born alive suffer stigmata of continuing intrauterine and neonatal rubella infection. The syndrome of congenital rubella includes one or more of the following abnormalities: (1) eye lesions including cataracts, glaucoma, microphthalmia, and various other abnormalities (2) heart disease, including patent ductus arteriosus, septal defects, and pulmonary artery stenosis; (3) auditory defects; (4) central nervous system defects

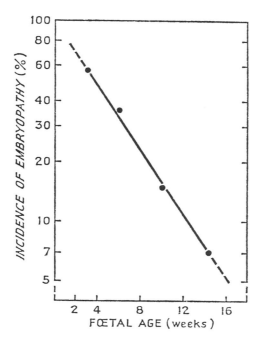

Fig. 7. Incidence of embryopathy in 200 reported cases of rubella. The dotted lines are hypothetical extrapolations. (From Rendle-Short. Lancet 2:373, 1964.)

including meningoencephalitis; (5) intrauterine growth retardation; (6) hematologic changes, including thrombocytopenia and anemia; (7) hepatosplenomegaly and jaundice; (8) chronic diffuse interstitial pneumonitis; (9) osseous changes; (10) chromosomal abnormalities, with an increased incidence of chromosomal breakage noted quite often. Infants born with congenital rubella may shed the virus for many months and thus be a threat to other infants, as well as to susceptible adults who come in contact with the affected infants.

The role of therapeutic abortion in cases of rubella occurring during the first 12 to 16 weeks of gestation has been one of the most difficult and controversial to define in modern times. We believe that abortion is justified when rubella has been acquired during the first trimester of pregnancy. In several states, however, it is still illegal to perform a therapeutic abortion because of the likelihood of severe fetal malformation.

After the first trimester the likelihood of major malformations from rubella is relatively slight. The infants whose mothers contracted the disease after the first trimester will not necessarily be perfectly healthy, however, as demonstrated by the investigations of Hardy and associates. Their long-term prospective epidemiologic inquiry to assess the impact of the extensive 1964 rubella epidemic in this country revealed 24 instances of serologic evidence of infection by rubella virus after the first trimester. Of the 22 liveborn infants, only 7 could be considered completely normal when followed for periods of up to 4 years.

Cytomegalovirus Disease. The virus responsible for cytomegalic inclusion disease may be harbored by a healthy mother and transmitted to the fetus, causing hydrocephaly, microcephaly, microphthalmia, seizures, encephalitis, blindness, hepatosplenomegaly, and hematologic changes including thrombocytopenia and hemolytic anemia. At autopsy cytomegalic inclusion bodies may be found in many organs of the body. The virus usually can be isolated in tissue culture of human cells.

Although about 3 per cent of women excrete the virus during pregnancy, few have offspring so afflicted. Since primary infection with cytomegalovirus is usually asymptomatic in the mother, the disease is seldom suspected. No effective therapy for mother or infant is available. Cytomegalovirus disease does not recur in subsequent fetuses of the mother of one so afflicted.

Herpesvirus Hominis Infections.   In common with rubella and cytomegalovirus disease, the infection caused by herpesvirus hominis in adults is usually mild, with only local manifestations such as "cold sores" or "fever blisters." Nonetheless, the virus may be lethal to the fetus and newborn infant. The so-called Type II virus may affect the genitalia, causing herpes genitalis characterized by vulvovaginitis and sometimes cervicitis. Characteristic intranuclear inclusion bodies may be identified in smears of cervical or vaginal epithelial cells stained by the Papanicolaou method.

Although transplacental transmission of herpesvirus has been documented, the mode of spread to the fetus is usually by direct contact with the virus in the genital tract during labor and delivery. To avoid a serious neonatal infection, cesarean section is recommended whenever the mother has had a herpetic infection involving the genitalia within three weeks of rupture of the membranes or labor. Idoxuridine has been found to be effective when applied locally to herpetic lesions. Parenteral use of the drug in infants with disseminated disease may be effective in some instances. Tuffli and Nahmias have reported the use of idoxuridine intravenously in two infants; one survived.

Coxsackie Virus Disease.   Coxsackie virus infection is a serious complication of pregnancy, since it may be fatal to the fetus although causing only symptoms of a minor illness in the mother (Benirschke and Pendleton). Myocarditis and encephalomyelitis are the primary lesions. Whether maternal Coxsackie infection ever causes sublethal injuries of the embryo and fetus, thus producing congenital anomalies, is not entirely certain.

Mumps (Epidemic Parotitis).   This uncommon disease during pregnancy occasionally causes abortion or premature labor and may result in fetal death if infection occurs late in pregnancy (Blattner and Heys). Hyatt reviewed 90 published cases and noted that 16 per cent of the infants were born with congenital defects. Manson and associates, however, in 501 cases found that major fetal anomalies were much more common than in the general population. Congenital mumps is very rare.

Measles (Rubeola).   Most women are immune to rubeola, and therefore this disease is seldom encountered during pregnancy. Measles may cause premature labor but it is very unlikely that the infection causes congential defects.

Influenza.   In the great influenza pandemic of 1918 the disease, particularly the pneumonic type, was an unusually serious complication of pregnancy. Harris, in a statistical study based on 1,350 cases, found a gross maternal mortality of 27 per cent, which increased to 50 per cent when pneumonia developed. The disease also had a most deleterious effect upon the pregnancy. The prognosis in uncomplicated epidemic influenza is excellent, however, and in cases with the less serious complications, such as sinusitis, laryngitis, and bronchitis, the prognosis is also good. But if pneumonia develops, the prognosis at once becomes serious. This complication should always be suspected when fever persists for more than four days. Although antibiotics are not effective against the virus of influenza, they are probably of value in the treatment of a secondary bacterial pneumonia.

The pandemic of so-called Asian influenza that swept the United States and other areas of the world in 1957 appeared to affect pregnant women with particular frequency and severity. In August and September of that year, for instance, 50 per cent of the women in the childbearing age who died of influenza in Minnesota were pregnant (Freeman and Barno). In the same year in that state the leading cause of maternal death was influenza. Similarly, in New York City, the incidence in pregnant women was 50 per cent higher than in nonpregnant controls, and the mortality rate also was higher (Bass and Molloshok). No convincing evidence has been derived that Asian influenza causes congenital malformations (Walker and McKee; Saxen and associates; Ebert; and Wilson and associates). Vaccination against influenza is probably of value during pregnancy, especially when an epidemic is anticipated.

Common Cold.   The pregnant woman appears to be slightly more susceptible to acute upper respiratory infections than the nonpregnant. Cases of pneumonia complicating pregnancy are often preceded by an acute cold. Hemolytic streptococcal puerperal infections may occur in patients who had acute respiratory infections at the time of delivery, and the incidence of hemolytic streptococci in the upper respiratory passages of such patients is much higher than in healthy women.

Smallpox.   Smallpox is so rare today that modern data are unavailable, but the older literature indicates that the mortality rate is higher in pregnant than in nonpregnant women, and that abortion and premature labor are exceedingly common, especially in the hemorrhagic form.

In general, vaccination for smallpox during pregnancy exerts no deleterious effect on the mother or fetus, according to Greenberg and associates. On rare occasions, vaccination or even contact with a recently vaccinated person, especially in the first half of pregnancy, may be followed by fetal vaccinia (Tucker and Sibson). This rare occurrence should not, however, prevent vaccination of pregnant women or their families when indicated.

Poliomyelitis.   Both the inactivated poliomyelitis vaccine (Salk) and the attenuated live vaccine (Sabin) are safe for immunization during pregnancy. With the widespread use of these vaccines, this disease is becoming a rarity in the United States. Siegel and Goldberg, in a carefully controlled study in New York City, have shown that pregnant women not only are more susceptible to the disease, but have a higher death rate. The perinatal loss was about 33 per cent; rarely, the fetus became infected. Cesarean section was not necessarily required even in the presence of extensive paralysis.

OTHER BACTERIAL INFECTIONS

Differing from some viruses, very few bacterial infections in the mother are likely to spread to the fetus, at least before labor and delivery.

Scarlet Fever.   Although the causative organism of scarlet fever, *Streptococcus pyogenes*, is sensitive to certain antibiotics, the disease in the early months of pregnancy has a tendency to cause abortion, presumably because of the high temperature of the mother. Regardless of antibiotics, rigid isolation must be instituted and maintained in the treatment of a pregnant, parturient, or puerperal patient with scarlet fever. For no obvious reasons, scarlet fever has become very uncommon in recent years.

Erysipelas.   Erysipelas is always a very serious disease, but is particularly dangerous in pregnant women because of the potential hazard of puerperal infection. The hemolytic streptococci associated with erysipelas may become more invasive, causing a septicemia and possibly producing fetal infection and even death. For the protection of other patients, strict isolation of women with erysipelas is absolutely essential. The disease should be actively treated with an appropriate antibiotic agent, which usually frees the patient of hemolytic streptococci in a relatively short time.

Typhoid Fever.   According to Alimurung and Manahan, pregnancy complicated by typhoid fever results in abortion or premature labor in 60 to 80 per cent of cases, with a fetal mortality of 75 per cent and a maternal mortality of 15 per cent. Chloramphenicol is usually quite effective in arresting the disease. Antityphoid vaccines appear to exert no harmful effects when administered to pregnant women and should be given in an epidemic or when otherwise definitely indicated.

Cholera.   Schütz stated that the mortality from cholera among pregnant women in the Hamburg epidemic of 1892 was 57 per cent, a figure much higher than that in nonpregnant women; 54 per cent of the cases, moreover, ended in abortion or premature labor.

PROTOZOAL, PARASITIC, AND FUNGAL INFECTIONS

Toxoplasmosis.   Toxoplasmosis is a protozoal disease carried asymptomatically in the adult population and may be transmitted to the fetus by transplacental migration of the protozoa. It causes serious damage to the fetus, often resulting in abortion or gross prematurity and death. According to Feldman, almost all surviving children have some disability, such as chorioetinitis, abnormality in the size of the head, mental retardation, and cerebral calcification. Thomascheck, Schmidtke, and Genz in an extensive study in West Berlin found serologic evidence of toxoplasmosis in 13 per cent of the pregnant women examined, and grave malformations in 4.6 per cent of their infants.

Malaria.   The incidence of abortion and premature labor is increased in malaria, although it depends on the severity of the disease and the promptness with which therapy is instituted. The increased fetal loss may be related to placental and fetal infection with malaria; but the evidence is somewhat contradictory, since parasites rarely cross the placenta to infect the fetus. Covell, who studied this question extensively, cites an incidence of neonatal malaria in Africa of 0.03 per cent. According to Jones, parasites have an affinity for the decidual vessels and may involve the placenta extensively without affecting the fetus. There is a marked tendency toward recrudescence of the disease during pregnancy and the puerperium, just as after surgical operations.

Pregnancy does not contraindicate the administration of any of the commonly used antimalarial drugs. Some of the newer antimalarial agents have antifolic acid activity, however, and may contribute to the development of megaloblastic anemia (Chanarin).

Amebiasis.   Dysentery caused by *Entamoeba histolytica*, especially with hepatic abscess, may be a quite serious illness during pregnancy. Therapy is similar to that for the nonpregnant woman.

Coccidioidomycosis. In the past, disseminated coccidioidomycosis during pregnancy commonly terminated in maternal death. In recent years treatment with amphotericin B has been employed successfully in a number of cases (Harris); the drug is likely to be toxic.

COLLAGEN DISEASES

The collagen diseases, a group of disorders of connective tissue, appear to have as their common denominator an autoimmune response. Since these diseases are relatively rare, their effect on pregnancy, and vice versa, is difficult to ascertain.

Systemic Lupus Erythematosus. Attempts at correlating the clinical course of systemic lupus erythematosus and pregnancy have been inconclusive (Madson and Anderson; McCombs and Patterson; Murray). The problem stems from the paucity of clinical experience and the protean nature of the disease, which predisposes to difficulty of uniform classification. Estes and Larson, in a comprehensive study, reviewed the experience with systemic lupus erythematosus at the Columbia-Presbyterian Medical Center. To obtain a uniform sample they included only patients with evidence of multiple system disease and a positive LE cell preparation. Of 213 women in whom the diagnosis of systemic lupus erythematosus was made, there were 36 who fulfilled the criteria and became pregnant during the course of their disease. Among this group of 36 there was a total of 25 pregnancies before and 79 pregnancies after the onset of the disease. The authors concluded that pregnancy did not alter the course of disease in the majority of patients studied. They noted that, in general, women in remission at the beginning of pregnancy remained in remission throughout the pregnancy and in the puerperium. They believe, furthermore, that in the absence of lupus nephritis or hypertension, pregnancy imposes no undue maternal risk, although fetal wastage is increased irrespective of the systems involved. The progression of renal involvement, and its accompanying high fetal loss, however, is a contraindication to pregnancy in patients with lupus nephritis or hypertension.

Since the course of the disease is more favorable when pregnancy occurs during a period of remission, patients are best advised to await such remissions before attempting to become pregnant. The duration of the remission before pregnancy, however, has no influence on either the course of the disease or the fetal outcome.

Some, but not all, observers have noted a high rate of recrudescence of activity postpartum, possibly related to the release of deoxynucleic acid from the involuting uterus. Therefore, close observation should be continued during the puerperium. In general, administration of adrenocorticosteroids remains the treatment of choice.

The LE factor has been found in cord blood and transiently in the newborn's blood, implying placental transmission (Burman and Oliver). None of the infants born of mothers with lupus erythematosus, however, has exhibited any clinical manifestations of the disease neonatally.

Rheumatoid Arthritis (Rheumatoid Disease). In 1938 Hench reported marked improvement in the inflammatory component of rheumatoid arthritis during 33 pregnancies in 20 women. The pattern of improvement involved gradual amelioration of the signs and symptoms of the rheumatoid process, as during a spontaneous remission. The cause of the remissions in pregnancy is uncertain. It may be related to slightly increased levels of free 17-hydroxycorticoids in the plasma, but some patients during remission may fail to show such an increase (Gould; Popert). The course may occasionally worsen during pregnancy, and sometimes the disease may first appear at that time.

Involvement of certain joints may interfere with delivery. Severe deformities of the hip, moreover, may preclude vaginal delivery.

The transmission of the rheumatoid factor, a macroglobulin, across the placenta is doubtful. Even when there have been high titers in the serum of the mother at the time of delivery, the factor has not been found in the newborn's blood.

Dermatomyositis.   Dermatomyositis is an uncommon acute, subacute, or chronic inflammatory disease of unknown cause involving skin and muscle. The disease may manifest itself as a severe generalized myositis with a cutaneous eruption and fever and a fatal outcome within a few days or weeks. It may also assume a chronic form, characterized by the gradual development of paresis with little, if any, cutaneous or systemic involvement.

About 20 per cent of adults developing dermatomyositis are found to have associated malignant tumor. The time of appearance of the two diseases, however, may be separated by several years. Extirpation of the malignant lesion is occasionally followed by a permanent remission of the dermatomyositis. The most common sites of the associated cancer are the breast, lung, stomach, and ovary. The uterus and cervix have also been reported as the primary sites.

There are so few reports of dermatomyositis in pregnancy that it is difficult to draw any definite conclusions about the effect of one upon the other (Glickman; Kaplan and Diamond).

Scleroderma.   Scleroderma occurs mostly in young women of childbearing age, but its rarity prevents an accumulation of extensive data (Hayes and associates; Tuffanelli and Winkelmann; Winkelmann; Slate and Graham). Scleroderma was formerly considered to have a markedly untoward effect upon pregnancy. Johnson, Banner, and Winkelmann were more encouraging in their report of 36 pregnancies in a group of 337 women in whom scleroderma had developed before the age of 45. They concluded that pregnancy had little or no effect on the course of the disease and that scleroderma had a minimal effect on the pregnancy. In our limited experience, however, dysphagia seems to be aggravated by pregnancy.

Vaginal delivery may generally be anticipated, unless the changes wrought by scleroderma in the soft tissues produce dystocia requiring abdominal delivery. There is no evidence that babies born of mothers with scleroderma are affected by the disease. The placenta, grossly and microscopically, is unremarkable.

Polyarteritis (Periarteritis) Nodosa.   Polyarteritis nodosa is a rare disease with protean manifestations. It is more frequent in men than in women and has its highest prevalence in the sixth and seventh decades. The disease may have a seasonal pattern with an increased frequency during the winter months.

The classic variety is a progressive illness characterized clinically by myalgia, neuropathy, gastrointestinal disorders, hypertension, and renal disease.

Only five documented cases of polyarteritis nodosa in association with pregnancy have been reported. In each instance the mother died postpartum; all had hypertension and renal involvement. Four of the infants survived, and in the fifth case a therapeutic abortion was performed. The etiologic factor in polyarteritis nodosa apparently does not affect the fetus, either because it fails to cross the placenta or because the fetus is either resistant or incapable of responding to it.

Cortisone or similar compounds remain the therapy of choice for polyarteritis nodosa, as for the other collagen diseases. Although symptomatic relief may be dramatic, there is little evidence that such therapy leads to ultimate recovery.

The experience is too scant to draw any definitive conclusions about polyarteritis nodosa and pregnancy other than that the combination is associated with unfavorable maternal outcome (Siegler and Spain).

Marfan's Syndrome. This disorder of connective tissue exhibits a mendelian autosomal pattern of inheritance that may be related to a dominant gene (McKusick). Both sexes are affected equally, and there appears to be no racial or ethnic basis for the syndrome. There are many mild cases (formes frustes) in which the intrinsic lesion of the connective tissue affects neither well-being nor longevity and consequently escapes detection. In young adults the syndrome may be a major cause of dissecting aortic aneurysm, which occurs much more commonly in pregnancy.

Although the specific defect is still controversial, there is a degeneration of the elastic lamina in the media of the aorta. The cardiovascular lesion is the most serious abnormality, involving most often the ascending portion of the aorta, and predisposing to aortic dilatation or dissecting aneurysm. Early death in Marfan's syndrome is thus ultimately caused by either congestive heart failure or rupture of a dissecting aneurysm. In Tricomi's review of the subject, dissection of the aneurysm occurred in 30 per cent of the cases before the onset of labor; thus, labor cannot be considered the predisposing factor.

Marfan's syndrome alone is not an indication for abdominal delivery, for cesarean section does not protect against excessive stress on the aorta before the onset of labor. The role of cardiovascular surgery in Marfan's syndrome is poorly defined.

Rheumatic Fever. Identifiable rheumatic fever, manifested by carditis or arthritis, is rare in pregnancy. At the Kings County Hospital a proven case occurs not more often than once a year, or about once in 6,000 to 7,000 deliveries. In pregnancy, the diagnosis of rheumatic activity is obscured by the normally elevated erythrocyte sedimentation rate and, according to Nesbitt, Hayes, and Mauro, the normally present C-reactive protein. Differential diagnosis must include gonococcal arthritis and the sickle-cell hemoglobinopathies.

DISEASES OF THE SKIN

The one serious dermatologic disease peculiar to pregnancy is herpes gestationis. Otherwise, diseases of the skin occur with about the same frequency in pregnant as in nonpregnant women.

Herpes Gestationis. This rare condition is characterized by multiform erythematous, vesicular, pustular, and bullous lesions, which cause severe burning and itching, occasionally of unbearable severity (Fig. 8). The forearms, legs, face, and trunk are most frequently involved. The disease usually develops during the second trimester. Although it is often regarded as a variant of dermatitis herpetiformis, the disease presents certain features that relate it specifically to pregnancy. The prognosis is good but the disease is likely to recur in subsequent pregnancies. A curious characteristic is the high incidence of congenital abnormalities; in 13 cases reported by Downing and Jillson, for example, 8 infants had anomalies. Another interesting feature is the eosinophilia that usually accompanies the disorder.

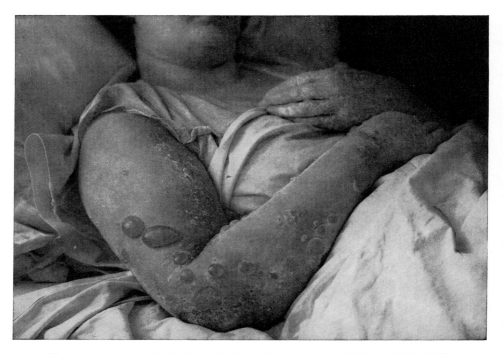

Fig. 8. Herpes gestationis. (From Hadley. J Obstet Gynaec Brit Emp 66:985, 1959.)

The frequency of herpes gestationis is probably less than 1 in 5,000 pregnancies. The disease may be controlled with corticosteroids, as indicated in the reports of Zakon and associates; Lindemann and associates; Hadley; and Mitchell and Jessop.

Melanoma.   Some benign nevi become malignant during pregnancy. The resulting melanoma may grow with unusual rapidity and may metastasize widely. The prognosis in pregnant women with melanoma is poor, for few cures have been obtained. Reynolds therefore recommended that all antepartum examinations include an evaluation of pigmented moles. Prophylactic removal of pigmented moles in pregnant women should be performed, according to Reynolds, in the following circumstances: (1) moles on the trunk that are subjected to irritation; (2) moles on the genitals or feet, locations more likely to undergo malignant change; (3) moles that are smooth, blue, black, or dark brown; (4) moles that exhibit increased pigmentation, elevation of growth, enlargement in diameter, or association with ulceration, bleeding, or pain. Transplacental metastasis of a melanoma from mother to fetus has been reported by Holland and by others. Despite its rarity, melanoma is the commonest tumor reported to metastasize to the placenta and fetus.

Pruritus.   Itching may occasionally be a distressing complication. It may extend over the greater part of the body or remain limited to the genitalia. It often gives rise to intense suffering, with itching sometimes to unrelenting that the patient is unable to sleep. Severe cases are best controlled by sedatives and general supportive treatment. Uncomplicated abdominal pruritus during pregnancy was found by Kasdon in 65 out of 365 pregnant women.

Abnormalities of Pigmentation.   During pregnancy, abnormalities in pigmentation are frequently noted and may be particularly marked along the linea alba and about the breasts. In other cases unsightly, more or less symmetric, brownish splotches (chloasma) appear upon the face. They are not amenable to treatment but usually disappear promptly after childbirth. Stilbestrol and several of the oral contraceptives may cause similar changes in pigmentation.

Diseases of the Nervous System

Epilepsy.   In general, epilepsy is not affected adversely by pregnancy. During early pregnancy, however, nausea and vomiting may interfere with the ingestion of anticonvulsant medication, increasing the likelihood of seizures. During labor, delivery, and the early puerperium, medication may be withheld inadvertently, similarly increasing the likelihood of convulsions.

Several of the anticonvulsant drugs in common use tend to precipitate or aggravate a deficiency of folic acid; and megaloblastic anemia has been described in these circumstances (Chanarin). In one recent study maternal folate deficiency was much more common than in the general obstetric population, although no cases of overt megaloblastic anemia were identified among the pregnant women treated with anticonvulsant drugs (Pritchard, Scott, and Whalley). Folic acid has been claimed by some to increase the likelihood of convulsions. Therefore, the benefits, if any, to be derived from folic acid supplements in these circumstances are not clear. It has recently been reported that the newborn infant whose mother has been taking anticonvulsant medication may develop serious deficiencies of several coagulation factors (Ch. 12, p. 343).

During the past 12 years at Parkland Memorial Hospital 77 pregnancies have been cared for in 43 women with epilepsy, all of whom were taking anticonvulsant medications throughout the period of gestation. The pregnancies were, for the most part, quite uncomplicated. The frequencies of spontaneous abortion, perinatal mortality, prematurity, and fetal malformation were similar to those in the general obstetric population (Pritchard, Scott, and Whalley). Each infant received 1 mg of vitamin K_1 (phytonadione) parenterally very soon after birth. None demonstrated abnormal bleeding including the male infants who were circumcised.

The treatment of epilepsy during pregnancy is the same as in the nonpregnant condition, and therapeutic abortion is seldom indicated. Because of the chronic nature of the illness and the hereditary features of several forms of the disease, and because some epileptics appear to undergo progressive mental deterioration, sterilization should be offered.

Intracranial Hemorrhage.   Intracranial hemorrhage is a much more common cause of maternal death than is generally believed. Among 170 maternal deaths reported by Barnes and Abbott, for example, 36 were caused by cerebral complications. Of these 36 deaths, 17, or about one half, were the result of intracranial hemorrhage. In Minnesota during the decade 1950–1959, the number of deaths of pregnant women from cerebral hemorrhage roughly equaled that from cardiac disease. Many of these deaths were the result of rupture of congenital aneurysms; but as emphasized by Pedowitz and Perell and by Laubstein, Kotz, and Herre, these accidents are probably not more frequent in pregnancy than in the general population. The main obstetric problem concerns the management of pregnancy and delivery in women who survive intracranial hemorrhage. Many, but certainly not all, authorities favor cesarean section for delivery, and in cases in which the cerebral hemorrhage occurred shortly before or very early in pregnancy, some believe that therapeutic abortion is indicated (Mack and associates; Gomberg).

Paraplegia.   Spinal cord lesions caused by trauma or tumor usually do not prevent conception. In women so affected the pregnancy is likely to be complicated by urinary infections and pressure necrosis of the skin. Labor often is easy and comparatively painless.

Multiple Sclerosis.   This disease is a rare complication of pregnancy, occurring about once in every 4,000 gravidas, as reported by Sweeney. In most cases pregnancy has no effect on the course of multiple sclerosis, which in itself is rarely an indication for therapeutic abortion. Although in many cases the condition seems to be aggravated in pregnancy, multiple sclerosis in pregnant women is often characterized by unexplained exacerbations and remissions.

Myasthenia Gravis.   With occasional exceptions women with myasthenia gravis go through pregnancy and labor without difficulty; but as pointed out by Fraser and Turner, there is some likelihood of a relapse during the first few weeks of the puerperium, necessitating increased doses of neostigmine or similar medications.

Transient symptomatic myasthenia gravis occurs in about 10 to 20 per cent of the newborn infants of mothers with the disease. The neonatal mysthenia responds to minute doses of neostigmine or similar drugs, subsiding completely within two or three weeks. Without prompt recognition and treatment, including good nursing care, the affected newborn infant may succumb to respiratory insufficiency caused by muscular weakness or the effects of aspiration.

Huntington's Chorea.   The obstetric importance of Huntington's chorea is chiefly eugenic, since this degenerative disease of the cerebral cortex and basal ganglia is inherited as a dominant autosomal trait. To attempt the elimination of this dread disease, therapeutic abortion is justifiable.

Sydenham's Chorea.   *Chorea gravidarum* is simply Sydenham's chorea occurring in pregnancy. It is an extremely rare complication of gestation today, only 1 mild case having been seen at the Johns Hopkins Hospital in a period of 20 years in the course of over 50,000 pregnancies, and none having occurred among 70,000 consecutive deliveries at the Kings County Hospital. It once carried a grave prognosis, but the study by Beresford and Graham revealed only 1 death among 127 cases as the direct result of chorea. The most serious complication is psychosis which may occasionally necessitate therapeutic abortion.

Psychiatric Aspects

Initial Reactions to Pregnancy.   To some women, the initial psychologic and emotional reactions to pregnancy and its associative implications for the immediate future are those of intense resentment, anger, fear, and panic. In the minds of these women, the continuation of the pregnancy is a serious, frightening, and dangerous personal threat to all their sources of emotional and physical security and to all their resources for adaptation. So real and life-threatening are the emotional reactions in these women that they not only reject the existence of the pregnancy, but urgently seek means to terminate the pregnancy before they, themselves, are engulfed and destroyed. Under the spell of this distorted thinking and reasoning, the medical hazards of instrumental abortions fade into insignificance.

Psychologically, the pregnancy at this early stage, possessing no objective, tangible evidence of reality, is identified in the minds of these women as an abstract concept or fantasy, which, if pleasant, can be accepted or, if unpleasant, rejected and eliminated without involving the censorship of the conscience. This thinking, in part, explains the absence of disturbing guilt feelings in many women following abortion (Ekblad). Other women, however, have been unable completely to convince their conscience that the pregnancy was only a fantasy, with the result that feelings of guilt and remorse continue to disturb them through subsequent years.

The obstetrician should be mindful of the following generalizations when confronted with decisions about interruption of pregnancy for psychiatric indications (Simon):

1. Unless the woman has been under psychiatric care before the pregnancy, the urgency of the situation created by the continuing growth of the fetus and the insistent demands for a decision made by the patient, and frequently her family, force the psychiatrist into a position in which he must render a judgment without adequate clinical observation. Unless the psychiatrist can maintain a scientifically objective point of view, he may find himself becoming the "unwitting accomplice" (Bolter), and the obstetrician will subsequently become the "unwilling executioner."

2. Serious psychotic decompensations requiring commitment in a psychiatric hospital are not common during pregnancy. Boyd, Gralnick, Cappon, Kline, and also White and associates discuss the clinical manifestations and management of these complications, pointing out the favorable response to conventional psychiatric treatment.

3. Asch has indicated that it is virtually impossible to ascertain accurately whether a woman is suicidal. However, the incidence of actual suicide during pregnancy is very low, considering the number of women seeking abortion.

It is sometimes wise obstetric practice to recommend that therapeutic sterilization accompany therapeutic abortion for psychiatric indications. Some well-educated married women seeking interruption of pregnancy because of psychiatric reasons admit their inability to utilize effectively contraceptive techniques even after careful medical instruction. Ekblad reported that 40 per cent of the Swedish married women who had had a legal abortion for psychiatric reasons became pregnant unintentionally again in less than two years, despite careful contraceptive instruction at the time of abortion.

Second and Third Trimester Complications. During the middle trimester, the identification of the pregnancy as an abstract concept becomes replaced, in the mind of the woman, by the identification with a real baby-to-be, whose growth is causing a progressive enlargement of the mother's abdomen, whose movements can be felt, and whose heart rate can be counted by the physician.

The third trimester is characterized, psychologically and emotionally, by thoughts and feelings about labor, delivery, and the subsequent responsibilities of motherhood. The reality of the impending arrival of the baby is evidenced by a variety of manifestations:

1. The majority of women who expressed ambivalent or rejecting attitudes toward the pregnancy in the early months of gestation now express positive, or at least more accepting, attitudes toward the baby.

2. Women in the lower socioeconomic group who seldom seek antepartum care begin to appear in the clinics, registering for delivery in the hospital.

3. The preparations are made in the home for the care of the baby after the mother returns from the hospital.

Fears expressed by two different groups of women in this trimester are worthy of mention:

1. Fears in those women who have had unfortunate experiences in previous pregnancies and fears in those primigravidas who have conversed with women whose pregnancies and deliveries have been associated with frightening and tragic experiences. These women require understanding and the opportunity to discuss their fears, as well as to gain confidence that the physician and hospital staff will do everything possible to ensure the comfort and safety of the mother and the safety of the babies.

2. Fears in older multiparous patients who have had successful pregnancies and deliveries. These women often express vague fears about the approaching delivery, remarking that they do not understand such fears, which they have never had before. Having been impressed with the vital importance of her own loving care and guidance for her children's normal growth and development, her fears are not for herself, but the result of her apprehension for her children. Who would take care of them and her baby if anything happened to her during delivery? With this orientation, these women are easily reassured, and the fears become only reasonable and understandable apprehensions.

Postpartum Problems. Gordon and associates have emphasized in their publication the importance of sociologic as well as psychologic factors in women's postpartum adjustments.

. . . it seems clear that in trying to treat or to prevent maternal emotional disorders, the physician will be more effective if he concentrates on helping the young woman adjust to the changes in her life associated with the maternal role. Her attitudes and activities (and those of her husband and family) that conflict with her maternal responsibilities are as effective in overwhelming her emotions as are insecurities derived from her past life. But she can reduce present-day role conflict quite readily, after listening to practical counsel in the obstetrician's office and reading literature about young mothers' responsibilities and problems, and their management. Women who modify their attitudes appropriately, learn the needed skills, and obtain practical guidance and dependable aid, adjust well in the immediate postpartum period and continue to do so for many years. As a rule, well-prepared mothers are happier and they have more successful marriages than women who receive no special orientation for the motherhood task.

Psychosomatic Therapy. Psychosomatic obstetric therapy requires that the obstetrician possess sound knowledge, training, and clinical experience in obstetric anatomy, physiology, and pathology. Moreover, it requires an interest on the part of the obstetrician in the normal emotional changes and adaptations associated with pregnancy, labor, and the puerperium; an interest in attempting to identify possible psychologic and emotional disturbances that may be etiologically related to the development or accentuation of various obstetric complications; and an interest in developing new and practical approaches, based upon the information, to therapeutic management.

In contrast to the "organic" approach to obstetric problems, in which the diagnosis is established by what the symptoms and signs mean to the obstetrician, the psychosomatic approach emphasizes that it is essential also for the obstetrician to learn the meaning and significance of the symptoms to the obstetric patient herself. What do these physiologic and pathologic changes and associated symptoms mean to the particular woman? What are the current and future implications of this pregnancy to the patient as a wife, a mother, a widow, a divorcee, or a single girl? What are the strengths of her resources for emotional stability? What is the degree of her emotional and psychosexual maturity? What are the characteristics of her interpersonal relations and responsibilities? What are her social and economic resources?

This information provides an additional dimension for clinical obstetrics, and the obstetrician finds himself in a more favorable and informed position from which to evaluate the clinical problems presented by his patients. He is able to achieve a greater understanding of the various etiologic factors involved and thus render more meaningful and helpful obstetric care to his patients.

Electroshock Treatment. Cooper reviewed the literature concerned with shock treatments in pregnant women and concluded that electroshock therapy may be carried out at any stage of gestation without injury to the fetus. Impastato, Gabriel, and Lardaro suggest that the administration of oxygen to the mother, and of succinylcholine to attenuate convulsions, provides additional protection to the fetus. Electroshock therapy early in pregnancy may possibly exert potentially teratogenic effects, presumably through hypoxia. It is therefore wise to defer such therapy, except when urgently indicated, until after the first trimester.

MISCELLANEOUS COMPLICATIONS

Carcinoma of the Breast. Pregnancy does not appear to exert much influence on the course of mammary cancer, and therapeutic abortion does not improve the prognosis of this disease. In the extensive investigation of Westberg, based on 224 cases of breast carcinoma in pregnant and nursing women and a control series of 3,000 nonpregnant women with mammary cancer, the difference in the survival rates was scarcely significant. Hochman and Schreiber contend that the five-year survival rate in cancer of the breast coexisting with pregnancy is primarily dependent on the stage of the disease at the time of diagnosis, and that interruption of pregnancy has no bearing on the course. The results to be anticipated correspond with the expected survival rates when the same stage of the disease is not complicated by pregnancy. As Hochman and Schreiber point out, the increased vascularity of the breast during pregnancy may result in rapid invasion of the lymph nodes and adjacent tissues and in distant hematogenous metastases. Provided that radical mastectomy is promptly performed, however, they maintain the increased vascularity has no effect on prognosis. Cooper and Butterfield similarly could find no evidence that pregnancy after mastectomy for cancer of the breast had an adverse effect on survival. They conclude that young patients with treated clinical Stage I lesions need not avoid pregnancy.

Diaphragmatic (Hiatal) Hernia.   Rigler and Eneboe performed upper gastro-intestinal radiologic examination on 195 unselected women in the last trimester of pregnancy. Among 116 multiparas, 21, or about 18 per cent, had hiatal hernias, and among 79 primigravidas, 4 had hiatal hernias. Ten of these 25 patients were reexamined 1 to 18 months postpartum, and hernias were observed in only 3. Hiatal hernias seen during pregnancy may be produced by intermittent but pro-longed increase in intraabdominal pressure. These hernias, which are an occa-sional cause of vomiting, epigastric pain, and even bleeding in the latter half of pregnancy, are discussed by Penman.

Rupture of the Spleen.   Rupture of the spleen is an uncommon obstetric com-plication, of which Barnett has collected 28 cases from the literature. The signs and symptoms are those of an acute abdominal catastrophe followed, after a vari-able interval, by those of internal hemorrhage. If the accident takes place in labor, it is usually mistaken for rupture of the uterus. Most cases, however, are attribu-table to a preexisting splenic lesion, such as malaria, leukemia, and Banti's disease. In the 28 cases studied by Barnett, 15 women died, but prompt operation and blood transfusions should give better results today.

Otosclerosis.   One out of every 10 adults in the United States has some osto-sclerotic damage, and it is a common belief that otosclerosis is aggravated by preg-nancy. Barton, for example, reports that of 133 cases of otosclerosis, 64 per cent were made worse by pregnancy. Such patients obviously limit their pregnancies, although, as pointed out by Pearson, otosclerosis is rarely an indication for thera-peutic abortion unless the disease is progressing rapidly.

Retinitis Gestationis.   Once in many thousand pregnancies, retinitis develops and progresses rather rapidly as gestation advances. It is characterized by blur-ring and impairment of vision, with scarring of the retina as the final result. Since the disease is very likely to recur in subsequent pregnancies, with no evidence of the disorder between gestations, and since it can be terminated promptly by therapeutic abortion, pregnancy must be assumed to play a causative role. Corti-sone and similar compounds are of value in controlling the disease, but thera-peutic abortion may be required.

Separation of the Symphysis Pubis.   Significant separations or ruptures of the symphysis pubis are associated with clinical symptoms in addition to roentgeno-logic findings. In general, only separations of more than 1.0 cm are symptomatic. Callahan reports an incidence of 1:2,200 deliveries at The New York Lying-In Hospital, whereas Waters cites a frequency of about only 1:20,000 at the Mar-garet Hague Maternity Hospital. Our experience is closer to that of Waters, in-dicating that the complication is extremely rare in this country today.

The symphysis may separate either during pregnancy or in the course of labor. If it occurs before labor, the separation may develop either spontaneously or after trauma. If the rupture takes place during labor, it is usually the result of a traumatic forceps delivery, but other cases have been attributed to forcibl abduction of the patient's thighs during positioning for delivery.

The symptoms are symphysial pain on motion, such as turning in bed, and tenderness over the symphysis or sacroiliac regions. Roentgenologic examination may reveal a slight separation or a widely gaping defect. Sacroiliac symptoms are noted in about a third of the cases.

Treatment is orthopedic, current opinion favoring simple strapping in most cases. Recovery of function is usually complete, although some separation and motion of the joint may persist. Subsequent vaginal delivery without recurrence of the original symptoms may be anticipated.

REFERENCES

Adams, R. H., and Combes, B. Viral hepatitis in pregnancy. JAMA 192:195, 1965.

Alimurung, M. M., and Manahan, C. P. Typhoid in pregnancy: report of a case treated with chloramphenicol and ACTH. J Philipp Med Ass 28:388, 1952.

Anderson, M. F. Pregnancy complicated by sickle cell disease. Blood 34:731, 1969.

Asch, S. S. Mental and emotional problems, in Medical, Surgical and Gynecological Complications of Pregnancy. A. F. Guttmacher and J. J. Rovinsky (ed.). Baltimore, The Williams & Wilkins Co., 1960, p. 375.

Bailey, J. E., and Giescke, A. H. Long term sequelae of aspiration of gastric contents. To be published.

Baker, D. P., Hutchison, J. R., and Vaughan, D. L. Comparison of standard oral and rapid intravenous glucose tolerance tests in pregnancy. Obstet Gynec 31:475, 1968.

Baker, L.R.I., and Brain, M. C. Heparin treatment of haemolytic anemia and thrombocytopenia in preeclampsia. Proc Roy Soc Med 60:477, 1967.

Ball, E. W., and Giles, C. Folic acid and vitamin B_{12} levels in pregnancy and their relation to megaloblastic anemia. J Clin Path 17:165, 1964.

Barnes, A. C. Discussion of paper by Cannell and Vernon. Amer J Obstet Gynec 85:744, 1963.
———— Discussion of paper by Greene. Amer J Obstet Gynec 91:688, 1965.

Barnes, J. L., and Abbott, K. H. Cerebral complications incurred during pregnancy and the puerperium. Calif Med 91:237, 1959.

Barnes, P. M., Hendrickse, J. P. deV., and Watson-Williams, E. J. Low-molecular weight dextran in treatment of bone-pain crises in sickle cell disease. A double blind trial. Lancet 2:1271, 1965.

Barnett, T. Rupture of the spleen in pregnancy: A review of recorded cases with a further case report. J Obstet Gynaec Brit Emp 59:795, 1953.

Barton, R. T. Influence of pregnancy on otosclerosis. New Eng J Med 233:433, 1945.

Bass, M. H., and Molloshok, R. E. In Medical, Surgical and Gynecological Complications of Pregnancy, A. F. Guttmacher and J. J. Rovinsky (eds.). Baltimore, The Williams & Wilkins Co., 1960, p. 526.

Bellina, J. H., Dougherty, C. M., and Mikal, A. Pyeloureteral dilation and pregnancy. Amer Obstet Gynec 108:356, 1970.

Bellingham, F., Mackey, R., and Winston, C. Pregnancy and intestinal obstruction: A dangerous combination. Med J Aust 2:318, 1949.

Bemiller, C. R., Forker, A. D., and Morgan, J. R. Complete heart block, prosthetic aortic valve, and successful pregnancy. JAMA 217:915, 1970.

Benirschke, K., and Pendleton, M. E. Coxsackie virus infection: an important complication in pregnancy. Obstet Gynec 12:305, 1958.

Benjamin, F., and Casper, D. J. Comparative validity of oral and intravenous glucose tolerance tests in pregnancy. Amer J Obstet Gynec 97:488, 1967.

Beresford, O. D., and Graham, A. M. Chorea gravidarum, J Obstet Gynaec Brit Emp 57:616, 1950.

Biglieri, E. G., and Slaton, P. E., Jr. Pregnancy and primary aldosteronism. J Clin Endocr 27:1628, 1967.

Blank, A. M., and Freedman, W. L. Sickle cell trait and pregnancy. Clin Obstet Gynec 12:123, 1969.

Blattner, R. J., and Heys, F. M. The role of viruses in the etiology of congenital malformations. Progr Med Virol 3:311, 1961.

Bolter, S. The psychiatrist's role in therapeutic abortion: the unwitting accomplice. Amer J Psychiat 119:312, 1962.

Borhanmanesh, F., and Haghighi, P. Pregnancy in patients with cirrhosis of the liver. Obstet Gynec 36:315, 1970.

Bowen, G. L., Grandin, D. J., Julien, E. E., and Krech, S., Jr.   Pheochromocytoma complicating pregnancy. Amer J Obstet Gynec 59:378, 1950.

Bowes, W. A., Jr., Gibson, J. L., Leibovitz, A., and Palin, W. J.   Rubella antibody screening in a prenatal clinic using the indirect fluorescent method. Obstet Gynec 35:7, 1970.

Boyd, D. A., Jr.   Mental disorders associated with childbearing. Amer J Obstet Gynec 43:148, 1942.

Brody, J. A., Sever, J. L., and Schiff, G. M.   Prevention of rubella by gamma globulin during an epidemic in Barrow, Alaska, in 1964. New Eng J Med 272:127, 1965.

Browne, F. J., and Browne, J.C.M.   Antenatal and Postnatal Care, 9th ed. London, Churchill, 1960.

Brumfitt, W., Davies, B. I., and Rosser, E.   Urethral catheter as a cause of urinary-tract infection in pregnancy and puerperium. Lancet 2:1059, 1961.

Bunim, J. J., and Appel, S. B.   A principle for determining prognosis of pregnancy in rheumatic heart disease. JAMA 142:90, 1950.

Burman, D., and Oliver, R. A. M.   Placental transfer of the lupus·erythematosus factor. J Clin Path 11:43, 1958.

Burrow, G. N., Bartsocas, C., Klatskin, E. H., and Grunt, J. A.   Children exposed in utero to propylthiouracil. Amer J Dis Child 116:161, 1968.

Burrows, S., and Bollman, C.   Rubella hemagglutination-inhibition test in an obstetric population. Obstet Gynec 33:703, 1969.

Burt, R. L., and Leake, N. H.   Oral glucose tolerance test during pregnancy and the early purperium. Obstet Gynec 33:48, 1969.

Burwell, C. S., and Metcalfe, J.   Heart Disease and Pregnancy. Boston, Little, Brown & Co., 1958.

Callahan, J. T.   Separation of the symphysis pubis.   Amer J Obstet Gynec 66:281, 1953.

Caplan, R. M., Dossetor, J. B., and Maughan, G. B.   Pregnancy following cadaver kidney homotransplantation. Amer J Obstet Gynec 106:644, 1970.

Cappon, D.   Some psychodynamic aspects of pregnancy. Canad Med Ass J 70:147, 1954.

Carswell, F., Kerr, M. M., and Hutchinson, J. H.   Congenital goitre and hypothyroidism produced by maternal ingestion of iodides. Lancet 1:1241, 1970.

Cave, V. G., Bloomfield, R. D., Hurdle, E. S., Gordon, E. W., and Hammock, D., Jr.   Gonorrhea in the obstetric and gynecologic clinic. JAMA 210:309, 1969.

Chanarin, I.   The Megaloblastic Anaemias. Oxford and Edinburgh, Blackwell Scientific Publications, 1969.

———— Rothman, D., Ward, A., and Perry, J.   Folate status and requirements in pregnancy. Brit Med J 2:390, 1968.

———— Rothman, D., and Watson-Williams, E. J.   Normal formiminoglutamic acid excretion in megaloblastic anemia in pregnancy. Studies on histidine metabolism in pregnancy. Lancet 1:1068, 1963.

Chau, S. S., Fitzpatrick, R. J., and Jamieson, B.   Diabetes insipidus and parturition. J Obstet Gynaec Brit Comm 76:444, 1969.

Cheek, D.   Personal communication.

Chesley, L. C.   The remote prognosis for pregnant women with rheumatic cardiac disease. Amer J Obstet Gynec 100:732, 1968.

Chisholm, D. M., and Sharp, A. A.   Formimino-glutamic acid excretion in anaemia of pregnancy. Brit Med J 2:1366, 1964.

Churchill, J. A., Berendes, H. W., and Nemore, J.   Neuropsychological deficits in children of diabetic mothers. Amer J Obstet Gynec 105:257, 1969.

Coblentz, D. R., Cimini, R., Mikity, V. G., and Rosen, R.   Roentgenographic diagnosis of congenital syphilis in the newborn. JAMA 212:1061, 1970.

Cooper, D. R., and Butterfield, J.   Pregnancy subsequent to mastectomy for cancer of the breast. Ann Surg 171:429, 1970.

Cooper, H. H.   Electroshock treatment of mental illness during pregnancy. S Afr Med J 26:366, 1952.

Cooper, L. Z., and Krugman, S.   Clinical manifestations of postnatal and congenital rubella. Arch Ophthal 71:434, 1967.

———— Matters, B., Rosenblum, J. K., and Krugman, S.   Experience with a modified rubella hemagglutination inhibition antibody test. JAMA 207:89, 1969.

Coopland, A. T., Friesen, W. J., and Galbraith, P. A. Acute leukemia in pregnancy. Amer J Obstet Gynec 105:1288, 1969.

Covell, G. Congenital malaria. Trop Dis Bull 47:1147, 1950.

Crohn, B. B., Yarnis, H., Walter, R. I., Gabrilov, J. L., and Crohn, E. B. Ulcerative colitis as affected by pregnancy. New York J Med 56:2651, 1956.

Curtis, E. M. Pregnancy in sickle cell anemia, sickle cell-hemoglobin C disease and variants thereof. Amer Obstet Gynec 77:1312, 1959.

Danforth, D. N., Kyser, F. A., and Boronow, R. C. Refractory anemia and thrombocytopenia due to pregnancy. JAMA 180:629, 1962.

D'Cruz, I. A., Balani, S. G., and Iyer, L. S. Infectious hepatitis in pregnancy. Obstet Gynec 31:449, 1968.

Delaney, J. J., and Ptacek, J. Three decades of experience with diabetic pregnancies. Amer J Obstet Gynec 106:550, 1970.

DeLeeuw, N.K.W., Lowenstein, L., and Hsieh, Y. Iron deficiency and hydremia in normal pregnancy. Medicine 45:291, 1966.

Del Prete, S., Doglia, M., Ajdukiewicz, A., Fox, R. A., Costantino, D., Graziina, A., Dudley, F. A., and Sherlock, S. Detection of a new serum-antigen in three epidemics of short-term hepatitis. Lancet 2:579, 1970.

Dines, D. E., and Banner, E. A. Sarcoidosis during pregnancy. JAMA 200:150, 1967.

Downing J. G., and Jillson, O. F. Herpes gestationis. New Eng J Med 241:906, 1949.

Driscoll, J. J., and Gillespie, L. Obstetrical considerations in diabetes in pregnancy. Med Clin N Amer 49:1025, 1965.

Ebert, J. D. First International Conference on Congenital Malformations. Summary and Evaluation. J Chron Dis 13:91, 1961.

Echt, C. R., and Doss, J. F. Myxedema in pregnancy. Obstet Gynec 22:615, 1963.

Ekblad, M. Induced abortion on psychiatric grounds. Acta Psychiat Neurol Scand, Suppl. 99, 1955.

Erf, L. A. Leukemia (summary of 100 cases) and lymphosarcoma complicated by pregnancy. Amer J Clin Path 17:268, 1947.

Estes, D., and Larson, D. L. Systemic lupus erythematosus and pregnancy. Clin Obstet Gynec 8:307, 1965.

Fairweather, D. Nausea and vomiting in pregnancy. Amer J Obstet Gynec 102:135, 1968.

Farquhar, J. D. Results with Cendehill rubella vaccine in postpartum women. Obstet Gynec 35:841, 1970.

Felding, C. Obstetric studies in women with renal disease in childhood. Acta Obstet Gynec Scand 45:141, 1964.

——— The obstetric prognosis in chronic renal disease. Acta Obstet Gynec Scand 47:166, 1968.

Feldman, H. A. Toxoplasmosis. Pediat Clin N Amer 1:169, 1955.

Felsen, J., and Wolarsky, W. Chronic ulcerative colitis and pregnancy. Amer J Obstet Gynec 56:751, 1948.

Fieldring, J. F., and Cooke, W. T. Pregnancy and Crohn's disease. Brit Med J 2:76, 1970.

Fleming, A. F. Hypoplastic anaemia in pregnancy. J Obstet Gynaec Brit Comm 75:138, 1968.

Forbes, J. A. International Conference on Rubella Immunization. I. Rubella as a disease. Amer J Dis Child 118:5, 1969.

Fox, L. P. Grandi, J., Johnson, A. H., Watrous, W. G., and Johnson, M. J. Pheochromocytoma associated with pregnancy. Amer J Obstet Gynec 104:288, 1969.

Fraser, D., and Turner, J.W.A. Myasthenia gravis and pregnancy. Lancet 2:417, 1953.

Freedman, L. R. Pyelonephritis and urinary tract infection, in M. B. Strauss and L. G. Welt (eds.), Diseases of the Kidney. Boston, Little, Brown & Co., 1963, Ch 14.

Freedman, W. L. Alpha and beta thalassemia and pregnancy. Clin Obstet Gynec 12:115, 1969.

Freeman, D. W., and Barno, A. Deaths from Asian influenza associated with pregnancy. Amer J Obstet Gynec 78:1172, 1959.

Freeth, A. Routine x-ray examination of the chest at an antenatal clinic. Lancet 1:287, 1953.

Freireich, E. J., Miller, A., Emerson, C. P., and Ross, J. F. The effect of inflammation on the utilization of erythrocyte and transferrin bound radioiron for red cell production. Blood 12:972, 1957.

Fullerton, W. T., Hendrickse, J. P. deV., and Watson-Williams, E. J.   Haemoglobin SC disease in pregnancy, in Abnormal Haemoglobins in Africa, A Symposium, J.H.P. Jonxis (ed). Philadelphia, F. A. Davis Co., 1965.

———— and Turner, A. G.   Exchange transfusion in treatment of severe anaemia in pregnancy. Lancet 1:75, 1962.

Ginz, B.   Myocardial infection in pregnancy. J Obstet Gynaec Brit Comm 77:610, 1970.

Glickman, F.   Dermatomyositis associated with pregnancy. U.S. Armed Forces Med J 9:417, 1958.

Gomberg, B.   Spontaneous subarachnoid hemorrhage in pregnancy not complicated by toxemia. Amer J Obstet Gynec 77:430, 1959.

Goodall, H. B.   Microscopic examination of the "buffy-coat" from the hematocrit in the investigation of anemia in pregnancy. J. Clin Path 10:248, 1957.

Gordon, R. E., Kapostons, E. E., and Gordon, K. K.   Factors in postpartum emotional adjustment. Obstet Gynec 25:158, 1965.

Gorenberg, H., and Chesley, L. C.   Rheumatic heart disease in pregnancy: the remote prognosis in patients with "functionally severe" disease. Ann Int Med 49:278, 1958.

Gould, I.   Rheumatoid arthritis aggravated by pregnancy and controlled by cortisone. New York J Med 55:1164, 1955.

Gralnick, A.   Shock therapy in psychoses complicated by pregnancy: report of two cases. Amer J Psychiat 102:780, 1946.

Greenberg, M., Yankauer, A., Jr., Krugman, S., Osborn, J. J., Ward, R. S., and Dancis, J.   The effect of smallpox vaccination during pregnancy on the incidence of fetal malformations. Pediatrics 3:456, 1949.

Greene, J. W., Jr., Smith, K., Kyle, G. C., Touchstone, J. C., and Duhring, J. L.   The use of estriol excretion in the management of pregnancies complicated by diabetes mellitus. Amer J Obstet Gynec 91:684, 1965.

Gregg, N. M.   Congenital cataract following German measles in the mother. Trans Ophthal Soc Aust 3:35, 1942.

Grüneberg, R. N., Leigh, D. A., and Brumfitt, W.   Relationship of bacteriuria in pregnancy to acute pyelonephritis, prematurity and fetal malformations. Lancet 2:3, 1969.

Hadley, J. A.   Herpes gestationis. A report of a case. J Obstet Gynaec Brit Emp 66:985, 1959.

Hallberg, L., Hallgren, J., Hollender, A., Hogdahl, A., and Tibblin, G.   Occurrence, causes and prevention of nutritional anaemias. Symposia of Swedish Nutrition Foundation, 6:19, 1968.

———— Solvell, L., and Brise, H.   Search for substances promoting the absorption of iron. Studies on absorption and side effects. Acta Med Scand, Suppl. 459:11, 1966.

Halstead, S. B., Char, D. F. B., and Diwan, A. R.   Evaluation of three rubella vaccines in adult women. JAMA 211:991, 1970.

Hamilton, B. E., and Thomson, K. J.   The Heart in Pregnancy and the Childbearing Age. Boston, Little, Brown & Co., 1941.

Hansen, H., and Rybo, G.   Folic acid dosage in prophylactic treatment during pregnancy. Acta Obstet Gynec Scand 46(Pt. 7):107, 1967.

Hardy, J. B., Hardy, P. H., Oppenheimer, E. H., Ryan, S. J., Jr., and Sheff, R. N.   Failure of penicillin in a newborn with congenital syphilis. JAMA 212:1345, 1970.

———— McCracken, G. H., Jr., Gilkeson, M. R., and Sever, J. L.   Adverse fetal outcome following maternal rubella after the first trimester of pregnancy. JAMA 207:2414, 1969.

Harer, W. B., Jr., and Harer, W. B., Sr.   Volvulus complicating pregnancy and the puerperium. A report of three cases and review of literature (37 references cited). Obstet Gynec 12:399, 1958.

Harrington, W. J., Sprague, C. C., Minnich, V., Moore, C. V., Aulvin, R. C., and Dubach, R.   Immunologic mechanism in idiopathic and neonatal thrombocytopenia purpura. Ann Int Med 38:433, 1953.

Harris, G.   Acute leukaemia in pregnancy. Brit Med J 2:101, 1955.

Harris, J. W.   Influenza occurring in pregnant women. JAMA 72:978, 1919.

Harris, R. E.   Coccidioidomycosis complicating pregnancy. Obstet Gynec 28:401, 1966.

———— and Dunnihoo, D. R.   The incidence and significance of urinary calculi in pregnancy. Amer J Obstet Gynec 99:237, 1967.

Harrison, K. A., Ajabor, L. N., and Lawson, J. B.   Ephacrynic acid and packed-blood cell transfusion in treatment of severe anaemia in pregnancy. Lancet 1:11, 1971.

Hartenstein, H., and Gardner, L. I.   Tetany of the newborn associated with maternal parathyroid adenoma. New Eng J Med 274:266, 1966.

Hayes, G. W., Walsh, C. R., and D'Alessandro, E. E.   Scleroderma in pregnancy. Obstet Gynec 19:273, 1962.

Hellegers, A., and Neill, C.   Personal communication.

Hench, P. G.   Ameliorating effect of pregnancy on chronic atrophic (infectious rheumatoid) arthritis, fibrositis and intermittent hydrarthrosis. Proc Mayo Clin 13:161, 1938.

Hendricks, C. H.   The neurohypophysis in pregnancy. Obstet Gynec Surv 9:323, 1954.

Hendrickse, J. P. deV., and Watson-Williams, E. J.   The influence of hemoglobinopathies on reproduction. Amer J Obstet Gynec 94:739, 1966.

Herbert, V.   Experimental nutritional folate deficiency in man. Trans Ass Amer Physicians 75:307, 1962.

―――― Cunneen, N., Jaskiel, L., and Kopff, C.   Minimal daily adult folate requirement. Arch Intern Med 110:649, 1962.

Hibbard, B. M.   The role of folic acid in pregnancy. J Obstet Gynaec Brit Comm 71:529, 1964.

―――― Hibbard, E. D., Hwa, T. S., and Tan, P.   Abruptio placentae and defective folate metabolism in Singapore women. J Obstet Gynaec Brit Comm 76:1003, 1969.

Hibbard, E. D.   The FIGLU excretion test and defective folic-acid metabolism in pregnancy. Lancet 2:1146, 1964.

―――― and Smithels, R. W.   Folic acid metabolism and human embryopathy. Lancet 1:1254, 1965.

Hochman, A., and Schreiber, H.   Pregnancy and cancer of the breast. Obstet Gynec 2:268, 1953.

Hoffman, E. S., and Suzuki, M.   Acute appendicitis in pregnancy, a 10-year survey. Amer J Obstet Gynec 67:1338, 1954.

Holland, E.   A case of transplacental metastasis of malignant melanoma from mother to foetus. J Obstet Gynaec Brit Emp 56:529, 1949.

Holly, R. G.   Hypoplastic anemia of pregnancy. Obstet Gynec 1:535, 1953.

Honiotes, G., Clark, P. J., and Cavanaugh, D.   Gastric ulcer perforation during pregnancy. Amer J Obstet Gynec 106:619, 1970.

Horger, E. O., III, Kellett, W. W., III, and Williamson, H. O.   Diabetes in pregnancy. Obstet Gynec 30:46, 1967.

Horstmann, D. M., Liebhaber, H., and Kohorn, E. I.   Post-partum vaccination of rubella–susceptible women. Lancet 2:1003, 1970.

Hunt, A. B., and McConahey, W. M.   Pregnancy associated with disease of the adrenal glands. Amer J Obstet Gynec 66:970, 1953.

Hutchinson, D.   Personal communication.

Hyatt, H. W., Sr.   The relationships of maternal mumps to congenital defects and fetal deaths and maternal mortality and morbidity. Amer Pract 12:359, 1961.

Impastato, D. J., Gabriel, A. R., and Lardaro, H. H.   Electric and insulin shock therapy during pregnancy. Dis Nerv Syst 25:542, 1964.

Jackson, W. P. U.   On Diabetes Mellitus. Springfield, Ill., Charles C Thomas, 1964.

Johnson, D. W., Krale, P. A., Afable, V. L., Stewart, S. D., Halverson, C. W., and Holmes, K. K.   Single-dose antibiotic treatment of asymptomatic gonorrhea in hospitalized women. New Eng J Med 283:1, 1970.

Johnson, T. R., Banner, E. A., and Winkelmann, R. K.   Scleroderma and pregnancy. Obstet Gynec 23:467, 1964.

Jones, B. S.   Congenital malaria: 3 cases. Brit Med J 2:439, 1950.

Kahil, M. E., Fred, H. L., Brown, H., and Davis, J. S.   Acute fatty liver of pregnancy. Report of two cases. Arch Intern Med 113:63, 1964.

Kaiser, L. H., and King, E. L.   Lymphopathia venereum complicating labor, Amer J Obstet Gynec 54:219, 1947.

Kaplan, D., and Diamond, H.   Dermatomyositis and pregnancy. Clin Obstet Gynec 8:304, 1965.

Kasdon, S. C.   Pregnancy and Hodgkin's disease. Amer J Obstet Gynec 57:282, 1949.

Kass, E. H.   Pyelonephritis and bacteriuria. Ann Intern Med 56:46, 1962.

―――― Progress in Pyelonephritis. Philadelphia, F. A. Davis Co., 1965. (Contains six articles by various authors on bacteriuria in pregnancy.)

Kellermeyer, R. W., Tarlov, A. R., Brewer, G. J., Carson, P. E., and Alving, A. S. Hemolytic effect of therapeutic drugs. Clinical considerations of the primaquine-type hemolysis. JAMA 180:388, 1962.

Kincaid-Smith, P., and Bullen, M. Bacteriuria in pregnancy. Lancet 1:395, 1965.

King, R. M., and Anderson, G. V. Appendicitis in pregnancy. Calif Med 97:158, 1962.

Kistner, R. W., Hertig, A. T., and Rock, J. Tubal pregnancy complicating tuberculous salpingitis. Amer J Obstet Gynec 62:1157, 1951.

Kleeman, C. R., Hewitt, W. L., and Guze, L. B. Pyelonephritis. Medicine 39:3, 1960.

Kline, C. L. Emotional illness associated with childbirth: A study of 52 patients and the literature, Amer J Obstet Gynec 69:748, 1955.

Klopper, A. The assessment of feto-placental function by estriol assay. Obstet Gynec Survey 23:813, 1968.

Kohn, S. G., Briele, H. A., and Douglass, L. H. Volvulus complicating pregnancy. Amer J Obstet Gynec 48:398, 1944.

Kraus, G. W., and Yen, S.S.C. Gonorrhea during pregnancy. Obstet Gynec 31:258, 1968.

Kreek, M. J., Weser, E., Sleisenger, M. H., and Jeffries, G. H. Idiopathic cholestasis of pregnancy. New Eng J Med 277:1391, 1967.

Krugman, S., and Giles, J. P. Viral hepatitis. New light on an old disease. JAMA 212:1019, 1970.

Kunelis, C. T., Peters, J. L., and Edmonson, H. A. The fatty liver of pregnancy and its relationship to tetracycline therapy. Amer J Med 38:359, 1965.

Landesman, R., and Scherr, L. Congenital polycystic kidney disease in pregnancy. Obstet Gynec 8:673, 1956.

Laros, R. K., Hage, M. L., and Hayashi, R. H. Pregnancy and heart valve prostheses. Obstet Gynec 35:291, 1970.

Laubstein, M. B., Kotz, H. L., and Herre, F. W. Obstetric and anesthetic management following spontaneous subarachnoid hemorrhage. Obstet Gynec 20:661, 1962.

Lazarow, A., Kim, J. N., and Wells, L. J. Birth weight and fetal mortality in pregnant subdiabetic rats. Diabetes 9:114, 1960.

Lehman, H., and Huntsman, R. G. Man's Haemoglobins. Philadelphia, J. B. Lippincott Co., 1966.

Lindemann, C., Engstrom, W. W., and Flynn, R. T. Herpes gestationis: Results of treatment with adrenocorticotropic hormones (ACTH) and cortisone. Amer J Obstet Gynec 63:167, 1952.

Little, P. J. The incidence of urinary infection in 5000 pregnant women. Lancet 2:925, 1966.

Lloyd, O. Pulmonary tuberculosis in pregnancy. Practitioner 173:32, 1954.

London, W. T., DiFiglia, M., and Rodgers, J. Failure of transplacental transmission of Australia antigen. Lancet 2:900, 1969.

Low, J. A., Johnston, E. E., McBride, R. L., and Tuffnell, P. G. The significance of asymptomatic bacteriuria in the normal obstetric patient. Amer J Obstet Gynec 90:897, 1964.

Lowenstein, L., Pick, C., and Philpott, N. Megaloblastic anemia of pregnancy and the puerperium. Amer J Obstet Gynec 70:1309, 1955.

Lucké, B. Pathology of fatal epidemic hepatitis. Amer J Path 20:471, 1944.

Lutz, E. E., and Margolis, A. J. Obstetric hepatosis: treatment with cholestyramine and interim response to steroids. Obstet Gynec 33:64, 1969.

MacDonald, H. N. Pregnancy following insertion of cardiac valve prostheses. J Obstet Gynaec Brit Comm 77:603, 1970.

Mack, H. C., Schreiber, F., Nielsen, A., and Huber, P. J. Intracranial hemorrhage associated with pregnancy. Harper Hosp Bull 14:249, 1956.

Mackay, E. V. Pregnancy and renal disease. A ten year survey. Aust New Zeal J Obstet Gynaec 3:21, 1963.

Mackenzie, J. Heart Disease and Pregnancy. London, Oxford Medical Publication, 1921.

Madson, J. R., and Anderson, G. V. Lupus erythematosus and pregnancy. Obstet Gynec 18:492, 1961.

Manson, M. M., Logan, W.P.D., and Loy, R. M. Rubella and other virus infections during pregnancy. London, Her Majesty's Stationery Office, 1960.

Marcus, S. L. The nephrotic syndrome during pregnancy. Obstet Gynec Survey 18:511, 1963.

Matthews, H. B. Pregnancy after nephrectomy. JAMA 77:1634, 1921.

McCombs, R. P., and Patterson, J. F.   Factors influencing course and prognosis of systemic lupus erythematosus. New Eng J Med 260:1195, 1959.

McCurdy, P. R.   Abnormal hemoglobins and pregnancy. Amer J Obstet Gynec 90:891, 1964.

McKusick, V. A.   Heritable Disorders of Connective Tissue. St. Louis, C. V. Mosby, 1956.

McLane, C. M.   Pyelitis of pregnancy, five year study. Amer J Obstet Gynec 38:117, 1939.

McLone, D. G., Billings, P. E., and Hardegree, W. E.   Gonorrhea in females treated with one oral dose of tetracycline. Brit J Vener Dis 44:218, 1968.

Mendelow, D. A., and Lewis, G. C., Jr.   Varicella pneumonia during pregnancy. Obstet Gynec 33:98, 1969.

Mendelson, C. L.   Aspiration of stomach contents into the lungs during obstetric anesthesia. Amer J Obstet Gynec 52:191, 1946.

———— Cardiac Disease in Pregnancy. Philadelphia, F. A. Davis, 1960.

Minkowitz, S., Soloway, H. B., Hall, J. E., and Yermankou, V.   Fatal hemorrhagic pancreatitis following chlorthiazide administration in pregnancy. Obstet Gynec 24:337, 1964.

Mitchell, D. M., and Jessop, J. C.   Herpes gestationis. Brit Med J 1:1425, 1964.

Montgomery, W. H., and Miller, F. C.   Pancreatitis and pregnancy. Obstet Gynec 35:658, 1970.

Monzon, O. T., Armstrong, D., Pion, R. J., Deigh, R., and Hewitt, W. L.   Bacteriuria during pregnancy. Amer J Obstet Gynec 85:511, 1963.

Murray, F. A.   Lupus erythematosus in pregnancy. J. Obstet Gynaec Brit Emp 65:401, 1958.

Murray, J. E., Reid, D. E., Harrison, J. H., and Merrill, J. P.   Successful pregnancies after human renal transplantation. New Eng J Med 269:341, 1963.

Nadler, N., Salinas-Madrigal, L., Charles, A. G., and Pollak, V. E.   Acute glomerulonephritis during late pregnancy. Obstet Gynec 34:277, 1969.

Nesbitt, R. E. L., Jr., Hayes, R. C., and Mauro, J.   The behavior of C-reactive protein in pregnant and puerperal women, fetal blood, and in the newborn infant under normal and abnormal conditions. Obstet Gynec 16:659, 1960.

Norden, C. W., and Kilpatrick, W. H.   In Kass E. H. (ed.), Progress in Pyelonephritis. Philadelphia, F. A. Davis Co., 1965, p. 64.

Oakley, W.   Prognosis in diabetic pregnancy. Brit Med J 1:1413, 1953.

Ober, W. B., and Le Compte, P. M.   Acute fatty metamorphosis of the liver associated with pregnancy; distinctive lesion. Amer J Med 19:743, 1955.

———— Reid, D. E., Romney, S. L., and Merrill, J. P.   Renal lesions and acute renal failure in pregnancy. Amer J Med 21:781, 1956.

O'Dwyer, J. P.   Acute idiopathic porphyria complicating pregnancy. J Obstet Gynaec Brit Emp 62:437, 1955.

O'Leary, J. A.   A continuing study of sarcoidosis and pregnancy. Amer J Obstet Gynec 101:610, 1968.

———— Klainer, L. M., and Neuworth, R. S.   The management of hypoparathyroidism in pregnancy. Amer J Obstet Gynec 94:1103, 1966.

Pearson, E.   The effect of pregnancy on otosclerosis. Ann West Med Surg 5:477, 1951.

Pedowitz, P., and Perell, A.   Aneurysms complicated by pregnancy. Part II. Aneurysms of cerebral vessels. Amer J Obstet Gynec 73:736, 1957 (64 references cited).

Penman, W. R.   Hiatal hernia: a cause of persistent gastrointestinal disturbances in pregnancy. West J Surg 59:622, 1951.

Penn, I., Makowski, E., Droegemueller, W., Halgrimson, C. G., and Starzl, T. E.   Parenthood in renal homograft recipients. JAMA (in press).

Peterson, O. H., Jr., and Larson, P.   Thrombocytopenic purpura in pregnancy. Obstet Gynec 4:454, 1954.

Pickard, R. E.   Varicella pneumonia in pregnancy. Amer J Obstet Gynec 101:504, 1968.

Popert, A. J.   Pregnancy and adrenal cortical hormone. Brit Med J 1:967, 1962.

Prather, G. C., and Crabtree, E. G.   Impressions relating to urinary tract stone in pregnancy. Urol Cutan Rev 38:17, 1934.

———— and Crabtree, E. G.   The lone kidney in pregnancy. Trans Amer Ass Genitourin Surg 26:313, 1933.

Pritchard, J. A.   Hereditary hypochromic microcytic anemia in obstetrics and gynecology. Amer J Obstet Gynec 83:1193, 1962.

———— Megaloblastic anemia during pregnancy and the puerperium. Amer J Obstet Gynec 83:1004, 1962.

———— Anemias complicating pregnancy and the puerperium, in Maternal Nutrition and the Course of Pregnancy, Report of the Committee on Maternal Nutrition, Food and Nutrition Board, National Research Council, National Academy of Sciences, Washington, 1970.

———— and Hunt, C. A comparison of the hematologic responses following the routine prenatal administration of intramuscular and oral iron. Surg Gynec Obstet 106:516, 1958.

———— and Mason, R. A. Iron stores of normal adults and replenishment with oral iron therapy. JAMA 190:897, 1964.

———— and Scott, D. E. Iron demands in pregnancy, in Iron Deficiency Pathogenesis, Clinical Aspects, Therapy. London and New York Academic Press, 1970.

———— Scott, D. E., and Whalley, P. J. Folic acid requirements in pregnancy-induced megaloblastic anemia. JAMA 208:1163, 1969.

———— Scott, D. E., Whalley, P. J., and Haling, R. F., Jr. Infants of mothers with megaloblastic anemia due to folate deficiency. JAMA 211:1982, 1970.

———— Scott, D. E., and Whalley, P. J. Maternal folate deficiency and pregnancy wastage. IV. Effects of folic acid supplements, anticonvulsants, and oral contraceptives. Amer J Obstet Gynec 110:375, 1971.

Radnich, R. H., and Jacobs, M. Prosthetic heart valves. Texas Med 66:58, 1970.

Reginster, A. (Five years of routine chest x-ray in the prenatal clinic of the University Hospital at Liège). Bull Soc Roy Belg Gynec Obstet 25:103, 1955.

Reynolds, A. G. Placental metastasis from malignant melanoma. Obstet Gynec 6:205, 1955.

Ricks, P. Sickle cell anemia and pregnancy. Obstet Gynec 17:513, 1961.

Rigler, L. G., and Eneboe, J. B. Incidence of hiatus hernia in pregnant women and its significance. J Thoracic Surg 4:262, 1935.

Robertson, H. E., and Dochat, G. R. Pregnancy and gallstones. Int Abst Surg (Surg Gynec Obstet) 78:193, 1944.

Robson, J. S., Martin, A. M., Ruckley, V. A., and Macdonald, M. K. Irreversible postpartum renal failure. Quart J Med 37:423, 1968.

Rose, D. Spontaneous hematoma of the abdominal wall in pregnancy. Report of a case. New Eng J Med 234:582, 1946.

Rovinsky, J. J. Primary refractory anemia complicating pregnancy and delivery. Obstet Gynec Survey 14:149, 1959.

Ruch, W. A., and Klein, R. L. Polycythemia vera and pregnancy. Obstet Gynec 23:107, 1964.

Savage, W. E., Hajj, S. N., and Kass, E. H. Demographic and prognostic characteristics of bacteriuria in pregnancy. Medicine 46:385, 1967.

Saxen, L., Hjelt, L., Sjostedt, J. E., Hakosalo, J., and Hakosalo, H. Asian influenza during pregnancy and congenital malformation. Acta Path Microbiol Scand 49:114, 1960.

Schaefer, G. Tuberculosis in Obstetrics and Gynecology. Boston, Little, Brown & Co., 1956.

———— Full term pregnancy following genital tuberculosis. Obstet Gynec Surv 19:81, 1964 (112 references cited).

———— and Silverman, F. Pregnancy complicated by asthma. Amer J Obstet Gynec 82:182, 1965.

Schenker, K. G., and Polishuk, W. Z. Pregnancy following mitral valvotomy. Obstet Gynec 32:214, 1968.

Schiffer, M. A. Fatty liver associated with administration of tetracycline in pregnant and non-pregnant women. Amer J Obstet Gynec 96:362, 1966.

Schmale, J. D., Martin, J. E., Jr., and Domescik, G. Observations on the culture diagnosis of gonorrhea in women. JAMA 210:312, 1969.

Schultz, J. C., Adamson, J. S., Jr., Workman, W. W., and Norma, T. D. Fatal liver disease after intravenous administration of tetracycline in high dosage. New Eng J Med 269:999, 1963.

Schütz. (The effect of cholera on menstruation, pregnancy, delivery and the puerperium). Zbl Gynäk 18:1138, 1894.

Schwarz, R. H., Fields, G. A., and Kyle, G. C. Timing of delivery in the pregnant diabetic patient. Obstet Gynec 34:787, 1969.

Schweitzer, I. L., and Spears, R. L. Hepatitis–associated antigen (Australia antigen) in mother and infant. New Eng J Med 283:570, 1970.

Scott, D. E., and Pritchard, J. A. Iron deficiency in healthy young college women. JAMA 199:147, 1967.

———— Whalley, P. J., and Pritchard, J. A.   Maternal folate deficiency and pregnancy wastage. II. Fetal malformation. Obstet Gynec 36:26, 1970.

Scudamore, H. H., Rogers, A. G., Bargen, J. A., and Banner, E. A.   Pregnancy after ileostomy for chronic ulcerative colitis. Gastroenterology 32:295, 1957.

Seftel, N. C., and Schewitz, L. J.   The nephrotic syndrome in pregnancy. J Obstet Gynaec Brit Emp 64:862, 1957.

Selikoff, I. J., and Dorfmann, H. L., in Surgical and Gynecological Complications of Pregnancy, 2nd ed., J. J. Rovinsky and A. F. Guttmacher (eds.). Baltimore, The Williams & Wilkins Co., 1965 (46 references cited).

Sever, J. L.   Viral teratogens: A status report. Hospital Practice, p. 75, April, 1970.

———— and White, L. R.   Intrauterine viral infections. Ann Rev Med 19:471, 1968.

Shapiro, L. H., and Lentz, J. W.   Kanamycin as treatment of acute gonorrhea in females. Obstet Gynec 35:794, 1970.

Sheehan, H. L.   Jaundice in pregnancy. Amer J Obstet Gynec 81:427, 1961.

———— The pathology of acute yellow atrophy and delayed chloroform poisoning. J Obstet Gynaec Brit Emp 47:597, 1940.

———— and Moore, H. C.   Renal Cortical Necrosis and the Kidney of Concealed Accidental Haemorrhage. Springfield, Ill., Charles C Thomas, 1953.

Shub, H., Black, M. M., and Speer, F. D.   Chronic granulocytic (myelogenous) leukemia and pregnancy. Blood 8:375, 1953.

Seigler, A. M., and Spain, D. M.   Periarteritis nodosa in pregnancy. Clin Obstet Gynec 8:280, 1965.

Siegel, M., and Goldberg, M.   Incidence of poliomyelitis in pregnancy. New Eng J Med 253:841, 1955.

Simon, A.   Psychiatric indications for therapeutic abortion and sterilization. Clin Obstet Gynec 7:67, 1964.

Skinner, W. E.   Routine rubella antibody titer determinations in pregnancy. Obstet Gynec 33:301, 1969.

Slate, W. G., and Graham, A. R.   Scleroderma and pregnancy. Amer J Obstet Gynec 101:335, 1968.

Sleigh, J. D., Robertson, J. F., and Isdale, M. H.   Asymptomatic bacteriuria in pregnancy. J Obstet Gynaec Brit Comm 71:74, 1964.

Smith, E. W., and Krevans, J. R.   Clinical manifestations of hemoglobin C disorders. Bull Johns Hopkins Hosp 104:17, 1959.

Stefanini, M., Chatterjea, J. M., and Adelson, E.   Immunologic aspects of idiopathic thrombocytopenic purpura. J Clin Invest 31:665, 1952.

Stokes, J., Jr., Wolman, I. J., Blanchard, M. C., and Farquhar, J. D.   Viral hepatitis in the newborn; clinical features, epidemiology and pathology. Amer J Dis Child 82:213, 1951.

Studd, J.W.W., and Blainey, J. D.   Pregnancy and the nephrotic syndrome. Brit Med J 1:276, 1969.

Studdiford, W. E.   Pregnancy and pelvic tuberculosis. Amer J Obstet Gynec 69:379, 1955.

Sutherland, H. W., Stowers, J. M., and McKenzie, C.   Simplifying the clinical problem of glycosuria in pregnancy. Lancet 1:1069, 1970.

Sweeney, W. J.   Pregnancy and multiple sclerosis. Amer J Obstet Gynec 66:124, 1953.

Talbert, L. M., Thomas, C. G., Jr., Holt, W. A., and Rankin, P.   Hyperthyroidism during pregnancy. Obstet Gynec 36: 779, 1970.

Thomascheck, G., Schmidtke, L., and Genz, H.   (Studies of Toxoplasma infection in pregnant subjects and morbidity of their progeny). Z Geburtsh Gynäk 156:182, 1961.

Tracy, T. A., and Miller, G. L.   Obstetric problems of the massively obese. Obstet Gynec 33:204, 1969.

Tricomi, V.   The Marfan syndrome and pregnancy. Clin Obstet Gynec 8:334, 1965.

———— and Baum, H.   Acute intermittent porphyria and pregnancy, Obstet Gynec Surv 13:307, 1958.

Tucker, S. M., and Sibson, D. E.   Foetal complication of vaccination in pregnancy. Brit Med J 2:237, 1962.

Tuffanelli, D. C., and Winklemann, R. K.   Systemic scleroderma: a clinical study of 727 cases. AMA Arch Dermat 87:359, 1961.

Tuffli, G. A., and Nahmias, A. J.   Neonatal herpetic infection. Amer J Dis Child 118:909, 1969.

Turck, M., and Petersdorf, R. G.   A study of chemoprophylaxis of postpartum urinary-tract infection. JAMA 182:899, 1962.

Vaheri, A., Vesikari, T., Oker-Blom, N., Seppala, M., Veronelli, J., Robbins, F. C., and Parkman, P. D.   Transmission of the rubella virus to the human fetus. Amer J Dis Child 118:243, 1969.

Vasicka, A., Lin, T. J., and Bright, R. H.   Peptic ulcer and pregnancy. Review of hormonal relationships and a report of one case of massive gastrointestinal hemorrhage. Obstet Gynec Surv 12:1, 1957 (56 references cited).

Wagoner, R. D., Holley, K. E., and Johnson, W. J.   Accelerated nephrosclerosis and postpartum acute renal failure in normotensive patients. Ann Intern Med 69:237, 1968.

Walker, W. M., and McKee, A. P.   Asian influenza in pregnancy. Relationship to fetal anomalies. Obstet Gynec 13:394, 1959.

Waters, E. G.   Discussion of paper by J. T. Callahan: Separation of symphysis pubis. Amer J Obstet Gynec 66:292, 1953.

———— and Fenimore, E. D.   Perforated carcinoma of the cecum in pregnancy. Obstet Gynec 3:263, 1954.

———— and McCall, W. H.   Fatal intestinal obstruction during pregnancy. Bull Margaret Hague Maternity Hosp 3:64, 1950.

Werkö, L., and Bucht, H.   Glomerular filtration rate and renal blood flow in patients with chronic diffuse glomerulonephritis during pregnancy. Acta Med Scand 153:177, 1956.

Westberg, S. V.   Prognosis of breast cancer for pregnant and nursing women. Acta Obstet Gynec Scand 25 (Suppl. 4), 1946.

Whalley, P. J.   Bacteriuria of pregnancy. Amer J Obstet Gynec 97:723, 1967.

———— Adams, R. H., and Combes, B.   Tetracycline toxicity in pregnancy. JAMA 189:357, 1964.

———— Martin, F. G., and Peters, P. C.   Significance of asymptomatic bacteriuria detected during pregnancy. JAMA 193:879, 1965.

———— Martin, F. G., Adams, R. H., and Combes, B.   Disposition of tetracycline by pregnant women with acute pyelonephritis. Obstet Gynec 36:821, 1970.

———— Martin, F. G., and Pritchard, J. A.   Sickle cell trait and urinary tract infection during pregnancy. JAMA 189:903, 1964.

———— Pritchard, J. A., and Richards, J. R., Jr.   Sickle cell trait and pregnancy. JAMA 186:1132, 1963.

———— Scott, D. E., and Pritchard, J. A.   Maternal folate deficiency and pregnancy wastage. I. Placental abruption. Amer J Obstet Gynec 105:670, 1969.

———— Scott, D. E., and Pritchard, J. A.   Maternal folate deficiency and pregnancy wastage. III. Pregnancy-induced hypertension. Obstet Gynec 36:29, 1970.

White, M. A., Prout, C. T., Fixsen, C., and Foundeur, M.   Obstetrician's role in postpartum mental illness. JAMA 165:138, 1957.

White, P.   Pregnancy and diabetes, medical aspects. Med Clin N Amer 49:1015, 1965.

Williams, D. A.   Asthma and pregnancy. Acta Allerg 22:311, 1967.

Williams, J. W.   The limitations and possibilities of prenatal care. JAMA 64:95, 1915.

Willoughby, M.L.N., and Jewell, F. G.   Folate status throughout pregnancy and in the postpartum period. Brit Med J 4:356, 1968.

Wilson, M. G., Heins, H. L., Imagawa, D. T., and Adams, J. M.   Teratogenic effects of Asian influenza. JAMA 171:638, 1959.

———— Hewitt, W. L., and Monzon, O. T.   Effect of bacteriuria on the fetus. New Eng J Med 274:115, 1966.

Winkelmann, R. K.   Scleroderma and pregnancy. Clin Obstet Gynec 8:280, 1965.

Wintrobe, M. M.   Clinical Hematology. Philadelphia, Lea & Febiger, 1967.

Zakon, S. J., Leader, L. O., and Siegel, I.   Herpes gestationis: Treatment with ACTH and cortisone. Obstet Gynec 2:78, 1953.

Zondek, B., and Bromberg, Y. M.   Infectious hepatitis in pregnancy. J Mt Sinai Hosp 14:222, 1947.

28

DYSTOCIA CAUSED BY ANOMALIES OF THE EXPULSIVE FORCES

Dystocia (difficult labor) may be defined as cessation of progress in parturition as the result of abnormalities in the mechanics involved. The causes of dystocia fall into three main groups:

1. **Subnormal or abnormal uterine forces that are not sufficiently strong to overcome the natural resistance offered to the birth of the baby by the maternal soft parts and the bony birth canal. Weakness of uterine action is called uterine dysfunction ("inertia").**
2. **Faulty presentation or abnormal development of the fetus of such a character that it cannot be extruded by the vis a tergo.**
3. **Abnormalities in the size or character of the birth canal that form an obstacle to the descent of the fetus. Pelvic contraction is often associated with uterine dysfunction, and the two together constitute the most common cause of dystocia.**

Certain complications during labor—such as abruptio placentae, placenta previa, and rupture of the uterus—may lead to various irregularities that interfere with the normal progress of labor. The issues involved in these complications, however, are quite different from those in the three groups listed above. Limiting discussion to those conditions connoting difficulty in the mechanics of labor will lead to clearer thinking about dystocia.

The expulsion of the fetus is brought about by contractions of the uterus, reinforced during the second stage of labor by the action of the muscles of the abdominal wall. Either of these factors may be lacking in intensity or, occasionally, may be abnormally strong.

Unfortunately there is no absolute standard by which the character of the labor pains can be gauged. In an exceptional primigravida, a rapid and successful termination of labor may follow a few relatively slight pains, which in the majority of normal primigravidas would prove quite inadequate to bring about the desired result. Clinically the efficiency of the uterine contractions may be measured by their effect upon the course and duration of labor, provided there is no serious mechanical obstacle to be overcome. Other things being equal, prolonged labor, on the one hand, and precipitate labor, on the other, occur as a result of abnormalities in the frequency and intensity of the contractions. Other than its effects, the best clinical index of the intensity of a labor pain is the degree to which the uterus can be indented by the palpating fingers at the acme of a contraction. If at the height of a contraction the uterine wall can be appreciably indented, the contraction is not of the best quality. The complaints of the patient regarding her pains do not, of course, always indicate the actual intensity of the contractions. Patients not only differ in their threshold of pain but complain particularly about the inefficient pains associated with incoordinate uterine action, as noted especially in posterior positions of the occiput.

Uterine dysfunction has always plagued obstetricians. It has resulted in innumerable maternal and perinatal deaths and in frequent tragic damage to children. In the delivery of Princess Charlotte of Wales, uterine inertia changed the course of history by causing her death and that of her son; the obstetrician later committed suicide (Holland). The oxytocic properties of extracts of the posterior pituitary were discovered by Dale in 1906. Use of pituitary extract followed the course of many potent drugs. At first it enjoyed unqualified acceptance. It was then overused, abused, and condemned. Finally, a half century after its introduction, its benefits, limitations, and risks were realized. Sogolow has written an excellent history of these developments. Although oxytocin was synthesized in 1953 by du Vigneaud and colleagues, and despite the knowledge that it is probably the specific hormone for initiation and potentiation of uterine contractions, very little is known about its crucial action at the cellular level. A beginning has been made by electrophysiologic studies of the action of oxytocin on individual myometrial cells (Kao; Kleinhaus and Kao).

UTERINE DYSFUNCTION

Friedman believes that an accurate picture of labor may be obtained from the progress of cervical dilatation. In normal labor there is first a latent phase of several hours' duration, during which the cervix becomes effaced but dilates only slightly. There follows an active phase of acceleration when the cervix dilates rather rapidly and, more important, progressively. A deceleration or slowing may occur just before full dilatation. Hendricks and associates present a slightly different graphic depiction of normal labor (Figs. 1 and 2). They believe that in the final weeks of pregnancy the mean dilatation of the cervix is 1.8 cm and 2.2 cm in nulliparas and primiparas respectively. They also find that in normal active labor there is a constant active acceleration with a "deceleration" phase and that cervical dilatation occurs at approximately the same rate in nulliparas and multiparas after 4 cm dilatation has been reached.

These seemingly divergent points of view do not alter the fact that any significant prolongation of any of the phases described by Friedman (Figs. 3 through 7) or any significant change in the curves presented by Hendricks, be it before or after 4 cm cervical dilatation, constitutes uterine dysfunction.

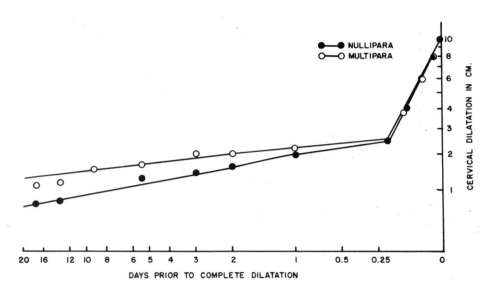

Fig. 1. Cervical dilatation through prelabor and labor. (From Hendricks, Brenner, and Kraus.)

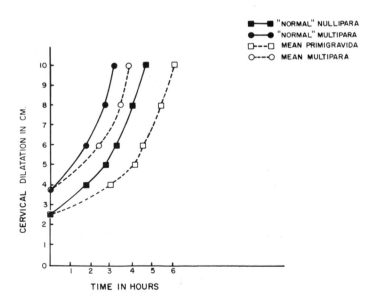

Fig. 2. Cervical dilatation in normal nulliparas and multiparas after the onset of true labor. (From Hendricks, Brenner, and Kraus.)

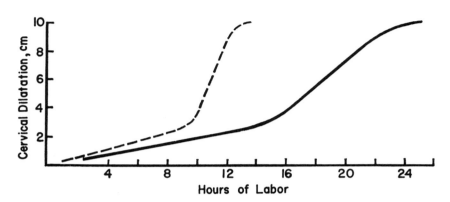

Fig. 3. Uterine dysfunction. Composite labor curve denoting prolongation of both the latent and the active phases. Broken line represents the mean curve. (After Friedman. Obstet Gynec 6:567, 1955.)

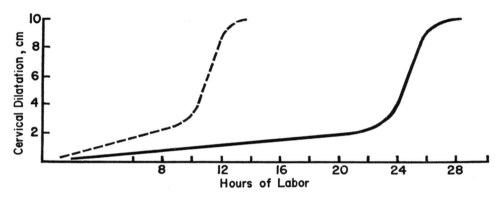

Fig. 4. Prolonged latent phase. Composite labor curve demonstrating prolongation of the latent phase, which is then followed by normal active phase. Prolongation of latent phase has been found to be closely associated with (1) "unripe" cervix, (2) early analgesic-sedative medication, and (3) early use of conduction anesthesia. (After Friedman. Obstet Gynec 6:567, 1955.)

Formerly dysfunction, or inertia, was classified as primary or secondary, the former occurring from the very onset of labor and of unknown cause, and the latter occurring somewhat later, following prolonged labor with maternal exhaustion. In modern practice great prolongation of labor with profound maternal exhaustion is not tolerated. Accordingly, secondary uterine inertia in the classical sense has become increasingly rare. Hellman, as well as Jeffcoate and others, has attempted to render the definitions of primary and secondary uterine inertia more precise, in accordance with modern obstetric diagnosis and therapy. In the main, these attempts have proved cumbersome and of little clinical value; the older terms thus continue in use, albeit with slightly altered meanings. Knowledge of uterine action provided by the research of Reynolds and his associates, Karlson, and others, and clarification by Moore and D'Esopo and by Friedman of the phases of labor just mentioned, render more logical a discussion of this subject

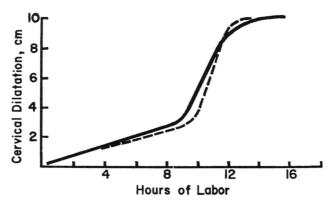

Fig. 5. Prolonged deceleration phase. Composite labor curve representing normal labor pattern except for prolonged deceleration. Prolongation of deceleration phase in an otherwise normal labor has been found most often in association with fetopelvic disproportion and malposition. (After Friedman. Obstet Gynec 6:567, 1955.)

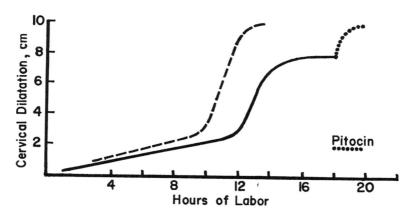

Fig. 6. Uterine dysfunction. Premature deceleration with arrest in the active phase following essentially normal latent and early active phases. Therapeutic effect of Pitocin infusion is indicated by dotted lines. (Data based on Moore and D'Esopo. Amer J Obstet Gynec 70:1338, 1955.)

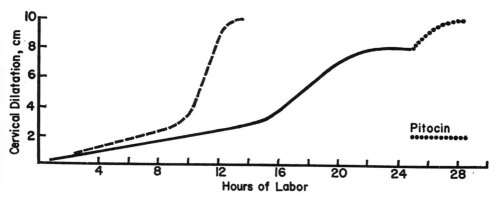

Fig. 7. Uterine dysfunction. Latent and active phases. The effect of Pitocin infusion is demonstrated (dotted lines). (Data based on Moore and D'Esopo. Amer J Obstet Gynec 70:1338, 1955.)

under the general heading of uterine dysfunction, since it involves the various phases of cervical dilatation. The term "uterine inertia" may be used interchangeably with "uterine dysfunction." If the former term is employed, primary uterine inertia refers to prolongation of the latent phase of labor, whereas secondary uterine inertia indicates an abnormality in the active phase.

Any extension of either the first or second stage of labor may result in an increased perinatal mortality. Whether it is the result of longer labor alone or whether it stems from other complications, such as heroic attempts to terminate labor or premature rupture of the membranes with infection, is still not clear. Hellman and Prystowsky have shown conclusively from data collected at the Johns Hopkins Hospital that the perinatal mortality increases as the first and, independently, as the second stage become prolonged (Fig. 8). These facts do

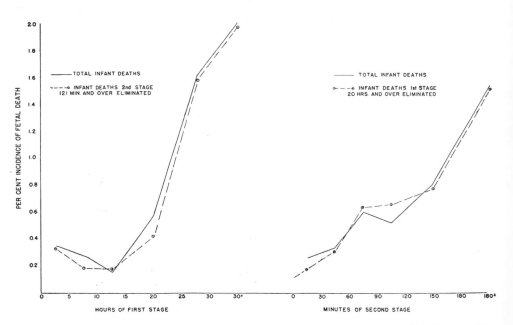

Fig. 8. The effect of the duration of the first and second stages of labor on infant mortality.

not justify hasty or radical intervention by the obstetrician, however, for the perinatal loss and subsequent damage to the infant are far greater in traumatic delivery than in desultory labor; nevertheless, delay in any of the phases of cervical dilatation or in the second stage should alert the obstetrician to possible danger. He must plan his course of action carefully and logically, step by step, aiming toward proper and timely therapy and delivery, as befit each individual case. Too often tragedies result from confused thinking or procrastination in the face of uterine dysfunction.

No arbitrary limit of time may be applied to either the definitions of uterine dysfunction or the proper period to initiate treatment. The onset of uterine dysfunction in any phase of cervical dilatation occurs when progress stops, for one of the prime characteristics of normal labor is its progression. Friedman, in an attempt at precision, defines prolongation of the latent phase as 20 hours and 14 hours in primigravidas and multigravidas, respectively, while cervical dilatation of less than 1.2 cm/hour in nulliparas and 1.5 cm/hour in multiparas represents a protracted active phase. Nevertheless, the diagnosis, especially in the latent phase, is difficult and sometimes can be made only in retrospect. The more experienced the obstetrician and the more astute his clinical judgment, the sooner will he detect this abnormality and the sooner and more successfully will be initiate treatment. The nicest obstetric judgment is required, for one of the commonest errors is to treat a patient for uterine inertia when she is not yet in labor.

There have been two significant advances in the treatment of uterine dysfunction. The first is philosophical and the second therapeutic:

1. The understanding that prolongation of labor contributes to perinatal mortality
2. The introduction of very dilute intravenous oxytocin in the treatment of certain types of uterine dysfunction

Types of Uterine Dysfunction. As indicated on page 356, Reynolds and his associates have shown that the uterine contractions of labor are characterized by a gradient of activity, greatest at the fundus and decreasing toward the cervix. Caldeyro-Barcia and his colleagues in Montevideo have advanced the work of Reynolds by inserting small balloons in the uterine muscle at various levels. With the balloons attached to strain-gauge transducers they have been able to show that there was, in addition to a gradient of activity, a time differential in the onset of the contractions in the fundus, midzone, and lower segment. Larks believes that he has confirmed the differential electronically, showing that the exciting stimulus starts in one cornu and then several milliseconds later in the other, the excitation waves then joining and sweeping over the fundus and down the uterus. Neither peristalsis nor simultaneous contraction is involved.

The group in Montevideo made another significant contribution to the understanding of uterine dysfunction. By inserting a polethylene catheter through the abdomen into the amniotic fluid they ascertained that the lower limit of pressure of contractions required to dilate the cervix is 15 mm Hg, a figure in keeping with the findings of Hendricks, which indicate that a normal uterine contraction may exert a much higher pressure of about 60 mm Hg. By combining the data of Reynolds, Caldeyro-Barcia, and Larks, it is possible to define two physiologic types of uterine dysfunction. In one, the hypotonic variety, the uterine contractions have a normal gradient pattern (synchronous) but a pressure of less than 15 mm Hg. in the other, the gradient is distorted, perhaps by contraction of the midsegment with more force than the fundus (reversal) or by complete asynchronism of the electrical impulses originating in each cornu. This variety is always accompanied by hypertonicity of the muscle.

Obviously the complicated instruments used to discover the various types of uterine malfunction are not universally available, nor are they adaptable to routine clinical differentiation between the two types of dysfunction. Fortunately, once the types had been clearly defined by research technics it became possible to distinguish them easily on a clinical basis. In the *hypotonic* variety, contractions become infrequent and of poor quality, and the uterus is easily indentable even at the acme of a contraction. Contractions of the *hypertonic* variety are clinically much more painful than palpation of the uterus would indicate.

Of almost equal importance is the fact that, by and large, hypertonic dysfunction occurs early in labor or in the latent phase, and therefore may be regarded as similar to primary uterine inertia, whereas hypotonic dysfunction occurs in the accelerated or active phase of labor or during the second stage and is similar to secondary uterine inertia. There are several other differences between the hypertonic and hypotonic types of dysfunction. Signs of fetal distress usually do not appear in hypotonic dysfunction until intrauterine infection has developed. On the contrary, in hypertonic dysfunction fetal distress may appear early. Finally, hypotonic dysfunction responds favorably to treatment with oxytocin, whereas the opposite is true of the hypertonic variety, in which the poor pattern of uterine contractions is more likely to become accentuated and the tension of the resting uterine muscle increased. At the risk of oversimplifying a rather complicated subject, Table 1 is presented. These criteria for differentiation of the

Table 1. Clinical Criteria for the Differentiation of the Two Types of Dysfunction

	Hypotonic	Hypertonic
Occurrence rate	4% of labors	1% of labors
Phase of labor	Active	Latent
Clinical symptom	Painless	Painful
Fetal distress	Late	Early
Reaction to oxytocin	Favorable	Unfavorable
Value of sedation	Little	Great

two types of uterine dysfunction are generalizations that do not invariably apply.
Etiology of Uterine Dysfunction.   Ill-timed and excessive administration of analgesia before the onset of true labor, minor degrees of pelvic contraction, and fetal malposition of even slight degree, such as extension of the head, are chief causes of uterine dysfunction. Friedman found some combination of these three factors in 95 per cent of dysfunctional nulliparous labors. That minor degrees of pelvic contraction may cause uterine inertia is of great clinical importance, for upon its recognition depends the success or failure of treatment. Overdistention of the uterus and an improper emotional approach to labor also may contribute to the condition. In many cases, however, the cause of uterine dysfunction is unknown.

The main fault rarely lies in a cervix that is too rigid to dilate or that shows a peculiar agglutination, as in conglutination of the external os. Often in such cases simple insertion and sweeping of the finger inside the cervix cause rapid dilatation. Such abnormalities of the cervix add but little to the problem of dysfunctional labor, for frequently the stimulation of effective labor by oxytocin causes the most rigid cervix to efface and dilate without difficulty. Occasionally in elderly primigravidas, however, excessive rigidity of the cervix and its consequent tardy and imperfect dilatation may be an important factor in the production of dystocia.

Complications of Uterine Dysfunction.   Perinatal loss and injury to the newborn infant are by far the most serious consequences of dysfunction. Loss of the fetal heart tones or impairment of the infant stems from undue prolongation of either the first or second stage of labor, or a combination of both, as indicated by Hellman and Prystowsky (Fig. 8). These unfortunate consequences are related to the duration of labor and are independent of the mode of delivery.

Both fetal and neonatal deaths are also frequent accompaniments of intrauterine infection, which commonly develops in dysfunctional labor. Although it may be wise for the mother's protection to treat these intrauterine infections with antibiotics, such therapy is of little value in protecting the fetus (Guilbeau and Eastman; Lebherz and associates). Unless the fetus is soon delivered, an unfortunate outcome may be expected in a high percentage of cases.

Maternal exhaustion and dehydration may occur if labor is greatly prolonged, particularly in hot, humid weather. Elevation of maternal pulse and temperature and acetonuria are the clinical signs of the syndrome. However, supportive therapy with adequate intravenous fluids should be initiated and delivery effected before these signs appear. Occasionally in neglected cases there are abdominal distention, perhaps the result of adynamic ileus, edema and even necrosis of the partially dilated cervix, and complete maternal exhaustion. Such situations require experienced clinical judgment whereby support, replacement of fluid and electrolytes, and rest are balanced against the passage of time to achieve delivery of a living undamaged child. Success in these cases is the pinnacle of obstetric art.

It has been the general impression of obstetricians that difficult labors and deliveries left few psychologic scars on the patients. Jeffcoate, as well as Steer, however, found that difficult labor exerted a definite deleterious effect upon future childbearing. The latter investigators showed that although more than about two thirds of their patients had further children after spontaneous delivery, only one third did so after midforceps operations. Every experienced obstetrician has had the problem of caring for patients with persistent, troublesome fear resulting from a previous difficult labor.

Treatment of Hypotonic Dysfunction (Secondary Uterine Inertia). Obstetricians in the past century taught that the safest treatment of uterine inertia was "tincture of time." Their view was naturally colored by the disastrous effects of instrumental and operative interference in those days. In modern obstetrics that concept retains only a modicum of truth, for the passage of time, if not well utilized, produces an ever increasing fetal loss, or as Jeffcoate writes, "Nature and time are unreliable allies." Once the diagnosis of hypotonic dysfunction has been made, time should be used to check the position and presentation of the fetus, the level of the presenting part, and the state of the cervix. A careful evaluation of the pelvis should be performed and supportive therapy initiated. In addition, the obstetrician should formulate a careful and orderly plan for the successful termination of a disordered labor. The passage of time should not be marked by hopeful procrastination or masterly inactivity.

The early diagnosis of uterine dysfunction is rewarded by an ever diminishing number of cases of fetal damage and death. It is not only the hallmark of the obstetrician who follows each mother carefully throughout her labor, but it is also the sign of a well-taught and well-disciplined house staff.

Uterine inertia is more often a protection against some degrees of pelvic contraction and abnormalities of position than a result of defective function of the uterus. Immediately upon suspecting interference with the progress of labor, therefore, the obstetrician should perform a vaginal examination to detect these factors. The vaginal examination should be carried out in an orderly fashion to assess the true state of the cervix and the position of the presenting part and to reevaluate the pelvis. If the diagnosis of hypotonic dysfunction in the active phase of labor is correct, the cervix will be at least 3 cm dilated.

X-ray pelvimetry in our experience, as well as that of Knapp and Warenski
The New York Lying-In Hospital, has been invaluable in the successful manag
ment of uterine dysfunction. It not only yields accurate measurements of t
pelvis, particularly the transverse diameters, but also may reveal abnormaliti
of fetal position. In hypotonic dysfunction the peculiar curvature of t
cervical spine of the fetus, termed "goosenecking" (Fig. 9), is pathognomonic
the condition, indicating the characteristically poor uterine forces. The pelvic e
amination and x-ray pelvimetry consume time, but this period may be used n
only to initiate supportive therapy but perhaps to give the patient an enema a
to allow her to walk. These essentially innocuous procedures may stimulate t
normal progress of labor.

At the time of the vaginal examination, assuming that the diagnosis is corre
the membranes may be ruptured. This procedure alone may effect satisfacto

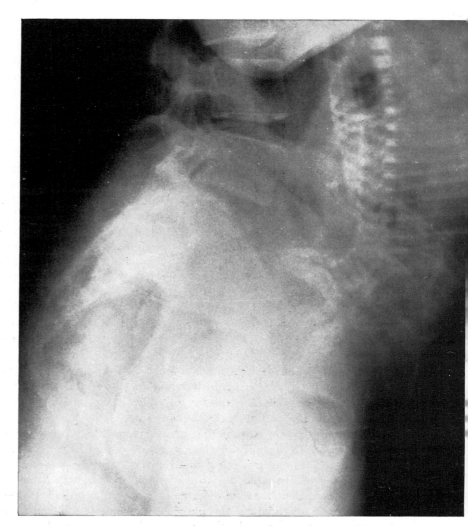

Fig. 9. Lateral roentgenogram of the pelvis showing peculiar curvature of the fetal nec
"goosenecking," indicative of hypotonic uterine dysfunction.

progress of labor. It is in no sense a "burning of bridges," for in the presence of hypotonic dysfunction, it is our belief that delivery must be accomplished reasonably soon to achieve a successful outcome for the mother and her child.

If any of the diameters of the pelvis fall below the critical levels mentioned on page 313, if the infant is unusually large, or if there is malposition, and simple rupture of the membranes does not effect progressive labor, delivery should be by the abdominal route. If none of these abnormalities is present, the proper administration of oxytocin is the specific treatment.

Intravenous Oxytocin.   Ten units of oxytocin are thoroughly mixed with 1 liter of 5 per cent glucose in water in a standard intravenous preparation. Although more dilute solutions have been found effective by numerous authors we believe this mixture is easy to prepare, safe, effective, and likely to cause least confusion. Since the solution contains 10 mU of oxytocin per ml, its rate of flow is easily calculated. The size of the drip apparatus in commercially available intravenous sets is not well standardized, however. Although sets from individual manufacturers deliver drops of a fairly constant size, sets from each company should be tested to ascertain the number of drops per milliliter. More dilute solutions that are equally easy to administer can be prepared by doubling the amount of diluent or halving the amount of oxytocin.

The oxytocin solution is usually mixed in a standard intravenous set. The needle, with the flow shut off, is inserted into an arm vein and the flow started at five drops (approximately 3 to 5 mU) per minute. In true hypotonic dysfunction, this amount of oxytocin will not initiate tetanic uterine contractions, although the physician should be prepared to cut off the flow in case the patient is overly sensitive to the drug. The flow can be gradually increased to yield 20 mU per minute. It is rarely necessary to exceed this rate. As a rule, if a flow of 30 mU per minute fails to initiate satisfactory uterine contractions, greater rates of infusion are unlikely to do so. At present, we administer about 0.3 unit of oxytocin during the first half hour. This small dose is frequently effective.

The patient should never be left alone while the infusion is running, because the best of clamps sometimes slip, necessitating intermittent checks on the rate of flow. Moreover, the uterine contractions must be observed continually and the flow shut off immediately if they exceed one minute in duration or if the fetal heart tones show any significant alterations. The event is rare in our experience, but when it occurs we have found that immediate discontinuation of the flow corrects the disturbances at once, preventing harm to mother or fetus.

Hendricks and associates, as well as Cohen, Danezis, and Burnhill, and others have refined the intravenous drip technic by use of a constant infusion pump. This method enhances the precision of the dosage, as required in experimental work.

Certain precautions should be followed in the use of oxytocin:

1. There must be true hypotonic dysfunction, with no progress and labor practically at a standstill.

2. The patient must be in true labor, not in false or prodromal labor. The only valid evidence of labor is progressive effacement and dilatation of the cervix. Although the process may have come to a standstill, it must have progressed to the extent of 3 or 4 cm dilatation. One of the most common mistakes in obstetrics is to try to stimulate labor in patients who have not been in labor at all. Oxytocin will lead only to trouble in such cases.

3. There must be no mechanical obstruction to safe delivery, as attested by all available evidence, including roentgenologic study of the pelvis and fetal skull. Unless radiologic examination is performed, an occasional instance of midpelvic contraction or of brow presentation may be overlooked.

4. Oxytocin should not be used in cases of overdistention of the uterus, such as those in which the infant appears to weigh in excess of 4,000 g. There have been recent good reports of its use with twins if the size of the babies is not excessive.

5. Patients of great parity (para V and over) in general must not be given oxytocin because their uteri rupture more readily than those of women of lower parity. For the same reason it usually should be withheld in patients over the age of 35.

6. The condition of the fetus must be good, as evidenced by regular heart rate and absence of meconium-stained liquor amnii. A dead fetus is, of course, no contraindication to oxytocin.

7. The obstetrician must note the time of the first contraction after administration of the drug and be prepared to discontinue its use if tetanic contractions occur.

8. When there is doubt whether a given case meets the above criteria, do not give oxytocin.

Hellman and co-workers have shown that when intramuscular oxytocin is used in 0.5 unit doses, there is a tendency for reversal of the normal gradient of uterine contractility, even in normal labor. The implication is that oxytocin has a tendency to produce hypertonia; the likelihood is materially lessened, however, if the dose is sufficiently small so that the amount in the circulation approaches physiologic values. Furthermore, if the intravenous method outlined here is used, the dosage can be nicely titrated against the action of the uterus; and if any untoward event occurs, the drug can be immediately discontinued and its effect thus obtunded. Therefore, in true hypotonic dysfunction the intravenous drip has every advantage and reduces some of the dangers inherent in other methods of administration. Although we believe the intravenous route is always surer and safer, there may be times, especially in the second stage of labor, when only a small increment in uterine force is needed to achieve delivery. Here, 0.5 to 1.0 unit of oxytocin injected intramuscularly or a nasal spray of oxytocin, as advocated by Hendricks and Gabel and by others, may be all that is necessary to terminate labor. Borglin in Sweden and Clement, Harwell, and McCain in Atlanta, Georgia, have reported good results with intranasal oxytocin.

Dillon and associates advocated oxytocin linguets, held under the tongue, as an aid to nursing mothers in causing milk ejection. These linguets may be satisfactory also in the treatment of terminal dysfunctional labor, but they have the disadvantage of an interval of 20 or 30 minutes before uterine activity becomes manifest. Methods of administration of oxytocin other than by the intravenous route are justified only because of the small increment of force and the short period of time necessary to conclude the labor. They are simple, mild, and less time-consuming than the intravenous method; however, the contraindications advocated for the intravenous methods apply to them also. Whether they are as safe as properly administered intravenous oxytocin is still debatable, but our own experience of many years and at least one report on uterine rupture with intranasal oxytocin (Green) call for skepticism.

Sparteine sulfate, the oxytocic action of which was first noted by Kleine more than 30 years ago, was reintroduced by Plentl and his associates in 1961. These investigators believed the drug was unique because of its safety and lack of side effects. Since then, Embrey and Yates have studied the effectiveness of sparteine sulfate with a tocograph and have confirmed its oxytocic properties, but have also demonstrated its lack of dose-related uniformity of action. They noted, furthermore, the occasional production of uterine tetany, although they used somewhat larger doses than usually recommended. Landesman and associates have confirmed the production of spasm with studies in vitro, and Goodno and associates, as well as Newton and colleagues and Aickin, have concluded that intramuscular sparteine sulfate lacks both the predictability and the susceptibility to control of oxytocin infusion.

The safety of sparteine has been questioned by Boysen and by others, who have reported cases of uterine rupture, and by Bedrosian and Gamble, who cite a case of uterine tetany with fetal distress. In summary, it seems that the oxytocic effect of sparteine sulfate is unpredictable and somewhat less than that of oxytocin; and its margin of safety, although difficult to quantitate, is probably not greater. As with all pharmacologically effective oxytocics, the inherent dangers of sparteine must not be ignored or underestimated.

Oxytocin is a powerful drug, which has killed or maimed many women in the past through rupture of the uterus and many more babies through tumultuous uterine contractions. The intravenous administration, however, as attested by many publications, has brought about a distinct advance in both its efficacy and safety. Failure to treat uterine dysfunction exposes the mother to the serious hazards of maternal exhaustion, intrapartum infection, and traumatic operative

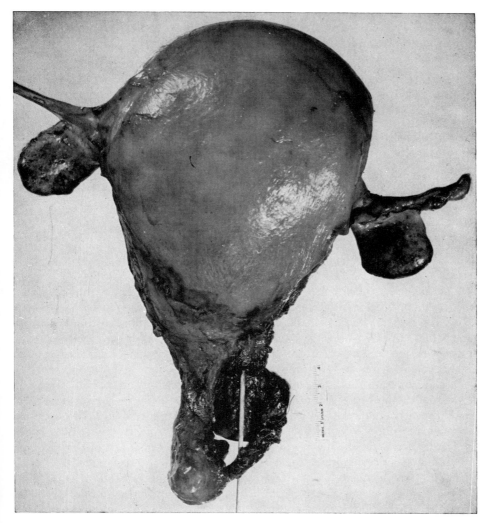

Fig. 10. Rupture of the lower uterine segment resulting from stimulation by dilute intravenous oxytocin in a 38-year-old multipara.

delivery. Furthermore, it may expose the infant to a risk of death as high as 20 per cent, whereas the risk of intravenous oxytocin in dilute solutions is considerably less. Serious accidents, nevertheless, can occur with its use unless the precautions mentioned here are rigidly observed. The ruptured uterus shown in Figure 10 emphasizes the need for these precautions. In that case, oxytocin was administered to a multipara about 38 years of age. Inasmuch as no other abnormalities were present, it must be assumed that the aging uterine muscle could no longer stand the stimulation produced by the oxytocin.

In our clinics, in nearly 100,000 deliveries oxytocin has been used to treat hypotonic uterine dysfunction in approximately 4 per cent of cases. One characteristic of intravenous oxytocin that we have come to recognize through the years is that, when successful, it acts surprisingly quickly, leading to noticeable progress without delay. Therefore, the drug should not be used for an indefinite period of time to stimulate labor. It may be well to employ it for a few hours with a period of rest and then to reemploy it but once again. If the cervix has failed to reach full dilatation by this time, and if easy delivery is not imminent, cesarean section should be performed. The ready resort to cesarean section is evident from the figures in Table 2.

Table 2. Method of Therapy and Perinatal Mortality in Hypotonic Uterine Dysfunction

	No	Per Cent	Perinatal Mortality
Oxytocin	812	52.8	2.9
Oxytocin and cesarean section	77	5.0	3.9
Cesarean section	155	10.1	1.9
Other (rupture of membranes, enemas, time, etc.)	494	32.1	3.5
Total	1,538	100.0	3.0

From Hellman, Kohl, and Schechter. Amer J Obstet Gynec 73:507, 1957.

In these 1,538 patients with hypotonic uterine dysfunction the failures of oxytocin represent 77 cases, or 5 per cent of the total. The 155 patients subjected to cesarean section obviously had some major contraindication to the successful use of oxytocin. This ready resort to cesarean section in patients in whom oxytocin fails or in patients with contraindications to its use has resulted in the diminution of the total perinatal mortality, as indicated in Table 2. A perinatal loss rate of 3 per cent in face of one of the most serious complications of labor reflects real progress in knowledge and treatment of uterine dysfunction.

Certain factors militate against the successful use of intravenous oxytocin: high station of the head, severe maternal exhaustion, and intrapartum fever. Although the drug may occasionally be successfully employed in such cases, the percentage of failure is somewhat higher.

Finally, oxytocin should never be used to test the adequacy of the pelvis or the soundness of a cesarean section scar.

Treatment of Hypertonic Uterine Dysfunction.   Coming at the onset of labor, this type of dysfunction is characterized by uterine pain out of proportion to the severity of contractions. Because of the relative infrequency of hypertonic dysfunctional labor, it has attracted little attention as a clinical entity, and its importance as a cause of fetal mortality has frequently been overlooked.

The unpredictability of oxytocin in augmenting hypertonia militates against its primary use in that situation. It is far better to stop the abnormal contractions with 16 mg of morphine and to produce relaxation and rest with 0.1 to 0.2 g of a short-acting barbiturate. In the vast majority of patients normal labor will ensue upon awaking. Occasionally, the ineffective and uncoordinated contractions continue. Van Praagh and Hendricks have shown that this deficiency may be corrected by amniotomy, but if these mothers develop intrapartum fever, the perinatal mortality rises. In this case or if sedation fails, oxytocin may be tried in about one half the usual dosage. It should, however, be discontinued and cesarean section employed if normal labor fails to supervene, if the fetal heart tones become abnormal, or if other signs of fetal distress occur. Abdominal delivery preceded by antibiotic therapy is advisable in cases complicated by intrapartum fever, particularly if the response to oxytocin, as in the usual case, is unsatisfactory.

PRECIPITATE LABOR

In certain multiparous women, and very rarely in primigravidas, precipitate labor may result from an abnormally low resistance of the soft parts, from abnormally strong uterine and abdominal contractions, or very rarely from the absence of painful sensations during labor. At The New York Lying-In Hospital, the incidence of precipitate labor, defined as lasting three hours or less, was 16.8 per cent in 7,643 labors.

In general, precipitate labor is rarely attended by serious maternal consequences, but the perinatal loss is appreciably increased for several reasons. First, the tumultuous uterine contractions, often with negligible intervals, prevent proper oxygenation of the fetal blood; second, the rapid transit of the baby through the bony pelvis sometimes produces cerebral trauma; and third, such infants are often born unattended and suffer from lack of proper care during the first few minutes of life. Chafetz indicates that rapid labor may be an etiologic factor in cerebral palsy. The mother is sometimes suddenly overtaken by intense labor pains and gives birth to the child before she can reach her bed. In such cases, amniotic fluid embolism may occur or the child may be injured by a fall to the ground. Laceration of the cord may result, but it rarely leads to fatal bleeding.

If tempestuous pains commence while the patient is under medical observation, the severity may be reduced by the administration of analgesia, although there is rarely time to achieve a satisfactory effect. It is unwise to employ physical force in holding back an impending birth. Attendants should be instructed not to lock the mother's legs in a futile attempt to delay delivery. These maneuvers may damage maternal soft parts and the infant's brain.

LOCALIZED ABNORMALITIES OF UTERINE ACTION

Pathologic Retraction and Constriction Rings. Very rarely, in association with prolonged rupture of the membranes and protracted labors, localized rings or constrictions of the uterus occur. Recent literature on the subject is virtually non-existent, and older publications fail to make clear whether there are in fact two types of pathologic rings (the pathologic retraction ring and the constriction ring) or only one. In all probability these rings represent varying degrees of the same abnormality. The most common type is the so-called pathologic retraction ring of Bandl, an exaggeration of the normal retraction ring described on page 355 and often but not always the result of obstructed labor with marked thinning and ballooning of the lower uterine segment. In such a situation, the ring is clearly evident as an abdominal indentation and signifies impending rupture of the lower uterine segment (Fig. 11). Rings may occur also in nonobstructed labor, as in the case first described by Smellie in 1730. In that case, as well as in those more recently described by Fields, the ring forms most commonly at the junction of the lower and upper uterine segments, encircling the fetal neck and impeding the progress of labor. These localized constrictions of the uterus are rarely seen today, when prolonged and obstructed labors are no longer compatible with good obstetric practice. They may, however, still occur as hourglass constrictions of

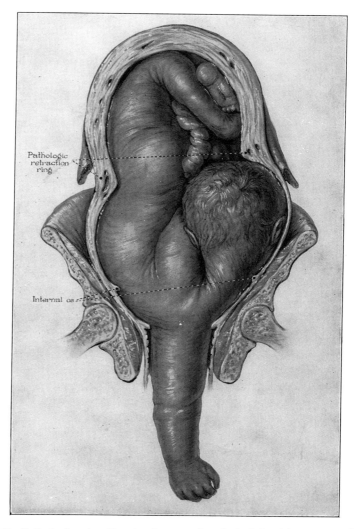

Fig. 11. Pathologic retraction ring in case of neglected shoulder presentation.

the uterus following the birth of the first of twins. In such a situation, they can usually be relaxed and delivery effected with deep general anesthesia.

Missed Labor. In very exceptional instances uterine contractions commence at or near term and, after continuing for a variable time, disappear without leading to the birth of the child. The fetus then dies and may be retained in utero for months, undergoing mummification or putrefaction, depending on whether the membranes have ruptured. This condition is known as *missed labor*. The term should not be applied to cases in which a living child is born, for they are probably only examples of prolonged gestation. True missed labor is extremely rare. If uterine contractions disappear without leading to the birth of the child, and especially if the infant dies and is retained, abdominal pregnancy is a much more likely diagnosis than missed labor.

REFERENCES

Aickin, D. R. Sparteine sulfate and synthetic oxytocin: a comparative study. Aust New Zeal J Obstet Gynaec 6:85, 1966.

Bandl, L. Über Ruptur der Gebärmutter. Wien, 1875.

Bedrosian, L., and Gamble, J. J. Uterine tetany and fetal distress coincidental with the administration of sparteine sulfate. Report of a case. Obstet Gynec 21:400, 1963.

Borglin, N. E. Intranasal administration of oxytocin for induction and stimulation of labor. Acta Obstet Gynec Scand 41:238, 1962.

Boysen, H. Sparteine sulfate and rupture of the uterus. Obstet Gynec 21:403, 1963.

Caldeyro-Barcia, R., Alvarez, H., and Reynolds, S. R. M. A better understanding of uterine contractility through simultaneous recording with an internal and a seven channel external method. Surg Obstet Gynec 91:641, 1950.

Chafetz, M. Etiology of cerebral palsy: role of reproductive insufficiency and the multiplicity of factors. Obstet Gynec 25:635, 1965.

Clement, J. E., Harwell, V. C., and McCain, J. R. Use of intranasal oxytocin for induction and/or stimulation of labor. Amer J Obstet Gynec 83:778, 1962.

Cohen, J., Danezis, J., and Burnhill, M. S. Response of the gravid uterus at term to intranasal oxytocin as determined by intra-amniotic fluid pressure recordings. Amer J Obstet Gynec 83:774, 1962.

Dale, H. H. On some physiological actions of ergot. J Physiol 34:163, 1906.

Dillon, T. F., Douglas, R. G., du Vigneaud, V., and Barber, M. L. Transbuccal administration of Pitocin for induction and stimulation of labor. Obstet Gynec 15:587, 1960.

du Vigneaud, V., Ressler, C., Swan, J. W., Roberts, C. W., Katsoyannis, P. G., and Gordon, S. The synthesis of an octapeptide amide with the hormonal activity of oxytocin. J Amer Chem Soc 75:4879, 1953.

Eastman, N. J. Editorial note. Obstet Gynec Survey 20:960, 1965.

Editorial. Buccal oxytocin. Brit Med J 2:705, 1964.

Embrey, M. P., and Yates, M. J. A tocographic study of the effects of sparteine sulfate on uterine contractility. J Obstet Gynaec Brit Comm 71:33, 1964.

Fields, C. Constriction ring dystocia. Amer J Obstet Gynec 65:960, 1953 (23 references cited).

Friedman, E. A. Labor: Clinical Evaluation and Management. New York, Appleton-Century-Crofts, 1967.

Goodno, J. A., Asoury, R., Dorsey, J. H., Barnes, A. C., and Kumar, D. In vitro and in vivo effects of sparteine sulfate on human uterine contractility—an objective evaluation. Amer J Obstet Gynec 86:288, 1963.

Green, G. H. Uterine rupture following intranasal oxytocin. New Zeal Med J 64:79, 1965.

Guilbeau, J. A., and Eastman, N. J. Unpublished data.

Hellman, L. M. Uterine inertia. Med Clin N Amer 35:791, 1951.

——— Pituitary extract in uterine inertia. Amer J Obstet Gynec (Suppl.) 61A:52, 1951.

———— Harris, J. S., and Reynolds, S. R. M.   Characteristics of the gradients of uterine contractility during the first stage of true labor. Bull Hopkins Hosp 86:234, 1950.

———— Kohl, S. G., and Schechter, H. R.   Pitocin—1955. Amer J Obstet Gynec 73:507, 1957.

———— and Prystowsky, H.   The duration of the second stage of labor. Amer J Obstet Gynec 63:1223, 1952.

Hendricks, C. H., and Gabel, R. A.   The use of intranasal oxytocin in obstetrics. Amer J. Obstet Gynec 79:780, 789, 1960.

———— Brenner, W. E., and Kraus, G.   The normal cervical dilatation pattern in late pregnancy and labor. Amer J Obstet Gynec 106:1065, 1970.

———— Quilligan, E. J., Tyler, A. B., and Tucker, G. J.   Pressure relationships between intervillous space and amniotic fluid in human term pregnancy. Amer J Obstet Gynec 77:1028, 1959.

Holland, E.   The Princess Charlotte of Wales: a triple obstetric tragedy. J Obstet Gynaec Brit Emp 58:905, 1951.

Jeffcoate, T. N. A.   Prolonged labour. Lancet 2:61, 1961.

———— Baker, K., and Martin, R. H.   Inefficient uterine action. Surg Gynec Obstet 95:257, 1952.

Kao, C. Y.   Ionic basis of electrical activity in uterine smooth muscle, in Wynn, R. M. (ed.), Cellular Biology of the Uterus. New York, Appleton-Century-Crofts, 1967, Ch. 11, pp. 386–448.

Karlson, S.   On the motility of the uterus during labour and the influence of the motility pattern on the duration of labour. Acta Obstet Gynec Scand 28:209, 1949.

Kleine, H. O.   (Sparteine—a new oxytocin). Klin Wschr 18:360, 1939.

Kleinhaus, A. L., and Kao, C. Y.   Electrophysiological actions of oxytocin on the rabbit myometrium. J Gen Physiol 53:758, 1969.

Knapp, R. C., and Warenski, J. C.   Clinical evaluation of dysfunctional labor. Obstet Gynec 21:627, 1963.

Landesman, R., Wilson, K. H., LaRussa, R., and Silverman, F.   Sparteine and oxytocin: in vitro comparison on pregnant uterus muscle. Obstet Gynec 23:2, 1964.

Larks, S. D.   Electrohysterography, Springfield, Ill., Charles C Thomas, 1960.

Lebherz, T. B., Hellman, L. P., Madding, R., Ancil, A., and Arje, S. L.   Double-blind study of premature rupture of the membranes. A report of 1896 cases. Amer J Obstet Gynec 87:218, 1963.

Moore, D. B., and D'Esopo, D. A.   The treatment of uterine inertia with dilute intravenous pituitrin. Amer J Obstet Gynec 70:1338, 1955.

Newton, B. W., Benson, R. C., and McCorriston, C. C.   Sparteine sulfate: a potent, capricious oxytocic. Amer J Obstet Gynec 94:234, 1966.

Plentl, A. A., and Friedman, E. A.   Sparteine sulfate: a clinical evaluation of its use for the induction of labor. Amer J Obstet Gynec 82:1332, 1961.

———— Friedman, E. A., and Gray, M. J.   Sparteine sulfate: a clinical evaluation of its use in the management of labor. Amer J Obstet Gynec 82:1332, 1961.

Reynolds, S. R. M., Heard, O. O., Bruns, P., and Hellman, L. M.   A multichannel strain-gauge tokodynamometer; an instrument for studying patterns of uterine contractions in pregnant women. Bull Hopkins Hosp 82:446, 1948.

Smellie, W.   The Theory and Practice of Midwifery, edited with annotations by Alfred H. McClintock. London, New Sydenham Society, 1877, Vol. II, case 220.

Sogolow, S. R.   An historical review of the use of oxytocin prior to delivery. Obstet Gynec Survey 21:155, 1966 (157 references).

Steer, C. M.   Effect of type of delivery on future childbearing. Amer J Obstet Gynec 60:395, 1950.

Van Praagh, I., and Hendricks, C. H.   The effect of amniotomy during labor in multiparas. Obstet Gynec 24:258, 1964.

29

DYSTOCIA CAUSED BY ABNORMALITIES IN POSITION, PRESENTATION, OR DEVELOPMENT OF THE FETUS

ABNORMALITIES OF POSITION OR PRESENTATION

PERSISTENT OCCIPUT POSTERIOR POSITIONS

In the great majority of cases, occiput posterior positions undergo spontaneous anterior rotation followed by either a spontaneous or an easy low forceps delivery. Since spontaneous outcome is the rule, labor with the occiput posterior should be regarded as simply a normal variant. Calkins found no prolongation of the first stage of labor and only a slight increase in duration of the second stage, whereas Bainbridge, Nixon, and Smythe found a slight prolongation in both stages for primigravidas but not for multiparas. This slight increase in duration of labor in occiput posterior position might be expected for two reasons: first, this position is commonly associated with android and anthropoid pelves, many of which are narrowed at the midpelvis; and second, internal rotation does not take place until the head is on the pelvic floor in about one third of these patients. Calkins believed that late rotation adds not more than a contraction or two to the entire length of labor.

In about 6 per cent of cases, rotation does not occur (*persistent occiput posterior*). Although the exact reasons for failure of rotation are not known, the narrowing of the forepelvis and midpelvis (common with android and anthropoid pelves) undoubtedly plays a prominent role. Many of these patients will deliver spontaneously with the occiput persistently posterior if given sufficient time (Fig. 1). In modern practice, however, with a tendency to shorten the second stage of labor, forceps delivery is frequent.

The best operative procedure to be employed will depend on the experience and training of the operator, the type of pelvis, the degree of molding of the fetal head, and the size of the infant. If the head is considerably molded (as it will often be if time is allowed for spontaneous rotation), delivery by forceps as an occiput posterior will usually prove the least traumatic measure to both mother and child. Delivery as an occiput posterior is probably indicated in anthropoid

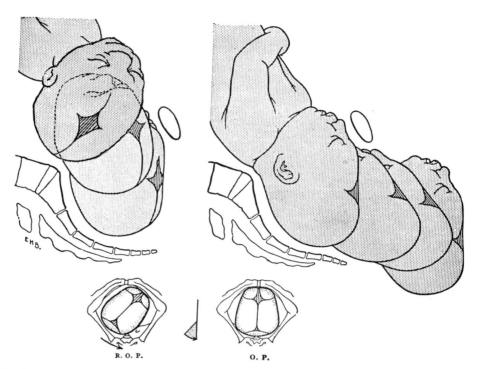

R. O. P.   O. P.

Fig. 1. Mechanism of labor for right occiput posterior position, posterior rotation. (From Steele and Javert. Surg Gynec Obstet 75:477, 1942.)

and android pelves and in the presence of a midpelvic contraction. Moreover, if the operator's experience with manual or forceps rotation is meager, delivery of the posterior occiput as such is usually the safest procedure. The decision to deliver the head as a posterior depends fundamentally on whether there are factors that threaten to make artificial rotation especially difficult. To ascertain whether such factors are present, some obstetricians attempt rotation gently either by the hand or by forceps. If it is easy, they carry it out; but if a molded head is so wedged in the pelvis as to interfere with easy rotation, they deliver the infant as an occiput posterior. In general, rotation is preferred to delivery of the occiput posterior as such, provided it can be done readily. In two parallel series of cases in our clinic, in one of which persistent occiput posterior positions were rotated either manually or by the Scanzoni maneuver (142 cases) and in the other of which forceps delivery was effected with the face to the pubis (216 cases), the total perinatal mortality was about the same in both groups—4.2 and 5.1 per cent, respectively.

If delivery of the occiput posterior as such is decided upon, a mediolateral episiotomy should be made and the forceps extraction performed slowly. Considerably more traction than usual is often required, and it should be spread over 5 or 10 minutes, with ample rest between pulls. Because of the longer duration of the operation, the baby should be spared the narcosis that might result from general anesthesia; instead, spinal, caudal, or pudendal block anesthesia should be used. If it is decided to carry out operative rotation of a persistent occiput posterior, several procedures are available: manual rotation followed by forceps extraction, rotation and delivery with the Kielland forceps, and the Scanzoni technic of rotation and extraction. If the head remains high in the pelvis in *deep transverse* arrest, however, there is a growing tendency to replace the required difficult and sometimes traumatic midforceps procedures with cesarean section. The deflection and molding of the posterior head may lead the obstetrician to believe that the presenting part is lower in the pelvis than it actually is. This error adds to the difficulty and danger of the extraction. These forceps operations are described in Chapter 40.

BREECH PRESENTATION

Incidence.   Breech presentation occurs in 3 to 4 per cent of deliveries. Hall, Kohl, and associates cite an incidence of 3.17 per cent of 190,661 deliveries of infants weighing over 1,000 g in the Obstetrical Statistical Cooperative. Morgan and Kane found 4 per cent in over 400,000 labors among the cooperating hospitals in the perinatal study of the Foundation for Medical Research; their incidence is slightly high because of the inclusion of twins and immature infants.

The varying relations between the lower extremities and buttocks of the fetus in breech presentations form the categories of frank breech, complete breech, and incomplete breech (foot and knee) presentations (Figs. 2, 3, and 4). The frank breech appears most common when the diagnosis is made radiologically near term.

Diagnosis.   On palpation, the first maneuver reveals the hard, round, readily ballottable fetal head occupying the fundus of the uterus. The second maneuver reveals the back on one side of the abdomen and the small parts on the other; position and variety are determined by the location of the sacrum. On the third maneuver, if engagement has not occurred, the irregular breech is freely movable above the superior strait. After engagement, the fourth maneuver shows that the pelvis is filled by a soft mass (Fig. 5).

In doubtful cases, diagnosis may be facilitated by radiologic examination, which shows that the head is usually less sharply flexed and the arms occupy a much freer position than generally thought.

On vaginal or rectal examination, the diagnosis of a frank breech presentation is made by palpating its characteristic portions. Both tubera ischii, the sacrum with its spinous processes, and the anus are usually palpable, and after further descent, the external genitalia may be distinguished. Especially when labor is prolonged, the buttocks may become markedly swollen, rendering differentiation of face and breech very difficult; the anus may be mistaken for the mouth, and the ischial tuberosities for the malar eminences. Careful examination, however, should prevent that error, for when the finger is introduced into the anus it encounters muscular resistance, whereas in the mouth the firmer, more unyielding jaws are felt. Furthermore, the finger upon removal from the anus is sometimes stained with meconium. The most accurate information, however, is based on the location of the sacrum and its spinous processes, which establish the diagnosis of position and variety.

In complete breech presentations the feet may be felt alongside the buttocks, and in footling presentations one or both feet may hang down into the vagina

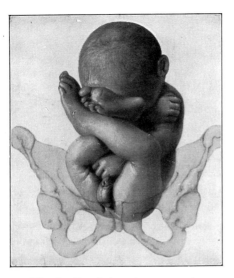

Fig. 2. Frank breech presentation.

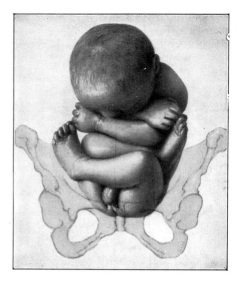

Fig. 3. Complete breech presentation.

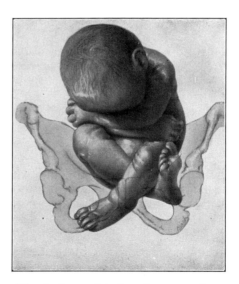

Fig. 4. Incomplete breech presentation.

(Fig. 6). In footlings, the foot can be readily identified as right or left on the basis of the relation of the great toe. When the breech has descended farther into the pelvic cavity, the genitalia may be felt; if not markedly edematous, they may permit identification of fetal sex. The heart sounds of the fetus are heard through its back, usually at or slightly above the umbilicus.

Etiology.   As the fetus approaches term, it tends to accommodate to the shape of the uterine cavity, assuming a longitudinal lie with the vertex presenting. When

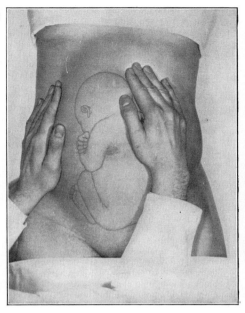
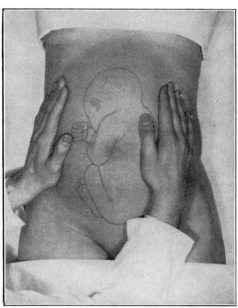

First maneuver   Second maneuver

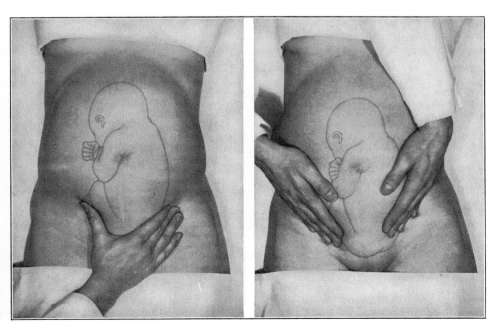

Third maneuver   Fourth maneuver

Fig. 5. Palpation in left sacroanterior position.

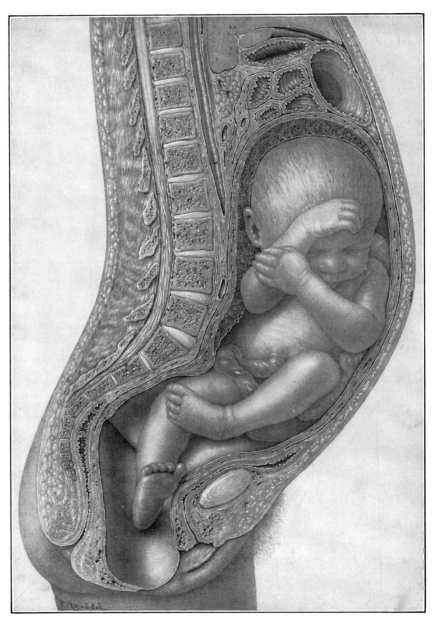

Fig. 6. Double footling breech presentation. Second stage of labor. Frozen section of Williams' case.

the fetus is premature, however, its small size naturally requires less accommodation, and breech presentation is much more frequent. As indicated in Table 2 (p. 324), breeches are nine times more common at the twenty-eighth week of pregnancy than at term. Factors other than prematurity that interfere with normal accommodation include uterine relaxation associated with great parity, twinning, hydramnios, hydrocephalus, and placenta previa. In all these conditions breech and other abnormal presentations are more common. Most recent studies show no positive correlation between breech presentation and contracted pelvis.

According to Hall and Kohl, about 14 per cent of breech presentations are preceded by breech presentations in previous pregnancies (*habitual breech*). A rate of recurrence of this magnitude might be expected because the commonest etiologic factor, prematurity, has a slight tendency to be repetitive. Furthermore, uterine relaxation related to high parity and the rarer uterine malformations are persistent factors that predispose to breech presentation.

Mechanism.   Unless there is disproportion between the size of the fetus and the pelvis, engagement and descent readily occur in one of the oblique diameters of the pelvis, with the anterior hip directed toward one iliopectineal eminence is encountered and the posterior hip toward the opposite sacroiliac synchondrosis. The anterior hip usually descends more rapidly than the posterior, and when the resistance of the pelvic floor, internal rotation usually occurs, bringing the anterior hip toward the pubic arch and allowing the fetal bitrochanteric diameter to occupy the anteroposterior diameter of the pelvic outlet. Rotation usually takes place from the iliopectineal eminence to the pubis through an arc of 45 degrees. If, however, the posterior extremity is prolapsed, it always rotates to the symphysis pubis, ordinarily through an arc of 135 degrees (Fig. 7), but

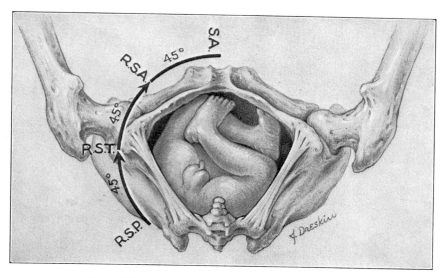

Fig. 7. Direction of internal rotation in RSP position.

occasionally in the opposite direction, past the sacrum and the opposite half of the pelvis through an arc of 225 degrees.

After rotation, descent continues until the perineum is distended by the advancing breech, while the anterior hip appears at the vulva and is stemmed against the pubic arch. By lateral flexion of the body, the posterior hip is then forced over the anterior margin of the perineum, which retracts over the buttocks, thus allowing the child to straighten out when the anterior hip is born. The legs and feet follow the breech and may be born spontaneously, although the aid of the obstetrician is sometimes required. After the birth of the breech there is slight *external rotation,* with the back turning anteriorly as the shoulders are brought into relation with one of the oblique diameters of the pelvis. The shoulders then descend rapidly and undergo internal rotation, with the bisacromial diameter occupying the anteroposterior diameter of the inferior strait. Immediately following the shoulders, the head, which is normally sharply flexed upon the thorax, enters the pelvis in one of the oblique diameters and then rotates in such a manner as to bring the posterior portion of the neck under the symphysis pubis; the head is then born in flexion, with the chin, mouth, nose, forehead, bregma, and occiput appearing in succession over the perineum. Not infrequently the breech engages in the transverse diameter of the pelvis, with the sacrum directed anteriorly or posteriorly. The mechanism of labor in the transverse position differs only in that internal rotation occurs through an arc of 90 degrees.

There is a fundamental difference between delivery in vertex and breech presentations. With a vertex, after the extrusion of the relatively voluminous head, the rest of the body follows without difficulty. With a breech, however, successively larger portions of the child are born; in practical terms there are three births—that of the buttocks, of the shoulders, and finally of the head, each of which is preceded by its own internal rotation.

In a small number of cases rotation occurs in such a manner that the back of the child is directed toward the vertebral column instead of toward the abdomen of the mother. Such rotation should be prevented if possible, for although the head may be delivered by allowing the chin and face to pass beneath the symphysis, the slightest traction on the body may cause extension of the head. Birth may then be traumatic or may necessitate forceps or manual rotation and extraction.

Prognosis. The prognosis for life of the mother differs but slightly in breech and vertex presentations. Because of the greater frequency of cesarean section, however, there may be a higher maternal morbidity. Labor, contrary to former teachings, is not prolonged. Hall and Kohl, in a large series of cases, showed the median duration of labor to be 9.2 hours for primigravidas and 6.1 hours for multiparas. The prognosis for the child, however, is considerably worse than in vertex presentations.

The uncorrected perinatal loss is about 12 per cent in current obstetric practice in the United States. Hall and colleagues cite an overall loss for infants over 1,000 g of 12 per cent, whereas Morgan and Kane report a total wastage of 15 per cent. Law cites a corresponding loss of 14.7 per cent for the Northwest Metropolitan Region (London, England). These high loss rates result not only from the abnormal presentation but from prematurity and other complicating factors, such as placenta previa, that play a highly significant role in the causation of the presentation. Thirty-four per cent of Hall's cases were premature, accounting for a little more than two thirds of the perinatal loss. Hall indicates a loss of 2.2 per cent of all infants alive at the onset of labor. Morgan and Kane cite a similar figure, indicating that the presentation alone is associated with a fetal risk three and a half to four times that of a normal vertex presentation.

The somber prognosis of the child is worsened by several mechanical factors associated with the delivery. In the first place, after the breech is born to the umbilicus, the cord is exposed to a varying degree of compression between the head and the pelvic brim. It is often stated that a maximum of eight minutes may elapse between the birth of the umbilicus and the delivery of the head if the child is to be born alive. Actually a longer time may elapse if the mouth has appeared at the vulva, and pulmonary exchange is unimpaired. Undue delay in delivery of the head, as well as excessive haste, will naturally increase the perinatal loss.

Holland and Capon indicated the predominant cause of fetal death in breech presentations in showing that tentorial tears and subsequent intracranial hemorrhage were twice as common as in cephalic presentations. Crothers and Putnam have emphasized the role of lesions of the spinal cord. Holland and Capon have shown, furthermore, that during breech extraction, especially when accompanied by suprapubic pressure upon the head, the medulla may protrude through the foramen magnum into the spinal canal. During attempts at premature extraction, moreover, descent of the head may be impeded by the imperfectly dilated cervix, and great force may be required to overcome the resistance.

Prolapse of the umbilical cord adds further to the risk, occurring in 3.8 per cent of Hall's cases, or about eight times the normally expected rate of 0.5 per cent. The weight of the baby appears to have no effect on the incidence of prolapse of the cord, but the type of breech is highly important. The incidence of this complication is about normal in frank breech, but is increased about twenty-fold in incomplete and complete breeches. The cause of the high frequency of prolapse of the cord in incomplete and complete varieties of breech is the failure of the presenting part to fill the lower uterine segment and cover the cervical os, as in frank breech and vertex presentations.

Prophylaxis. In view of the serious fetal prognosis attending breech presentations, the obstetrician should aim at preventing them as far as possible. Whenever they are recognized in the later weeks of pregnancy, an attempt may be made by *external version* to substitute a vertex presentation. This procedure, if properly and gently performed, carries little danger. Little is usually accomplished, however, since in most series the final incidence of breech presentation at delivery is not much less following external version than in a control group. The explanation is based on several facts. First, if nothing is done, spontaneous conversion often occurs, especially in cases in which external version is readily performed. Furthermore, although version may be temporarily successful, the breech presentation often recurs. Finally, in the common frank variety of breech, version is especially difficult. Since a gentle attempt should do no harm, however, many authorities recommend the procedure. Because of possible trauma, anesthesia should never be used. External version is readily accomplished in multiparas with lax abdominal walls but is more difficult in primigravidas. If the head can be forced into the pelvis after conversion has been effected, the new position becomes permanent; if impossible, however, the fetus will frequently revert to its original position despite the application of a properly fitting bandage or abdominal binder. In MacArthur's series the optimal time for version was found to be between the twenty-eighth and thirty-sixth weeks of gestation, with over 50 per cent of the conversions accomplished by the thirty-third week. Various authors advise that in all breech presentations an attempt at version should be made during the last two months. The procedure may also be attempted in the first stage of labor provided the breech has not descended well into the pelvis; once it becomes fixed, all such efforts are futile. The procedure is not advisable after rupture of the membranes because of the possibility of prolapse of the umbilical cord. The fetal heart should be auscultated before and after the maneuver. Despite optimistic reports of the value of this maneuver, critical evaluation of many papers fails to show a significant increase in fetal salvage. Ellis recently examined the results in 312 gravidas on whom external version was attempted under anesthesia after the thirty-fourth week of gestation. Eighty-two per cent of the gravidas presented in labor with vertex presentations The overall perinatal loss in infants over 4½ pounds was 2.6 per cent, not a significant improvement over the general rate in modern obstetric practice. External version, furthermore, is not a totally innocuous procedure. To the known cases of coincidental fetal death, Pollock has recently added a report of fetal hemorrhage into the maternal bloodstream immediately after version.

Management.   In most breech presentations spontaneous delivery to the umbilicus occurs, and the attitude of the obstetrician should be merely expectant, although he should be ready to intervene at a moment's notice. As soon as the breech appears at the vulva, therefore, the patient should be prepared for delivery in order that not a moment be lost in performing extraction should it become necessary. The breech should be allowed to advance spontaneously until the umbilicus has been born. Completion of labor is materially facilitated by the arms' retaining their normal crossed position over the thorax, as well as by sharp flexion of the head. These anatomic relations are best attained by avoiding traction as far as possible and any fundal pressure that may push the head between the arms.

The frank breech generally forms a better dilating wedge than the complete variety, since it provides closer application to the margins of the partially dilated os. If interference becomes necessary, however, the complete breech offers more satisfactory conditions for immediate delivery, since a foot can be brought down for traction. As soon as the cervix is fully dilated, some obstetricians prefer to rupture the membranes and bring both feet down into the vagina so that extraction can be promptly effected when necessary. The technic of this manipulation and the rules for extraction are discussed in Chapter 41.

In the past, some authors have advocated bringing down the feet and extraction as soon as full dilatation has occurred, but this radical policy no longer has many advocates. Decomposition should be reserved until it becomes evident that the second stage is going to be prolonged to the detriment of the mother and child. This practice will result in the spontaneous delivery of many frank breeches; only in the exceptional case will it be necessary to decompose the breech. The prompt elective application of Piper forceps to the aftercoming head offers many advantages; it may often be less traumatic than difficult manual procedures. Cesarean section also is a safer approach, which yields better results for the infant than does a difficult extraction. The incidence of cesarean section is shown in Table 1. It should be freely employed in the presence of pelvic contraction, oversized infant, and uterine dysfunction, and in primigravidas over the age of 35 years. Lanka and Nelson believe that cesarean section should be seriously considered in term footling breech presentation, an especially hazardous complication because of the frequency of prolapse of the umbilical cord. There is no justification, however, for abdominal delivery of all term breeches even in primigravidas, for cesarean section in the best hands carries a maternal risk

Table 1. Cesarean Section Incidence in Breech Presentation

Weight in Grams	Nulliparas (Per Cent)	Multiparas (Per Cent)	Total (Per Cent)
2,000–2,499	12.5	6.8	8.7
2,500–2,999	8.8	10.9	10.1
3,000–3,499	13.5	7.2	9.9
3,500–3,999	24.6	13.7	18.2
4,000–4,499	36.3	8.7	17.6
4,500–4,999	50.0	25.0	33.3
Entire series	12.7	9.5	10.7

From Hall and Kohl. Amer J Obstet Gynec 72:974, 1956.

of at least 0.1 per cent (p. 1187) and imposes upon the mother the likelihood of abdominal delivery in all future pregnancies.

Premature Rupture of the Membranes. For reasons not entirely clear, premature rupture of the membranes occurs more frequently with breech presentation. If the membranes rupture before the onset of labor, an additional hazard is imposed upon the infant, as indicated by the studies of Hall and those of Hawkes (unpublished data) at The New York Lying-In Hospital. In Hall's series nearly one third of the patients with premature rupture of the membranes failed to go into labor for 12 hours or more after the event. Because the perinatal loss was more than double that in patients who went into labor more promptly, we now frequently perform cesarean section in term pregnancies if labor does not ensue by 12 hours after rupture of the membranes.

Uterine Dysfunction. Hypotonic uterine dysfunction associated with breech presentation compounds the fetal risk. Several authorities have advocated the use of oxytocin in treatment of uterine inertia in this situation. The reported results have been encouraging, but the hazard of this complication added to the increased fetal risk inherent in breech presentation should orient the obstetrician toward abdominal delivery in most instances.

Hyperextension of the Fetal Head. In rare cases of breech presentation, a scout film of the abdomen may show that the fetal head is in extreme hyperextension. If this attitude of the fetus persists, a very large diameter of the head will present during labor, with resulting difficulty in extraction. In such cases the consensus favors cesarean section (Lazar and Salvaggio).

FACE PRESENTATION

In face presentations the head is sharply extended so that the occiput is in contact with the back, while the face looks downward. Posner, Rubin, and Posner report an incidence of 1 in 380 or 0.26 per cent of 19,766 deliveries, and the Obstetrical Statistical Cooperative shows a similar rate of 0.2 per cent. The incidences in nonwhite and white women are approximately equal.

It is commonly stated that the face most frequently occupies the right oblique diameter of the pelvis, resulting in either LMA or RMP positions (Fig. 8). These two positions, however, accounted for only 31.7 per cent of our cases, the right mentoanterior variety being the most frequent (25 per cent). The initial position of the chin is posterior in about 30 per cent of cases.

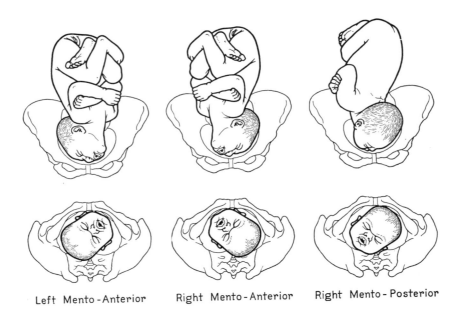

Left Mento-Anterior   Right Mento-Anterior   Right Mento-Posterior

Fig. 8. Left and right positions in face presentations.

Diagnosis. In the right mentoanterior variety, the findings on palpation are as follows:

First maneuver: Breech in fundus
Second maneuver: Back in the left and posterior portion of the abdomen and felt distinctly only in its upper portion; small parts in right and anterior portion of the abdomen
Third maneuver: Head may be detected above superior strait
Fourth maneuver: Marked cephalic prominence on left side; fingers can be depressed deeply on right

In the case of engagement in the transverse diameter, right and left mentotransverse, the findings differ from the corresponding anterior positions only in that the back is directed to the side of the abdomen, and the small parts are directed laterally on the opposite side. The characteristic sign is palpation of the cephalic prominence on the same side as the back instead of on the side of the small parts, as in vertex presentations. The back is felt distinctly only near the breech.

Although these abdominal findings may be suggestive, the diagnosis of face presentation must rest on vaginal examination. Since x-ray pelvimetry in the presence of a term-sized face presentation is indicated in most cases, the vaginal findings should be confirmed or refuted by radiologic examination. If a face presentation is suspected, vaginal examination is much more informative than rectal.

On vaginal palpation, the distinctive features of the face are the mouth and nose, the malar bones, and particularly the orbital ridges. It is possible to mistake a breech presentation for a face, since the anus may be mistaken for the mouth and the ischial tuberosities for the malar prominences. The anus is always on a line with the ischial tuberosities, however, whereas the mouth and malar prominences form the corners of a triangle.

Since the heart sounds are transmitted through the thorax, they are heard through the side of the abdomen that contains the small parts, and generally below the umbilicus. The only other conditions with similar auscultatory characteristics are brow presentations and occipitoposterior positions in which the head is partially extended. All are extended positions of the head.

Etiology. The causes of face presentations are manifold, generally stemming from any factor that favors extension or prevents flexion of the head. Extended positions of the head, therefore, occur more frequently when the pelvis is contracted or the child is very large. In a series of 141 face presentations studied by Hellman, Epperson, and Connally, the incidence of inlet contraction was 39.4 per cent. This high incidence of pelvic contraction and large infants is most important to consider in the management of face presentation, usually necessitating x-ray pelvimetry before deciding on the method of delivery.

In multiparas the pendulous abdomen is another factor that predisposes to face presentation. It permits the back of the fetus to sag forward or laterally and often in the same direction in which the occiput points, thus promoting extension of the cervical and thoracic spine (Fig. 9); at the same time, the fetal axis is displaced from that of the birth canal.

In exceptional instances, marked enlargement of the neck or thorax, coils of cord about the neck, spastic contraction, or congenital shortening of the fetal cervical muscles may cause extension. Anencephalic fetuses naturally present by the face as a rule because of faulty development of the cranium.

Mechanism. Since face presentations are usually derived from vertex presentations, they are but rarely observed at the pelvic inlet, where the brow generally engages, while the face descends only after further extension.

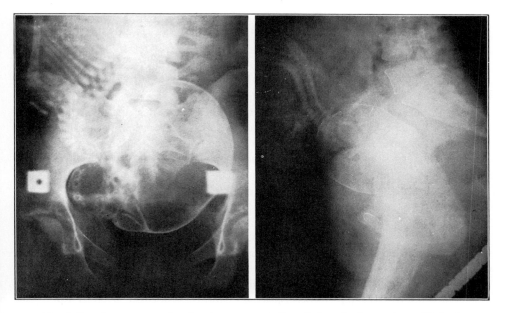

Fig. 9. Roentgenograms showing face presentation. Note spinal curvature of infant.

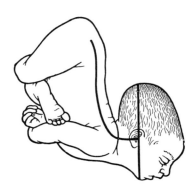

Fig. 10. Face presentation. Occiput on the long end of head lever.

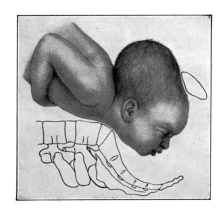

Fig. 11. Face presentation. Chin directly posterior, showing impossibility of spontaneous delivery unless rotation occurs.

The mechanism in these cases consists of the *cardinal movements* of descent, internal rotation, and flexion, and the *accessory movements* of extension and external rotation. Descent is brought about by the same factors as in vertex presentations. Extension results from the relation of the fetal body to the deflected head, which is converted into a two-armed lever, the longer arm of which extends from the occipital condyles to the occiput. When resistance is then encountered, the occiput must be pushed upward, while the chin descends (Fig. 10).

The object of internal rotation of the face is to bring the chin under the symphysis pubis; natural delivery cannot otherwise be accomplished. Only in this way can the neck subtend the posterior surface of the symphysis pubis. If the chin rotates directly posteriorly, the relatively short neck cannot span the anterior surface of the sacrum, which measures 12 cm in length. Hence, the birth of the head is manifestly impossible unless the shoulders enter the pelvis at the same time, an event that is out of the question except when the fetus is markedly premature or macerated (Fig. 11). Internal rotation in a face presentation results from the same factors as in vertex presentations.

After anterior rotation and descent, the chin and mouth appear at the vulva, the undersurface of the chin presses against the symphysis, and the head is delivered by flexion. The nose, eyes, brows, bregma, and occiput then appear in succession over the anterior margin of the perineum (Fig. 12). After the birth of the head the occiput sags backward toward the anus. In a few moments the chin rotates externally to the side toward which it was originally directed, and the shoulders are born as in vertex presentations.

Edema may sometimes distort the face sufficiently to obliterate the features and lead to erroneous diagnosis of breech presentation (Fig. 13). At the same time, the skull undergoes considerable molding, manifested by increase in length of the vertical diameter of the head.

Prognosis.   Until the latter part of the eighteenth century, face presentations were considered extremely unfavorable, and most authorities advised their conversion into some other variety. About that time, however, a number of obste-

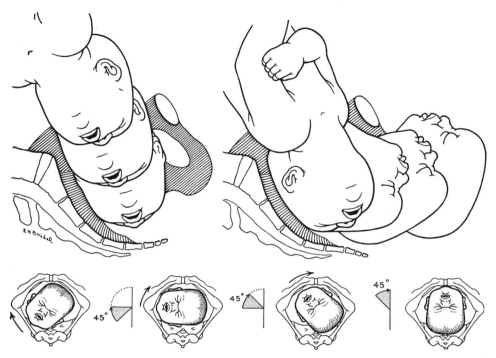

Fig. 12. Mechanism of labor for right mentoposterior position.

Fig. 13. Edema and discoloration in face presentation.

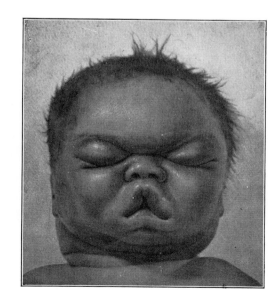

tricians in France and Austria pointed out that most of them would deliver spontaneously in time. A conservative policy was definitely established by Boer, who reported spontaneous labor in 79 out of 80 face presentations, with forceps required only once.

Deep tears in the perineum may occur unless avoided by episiotomy. They are often erroneously attributed to excessive distention of the vulvar outlet by the largest circumference of the head, the mentooccipital. In reality, however, the trachelobregmatic is the circumference concerned. Since it is only slightly larger than the suboccipitofrontal of vertex presentations, some other factor must be involved in the greater incidence of perineal tears. The explanation is probably the greater downward protrusion of the pelvic floor during face presentations, since the presenting part must descend very far before flexion of the neck under the symphysis can occur (Fig. 14).

Because of the prolongation of labor and the high incidence of prematurity

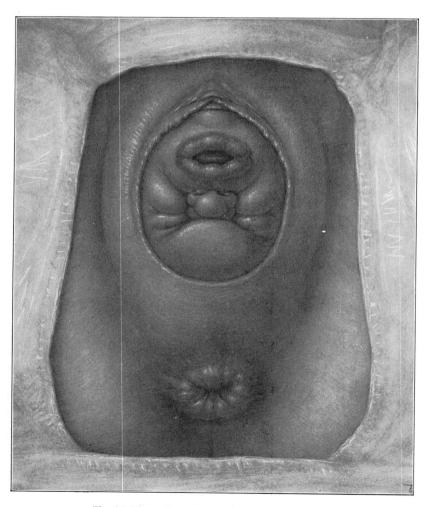

Fig. 14. Distention of vulva in face presentation.

and immaturity, perinatal loss is usually increased to between 15 and 20 per cent. It varies from 2.5 (Prevedourakis) to 5.0 (Salzman and co-workers) per cent for term infants.

In face presentations internal rotation does not occur until the pelvic floor is well distended by the advancing face. Frequently, when the chin is obliquely posterior, it may not take place until the obstetrician has almost abandoned hope of its occurrence. Figures 15 and 16 show that the face must occupy a lower level

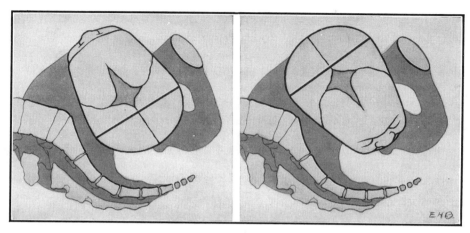

Fig. 15. Diagram showing that when the vertex is on the line joining the ischial spines, the greatest diameter of the head has passed the superior strait.

Fig. 16. Diagram showing that when the face is on the level of the ischial spines, the greater diameter of the head is still above the superior strait.

than the vertex before there may be assurance that the greatest circumference of the head has passed through the superior strait. The distance from the parietal boss to the vertex is only 3 cm, whereas a line drawn from the same point to the face measures 7 cm.

Treatment. The management of face presentations comprises the following principles. (1) X-ray pelvimetry is essential to prove or rule out pelvic contraction. (2) If any significant degree of pelvic contraction with disproportion is present, cesarean section is indicated. (3) If the pelvis is normal and the chin anterior, spontaneous delivery or an easy low forceps delivery should be expected. (4) If the pelvis is normal and the chin posterior, spontaneous rotation and an easy vaginal delivery should be expected in two thirds of these cases. Since only about one third of all face presentations have the chin posterior, and since two thirds of this one third undergo spontaneous rotation, a case of persistent mentum posterior is encountered only once in about ten face presentations. (5) If the chin persists as a posterior, whether in a primigravida or multipara, cesarean section is usually indicated if the fetus is alive. (6) If the fetus is dead, perforation of its skull is often the procedure of choice.

Other methods of management of persistent face presentations are rarely indicated in modern obstetrics. They include manual conversion of the face to a vertex presentation, manual or forceps rotation of a posterior chin to a mentum anterior position, and version and extraction. The conversion operations are likely to be traumatic to both fetus and mother and are successful in only about half the cases. If the fetus is alive, the only recourse after unsuccessful attempts at conversion is cesarean section. The operation is made more hazardous by the manipulations inherent in the attempted conversion. The risk for the infant in version and extraction is great. In Reddoch's large series of face presentations, the perinatal mortality associated with version and extraction was extremely high. Reinke cited the loss of 5 infants in 12 versions, and Kenwick lost 7 in 48. Even though better results have been reported by Hellman, Epperson, and Connally in patients with normal pelves, this operation is potentially so hazardous for both mother and infant that it is no longer acceptable in modern obstetric practice for the delivery of patients with face presentations.

BROW PRESENTATION

Incidence.   In brow presentations the head occupies a position midway between full flexion and full extension, and the portion between the orbital ridge and the large fontanel presents at the pelvic inlet. Since most face presentations are preceded by a stage at which the brow presents, it is clear that most brows subsequently convert spontaneously by flexion to a vertex or by extension to a face. Persistent brows occur only once in 1,314 labors, according to Meltzer and co-workers. The rate is 0.1 per cent in the Obstetrical Statistical Cooperative.

Etiology.   The causes of brow presentation are essentially the same as those of face presentation. Meltzer indicates that 21 per cent of cases are related to prematurity or a contracted pelvis.

Diagnosis.   The presentation can occasionally be recognized by abdominal palpation, but vaginal examination is usually necessary. The palpatory findings are similar to those in face presentations, except that the cephalic prominence is less marked on the side of the back, whereas the resistance offered by the chin can be felt on the same side as the small parts. On vaginal or rectal examination, the frontal suture and part of the sagittal sutures are felt. In addition, part of the large fontanel, orbital ridges, eyes, and root of the nose can be identified, but neither nose, mouth, nor chin is within reach (Figs. 17 and 18).

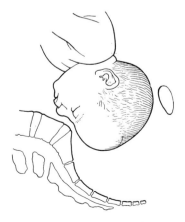

Fig. 17. Brow posterior presentation.

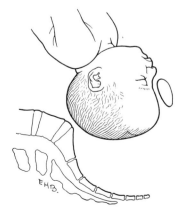

Fig. 18. Brow anterior presentation.

Mechanism. The mechanism of labor in brow presentations varies greatly with the size of the fetus, which most observers have stated to be frequently below normal. The rate of prematurity was almost 70 per cent in Posner, Rubin, and Posner's series, although it was only 18.7 per cent in the Obstetrical Statistical Cooperative. With small infants labor is generally easy, but with larger babies it is usually very difficult. The cause of the difficulty is the engagement at the superior strait of the mentooccipital circumference, the greatest diameter of which averages 13.5 cm. Consequently, engagement is impossible until after marked molding, by means of which the mentooccipital diameter is diminished and the frontooccipital increased.

After molding and descent the brow sometimes rotates anteriorly, with the forehead, orbital ridges, and root of the nose appearing at the vulva. One of the superior maxillary bones then becomes stemmed against the inferior margin of the symphysis. The rest of the head is then born by extreme flexion, with the brow, bregma, and occiput appearing in succession over the anterior margin of the perineum. After the birth of the occiput, the mouth and chin descend from behind the pubic arch by extension. The mechanism is thus somewhat similar to that of posterior occipital positions that rotate into the hollow of the sacrum. Sometimes, however, the brow descends to the outlet with the frontal suture directly transverse and is born in that position. Alternatively, partial anterior rotation may occur, bringing the root of the nose to about the middle of the ischiopubic ramus. The occiput is then delivered posteriorly by extreme flexion, after which the face escapes, following extreme extension. In either event, the second stage tends to be prolonged.

A large fetus cannot enter the birth canal without considerable molding, which adds materially to the length of labor and results in the characteristically deformed heads at birth. The caput succedaneum is found over the forehead, extending from the orbital ridges to the large fontanel. It is often so marked that diagnosis by vaginal touch is almost impossible. In these cases, the forehead is very prominent and square, the mentooccipital diameter is diminished, and the frontooccipital diameter is increased in length.

Prognosis. In the transient varieties of brow presentation, the prognosis depends upon the ultimate presentation. In persistent brow the outlook is generally poor unless the fetus is small. Disproportion between the size of the head and the pelvis is an important factor in extension of the head, and under identical mechanical conditions the possibility of a spontaneous outcome is always much smaller in a brow than in a vertex presentation. Because many brow presentations occur with premature infants and because the presentation is transient in a significant proportion of the remainder, spontaneous or forceps deliveries can be expected. Posner, Rubin, and Posner's 11 cases were all delivered vaginally. Persistent brow at term, however, demands cesarean section. Abdominal delivery was necessary in 17 of 64 brow presentations in the Obstetrical Statistical Cooperative. Formerly, because of traumatic procedures used for delivery, the perinatal mortality exceeded 20 per cent and maternal deaths were frequent. In modern practice, the perinatal loss, excluding premature infants and congenital malformations, is about 12 per 1,000 births (Meltzer).

Treatment. The principles underlying the treatment of brow presentations are much the same as those for face presentation. If labor is progressing, especially with a small infant, no interference is necessary, but if delay occurs with a term-size infant, cesarean section is preferable. The increasing prevalence of cesarean section in such circumstances is perhaps reflected in the improved perinatal mortality rates.

SHOULDER PRESENTATION

In this condition the long axis of the fetus crosses that of the mother at about a right angle. When it forms an acute angle an *oblique lie* results. This presentation is usually only transitory, however, for either a longitudinal or transverse lie commonly results when labor supervenes. For this reason, the oblique lie is termed *unstable* in Great Britain.

In transverse lies the shoulder usually occupies the superior strait, the head lying in one iliac fossa and the breech in the other. This condition is referred to as a *shoulder* or an *acromion* presentation. The side of the mother toward which the acromion is directed determines the designation of the lie as right or left acromial. Moreover, since in either position the back may be directed anteriorly or posteriorly, superiorly or inferiorly, it is customary to distinguish varieties as *dorsoanterior* and *dorsoposterior*. The shoulder is directed toward the left side of the mother more frequently than toward the right, and the back is more often anterior than posterior (Greenhill).

Incidence. Transverse lie occurred once in 322 deliveries at the Mayo Clinic according to Johnson, and in 0.5 per cent of labors according to Yates.

Etiology. The common causes of transverse lie are (1) abnormal relaxation of the abdominal wall resulting from great multiparity, (2) pelvic contraction, and (3) placenta previa. The incidence of transverse lie increases with parity, occurring ten times more frequently in patients of parity of four or more than in primigravidas. Relaxation of the abdominal wall with a pendulous abdomen allows the uterus to fall forward, deflecting the long axis of the fetus away from the axis of the birth canal into an oblique or transverse position. Placenta previa and pelvic contraction act similarly by preventing engagement. A transverse or oblique lie occasionally develops in labor from an initial longitudinal presentation, the head or breech migrating to one of the iliac fossas. Pelvic contraction is almost always the cause.

Diagnosis. The diagnosis of a shoulder presentation is usually readily made, often by inspection alone. The abdomen is unusually wide from side to side, whereas the fundus of the uterus extends scarcely above the umbilicus.

On palpation, the first maneuver reveals no fetal pole in the fundus. On the second maneuver a ballottable head is found in one iliac fossa and the breech in the other. The third and fourth maneuvers are negative unless labor is well advanced and the shoulder has become impacted in the pelvis. At the same time, the position of the back is readily identified. When it is anterior, a hard resistant plane extends across the front of the abdomen; when it lies posteriorly irregular nodulations, representing the small parts, are felt in the same location (Fig. 19).

On vaginal examination in the early stages of labor, the side of the thorax is recognized by the "gridiron" feel of the ribs at the superior strait. When dilatation is further advanced, the scapula and the clavicle are distinguished on opposite sides of the thorax. The position of the axilla indicates the side of the mother toward which the shoulder is directed. Later in labor the shoulder becomes tightly wedged in the pelvic canal, and a hand and arm frequently pro-

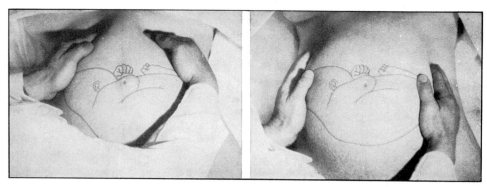

First maneuver   Second maneuver

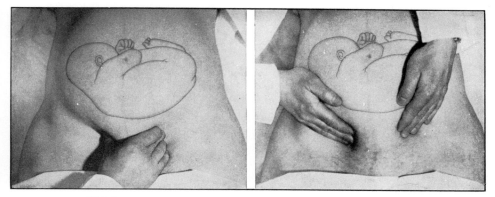

Third maneuver   Fourth maneuver

Palpation in right acromiodorsoanterior position.

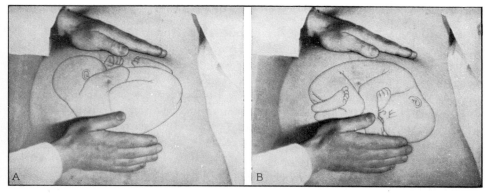

Palpation of back in dorsoanterior (A) and in dorsoposterior (B) positions.

Fig. 19. Palpation in transverse lie.

lapse into the vagina and through the vulva. Whether it is the right or left hand can be ascertained by noting to which of the obstetrician's it corresponds in shaking hands. Confirmation is available radiologically (Fig. 20).

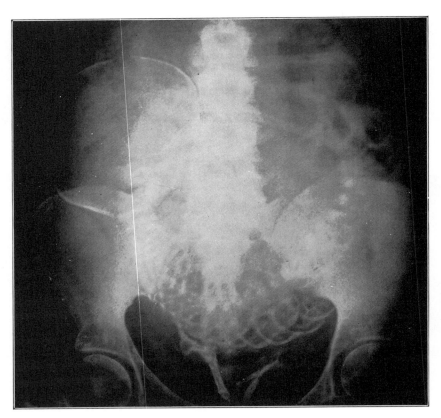

Fig. 20. Roentgenogram of transverse lie showing posterior elbow in the cervix.

Course of Labor.   With very rare exceptions, the spontaneous birth of a fully developed child is manifestly impossible in persistent transverse lies, since expulsion cannot be effected unless both the head and trunk of the fetus enter the pelvis at the same time. At term, therefore, both the fetus and mother will die unless appropriate measures are instituted. Very small, premature, and, particularly, macerated fetuses are, however, frequently born spontaneously.

Throughout the first stage and particularly during the early part of the second stage of labor, preliminary but futile preparations are made for spontaneous delivery. The fetal head and ventral surface are approximated, with decrease in the transverse diameter of the fetal ovoid and increase in the vertical diameter. After rupture of the membranes, if the patient is left to herself, the shoulder is forced into the pelvis, and the corresponding arm frequently prolapses (Fig. 21). After some descent, the shoulder is arrested by the margins of the pelvic inlet, with the head in one iliac fossa and the breech in the other. As labor continues, the shoulder is firmly impacted in the upper part of the pelvis. The uterus then contracts vigorously in an unsuccessful attempt to overcome the obstacle. After a certain time the retraction ring rises increasingly higher and becomes more marked. As the lower segment undergoes increasing stretch, the fetus dies and the patient becomes febrile. The situation is referred to as *neglected transverse lie*. If not vigorously and properly treated, the uterus eventually ruptures and the mother dies.

Very rarely the uterus may cease to contract before the membranes rupture, and retention of the fetus within the uterus may eventually lead to mummification. Such *missed labor* is very rare in human beings, though it is better known to veterinarians.

In very exceptional instances, if the child is quite small and the pelvis large, spontaneous delivery may eventuate despite persistence of the abnormal lie. In such cases the fetus is compressed with its head forced against its abdomen. A portion of the thoracic wall below the shoulder thus becomes the most dependent part, appearing at the vulva. The head and thorax then pass through the pelvic cavity at the same time, and the fetus, which is doubled upon itself (*conduplicato corpore*), is expelled (Fig. 22). Such a mechanism obviously is possible only in the case of very small infants and occasionally when the second fetus in a twin pregnancy is prematurely born.

Rarely, a dead fetus of average size may be expelled spontaneously by another mechanism designated *spontaneous evolution*, which requires such unusual conditions that most modern obstetricians will never encounter it. Attended by great risks to the mother, it occurs in neglected cases, in which it may appear suddenly. Several cases have been observed at the Johns Hopkins Hospital, two of which are described in Stephenson's article; in one of them a 2,700 g child was

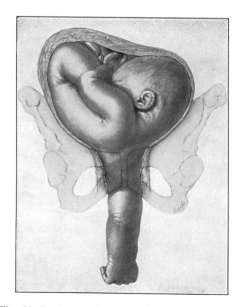

Fig. 21. Prolapse of an arm in transverse lie.

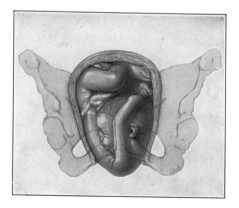

Fig. 22. Conduplicato corpore.

born eight hours after the onset of labor. Eastman described three additional cases and reported an incidence of spontaneous evolution at the Johns Hopkins Hospital of 5 in 147 consecutive cases of transverse lie, or 3.4 per cent.

Spontaneous evolution was first mentioned by Denman in 1784; its mechanism was accurately described by Douglas in 1819. In Denman's method of spontaneous evolution the breech appears immediately after the prolapsed shoulder. According to the mechanism of Douglas, the lateral aspect of the thorax follows the prolapsed shoulder, and the breech is born after the thorax and abdomen have been delivered (Figs. 23 and 24).

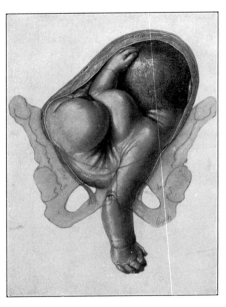 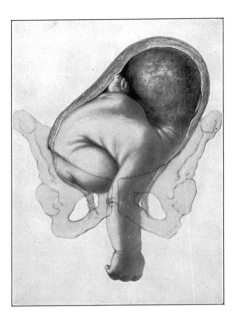

Fig. 23. Douglas' method of spontaneous evolution in transverse lie. Extreme lateral flexion of vertebral column with birth of lateral aspect of thorax before buttocks.

Fig. 24. Denman's method of spontaneous evolution in transverse lie. Same extreme lateral flexion of vertebral column as in Figure 23 but in opposite direction, so that buttocks are born before thorax.

In both mechanisms, the first stage consists in molding of the fetus and impaction of the shoulder with prolapse of the arm. Then, under the influence of strong uterine contractions, the fetus rotates about its vertical axis. As a result, one side of the head comes to lie over the horizontal ramus of the pubis, with the breech in the region of the opposite sacroiliac joint, while the neck subtends the inner surface of the symphysis pubis (Fig. 23). Coincident with excessive stretching of the neck, the prolapsed arm continues to descend until the corresponding shoulder eventually emerges under the pubic arch. The escape of the arm and shoulder affords room for the entrance of the rest of the body into the pelvic cavity. At this juncture in the mechanism, the crucial process of extreme lateral flexion of the spinal column occurs. Lateral flexion may force the breech either toward or away from the prolapsed arm. If the breech is forced in the direction of the prolapsed shoulder, it is born before the lateral aspect of the thorax. If lateral flexion takes place in the opposite direction, the breech cannot be delivered until the lateral aspect of the thorax is born (the mechanism of Douglas). The mechanism by which the breech is born before the lateral aspect of the thorax is not what Denman actually described, for he reported only that the "breech and inferior extremities are expelled before the head." The two methods are probably merely variations of one mechanism, basically lateral flexion of the spine. Following the breech or the side of the thorax, the remaining arm is delivered, and finally the head is born spontaneously or extracted manually.

In such cases the prolapsed arm is immensely swollen, with marked edema of the presenting shoulder. Our studies indicate that spontaneous evolution is possible only when the fetus is relatively small, uterine contractions are strong, and the fetal neck is unusually elastic. Herrgott, however, reported a case in which the child weighed 3,300 g.

Prognosis. Shoulder presentations, even in competent hands, increase somewhat the maternal risk and add tremendously to the fetal hazard. Most maternal deaths from this complication occur in neglected cases, from spontaneous rupture of the uterus or traumatic rupture consequent upon late and ill-advised version and extraction. Even with the best care, however, the maternal mortality will be increased slightly for three reasons: (1) the frequent association of transverse lie with placenta previa; (2) its greater incidence in older women in whom other complications, such as hypertension and myomas, may worsen the outlook; and (3) the almost inevitable necessity of major operative interference.

With vaginal delivery the perinatal mortality is extremely high, approximately 30 per cent for term infants whose fetal heart tones are heard on admittance to the hospital. The main causes of these infant deaths are prolapse of the umbilical cord, trauma in association with version and extraction, and hypoxia consequent upon uterine tetany. Furthermore, the extreme flexion of the infant during labor so interferes with the fetal venous return that intrauterine cardiac embarrassment occurs. The hazard for the fetus increases directly with the duration of time between rupture of the membranes and delivery. If the membranes remain intact until complete dilatation, and if delivery by version and extraction can be effected shortly thereafter, the prognosis for a term infant is relatively good (less than 10 per cent mortality). If, however, the membranes rupture before or at the onset of labor, the perinatal mortality soars to above 60 per cent. Since the shoulder of a fetus in transverse lie occludes the inlet very imperfectly, premature rupture of the membranes is quite common.

Treatment. Transverse lie in a primigravida should always suggest pelvic contraction and require x-ray pelvimetry. Any significant pelvic contraction in a primigravida with a persistent transverse lie is an indication for elective cesarean section several days before term. Moreover, any primigravida with a normal pelvis whose fetus at the onset of labor is in transverse lie should be delivered abdominally. The management of transverse lie in a primigravida is based on several facts. First, the shoulder is a poor dilating wedge; and especially in a primigravida, the first stage is likely to be prolonged as well as incomplete. During the prolonged interval, rupture of the membranes with its danger to the fetus is very likely. Version and extraction, furthermore, may be dangerous to both mother and infant because of incomplete cervical dilatation. In primigravidas attempts at conversion to a longitudinal lie by abdominal manipulation or postural therapy are rarely successful.

The management of transverse lie in multiparas may be slightly more flexible. Attempts at external version both late in pregnancy and early in labor are occasionally successful and worthy of trial. If during early labor the head can be brought into the pelvis by abdominal manipulation, it should be held there during the next six contractions, a measure that tends to prevent return to the previous position. If that measure fails, as it often does, subsequent management will depend chiefly on the state of the membranes. Because of the extremely high perinatal mortality in shoulder presentations in term infants, virtually all of these infants should be delivered by cesarean section. Similarly, in any patient with rupture of the membranes before the onset of labor, cesarean section is the wisest method of delivery. Harris and Epperson have shown a reduction in term perinatal mortality from 33.3 per cent to 2 per cent by this means. Rarely, perhaps in the multipara with a small fetus, normal pelvis, intact membranes, and cervix fully dilated, internal podalic version and extraction may be justified, but the hazards of the procedure are such that it ranks as the second most common cause of rupture of the uterus. Gareis and Ritzenthaler report 3 uterine ruptures in 81 versions and breech extractions for shoulder presentations. Furthermore, the perinatal loss is unconscionable. Harris and Epperson report a figure of 39 per cent; Wood and Forster give a corrected rate of 40 per cent; and Yates reports 50 per cent.

The increasing use of cesarean section in most transverse lies is justified by the very low perinatal losses recently reported. Wilson and associates cite a cesarean rate of 87 per cent with a loss of infants over 1,500 g of 5.6 per cent. In the Obstetrical Statistical Cooperative, as quoted by Hall and colleagues, the incidence of cesarean section was almost 78 per cent, with a 4.5 per cent loss of term infants.

Type of Cesarean Section.   Cesarean hysterectomy has a definite place in the treatment of certain types of transverse lie, particularly the neglected or infected cases. These situations are rare, however, in the United States today. In most instances simple cesarean section is performed on afebrile patients in good condition. Because neither the fetal feet nor the vertex occupies the lower uterine segment, the low transverse incision may cause difficulty in extraction of the fetus. A vertical incision may therefore be more expeditious when the fetal back faces the mother's abdominal wall. Either the Kroenig incision, which may be extended into the upper segment, or the classical operation may be used in these circumstances.

The treatment of neglected transverse lie at first entails support in the form of antibiotics, hydration, and transfusion if needed. Delivery may be accomplished abdominally by cesarean section or cesarean section–hysterectomy, as the situation demands (p. 1176). If the cervix is fully dilated and the fetus is dead, decapitation by means of a blunt hook and scissors or sickle knife may permit vaginal delivery (Fig. 25). Since the destructive procedures may rupture the uterus, cesarean section–hysterectomy is often preferable, even with a dead baby. Version and extraction should never be attempted in the presence of a thinned-out, easily ruptured lower uterine segment.

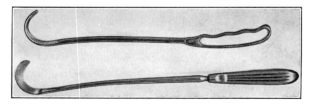

Fig. 25. Blunt hook, above. Sickle knife, below.

COMPOUND PRESENTATION

In compound presentations an extremity prolapses alongside the presenting part, both entering the pelvic canal simultaneously (Fig. 26). In a study of com-

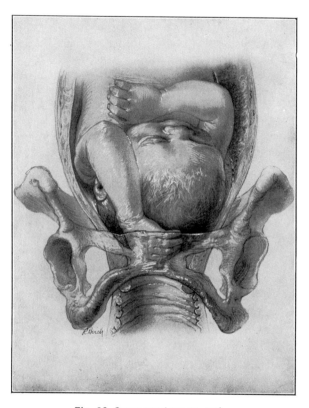

Fig. 26. Compound presentation.

pound presentations by Goplerud and Eastman at the Johns Hopkins Hospital, in the course of 42,410 viable deliveries 55 cases occurred in which a hand or arm prolapsed alongside the vertex, an incidence of once in every 744 deliveries. Much less common is prolapse of one or more lower extremities alongside a vertex presentation, only 6 cases having been observed in Goplerud and Eastman's series, or 1 in 7,068 deliveries. In addition to these 61 cases, there were 4 in which a hand prolapsed alongside a breech presentation. In similar studies at The New York Lying-In Hospital, Sweeney and Knapp found 74 instances of compound presentation in a 30-year period, or 1 in every 1,293 labors; Chan in Hong Kong cites an incidence of 1 in 1,321 deliveries. Compound presentations are frequently accompanied by prolapse of the umbilical cord, which determines the fetal prognosis. The cord prolapsed in 17 per cent of the total cases in the three series cited.

As expected, the causes of compound presentation are conditions that prevent complete occlusion of the pelvic inlet by the presenting part. They include multiparity (through lax abdominal walls and a high head), pelvic contraction, and small infants. In Goplerud and Eastman's series the incidence of prematurity was twice the expected rate. Often, however, no cause is demonstrable.

In most cases the prolapsed part should be left alone, since it will rarely interfere with labor. In Goplerud and Eastman's series of 50 cases not associated with prolapse of the cord, 24, or approximately half, had no treatment; normal delivery ensued in all, with the loss of only one infant. If the entire arm is prolapsed alongside the head, replacement may become necessary. In such circumstances, the condition should be observed closely to ascertain whether the arm rises out of the way with descent of the presenting part. If it fails to do so and if it appears to prevent descent of the head, the prolapsed arm should be pushed upward and the head simultaneously pushed downward by fundal pressure.

Although the reported perinatal loss is above 25 per cent, a major portion of the wastage is contributed by prematurity, prolapsed cord, and traumatic obstetric procedures. The loss for term infants in the absence of prolapsed cord and traumatic operative deliveries was 3.2 per cent in Goplerud and Eastman's series and 4.4 in Sweeney and Knapp's.

ABNORMALITIES OF DEVELOPMENT

EXCESSIVE DEVELOPMENT

The child at birth rarely exceeds 11 pounds (5,000 g) in weight, although authentic accounts of much larger infants are found in the literature. The largest infant on record weighed 23¾ pounds (10,800 g), as reported by Beach of Selville, Ohio in 1879 (Barnes).

Provided the pelvis is not contracted, it is unusual for a normally formed child weighing less than 10 pounds (4,500 g) to give rise to dystocia on the basis of its size alone. In overdeveloped fetuses the difficulty generally arises because the head becomes not only larger but harder and less malleable with increasing weight. After the head has passed through the pelvic canal without difficulty, the dystocia may be caused by the arrest of the unusually large shoulders at either the pelvic brim or outlet. Excessive size of the fetus can usually be traced to one of three causes: large size of one or both parents, multiparity, or diabetes in the mother.

Koff and Potter in a study of 20,219 births found that 0.94 per cent of the infants weighed more than 4,500 g and that the duration of pregnancy, calculated from the first day of the last menstrual period, averaged 288 days, or only 8 days more than the average. This study and others indicate that so-called postmaturity is not an important cause of excessive size of the infant. It is our practice to designate all newborn infants weighing 4,000 g or more as "excessive-sized." The incidence of these infants in more than 104,000 deliveries in the Obstetrical Statistical Cooperative was 5.3 per cent, and the incidence of children weighing 4,500 g or more was 0.4 per cent. Although studies by Smith, Worcester, and Burke, and many others have shown a relation between maternal diet and growth and survival of the fetus, it is dubious whether strict dietary control can materially reduce excessive growth of the infant. There is, however, an association between large women and large babies, heavy mothers and excessive weight gain during pregnancy, and thus, excessive prenatal weight gain and large babies (Sheldon; Nelson, Rovner, and Barter).

Although with a normal pelvis a moderate increase in the size of the fetus is usually without practical significance, in the presence of contraction a very large fetus may convert an easy into a very difficult labor. At the same time, dystocia in multiparas often results in great part from the loss of tone of the uterine musculature. Similarly, serious dystocia may arise when an excessively large head attempts to pass through a normal pelvis, just as when a head of average size is arrested by a definitely contracted pelvic inlet.

Inasmuch as our clinical estimation of the size of the fetus, particularly of its head, is often still inaccurate, the diagnosis of excessive size is often not made until after fruitless attempts at delivery. Nevertheless, thorough examination, including careful palpation and Müller's method of impression, enables the trained obstetrician to arrive at fairly accurate conclusions. Ultrasonic cephalometry greatly increases the accuracy of the measurement.

Treatment. In general, regulation of the mother's diet has little or no effect on the size of her offspring. These mothers should always be investigated for diabetes. If the fetus of a diabetic mother is obviously large in the last three weeks of pregnancy, cesarean section is usually indicated for other reasons (Ch. 27, p. 795).

Prognosis. Since excessive-sized infants are often born to obese multiparous mothers who are subject to a host of complications, such as diabetes, hypertension, and prolonged labor, both the maternal and fetal risks are increased. In Nelson, Rovner, and Barter's series of 231 gravidas who delivered infants weighing more than 4,500 g, there was 1 maternal death and a 13 per cent perinatal loss. In a thoughtful report of 766 infants weighing over 4,500 g, Sack cites a perinatal loss of 7.2 per cent. More distressing, 16 per cent of the infants were severely depressed at birth, 11.4 per cent had severe neurologic complications, and 4.5 per cent were dead before the age of 7 years.

SHOULDER DYSTOCIA

Shoulder dystocia is a serious complication of delivery, hitherto insufficiently emphasized. The problem is that the head is delivered before the obstetrician realizes that he cannot deliver the shoulders. Morris has described this potentially hazardous situation in colorful language.

Schwartz reviewed the experience with shoulder girdle dystocia at the Johns Hopkins Hospital, as summarized in Table 2. The total incidence is 0.15 per cent of term deliveries; the incidence in infants over 4,000 g, however, rises to 1.7 per cent. In Swartz' series, the mortality was approximately 16 per cent. Reduction of the interval of time from delivery of the head to delivery of the body is of great importance to survival, but overly vigorous traction on the head or neck, or excessive rotation of the body, may cause serious damage to the infant. The obstetrician is thus caught on the horns of a dilemma. Very infrequently, deliberate fracture of the clavicle may be necessary and lifesaving to the infant. Fundal pressure may compound the difficulties, but a mediolateral episiotomy and adequate anesthesia are helpful.

The first step is to clear the child's mouth and nose. Avoiding unnecessary haste and force, the operator sweeps the posterior arm across the chest and delivers it. The shoulder girdle is then rotated into one of the oblique diameters of the pelvis. The anterior shoulder can usually be delivered at this point. Woods

Table 2. Complications of Shoulder Dystocia in 31 Cases

	Total No of Cases	No of Cases Infants 4,000 g or More
Stillborn (died during delivery)	3	3
Neonatal death	2	2
Total Deaths	5	5
Brachial plexus palsy (7 left, 2 right)	9	5
Fractured clavicle (1 left, 2 right)	3	2
Total Upper Extremity Injury	12	7
Prolonged infant morbidity (29 days) Survival	1	1
Maternal lacerations, 3°	3	3
4°	3	1
Total Maternal Injury	6	4

suggests another method, which utilizes the principle of a screw. The operator applies pressure to the infant's posterior scapula, rotating it laterally and upward. The posterior shoulder then passes beneath the symphysis in a screwlike motion and is delivered as an anterior shoulder.

MALFORMATIONS OF THE FETUS AS A CAUSE OF DYSTOCIA

Double Monsters. For practical purposes three groups of double monsters may be distinguished: (1) incomplete double formations at the upper or lower half of the body (*diprosopus dipagus*); (2) twins that are united at the upper or lower end of the body (*craniopagus, ischiopagus,* or *pygopagus*); and (3) double monsters united at the trunk (*thoracopagus* and *dicephalus*).

Although multiple pregnancy may be suspected, the diagnosis of these conditions is rarely made unless difficulty in attempting delivery has led to careful exploration of the uterus under anesthesia with the entire hand. Since such monstrosities frequently present minor deformities as well, the detection of a clubfoot or harelip, for example, should direct attention to the possibility of a more serious abnormality.

Fortunately, the delivery of many monstrosities is sometimes much easier than expected, for two reasons: First, since such pregnancies rarely go to term, the monstrosity may not exceed the size of a normal child. Second, the connection between the halves is often sufficiently flexible to allow successful delivery.

In the first group, however, the large size of the double portion of the monster may lead to serious mechanical obstacles. The fused head in a *diprosopus* is, as a rule, much more readily delivered when it forms the aftercoming part than when it presents primarily. In the second group, a *craniopagus* presenting by the head usually causes only moderate difficulty, whereas *ischiopagi* and *pygopagi,* as a rule, require complicated maneuvers for delivery. In the third group, the delivery of *dicephalic* monsters is facilitated when they present by the breech, since in many cases the heads may be successively extracted.

In cephalic presentations, the two heads may interfere with each other and thus prevent engagement until one has been diminished in size by craniotomy. When engagement of one head occurs, delivery can be partially effected by forceps, but as a rule the head cannot be delivered beyond the pubic arch, since further descent is prevented by the arrest of the second head at the pelvic inlet. In such circumstances, amputation of the first head is advisable. Delivery of the rest of the monster is, as a rule, then best accomplished by version, unless the uterus is too firmly contracted to avoid danger of rupture.

Thoracopagi (Figs. 27 and 28) usually present a less serious obstacle to delivery because they are frequently very loosely connected. Indeed, it is not unusual for the two fetuses to present differently. When possible, it is advisable to bring down all four feet at the same time and to effect extraction in such a way that the posterior head is delivered first. In cephalic presentations the head and body of the first child are expelled, and the second child is then born very much as in an ordinary twin pregnancy. If, however, the second presents by the

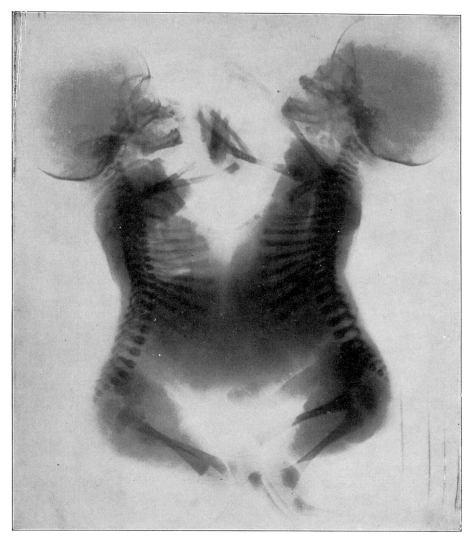

Fig. 27. Roentgenogram of thoracopagus monster. (From Shaw, Brumbaugh, and Novey. Amer J Obstet Gynec 27:655, 1934.)

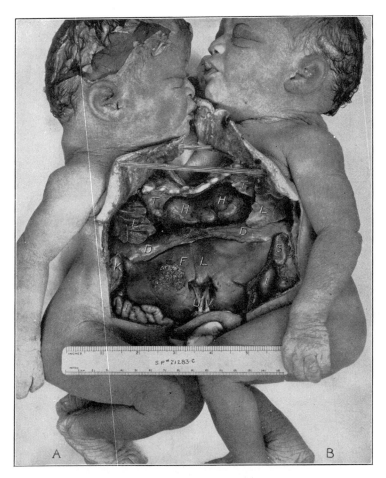

Fig. 28. Dissection in situ of monster shown in Figure 27. The conjoined heart (H), lungs (L), and the thymus glands (T) lie above the common diaphragm (D). The fused liver (F.L.), a portion of intestine (I), the right kidney (K) of twin A and the spleen (S) of twin B are seen lying in the peritoneal cavity. The umbilical veins (U.V.) enter the anterior surface of the liver. (From Shaw, Brumbaugh, and Novey. Amer J Obstet Gynec 27:655, 1934.)

shoulder, its delivery can be effected only by version and extraction. Easy vaginal delivery is not always possible, as demonstrated by Freedman, Tafeen, and Harris. In their report a pair of thoracopagus twins together weighed 7,200 g and were so closely joined that the first twin could be delivered only as far as the shoulders. Both twins were finally delivered by cesarean section.

OTHER DEFORMITIES OF THE FETUS

Attention is here directed only to those abnormalities in fetal development that may give rise to difficult labor; other deformities are discussed in Chapter 38. An *acardius* is a monster that sometimes develops in single-ovum twin pregnancies as the result of inequalities in the communicating placental circulation. One twin is well developed and normal, whereas the other is imperfectly formed, with either a rudimentary (hemiacardius) or an absent (holoacardius) heart.

The holoacardiac monsters may occur as acephali, amorphi, or acormi. The most common variety is the *acephalus*, or headless fetus. Less common is the *amorphus* monster, a roundish mass with numerous nodules on its surface but without either head or extremities. The umbilical cord may be attached to any portion of its surface. The monster contains a rudimentary intestinal tract and vertebrae but no trace of a heart. The rarest variety of acardius is the *acormus*, or trunkless monster, which consists of an imperfectly developed head and a rudimentary body, with the umbilical cord attached to the cervical region.

As a rule, such monsters do not attain large size, although, exceptionally, as the result of obstruction of the umbilical vein, they may become edematous and give rise to dystocia.

HYDROCEPHALUS

Hydrocephalus internus, or excessive accumulation of cerebrospinal fluid in the ventricles of the brain with consequent enlargement of the cranium, occurs in about 1 fetus in 2,000, accounting for about 12 per cent of all malformations found at birth (Fig. 29). Associated defects are common, spina bifida occurring in about one third of the cases. Not infrequently the circumference of the head exceeds 50 cm, and sometimes reaches 80 cm. The volume of fluid is usually between 500 and 1,500 ml, but as much as 5 liters can accumulate. Since the distended cranium is too large to enter the pelvis, breech presentations are common, occurring in about one third of such cases. Whatever the presentation,

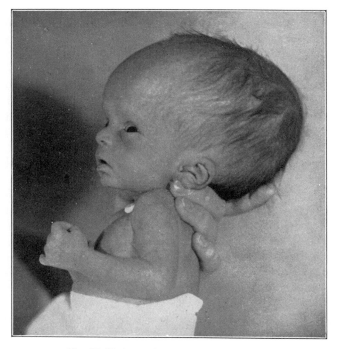

Fig. 29. Hydrocephalus of newborn child.

gross cephalopelvic disproportion is the rule and serious dystocia the usual consequence (Fig. 30).

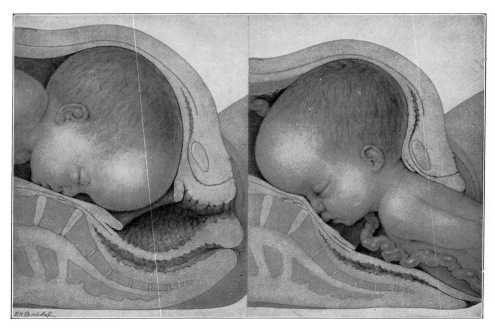

Fig. 30. Hydrocephalus causing dystocia. Left, in vertex presentation. Right, in aftercoming head of breech presentation.

Diagnosis.   Since the treatment of this complication of labor is straightforward, early diagnosis is the key to success, upon which may rest the life of the mother. In this condition particularly, an empty bladder facilitates both abdominal and vaginal examination; catheterization, therefore, is desirable prior to examination in suspected cases. In vertex presentations, abdominal palpation reveals a broad, hard mass above the symphysis; the thickness of the abdominal wall usually prevents detection of the thin, elastic, hydrocephalic cranium. The high head forces the body of the infant upward, with the result that the fetal heart is often loudest above the umbilicus, a circumstance not infrequently leading to suspicion of a breech. As labor advances, the lower uterine segment becomes rigid and tender. Rectal examination reveals an empty pelvis. Vaginally, the broader dome of the head feels tense, but more careful palpation may reveal the wide fontanels, the stretched suture lines, and the indentable, thin cranium characteristic of hydrocephalus. It is occasionally necessary to introduce the entire hand into the uterus to confirm the diagnosis, but the greatest care must be taken to avoid further stretching of the already distended lower uterine segment. In vertex presentations (but not in breech), roentgenography provides confirmation in the demonstration of a large, globular head with a thin, sometimes scarcely visible cranial outline (Figs. 31 and 32).

In breech presentations, the diagnosis is usually overlooked until it is found that the head cannot be extracted. Outlines of the head obtained roentgenologically with the fetus in breech position are misleading unless distortion is cor-

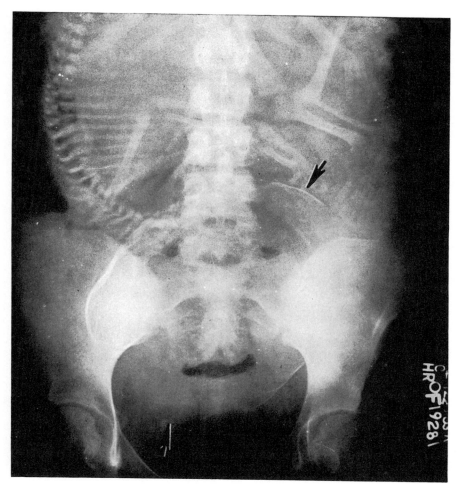

Fig. 31. Roentgenogram showing hydrocephalic fetus in vertex presentation.

rected. In ordinary scout films, the normal head in the upper pole of the uterus may appear huge, causing, according to Dippel, grave errors. The mistake may be avoided by particular attention to the following criteria: (1) the face of the hydrocephalic infant is very small in relation to the large head; (2) the hydrocephalic cranium tends to be globular, whereas the normal head is ovoid; and (3) the shadow of the hydrocephalic cranium is often very thin or scarcely visible. These difficulties in radiologic diagnosis are obviated by the use of compound scanning by ultrasound. In Figure 32 the large size of the head and thinness of the bones are readily seen.

Failure to recognize dystocia from fetal hydrocephalus is more often the result of negligence than of ignorance. Hydrocephalus will rarely be missed if the obstetrician is alerted to the possibility whenever (1) the head remains high, despite a normal pelvis and good contractions; (2) a floating head feels unusually broad; and (3) spina bifida is encountered as the trunk of a breech is extracted.

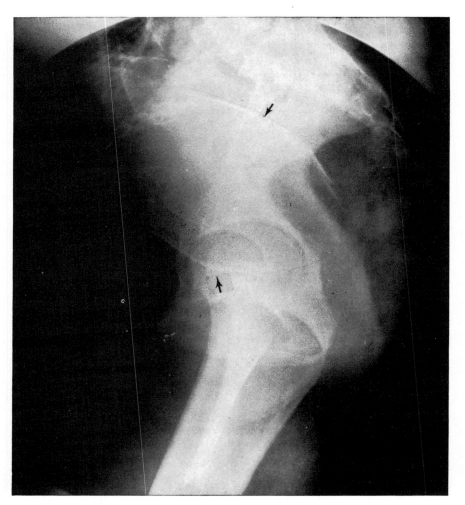

Fig. 32. Same patient as in Figure 31, showing infant's head after 1,000 ml of fluid had been removed by needle.

Prognosis.   Rupture of the uterus is the great danger and is the outcome of almost all untreated cases (Fig. 33). This risk was well illustrated many years ago by Schuchard, who collected 73 examples of the condition, with uterine ruptures in 14; 8 were spontaneous and 6 were the result of attempted forceps operation; 12 of the mothers died.

Hydrocephalus predisposes to rupture not only because of the obvious disproportion but also because the great transverse diameter of the cranium overdistends the lower uterine segment. Rupture not infrequently occurs before complete dilatation of the cervix and may occasionally occur even though the cervix is only 7 cm dilated. Because fetal hydrocephalus is frequently overlooked, the maternal mortality has been lamentably high. In Kleinhaus' data collected from 254 cases there were 46 maternal deaths, a mortality rate of 18 per cent. Even in Feeney and Barry's more recent series of 304 cases there were 9 maternal deaths.

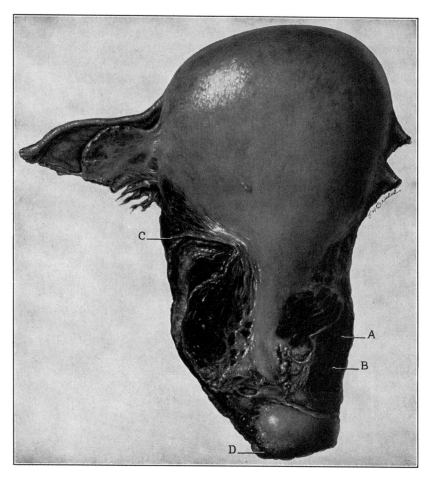

Fig. 33. Rupture of uterus caused by hydrocephalus. Right tear, A–B, is 3 cm long; left tear, C–D, extends through cervix into vagina.

There are cases on record in which the force of the uterine contractions caused the hydrocephalic head to burst, with the result that spontaneous delivery ensued. Almost always, however, the uterus rather than the cranium ruptures. Minor degrees of hydrocephalus may cause no dystocia, but such cases are usually incipient, and the diagnosis of frank hydrocephalus is not made until several days after birth.

Treatment. The progress of labor should be followed with utmost care, always considering the possibility of rupture of the uterus. In unequivocal examples of this disorder, the size of the head must be reduced to allow passage through a normal birth canal. Drainage of excess cerebrospinal fluid is easily accomplished by simple puncture of the head with a spinal needle, as advocated by O'Connor and Gorman. The head retains its rotundity, and labor usually progresses swiftly and easily. The great advantage of this method is that it can be done early in labor when the cervix is only 3 cm dilated and the lower segment has not thinned to the point of rupture (Fig. 32).

The hydrocephalic aftercoming head of a breech presentation is ideally treated by decompression with a metal catheter through the spinal canal. In the presence of a spina bifida the natural hiatus conveniently admits the passage of a metal catheter up the spinal canal into the skull. With the release of cerebrospinal fluid the fetal skull collapses and rapid delivery follows.

In the absence of a spina bifida, an artificial hiatus can be created by incising the tissues between two vertebral spinous processes in the upper dorsal region. Using a pair of strong scissors the following layers are cut through: skin and subcutaneous tissue, erector spinae muscles, ligamentum flavum, and interspinous ligament. The gap thus created is enlarged to allow the introduction of a metal catheter. This method is recommended by S. H. Tow in a personal communication based on his vast experience in Singapore. Unlike perforation of the aftercoming head, it carries no risk of injury to the maternal tissues. If the maternal abdominal wall is not too thick and the sutures are widely separated, fluid can be removed under fluoroscopy using a long needle.

Feeney and Barry have shown that the infant mortality in hydrocephalus, including the mildest forms of the disorder, is 70 per cent. Although cures have been reported, the prognosis for the child is exceedingly poor when hydrocephalus is severe enough to require drainage.

ENLARGEMENT OF THE BODY OF THE FETUS

Enlargement of the abdomen sufficient to cause grave dystocia is usually the result of ascites, a greatly distended bladder, or tumors of the kidneys or liver. Whenever the abdominal distention is so massive that it prevents spontaneous delivery, its cause is naturally investigated. The condition frequently escapes detection, however, until fruitless attempts at delivery have demonstrated an obstruction and led the obstetrician to introduce his entire hand into the uterus to ascertain its nature. Occasionally a fetus affected with generalized edema may attain such immense proportions that spontaneous delivery is impossible. Several such cases are recorded in the monographs of Ballantyne and of Dorland. They may well be examples of the hydropic form of erythroblastosis. In very rare instances a fetus with *chondrodystrophia fetalis* may become sufficiently edematous to cause dystocia.

As the result of dilatation of the lymphatics and subcutaneous edema, the fetus may assume immense proportions and a bizarre shape. This condition, *elephantiasis congenita cystica*, studied in detail by Ballantyne, is a very rare cause of difficult labor.

Defective development of the lower portion of the urinary tract may lead to *retention of urine*, accompanied by distention of the abdomen sufficient to render normal delivery impossible (Fig. 34). At the Kings County Hospital diagnosis of a similar case has been recently made prenatally by ultrasonography.

A more frequent cause of abdominal enlargement is *congenital cystic kidneys*, which may involve one or both organs and give rise to immense tumors. The condition is frequently associated with dilatation of the ureters and with massive ascites. Congenital cystic kidneys may cause great abdominal enlargement, as in the case described by Lynch.

In rare circumstances abdominal enlargement may be caused by *tumors of the liver*. Large tumors arising from any of the other abdominal organs may

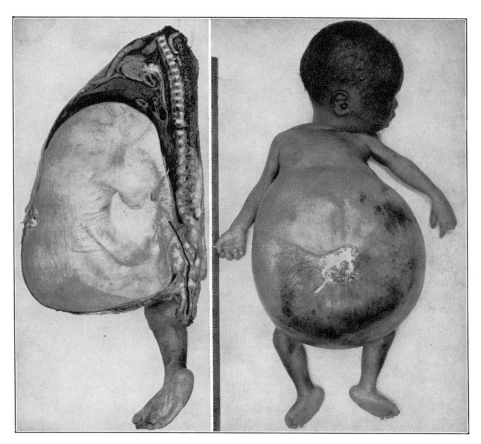

Fig. 34. Twenty-eight weeks fetus with immensely distended bladder. Delivery made possible by expression of fluid from bladder through perforation at umbilicus. Median sagittal section shows interior of bladder and compression of organs of abdominal and thoracic cavities. A black thread has been laid in the ureter. (From Savage. Amer J Obstet Gynec 29:276, 1935.)

also give rise to dystocia. Rarely, infection by *Clostridium perfringens* may be followed by such extensive production of gas that the size of the fetus is more than doubled and spontaneous delivery is impossible.

In all of these conditions, if the dystocia is marked, delivery can be accomplished only after allowing the fluid to escape from the body of the fetus, or by removing part or all of the obstructing tumor. These procedures are often so difficult and traumatic that cesarean section becomes the preferred method of delivery. In rare instances other abnormal growths may interfere with delivery. Lipomas, carcinomas, angiomas, and various teratomas, particularly those of the sacrum, are known to produce obstruction.

REFERENCES

Bainbridge, M. N., Nixon, W. C., and Smythe, C. N. Foetal weight, presentation and the progress of labour. Part II. Breech and occipito-posterior presentation related to the baby's weight and length of the first stage of labour. J Obstet Gynaec Brit Comm 68:748, 1961.

Ballantyne, J. W.   General cystic elephantiasis of the foetus, in Diseases and Deformities of the Fetus. Edinburgh, 1892, Vol. I, pp. 182–219.

Barnes, A. C.   An obstetric record from The Medical Record. Obstet Gynec 9:237, 1957.

Baudelocque.   L'art des accouchements, 1796, Vol. II, p. 36.

Beach, A. P.   A giant birth—the child weighing twenty-three and three-quarters pounds. Medical Record 15:271, 1879.

Boer, L. J.   Sieben Bücher über natürliche Geburtshülfe. Vienna, 1834 (7 books about natural childbirth).

Calkins, L. A.   Occiput posterior—a normal presentation. Amer J Obstet Gynec 43:277, 1942.

——— Occiput posterior presentation. Obstet Gynec 1:466, 1953.

Capon, N. B.   Intracranial traumata in the newborn. J Obstet Gynaec Brit Emp 29:572, 1922.

Chan, D. P. C.   A study of 65 cases of compound presentation. Brit Med J 2:560, 1961.

Crothers, B., and Putnam, M. C.   Obstetrical injuries of the spinal cord. Medicine 6:41, 1927.

Dede, J. A., and Friedman, E. A.   Standard practices at Sloane Hospital. Management of face presentation. Bull Sloane Hosp 9:118, 1963.

Denman, T.   Essays and observations. London Medical Journal 5:64, 1784.

——— Letter. Further remarks on the spontaneous evolution of children, presenting with the arm at the time of birth. London Medical Journal 5:301, 1784.

Dippel, A. I., and King, A. B.   Errors in diagnosis of hydrocephalus in the breech presentation. Amer J Obstet Gynec 38:1047, 1939.

Dorland, W. A. N.   Watery accumulations in the fetal abdomen obstructing labor. Amer J Obstet Gynec 79:474, 1919.

Douglas, J. C.   An Explanation of the Real Process of the Spontaneous Evolution of the Foetus, 2nd ed. Dublin, Hodges and MacArthur, 1819, 45 pp.

Duncan, J. M.   On the production of presentation of the face, in Contributions to the Mechanism of Natural and Morbid Parturition. Edinburgh, Adam & Charles Black, 1875, Ch. 14, pp. 218–231.

Eastman, N. J.   Spontaneous evolution of the fetus in transverse presentation. Amer J Obstet Gynec 25:382, 1933.

Ellis, R.   External cephalic version under anaesthesia. J Obstet Gynaec Brit Comm 75:865, 1968.

Feeney, J. K., and Barry, A. P.   Hydrocephaly as a cause of maternal mortality and morbidity; a clinical study of 304 cases. J Obstet Gynaec Brit Emp 61:652, 1954.

Freedman, H. L., Tafeen, C. H., and Harris, H.   Conjoined thoracopagus twins. Amer J Obstet Gynec 84:1904, 1962.

Gareis, L. C., and Ritzenthaler, J. C.   Transverse presentation. Amer J Obstet Gynec 63:583, 1952.

Goplerud, J., and Eastman, N. J.   Compound presentation. Survey of 65 cases. Obstet Gynec 1:59, 1953.

Greenhill, J. P.   Editorial comment. Year Book of Obstetrics and Gynecology, 1964–1965. Chicago, Year Book Publishing Co., 1964, p. 192.

Hall, J. E., and Kohl, S. G.   Breech presentation. A study of 1456 cases. Amer J Obstet Gynec 72:977, 1956.

——— Kohl, S. G., and Kavaler, F.   Transverse lie and perinatal mortality, New York J Med 62:2186, 1962.

——— Kohl, S. G., O'Brien, F., and Ginsburg, M.   Breech presentation and perinatal mortality. Amer J Obstet Gynec 91:665, 1965.

Harris, B. A., and Epperson, J. W. W.   An analysis of 131 cases of transverse presentation. Amer J Obstet Gynec 59:1105, 1950.

Hellman, L. M., Epperson, J. W. W., and Connally, F.   Face and brow presentation. The experience of the Johns Hopkins Hospital, 1896 to 1948. Amer J Obstet Gynec 59:831, 1950.

Herrgott, A.   (A case of spontaneous evolution). Ann Gynec Obstet 13:series 2, 193, 1918.

Holland, E.   Cranial stress in the foetus during labour, and on the effects of excessive stress on the intracranial contents; with an analysis of 81 cases of torn tentorium cerebelli and subdural cerebral haemorrhage. J. Obstet Gynaec Brit Emp 29:549, 1922.

Hughes, K. B., and Robbins, J.   Spontaneous evolution of a shoulder presentation. Lancet 1:825, 1968.

Johnson, C. E. Transverse presentation of the fetus. JAMA 187:642, 1964.

Kenwick, A. Face and brow presentations. Amer J Obstet Gynec 66:67, 1953.

Kleinhaus, F. Winckel's Handbuch, Bd. 2, Teil 3, p. 1631.

Koff, A. K., and Potter, E. L. The complications associated with excessive development of the fetus. Amer J Obstet Gynec 38:412, 1939.

Lanka, D. D., and Nelson, H. B. Breech presentation with low fetal mortality. Amer J Obstet Gynec 104:879, 1969.

Law, R. G. Standards of Obstetric Care. Edinburgh, Livingstone, 1967.

Lazar, M. R., and Salvaggio, A. T. Hyperextension of the fetal head in breech presentation. Obstet Gynec 14:198, 1959.

Lynch, F. W. Dystocia from congenital cystic kidney of the foetus, with report of a case. Surg Gynec Obstet 3:628, 1906.

MacArthur, J. L. Reduction of the hazard of the breech presentation by external cephalic version. Amer J Obstet Gynec 88:302, 1964.

Meltzer, R. M., Sachtleben, M. R., and Friedman, E. A. Brow presentation. Amer J Obstet Gynec 100:255, 1968.

Morgan, H. S., and Kane, S. H. Analysis of 16,327 breech births. JAMA 187:262, 1964.

Morris, W. I. C. Shoulder dystocia. J Obstet Gynaec Brit Emp 62:302, 1955.

Nelson, J. H., Rovner, I. W., and Barter, R. H. The large baby. South Med J 51:23, 1958.

O'Connor, C. T., and Gorman, A. J. The treatment of hydrocephalus in cephalic presentation. Amer J Obstet Gynec 43:521, 1942.

Pollock, A. Transplacental hemorrhage after external cephalic version. Lancet 1:612, 1969.

Posner, L. B., Rubin, E. J., and Posner, A. C. Face and brow presentations. Obstet Gynec 21:745, 1963.

Prevedourakis, C. N. Face presentation. Amer J Obstet Gynec 94:1092, 1966.

Reddoch, J. W. Face presentation, a study of 160 cases. Amer J Obstet Gynec 56:86, 1948.

Reinke, T. Face presentation, a review of 94 cases. Amer J Obstet Gynec 66:1185, 1953.

Sack, R. A. The large infant. A study of maternal, obstetric and newborn characteristics; including a long-term pediatric follow-up. Amer J Obstet Gynec 104:195, 1969.

Salzman, B., Soled, M., and Gilmour, T. Face presentation. Obstet Gynec 16:106, 1960.

Savage, J. E. Dystocia due to dilatation of fetal urinary bladder. Amer J Obstet Gynec 29:276, 1935.

Schuchard, R. Ueber die Schwierigkeit der Diagnose und die Häufigkeit der Uterusruptur bei fötaler Hydrocephalie. Berlin, H. S. Heimann, 1884, 36 pp.

Shaw, C. C., Brumbaugh, B. B., and Novey, M. A. An anatomical and clinical study of a thoracopagus monster delivered alive at full term. Amer J Obstet Gynec 27:655, 1934.

Sheldon, J. H. Maternal obesity. Lancet 2:869, 1949.

Skalley, T. W., and Kramer, T. F. Brow presentation. Obstet Gynec 15:616, 1960.

Smith, C. A., Worcester, J., and Burke, B. S. Maternal-fetal nutritional relationships; effect of maternal diet on size and content of fetal liver. Obstet Gynec 1:46, 1953.

Stephenson, H. A. The mechanism of labor in spontaneous evolution. Bull Hopkins Hosp 26:331, 1915.

Swartz, D. P. Shoulder girdle dystocia in vertex delivery, clinical study and review. Obstet Gynec 15:194, 1960.

Sweeney, W. J., and Knapp, R. C. Compound presentations. Obstet Gynec 17:333, 1961.

Thorn, W. (On the manual conversion of face presentations into occiput posteriors). Z Geburtsh Gynaek 13:186, 1886.

von Weiss, O. (On the management of face and brow presentations). Samml Klin Vortr n.f. Leipz, 1–33:601, 1892.

Wilson, L. A., Updike, G. B., Thornton, W. N., and Brown, D. J. The management of transverse presentation. Amer J Obstet Gynec 74:1257, 1957.

Wood, E. C., and Forster, F. M. C. Oblique and transverse foetal lie. J Obstet Gynaec Brit Emp 66:75, 1959.

Woods, C. E. A principle of physics as applicable to shoulder delivery. Amer J Obstet Gynec 45:796, 1943.

Yates, M. J. Transverse foetal lie in labour. J Obstet Gynaec Brit Comm 71:245, 1964.

30

DYSTOCIA CAUSED BY PELVIC CONTRACTION

Any contraction of the pelvic diameters or any morphologic distortion that diminishes the capacity of the pelvis can create dystocia during labor. Pelvic contractions may be classified as follows:

1. Contraction of the inlet
2. Contraction of the midpelvis
3. Contraction of the outlet
4. Combinations of inlet, midpelvic, and outlet contraction

INLET CONTRACTION

The inlet is considered to be contracted if its shortest anteroposterior diameter is *10.0 cm or less,* or if the greatest transverse diameter is *12.0 cm or less.* Since the anteroposterior diameter of the pelvis is frequently measured by the diagonal conjugate (roughly 1.5 cm greater than the obstetric conjugate), inlet contraction is also defined as diminution of the diagonal conjugate measurement to *11.5 cm* or less. The errors inherent in the use of this measurement have been discussed in Chapter 10. These figures are not arbitrary but are based on the fact that since the biparietal diameter of an infant's head is occasionally as large as 10.0 cm (average 9.25 cm), it might prove difficult or even impossible for such an infant to pass through an inlet with an anteroposterior diameter of less than 10.0 cm. The investigations of Mengert and of Kaltreider in x-ray pelvimetry have clearly shown that the incidence of "difficult" deliveries is increased to the same degree when either the anteroposterior diameter is decreased below 10.0 cm or the transverse diameter is decreased below 12.0 cm. The configuration of the plane of the inlet is also of great significance in determining the adequacy of any pelvis, independent of actual measurements (Ch. 10). When both diameters are contracted, the incidence of obstetric difficulty is increased threefold over that which obtains when only one of them is contracted.

The configuration is important at any plane, moreover, because the functional capacity of a pelvis is directly related to its structure. Consequently, a pelvis that appears adequate by measurement may offer obstruction, while a pelvis with smaller measurements may prove adequate.

Etiology. Although no longer the case, it was formerly estimated that about 2 per cent of white women and about 15 per cent of Negro women have pelvic contraction as the result of rickets suffered in infancy or early childhood (Fig. 1).

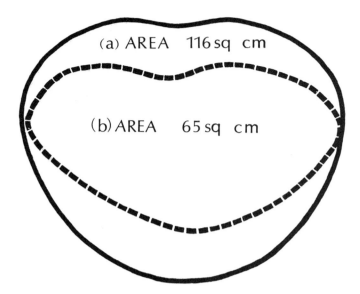

Fig. 1. "Areas" of normal pelvic inlet (a) and contracted inlet (b). The extreme degree of inlet contraction in (b) occurred in a 26-year-old black woman who had severe rickets in childhood (J.H.H. 283193).

Because of the mechanical action of various forces upon the softened bones and the traction or compression exerted by various muscles and ligaments, the rachitic pelvis shows characteristic changes, the most important of which are in the sacrum. The rachitic sacrum differs from the normal in that it is broader and less concave from side to side, thinner from behind forward, and shorter from above downward. The longitudinal axis of the bone is so altered as to form a greater angle with the obstetric conjugate; consequently, the promontory lies at a level lower than usual, approaches the symphysis pubis, and encroaches markedly upon the pelvic inlet. Usually the entire sacrum is sharply bent upon itself near its third vertebra, so that its vertical concavity becomes markedly accentuated. The bodies of the individual vertebrae, moreover, extend beyond the level of their alae, thereby diminishing the lateral concavity of the sacrum and generally converting it into a pronounced convexity. In that case the spinous processes project less than usual beyond the posterior surface, which tends to become concave. Occasionally, however, the increase in vertical concavity does not occur, in which case the sacrum may be quite straight from base to tip. The final result of rachitic changes in a particular pelvis, of course, is related to the basic pelvic configuration.

Occasionally the body of the first sacral vertebra is displaced farther forward than those below it, so that its lower margin projects beyond the general surface, and can be felt as a *false* or *double promontory*. In such circumstances the distance between this false promontory and the symphysis pubis may be shorter than the obstetric conjugate. In that case the distance to the false promontory is taken as the measurement of clinical importance, since interest always centers on the smallest diameter through which the infant must pass. The presence of a false promontory is usually indicative of the assimilation of an extra vertebra of the sacrum.

The overall change in the rachitic pelvis is a flattening of the inlet. Not infrequently, however, if the anteroposterior flattening is not pronounced, the capacity of the inlet is improved, since more of the forepelvis becomes utilizable.

In extreme cases the pubic arch may be relatively, and sometimes actually, wider than normal, and the tubera ischii may be so everted that the transverse diameter of the outlet appears to be exaggerated. In view of the upward and backward dislocation of the tip of the sacrum, the anteroposterior diameter of the outlet is also either relatively or absolutely increased in length. Consequently, in contrast to the flattened pelvic inlet, the pelvic outlet may appear wide and gaping, but occasionally a rachitic inlet is associated with a contracted outlet.

Currently in the United States rickets is extremely rare, and contraction of the pelvic inlet more often results from poor development. In such cases, since all of the pelvic measurements are more or less proportionately shortened, a miniature pelvis results. Such a "generally contracted pelvis" is often found in short women.

With the disappearance of rickets, transverse narrowing of the inlet accompanied by a normal or even elongated anteroposterior diameter of the inlet, as in android or anthropoid pelves, has assumed increasing importance. According to Manahan, Connally, and Eastman, such pelves are particularly treacherous, for the transverse diameters defy accurate clinical mensuration. Even with x-ray pelvimetry, moreover, the inexperienced obstetrician may underestimate the problems inherent in minor degrees of transverse contraction (McLane).

Effect on the Course of Pregnancy.   Marked degrees of pelvic deformity exert a pronounced influence upon the course of pregnancy as well as upon the mechanism of labor.

Position of the Uterus.   Rarely, in the early months of pregnancy a pronounced degree of pelvic malformation may interfere with the normal rise of the uterus, particularly if the promontory of the sacrum projects far into the pelvic inlet. In these rare cases, as the uterus increases in size it may assume a position of pronounced retroflexion, which may rarely lead to incarceration.

Later in pregnancy, if the deformity is sufficient to interfere with the descent of the presenting part into the pelvis, marked abnormalities in the position of the uterus may occur. Particularly in primigravidas, the fundus may occupy a higher position than usual. At the same time, because the lower portion of the uterus is not fixed by the engaged head, the entire organ is frequently more freely movable than usual.

More important, however, is the sharply anteflexed position that the uterus may assume, particularly in small women with marked lumbar lordosis. In such cases the capacity of the abdomen is so diminished that the growing uterus gains room by pushing forward the anterior abdominal wall. Consequently, a pendulous abdomen is a sign of considerable importance in primigravidas and should always lead to suspicion of marked pelvic deformity. The converse, however, does not necessarily indicate the absence of disproportion. The same condition may have no great significance in multiparas, however, since it generally results from a loss of tonicity of the uterine and abdominal walls caused by previous pregnancies.

Position and Presentation of the Fetus.   A contracted pelvis plays an important part in the production of abnormal presentations. In normal primigravidas, the presenting part, as a rule, descends into the pelvic cavity during the last few weeks of pregnancy. When the pelvic inlet is considerably contracted, however, descent does not occur at all, or not until after the onset of labor. Vertex presentations still predominate, but since the head floats freely above the pelvic inlet or rests in one of the iliac fossae, very slight influences may cause the fetus to assume other positions. According to Michaelis, vertex presentations are rarer by 10 per cent in contracted than in normal pelves, whereas face, breech, and shoulder presentations occur two or three times, and prolapse of the cord and the extremities four to six times, more frequently in contracted pelves.

Of 47,671 cases in the Obstetrical Statistical Cooperative there were 2,378 term deliveries complicated by contracted pelvis, an incidence of almost exactly 5 per cent. The distribution by position and presentation in both normal and contracted pelves is shown in Table 1.

Table 1. Fetal Presentation in Normal and Contracted Pelves

Position	Normal Pelvis (Per Cent)		Contracted Pelvis (Per Cent)	
OA	86.4	⎫	64.2	⎫
OT	5.1	⎬96.4	15.1	⎬89.7
OP	4.9	⎭	10.4	⎭
Breech	2.4		6.3	
Face, brow	0.3		0.8	
Transverse lie, compound	0.3		0.4	
Unknown	0.6		2.8	
	100.0		100.0	

Abnormal presentations occur more frequently in multiparas than in primigravidas, even under favorable conditions, and are still more common when the pelvis is contracted. Schauta estimated that they are three times more frequent in the fifth than in the first pregnancy.

In primigravidas, face and shoulder presentations are especially significant, since they are often associated with serious disproportion between the size of the head and the pelvis. Whenever face or shoulder presentations are encountered, therefore, the suspicion is justified that the head is unusually large or the pelvis abnormally small.

Size of the Fetus. Women with inlet contraction tend to have smaller children than those with normal pelves, probably because the contracted pelvis is only one of the many stigmata of underdevelopment that characterize the patient. Thoms, in a study of 362 white primigravidas, found the average weight of the offspring to be 278 g lower in women with small pelves than in those with medium or large pelves. He observed, furthermore, that the relation between maternal height and the weight of the newborn parallels that between the size of the pelvic inlet and the weight of the newborn. In veterinary obstetrics it has been frequently observed that in most species the maternal size determines the fetal size.

Mechanism of Labor. In a simple platypelloid pelvis the obstacle to the passage of the child's head is presented by the shortened anteroposterior diameter of the inlet. When it measures less than 9 cm it is impossible for the biparietal diameter of the normal head to pass through it without undergoing diminution in size (Fig. 2). Accordingly, when engagement occurs the head may gradually move to one side to bring the shorter bitemporal diameter into relation with the anteroposterior diameter of the inlet. As a result, the long arm of the head lever is displaced to the side of the occiput so that, under the influence of the uterine contractions, the anterior portion of the head descends while the occipital portion rises, resulting in some extension of the head. This mechanism leads to the increased frequency of face presentation in inlet contraction. The large fontanel becomes more readily accessible to the examining finger on one side of the pelvis,

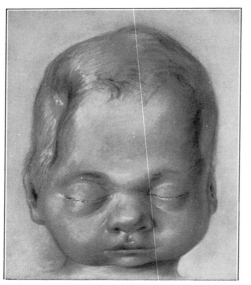

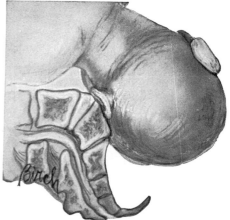

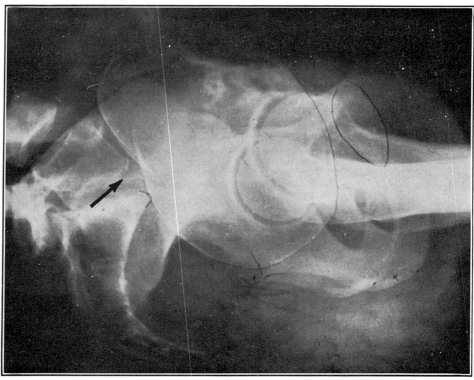

Fig. 2. Depression of skull caused by labor in a contracted pelvis.

and the small fontanel less so on the other. At the same time, the head tends to accommodate itself to the transverse diameter of the superior strait, so that its long axis, as indicated by the sagittal suture, comes to lie transversely.

As discussed on page 376 and illustrated in Figure 1 of Chapter 14, a certain degree of asynclitism is part of the mechanism of every labor. The successive posterior and anterior asynclitism may facilitate descent by permitting the fetal head to occupy the roomiest diameters of the pelvis at successive levels. It seems probable that asynclitism is exaggerated when the head passes through an anteroposteriorly contracted pelvis.

Breech presentations complicate inlet contraction to some extent, since the imperfect adaptation of the breech to the pelvic inlet facilitates prolapse of the cord. In such circumstances, although the prognosis for the mother remains favorable, the child's life is seriously endangered. In breech presentations, unfortunately, Müller's method of impression of the head cannot be used to estimate the extent of any marked disproportion between the fetal head and the pelvis. In the presence of pelvic contraction, there may be great difficulty in extracting the aftercoming head, since there is no opportunity for molding.

The effect of the generally contracted pelvis upon the course of labor is characteristic. Because all of the diameters of the inlet are shortened, the head encounters approximately equal resistance from all sides of the pelvic inlet. Consequently, the head enters the pelvis obliquely and in a sharply flexed position, with the result that on vaginal examination the small fontanel is readily felt, while the large fontanel is almost or quite out of reach. Since the contraction involves all portions of the pelvic canal, furthermore, labor is not rapidly completed after the head has passed the pelvic inlet. The prolongation is caused not only by the resistance offered by the pelvis but also in many instances by the faulty uterine contractions that frequently accompany diminution in the size of the pelvis.

Course of Labor. When the pelvic deformity is sufficiently pronounced to prevent the head from entering the inlet during the last few weeks of pregnancy or at the onset of uterine contractions, the course of labor is usually prolonged. The prolongation of the second stage of labor results from the time required for sufficient molding of the head to allow passage through the contracted pelvis.

Abnormalities in Dilatation of the Cervix. Dilatation of the cervix is normally facilitated by the hydrostatic action of the unruptured membranes or, after their rupture, by the direct action of the presenting part. In contracted pelves, however, when the head is arrested at the pelvic inlet the entire force exerted by the uterus acts directly upon the portion of membranes in contact with the internal os. Consequently, premature rupture of the membranes is more likely to result.

After rupture of the membranes, the absence of pressure by the fetal head against the cervix and lower uterine segment predisposes to ineffective contractions. Hence, further dilatation of the cervix may proceed very slowly or not at all. In our experience, the cervix fails to dilate to more than 5 cm in about one half the patients with pelvic contraction. In degrees of contracted pelvis incompatible with vaginal delivery, the cervix rarely dilates satisfactorily. The behavior of the cervix thus has a certain prognostic value in regard to the outcome of labor in women with inlet contraction.

Cibils and Hendricks have shown that the mechanical adaptation of the passenger to the bony passage plays an important part in determining the efficiency of uterine contractions. The better the adaptation, the more efficient are the contractions. Since adaptation is poor in the presence of a contracted pelvis, prolongation of labor often results.

Danger of Uterine Rupture. Abnormal thinning of the lower uterine segment creates a serious danger during a prolonged second stage. When the disproportion between the head and the pelvis is so pronounced that engagement and descent do not occur, the lower uterine segment becomes increasingly stretched, and the danger of rupture becomes imminent. In such cases the *retraction ring* may be felt as a transverse or oblique ridge extending across the uterus somewhere between the symphysis and the umbilicus. Whenever this condition is noted, prompt delivery is urgently indicated. Unless cesarean section is employed, there is the great danger of traumatic rupture caused by intrauterine maneuvers.

Production of Fistulas. When the presenting part is firmly wedged into the pelvic inlet but does not advance for a long time, portions of the birth canal lying between it and the pelvic wall may be subjected to excessive pressure. As the circulation is impaired, the resulting necrosis may manifest itself several days after delivery by the appearance of *vesicovaginal, vesicocervical,* or *rectovaginal fistulas.* Formerly, when operative delivery was deferred as long as possible, such complications were frequent, but today they are rarely seen except in neglected cases. In general, pressure necrosis follows a very prolonged second stage.

Intrapartum Infection. Infection is another serious danger to which the mother and the fetus are exposed in prolonged labors complicated by premature rupture of the membranes. The danger of infection is increased by repeated rectal and vaginal examinations. If the amniotic fluid becomes infected, fever may appear during labor, whereas in other cases puerperal infection later results. Intrapartum infection is a serious complication for the mother and an important cause of fetal death, since bacteria can make their way through the amnion and invade the walls of the chorionic vessels, thus giving rise to fetal bacteremia. Fetal pneumonia is often associated with intrauterine infection.

Effect of Labor upon the Child. Prolonged labor in itself is deleterious to the child. In labors of more than 20 hours or a second stage of more than 3 hours, Hellman and Prystowsky found a significant increase in perinatal mortality. In cases of contracted pelvis with associated premature rupture of membranes and intrauterine infection, the risk to the infant is compounded.

Prolapse of the Cord. A serious complication for the fetus is prolapse of the cord, the occurrence of which is facilitated by imperfect adaptation between the presenting part and the pelvic inlet. The condition exerts no influence upon the course of labor, but unless prompt delivery is accomplished, fetal death results from compression of the cord between the presenting part and the margin of the pelvic inlet.

Changes in Scalp and Skull. A large caput is frequently developed upon the most dependent part of the head in the presence of a contracted pelvis. It may assume considerable proportions and lead to serious diagnostic errors. *It may reach almost to the pelvic floor while the head is still not engaged. An inexperienced physician may thus mistake it for the head itself and attempt premature and unwise operative measures.* After delivery, the large caput has no effect upon the child's well-being, since it disappears within a few days after birth.

When the disproportion between the size of the head and the pelvis is considerable, the head can pass through only after *molding* and accommodation. In exceptional cases the head may descend into the pelvic cavity comparatively early in pregnancy. Since it cannot escape, it undergoes further development in that position. As a result, it presents characteristic deformities at birth, with the part within the pelvis markedly flattened and that above unusually large.

Under the influence of the strong uterine contractions the bones of the skull overlap one another at the major sutures. As a rule, the median margin of the parietal bone, which is in contact with the promontory, is overlapped by that of its fellow; the same result occurs with the frontal bones. The occipital bone, however, is pushed under the parietal bones, the posterior margins of which frequently overlap it. These changes are frequently accomplished without obvious detriment to the child, although when the distortion is marked they may lead to tentorial tears and, when vessels are involved, to fatal intracranial hemorrhage. Molding of the fetal head may produce diminution of 0.5 in the biparietal diameter without detriment to the brain, but when greater degrees of compression are demanded, the likelihood of cerebral injury increases.

Coincident with the molding of the head, the parietal bone, which was in contact with the promontory, may show signs of having been subjected to marked pressure, sometimes becoming very much flattened. Accommodation is more readily accomplished when the bones of the head are imperfectly ossified. In rare instances the skull is so soft that it yields to pressure far more readily than does the normal fetal head. This important process explains the differences in the course of labor in two apparently similar cases in which the pelvis and the head present identical measurements. In one case, the head is soft and readily molded, and spontaneous labor results; in the other, the more resistant head retains its original shape, and operative interference is required for its delivery.

Characteristic pressure marks form upon the scalp covering the portion of the head that passes over the promontory of the sacrum. From their location it is frequently possible to ascertain the movements that the head has undergone in passing through the superior strait. Much more rarely, similar marks appear on the portion of the head that has been in contact with the symphysis pubis. Such marks have no influence upon the well-being of the child and usually disappear a few days after birth, although in exceptional instances severe pressure may lead to necrosis of the scalp.

Fractures of the skull are occasionally encountered, usually following forcible attempts at delivery, though sometimes they may occur spontaneously. The fractures are of two varieties, appearing either as a shallow groove or as a spoon-shaped depression just posterior to the coronal suture. The former is relatively common; since it involves only the external plate of the bone, it is not very dangerous. The latter, however, if not operated upon, leads to the death of the child in over one half of the cases, since it extends through the entire thickness of the skull and gives rise upon its inner surface to projections that exert injurious pressure upon the brain (Fig. 3). Accordingly, as soon as feasible after delivery, it is advisable to elevate or remove the depressed portion of the skull in an attempt to prevent pressure symptoms and relieve the effects of hemorrhage.

Prognosis. The term "prognosis of labor" in inlet contraction refers essen-

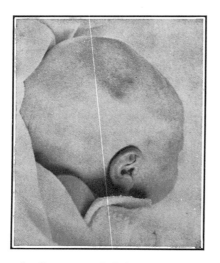

Fig. 3. Depressed fracture of skull caused by labor in a contracted pelvis. The infant did well after immediate neurosurgical elevation of the depressed bone (J.H.H. 23443).

tially to whether vaginal delivery can be effected safely for mother and child, and with relative ease. The outlook depends on many factors in addition to the absolute size of the pelvis. Among them are the size and position of the fetus, the outcome of past labors, the quality of the uterine contractions, the condition of the cervix, the extent to which the head descends in given periods of time, the mobility of the head, and whether it can be pushed manually through the inlet. Although pelvic size is but one of many factors that determine prognosis, it is the only factor that can be assessed with any degree of precision before labor. No mature infant can be delivered safely vaginally if the obstetric conjugate is 8.5 cm or less, regardless of other factors.

In general, about 90 per cent of patients who have contraction of the inlet, according to numerical definition, may be expected to deliver vaginally without great increase in risk to mother and child. In 2,316 cases of inlet contraction managed at the Johns Hopkins Hospital and studied by Manahan, Connally, and Eastman, 89.6 per cent were delivered vaginally, with a total loss of 4.6 per cent. This loss represents an increase of 20 per cent over the perinatal mortality rate obtained in the clinic over the period of study. There was, however, one maternal death in this series, which was the direct result of pelvic contraction. In the early years of the century the relatively high mortality of cesarean section justified taking such a great risk with the baby. At the Kings County Hospital, a cesarean section incidence of 32 per cent in contracted inlet was associated with a perinatal mortality of 1.5 per cent for white patients and 3.7 per cent for nonwhite patients. The diagnosis of contracted pelvis in these cases was based on roentgenography only.

As discussed in Chapter 10, the transverse diameter of the pelvis appears to be of equal significance to the anteroposterior in determining the success of engagement and subsequent vaginal delivery, although the data are not available to prove its importance, as in the case of the anteroposterior diameter. As shown by Mengert, by Kaltreider, and by others, contractions of the anteroposterior or transverse diameters are of equal importance in prognosis for safe vaginal delivery. Since the transverse diameter cannot be estimated clinically, x-ray pelvimetry is essential for the recognition of transverse contraction. (Tricomi and Kohl).

An obstetric conjugate of 8.5 cm is taken as the limit below which cesarean section is mandatory for the delivery of an undamaged term infant. Conversely, when the obstetric conjugate is 9.5 cm or above, successful vaginal delivery can be anticipated in most instances. In summary, the prognosis of labor in cases of severe contraction (obstetric conjugate under 8.5 cm) and cases of very mild contraction (obstetric conjugate of at least 9.5 cm) can be stated as almost hopeless in the former and excellent in the latter. There remains the borderline group in which the obstetric conjugate lies between 8.5 and 9.5 cm and in which the prognosis is often difficult to establish. Of patients with an obstetric conjugate of 9.0 cm, about one half require abdominal delivery.

In this borderline category the prognosis of labor must be established on the basis of a number of associated circumstances, as follows: (1) If, on the one hand, the patient has had a previous term labor (a small minority of cases), the outcome of that previous labor is of substantial significance. On the other hand, it may be misleading, since if it was easy, the happy outcome may have been attributable to a much smaller baby in the previous labor; or if it was difficult, the dystocia may have reflected poor management of labor rather than a small pelvis. (2) The size of the infant is naturally of extreme importance. (3) Premature rupture of the membranes in inlet contraction (but not otherwise) is an unfavorable prognostic sign, since it suggests considerable overriding of the head. (4) The quality of the uterine contractions is a determining factor, and uterine dysfunction is common. (5) Again, the behavior of the cervix in labor has great prognostic significance; satisfactory progress in dilatation usually indicates that vaginal delivery will be feasible, whereas an undilating cervix usually means that vaginal delivery cannot be accomplished with safety. (6) The architecture of the pelvis plays a role; in the android type there is less available space in the inlet for any given obstetric conjugate measurement than in other types. (7) Intrapartum infection seems to inhibit uterine contractility and is a bad sign. (8) Extreme asynclitism is unfavorable. (9) Naturally, cases in which the obstetric conjugate is nearer to 8.5 than to 9.5 cm carry a poorer prognosis. (10) A lateral x-ray film of the pelvis obtained during labor with the patient standing often demonstrates whether the head is engaged or is likely to engage.

Other methods of ascertaining whether the fetal head will pass through the pelvis are discussed in the ensuing paragraphs.

Methods of Estimating Size of the Head. Müller's method of impression often affords material aid. In this procedure the obstetrician grasps the brow and occiput of the child through the abdominal wall with his fingers and makes firm pressure downward in the axis of the pelvic inlet. The effect of the pressure may be ascertained by a finger in the rectum or vagina. If there is no disproportion, the head readily enters the pelvis and spontaneous delivery may be predicted. Inability to force the head into the pelvis, however, does not necessarily indicate that spontaneous delivery is impossible. Demonstration of overriding of the fetal head (Fig. 4) is of value if the findings are positive, but absence of overriding is of little significance, since it may be the result of asynclitism. Pressure upon the fundus by an assistant at the same time is often of great additional help.

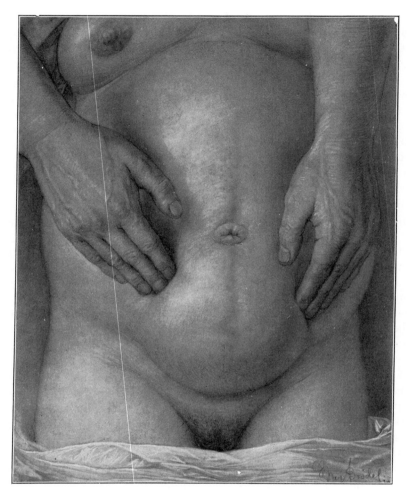

Fig. 4. Method of ascertaining degree of disproportion by noting the extent to which the head overrides the symphysis.

In general, radiologic measurements of the absolute diameters of the fetal head have proved disappointing. The precision of roentgencephalometry is decidedly less than that of pelvimetry, with an error of plus or minus 0.5 cm in most hands.

The ultrasonic demonstration of fetal structures has provided a method of cephalometry that has proved to be more accurate (Donald and colleagues; Hellman and co-workers; Taylor and associates). This technic not only offers a rapid method of ascertaining the biparietal diameter but also can be used to measure the occipitofrontal diameter and circumference as well (Figs. 5 and 6).

In many cases of borderline inlet contraction, it is desirable to allow a "trial labor," or a period of labor long enough to afford evidence, on the basis of the prognostic criteria enumerated, as to whether vaginal delivery may be anticipated with safety to mother and child. The period of time required for such evidence

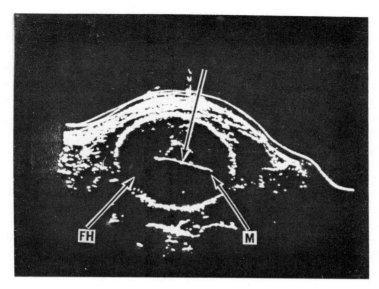

Fig. 5. Ultrasonic transverse scan of the fetal head, showing midline (B-mode cephalometry). The arrow is perpendicular to the linear midline structures of the fetal head. With this line as reference, the various measurements of the head can be made. FH, fetal head; M, midline of the fetal head.

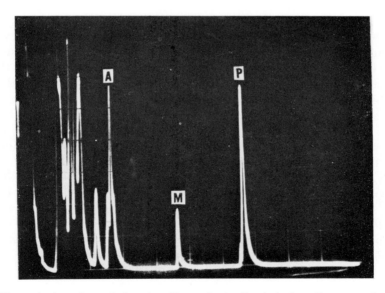

Fig. 6. Ultrasonic A-mode cephalometry. The probe is directed along the arrow shown in the B-mode presentation (Fig. 5). The anterior (A) and posterior (P) skull echoes are clearly seen with a midline echo (M) between them. The biparietal diameter of the fetal head is the distance between these two peaks (A and P).

to accrue varies, though it probably should not exceed four to six hours. Formerly, a so-called *test of labor* was often used, which entailed allowing labor to continue until complete dilatation and two hours thereafter. This "test" has no place in the modern management of pelvic contraction for two reasons: First, many labors with advanced inlet contraction do not reach complete dilatation even after 30 hours. Second, the perinatal mortality resulting from this practice is appalling, exceeding 30 per cent in the days when it was employed. The proper utilization of "trial labor" will safely decrease the number of unnecessary cesarean sections. The most important concept in its proper use is as *a definite timetable*. The trial must not be allowed to continue indefinitely, nor should it be used perfunctorily to justify cesarean section. The problem should be analyzed and a definite plan of management established. The timetable should then be decisively followed.

Breech and Face Presentations in Contracted Pelves. A breech presentation with moderate degrees of pelvic deformity should be regarded as a complication especially unfavorable for the child, inasmuch as in the early stages of labor prolapse of the cord is facilitated, and in the later stages serious delay may be encountered in extraction of the aftercoming head. The result may often be loss of the child or at least serious damage (see Ch. 10). Since the head, moreover, is not in contact with the pelvic inlet, it is difficult to ascertain the degree of disproportion. For these reasons, more liberal use of elective cesarean section is justified. Face and brow presentations should be regarded as much more serious complications, for they often indicate, except in certain cases in which the fetus is very small or dead, a considerable degree of disproportion. Cesarean section is almost always indicated in face or brow presentations at term with a contracted pelvis.

Treatment. The management of inlet contraction is essentially determined by the prognosis for safe vaginal delivery. If, on the basis of the criteria reviewed, a delivery that is safe for both mother and child cannot be anticipated, cesarean section should be done. Today it is so rare to employ craniotomy that even dead fetuses are often delivered by cesarean section in cases of frank contraction. In very rare instances, the prognosis in a given case can be reached before the onset of labor, and section can be done electively at an appointed time. A trial of labor is desirable in most instances, however. Patients with inlet contraction are particularly likely to have weak uterine contractions. The type of analgesia and the timing of its initiation should be carefully selected lest they further decrease effective uterine action. The course of labor should be followed carefully from hour to hour, and the prognosis established as soon as reasonably possible. Although signs of impending uterine rupture should always be looked for if the contractions are strong, the danger of the accident is very remote in primigravidas. With greater parity, however, the likelihood of the accident increases. Finally, *the administration of oxytocin in the presence of any form of pelvic contraction, unless the fetal head has passed the point of obstruction, can be catastrophic for the child and may rupture the mother's uterus.*

MIDPELVIC CONTRACTION

Definitions. The so-called plane of the obstetric midpelvis extends from the inferior margin of the symphysis pubis, passes through the ischial spines, and touches the sacrum near the junction of the fourth and fifth vertebrae (Mengert). The anatomic description places the posterior limits at the tip of the sacrum. The interspinous line divides the midpelvis into a fore and hind portion. The former is bounded anteriorly by the lower border of the symphysis pubis and laterally by the ischiopubic rami. The hind portion is bounded posteriorly by the sacrum and laterally by the sacrospinous ligament, forming the lower limits of the sacrosciatic notch. Average midpelvic measurements are as follows: transverse (interspinous), 10.5 cm; anteroposterior (from the lower border of the symphysis pubis to the junction of the fourth and fifth sacral vertebrae), 11.5 cm; and posterior sagittal (from the midpoint of the interspinous line to the same point on the sacrum), 5.0 cm. Although the definition of midpelvic contraction has not been established with the precision possible in inlet contraction, the midpelvis may be considered contracted when the sum of the interischial spinous and posterior sagittal diameters of the midpelvis (normally, 10.5 cm plus 5.0 cm, or 15.5 cm) falls to 13.5 cm or below (Guerriero, Arnell, and Irwin). There is reason to suspect midpelvic contraction whenever the interischial spinous diameter falls below 9.5 cm. When it is lower than 9.0 cm, the pelvis is most likely contracted.

The preceding definition of midpelvic contraction does not, of course, imply that dystocia will necessarily occur in such a pelvis, but simply that it may develop, depending upon the size and shape of the forepelvis, the degree of the midpelvic contraction, and the size of the baby.

Since there is no satisfactory manual method of ascertaining midpelvic contraction, x-ray pelvimetry is necessary. A suggestion of midpelvic contraction, however, is sometimes obtainable by ascertaining on vaginal examination that the spines are prominent, that the side walls converge, or that the sacrosciatic notch is narrow. Eller and Mengert, moreover, point out that the relation between the intertuberous and interspinous diameters of the ischium is sufficiently constant that interspinous contractions will seldom be missed if x-ray pelvimetry is limited to patients whose intertuberous diameter is 8.5 cm or less.

Prognosis. Midpelvic contraction is probably more common than inlet contraction and is frequently a cause of transverse arrest of the head and, consequently, of difficult midforceps operations. Although extreme dystocia in midpelvic contraction is rare, an interspinous diameter of 9.0 cm or less often results in uterine inertia and thus may lead to a cesarean section.

Treatment. In the management of labor complicated by midpelvic contraction, the main injunction is to allow the natural forces to push the biparietal diameter through the interspinous obstruction. Forceps operations may be very difficult when applied to a head whose greatest diameter has not yet passed a contracted midpelvis. This difficulty may be explained on two grounds: (1) forceps pull destroys flexion, whereas pressure from above increases it; (2) the few millimeters occupied by the thickness of the forceps blades diminish further the available space for passage of the fetal head. Only when the head has been allowed to descend until the perineum is bulging and the vertex is actually visible is it reasonably certain that the head has passed the obstruction; only then is it safe to apply forceps. Strong suprafundal pressure should not be used to force the head past the obstruction.

The use of the obstetric forceps to effect delivery in midpelvic contraction, usually undiagnosed, has been responsible for the stigma attached to the midforceps operation. The perinatal mortality associated with the operation is prohibitive; midforceps delivery is, therefore, usually contraindicated in any midpelvic contraction. It is assumed that x-ray pelvimetry has been obtained and evaluated before a final decision about method of delivery is made. Unless the leading point of a flexed fetal skull is at least at the level of the ischial spines, furthermore, the greatest transverse diameter of the head may not yet have negotiated the plane of the inlet. The forceps opration is then not a midforceps procedure but rather a "high forceps."

The vacuum extractor (p. 1139) has been employed to good advantage in some cases of midpelvic contraction. It does not cause deflection, nor does it occupy space, as do forceps. Oxytocin, of course, has no place in the treatment of dystocia caused by midpelvic contraction.

Outlet Contraction

Definitions.   Contraction of the pelvic outlet is defined as diminution of the interischial tuberous diameter to 8.0 cm or less. Figures 7 and 8 indicate that

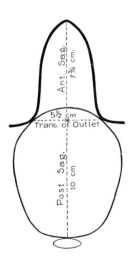

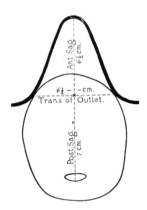

Fig. 7. Diagram of pelvic outlet of case shown in Figure 9, illustrating possibility of spontaneous labor because of long posterior sagittal diameter.

Fig. 8. Diagram of pelvic outlet of case shown in Figure 10, illustrating necessity for cesarean section.

the area of the outlet (not actually a plane) may be likened to two triangles. The interischial tuberous diameter constitutes the base of both. The sides of the anterior triangle are the pubic rami, and its apex the inferior posterior surface of the symphysis pubis. The posterior triangle has no bony sides but is limited at its apex by the tip of the last sacral vertebra (not the tip of the coccyx). It is thus apparent that diminution in the intertuberous diameter with consequent narrowing of the anterior triangle must inevitably force the fetal head posteriorly; whether delivery can take place, therefore, depends partly on the size of the latter triangle. Since, moreover, the posterior triangle has no bony sides, the possibility of delivery depends, in good part, on the altitude of the posterior triangle. In other words, the degree to which outlet contraction may cause dystocia depends not on one measurement alone but on two, the interischial tuberous diameter and the posterior sagittal diameter of the outlet (Figs. 9 and 10).

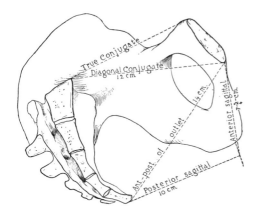

Fig. 9. Diagram showing the significance of anterior and posterior sagittal diameters. Spontaneous labor through a transverse diameter of 5.5 cm. (See Figure 7.)

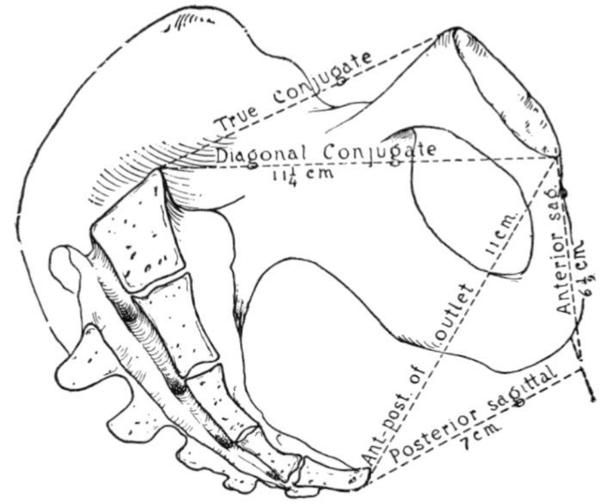

Fig. 10. Diagram showing the significance of anterior and posterior sagittal diameters. Cesarean section with a transverse diameter of 6.5 cm.) See Figure 8.)

Thoms believed that whenever the sum of the interischial tuberous diameter and the posterior sagittal diameter of the outlet is less than 15.0 cm, dystocia may result. It does not necessarily develop, of course, since it is quite possible for a mature infant to be delivered easily through an outlet in which the sum of these two diameters is only 13.0 cm. With a large baby, however, and other unfavorable pelvic factors, dystocia may very likely develop if the sum of these two diameters falls appreciably below 15 cm. There is usually a positive correlation between the size of the outlet and that of the midpelvis. A contracted outlet may cause dystocia not so much by itself as through the often associated *midpelvic contraction*. In our combined experience with x-ray pelvimetric studies, we have observed outlet contraction without concomitant midplane contraction only very rarely.

Contractions of the pelvic outlet occur in 3 to 5 per cent of women. Even when the disproportion is not sufficiently great to give rise to serious dystocia, it may play an important part in the production of perineal tears. In such cases, with the increasing narrowing of the pubic arch, the occiput cannot emerge directly beneath the symphysis pubis but is forced increasingly farther down upon the ischiopubic rami. In extreme cases, it must rotate around a line joining the ischial tuberosities. The perineum, consequently, must become increasingly distended and thus exposed to great danger of disruption. Schumacher believed that this type of pelvis has a serious effect upon the mechanism of labor by hindering the anterior rotation of the obliquely posterior occiput.

In view of potential significance of outlet contractions, palpation of the pubic arch should form an integral part of the preliminary examinations of every pregnant woman. If any abnormality is detected, x-ray pelvimetry is often indicated.

Generally, in multiparas with a history of previous severe outlet dystocia, unequivocal contraction of the outlet may afford an indication for cesarean section. In women not previously subjected to the final test of delivery through the birth canal, intelligent conduct of the second stage of labor is of the utmost importance. As the head is brought under the pubic rami, a deep episiotomy facilitates delivery and prevents the third-degree lacerations of the perineum that so frequently develop in patients with funnel pelves. In very rare instances an elective cesarean section may be indicated.

COMBINATIONS OF INLET, MIDPELVIC, AND OUTLET CONTRACTION

Combinations of inlet, midpelvic, and outlet contraction are common. They tend to aggravate the prognosis of labor in proportion to the additive effects that the several individual contractions produce.

RARE PELVIC CONTRACTIONS*

Kyphotic Pelvis. Kyphosis, or humpback, the result of spinal caries, plays an important part in the production of pelvic abnormalities, for when involving the lower portion of the vertebral column, it is usually associated with a characteristically funnel-shaped distortion. The effect exerted upon the pelvis by kyphosis differs acording to its location. When the gibbus, or hump, is situated in the thoracic region, there is usually a compensatory pronounced lordosis beneath it, so that the pelvis itself is but little changed. When situated at the junction of the thoracic and lumbar portions of the vertical column, however, its effect upon the pelvis becomes manifest. It is further accentuated when the kyphosis is lower down and is most marked when it is at the lumbosacral junction (Fig. 11). If the vertebral defect is in the lumbosacral region, the upper arm of the gibbus may overlie the inlet (*pelvis obtecta*).

CHARACTERISTICS.   The characteristic feature of the kyphotic pelvis is a retropulsion and rotation of the sacrum, by which the promontory becomes displaced backward and the tip forward. At the same time, the entire bone becomes elongated vertically and narrowed from side to side. These changes are associated with a rotation of each innominate bone about an axis extending through the symphysis pubis and either sacroiliac articulation. As a result the iliac fossae flare outward, and the lower portions of the ischial bones are turned in toward the midline.

When the kyphosis is in the dorsolumbar region, marked lordosis below it indicates an attempt at compensation, which, since it is imperfect, transmits the weight of the body in such a way that the sacrum is retroposed and lengthened. The sacral promontory is thus farther backward and at a higher level than usual. At the same time, the anterior surface of the sacrum loses its normal vertical concavity and becomes straight or even convex, whereas its lateral concavity is obliterated by the projection of the vertical bodies beyond the alae. The bodies themselves are considerably narrower than usual, and the alae of the first sacral vertebra appear to be drawn out and to extend obliquely upward to the promontory.

Because of its backward displacement the posterior surface of the sacrum approaches the superior posterior spines of the ilium, thereby relaxing the iliosacral liga-

---

* Illustrations of several rare pelvic contractions appear in earlier editions of this textbook.

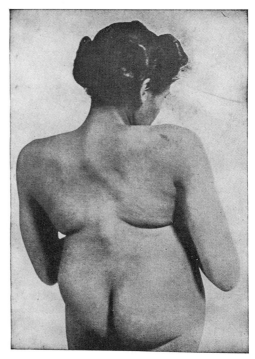

Fig. 11. Patient with obliquely contracted, kyphotic, funnel pelvis. Note presence of double gibbus. The lumbosacral deformity produces the funnel pelvis.

ments. As a result, the posterior extremities of the innominate bones are pushed apart, and their upper portions rotate outward and the lower portions inward. The crests are thereby flared out, occupying a lower level than usual, and the ischial spines and tuberosities approach the midline. This tendency is further accentuated by the increased tension exerted by the iliofemoral ligaments resulting from a diminution of the pelvic inclination. The acetabula also are shifted slightly and are directed more to the front than usual. With the displacement of the sacrum, the iliopectineal line becomes longer, particularly in its iliac portion.

These changes give rise to a funnel-shaped pelvis, in which, as the result of the increased length of the conjugata vera, the pelvic inlet becomes round or oval, with the long diameter running anteroposteriorly, whereas the transverse diameter remains unchanged or may even be shorter than usual. There is also a gradual diminution of all the anteroposterior diameters of the pelvis below the superior strait, but the most characteristic change is the shortening of the distance between the ischial spines and, to a somewhat lesser extent, of that between the ischial tuberosities.

MODE OF PRODUCTION. A kyphosis in the dorsal region is usually accompanied by a compensatory marked lordosis below it, so that the body weight is transmitted to the sacrum in the usual manner. When the hump is situated lower down, however, the body weight is transmitted through its upper limb. On reaching the gibbus, it is resolved into two components, one of which is directed downward and the other backward. This latter force draws the promontory of the sacrum backward and upward, thus leading to rotation and elongation of the entire bone.

DIAGNOSIS. The diagnosis is usually easy, for the external deformity is readily visible and should at once suggest the possibility of a funnel pelvis.

External pelvimetry is of great value, for in pronounced cases it shows that the distance between the iliac crests is equal to or exceeds that between the trochanters, whereas normally the reverse obtains. Consequently, in a patient suffering from this deformity, lines drawn through the iliac crests and trochanters meet somewhere near the feet, instead of near the head, as is the case in normal women.

On palpation of the pubic arch the transverse narrowing of the pelvic outlet is noted, whereas internal examination reveals the lengthening of the conjugate vera. In lumbosacral kyphosis there is no longer a promontory, and the bodies of the lower lumbar vertebrae overhang the superior strait. In this type of deformity, therefore, particular attention should be devoted to the length of the "pseudoconjugate," the distance from the upper margin of the symphysis pubis to the nearest portion of the vertebral column. Occasionally the condition may be mistaken for spondylolisthesis.

EFFECT UPON LABOR.   The mechanical conditions favor abnormal positions of the fetus. Klien, in a study of 100 longitudinal presentations, found 90 vertex, 4 face, and 6 breech presentations. The right anterior position of the occiput is said to be unusually common.

Except in pelvis obtecta or in patients with a very pendulous abdomen, the presenting part is unobstructed in entering the superior strait at the time of labor, and it meets no obstacle until it reaches the vicinity of the ischial spines. If the transverse contraction there is not too marked to prevent descent, further difficulty is encountered when the head reaches the pelvic outlet. Because of the approach of the tubera ischii, the pubic arch becomes more angular than usual, so that the head is prevented from filling it out and must descend lower than usual to be born. This fact readily explains the deep perineal tears so frequently observed.

Generally when the distance between the tubera ischii is less than 8 cm, labor becomes difficult or impossible, according to the degree of transverse contraction of the outlet. In such cases the dystocia is more pronounced than in typical funnel pelves presenting identical measurements, because the anterior displacement of the tip of the sacrum is inevitably associated with shortening of the posterior sagittal diameter. Because of the narrowing of the pubic arch, occipitoanterior presentations are less favorable than occipitoposteriors, in which the smaller brow, instead of the wider biparietal, accommodates itself to the pubic arch. According to Klien and others, face presentations are still more favorable for the same reason.

EFFECT UPON THE HEART.   In 50 fatal cases of kyphoscoliosis associated with pregnancy that were collected by Jensen, at least 31 were caused by heart failure, far more than resulted from pelvic dystocia. Because of the collapse of the vertebral column, the volume of the thoracic cage in thoracic kyphoscoliosis is diminished, with consequent pressure exerted on the lungs and heart. As a result, the vital capacity is decreased to one half the normal value, as shown by the studies of Chapman, Dill, and Graybiel. This reduction applies to both the absolute and relative vital capacities. In five patients with thoracic kyphoscoliosis studied by them, the vital capacity was from 35 to 53 per cent of the total pulmonary volume, whereas in the normal women studied, the fraction was 57 to 69 per cent of the total. The ratio of residual air to vital capacity was 1.3 in kyphoscoliotic patients and 0.6 in the normal subjects. In other words, in these deformed women the usual mechanism of respiration is altered by the great limitation of costal movement. The ribs move only ineffectively, and breathing is accomplished largely by movements of the diaphragm. Partial collapse and infection are but natural results of these poorly aerated lungs.

Chapman, Dill, and Graybiel believe that the hypertrophy and ultimate failure of the right ventricle observed in these patients result from the increased work and pressure that must be maintained by the right ventricle to support arterial blood flow through the lungs. The hazard that these patients face in pregnancy demands special cardiac evaluation.

PROGNOSIS AND TREATMENT.   The kyphoscoliotic patient is severely handicapped in childbearing. If the condition is entirely thoracic, cardiac complications are a threat; if entirely lumbar, midpelvic contraction is common, and if low down, may be extreme. When the gibbus is thoracolumbar, both heart and pelvis may be sources of difficulty.

The prognosis here, as in all other types of contracted pelves, depends not only upon the dimensions of the pelvis but upon the progress of labor. If labor is prolonged with dimensions below the critical levels, delivery is best accomplished by cesarean section.

Kyphorachitic Pelvis.   Kyphosis is nearly always of carious origin, but when caused by rachitis it is usually associated with scoliosis. In the rare cases of pure rachitic kyphosis, however, the pelvic changes are slight, for the effect of the kyphosis is counterbalanced to a great extent by that of the rachitis, the former leading to an elongation and the latter to a shortening of the conjugata vera. The kyphosis tends to narrow, and the rachitis to widen, the inferior strait. Thus it may happen that a woman presenting a markedly deformed vertebral column of this character may have a practically normal pelvis. The two processes, however, do not always counteract each other; and as a rule, when the kyphosis is high up, the pelvic changes are predominantly rachitic.

Scoliotic Pelvis.   Pronounced scoliosis, or lateral curvature of the spine, is usually of rachitic origin, but minor degrees of the deformity are often observed unrelated to rickets. With scoliosis involving the upper portion of the vertebral column, there is usually a compensatory corresponding curvature in the opposite direction lower down, thus giving rise to a double or S-shaped curve. In such cases the body weight is transmitted to the sacrum in the usual manner, so that the pelvis is not involved. When the scoliosis is lower down and involves the lumbar region, however, the sacrum takes part in the compensatory process and assumes an abnormal position, leading to slight asymmetry of the pelvis.

Kyphoscoliotic Pelvis.   In this type of deformity, the distortion of the pelvis varies according to whether the kyphosis or the scoliosis is predominant. When the extent of the two deformities is approximately equal, however, the kyphotic changes in the pelvis predominate, although the influence of the scoliosis tends to counteract, to a certain extent, the transverse narrowing of the inferior strait.

Kyphoscoliorachitic Pelvis.   Kyphosis resulting from rachitis is nearly always complicated by scoliosis, which usually predominates in the production of the pelvic deformity, because the kyphosis and the rachitis tend to counteract each other in their effect on the pelvis. The resulting pelvis, therefore, does not differ materially from that observed in scoliorachitis, except that the tendency to anteroposterior flattening is partially counteracted by the action of the kyphotic vertebral column. Because of the scoliosis, the oblique deformity of the superior strait is usually quite marked. Generally, however, this type of pelvis is more favorable, from an obstetric standpoint, than that resulting from scoliorachitis alone.

EXTREMELY RARE PELVIC CONTRACTIONS

In the past century and a half, descriptions of the seven following extremely rare contracted pelves have appeared in the obstetric literature. A busy obstetrician or even a large obstetric service in this country may in many years encounter none of them. Osteomalacia, for example, although seen in the Far East, is virtually absent from this country. (For details see *Williams Obstetrics*, 10th edition, 1950.)

1. Robert pelvis
2. Split pelvis
3. Litzmann pelvis
4. Assimilation pelvis
5. Naegele pelvis
6. Osteomalacic pelvis
7. Spondylolisthetic pelvis (Fig. 12)

PELVIC ANOMALIES RESULTING FROM ABNORMAL FORCES EXERTED BY FEMURS

Normally, when a woman stands erect, the upward and inward force exerted by the femurs is of equal intensity on either side and is transmitted to the pelvis through the acetabula. In walking or running, the entire body weight is transmitted alternately first to one and then to the other leg. In a person suffering from disease affecting one leg, the sound extremity must bear more than its share of the body weight; consequently,

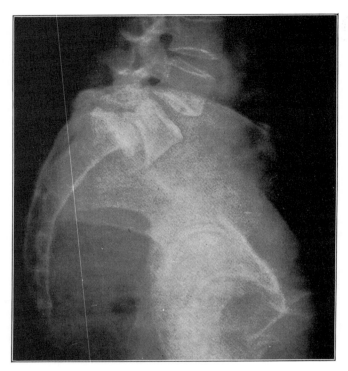

Fig. 12. Roentgenogram of spondylolisthesis, lateral view, showing forward displacement of lower lumbar vertebrae.

the upward and inward force exerted by the femur is generally greater upon that side of the pelvis. To these mechanical factors are attributed the changes in shape that accompany certain forms of lameness, provided the lesion appears early in life.

The defect may be either unilateral or bilateral; the former is usually caused by coxitis, luxation of the femur, poliomyelitis, or shortening of one leg from various causes. Common causes of the bilateral defect include luxation of both femurs and double clubfoot.

PELVIC DEFORMITIES CAUSED BY UNILATERAL LAMENESS

Coxalgic Pelvis. Coxitis occurring in early life nearly always gives rise to an obliquely contracted pelvis. If the disease appears before the patient learns to walk, or if the child is obliged to keep to its bed for a prolonged period, there may be imperfect development of the pelvis. It produces the generally contracted type, to which are added the mechanical effects and atrophic changes resulting from the unilateral disease (Fig. 13). They are manifested by imperfect development of the diseased side of the pelvis. The affected innominate bone is smaller than its fellow, and the iliopectineal line forming the arc of a circle has a smaller radius than that of the other side. At the same time, the sacral alae are more poorly developed on the affected side. The entire bone is somewhat rotated about its vertical axis, so that its anterior surface looks toward the normal side.

When the woman begins to stand, the body weight is transmitted in great part to the unaffected leg, because of the actual shortening of the diseased leg or because of fear of placing it firmly upon the ground. As a result, the pelvis becomes obliquely tilted. It is higher on the well side, and a compensatory scoliosis appears. At the same time,

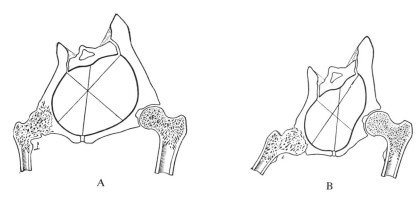

Fig. 13. Diagram showing coxalgic pelvis, before (A) and after (B) the subject has walked.

the upward and inward force exerted by the normal femur tends to push that side of the pelvis upward, inward, and backward. The iliopectineal line is thereby markedly flattened and the asymmetry of the sacrum further increased, thus giving rise to an obliquely contracted pelvis. The contraction is not limited to the superior strait, for there is an oblique contraction of the midplane and outlet as well.

Occasionally these changes are accompanied by irritation at the sacroiliac articulations, which sometimes leads to ankylosis. As a rule, the oblique contraction is found on the normal side of the pelvis, but according to Tarnier and Budin, the reverse obtains when the affected leg is ankylosed in a position of adduction and internal rotation.

Oblique contraction of the pelvis may also develop when *unilateral luxation* of the femur occurs in early life, although it is usually less pronounced than that following coxitis. In such circumstances the head of the bone is displaced backward and upward upon the outer surface of the ilium, where a new articular surface may occasionally be formed. The affected leg becomes considerably shortened, and a disproportionate share of the body weight is transmitted through the normal leg, forcing the healthy side of the pelvis upward, inward, and backward, and resulting in the same oblique contraction seen in coxalgia.

Unless the patient has had the benefit of proper orthopedic treatment in unilateral poliomyelitis, as well as in those cases in which disease at the knee or ankle or amputation early in life has caused shortening of one leg, similar changes occur in the pelvis, though they rarely assume the extreme obliquity that characterizes the coxalgic variety.

DIAGNOSIS. A limp at once suggests an obliquely contracted pelvis. When the condition has been present since early childhood, a pelvic deformity on the side corresponding to the unaffected leg is likely.

More accurate information can be obtained by careful examination of the unclothed patient, when the posture of the involved leg as well as the relative positions of the posterior or superior spines and the crests of the ilia may be ascertained. At the same time, the presence or absence of compensatory scoliosis may be noted. An accurate estimation of the degree of contraction, however, is obtainable only by careful pelvic examination. X-ray pelvimetry is, of course, of particular value in such cases.

EFFECT UPON LABOR. The effect of this type of pelvis upon labor varies with the extent and position of the deformity. If the affected side is so contracted that it prevents its being occupied by a portion of the presenting part, for all practical purposes a generally contracted pelvis results. Engagement, if it can occur at all, will take place more readily when the biparietal diameter of the head is aligned with the long oblique diameter of the superior strait. Even after descent has occurred, however, not all obstacles to labor have been overcome, since in many cases the inward projection of the ischium may lead to abnormalities in rotation. Generally these pelves are not excessively contracted. Prouvost reported that 40 out of 50 cases of labor complicated by them ended spontaneously.

TREATMENT.   Although the pelvic contraction is usually not markedly pronounced, serious dystocia may occur. If, therefore, engagement has not occurred during the last weeks of pregnancy, the patient should be examined, and if possible, the entire interior of the pelvis carefully palpated. If facilities are available, careful roentgenologic examination of the pelvis should, of course, be carried out in all cases. If it appears probable that engagement will not occur, cesarean section should be performed before the onset of labor. Fortunately, it is rarely indicated unless the fetus is excessively large or the history of previous labors has shown that the birth of a living child is impossible. The awkward position of the ankylosed leg may make the application of forceps very difficult, a factor that must be considered when deciding on the conduct of labor.

Coxarthrolisthetic Pelvis.   Very exceptionally, as the result of localized softening near the acetabulum, the base of one or both acetubula yields to the pressure exerted by the head of the femur, projecting into the pelvic cavity and leading to a unilateral or bilateral transverse contraction. Eppinger designated such pelves as coxarthrolisthetic and attributed their production to delayed and deficient ossification of the base of the acetabulum. Breus and Kolisko stated that the deformity is usually related to gonorrheal coxitis, rather than to arthritis deformans or tuberculosis, as was formerly believed. Chiari, however, described a specimen that he believed to have resulted from tabetic arthritis. Benda collected cases of this rare condition reported up to 1926 and critically considered their mode of production.

PELVIC DEFORMITIES RESULTING FROM BILATERAL LAMENESS

Children occasionally are born with *luxation of both femurs*, the heads of the bones lying, as a rule, upon the outer surfaces of the iliac bones, above and posterior to their usual location. In some cases the acetabula are entirely absent, but more frequently they are rudimentary; new but imperfect substitutes then form higher up. The condition does not usually interfere seriously with learning to walk at the usual age, though the gait is more or less wobbly.

Because the upward and inward force exerted by the femurs is not applied in its usual direction through the acetabula, the pelvis becomes excessively wide and more or less flattened anteroposteriorly. The transverse widening is particularly marked at the inferior strait, while the flattening, as a rule, is not very pronounced. This pelvis, therefore, rarely offers any serious obstacle to labor.

Verning pointed out that when the patient is placed in the obstetric position, the heads of the femurs may slip through the sacrosciatic notches and so encroach upon the pelvic cavity as to cause dystocia. This accident should not lead to serious trouble, for a change in the position of the legs effects reduction of the luxation.

The patient presents a characteristic appearance suggestive of that observed in spondylolisthesis. Because of the displacement of the femurs, the trochanters are more prominent than usual, and the width of the buttocks is increased. At the same time, because of the increase in pelvic inclination, there is marked lordosis, the back of the patient appearing considerably shortened and presenting a marked saddle-shaped depression just above the sacrum.

ATYPICAL DEFORMITIES OF THE PELVIS

The pelvis may rarely be deformed by bony outgrowths at various points and even less frequently by tumors. *Exostoses* are most frequently found on the posterior surface of the symphysis, in front of the sacroiliac joints, and on the anterior surface of the sacrum, although occasionally they may be formed along the course of the iliopectineal line.

Kilian indicated that such structures may form sharp, knifelike projections. He designated the condition *acanthopelyx* or *pelvis spinosa*. Such formations are rarely sufficiently large to present any obstacle to labor, but because of their peculiar structure may cause considerable injury to the maternal soft parts.

Tumors of various kinds may arise from the walls of the false or true pelvis and so obstruct its cavity as to render labor impossible. Fibromas, osteomas, chondromas, carcinomas, and sarcomas of the pelvis have been described. They sometimes grow large and occasionally become cystic. Chondromas are the most common variety.

Unless cesarean section is performed, the prognosis is very grave when the pelvis is obstructed by tumors from its walls; 50 per cent of the mothers and 89 per cent of the infants were lost in the cases collected by Stadfeld.

Occasionally healed fractures of the pelvis pose an insuperable obstacle to the birth of the child. Voegelin and McCall directed attention to the increasing incidence of fractures of the female pelvis as a result of several factors, such as automobile accidents, and the decreased mortality in such cases. According to Speed, they account for 3 per cent of all fractures. The effect upon labor depends upon the location of the fracture and its manner of healing. Figure 14 shows the pelvis of an 8-year-old child with a fracture of

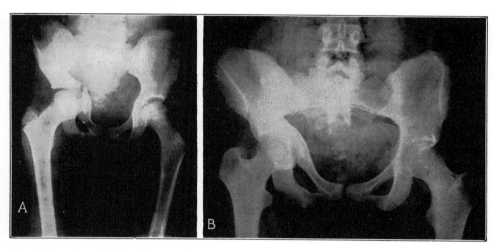

Fig. 14. Fracture of right ilium, pubic ramus, and acetabulum. A, age 8 years; B age 22 years, showing residual asymmetry of pelvis. (Courtesy of Dr. L. A. Wing.)

the right acetabulum, ilium, and pubic ramus and indicates the extent of the changes that sometimes result and the residual deformity 14 years later. Each case of fracture of the pelvis must be evaluated clinically as well as radiologically before the onset of labor, and a decision reached about the type of delivery. As Voegelin and McCall point out, operative delivery is the exception rather than the rule in such acquired deformities of the pelvis.

DWARF PELVIS

According to Breus and Kolisko, several varieties of dwarfs must be distinguished: the "true," the hypoplastic, the chondrodystrophic, the cretin, and the rachitic dwarf.

In the *true dwarf* there is a proportionate lack of general development in which epiphyses do not ossify but remain cartilaginous until an advanced age.

In the *hypoplastic dwarf* the changes are quantitative rather than qualitative, the individual differing from the normal only in her miniature appearance.

In the *chondrodystrophic dwarf* the deformity results from chondrodystrophia fetalis or achondroplasia. It is characterized by changes in the epiphysial cartilage, which interfere with the normal apposition of bone, with the result that the shafts of the long bones are imperfectly developed. The individual therefore has a normally formed trunk, but the extremities are short and stumpy. The head is often brachycephalic, with a prominent forehead and saddle nose. Since the musculature is often excessively developed, chondrodystrophic dwarfs may be unusually strong. Such dwarfs are fertile, in contrast to the cretins, in whom sterility is the rule.

In the *cretin dwarf* the lack of development is general. The bony changes are allied to those observed in the true dwarf but are less marked.

The term *rachitic dwarf* should not be applied to people whose short stature results from skeletal deformities but should be restricted to those who would fall far below the normal height even if the deformities were straightened out.

Each of these varieties of dwarf has a characteristically shaped pelvis, which is more or less generally contracted.

True Dwarf (Pelvis Nana).   This extremely rare variety of pelvis is generally contracted and tends toward the infantile type, but its most characteristic feature is the persistence of cartilage at all the epiphyses.

Hypoplastic Dwarf Pelvis.   According to Breus and Kolisko, this variety of pelvis is found in very small adults and is simply a normal pelvis in miniature. It differs significantly from that of the true dwarf in that it is completely ossified.

Chondrodystrophic Dwarf Pelvis.   This variety of pelvis is characterized by an extreme anteroposterior flattening, which appears at first to resemble that of a rachitic pelvis. On closer examination, however, the flattening is seen to result from the imperfect development of the portion of the iliac bone entering into the formation of the iliopectineal line. As a result the sacral articulation is brought much nearer the pubic bone than usual. In six pelves of this type described by Breus and Kolisko the conjugata vera varied from 4 to 7 cm, whereas the transverse diameter of the superior strait was only slightly shortened, varying from 11 to 12 cm.

Cretin Dwarf Pelvis.   This generally contracted pelvis is formed of imperfectly developed bones. Unlike that of the true dwarf, it does not present infantile characteristics but shows signs of a steady though imperfect growth throughout early life. Unossified cartilage may be present focally in young subjects, but it disappears with advancing age and is never found in all the epiphyses as in the true dwarf pelvis.

Rachitic Dwarf Pelvis.   True rachitic dwarfs are rare and possess generally contracted rachitic pelves, which do not differ, except by their small size, from other rachitic pelves.

References*

Barbour, A. H.   Spinal Deformity in Relation to Obstetrics. Edinburgh, 1883.

Benda, R.   (Contribution to the etiology and pathogenesis of coxitic protusion of the acetabulum). Arch Gynaek 129:186, 1927.

Breus, C., and Kolisko, A.   Die pathologischen Beckenformen. Leipzig und Wien, 1904, Bd. I: Spaltbecken, ff. 107–139; Assimilationsbecken, ff. 169–256; Zwergbecken, ff. 259–366.

———— and Kolisko, A.   Die pathologischen Beckenformen, Leipzig und Wien, 1900. Bd. III:I. Teil Spondylolisthesis, ff. 17–159; Kyphosen-Becken, ff. 163–307; Skoliosen-Becken, ff. 311–352; Kyphoskoliosen-Becken, ff. 355–359.

———— and Kolisko, A.   Rachitis-Becken, Die pathologischen Beckenformen. Leipzig und Wien, 1904, Bd. I, Teil 2, ff. 435–636.

———— and Kolisko, A.   Coxitis-Becken, Die pathologischen Beckenformen. Leipzig und Wien, 1912, Bd. III, ff. 474–593.

Caldwell, W. E., and Moloy, H. C.   Anatomical variations in the female pelvis and their effect in labor with a suggested classification. Amer J Obstet Gynec 26:479, 1933.

———— Moloy, H. C., and D'Esopo, D. A.   Studies on pelvic arrests. Amer J Obstet Gynec 36:928, 1938.

———— Moloy, H. C., and Swenson, P. C.   The use of the roentgen ray in obstetrics. Amer J Roentgen 41:305, 1939.

Callahan, J. T.   Separation of the symphysis pubis. Amer J Obstet Gynec 66:281, 1953.

Campbell, S.   An improved method of fetal cephalometry by ultrasound. J Obstet Gynaec Brit Comm 75:568, 1968.

* In this chapter, many historical references are included. Further information may be found in earlier editions of this textbook.

Chapman, E. M., Dill, D. B., and Graybiel, A. Decrease in functional capacity of lungs and heart resulting from deformities of chest: pulmonocardiac failure. Medicine, 18:167, 1939.

Chiari, H. Spondylolisthesis. Bull Hopkins Hosp 22:41, 1911.

Cibils, L. A., and Hendricks, C. H. Normal labor in vertex presentation. Amer J Obstet Gynec 91:385, 1965.

DeLee, J. B. Two cases of rupture of the symphysis pubis during labor. Amer J Obstet 38:483, 1898.

Donald, I., MacVicar, J., and Willocks, J. Sonar: A new diagnostic echo-sounding technique. Proc Roy Soc Med 55:637, 1962.

Eastman, N. J. Pelvic mensuration: a study in the perpetuation of error. Obstet Gynec Survey 3:301, 1948.

———— Williams Obstetrics, 10th ed. New York, Appleton-Century-Crofts, Inc., 1950.

Eller, W. C., and Mengert, W. F. Recognition of midpelvic contraction. Amer J Obstet Gynec 53:252, 1947.

Eppinger. Pelvis-Chrobak (Coxarthrolisthesis-Becken). Beiträge, Geb. u. Gyn. Wien, 2:173, 1903.

Fehling, H. Pelvis obtecta. Arch Gynaek 4:1, 1872.

——— (The origin of rachitic pelvic configuration). Arch Gynaek 11:173, 1877.

Guerriero, W. F., Arnell, R. E., and Irwin, J. B. Pelvicephalography; analysis of 503 selected cases. Southern Med J 33:840, 1940.

Hellman, L. M., Kobayashi, M., Fillisti, L. and Lavenhar, M. Sources of error in sonographic fetal mensuration and estimation of growth. Amer J Obstet Gynec 99:662, 1967.

——— and Prystowsky, H. Duration of the second stage of labor. Amer J Obstet Gynec 63:1223, 1952.

Jensen, J. The Heart in Pregnancy. St. Louis, C. V. Mosby Co., 1938, pp. 333–341.

Kaltreider, D. F. The diagonal conjugate. Amer J Obstet Gynec 61:1075, 1951.

——— Criteria of midplane contradiction. Amer J Obstet Gynec 63:392, 1952.

Kilian, H. S. Das Stachelbecken (Akanthopelys). Mannheim, Schilderungen neuer Becken-formen, 1854.

Klien, R. (Delivery with a kyphotic pelvis). Arch Gynaek 50:1, 1896.

Leopold, C. G. Das skoliotische und kypho-skoliotische rachitische Becken. Leipzig, 1879.

Litzmann, C. C. T. Die Formen des Beckens, nebst einem Anhang über Osteomalacie. Berlin, 1861.

——— Ueber die Behandlung der Geburt. Leipzig, 1884, f. 36.

Manahan, C. P., Connally, H. F., and Eastman, N. J. The experience of the Johns Hopkins Hospital with cesarean section. Amer J Obstet Gynec 44:999, 1942.

——— Marquez, C., and Mangay, H. S. A roentgenologic study of the Filipino female pelvis. Amer J. Obstet Gynec 68:228, 1954.

McLane, C. M. Obstetric significance of the narrow transverse diameter of the pelvic inlet. Amer J Obstet Gynec 84:1887, 1962.

Mengert, W. F. Pelvic measurements of 4144 Iowa women. Amer J Obstet Gynec 36:260, 1938.

——— Estimation of pelvic capacity. JAMA 138:169, 1948.

——— and Eller, W. C. Graphic portrayal of relative pelvic size. Amer J Obstet Gynec 52:1032, 1946.

Michaelis, G. A. Das enge Becken. Leipzig, 1865.

Müller. (On the frequency and etiology of general pelvic contraction). Arch Gynaek 16:155, 1880.

Naegele, F. C. Das schrägverengte Becken. Mainz, 1839.

Prouvost, E. Etudes sur les bassins viciés par boiterie. Thèse de Paris, 1891.

Rischbeith and Barrington. Dwarfism. London, Eugenic Laboratory Memoirs, Vol. 15, 1912.

Robert, F. Beschreibung eines im höchsten Grade querverengten Beckens. Karlsruhe und Freiburg, 1842.

Schauta, F. Die Beckenanomalien, Müllers Handbuch der Geburtshülfe, 1889, ii.

Schumacher. (On etiology, mechanism of delivery and management of persistent deep transverse position). Arch Gynaek 131:262, 1927.

Speed, K. A Textbook of Fractures and Dislocations, Covering Pathology, Diagnosis and Treatment, 3rd ed. Philadelphia, Lea & Febiger, 1935, p. 597.

Stadfeld, A.   (Delivery with tumors of the pelvis). Zbl Gynaek 4:No. 221:417, 1880.

Tarnier and Budin.   Traité de l'art des accouchements. T. III, pp. 314–318, 1898.

Taylor, E. S., Holmes, J. H., Thompson, H. E., and Gottesfeld, K. R.   Ultrasound diagnostic techniques in obstetrics and gynecology. Amer J Obstet Gynec 90:655, 1964.

Thompson, H. E.   The clinical use of pulsed echo ultrasound in obstetrics and gynecology. Obstet Gynec Survey 23:903, 1968.

Thoms, H.   A statistical study of the frequency of funnel pelves and the description of a new outlet pelvimeter. Amer J Obstet 72:121, 1915.

———   The obstetrical significance of pelvic variations. A study of 450 primiparous women. Brit Med J 2:210, 1937.

———   Outlet pelvimetry: a commentary, and the presentation of a pelvimeter for measuring the "symphysis and sacral biparietal distance." Surg Gynec Obstet 83:399, 1946.

———   and Schumacher, P. C.   The clinical significance of midplane pelvic contraction. Amer J Obstet Gynec 48:52, 1944.

Tricomi, V., and Kohl, S. G.   Pelvimetry—a contemporary view. Clin Obstet Gynec 9:44, 1966.

Verning, P.   (Research on bilateral congenital coxofemoral luxation). Gynec Obstet (Paris) 17:292, 1928.

Voegelin, A. W., and McCall, M. L.   Some acquired bony abnormalities influencing the conduct of labor. Amer J Obstet Gynec 48:361, 1944.

31

DYSTOCIA CAUSED BY ABNORMALITIES
OF THE GENERATIVE TRACT

Vulva.   Complete atresia of the vulva or the lower portion of the vagina is usually congenital and, unless corrected by operative measures, constitutes an insuperable obstacle to conception. More frequently vulvar atresia is incomplete, resulting from adhesions or scars following injury or inflammation. The defect may present a considerable obstacle to labor, but the resistance is usually overcome by the continued pressure exerted by the head, though frequently only after deep perineal tears.

Especially in elderly primigravidas, the vulvar outlet may be very small, rigid, and inelastic. Dystocia and extensive laceration may result unless prevented by deep episiotomy. Because of various factors, the vulva may become extremely edematous, but dystocia rarely results therefrom. Thrombi and hematomas about the vulva, although more common during the puerperium, occasionally form during the latter part of pregnancy or at the time of labor and may give rise to difficulty (p. 999). Inflammatory lesions or tumors near the vulva may have a similar effect. Rarely, condylomata acuminata may be so extensive as to make vaginal delivery undesirable, although it can usually be accomplished without extensive lacerations or hemorrhage. The danger of infection is increased, however.

Vagina.   Complete vaginal atresia is nearly always congenital and, unless corrected operatively, forms an effective bar to pregnancy. Solomons delivered a patient of a term pregnancy by cesarean section after plastic reconstruction of the vagina. Similar cases are reported by Whittemore, and by Baer and DeCosta. Incomplete atresia, on the other hand, is sometimes a manifestation of faulty development, but more frequently results from postnatal accidents (Fig. 4 in Ch. 24).

Occasionally the vagina is divided by a longitudinal septum, which may be complete, extending from the vulva to the cervix, or more often incomplete, limited to either the upper or lower portion of the canal. Since such conditions are frequently associated with other abnormalities in development of the generative tract, their detection should always prompt careful examination to ascertain whether there is a coexistent uterine deformity.

A complete longitudinal septum rarely gives rise to dystocia, since the half of the vagina through which the child descends gradually undergoes satisfactory dilatation. An incomplete septum, however, occasionally interferes with descent of the head, over which it becomes stretched as a fleshy band of varying thickness. Such structures are usually torn through spontaneously but occasionally are so resistant that they must be divided by the obstetrician.

Occasionally the vagina may be obstructed by annular strictures or bands of congenital origin. They rarely interfere seriously with delivery, however, since they usually yield before the oncoming head, requiring incision in only extreme cases.

Sometimes the upper portion of the vagina is separated from the rest of the canal by a transverse septum with a small central opening. Such a stricture is occasionally mistaken for the vaginal fornix and, at the time of labor, for the undilated external os. On careful examination, however, the obstetrician can pass a finger through the opening and feel the cervix above. After the external os has become completely dilated, the head impinges upon the septum and causes it to bulge downward. If it does not yield, slight pressure upon its opening will usually lead to further dilatation, but crucial incisions may occasionally be required to permit delivery.

Accidental atresia results from cicatrices following injury or inflammation. It sometimes follows severe puerperal or systemic infections in the course of which much of the lining of the vagina sloughs, with the result that during healing its lumen is almost entirely obliterated. In other instances, it may result from the corrosive action of abortifacients inserted into the vagina.

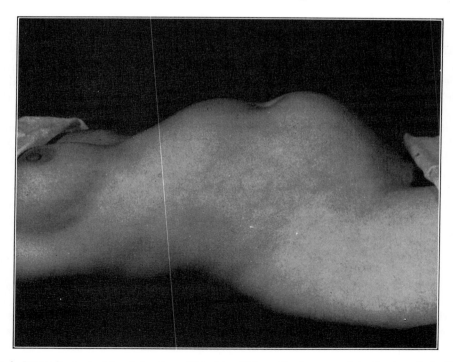

Fig. 1. Dystocia caused by distention of bladder. This patient was sent to the hospital after three days of ineffectual labor at home. The cervix was thought to have been dilated for 24 hours. After catheterization of the greatly distended bladder, which yielded over a 1,000 ml of urine, the baby's head descended at once and delivery was easy. (J.H.H. 217811.)

The effects of atresia vary greatly. In most cases, because of the softening of the tissues incident to pregnancy, the obstruction is gradually overcome by the pressure exerted by the presenting part; less often, manual or hydrostatic dilatation or incisions may become necessary. If, however, the structure is so resistant that spontaneous dilatation appears improbable, cesarean section should be performed at the onset of labor.

Among the rare causes of serious dystocia are large cysts of the vagina or Gartner's ducts and neoplasms such as fibromas, carcinomas, sarcomas, or hematomas, arising from the vaginal walls or the surrounding tissues.

Exceptionally, tetanic contraction of the levator ani may seriously interfere with descent of the head. In that condition, analogous to vaginismus in nonpregnant women, a thick, ringlike structure completely encircles and markedly contricts the vagina several centimeters above the vulva. Ordinarily the obstruction yields under anesthesia. A markedly distended bladder is another cause of arrested labor (Fig. 1).

Cervix.   Complete atresia of the cervix is incompatible with conception. In pregnancy, therefore, cervical atresia must be incomplete unless it occurs after conception.

In cases of *conglutination of the cervical os* the cervical canal undergoes complete obliteration at the time of labor, while the os remains extremely small with very thin margins, the presenting part separated from the vagina by only a thin layer of cervical tissue. Cervical conglutination is probably the result of a very small and resistant external os. Ordinarily, complete dilatation promptly follows pressure with a fingertip, although in rare instances manual dilatation or crucial incisions may be required.

Cicatricial stenosis of the cervix may follow cauterization or difficult labor associated with infection and considerable destruction of tissue. Rarely, it is caused by extensive infiltration by carcinoma or by syphilitic ulceration and induration. Occasionally, it results from corrosives used in an attempt to produce abortion or from the sequelae of gynecologic operations. Gibbs and Moore have recently reported 10 cases of severe cervical dystocia following treatment of the cervix. In 6 instances, previous conization was responsible. The increasing frequency of this operation will probably lead to occasional abdominal deliveries because of cervical scarring.

Ordinarily, because of the softening of the tissues during pregnancy, the stenosis gradually yields during labor. In rare instances, however, the stenosis may be so pronounced that dilatation appears improbable, and elective cesarean section is the procedure of choice. Such marked atresia may be associated with high amputation of the cervix, although cervical incompetency is more likely to occur. Gordon and Gordon, as well as others, have shown, however, that the Manchester-Fothergill operation to correct uterine prolapse, although much less commonly recommended in this country than in the United Kingdom, is not necessarily incompatible with future pregnancy.

Rigidity of Cervix. Reference has already been made to the unyielding cervix that causes *cervical dystocia*, as well as to the cervical rigidity often seen in elderly primigravidas. Occasionally, still greater rigidity is encountered following severe inflammation, though it rarely gives rise to serious dystocia. In certain cases of hypertrophic elongation of the cervix, spontaneous dilatation does not occur, although, as a rule, even the abnormally elongated cervix is completely effaced during the course of pregnancy.

Uterine Displacements.   *Anteflexion.*   Marked anteflexion of the uterus is usually associated with a pendulous abdomen. When the abnormal position of the uterus prevents the proper transmission of the force of the contractions to the cervix, cervical dilatation is impeded. Marked improvement may follow maintenance of the uterus in an approximately normal position by means of a properly fitting abdominal binder.

Retroflexion.   As stated on page 650, persistent retroflexion of the pregnant uterus is usually incompatible with advanced pregnancy, since if spontaneous or artificial reposition does not occur, the patient either aborts or presents symptoms of incarceration before the end of the fourth month. In very exceptional instances, however, pregnancy may proceed, in which event the adherent fundus remains applied to the floor of the pelvis, while the anterior wall stretches to accommodate the product of conception. In this condition, known as *sacculation,* the head of the fetus may occupy the displaced fundus, while the cervix is drawn up so high that the external os lies above the upper margin of the symphysis pubis. Consequently, during labor the contractions tend to force the infant through the most dependent portion of the uterus, while the cervix dilates only partially. Spontaneous delivery is thus impossible and rupture of the uterus may occur. For these reasons cesarean section affords the best method of delivery and at the same time facilitates possible reposition of the organ.

DYSTOCIA RESULTING FROM OPERATIONS FOR RETROFLEXION OF THE UTERUS.   Fortunately the operative correction of uterine displacement has fallen into disrepute, but even today some retroflexed uteri are brought into the anterior position as part of an operation for another pelvic abnormality. With the exception of certain obsolescent procedures, such as the interposition operation and ventral fixation of the uterus, operations to correct uterine retroflexion rarely give rise to serious dystocia.

Prolapse.   Conception rarely occurs with complete prolapse, and term pregnancy in a uterus completely outside the vulva is probably impossible. Naidu, on the basis of a very large experience in India, reported eight cases of prolapse, one of which was complete and complicated by abortion at 22 weeks. Term pregnancy may occur with incomplete prolapse, although abortion is the more frequent termination. In partial prolapse the fundus occupies the usual position, while the hypertrophied and elongated cervix protrudes from the vagina. As a rule the cervix retracts as pregnancy progresses, and if supported by a suitable pessary until near term, the danger of infection may be decreased. Occasionally hysterotomy may be necessary, as in one of Naidu's cases, or the cervix may be so edematous and hypertrophied that cesarean section is required. Such prolapsed cervices are generally not suitable for incision, although Keettel cites a case in which that procedure was successfully performed. Even in the absence of dystocia, the condition greatly increases the danger of infection in labor.

Pelvic Tumors.   *Carcinoma of the Cervix.*   The effect of this condition upon pregnancy and labor and its appropriate treatment are discussed on page 649.

Myomas of the Uterus.   Myomas are reported to occur in between 0.1 and 2.1 per cent of labors. The incidence is higher in black than in white women. Moderate and large-sized myomas deforming the uterine cavity may often cause relative sterility. This subject has been reviewed by Parks and Barter.

In many instances the association of myomas and pregnancy is without significance, whereas in others the tumors may be of considerable obstetric importance for the following reasons: (1) they may diminish the chances of conception; (2) they increase the probability of abortion; (3) under the influence of pregnancy, they may increase so rapidly in size as to produce serious symptoms from pressure; (4) if situated in the lower segment or cervix, they may give rise to serious dystocia; (5) they favor the occurrence of abnormal presentations; (6) infrequently they may so interfere with the efficiency of the uterine contractions as to give rise to inertia; (7) if submucous or interstitial, they may so interfere with the separation of the placenta as to render radical operative interference necessary; and finally (8) they may undergo degenerative changes (red or carneous degeneration) during pregnancy or the puerperium (Fig. 2).

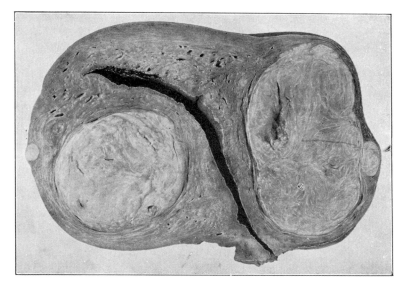

Fig. 2. Intramural myomas. Puerperal uterus containing large myomas removed because of uterine infection on third postpartum day, following spontaneous delivery at term. (From Traut and Kuder. New International Clinics. Philadelphia, J. B. Lippincott Co.)

The obstacle to conception is most marked in the submucous and interstitial varieties of myomas, partly as a result of changes in the endometrium that interfere with implantation of the ovum. Ingersol states that removal of such tumors results in pregnancy in 50 per cent of patients who desire children. In our own experience the success rate in these patients is less than 30 per cent. When pregnancy occurs, however, the incidence of abortion is considerably increased because of pathologic changes in the decidua that may be associated with imperfect nidation. In very unusual circumstances, when the tumor projects markedly into the uterine cavity and the placenta is located above it, spontaneous separation may be impossible and manual removal so difficult that hysterectomy may be necessary.

Conversely, pregnancy may influence the tumors themselves. Myomas usually increase rapidly in size because of both hypertrophy and edema and may give rise to serious symptoms of pressure. Furthermore, the softened tumors may undergo considerable changes in shape and hemorrhagic, red, or *carneous, degeneration.* When it is the cause of pain, low-grade fever, and leukocytosis, carneous degeneration may very infrequently necessitate operative removal; but as a rule, the signs and symptoms subside after two or three days of mild sedation and rest in bed. Occasionally the pedicle of a subserous myoma may become twisted, leading to gangrene and peritonitis.

During labor the effect of the myomas depends entirely upon their size and situation. Subserous tumors are generally without great significance, except when large enough to cause symptoms of pressure or when a pedunculated tumor undergoes torsion. Interstitial myomas situated in the cervix or lower uterine segment, however, may obstruct the pelvis, preventing normal delivery. A submucous myoma may protrude through the cervix as a polypoid mass and prevent descent of the head unless the tumor is removed by cutting through its pedicle.

Myomas may predispose to abnormal presentations. In 180 cases at The New York Lying-In Hospital there were 26 abnormal presentations, comprising 2 face, 8 shoulder, and 16 breech presentations (Douglas). Infrequently the tumors may sufficiently interfere with normal uterine contrations to cause dysfunctional labor or uterine atony with consequent postpartum hemorrhage. Additional hemorrhage may occur during the third stage from mechanical interference with separation or expulsion of the placenta or possibly from the myoma itself.

In the puerperium, myomas sometimes undergo degeneration and, if subjected to prolonged pressure, may become gangrenous. In other cases the tumors may undergo puerperal involution or occasionally disappear.

The diagnosis of pregnancy complicated by myomas is not always easy. Intermittent hemorrhage, as a result of poor implantation, may be mistaken by the patient for menstrual flow, and pregnancy may not be considered for several months or until an abortion occurs. A sudden increase in growth of the uterine tumor, however, should suggest the possibility of pregnancy; the suspicion is strengthened by palpation of soft areas between the firmer myomatous nodules. Subserous myomas occasionally escape detection or are mistaken for the small parts or head of the fetus, occasionally even leading to a diagnosis of multiple pregnancy.

Myomectomy is frequently but not necessarily followed by abortion. The duration of pregnancy; the size, number, and location of the myomas; the age and obstetric history of the patient; and the type and severity of symptoms are among the factors that determine the procedure of choice in a given case. Child and Douglas reported that among 40,000 pregnant women admitted to The New York Lying-In Hospital over an 11-year period, there were 120, or 0.3 per cent, who required surgical or gynecologic operations during gestation. Among the cases in which myomas were the indication for operation there were 9 patients in whom myomectomy was performed during the antenatal period, 7 who had a cesarean section and hysterectomy (Fig. 3), and 7 who underwent cesarean section and myomectomy at term. Of the 9 patients subjected to myomectomy during pregnancy, 4 aborted after the operation. In addition to the 23 patients in whom the myomas were removed either before or at the time of delivery, there were 8 in whom a cesarean section was performed and the tumor not removed. Of these patients one died of peritonitis, the only maternal death in the entire group of operative cases.

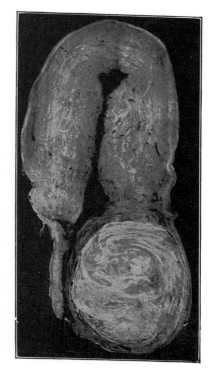

Fig. 3. Uterus removed by supravaginal amputation following cesarean section necessitated by myoma in posterior wall of cervix.

If serious symptoms do not supervene during pregnancy, operative interference should be deferred until shortly before the expected onset of labor, since the tumor may so change its shape or position as to render an operation unnecessary on obstetric grounds. In one of our patients, a large tumor in the lower uterine segment at the fifth month appeared to present a serious obstacle to delivery. At term, however, when the patient returned for a cesarean section, the tumor had risen out of the pelvis, rendering operation unnecessary and permitting easy spontaneous delivery.

So fortunate an outcome cannot always be expected. In any event, the patient should be examined thoroughly, under anesthesia if necessary, shortly before the expected date of confinement. If the tumor is found to be firmly wedged in the pelvis, cesarean section should be performed before the onset of labor, followed by hysterectomy when indicated. Huge or extensively degenerated myomas often necessitate hysterectomy, but we do not favor extensive myomectomy at the time of cesarean section because of the increased incidence of hemorrhage and puerperal infection. A pedunculated myoma may, of course, be removed with impunity, but any dissection in the uterine wall should be avoided. If, however, there is no apparent danger of impaction, and spontaneous delivery is likely, the patient should be allowed to go into labor. If the prognosis proves wrong and obstruction occurs, cesarean section should be promptly performed.

The completion of labor does not necessarily indicate that all danger is passed, since the tumor may degenerate during the puerperium. Fever and abdominal pain should suggest such a diagnosis and the possible necessity of laparotomy.

Benign Ovarian Tumors. Ovarian tumors may be serious complications of pregnancy, may undergo torsion, and may pose insuperable obstacles to vaginal delivery. Moreover, even after a spontaneous labor, they may give rise to disturbances during the puerperium.

Although all varieties of ovarian tumors may complicate pregnancy and labor the most common are cystic (Fig. 4), occurring once in every 81 pregnancies, ac-

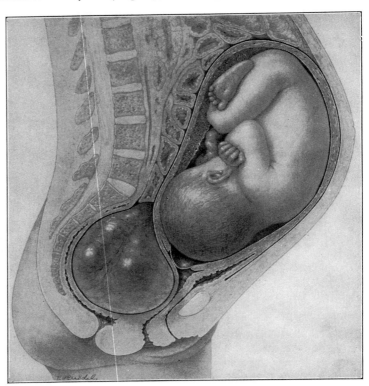

Fig. 4. Ovarian cyst producing dystocia.

cording to Grimes and associates. If, however, only cysts sufficiently large to be hazardous to pregnancy are considered, the incidence is reduced to 1 in 328. Dermoid cysts (benign cystic teratomas) have been described fairly frequently in this connection, forming between a quarter and a half of all these tumors. Similar data have been reported by Booth from Queen Charlotte's Hospital. The most frequent and serious complication of ovarian cysts is torsion. The incidence of the accident was 12 per cent in Booth's series. Torsion usually occurs in the first trimester, most frequently after the ninth week. Moreover, the cyst may rupture and extrude its contents into the peritoneal cavity during spontaneous labor or as the result of operative interference. This event is not so significant with serous cystomas as with dermoids, rupture of which may be followed by fatal peritonitis. When the tumor blocks the pelvis it may lead to rupture of the uterus or may be forced into the vagina and occasionally even into the rectum. It is surprising that spontaneous rupture of an ovarian cystoma is not more common. In one patient at The New York Lying-In Hospital, a thin-walled unilocular cyst impacted in the pelvis led to rupture of the uterus, but itself remained intact although its walls did not exceed 1 mm in thickness.

Unfortunately, an ovarian tumor complicating pregnancy is often entirely unsuspected. Careful examination of all pregnant women, however, particularly at the first visit and again four to six weeks before the calculated date of confinement, should eliminate a large proportion of these errors. Failure of the presenting part to engage in a normal pelvis further suggests an obstructing mass. If, however, the tumor does not occupy the pelvis, the diagnosis may be extremely difficult, since the abdominal enlargement may be attributed to a multiple pregnancy or hydramnios, and the true condition not recognized until after labor.

In view of the relatively high incidence of abortion following excision of an ovarian cyst during early pregnancy, Child and Douglas concluded that the safest time to perform the operation is during or after the fourth month of gestation, provided operation can be postponed until that time. Although the chances of abortion or premature labor may be increased by the operation, that danger is minimal compared with that of possible torsion or rupture of the cyst. Furthermore, the likelihood of abortion is decreased by postponing the operation until later in pregnancy. Progesterone is sometimes given for the purpose of "quieting" the myometrium, although its efficacy in these circumstances is questionable.

When the diagnosis is not made until late in pregnancy, it is usually advisable, except in the case of known or suspected malignant tumors, to postpone operation until term, to avoid stressing the fresh abdominal cicatrix during parturition. If the tumor is impacted in the pelvis, cesarean section should be performed, followed by removal of the tumor. If it is not impacted, it is preferable to permit spontaneous labor and remove the tumor late in the puerperium.

Carcinoma of the Ovary. Malignant ovarian neoplasms are rare in pregnancy. Only 41 cases were collected from the literature by Valenti, who, along with Amico, believes that the natural course of the disease is uninfluenced by pregnancy. If the tumor is discovered at the time of laparotomy or if the disease is widespread, the treatment should be the same as in the nonpregnant patient. Only if the tumor is discovered when the fetus is viable is it justifiable to remove only the ovary and allow the pregnancy to continue. Even then delivery should usually be by cesarean section, with decision regarding further surgical and radiologic treatment based on the clinical and pathologic findings.

Tumors of Other Origin. Labor is occasionally obstructed by masses of various origin sufficiently large to render delivery difficult or even impossible. Among these masses, *pelvic ectopic kidney* is a rare complication of pregnancy. Anderson, Rice, and Harris were able to collect only 98 cases from the literature, to which they added 14 more. Since such a kidney may occasionally block the birth canal and sustain injury during passage of the child, the condition is important obstetrically. In the 209 full-term deliveries recorded in the foregoing series, spontaneous vaginal delivery occurred in 153, or in about three quarters; cesarean section was employed in 32 cases, the remainder having terminated in vaginal operative procedures. The maternal mortality was 8.9 per cent and the total fetal loss 14.3 per cent. Both these figures are high, but no maternal death attributable to a pelvic kidney has been recorded since 1927. In the 14 deliveries in 7 mothers in our clinic, no maternal or fetal deaths occurred. Anderson, Rice, and Harris, as well as Bergqvist, believe that most of these patients will deliver vaginally without hazard, but if one or both of the kidneys are entirely intrapelvic, abdominal delivery is probably safer.

In rare instances a normal-sized or enlarged spleen may prolapse into the pelvic cavity and obstruct labor. Echinococcal cysts are occasionally found in the pelvis. An old extrauterine gestation may obstruct the pelvic canal, interfering with the delivery of a subsequent intrauterine fetus. Enterocele occasionally gives rise to dystocia, though in the majority of cases the herniated intestine can be replaced and the obstacle temporarily overcome. When reduction is impossible, cesarean section is indicated as a procedure more conservative than forcing the child over a large irreducible hernia. A large rectocele or cystocele, though occasionally offering slight obstacle to labor, can generally be replaced during delivery.

Occasionally tumors of the bladder may impede passage of the child, though rarely seriously enough to demand operative interference. It is sometimes necessary, however, to remove a large calculus from the bladder before delivery can be effected. Tumors arising from the lower part of the rectum or pelvic connective tissue also may give rise to serious dystocia, as reported by Pederson, who collected a series of cases in which carcinoma of the rectum necessitated cesarean section.

References

Amico, J. C.   Pregnancy complicated by primary carcinoma of the ovary. Amer J Obstet Gynec 74:920, 1957.

Anderson, G. W., Rice, G., and Harris, B.   Pregnancy and labor complicated by pelvic ectopic kidney anomalies; review of literature. Obstet Gynec Survey 4:737, 1949.

Baer, J. L., and DeCosta, E. J.   Full term pregnancy following operation for congenital absence of vagina. Amer J Obstet Gynec 54:696, 1947.

Bergqvist, A.   Ectopic kidney as a complication of pregnancy and labour. Acta Obstet Gynec Scand 44:289, 1965.

Booth, R. T.   Ovarian tumors in pregnancy. Obstet Gynec 21:189, 1963.

Child, C. G., and Douglas, R. G.   Surgical problems arising during pregnancy. Amer J Obstet Gynec 47:213, 1944.

Douglas, R. G.   Personal communication.

Gibbs, C. E., and Moore, S. F.   The scarred cervix in pregnancy and labor. Gen Pract 37:85, 1968.

Gordon, C. A., and Gordon, R. E.   Discussion of Manchester operation. Amer J Obstet Gynec 74:392, 1957.

Grimes, W. H., Bartholomew, R. A., Colvin, E. D., Fish, J. S., and Lester, W. M.   Ovarian cyst complicating pregnancy. Amer J Obstet Gynec 68:594, 1954.

Ingersol, F. B.   Fertility following myomectomy. Fertil Steril 14:596, 1963.

Keettel, W. C.   Prolapse of the uterus during pregnancy. Amer J Obstet Gynec 42:121, 1941.

Lock, F. R.   Multiple myomectomy. Amer J Obstet Gynec 104:642, 1969.

Naidu, P. M.   Prolapse of the uterus complicating pregnancy and labour. A report of 8 cases. J Obstet Gynaec Brit Comm 68:1041, 1961.

Parks, J., and Barter, R. H.   The myomatous uterus complicated by pregnancy. Amer J Obstet Gynec 63:260, 1952.

Pederson, A.   Dystocia caused by diseases of the rectum. Acta Obstet Gynec Scand 1:445, 1922.

Schauta, M.   (Myoma and birth.) Compt. rend. du XVIe Cong. internat. de médecine, 7:8, Budapest. Vol. 2, 1909.

Solomons, E.   Conception and delivery following construction of an artificial vagina. Obstet Gynec 7:329, 1956.

Valenti, C.   (On carcinoma of the ovary in pregnancy). Minerva Ginec 9:4, 1960.

Whittemore, W. S.   Pregnancy following operation for congenital absence of vagina. Amer
J Obstet Gynec 44:516, 1942.

32

INJURIES TO THE BIRTH CANAL

VAGINA AND VULVA

All except the most superficial perineal lacerations are accompanied by varying degrees of injury to the lower portion of the vagina. Such tears rarely occur in the midline but extend up one or both vaginal sulci, often of sufficient depth to involve fibers of the levator ani. Bilateral lacerations of this variety are usually unequal in length and separated by a tongue-shaped portion of vaginal mucosa (Figs. 18 and 19 in Ch. 16).

These injuries should always be looked for, and their repair should form part of every operation for the restoration of a lacerated perineum. If only the external wound is sutured, the patient may eventually develop symptoms related to relaxation of the vaginal outlet, even in the presence of an apparently normal perineum. Isolated tears involving the middle or upper third of the vagina but unassociated with lacerations of the perineum or cervix are rarely observed. They are usually longitudinal, resulting from injuries sustained during a forceps operation, though occasionally they follow spontaneous delivery. They frequently extend deeply into the underlying tissues and may give rise to copious hemorrhage, which, however, is usually readily controlled by appropriate suturing. They may be overlooked unless deep vaginal inspection is performed.

More important are injuries to the levator ani that are unassociated with tears through the vaginal mucosa and consequently often escape detection. As a result of overdistention of the birth canal, a submucosal separation of certain muscular fibers may occur, or a diminution in their tonicity sufficient to interfere with the function of the pelvic diaphragm. In such cases the patient may eventually develop pelvic relaxation. If these injuries involve pubococcygeus muscle, urinary incontinence may supervene. Although the accident may sometimes be avoided by intelligent use of forceps and episiotomy, it may follow spontaneous and rapid delivery, as in the case reported by Brander and Buchman, in which complete spontaneous rupture of the posterior wall of the vagina caused the rectosigmoid to protrude from the site (Fig. 1). The rarity of such severe instances of spontaneous *colporrhexis* is attested by Brander and Buchman's inability to collect more than 15 cases from the literature of the past 25 years.

Traumatic lesions of the upper third of the vagina are uncommon by themselves but are often associated with extensions of deep cervical tears. In rare in-

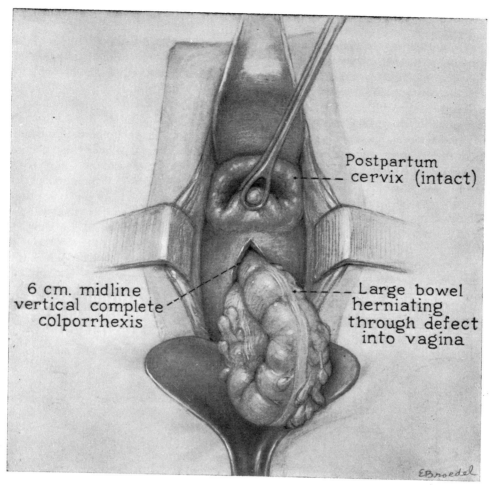

Postpartum
cervix (intact)

6 cm. midline
vertical complete
colporrhexis

Large bowel
herniating
through defect
into vagina

E.Broedel

Fig. 1. Rupture of the posterior cul-de-sac with protrusion of large bowel through the defect. (From Brander and Buchman. Obstet Gynec 24:151, 1964.)

stances, however, the cervix may be entirely or partially avulsed from the vagina, with colporrhexis in the anterior, posterior, or lateral fornices. Such lesions usually follow difficult forceps deliveries and may extend through the peritoneum, sometimes involving even the uterine artery and the lower uterine segment. Gamble has made an extensive survey of the literature on this subject up to 1927. Fortunately, such extensive traumatic lesions are rare in modern obstetrics. They may be totally unsuspected or may manifest themselves by excessive external hemorrhage or by the formation of a retroperitoneal hematoma. These extensive tears of the vaginal vault should be carefully explored. If there is the slightest question of perforation of the peritoneum or retroperitoneal or intraperitoneal hemorrhage, laparotomy should be performed. In the presence of damage of this severity, intrauterine exploration for possible rupture is, of course, mandatory. Whereas treatment of these lacerations by packing was formerly recommended, surgical repair is, in general, more effective.

Cervix

Slight degrees of cervical lacerations must be regarded as inevitable in child-birth. Such tears, however, heal rapidly and are rarely symptomatic. In healing they cause a significant change in the shape of the external os and thereby afford a means of ascertaining whether a woman has borne children.

In other cases the tears are deeper, involving one or both sides of the cervix and possibly extending up to or beyond the vaginal junction. In rarer instances the laceration may extend across the vaginal fornix or into the lower uterine seg-ment or the broad ligament. Such extensive lesions frequently involve vessels of considerable size and are then asssociated with profuse hemorrhage.

Deep cervical tears occasionally occur during the course of spontaneous la-bor. In such circumstances their genesis is not always clear. In the past, they often followed manual or instrumental dilatation of the cervix. In modern ob-stetrics, however, they most often result from traumatic deliveries through an incompletely dilated cervix.

Occasionally, even in spontaneous labors, the edematous anterior lip of the cervix may be caught between the head and the symphysis pubis and compressed until it undergoes necrosis and separation. In still rarer instances, the entire vag-inal portion may be avulsed from the rest of the cervix. Such *annular* or *circular*

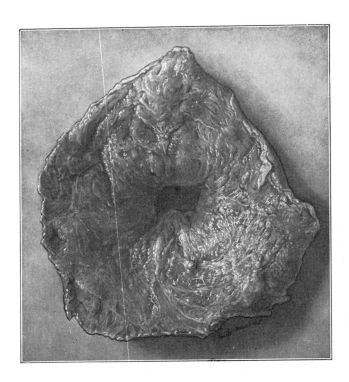

Fig. 2. Annular detachment of cervix. Specimen, cast off before the birth of child, shows undilated and rigid external os and obliterated cervical canal seen from within.

detachments of the cervix probably occur only in neglected labors or in gravidas receiving massive, unphysiologic doses of oxytocin (Fig. 2). Spritzer reported a case that implicated both the vacuum extractor, employed in the first stage of labor, and necrosis of the edematous cervix.

Symptoms. In all lesions involving the cervix there is usually no bleeding until after birth of the child, when hemorrhage may be profuse. In many cases, however, the bleeding is so slight that the lesion would pass unrecognized were it not detected upon vaginal examination. When one lip of the vaginal portion of the cervix is torn off, there may be very little hemorrhage, since the tissues have been so compressed before the accident that the vessels have undergone thrombosis. In our case of circular detachment of the cervix (Fig. 2) there was no bleeding, and the nature of the detached tissue was not recognized until after examination in the laboratory. Slight cervical tears heal spontaneously; extensive lacerations have a similar tendency, but perfect union rarely results. They provide for pathogenic microorganisms a portal of entry into the lymphatics at the base of the broad ligament. Erosions developing at the site of the tears are frequently the cause of persistent leukorrhea. At the end of the puerperium, therefore, it is advisable routinely to examine the cervix with a speculum and to cauterize such erosions prophylactically. If a Papanicolaou smear had not been obtained during pregnancy, it should be done at this time.

Diagnosis. A deep cervical tear should always be suspected in cases of profuse hemorrhage during the third stage of labor, particularly if the uterus is firmly contracted. For a positive diagnosis, however, a thorough examination is necessary. Because of the flabbiness of the cervix immediately after delivery, mere digital examination is often unsatisfactory. The extent of the injury can be fully appreciated only after adequate exposure and direct inspection of the cervix.

In view of the frequency with which deep tears follow major operative procedures, the cervix should be inspected routinely at the conclusion of the third stage, even if there is no bleeding, after all difficult deliveries. If a tear is discovered it should be sutured promptly. Annular detachment of the vaginal portion of the cervix should be suspected whenever an irregular mass of tissue with a circular central opening is cast off before or after birth of the child.

Treatment. Deep cervical tears accompanied by hemorrhage should be immediately repaired; a few sutures usually effect hemostasis. Their treatment varies with the extent of the lesion. When the laceration is limited to the cervix, or even when it extends well into the vaginal fornix, satisfactory results are obtained by suturing the cervix after bringing it into view at the vulva. Visualization is best accomplished when an assistant makes firm downward pressure on the uterus while the operator exerts traction with fenestrated ovum or sponge forceps on the lips of the cervix, and the vaginal walls are held apart with retractors (Fig. 3). As the hemorrhage usually comes from the upper angle of the wound, it is advisable to apply the first suture there; if the suturing is begun at the free end of the tear, a dead space is often left toward its upper extremity, from which subsequent hemorrhage may occur. Interrupted chromic catgut sutures should be employed, since they do not have to be removed. The beginner is cautioned against overzealous attempts to restore the normal appearance of the cervix, for involution during the following few days may lead to stenosis and retention of the lochia.

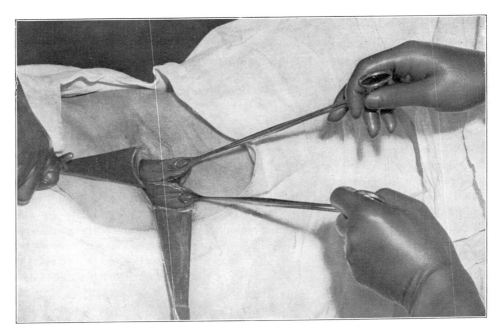

Fig. 3. Cervical laceration exposed for repair.

RUPTURE OF THE UTERUS

The term *rupture of the uterus* is usually employed to denote rupture after the period of viability of the fetus. This definition eliminates such conditions as rupture of interstitial pregnancies and traumatic perforations in the course of abortion in the early months of pregnancy.

Incidence.   This accident is one of the most serious in obstetrics. Its actual incidence among pregnant and parturient women is difficult to assess, since published hospital data vary greatly and are affected by the type of patient and number of referred cases received. The combined figures from many countries (430,471 births) reported by Krishna Menon give an incidence of 1 in 760 deliveries. This figure is probably too high, reflecting the influence of such clinics as Menon's, where many neglected cases are treated, and raising the incidence there to 1 in 415 deliveries. There are parts of the world where obstetric neglect coupled with a prevalence of contracted pelves creates even higher rates; for example, a rate over 1 per cent is reported by Rendle Short from Kampala, Uganda. The incidence in the United States is difficult to estimate, but is probably between 1 in 1,000 and 1 in 1,500 births, according to Garnet. Despite its infrequency, rupture of the uterus looms as a major cause of death in modern obstetrics; it is responsible for at least 5 per cent of all maternal deaths.

Of the various classifications of rupture of the uterus, one of the most useful clinically, based upon the time of rupture, is as follows:

    A. Rupture before labor
        1. Spontaneous rupture of
            a. Previous cesarean section scar
            b. Previous operative scar
            c. The intact uterus
        2. Traumatic rupture
    B. Rupture during labor
        1. Spontaneous rupture of
            a. Previous cesarean section scar
            b. Previous operative scar
            c. The intact uterus
        2. Traumatic rupture

More simply, for all practical purposes, ruptures may be etiologically classified as follows:

1. Rupture of previous uterine scar
2. Spontaneous rupture of the intact uterus
3. Traumatic rupture of the intact uterus

RUPTURE OF PREVIOUS CESAREAN SCAR

With the increasing incidence of cesarean section, rupture of the scar in subsequent pregnancy has become a matter of much concern. As shown in Table 1, in 624 pregancies subsequent to cesarean section that were managed at the Johns Hopkins Hospital between 1900 and 1942, the frequency of rupture was 1.0 per cent in pregnancy and 1.1 per cent in labor, a total incidence of 2.1 per cent, as reported by Delfs and Eastman. Almost all these sections were of the classical variety; furthermore, since improved surgical management should yield stronger scars today than in the period covered, the figure of 2.0 per cent may reasonably be taken as the maximal figure in modern obstetrics for the incidence of rupture of an infraumbilical classical scar. The higher the incision in the fundus the greater is the likelihood of rupture. In an analysis during 1961 by Hellegers and Eastman at the same hospital, in 699 pregnancies following cesarean section, mostly of the lower segment type, the frequency of rupture* of the lower segment was about 0.5 per cent. In 310 labors following lower segment operations with transverse uterine incisions, as reported by Lawrence, two ruptures occurred, giving an incidence of 0.6 per cent.

Comparison of Classical Cesarean Section and Lower Segment Scars. The behavior of a classical scar in any subsequent pregnancy differs from that of a scar confined to the lower uterine segment. First, the probability of rupture of a classical scar is three or four times greater than that of a lower segment scar. Second,

---

* It is essential to differentiate between *rupture* of a cesarean section scar and *dehiscence*, or occult rupture. For the purposes of the present discussion, the word "rupture" means separation of the edges of the old scar throughout its length and rupture of the fetal membranes, with connection between the uterine and peritoneal cavities. In these circumstances, all or part of the fetus is usually extruded into the peritoneal cavity; in addition, there is bleeding, often massive, either from the edges of the scar or from extension of the scar into fresh muscle. Dehiscence differs from rupture in that the fetal membranes are not ruptured, and no part of the fetus therefore is extruded from the uterine cavity. Bleeding is absent or minimal, and in most cases the separation does not extend throughout the entire length of the scar. Occult ruptures occur gradually and are painless, whereas true ruptures are sudden, explosive, and almost always associated with severe pain and shock (Fig. 4).

Table 1. Incidence of Rupture of Cesarean Section Scar in Patients
Who Had Had One or More Abdominal Deliveries

	No.	%
Total deliveries	624	
Cesarean section because of disproportion and scar	316	50.7
Cesarean section, scar only indication	120	19.2
Delivered vaginally	188	30.1
Total pregnancies	624	
Ruptures in pregnancy	6	1.0
Total labors	188	
Ruptures in labor	2	1.1

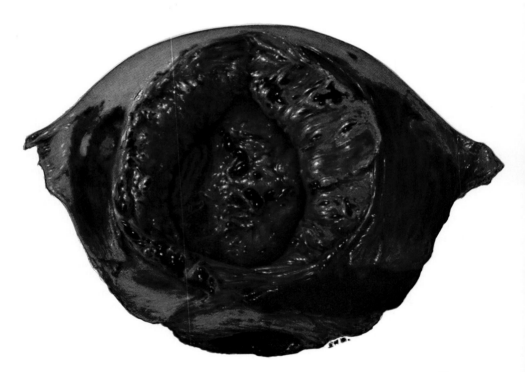

Fig. 4. Rupture of uterus through scar of previous classical cesarean section.

if a classical scar does rupture, the accident takes place in the latter part of pregnancy rather than in labor in about one third of the cases. With very rare exceptions, rupture of a lower segment scar occurs only in the course of labor. This difference is a considerable disadvantage of the classical operation, following which rupture not infrequently takes place several weeks before term, before a cesarean section is ordinarily repeated. Delivery by subsequent section cannot therefore prevent all those ruptures. Lower segment scars that are confined to the noncontractile portion of the uterus do not rupture before labor, however, and rarely do so in labor. Thus, the policy of repeating cesarean sections would be expected to forestall almost all ruptures of well-healed, lower segment scars. The available statistics are insufficient to permit an accurate calculation of the maternal mortality that attends rupture of a cesarean section scar; it is probably less than 5 per cent, but the perinatal mortality is about 50 per cent. Rupture of a lower segment scar may produce extensive damage and even rupture of the bladder.

Dehiscence of a cesarean section scar is much more frequent than actual rupture, occurring, according to Lane and Reid, in 2.7 per cent of 583 patients delivered by subsequent section. Pedowitz and Schwartz report an even higher figure of 8 per cent following the lower segment operation. Dehiscence may occur after both types of operation but seems to be somewhat more frequent with the lower segment scar. It is remarkable that these separated scars, covered only by the peritoneum, frequently appear to cause no difficulty in labor or subsequently. Their frequency, however, and the possible associated risk, lends support to the dictum: "Once a cesarean, always a cesarean."

Healing of the Cesarean Section Scar.   Little information on this subject has been garnered from studies of cesarean section scars. Williams believed that the uterus heals by regeneration of the muscular fibers and not by scar tissue. He based his conclusions on histologic examination of the site of the incision and on the two principal observations: First, inspection of the unopened uterus at the time of repeated sections usually shows no trace of the former incision or, at most, an almost invisible linear scar. Second, when the body of the uterus has been amputated, no scar is visible after fixation, or only a shallow vertical furrow in the external and internal surfaces of the anterior uterine wall, with no trace of scar tissue between them. Schwarz, Paddock, and Bortnick, however, conclude that healing occurs mainly by the proliferation of fibroblasts. They studied the site of the incision in the human uterus some days after cesarean section, as well as in the uteri of experimental guinea pigs, rabbits, and dogs. They observed that as the scar shrinks, the proliferation of connective tissue becomes less obvious. Schwarz, Paddock, and Bortnick's conclusions appear justified by their histologic studies, particularly in cases of adequate approximation of the myometrial edges (Fig. 5). If the cut surfaces are closely apposed, the proliferation of connective tissue is minimal, and the normal relation of smooth muscle to connective tissue is gradually reestablished, accounting for the occasional absence of even a trace of a former incision. Even when the healing is so poor that marked thinning has resulted, the remaining tissue is often almost entirely muscular (Fig. 6). The fundamental weakness stems from failure to approximate carefully the inner margins of the incision or from formation of a hematoma in the area. Additional factors affecting the healing of wounds in general are likely to play a role in the final result. In an effort to assay the effect of steroids, Poidevin injected large doses of hydrocortisone and cortisone acetate into cats for over a month after cesarean section. On examination of the uteri, he could find no difference in healing between the treated cats and controls.

Delivery Subsequent to a Cesarean Section.   In most American clinics, previous cesarean section is the most common indication for cesarean section. At the Kings County Hospital, for instance, it was the indication in 47.2 per cent of 1,000 consecutive sections, while in Hartford, Connecticut, it was an indication in 49.7 per cent (Kohl). At Kings County Hospital a patient is infrequently delivered vaginally after a previous abdominal delivery, and in Hartford only 4.3 per cent of such patients had a subsequent vaginal delivery. At the Margaret Hague Hospital and on the ward service of The New York Lying-In Hospital, however, at

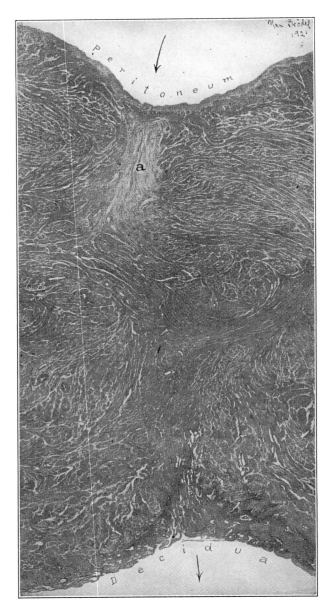

Fig. 5. Ideal healing of cesarean section scar. Scar tissue at a.

least half of the patients with previous cesarean sections have been delivered vaginally (Donnelly and Franzoni; Douglas, Birnbaum, and MacDonald). Pedowitz and Felmus have reported the incidence of rupture of a *myomectomy scar* reaching the endometrial cavity to be about the same as that of classical cesarean section scar.

If the previous cesarean section was done for pelvic contraction, section is, of course, repeated, not only because the pelvic indication is still present but also

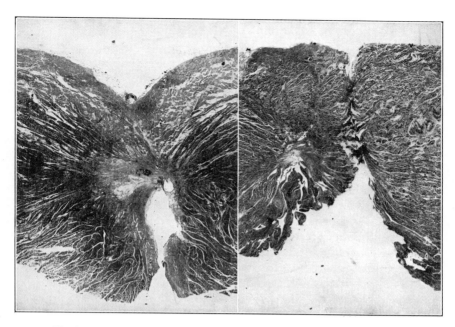

Fig. 6. Photomicrographs of two poorly healed cesarean section scars.

because of the increased strain that may be placed upon the scar. Gravidas who have undergone two or more previous sections of any type should also be delivered abdominally. Patients with a previous classical section also should have section repeated unless they go into labor prematurely with a fetus that is quite small.

The danger of rupture of a transverse lower segment scar is small, however. It is thus logical that many well-qualified obstetricians believe that if the indications for the first section are not recurrent and if the patient has already delivered a term-sized baby vaginally, then with careful observation vaginal delivery may be permitted. Silent weaknesses of the scar are common, however. They can sometimes be detected by hysterography in the nonpregnant state (Fig. 7) (also see Lepage and associates). Neither radiologic technics nor any clinical findings, such as the patient's course following the first operation, the location of the placenta in the present pregnancy, the type of previous operation or incision, the skill of the previous operator, *or even the fact of an intervening vaginal delivery,* provide incontrovertible proof of the integrity of the scar under the stress of labor. Many reliable institutions, however, report 30 to 40 per cent of vaginal deliveries following cesarean section without difficulty.

There is a fetal consideration that bears on this decision as well. Elective repeated cesarean section carries a perinatal loss slightly in excess of that in normal gravidas after a normal labor at term. This excess loss is largely the result of unexpected and undiagnosed prematurity, which, theoretically, could be eliminated by allowing the spontaneous onset of labor. Hall, Kohl, and Schechter, however, could show no such improved salvage in a study of 1,172 normal gravidas with repeated cesarean sections in which one group was allowed to begin

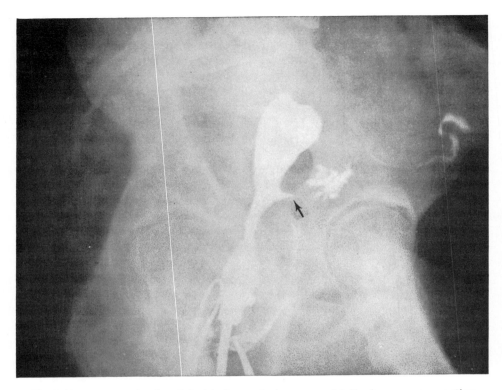

Fig. 7. Hysterogram showing defect in lower uterine segment following cesarean section.

labor and a control group was sectioned electively. The hazards of prematurity may possibly be reduced through the newer diagnostic technics described in Chapter 37 (p. 1029).

The difficulties inherent in formulating an inflexible policy concerning the mode of delivery after cesarean section are obvious. Although there is a greater tendency toward individualization in the United States today, most patients with cesarean section scars are delivered abdominally. The current concern with "fewer but better babies" leads to the avoidance of all unnecessary risks. In the United Kingdom, however, a greater willingness to perform vaginal delivery after cesarean section is prevalent. The subject is discussed further in Chapter 42. An occult rupture discovered at a subsequent cesarean section does not necessitate hysterectomy, for the edges of the scar may be reapproximated with good healing of the new wound. In a patient scheduled for cesarean section and tubal ligation, however, a separation of the uterine scar may suggest cesarean section–hysterectomy as a preferable method of sterilization.

SPONTANEOUS RUPTURE OF INTACT UTERUS

Spontaneous rupture of the uterus is one of the gravest complications in all obstetrics, carrying a very high maternal and perinatal mortality. Its frequency approximates or exceeds that of rupture of a cesarean section scar and today is probably more common than traumatic rupture. In three series cited by Eastman, there were 68 overt ruptures of cesarean section scar and 89 ruptures of the intact uterus, either spontaneous or traumatic. In our experience spontaneous rupture is about three times as frequent as rupture of a transverse lower segment scar. Spontaneous rupture of the uterus is especially likely to occur in women of great parity and is almost never seen in a primigravida. For this reason, of course, oxytocin should rarely be given to patients of great parity, as discussed on page 845. Disproportion, sometimes of only minor degree, is an additional factor in about half the cases.

In the past, spontaneous rupture during labor was somewhat less common than traumatic rupture, but with the modern trend away from difficult vaginal procedures, the situation no longer obtains. Delfs and Eastman found 40 per cent of the ruptures during labor to be spontaneous, and Pedowitz and Perell found a 50 per cent frequency. In both series, the patients were in the higher age groups and of high parity. The second most common contributing factor was cephalopelvic disproportion. Even slight mechanical difficulties may jeopardize a uterus weakened by repeated childbearing and aging. This point is emphasized here because it has been customary to stress as causes of spontaneous rupture only the more obvious factors in dystocia, such as pelvic contraction, transverse lie, hydrocephalus, impacted tumors, and brow or face presentation.

Spontaneous rupture of the intact uterus during pregnancy before the onset of labor is exceedingly rare. Felmus, Pedowitz, and Nassberg in a complete review were able to find only 116 such cases, to which they added 5 of their own. They found the most common causes to be previous curettage, manual removal of the placenta, and postabortal or postpartum sepsis. Pregnancy in a maldeveloped horn of a bicornuate uterus and adenomyosis of the corpus have also been implicated, but in some cases there is no discernible cause. Bateman has reported a patient with a twin pregnancy whose uterus ruptured spontaneously at 22 weeks. In rupture during pregnancy the lesion is almost always in the body of the uterus, either fundal or on the anterior or posterior wall, in contrast to ruptures during labor, which are characteristically in the lower uterine segment.

The symptoms and signs of rupture during pregnancy are the same as those of ruptures during labor. A few cases have been reported, however, in which intraperitoneal hemorrhage was slight and symptoms minimal, with hours or even days elapsing before the patient sought medical attention. In very rare cases the fetus may be extruded into the peritoneal cavity while the placenta remains in the uterus, the gestation continuing as a uteroabdominal pregnancy (Gepfert; Badawy). Escape into the abdomen is almost always accompanied by death of the fetus because the contraction of the uterus critically reduces the circulation to the placenta.

TRAUMATIC RUPTURE OF INTACT UTERUS

Traumatic rupture of the uterus during pregnancy is quite uncommon but may occur at any stage beyond the early months. A blow or fall on the abdomen or an automobile accident may cause rupture. The tear may occur at the site of the blow or elsewhere in the body of the uterus by contrecoup. Although the uterus is surprisingly resistant to external trauma, occasionally an apparently slight force causes rupture. Any pregnant woman involved in an automobile accident should be watched carefully for signs of ruptured uterus.

Traumatic rupture during labor is most commonly produced by version and extraction. Although the accident is most likely to occur when version is attempted after rupture of the membranes or with impaction of a shoulder presentation, it may also happen in more favorable cases managed with great care and gentleness. Other causes of traumatic rupture are Braxton Hicks version, breech extraction, and difficult or unsuccessful forceps. Unfortunately, administration of oxytocin (Ch. 28, Fig. 10) in the first or second stage of labor continues to be a rather common cause of traumatic rupture especially in women of high parity (Awais and Lebherz). Particularly reprehensible as a cause of ruptured uterus is strong fundal pressure to accomplish spontaneous delivery or to push the head deeply into the pelvis. Fundal pressure is a more important cause of uterine rupture than its relatively infrequent mention in the recent obstetric literature would indicate. If this procedure is used at all in modern obstetrics, the pressure should be gently applied with full appreciation of its dangers.

Pathologic Anatomy.   The important role in uterine rupture of excessive stretching of the lower uterine segment with the development of a pathologic retraction ring has already been stressed in Chapter 28. Rupture of the uterus at the time of labor is limited almost entirely to the lower uterine segment; the rent usually extends obliquely, although when it is in the immediate vicinity of the cervix, it frequently extends transversely. It is usually longitudinal, however, when it occurs in the portion of the uterus adjacent to the broad ligament. Although occurring primarily in the lower uterine segment, it is not unusual for the laceration to extend farther upward into the body of the uterus or downward through the cervix into the vagina. The tear itself usually presents jagged, irregular margins that are stained with blood (Fig. 8).

It is customary to distinguish between *complete* and *incomplete* ruptures, depending on whether the laceration communicates directly with the abdominal cavity or is separated from it by the peritoneum of the uterus or broad ligament. Incomplete ruptures frequently extend into the broad ligament; in such circumstances the hemorrhage often occurs less rapidly than in the complete variety, the blood slowly accumulating between the leaves and separating the peritoneum from the surrounding viscera, with the consequent formation of a large retroperitoneal hematoma, occasionally sufficiently large to cause death. More frequently, however, the fatal outcome supervenes only after secondary rupture of the hematoma relieves the pressure, which had previously to some extent restrained the bleeding, and leads to resumption of intraperitoneal bleeding. After complete rupture, the uterine contents may escape into the peritoneal cavity, but when the presenting part is firmly engaged, only a portion of the fetus may escape, the rest remaining in the uterine cavity. In the incomplete variety, however, the products of conception may remain within the uterus or assume a position beneath the serosa of the uterus or between the leaves of the broad ligament. Despite its close relation to the uterus, the bladder is injured in only 13 per cent of cases (Hassim).

Clinical Course.   If the accident occurs during labor, the patient, after a period of premonitory signs, at the height of an intense uterine contraction suddenly complains of a sharp, shooting pain in the lower abdomen and frequently cries out that "something has given way" inside her. At the same time the lower uterine segment becomes much more sensitive to pressure. Immediately after these symp-

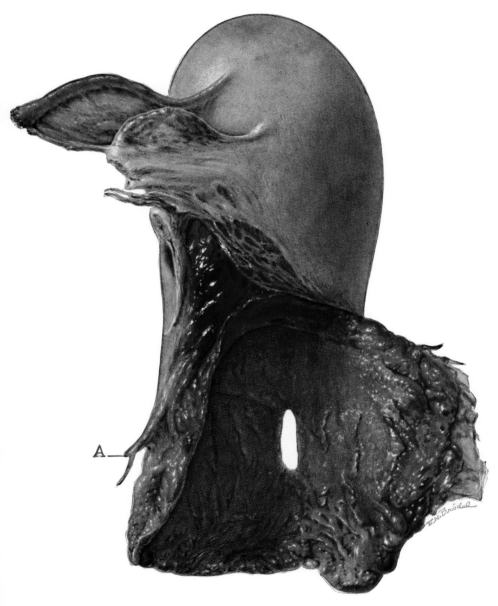

Fig. 8. Rupture of uterus, bilateral. A, laceration extends through left uterine artery. (Same case as Fig. 33 in Ch. 29.)

toms appear, there is cessation of uterine contractions, and the patient, previously in intense agony, suddenly experiences great relief. At the same time there is usually external hemorrhage, although it is often very slight.

Palpation or vaginal examination indicates that the presenting part has slipped away from the pelvic inlet and has become movable, while a hard, round body (the firmly contracted uterus) may be felt alongside the fetus, which is often more easily palpated than usual. Naturally, if the uterine contents have escaped into the abdominal cavity, the presenting part cannot be felt on vaginal examination. Vaginal examination sometimes reveals a tear in the uterine wall through which the fingers can be passed into the abdominal cavity, where the viscera may be felt. Failure to detect the tear, however, by no means proves its absence.

As a rule, shortly after complete rupture the patient presents signs and symptoms of shock. The pulse increases in rapidity and loses tone, the face becomes pallid, drawn, and often covered with sweat. Copious hemorrhage may be followed by chills, disturbance of vision, air hunger, and eventually unconsciousness. Shock, however, is sometimes delayed for several hours after rupture and is usually less marked when the fetus remains partially within the uterus. After incomplete rupture, moreover, the immediate symptoms are sometimes very slight and labor may even continue. The tendency of uterine ruptures to remain asymptomatic often for many hours is the cause of many deaths. In general, the most constant clinical symptom is pain coupled with abdominal tenderness, rather than overt shock. In cases in which there is any possibility of uterine rupture, a specimen of urine obtained by catheterization is valuable. If the urine is grossly bloody, strong support is lent to the diagnosis of rupture, but a clear specimen, of course, by no means rules out the accident. When rupture during labor is overlooked, its first sign may be abdominal distention in the puerperium consequent upon irritation produced by retroperitoneal blood. Since patients who suffer traumatic rupture in labor are usually under analgesia, pain and tenderness are not immediately evident, and the condition manifests itself by the bleeding and shock. In this situation, also, blood in the urine is an important finding.

Prognosis.   The chances for the child are almost uniformly bad, the mortality rates in various reports ranging between 50 and 75 per cent. If, however, the fetus is alive at the time of the accident, its only chance of further survival is afforded by immediate laparotomy; otherwise, hypoxia, the result of the separation of the placenta, is inevitable. If untreated, most of the mothers die from hemorrhage or infection, although spontaneous recovery has been noted in exceptional cases. The maternal mortality rate following rupture of a cesarean section scar is about 5 per cent. By combining four modern reports, Eastman found that in 97 ruptures of a cesarean section scar, there were 3 deaths. The death rate after rupture of the intact, unscarred uterus, whether spontaneous or traumatic, is much higher. In Eastman's report, for instance, the mortality rate ranged between 20 and 40 per cent. Death is almost always the result of shock and hemorrhage, but pulmonary embolism is occasionally an additional factor. Earlier diagnosis, immediate operation, the availability of large amounts of blood, and chemotherapy have greatly improved the maternal prognosis in rupture of the uterus.

Treatment.   *Prophylactic.*   Intelligent obstetric care during labor should largely eliminate this accident. Whenever there is a possible obstacle to the birth of the child, the obstetrician should be on the alert for an impending uterine rupture. He should be especially cautious in labors complicated by transverse lie or hydrocephalus. In vertex presentations, failure of progress in engagement and labor requires very careful study of the presentation and estimation of fetal and pelvic size by the most accurate technics available.

Curative.   Whether the fetus is alive or dead or whether it is still within the ruptured uterus or has already escaped into the abdominal cavity, no attempt should be made to extract it per vaginam, but laparotomy should be performed immediately. After removal of the child, the necessary operative procedures may then be carried out. Hysterectomy is usually required, but in selected cases suture of the wound may be performed. Seth has recently reported a series of 66 cases of repair of a uterine rupture. In 25 the repair was accompanied by tubal ligation. Thirteen of the 41 mothers who did not have tubal ligation had a total of 21 subsequent pregnancies. Rupture recurred in 4 patients.

In the presence of a large hematoma in the broad ligament, identification and ligation of the uterine artery is often extremely difficult. Repeated efforts to con-

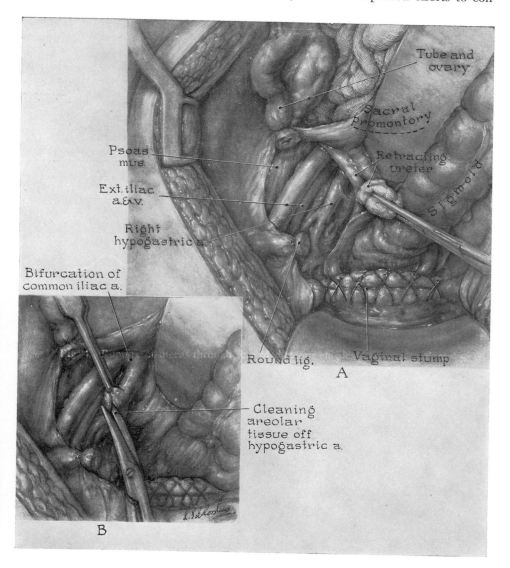

Fig. 9. Technic of ligation of hypogastric artery. A, identification of right iliac vessels in retroperitoneum and isolation or right ureter. B, identification of bifurcation of right common iliac artery and removal of areolar tissue from right hypogastric artery.

trol the hemorrhage are fruitless, time-consuming, and dangerous to the underlying ureter. It is often far simpler and more effective to ligate the hypogastric artery on the affected side. Hypogastric ligation may be quickly accomplished by opening first the peritoneum over the common iliac artery and then the arterial sheath by sharp dissection down to the origin of the hypogastric and then along the hypogastric artery. A clamp may then be passed beneath the hypogastric artery and the vessel ligated with silk sutures (Figs. 9, 10, and 11). It is of interest that bilateral ligation of the hypogastric arteries per se does not seem to interfere seriously with subsequent reproduction. Mengert and associates have documented successful pregnancies in 5 women after bilateral hypogastric artery ligation. In 3 both ovarian arteries were also ligated.

Blood transfusion is lifesaving in the treatment of a ruptured uterus. It should be started at once in the presence of shock. In any case, blood should be running throughout the operation. The operation should not be delayed because of shock, which may persist until the hemorrhage is controlled. Adequate replacement in many cases requires massive transfusion. Broad-spectrum antibiotics are used in the presence of infection.

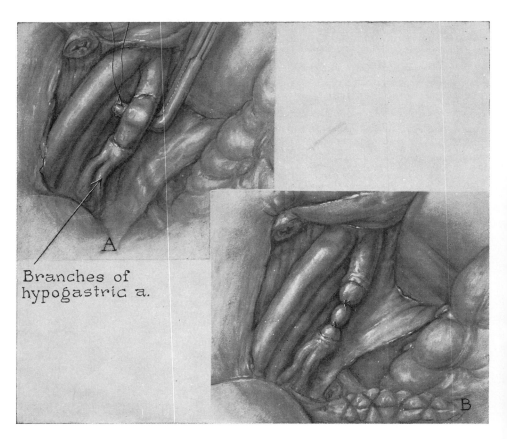

Fig. 10. Technic of ligation of hypogastric artery (cont.). A, ligature passed beneath isolated right hypogastric artery. B, right hypogastric artery doubly ligated but not divided.

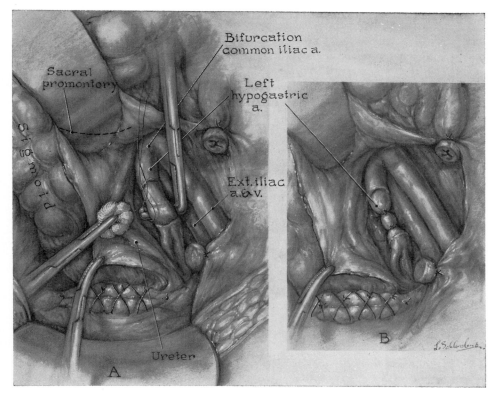

Fig. 11. Technic of ligation of hypogastric artery (cont.). A, ligature passed beneath left hypogastric artery. Sigmoid retracted to expose left retroperitoneum. B, completion of bilateral operation with double ligation of left hypogastric artery.

Instrumental Perforation of the Uterus

Reference has already been made to perforation of the uterus after attempts at criminal abortion or removal of placental tissue with a curette or ovum forceps after an incomplete abortion. Similar accidents occasionally are the result of poor obstetric management of labor at term, when either the uterus or the vaginal vault may be perforated. In these accidents, loops of intestine may prolapse through the site of rupture. In such circumstances laparotomy is the ideal treatment, though, in the absence of prolapse of the intestines, cases are recorded in which recovery occurred spontaneously under what were apparently most unfavorable conditions. The variety and extent of these injuries are illustrated in Liepmann's book on criminal abortion and described in Taussig's volume.

Accidental Injury to the Uterus and Genital Tract

The increase of automobile accidents and violence has resulted in an increase in the number of traumatic accidents during pregnancy. In most instances, these accidents involve parts of the body other than the genital tract. An extensive experience at Charity Hospital in New Orleans has been reported by Dyer and Barclay. Gunshot wounds of the uterus have been summarized by Buchsbaum and Caruso. Genital trauma resulting from automobile accidents has been studied by Elliot in Australia as well as by Crosby and co-workers and Buchsbaum in this country.

In any severe injury to a pregnant woman the resulting shock should be vigorously treated. The fetus cannot survive a prolonged period of maternal hypotension. If there is any question of uterine rupture or perforation, laparotomy should be performed.

Perforation of the Genital Tract Following Necrosis

In obstructed labor the tissues of various portions of the genital tract may be compressed between the head and the bony pelvis. If the pressure is transitory, it is without significance; but if it is prolonged, necrosis results, followed in a few days by sloughing and perforation.

In most such cases, the perforation occurs between the vagina and the bladder, giving rise to a *vesicovaginal fistula*. Less frequently, the anterior lip of the cervix is compressed against the symphysis pubis, and an abnormal communication is eventually established between the cervical canal and the bladder, a *vesicocervical fistula*. If the patient has no infection, the fistula may heal without further treatment. In other cases, however, it may persist, requiring subsequent plastic operations.

Occasionally the posterior wall of the uterus may be subjected to so much pressure against the promontory of the sacrum that necrosis results, with a fistula communicating with the cul-de-sac. If infection occurs, the accident is usually followed by septic peritonitis. Localized peritonitis may lead to the formation of adhesions between the posterior wall of the uterus and the pelvic peritoneum, however, thereby preventing general peritonitis. Similar lesions may occur in the rare cases in which exostoses or bony spicules protrude from the walls of the birth canal, as in *pelvis spinosa*.

Amniotic Fluid Embolism

Amniotic fluid embolism is included in this section because it is an accident that often results from tumultuous labor and sometimes accompanies rupture of the uterus.

At any time after the membranes have ruptured, the amniotic fluid may enter the gaping venous sinuses of the placental site as well as the endocervical vein and be drawn into the general circulation, and thus into the pulmonary capillaries. Leary and Hertig suggest that amniotic fluid might enter the maternal circulation through a break in the chorionic plate of the placenta, without overt leakage of amniotic fluid. Since the amniotic fluid commonly contains particulate matter, such as lanugo hair and particles of vernix caseosa and meconium, multiple emboli may reach the lungs in this manner.

First described by Meyer in 1926 and later documented with a mass of clinical evidence by Lushbaugh and Steiner, this accident is an occasional cause of death during or shortly after the completion of labor. The clinical characteristics of amniotic fluid embolism are sudden dyspnea, cyanosis, pulmonary edema, shock, and uterine relaxation with postpartum hemorrhage. A frequent complication is failure of the blood to coagulate. Lushbaugh and Steiner advanced the idea that the phenomena following amniotic fluid emboli result from anaphylactoid shock from the sudden deposition of the amniotic material in the pulmonary arterioles. This anaphylactoid reaction in turn causes the vascular collapse, which leads to the postpartum atony and hemorrhage. Experimental studies by Hanzlik and Karsner indicate that the injection of finely divided particulate matter, such as suspensions of charcoal particles or India ink, produces not only altered coagulability of the blood but also dramatic systemic phenomena, such as restlessness, tremors, marked dyspnea, convulsions, and often death. Additional support is provided by the experiments of Halmagyi, Starzecki, and Shearman. After injecting human amniotic fluid into sheep, they noted pulmonary hypertension, arterial hypoxia, and a marked fall in pulmonary compliance. These changes, however, are similar to those found in pulmonary embolism of other cause and failed to occur when the amniotic fluid was filtered. Attwood caused the death of only 5 of 15 dogs by the intravenous injection of 50 ml of amniotic fluid. In those that survived he found squamous cells in the pulmonary circulation up to 3 weeks after injection. Stolte and co-workers could not produce the syndrome in monkeys.

There is evidence, therefore, both clinical and experimental, that sudden pulmonary blockage by extremely small particles may cause a wide variety of grave signs and symptoms. The condition is fortunately very rare, occurring only once in about 22,000 labors, according to Relyveld's study from Rotterdam. There were 101 maternal deaths during the period under investigation. As pointed out by Kistner, Graf, and Johnstone, amniotic fluid embolism appears to occur most frequently in the white multipara in her midthirties, of parity two or three, at term or slightly past term. It is observed most frequently near the end of the first stage of labor. The syndrome is seen more often, furthermore, in rapid labors with tumultuous uterine contractions. In a disproportionately large number of cases, oxytocin has been given either to initiate or to stimulate labor. The clinical picture is usually catastrophic; death may occur within a few minutes after the first symptom. Two instances have been reported accompanying cesarean section (Barno and Freeman; Willocks and co-workers) and possibly after intraamniotic injection of saline to produce abortion (Goldstein).

An important feature of most cases of amniotic fluid embolism is fibrinogenopenia and other alterations in coagulation mechanics. The mechanism by which hypofibrinogenemia is produced may be identical with that in abruptio placentae, as described on page 629. The profound shock that characterizes amniotic fluid embolism, moreover, may be related to obstruction of the pulmonary vasculature as well as intravascular clotting with defibrination rather than to the anaphylactoid reaction previously described. In the studies of Halmagyi and co-workers, prior heparinization failed to protect experimental animals completely against pulmonary hypertension when human amniotic fluid was injected intravenously. The shock may then be augmented by uterine bleeding due to the incoagulability of the blood. If the amniotic fluid is filtered to free it of particulate matter, experimental animals show no effect when it is injected intravenously. On the other hand, if meconium is added to amniotic fluid, it is much more likely to be lethal when so injected. The clinical significance of the presence of meconium in the amniotic fluid is borne out by the recent report of Peterson and Taylor. They identified meconium in amniotic fluid of one third of 40 women before fatal amniotic fluid embolism.

Although few presumptive cases of amniotic fluid embolism with recovery have been reported, the accident is usually fatal. To establish an incontrovertible diagnosis, it is necessary to demonstrate amniotic debris in the pulmonary vessels, as shown in Figure 12. Without such proof, death, according to Thompson and Budd, is far more likely to have some other cause.

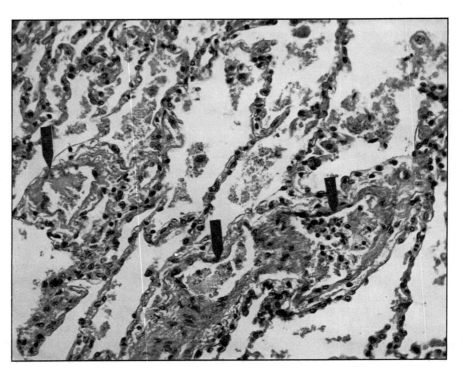

Fig. 12. Photomicrograph of lung of patient dying from amniotic fluid embolism, showing squames and other amniotic debris in small vessels.

To date, the treatment of amniotic fluid embolism most often has proved to be unsatisfactory. The coexistence of pulmonary vascular obstruction causing acute cor pulmonale and systemic hypotension from hemorrhage compounds the problem of appropriate blood replacement. Severe bleeding caused by a grossly defective coagulation mechanism appears to result in some instances, from intense intravascular coagulation coupled with intense fibrinolytic activity. Since the mortality rate is so high, perhaps amniotic fluid embolism is one of the few situations in obstetrics that might warrant the use simultaneously of fresh blood to provide clotting factors as well as restore blood volume and heparin to try to control further intravascular coagulation, especially in the pulmonary circulation. Clinical observations to establish the merit of such therapy are lacking, however. Certainly if hemorrhage appears to be the major threat while cardiopulmonary signs and symptoms are minimal, therapy with fresh whole blood and fibrinogen is more rational.

By carefully monitoring central venous pressure, the arterial blood pressure, and urine flow, we try to administer a volume of fluids sufficient to allow adequate perfusion of vital organs without contributing to fatal cor pulmonale. Oxygen should be administered in high concentration, and in some instances assisted ventilation is of value to try to overcome loss of pulmonary compliance.

REFERENCES

Aguillon, A., Andjus, T., Grayson, A., and Race, G. J. Amniotic fluid embolism: a review. Obstet Gynec Survey 17:619, 1962.

Attwood, H. D. A histological study of experimental amniotic-fluid and meconium embolism in dogs. J Path Bact 88:285, 1964.

Awais, G. M., and Lebherz, T. B. Ruptured uterus, a complication of oxytocin induction and high parity. Obstet Gynec 36:465, 1970.

Badawy, A. H. Abdominal pregnancy in a previously ruptured uterus. Lancet 1:510, 1962.

Barno, A., and Freeman, D. W. Amniotic fluid embolism. Amer J Obstet Gynec 77:1199, 1959.

Bateman, D. E. Spontaneous rupture of uterus at 22 weeks' pregnancy. Brit Med J 3:844, 1967.

Brander, J. H., and Buchman, M. I. Rupture of the vagina during spontaneous delivery. Obstet Gynec 24:151, 1964 (31 references cited).

Buchsbaum, H. J. Accidental injury complicating pregnancy. Amer J Obstet Gynec 102:752, 1968.

———— and Caruso, P. A. Gunshot wound of the pregnant uterus. Obstet Gynec 33:673, 1969.

Crosby, W. M., Snyder, R. G., Snow, C. C., and Hanson, P. G. Impact injuries in pregnancy. I. Experimental Studies. Amer J Obstet Gynec 101:100, 1968.

Delfs, E., and Eastman, N. J. Rupture of the uterus (an analysis of 53 cases). Canad Med Ass J 52:376, 1945.

Donnelly, J. P., and Franzoni, K. T. Uterine rupture. A 30-year survey. Obstet Gynec 23:774, 1964.

Douglas, R. G., Birnbaum, S. J., and MacDonald, F. A. Pregnancy and labor following cesarean section. Amer J Obstet Gynec 86:961, 1963.

Dyer, F., and Barclay, D. L. Accidental trauma complicating pregnancy and delivery. Amer J Obstet Gynec 83:907, 1962.

Eastman, N. J. Editorial note: Rupture of the uterus due to placenta accreta at the site of a previous cornual resection. Obstet Gynec Survey 13:833, 1958.

Elliot, M. Vehicular accidents and pregnancy. Aust New Zeal J Obstet Gynaec 6:279, 1966.

Fainstat, T. Changes in uterine connective tissue during pregnancy (the uterine stromal phenomenon). Biochem Pharmacol, Supplement, p. 60, March 1968.

Felmus, L. B., Pedowitz, P., and Nassberg, S. Spontaneous rupture of an apparently normal uterus during pregnancy. Obstet Gynec Survey 8:155, 1953.

Gamble, T. O. Colporrhexis, or rupture of the vault of the vagina. Amer J Obstet Gynec 14:766, 1927.

Garnet, J. D. Uterine rupture during pregnancy. An analysis of 133 patients. Obstet Gynec 23:898, 1964.

Gepfert, J. R. Ante-partum rupture of the uterine scar following low flap cesarean section, with a report of a case giving rise to a secondary abdominal pregnancy. Amer J Obstet Gynec 37:466, 1939.

Goldstein, P. J. Amniotic fluid embolism complicating intrauterine saline abortion. Amer J Obstet Gynec 101:858, 1968.

Hall, J. E., Kohl, S. G., and Schechter, H. R. Current aspects of cesarean section and perinatal mortality. Amer J Obstet Gynec 75:387, 1958.

Halmagyi, D. F., Starzecki, B., and Shearman, R. P. Experimental amniotic fluid embolism: mechanism and treatment. Amer J Obstet Gynec 84:251, 1962.

Hanzlik, P. J., and Karsner, H. T. Anaphylactoid phenomena from the intravenous administration of various colloids, arsenicals and other agents. J Pharmacol Exp Ther 14:379, 1920; 23:173, 1924.

Hassim, A. M. Uterine rupture with extrusion of the fetus into the bladder. Int Surg 49:130, 1968.

Hellegers, A. E., and Eastman, N. J. The problem of prematurity in gravidas with cesarean section scars. Amer J Obstet Gynec 82:679, 1961.

Kistner, R. W., Graf, W. R., and Johnstone, R. E. Pulmonary embolism by particulate matter of the amniotic fluid. Obstet Gynec Survey 5:629, 1950 (60 references cited).

Kohl, S. G. Community Obstetrical Study. Progress Report, 1960.

Lane, F. R., and Reid, D. E. Dehiscence of previous uterine incision at repeat cesarean section. Obstet Gynec 2:54, 1953.

Lawrence, R. F. Vaginal delivery after Cesarean section. J Obstet Gynaec Brit Emp 60:237, 1953.

Leary, O. C., and Hertig, A. T. The pathogenesis of amniotic-fluid embolism. I. Possible placental factors—aberrant squamous cells in placentas. New Eng J Med 243:588, 1950.

Leopold, G. (Delivered secondary abdominal pregnancy after traumatic rupture of the uterus). Arch Gynaek 52:376, 1896.

Lepage, F., Noël, B., Lemerre, L., and Schramm, B. (Hysterographic study of scars of segmental cesarean). Gynec Obstet (Paris) 58:506, 1959.

Liepmann, W. Die Abtreibung, Berlin und Wien, 1927.

Lushbaugh, C. C., and Steiner, P. E. Additional observations on maternal pulmonary embolism by amniotic fluid. Amer J Obstet Gynec 43:833, 1942.

Mengert, W. J., Burchell, R. C., Blumstein, R. W., and Daskal, J. L. Pregnancy after bilateral ligation of the internal iliac and ovarian arteries. Obstet Gynec 34:664, 1969.

Menon, M. K. K. Rupture of the uterus. J Obstet Gynaec Brit Comm 69:18, 1962.

Meyer, J. R. (Amniotic fluid pulmonary embolism). Brasil-Medico 40:No. 2, 301, 1926.

Pedowitz, P., and Felmus, L. B. Rupture of myomectomy scars during subsequent pregnancies: a review. Obstet Gynec Survey 7:305, 1952.

———— and Perell, A. Rupture of the uterus. Amer J Obstet Gynec 76:161, 1958.

———— and Schwartz, R. M. The true incidence of silent rupture of cesarean section scars: a prospective analysis of 403 cases. Amer J Obstet Gynec 74:1071, 1957.

Peterson, E. P., and Taylor, H. B. Amniotic fluid embolism. Obstet Gynec 35:787, 1970.

Poidevin, L. O. S. Histopathology of cesarean section wound. An experimental study. J Obstet Gynaec Brit Comm 68:1025, 1961.

Reid, D. E., Weiner, A. E., and Roby, C. C. I. Intravascular clotting and afibrinogenemia, the presumptive lethal factors in the syndrome of amniotic fluid embolism. Amer J Obstet Gynec 66:465, 1953.

Relyveld, R. W. (The frequency of amniotic fluid embolism) Nederl T Verlosk 64:17, 1964.

Rendle Short, C. W. Causes of maternal death among Africans in Kampala, Uganda. J Obstet Gynaec Brit Comm 68:44, 1961.

———— Personal communication.

Schwarz, O., Paddock, R., and Bortnick, A. R. The cesarean scar. An experimental study. Amer J Obstet Gynec 36:962, 1938.

Seth, R. S. Results of treatment of rupture of the uterus by suturing. J Obstet Gynaec Brit Comm 75:55, 1968.

Spritzer, T. D. Annular detachment of the cervix during labor and delivery by vacuum extractor. Amer J Obstet Gynec 83:247, 1962.

Stolte, L., Seelen, J., Eskes, T., and Wagatsuma, T. Failure to produce the syndrome of amniotic fluid embolism by infusion of amniotic fluid and meconium into monkeys. Amer J Obstet Gynec 98:694, 1967.

Taussig, F. J. Abortion. Spontaneous and Induced, Medical and Social Aspects. St. Louis, C. V. Mosby Co., 1936.

Thompson, W. B., and Budd, J. W. Erroneous diagnoses of amniotic fluid embolism. Amer J Obstet Gynec 91:606, 1965.

Williams, J. W.   A critical analysis of 21 years' experience with cesarean section. Bull Hopkins Hosp 32:173, 1921.

Willocks, J., Mone, J. G., and Thomson, W. J.   Amniotic fluid embolism: case with biochemical findings. Brit Med J 2:1181, 1966.

33

ABNORMALITIES OF THE THIRD STAGE OF LABOR

POSTPARTUM HEMORRHAGE

Postpartum hemorrhage has most often been defined as loss of blood in excess of 500 ml during the first 24 hours after birth. More recent studies, however, demonstrate quite clearly that blood loss as the consequence of vaginal delivery frequently is somewhat more than 500 ml. Newton, for example, measured the amount of hemoglobin shed by 105 women from the time of vaginal delivery through the next 24 hours and ascertained that the average blood loss was at least 546 ml. If appropriate allowance was made for the maternal blood discarded with the placenta, as well as that not measured because of incomplete recovery of shed hemoglobin, the blood loss during the first 24 hours averaged about 650 ml. Moreover, Pritchard and associates and DeLeeuw and co-workers have demonstrated that red cells equivalent to approximately 600 ml of blood are lost from the maternal circulation during vaginal delivery and the next several hours. Therefore, a blood loss somewhat in excess of 500 ml by accurate measurement is not necessarily an abnormal event for vaginal delivery. Pritchard and associates noted that about 5 per cent of women delivering vaginally lost more than 1,000 ml according to measurements. At the same time, their studies confirmed that the estimated blood loss commonly is only about one half the actual loss. Moreover, on the basis of an estimated blood loss greater than 500 ml, postpartum hemorrhage has been found in many hospitals to occur in about 5 per cent of the deliveries. An *estimated* blood loss in excess of 500 ml in most instances, therefore, will call attention to patients who are bleeding or have bled excessively and will warn the physician that dangerous hemorrhage is likely. Hemorrhage after the first 24 hours is designated as late postpartum hemorrhage and is discussed under disorders of the puerperium on page 998.

Postpartum hemorrhage is the most common cause of serious blood loss in obstetrics. As a direct factor in maternal mortality it is the cause of about one quarter of the deaths from obstetric hemorrhage in the group that includes postpartum hemorrhage, placenta previa, abruptio placentae, ectopic pregnancy, hemorrhage from abortion, and rupture of the uterus. In addition, loss of excessive amounts of blood has a general debilitating effect, especially on women of the childbearing age, whose stores of iron may be marginal. In the past, as pointed out by Douglas and Davis in an analysis of 183 cases of puerperal infection at

The New York Lying-In Hospital, this debilitation was associated with puerperal infection.

Immediate Causes. There are three major immediate causes of postpartum hemorrhage: (1) uterine atony, (2) vaginal and cervical lacerations, and (3) retention of placental fragments. The most frequent cause is uterine atony, which accounts for over 90 per cent of the cases. Vaginal and cervical lacerations are the main source of postpartum bleeding in about 6 per cent. Retention of a placental fragment is an uncommon cause of immediate postpartum hemorrhage but is frequently associated with late bleeding. A much less common cause relates to defects of clotting.

Somewhat akin to bleeding vaginal lacerations at delivery is blood loss from the episiotomy site. Although much of the bleeding from the incision occurs before the birth of the child, it is not generally feasible to measure that blood separately, and it is usually regarded as part of the total blood lost postpartum. Although it is uncommon for an episiotomy alone to cause postpartum hemorrhage, blood so lost averages about 200 ml. Odell and Seski found the average blood loss from episiotomy to be 253 ml and believe that it is probably the chief source of bleeding in most primigravidas.

Predisposing Causes. The factors predisposing to postpartum hemorrhage fall into two main groups: (1) those that are predetermined and beyond the control of the obstetrician and (2) those that are directly under his surveillance. A most important predetermined factor in postpartum hemorrhage is large size of the baby. This relation was noted by Ahlfeld and Aschoff as early as 1904 and has since been substantiated by the statistical study of Calkins, Litzenberg, and Plass, and by Reich. The likelihood of postpartum hemorrhage with a baby of 2,200 g or less was 1 in 21, according to Reich, whereas with a baby of 4,000 g or more the chances of excessive bleeding were 1 in 4.

Multiple pregnancy is associated with an increased frequency of postpartum hemorrhage. In cases of twinning three factors predisposing to hemorrhage occur: overdistention of the uterus, an increased use of surgical anesthesia for operative delivery of the second twin, and a larger placental area. Kurtz, Keating, and Loftus claimed that with careful use of oxytocin in the placental stage, the incidence of postpartum hemorrhage at the Margaret Hague Maternity Hospital in 500 consecutive twin deliveries was only 3 per cent. Pritchard, however, found that blood loss during vaginal delivery and the next few hours was on the average close to one liter, or nearly twice the value for vaginal delivery of singletons.

High parity is another factor associated with increased blood loss during delivery. Other conditions in which hemorrhage is extremely frequent are abruptio placentae and placenta previa. According to Doran, O'Brien, and Randall, a woman who has had one postpartum hemorrhage stands a slightly greater chance of having another hemorrhage in a subsequent pregnancy.

The most important controllable causes of postpartum hemorrhage are operative delivery, deep anesthesia, prolonged labor with maternal exhaustion, and mismanagement of the third stage. The data of Pastore, Reich, and others indicate that excessive bleeding is about three times more common after operative delivery than after spontaneous termination of labor. Anesthesia, particularly ether, and lacerations contribute to this result. Internal podalic version is followed by serious postpartum hemorrhage in such a high percentage of cases that blood should be ready for transfusion whenever version is contemplated.

In prolonged labor with maternal exhaustion, the uterus does not contract satisfactorily. In such cases the triad of exhaustion, infection, and hemorrhage sometimes spells maternal death. The most common mismanagement of the third stage of labor involves an attempt to hasten it. Constant kneading and squeezing of the uterus that is already contracted are likely to cause incomplete placental separation and interference with the physiologic mechanism of placental detachment.

Clinical Picture.   Postpartum hemorrhage before delivery of the placenta is called *third-stage hemorrhage.* Whether bleeding occurs before or after delivery of the placenta, or at both times, contrary to general opinion there is usually no sudden massive hemorrhage but rather a steady, moderate bleeding. Especially in hemorrhage after delivery of the placenta, the constant seepage may, over a period of an hour or two, lead to enormous loss of blood, as emphasized by Beecham. The average interval between delivery and death in his series was 5 hours and 20 minutes. Only 6 patients died within 2 hours of delivery, and none in less than one and one-half hours. In other words, there was ample time for intensive treatment in all these patients, but the extent of blood loss was obviously not recognized. The other factor, of course, is the ability to tolerate a *large* hemorrhage.

The effect of hemorrhage depends upon the maternal blood volume and the degree of anemia at the time the patient arrives in the labor room. A woman already exhausted by prolonged labor or weakened by antecedent anemia or chronic disease may succumb after the loss of 1,000 ml, a hemorrhage well tolerated by patients in good physical condition. Moderate loss of blood is not ordinarily attended by serious signs and symptoms, but with profuse hemorrhage the pulse becomes rapid and thready, the face becomes pallid and drawn, and chills, shortness of breath, and disturbed vision appear. As shock deepens, air hunger develops and not infrequently restlessness and sweating. The patient becomes unconscious and death may follow.

A treacherous feature of postpartum hemorrhage is the failure of the pulse and blood pressure to undergo more than moderate alterations until large amounts of blood have been lost. With subsequent failure of compensatory vascular mechanisms, the pulse suddenly soars and soon becomes impalpable, while the blood pressure falls precipitously.

In rare instances, in which the fundus has not been adequately monitored after delivery, the blood may not escape vaginally but may instead collect within the uterus. The uterine cavity may thus become distended by 1,000 ml or more of blood while an incompetent attendant massages a roll of abdominal fat. The care of the postpartum uterus must not, therefore, be left to an inexperienced person.

Diagnosis.   Except possibly when an intrauterine accumulation of blood is not recognized, the diagnosis of postpartum hemorrhage should be obvious. The differentiation between bleeding from uterine atony and from lacerations is tentatively made on the condition of the fundus. If bleeding persists, despite a firm, well-contracted uterine corpus, the cause of the hemorrhage is probably laceration. Bright red blood also suggests lacerations. To ascertain the role of lacerations as a cause of bleeding, careful inspection of the cervix and vagina is essential. Sometimes bleeding may occur from both atony and trauma, especially after major operative delivery. Routine inspection of the cervix and all of the vagina should be done after forceps, version and breech extraction, or other vaginal operations, as well as when unusual bleeding occurs during the second stage or immediately after birth of the child. Many authorities believe that routine inspection of the cervix and vagina should be performed after every delivery—to prevent hemorrhage from cervical or vaginal lacerations and to ensure restoration of cervical integrity.

Prognosis. In modern obstetrics, with blood readily available for transfusion, no woman should die from postpartum hemorrhage. Although once in several thousand deliveries a hemorrhage of 2,000 to 2,500 ml may be encountered, long before this amount of blood is lost transfusion should be started into one or more of the patient's veins. At no time should the deficit of blood be more than 1,000 ml. It should be possible to save the life of every woman with postpartum hemorrhage, even though hysterectomy may be required in some instances. To obtain this objective, however, requires assiduous attention to all patients immediately postpartum, a good blood bank, and alert action by an experienced obstetric team. In the past 10 years at the Kings County Hospital in more than 50,000 deliveries, we have had only 1 death from postpartum hemorrhage associated with atony and 1 associated with a clotting deficit. Although death from postpartum hemorrhage is extremely rare in current obstetric practice in modern hospitals, it is not uncommon under less favorable conditions. For example, Menon indicates that postpartum hemorrhage accounts for nearly 95 per cent of the hemorrhagic deaths in India. There are other hazards imposed by postpartum hemorrhage, not the least of which are transfusion reactions and hepatitis. The mortality of transfusion reaction today equals that of appendectomy. Postpartum hemorrhage, furthermore, is on rare occasion followed by *Sheehan's syndrome*, which is characterized by varying degrees of anterior pituitary necrosis. In a typical case, there are failure of lactation, amenorrhea, atrophy of the breasts, loss of pubic and axillary hair, superinvolution of the uterus, hypothyroidism, and adrenal cortical insufficiency. Schneeberg, Perloff, and Israel found 4 patients with the syndrome among 35 women who survived a major postpartum hemorrhage. The severity of the hemorrhage does not always bear a close relation to the occurrence of Sheehan's syndrome.

Management of Third-Stage Bleeding. A certain amount of bleeding is inevitable during the third stage of every labor as the result of transient partial separation of the placenta. When the placenta is extruded by the Schultze mechanism, the blood follows delivery of the placenta, but in the Duncan mechanism, hemorrhage occurs immediately. Losses of 50 to 200 ml of blood during the third stage of labor should therefore not be regarded as necessarily pathologic.

The routine use of oxytocics after delivery has been of great aid in minimizing postpartum hemorrhage. Ten units of oxytocin intramuscularly as soon as the baby is born may expedite placental separation, although a slightly increased incidence of retention of the placenta may occur. Alternatively, the oxytocin may be administered intravenously immediately after delivery of the placenta. A third effective regimen includes intramuscular oxytocin after completion of the second stage and intravenous administration of an ergot derivative after the third stage.

In the presence of any external hemorrhage during the third stage, the uterus should be massaged if it is not firmly contracted. If the signs of placental separation have appeared, expression of the placenta should be attempted by pressure with the palm of the hand, pushing the fundus of the uterus toward the vagina.

The organ should not, however, be squeezed as in the classical Credé procedure. If, with the placenta undelivered, bleeding continues, manual removal of the placenta is indicated. Attempts to deliver the placenta by squeezing and kneading the uterus through the abdomen not only are futile as a rule but often traumatize the myometrium and aggravate the difficulties.

Management After Placental Delivery.   After the delivery of the placenta, the fundus should always be palpated to make certain that it is well contracted. If it is not firm, massage with the fingertips is indicated. In many institutions 0.2 mg of ergonovine is administered routinely, by either the intravenous or intramuscular route. On other services, however, ergonovine is given only if the uterus is atonic or there is excessive bleeding. Some authors recommend ergonovine with the birth of the anterior shoulder to reduce the incidence of postpartum hemorrhage. In our experience, this technic has shown no particular advantage over the use of oxytocin and is far more likely to cause retention of the placenta. If bleeding persists, 0.2 mg of ergonovine may be given intravenously. In addition, 10 or 20 units of oxytocin in 1,000 ml of lactated Ringer's solution or normal saline in water may be administered by intravenous drip. Meanwhile, massage of the uterus is continued. These simple measures will control postpartum hemorrhage in the great majority of cases. If bleeding persists despite these procedures, no time should be lost in haphazard efforts to control hemorrhage, but the following orderly routine should be initiated:

1. Begin transfusion of blood (*the blood group of every obstetric patient should be known before labor, and crossmatched blood should be available for those in whom hemorrhage is anticipated*).
2. Employ bimanual uterine compression while an associate scrubs. This procedure will control most hemorrhage, but if not, proceed to the next two steps.
3. Explore the uterine cavity manually for retained placental fragments or lacerations.
4. Inspect the cervix after adequate exposure, using a special cervical set containing two vaginal retractors and at least four ring forceps sponge sticks for traction.

The technic of bimanual compression (Fig. 1) consists simply of massage of the posterior aspect of the uterus with the abdominal hand and massage of the anterior uterine aspect with the other fist, the knuckles of which contact the uterine wall. The effect of additional uterine stimulation is thus added to that of direct compression of the uterine veins. This procedure was described by Hamilton in 1861 and has enjoyed wide usage in England and continental Europe. Packing the uterus was an alternative procedure that formerly enjoyed greater popularity. The uterus cannot be satisfactorily packed immediately after delivery, however, since it dilates under the packing. An additional disadvantage is infection. Donald of Glasgow has described the method as a desperate procedure that is seldom used in Scotland.

After extensive experience with both bimanual compression and packing of the uterus, we are convinced that the former procedure is, aside from hysterectomy, the most efficacious method of combating postpartum hemorrhage. Despite the time-honored place of uterine packing in American obstetrics, its efficacy is questionable and its disadvantages many. The drawbacks to packing the uterus

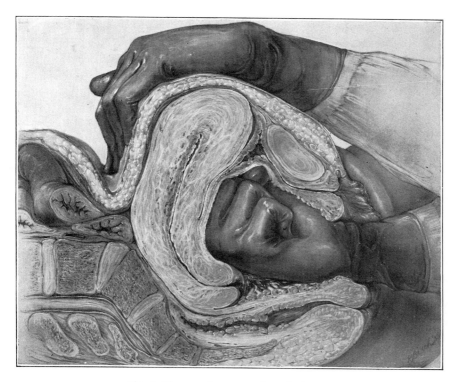

Fig. 1. Bimanual compression of uterus.

were set forth lucidly by Cosgrove in a verbatim quotation that appeared in the preceding edition of this textbook. In essence, it is an unphysiologic procedure that may increase rather than diminish uterine bleeding by preventing effective myometrial contraction.

In any case of postpartum hemorrhage in which abdominal massage of the uterus and oxytocic agents fail to control the bleeding, blood transfusion should be initiated immediately. Blood should always be ready for transfusion whenever 500 ml or more appear to have been lost. With transfusion and simultaneous manual compression of the uterus, additional measures are rarely required. If the operator's hand tires, an assistant can relieve the operator.

Rarely, when all other measures to combat postpartum hemorrhage fail, the question of hysterectomy arises. If performed without adequate blood available on a woman in shock, hysterectomy may hasten death. If the operation has not been too long delayed, however, and if adequate blood transfusions are given, it will prevent many deaths in cases in which all other measures to check the hemorrhage fail.

Waters and also O'Leary and O'Leary have indicated that such bleeding might be controlled by transabdominal ligation of the uterine arteries, thus saving the uterus. In our opinion it is usually easier and less dangerous to the ureters to interrupt the uterine blood supply by ligation of the hypogastric arteries.

Bleeding from Cervical Lacerations. In any case in which bleeding persists in the presence of a tightly contracted uterus, or in which the blood appears to be arterial, inspection of the cervix should be performed and any cervical lacerations greater than 1 cm in extent repaired. In any case of protracted hemorrhage, moreover, even though the obstetrician is certain that uterine atony is the cause, inspection of the cervix is a wise precaution to avoid overlooking a laceration. Proper exposure of the cervix and repair of such lacerations usually require an assistant. Two retractors are inserted into the vagina, the walls of which are separated widely. Sponge forceps are then placed on the anterior and posterior lips of the cervix. Lacerations that are obviously bleeding or are longer than 1 cm should be promptly repaired. Interrupted sutures are employed, with the highest one placed slightly above the apex of the tear, because bleeding from cervical lacerations usually arises from a vessel at this point. Cervical lacerations as a cause of postpartum hemorrhage sometimes cause profuse bleeding; if extensive and multiple, they may prove fatal.

Postpartum Hemorrhage from Retained Placental Fragments.   Immediate postpartum hemorrhage is rarely caused by retained placental fragments, but a remaining piece of placenta is the most common cause of late bleeding in the puerperium. Inspection of the placenta after delivery must be routine. If a portion of placenta is missing, the uterus should be explored and the placental fragment removed, particularly in the face of continuing postpartum bleeding. Retention of a succenturiate lobe, moreover, is an occasional cause of postpartum hemorrhage. Diagnosis and management, similarly, entail manual exploration of the uterus. The late bleeding that may result from a placental polyp is discussed in Chapter 35.

RETENTION OF THE PLACENTA

The placenta separates spontaneously from its site in most instances during the first few minutes after delivery of the infant. The precise reason for delay in detachment beyond this time is not always obvious, but quite often it seems to be inadequate uterine contraction and retraction. Very infrequently, the placenta is unusually adherent to its site because of scanty or absent decidua, so that the physiologic line of cleavage through the spongy layer is lacking. As a consequence, one or more cotyledons of the placenta are firmly bound to the defective decidua basalis or even to the myometrium. When the placenta is thus densely anchored the condition is called *placenta accreta*.

Manual Removal of the Placenta.   Management of the retained placenta varies considerably. In recent years manual removal of the placenta has been practiced much more often than in the past. In fact, some obstetricians practice routine manual removal of any placenta that has not separated spontaneously by the time they have completed delivery of the infant and care of the cord. The majority, however, do not resort so promptly to manual removal of the placenta, although currently the procedure is nearly always performed within 30 minutes of the time of delivery of the infant.

Manual removal of the placenta has proved to be a safe procedure for patients in the following circumstances: if few vaginal examinations were performed during labor and if they were accompanied by a minimum of bacterial contamination; if the vulva, perineum, and adjacent areas were carefully prepared and draped prior to delivery; if delivery was accomplished without contaminating the lower genital tract or the obstetrician; and if satisfactory regional or general anesthesia is available. In other circumstances, since the risks of immediate manual removal of the placenta outweigh the advantages, the procedure should be limited to instances in which hemorrhage threatens.

Technic of Manual Removal. When this operation is required, aseptic surgical technic should be employed. After grasping the uterus through the abdominal wall with one hand, the other hand is introduced into the vagina and passed into the uterus, along the umbilical cord. As soon as the placenta is reached, its margin should be located, and the ulnar border of the hand insinuated between it and the uterine wall (Fig. 2). Then, with the back of the hand in contact with

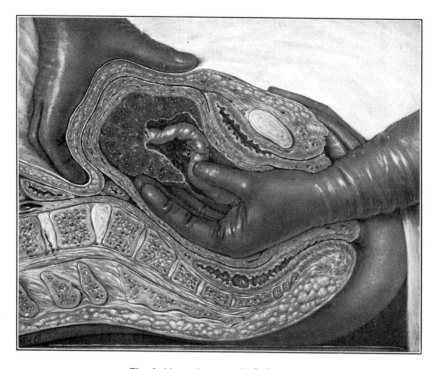

Fig. 2. Manual removal of placenta.

the uterus, the placenta should be peeled off its attachment by a motion similar to that employed in separating the leaves of a book. After its complete separation, the placenta should be grasped with the entire hand, but not extracted immediately. The operator should wait until the uterus contracts down firmly over his hand, which is then gradually withdrawn.

Placenta Accreta. Placenta accreta is an abnormal adherence of the placenta to the uterine wall, resulting from defective formation of decidua, with chorionic villi in direct contact with the uterine muscle (Fig. 3). In *placenta increta* the chorionic villi not only contact but actually penetrate the uterine muscle; in *placenta percreta* the chorionic villi penetrate the entire thickness of the uterine wall, reaching its serosa and sometimes rupturing into the peritoneal cavity. Placenta accreta may be complete or partial. The partial variety has been described in the preceding section of this chapter. Total placenta accreta is an extremely

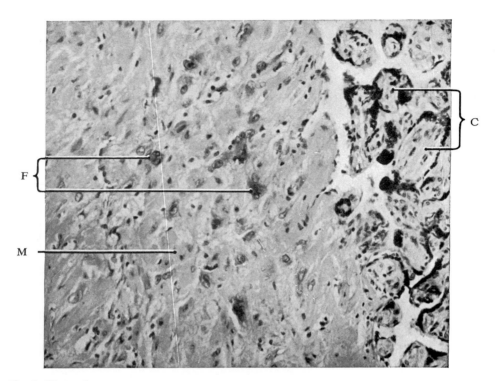

Fig. 3. Photomicrograph of uterine wall in case of placenta accreta, showing absence of decidua and invasion of myometrium by trophoblast. C, chorionic villi; F, trophoblastic giant cells; M, myometrium.

rare complication of the third stage. Kaltreider found only 177 cases in the literature up to 1945. In the course of over 70,000 deliveries at the Johns Hopkins Hospital, not a single case of complete placenta accreta was observed. Placenta increta and percreta are still more rare. Kistner, Hertig, and Reid, as well as James and Misch, reported several cases of placenta previa occurring with placenta accreta. Malkasian and Welsh have cited a case of placenta previa percreta.

Millar, as well as others, points up the salient histologic features of placenta accreta: (1) defective decidua, (2) a dense fibrin layer representing fusion of Nitabuch's and Rohr's striae, and (3) hyalinization of uterine muscle. The clinical characteristic of placenta accreta is its failure to separate from the uterus, unaccompanied by hemorrhage. Attempts to separate the placenta manually are futile. If persistent, they lead only to gouging the uterine muscle, with the obvious hazard of perforation. The usual treatment is immediate hysterectomy. It has recently again been suggested that no treatment be instituted in cases of placenta accreta and that the placenta be allowed to slough out. The results of this practice several decades ago were very unfavorable, but with modern antibiotics it may well have a place in the management of placenta accreta, especially in primiparas. McKeogh and D'Errico reported 13 patients with placenta accreta, 4 of whom were treated by hysterectomy and the other 9 conservatively. The only fatality occurred in the former group.

INVERSION OF THE UTERUS

This condition is a very rare but serious cause of postpartum shock. McCullagh estimates that it occurs about once in 30,000 labors. In our patients it has occurred once in the last 20,000 cases. Many obstetricians with large practices have never seen a case, but it is a much more frequent complication in areas of the world where obstetrics is practiced by ignorant midwives.

Occasionally the fundus of the uterus becomes inverted, contacting or protruding through the external os. Rarely, the entire organ appears outside of the vulva. The conditions are designated, *incomplete* and *complete inversion,* and *prolapse of the inverted uterus,* respectively (Figs. 4, 5, and 6). In certain cases the placenta remains attached to the inverted organ.

Etiology. Three factors are usually required to produce the accident: (1) markedly lax or thin uterine walls, particularly at the placental site; (2) pressure from above or traction on the cord or placenta; and (3) a patulous cervical canal. Fundal location of the placenta is said to be another predisposing factor (Das). Inversion may occur spontaneously as the result of increased intraabdomi-

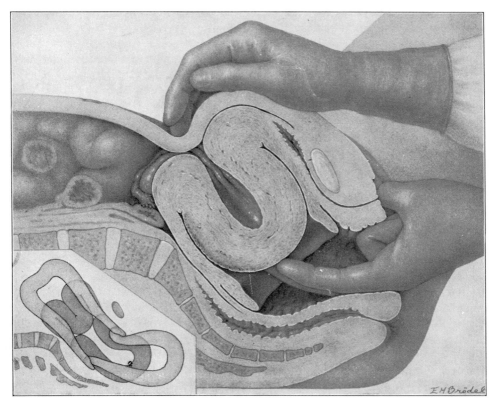

Fig. 4. Incomplete inversion of the uterus. Diagnosis by abdominal palpation of craterlike depression and vaginal palpation of tumor in the cervix. Insert shows progressive degrees of inversion.

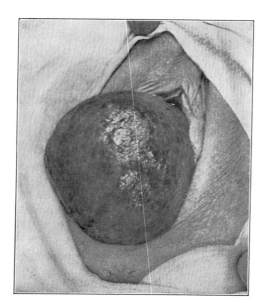

Fig. 5. Prolapse of the completely inverted uterus.

nal pressure, but in most cases it results from overly vigorous use of Credé's maneuver or traction upon the cord. Occasionally, inversion may recur in subsequent deliveries.

Although inversion of the uterus may rarely occur spontaneously, the accident usually results from faulty management of the third stage of labor. The complication usually follows labor at term, although certain cases are noted after abortion. More than 58 per cent of the cases collected by Bell, Wilson, and Wilson occurred in primigravidas.

Symptoms.   Inversion of the uterus is usually followed promptly by shock and a tendency to syncope. In many cases there are severe uterine pain and profuse hemorrhage. Signs and symptoms may sometimes be mild, however, and in rare instances the condition may continue for several days without serious annoyance to the patient. The commonly held view that the shock is out of proportion to the blood loss is probably incorrect. The patients we have observed with acute uterine inversion and shock have all suffered from severe postpartum hemorrhage.

Occasionally the cervix may contract so tightly about the completely inverted uterus that strangulation occurs, followed by gangrene. In other cases the condition becomes chronic, necessitating subsequent operative procedures.

Diagnosis.   The diagnosis of complete inversion of the uterus is usually simple, since the organ frequently protrudes through the vaginal orifice. Incomplete inversion, however, may remain unrecognized, unless careful abdominal palpation fails to reveal the fundus or shows a craterlike depression above or behind the symphysis. Unexplained shock following delivery should suggest inversion of the uterus and immediate vaginal examination to make the diagnosis.

Prognosis.   If the condition is detected promptly and the uterus replaced immediately, the prognosis is good. Bell, Wilson, and Wilson, in reviewing the American and British literature from 1940 to mid-1952, found 76 cases of puerperal inversion of the uterus, excluding their own 2 cases, and concluded that mortality seems to rise steadily as recognition is delayed up to 48 hours. If the

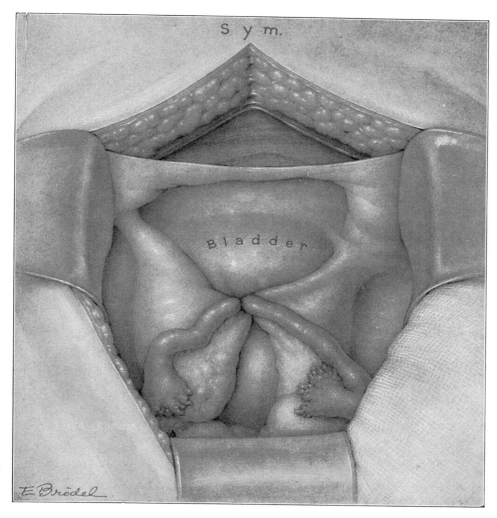

Fig. 6. Prolapse of the completely inverted uterus. Operative findings in same patient as shown in Figure 5.

patient with unrecognized inversion survives beyond 48 hours, however, the mortality rate declines sharply. There were 14 deaths in the series of 78 cases reviewed, an uncorrected maternal mortality rate of 17.9 per cent. In only 9 of the 14 deaths, however, was the inversion recognized. When effective therapy was instituted, the corrected mortality rate dropped to 12.3 per cent. With blood transfusion and antibiotics available, it appears that delay or failure in diagnosis is the major obstacle to further reduction of mortality.

Treatment.   Immediately following inversion, reposition can frequently be effected without difficulty according to the method of Johnson. He advises placing the entire hand in the vagina and making pressure at the junction of cervix and corpus with the tips of the fingers, and on the fundus with the palm. The entire uterus is then lifted out of the pelvis and kept above the level of the umbilicus. It is sometimes necessary to hold the uterus in this position from three to five minutes, but in any event the tension thus applied to the uterine ligaments will serve to reinvert the uterus. Since the procedure is generally painful, anesthesia should be employed. If several hours have elapsed, reposition may be difficult or impossible. In that event, the patient is usually in profound shock. It is advisable to begin treatment of shock before attempting any operative replacement of the inverted uterus. If at this stage the placenta is still attached to the fundus, it should be removed. Earlier removal of the placenta may, however, increase postpartum hemorrhage.

There are two principal types of corrective operations. The vaginal approach, for chronic inversion, credited to Spinelli, was actually described earlier by Küstner and by Kehrer. Vaginal correction of uterine inversion was reported even 10 years earlier by Browne from Baltimore. An abdominal approach, for both acute and chronic inversion, was devised by Haultain. In the abdominal operations, an incision is made through the posterior wall of the uterus at the site of the constricting ring. After the round ligaments are grasped with clamps, the uterus can generally be reinverted by gentle traction. The posterior defect in the uterine wall is then repaired. In Spinelli's operation for chronic inversion the bladder is dissected off the anterior uterine wall and cervix, and the anterior peritoneum is opened. The cervix and anterior uterine wall are then incised and the inversion corrected. After repair of the cervical and uterine defects, the body of the uterus is reposited in the peritoneal cavity, and the anterior vaginal wall is repaired.

References

Ahlfeld and Aschoff. (New studies of the etiology of placenta previa). Z Geburtsh Gynaek 51:544, 1904.

Beecham, C. T. Postpartum hemorrhage as a cause of death. Amer J Obstet Gynec 37:258, 1939.

Bell, J. E., Wilson, G. F., and Wilson, L. A. Puerperal inversion of the uterus. Amer J Obstet Gynec 66:767, 1953.

Browne, B. B. A new operation for the reduction of chronic inversion of the uterus. New York Med J 38:577, 1883.

Calkins, L. A., Litzenberg, J. C., and Plass, E. D. Management of the third stage of labor with special reference to blood loss. Amer J Obstet Gynec 21:175, 1931.

Cosgrove, S. A. Obstetric hemorrhage and its management. Southern Med J 29:1219, 1936.

Das, P. Inversion of the uterus. J Obstet Gynaec Brit Emp 47:525, 1940.

De Leeuw, N. K. M., Lowenstein, L., Tucker, E. C., and Dayal, S. Correlation of red cell loss at delivery with changes in red cell mass. Amer J Obstet Gynec 84:1271, 1962.

Donald, I. Practical Obstetric Problems, 3rd ed. Chicago, Year Book Publishers, 1964.

Doran, J. R., O'Brien, S. A., and Randall, J. H. Repeated postpartum hemorrhage. Obstet Gynec 5:186, 1955.

Douglas, R. G., and Davis, I. F. Puerperal infection. Etiologic, prophylactic and therapeutic considerations. Amer J Obstet Gynec 51:352, 1946.

Hamilton, G. Postpartum haemorrhage. Edinburgh Med J 7:313, 1861.

Haultain, F. W. N. The treatment of chronic uterine inversion by abdominal hysterectomy with a successful case. Brit Med J 2:974, 1901.

James, D. W., and Misch, K. A. Placenta accreta associated with placenta praevia. J Obstet Gynaec Brit Emp 62:551, 1955.

Johnson, A. B. A new concept in the replacement of the inverted uterus and a report of nine cases. Amer J Obstet Gynec 57:557, 1949.

Kaltreider, D. F.   Placenta accreta; report of a case. Bull Sch Med Univ Maryland, 30:1, 1945.

Kehrer, F. A.   (On the conservative surgical management of chronic inversion of the uterus.) Zbl Gynaek 22:297, 1898.

Kistner, R. W., Hertig, A. T., and Reid, D. E.   Simultaneously occurring placenta previa and placenta accreta. Surg Gynec Obstet 94:141, 1952.

Kurtz, G. R., Keating, W. J., and Loftus, J. B.   Twin pregnancy and delivery; analysis of 500 twin pregnancies. Obstet Gynec 6:370, 1955.

Küstner, O.   (Method of conservative management of chronic inversion of the puerperal uterus.) Zbl Gynaek 17:945, 1893.

Malkasian, G. D., and Welch, J. S.   Placenta previa percreta. Obstet Gynec 24:298, 1964.

McCullagh, W. McK. H.   Inversion of the uterus: a report of three cases and an analysis of 233 recently recorded cases. J Obstet Gynaec Brit Emp 32:280, 1925.

McKeogh, R. P., and D'Errico, E.   Placenta accreta: clinical manifestations and conservative management. New Eng J Med 245:159, 1951.

Menon, M. K. K.   A letter from India. Obstet Gynec Survey 23:407, 1968.

Millar, W. G.   A clinical and pathological study of placenta accreta. J Obstet Gynaec Brit Emp 66:353, 1959.

Newton, M.   Postpartum hemorrhage. Amer J Obstet Gynec 94:711, 1966.

Odell, L. D., and Seski, A.   Episiotomy blood loss. Amer J Obstet Gynec 54:51, 1947.

O'Leary, J. L., and O'Leary, J. A.   Uterine artery ligation in control of intractable postpartum hemorrhage. Amer J Obstet Gynec 94:920, 1966.

Pastore, J. B.   A study of the blood loss in the third stage of labor and the factors involved. Amer J Obstet Gynec 31:78, 1936.

Pritchard, J. A., Baldwin, R. M., Dickey, J. C., and Wiggins, K. M.   Blood volume changes in pregnancy and the puerperium. II. Red blood cell loss and changes in apparent blood volume during and following vaginal delivery, cesarean section, and cesarean section plus total hysterectomy. Amer J Obstet Gynec 84:1271, 1962.

Reich, A. M.   A critical analysis of blood loss following delivery with special reference to the value of ergotrate. Amer J Obstet Gynec 37:224, 1939.

Schneeberg, N. G., Perloff, W. H., and Israel, S. L.   Incidence of unsuspected "Sheehan's syndrome": hypopituitarism after postpartum hemorrhage and/or shock; clinical and laboratory study. JAMA 172:20, 1960.

Spinelli, P. G.   (Inversion of the uterus). Riv di Ginec Contemp 1:1, 1897.

Thomas, W. O.   Manual removal of the placenta. Amer J Obstet Gynec 86:600, 1963.

Waters, E. G.   Surgical management of postpartum hemorrhage with particular reference to ligation of uterine arteries. Amer J Obstet Gynec 64:1143, 1952.

34

PUERPERAL INFECTION

Definition. Puerperal infection is postpartum infection of the genital tract, usually of the endometrium, which may remain localized to the endometrium but often extends along various avenues to produce diverse clinical and pathologic pictures. Febrile reactions are the rule. The outcome varies according to the portal of entry; the type, virulence, and number of the invading organisms; the reaction of the tissues; and the general resistance of the patient. Commonly used but less satisfactory synonyms are puerperal fever, puerperal sepsis, puerperal septicemia, and childbed fever.

Since many elevations of temperature in the puerperium are caused by puerperal infection, the incidence of fever after childbirth is a reliable index of the incidence of the disease. For this reason it has been customary to group all puerperal fevers under the general term *puerperal morbidity* and to estimate the frequency of puerperal infection on this basis. Several definitions of puerperal morbidity have been established on the basis of the degree of pyrexia reached. The Joint Committee on Maternal Welfare, United States, has defined morbidity as a *"temperature of 100.4°F (38.0°C or higher), the temperature to occur on any two of the first ten days postpartum, exclusive of the first 24 hours, and to be taken by mouth by a standard technic at least four times daily."* This is probably the most commonly employed standard in the United States, but early discharge of puerperas from the hospital renders it less valuable today from the statistical standpoint.

This definition may suggest that all fever in the puerperium is caused by puerperal infection. Elevations in temperature may, however, be the result of extraneous causes, such as pyelonephritis and upper respiratory infections; for that reason, therefore, "corrected morbidity statistics" are sometimes reported. The practical difficulties of differentiating extraneous causes of fever from puerperal infection, however, are often great, depending upon a variable subjective factor. For this reason, total morbidity figures are unquestionably the most reliable index of the incidence of the disease. It should be the rule, moreover, to regard every fever in the puerperium as caused by puerperal infection unless positive proof can be advanced that it is the result of some extraneous cause.

History. Puerperal infection is referred to in the works of Hippocrates and Galen. In the seventeenth century, Willis wrote on the subject of *febris puerperarum*, although the English term "puerperal fever" was probably first employed by Strother in 1716.

The ancients regarded the affection as the result of retention of the lochia, and for centuries this explanation was universally accepted. In the early part of the seventeenth century metritis was thought to be the essential cause; the theory of "milk metastasis" of Puzos followed next. Until Semmelweis proved the identity of puerperal sepsis with wound infection and until Pasteur cultivated the streptococcus, and Lister demonstrated the value of antiseptic methods, many theories were suggested concerning the origin and nature of childbed fever. They are comprehensively discussed in the monographs of Eisenmann, Burtenshaw, and Peckham.

Although John Leake (1772) first made the suggestion of the contagiousness of puerperal infection, it remained for Alexander Hamilton to make the earliest positive statement on this subject in 1781. Alexander Gordon of Aberdeen clearly stated in a treatise on epidemic puerperal fever in 1795 the idea of the infectious and contagious nature of the disease, antedating the papers of Holmes and Semmelweis by a half-century. Charles White (1773) of Manchester believed puerperal fever to be an absorption fever dependent on stagnation of the lochia. He advised the semirecumbent posture to facilitate drainage and insisted on rigorous cleanliness and ventilation of the lying-in room and complete isolation of infected patients. Although many other British observers had vague ideas upon the subject, it was not until the middle of the nineteenth century that such views were strongly urged. In 1843, Oliver Wendell Holmes read a paper before the Boston Society for Medical Improvement, entitled "The Contagiousness of Puerperal Fever," in which he clearly showed that at least the epidemic forms of the affection could always be traced to the lack of proper precautions on the part of the physician or nurse. Four years later Semmelweis, then an assistant in the Vienna Lying-In Hospital, began a careful inquiry into the causes of the frightful mortality attending labor in that institution, as compared with the relatively small number of women succumbing to puerperal infection when delivered in their own homes. As a result of his investigations he concluded that the morbid process was essentially a wound infection caused by the introduction of septic material by the examining finger. Acting upon this idea he issued stringent orders that the physicians, students, and midwives disinfect their hands with chlorine water, the forerunner of Dakin's solution, before examining parturient women. In spite of immediate surprising results, the mortality falling from over 10 to 1 per cent, both his work and that of Holmes were scoffed at by many of the most prominent men of the time, and his discovery remained unappreciated until the influence of Lister's teachings and the development of bacteriology had brought about a revolution in the treatment of wounds.

Although epidemics of puerperal infection have occurred in hospitals of the United States in recent times (Watson, 1927; Jewett and colleagues, 1968), the advent of effective antimicrobial therapy and prophylaxis has rendered serious infections uncommon today. For example, Douglas and Stromme reported a decline in the total frequency of puerperal infection in the New York Hospital from 11.2 per cent in 1934 to 1.4 per cent in 1956. Hill indicated that the incidence of death from puerperal infection in Melbourne, Australia, declined from 1 in 340 deliveries in 1931 to 1 in 36,000 in 1960. Many factors other than antimicrobial drugs have played a role in this salutary change. The following changes in practice have doubtless contributed as much as or more than drug therapy to the virtual conquest of this former scourge: marked reduction in traumatic operative delivery and excessively long labors, aseptic technic, effective use of blood transfusions, and better general health of parturients.

In view of the increasing number and prevalence of virulent, antibiotic-resistant strains of bacteria, it is important for all personnel attending obstetric patients to be familiar with the bacteriology of puerperal infection. The 1968 epidemic at the Boston Hospital for Women (Lying-in Division) is an example. As the fear of infecting a parturient by cross-contamination (once considered the most likely source of epidemic) has given way to overconfidence in antibiotics, aseptic technics have too often been replaced by carelessness.

BACTERIOLOGY

Organisms responsible for puerperal infection may be introduced from exogenous sources or may be normal inhabitants of the genital tract. The endogenous infections constitute by far the largest group. Table 1 shows the incidence of the organisms cultured from 241 cases of puerperal infection in which the patients were delivered operatively. In this series the anaerobic streptococcus, a normal inhabitant of the birth canal, was the causative organism in over half the cases.

Table 1. Organisms Cultured in Postoperative Puerperal Infection

Organism	Number	Per Cent
Anaerobic streptococcus	144	60.0
Aerobic nonhemolytic streptococcus	58	24.0
Escherichia coli	55	22.8
Staphylococcus albus	43	18.0
Anaerobic staphylococcus	29	12.0
Streptococcus viridans	29	12.0
Anaerobic diphtheroid	24	9.9
Aerobic diphtheroid	19	7.8
Alpha[1] streptococcus	14	5.8
Staphylococcus aureus	8	3.3
Anaerobic gram-negative rods	7	2.9
Clostridium perfringens (welchii)	6	2.4
Aerobacter aerogenes	4	1.6
Proteus vulgaris	4	1.6
Beta hemolytic streptococcus	4	1.6
Enterococcus	2	0.8
Candida albicans	2	0.8
Gonococcus	1	0.4
Klebsiella pneumoniae	1	0.4
Pneumococcus, Type IV	1	0.4
No growth	14	5.8

Modified from Douglas and Stromme. Operative Obstetrics, 2nd ed. New York, Appleton-Century-Crofts, 1965.

Anaerobic Streptococcus.   The most common cause of puerperal infection in general is the anaerobic streptococcus, an organism frequently found in the vaginas of normal pregnant women. Weinstein, using special culture media (cystine-glucose agar), found anaerobic streptococci in the vagina of 93 per cent of normal pregnant women. They are encountered very frequently also in uterine cultures from normal, afebrile puerperas. Guilbeau and Schaub demonstrated them in 81.3 per cent of patients during the first three days of the puerperium, and Wierdsma and Clayton in 34 per cent. The anaerobic streptococcus is ordinarily nonpathogenic; the determining factor in its becoming pathogenic and invading the maternal tissues appears to be traumatized, devitalized tissues, which provide an environment of low oxidation-reduction potential, where the organisms can multiply rapidly. This circumstance should logically lead to greater restraint and greater gentleness in operative interference.

Beta Hemolytic Streptococcus. As seen in Table 1, the beta hemolytic streptococcus, despite its virulence in the past, is now rarely a cause of puerperal infection. It is a relatively uncommon inhabitant of the vagina of pregnant women according to Slotnick, Hildebrandt, and Prystowsky, who found it 4 times in 79 cervical cultures of 10 women at various times during pregnancy, and in about 15 per cent of their patients in labor. Probably the past epidemics of puerperal infection were caused by virulent beta hemolytic streptococci introduced from an outside source. The reservoir of such organisms has no doubt been reduced during the years of widespread antibiotic therapy.

Streptococcus faecalis (Enterococcus). These bacteria are normally found in the gastrointestinal tract and may be harbored in the vagina. Slotnick, Hildebrandt, and Prystowsky cultured enterococcus from the cervix of 3 per cent of patients in labor and 11 per cent of parturients during the first 48 hours following delivery. In cases of puerperal infection the enterococcus usually occurs in combination with other organisms.

Staphylococcus. Staphylococci are becoming an increasingly common cause of puerperal infection, including stitch abscesses in perineal and vaginal wounds. Douglas and Stromme found it to be the fourth commonest organism in puerperal infection, and Slotnick, Hildebrandt, and Prystowsky found coagulase-positive staphylococci in 4 per cent of normal patients on admittance in labor and 2 per cent of postpartum patients. Similar findings are cited by Calman and Gibson.

Coliform Organisms. *Escherichia coli* and related gram-negative bacilli, including *Aerobacter and Klebsiella*, are increasingly common organisms associated with puerperal infections. Often other bacteria are found with the coliform organisms. The misconception prevails that a very foul smell to pus indicates a coliform infection, but the odor is often caused by other bacteria, most likely anaerobic streptococci or bacteroides. Bacteremia resulting from these organisms can lead to classic endotoxin shock.

Bacteroides. These strictly anaerobic gram-negative bacteria are normally found in the intestinal tract and are present in large numbers in the feces. They are not highly invasive organisms but may cause infection at the site of trauma or a surgical procedure. When bacteroides are identified during the puerperium or following abortion, they are often part of a mixed infection, which includes anaerobic streptococci. Characteristically fetid pus is formed, at times in large amounts; bacteroides infection should therefore be considered whenever pus with a very foul odor is encountered. Without appropriate therapy suppurative thrombophlebitis adjacent to the site of the initial infection is likely to occur. It may, in turn, cause septic emboli and abscesses in the lung, brain, kidney, liver, joints, and elsewhere. Pearson and Anderson have recently reported their extensive experiences with bacteroides infections complicating pregnancy. Bacteremia was identified in half of the cases in which bacteroides infected the genital tract.

Clostridium perfringens. The clostridia are a rare cause of puerperal infection, but the striking course and the high mortality that usually attend such infections in the puerperium make these organisms of signal interest to the obstetrician. Clostridia are normal inhabitants of the intestinal tract. Difference of opinion has been expressed concerning the presence of the clostridia in the birth canal of healthy pregnant women, but some studies indicate that about 1 gravida in 20 harbors the organism in the vagina. Sadusk and Manahan studied the prevalence of *Clostridium perfringens* in the vaginas of normal pregnant women and attempted to ascertain its virulence. In 219 patients the organism was isolated in 19, or 8.7 per cent; in 9 of these 19 cases the organism was lethal to a guinea pig in less than 48 hours.

The variation in pathogenicity of the organism is enormous. On the one hand, it may produce a catastrophic clinical picture: rapid hemolysis, profound vasomotor collapse, metastatic gas gangrene, and sometimes death within 24 hours. On the other hand, it is sometimes harmless. Although the virulences of different strains of *Clostridium perfringens* vary greatly, the most important determining factor in the production of an infection is traumatized and devitalized tissue, which provides the anaerobic environment necessary for this organism to multiply. Most serious infections associated with pregnancy, therefore, follow criminal abortion or traumatic operative delivery. The organism liberates a number of exotoxins and enzymes. The major alpha-toxin is a lecithinase that causes local necrosis of muscle as well as intense intravascular hemolysis. Saccharolytic enzymes break down muscle glycogen with release of hydrogen, causing the characteristic clinical picture of gas gangrene.

Gonococcus. The gonococcus is a rare cause of puerperal infection, producing acute or subacute salpingitis. Even then, the process is usually an exacerbation of chronic pelvic inflammatory disease rather than an initial infection.

Pneumococcus. Formerly the pneumococcus was an occasional cause of a lethal type of puerperal infection, as reported by Nuckols and Hertig. Most cases were secondary to pneumococcal infections elsewhere in the body, such as lobar pneumonia, otitis media, or nasopharyngitis. Antimicrobial therapy has virtually eliminated this form of puerperal infection.

Salmonella typhosa. Although the typhoid bacillus is occasionally found in uterine cultures, it is almost always associated with some other organism, often an anaerobic streptococcus. It is much less virulent in the birth canal than in the intestinal tract.

Clostridium tetani. Puerperal tetanus is very rare today, but 210 cases of postabortal tetanus and 114 cases of postpartum tetanus were reported in the review by Adams and Morton in 1955.

Diphtheroids. Diphtheroid organisms may be found in the lochia, particularly in mixed cultures. They appear to be normal, nonpathogenic inhabitants of the birth canal.

MODES OF INFECTION

Often the physician himself carries infection to the parturient uterus. He may do so in two ways. First, although his hands may be covered with sterile gloves, he may carry the already present anaerobic streptococcus from the vagina to the uterus through vaginal examinations or operative manipulations. Second, his hands and instruments may become contaminated by virulent organisms as the result of droplet infection, dispersed by himself or some of the attendants. The nose and mouth of all attendants in the delivery room should therefore be covered, and all persons with upper respiratory infection should be excluded. It is still possible for the careless attendant to carry infections from one patient (or from himself) to another.

Coitus late in pregnancy may rupture the membranes and introduce bacteria into the birth canal. Some serious cases of puerperal infection begin in this way.

Predisposing Causes

The most important predisposing causes of puerperal infection are hemorrhage and trauma during labor. Spontaneous delivery with minimal blood loss is rarely followed by fever, but women who have suffered serious hemorrhage become infected more easily. The treatment of obstetric hemorrhage, furthermore, may entail intrauterine manipulations, which often introduce infection. Trauma may potentiate the effects of hemorrhage by creating additional portals of entry for bacteria and by leading to necrosis of tissue.

Labors lasting more than 24 hours, particularly if the membranes have been ruptured throughout most of the period, provide vaginal bacteria with readier and more prolonged access to the uterus, promote exhaustion, and are followed by an increased incidence of puerperal infection. Since such cases are often terminated by difficult operative means, the triad of exhaustion, trauma, and hemorrhage creates optimal conditions for bacterial growth.

Retention of the placenta, in whole or in part, predisposes to infection in a number of ways. First, vigorous and repeated efforts to express the placenta may traumatize the uterus. Second, manual removal of the placenta may convey bacteria to the most vulnerable site in the uterus. Finally, if small fragments of placenta and membranes are retained, they may undergo necrosis and readily become infected. Usually superimposed on these accidents of the third stage is hemorrhage.

Severe anemia, undernutrition, and debilitation in general make puerperal infection more likely. Bickerstaff has shown that the incidence of puerperal morbidity is in direct proportion to the degree of anemia in the last month of pregnancy.

Although it is important to avoid as many of the preceding complications as possible and adequately to replace blood when indicated, nothing is gained by prophylactic antibiotics. On the contrary, indiscriminate use of these drugs may encourage the growth of virulent, resistant strains of organisms. Furthermore, the patient may be needlessly sensitized, or she may develop a fungal infection. Fatal monilial septicemia has been reported (Masterson, Nelson, and Valenti) in gynecologic patients.

Pathology

After completion of the third stage of labor, the area of placental attachment is raw and elevated, deep red, and about 4 cm in diameter. Its surface is made nodular by the numerous veins, many of which are occluded by thrombi. This area is an excellent culture medium for bacteria and the most common portal of entry for pathogenic organisms. At this time, furthermore, the entire decidua is peculiarly susceptible to bacterial invasion, since it is less than 2 mm in thickness, is infiltrated with blood, and presents numerous small openings. Since the cervix rarely escapes some degree of laceration in labor, it is another ready site for bacterial invasion. Vulvar, vaginal, and perineal wounds provide additional portals of entry.

The lesions of puerperal infection are basically wound infections. The inflammatory process may remain localized in these wounds or may extend through the blood or lymphatics to tissues far beyond the initial lesion. Whether such extension occurs is the determining factor in the pathologic changes and in the whole clinical course, prognosis, and treatment of the disease. Puerperal infection is divided into two main categories according to the means of extension:

1. Local inflammatory lesions of the perineum, vulva, vagina, cervix, and endometrium.
2. Extensions of the original process along the veins to produce thrombophlebitis and pyemia, through the lymph vessels to produce peritonitis and parametritis, and along the surface of the endometrium and endosalpinx to produce salpingitis.

Lesions of the Perineum, Vulva, Vagina, and Cervix. A common puerperal lesion of the external genitalia is a localized infection of a repaired laceration or episiotomy wound. The opposing wound edges become red, brawny, and swollen; the sutures cut through the edematous tissues, allowing the necrotic edges of the wound to gape, with the result that greenish yellow pus exudes from the wound. In this manner, complete breakdown of the wound may occur, with profuse serous and purulent discharge. After traumatic operative delivery, wounds and contusions of the vulva are common; the entire vulva may become edematous, ulcerated, and covered with a grayish exudate. Lacerations of the vagina are very common after operative delivery and may become infected directly or by extension from the perineum. The mucous membrane becomes swollen and intensely red; slough and necrotic debris result, and purulent secretions are discharged in large amounts from ulcerated areas. A pseudodiphtheritic membrane occasionally forms, as in vulvar lesions. Extension may occur by infiltration, resulting in lymphangitis, but as a rule the infection remains local. It is, however, occasionally followed by large cicatrices of the vagina.

Cervical infection is probably rather common. Moreover, since deep lacerations of the cervix often extend directly into the tissue at the base of the broad ligament, infection of such wounds may form the starting point for lymphatic infection, parametritis, and bacteremia.

Endometritis. The most common manifestation of puerperal infection is endometritis. After an incubation period of a few hours to several days, the bacteria invade the tissues of an endometrial wound, usually at the placental site. The blood vessels and lymphatics in the vicinity of the infected area become engorged and infection spreads rapidly to involve the entire endometrium. If the process is limited to the endometrium, the superficial necrotic tissues are cast off within about a week.

The appearance of the endometrium varies widely. In some cases the necrotic mucosa sloughs, the debris is abundant, and the discharge is foul, profuse, bloody, and sometimes frothy. The necrotic material covering the endometrium is yellowish green, as a rule, but may be black from decomposed blood. The cervix is usually involved, and its lacerations may ulcerate and slough. As a rule, involution is greatly retarded. Microscopic sections show a thick superficial layer of necrotic material containing bacteria, and a thick zone of leukocytic infiltration above the normal tissue. In puerperal infection of long duration, secondary abscesses in the lungs and elsewhere may lead to death, although the endometrium in such cases appears normal at autopsy.

Thrombophlebitis and Pyemia.   In modern obstetrics the most common mode of extension of puerperal infection is along the veins, with resultant thrombophlebitis (Fig. 1). From 30 to 50 per cent of all deaths from puerperal infection are attributable to this type of extension. At the Johns Hopkins Hospital, 41 per cent of the fatal cases of puerperal infection were associated with thrombophlebitis. Halban and Köhler, in autopsies of 163 women who died from puerperal infection, found 82 instances of thrombophlebitis; in 36, it was the only mode of extension, whereas in 46 there was a coexisting lymphatic involvement. Thrombophlebitis results because the placental site is a mass of thrombosed veins and because the anaerobic streptococcus, which is frequently a normal inhabitant of the vagina, thrives in the anaerobic medium provided by venous thrombi.

Two groups of veins are principally involved: (1) the veins of the uterine wall and broad ligament (the ovarian, uterine, and hypogastric veins) and (2) the veins of the leg (femoral, popliteal, and saphenous). Inflammation of the former is *pelvic thrombophlebitis,* and of the latter *femoral thrombophlebitis.* The pathology, clinical course, and treatment of the two conditions differ widely. Femoral thrombophlebitis is discussed in Chapter 35 (p. 1001).

The vein most commonly involved in pelvic thrombophlebitis is the ovarian, since it drains the upper part of the uterus, which most often includes the veins of the placental site. The process is usually unilateral, with one side affected as often as the other. Extension of the process into the left ovarian vein may reach its junction with the renal vein with involvement of that vessel and consequent renal complications. If the right ovarian vein is affected, the thrombosis may extend well into the inferior vena cava. Not infrequently, thrombosis of uterine veins eventually extends far into the common iliac vessels.

As the inflammation progresses, the thrombosis extends higher, a mechanism designed to prevent wide dissemination of the infecting organisms. Thrombosis of the infected vein may limit the advance of the infection, and the thrombus may undergo organization. In other cases, the thrombus may suppurate, while the surrounding venous wall becomes edematous and necrotic. As the process continues, small emboli are hematogenously disseminated to various parts of the body, giving rise to *pyemia.* The most common secondary sites in pelvic thrombophlebitis are the lungs, the kidneys, and the cardiac valves. Rarely, large emboli may reach the pulmonary artery and cause sudden death. More often, small emboli reach the terminal branches of the pulmonary vessels and produce infected hemorrhagic infarcts. Pulmonary abscesses are frequent sequelae, found at autopsy in more than one half of such cases. Pleurisy and pneumonia are also common.

Peritonitis.   Puerperal infection may extend by way of the lymphatics of the uterine wall to reach either the peritoneum or the loose cellular tissues between the leaves of the broad ligaments (Fig. 2), in the former instance producing a peritonitis and in the latter a parametritis. The peritonitis may be localized to the pelvis or generalized. In either case the peritonitis may result either from direct involvement of the peritoneum through the lymphatics of the uterine wall, or from secondary extension to the peritoneum of thrombophlebitis or parametritis.

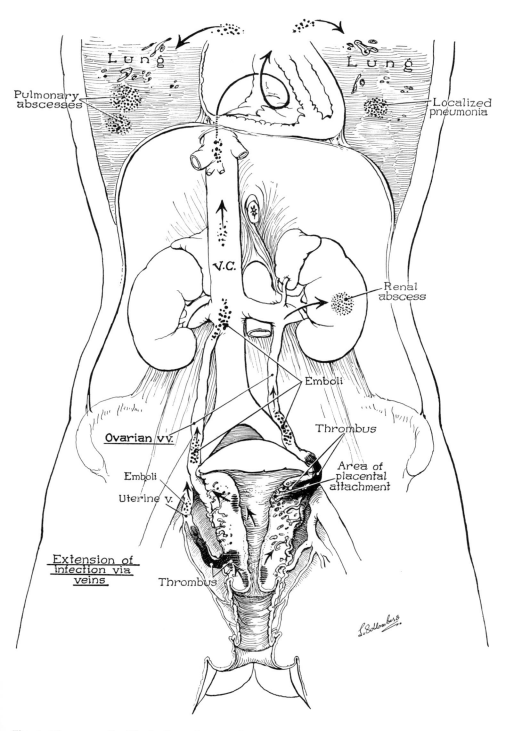

Fig. 1. Diagrammatic illustration of extension of puerperal infection in uterine thrombophlebitis.

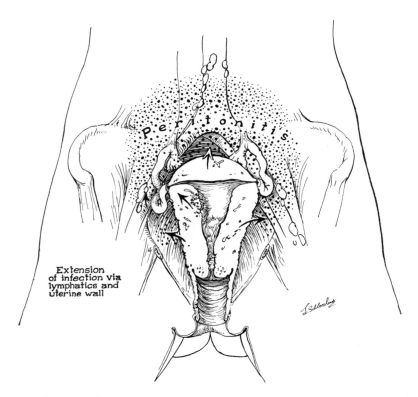

Fig. 2. Diagrammatic illustration of extension of puerperal infection in peritonitis.

Rarely, in these circumstances, pelvic peritonitis may be produced by escape of pus from the lumen of a fallopian tube.

Generalized peritonitis, one of the gravest complications of childbearing, is the cause of death in about one third of the fatal cases of infection. Fibrinopurulent exudate binds loops of bowel to one another, and locules of pus may form between the loops or in the pelvis. The pouch of Douglas, the subdiaphragmatic space, and the fold between the infundibulopelvic and broad ligaments are common sites for such accumulations. In general, the more virulent the causative organism, the less is the peritoneal reaction. For example, in peritonitis caused by the beta hemolytic streptococcus, the peritoneum may be only reddened with little exudate, whereas with organisms of lower virulence the peritoneal cavity may become filled with pus. In such cases frank bacteremia may result.

Pelvic Cellulitis (Parametritis).   Infection of the loose fibroareolar pelvic connective tissue may occur in three main ways. (1) It is most commonly caused by the lymphatic transmission of organisms from an infected cervical laceration. Similar lymphatic extension from an endometritis may also be responsible but is probably less frequent. Although lacerations of the perineum or vagina may be a cause of localized cellulitis, the process is usually limited to the paravaginal cellular tissue, rarely extending deeply into the pelvis (Fig. 3). (2) Since cervical

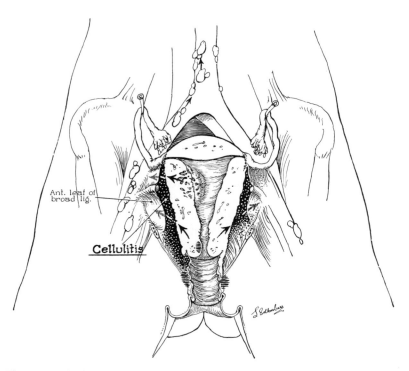

Fig. 3. Diagrammatic illustration of extension of puerperal infection in pelvic cellulitis (parametritis).

lacerations not infrequently extend well into the connective tissue at the base of the broad ligaments, this tissue may be laid bare to direct invasion by pathogenic organisms in the vagina. Similar results are frequently seen in cases of criminal abortion in which a sharp instrument has created a false passage into the para-cervical connective tissue. (3) Pelvic cellulitis may be secondary to pelvic thrombophlebitis, which is rarely unaccompanied by some degree of cellulitis. If the thrombi become purulent, the venous wall may undergo necrosis and large numbers of organisms may be discharged into the surrounding connective tissue. As a rule, the organisms involved are either the coliform bacillus, the anaerobic streptococcus, or coagulase-positive staphylococci.

The process may remain limited to the base of the broad ligament, but if the inflammatory reaction is more intense, the exudate may be forced along natural lines of cleavage. The most common form of extension is directly laterally, along the base of the broad ligament, with a tendency to extend to the lateral pelvic wall. As the mass increases in size, it distends the leaves of the broad ligament and, raising the anterior leaf upward, dissects its way forward to reach the abdominal wall just above Poupart's ligament. The uterus is pushed toward the opposite side and fixed. In other cases, high intraligamentous exudates spread from the region of the uterine cornua to the iliac fossae. Retrocervical exudates tend to involve the rectovaginal septum with the development of a firm mass posterior to the cervix. Occasionally, involvement of the connective tissue anterior to the cervix results in a cellulitis of the space of Retzius with extension upward, beneath the anterior abdominal wall, as high as the umbilicus. Rarely the process may extend out through the sciatic foramen into the thigh.

Inflammatory exudates in the pelvic connective tissue follow an indolent course but ultimately undergo either suppuration or, more commonly, resolution. If suppuration occurs, the most frequent outcome is "pointing" just above Poupart's ligament. The skin over the inguinal region becomes edematous, red, and tender, until fluctuation indicates that the abscess is ready for incision or rupture. A somewhat less common outcome is "pointing" in the posterior cul-de-sac. A high intraligamentous abscess may also rupture directly into the peritoneal cavity.

Pelvic cellulitis is usually unilateral, but it involves both sides in about one case in four. It is encountered at autopsy in about one third of all fatal cases of puerperal infection, sometimes alone but more often in association with thrombophlebitis or peritonitis.

Other Modes of Extension.   Bacteremia frequently accompanies pelvic thrombophlebitis, peritonitis, and, to a lesser extent, pelvic cellulitis. Whenever bloodstream infection complicates puerperal infection, it almost invariably results from one of these three processes. In rare instances, however, when the organisms are exceedingly virulent and the resistance of the host very weak, the patient may be overwhelmed by rapidly invading bacteria, and death may follow quickly. Occasionally, small abscesses in the myometrium develop, secondary to either thrombophlebitis or lymphatic infection. Extension to the peritoneal surface often occurs with the formation of adhesions to surrounding structures; less commonly, direct perforation into the peritoneal cavity ensues with resulting peritonitis. *Metritis dissecans,* or *gangrene of the uterus,* is a rare and grave form of puerperal infection in which not only the endometrium but also part of the myometrium may undergo necrosis. In some cases the entire endometrium is detached and expelled as a complete cast of the uterine cavity. Clinically the condition is characterized by the expulsion of large pieces of necrotic tissue, usually during the second or third week of the puerperium.

CLINICAL COURSE

Lesions of the Perineum, Vulva, Vagina, and Cervix.   Pain, burning on urination, and a sensation of local heat are the common symptoms. Provided drainage is good, the reaction in these local conditions is seldom severe, the temperature remaining below 101°F and the pulse rate under 100. If, however, purulent material is dammed back by perineal or vaginal suture, the complication may be signalized by a chill and a sharp rise of fever to 104°F or 105°F.

Endometritis.   The clinical picture of puerperal endometritis varies with the type and virulence of the offending organism, the resistance of the host, the degree of trauma to the genital tract, and the freedom of drainage of the uterine cavity. Often the cases are mild with only moderate malaise and slight elevation of temperature. There is usually retention of lochia and possibly of fragments of placenta or membrane. When there is free drainage or artificial removal of this culture material, the signs and symptoms disappear rapidly. Other cases are ushered in by a chill, fever between 104°F and 105°F, and other evidence of a fulminating infection. In the average case, the temperature begins to rise about 48 hours postpartum and mounts with morning remissions, in sawtooth fashion, to reach levels between 101°F and 103°F on the fourth or fifth day. The pulse rate tends to follow the temperature curve, but in grave infections it is usually rapid from the first. The uterus is almost always large, but occasionally it may involute satisfactorily despite frank endometritis. There is tenderness over the uterus, and afterpains are frequently severe and prolonged. Even in the early stages there are changes in the lochia, from which the infecting organism may often be cultured. As a rule, the discharge is increased and hemorrhagic or dark brown. An offensive smell, long regarded as an important sign of endometrial infection, results from invasion of the uterine cavity by putrefactive bacteria, particularly certain strains of anaerobic streptococci and bacteroides. Some infections, however, notably beta hemolytic streptococcal endometritis, are frequently associated with scanty, odorless lochia. Indeed, the gravity of a case of endometritis may sometimes be in almost *inverse* proportion to the amount and putridity of the lochia. Leukocytosis may range from 15,000 to 30,000 cells per cubic millimeter, but in view of the physiologic leukocytosis of the puerperium these figures are difficult to interpret. In simple endometritis, blood cultures are almost invariably negative; a positive culture points to lymphatic or thrombophlebitic extension.

The symptoms of endometritis are variable. Many patients feel well, with no complaints whatsoever. The common symptoms are headache, varying degrees of insomnia, and anorexia. Except in very mild cases, secretion of milk may be suppressed. Chills may occur at the onset of endometritis, but after the first day or two they invariably mean extension, usually thrombophlebitis. If the process remains localized in the endometrium, the temperature falls by lysis, the uterine discharge diminishes, and by the end of a week, or at the most ten days, the infection is over. Simple endometritis is often misdiagnosed as a urinary tract infection.

Pelvic Cellulitis. Minor degrees of pelvic cellulitis (parametritis) are a very common cause of prolonged, sustained fever in the puerperium; whenever steady elevations of temperature persist for longer than a week, the condition should be suspected. In mild cases the findings are limited to moderate but persistent elevations of temperature in association with local tenderness. The involvement of the parametrium may be marked by a chill, but more often it is difficult to ascertain precisely when the extension occurred, the course apparently representing merely the continuation of the original endometrial infection. The height of the temperature varies with the degree of cellulitis but, in the average case, runs around 102°F with moderate morning remission. There is pain or tenderness in one or both sides of the abdomen and marked tenderness on vaginal examination. As the process advances, other findings on vaginal examination become more characteristic, such as fixation of the uterus by the parametrial exudate or induration in the fornices, and the development of a hard, unyielding mass in the broad ligament. The exudate may extend upward and an area of resistance may be felt along the upper border of Poupart's ligament. Not infrequently it extends backward into the lower part of the broad ligament along the sacrouterine folds and into the cellular tissue surrounding the uterus. In these cases a rectal examination is very helpful in diagnosis.

Absorption of the exudate occurs in about two thirds of the cases, but it may require several weeks. In this process the swelling often becomes stony hard and gradually diminishes in size from week to week. Not infrequently the final result is dense scar tissue in the parametrium. Suppuration of the parametrial mass occurs in the remaining third of the cases; it too is a slow process. Pointing of the abscess may not occur until six or eight weeks after the commencement of the illness. Suppuration may be suspected in the following circumstances: a change to a steady temperature curve, often in association with chills; spontaneous, intense pain; leukocytosis in excess of 20,000; and general deterioration of the patient, with rapid loss of weight and a characteristic sallow complexion. As the abscess points above Poupart's ligament, the skin becomes red and edematous. After the abscess has been drained, recovery is usually prompt.

Pelvic Thrombophlebitis.   The clinical picture of pelvic thrombophlebitis is characterized by repeated, severe chills, hectic temperature swings, a tendency toward distant spread (particularly in the lungs), and a prolonged course. Chills are a constant feature of the disease; the initial chill is likely to be very severe, lasting 30 or 40 minutes; the interval between chills may be only a few hours but is sometimes as long as three days. The swings in temperature are often enormous, with steep climbs from 96.0°F to 105.0°F, followed by a precipitous fall within an hour. Although the onset is ordinarily in the second week, a survey of the temperature chart will almost always show that the condition has been preceded by a low-grade fever. Between the episodes of chills and high fever, the patient may look and feel well. Pelvic examination helps little, as a rule, since the vein most commonly affected, the ovarian, is not reached on palpation. Although leukocytosis is sometimes present, in our experience these patients may have white counts under 10,000. Bacteria are present in the bloodstream during the chills, but positive blood cultures are notoriously hard to obtain because the offending organisms are often anaerobic and, therefore, difficult to culture. The optimal time to take the blood is early in the chill or, if possible, just before the chill begins.

Pulmonary complications are common, particularly infarction, abscesses, pleurisy, and pneumonia. The next most common site is the left kidney, involvement of which is marked, as a rule, by sudden renal pain followed by proteinuria and hematuria. The joints, eyes, subcutaneous tissues, and bone may also be affected by mycotic emboli. As these infections are established, the temperature curve becomes steadier.

The typical case of pelvic thrombophlebitis formerly lasted between one and three months, with a fatal outcome in about half the cases. With modern antimicrobial therapy both the mortality and the duration of the disease have been reduced. The common cause of death was a pulmonary complication, usually a combination of vascular blockade by septic emboli, infarction, pneumonitis, and abscesses.

Peritonitis.   Puerperal peritonitis resembles surgical peritonitis in general, except that abdominal rigidity is slight or absent. In general peritonitis the symptoms seldom appear later than the third day. These are a definite chill, a temperature from 103°F to 105°F or over without marked remissions, and a pulse rate of 140 per minute or more, which soon becomes weak and compressible. Pain may be excruciating; tympanites is frequently associated with paralytic ileus, but intractable and exhausting diarrhea may occur. Vomiting is frequent, eventually stercoraceous, and often projectile. Bacteremia is invariable, and consequent pulmonary involvement frequent. Delirium and coma usually precede death. Sometimes, shortly before death, the temperature drops from 105°F or over to below normal, crossing on the chart the rapidly mounting pulse line, and thereby forming the so-called cross of death. Occasionally, grave symptoms may be entirely absent; the patient seems euphoric, and only from the facies and the rapid and thready pulse may the true gravity of the situation be deduced. Rarely in the course of pelvic cellulitis an abscess may rupture into the peritoneal cavity and catastrophically produce general peritonitis. Septic shock may occur in the puerperium, as it does after abortion (see Ch. 20, p. 521).

Salpingitis.   Initial attacks of gonorrheal salpingitis during the puerperium are rare, most instances of puerperal salpingitis representing exacerbations of old infections. The onset occurs late, ordinarily between the ninth and fifteenth days, and is characterized by pain and tenderness in the lower abdomen, usually bilateral, together with fever around 103°F or 104°F. Rebound tenderness is likely to occur as the result of pelvic peritonitis. Chills are uncommon. Involvement of a joint, usually a knee or a wrist, may clinch the diagnosis in the small number of cases in which it is found.

The life of the patient is rarely jeopardized, the acute symptoms subsiding within a week or two as a rule. Residual changes in the tubes frequently lead to chronic gynecologic symptoms. Sterility may ensue as the result of tubal closure, the so-called one-child sterility. Such sterility, however, is much more frequently the result of gonorrhea contracted subsequently than of gonorrheal salpingitis developing in the puerperium.

Clostridium perfringens.   The classical picture of puerperal infection caused by *Cl. perfringens* is catastrophic. Within two or three days after delivery, or much more commonly after abortion, the patient develops jaundice, which is accompanied by slightly dusky cyanosis of the fingers and toes. Within a few hours the skin and conjunctivae may become darkened to a bronze or mahogany color. The temperature averages between 101°F and 102°F, but it may be elevated, normal, or even subnormal. The pulse rate, however, is 140 or above. The patient sinks into extreme prostration, and within a few hours to a day or two, the cyanosis deepens, circulatory collapse ensues, and the respirations become rapid and shallow. Consciousness, however, is usually remarkably clear to the end. Catheterization yields but scant port-wine-colored urine, which contains hemoglobin. Anemia often progresses with enormous rapidity. A fall in the erythrocyte count of over two million may occur within six hours. Leukocytosis, which is the rule, is often extreme. Renal failure is a virtually constant finding, with a great rise in the blood urea nitrogen, if the patient survives long enough. Although gas in the subcutaneous tissues or uterus has long been regarded as an important diagnostic sign, it is demonstrable antemortem in only one fourth or one fifth of cases. Not infrequently the gas manifests itself by excruciating pain in skeletal muscles before crepitus can be elicited. When it is widespread ("metastatic gas gangrene"), the course is extremely rapid; death may ensue within ten hours after the onset of the pain in the muscles. Before modern antimicrobial agents were available, the severer forms of puerperal clostridial infection were almost uniformly fatal within five or six days; even the "milder" types carried a mortality of about 20 per cent. Today the results are good, unless hemolysis and oliguria have supervened. Antitoxin has not proved valuable in this infection.

Most fevers occurring after childbirth are caused by puerperal infection. This diagnosis should be assigned to all puerperal elevations of temperature unless there is incontrovertible proof that the fever is the result of an extragenital infection.

The diagnosis of puerperal infection can often be made without difficulty, especially if the preceding labor has been attended by extensive vaginal or uterine manipulation. In mild cases, however, fever may be the only sign. In any event, every puerperal woman whose temperature rises to 100.4°F should be given a complete examination to rule out extrapelvic causes of fever and to establish the diagnosis by exclusion.

The most common extragenital causes of fever in the puerperium are respiratory infections (influenza, tonsillitis, and pneumonia), pyelonephritis, and mastitis. Pyelonephritis presents the most difficult problem in differential diagnosis; occasionally it may be almost impossible to rule it out. In the typical case, pyuria, bacteremia, costovertebral angle tenderness, and spiking temperature point clearly to pyelonephritis. The clinical picture varies, however. A slight pyuria and bacilluria may characterize the urine of even normal puerperal women; moreover, chills and fever are common to both puerperal infection and pyelonephritis. The diagnosis of pyelonephritis in the puerperium should, therefore, be limited to cases in which there are more than 50 clumped white cells per high-power field in addition to the usual clinical syndrome of spiking fever and costovertebral angle tenderness. Finally it should be confirmed by a positive urine culture that identifies quantitatively a significant number of organisms. Mammary engorgement may occasionally give rise to a single brief temperature spike at any time during the first 10 days, which characteristically never lasts longer than 24 hours. The temperature curve of true mastitis is usually sustained and associated with mammary signs and symptoms that become overt within 24 hours.

One of the most important diagnostic procedures is the uterine culture. For purposes of research, elaborate technics for taking these cultures from the uterine cavity without contamination have been developed (Guilbeau and Schaub). In clinical practice, however, transfer of a sterile swab passed carefully into the cervical canal to an appropriately enriched culture medium provides for satisfactory growth of the major offending organisms.

Blood cultures should be obtained when the temperature reaches 102°F. In pelvic thrombophlebitis and in all anaerobic infections, positive blood cultures are notoriously difficult to obtain; repeated attempts are usually necessary. The optimal time to draw the blood is at the very beginning of the chill or, whenever possible, shortly before.

During Pregnancy. Since severe anemia predisposes to puerperal infection, low hemoglobin levels should be raised by appropriate means. Since the general nutritional status of the patient is an important factor, the necessity of a well-balanced diet should be emphasized to every expectant mother. Since sexual intercourse shortly before the onset of labor may rupture the membranes and thus introduce infection, it is considered by some inadvisable late in pregnancy.

During Labor. The three main principles are minimization of the number of bacteria introduced into the birth canal, limitation of trauma, and prevention of loss of blood.

The first of these principles demands, of course, aseptic technic. It was formerly taught that vaginal examination during labor should be carried out only when strictly indicated and always with rigid aseptic technic. Cervical dilatation was routinely assessed by rectal examination. Slotnick, Hildebrandt, and Prystowsky, as well as many others, have shown that vaginal examinations during labor performed with aseptic technic do not increase the likelihood of puerperal infection. Whether these conclusions can be applied universally of even extensively on a service with a high incidence of obstetric complications is still open to question. Today vaginal examinations in labor are certainly used with increasing frequency, casualness, and lack of preparation of the patient.

Since the nasopharynx is the most common source of extraneous bacteria brought to the birth canal, all obstetric personnel in the delivery room must wear masks that cover the nose and mouth. Attendants with upper respiratory infections should be excluded from the delivery suite.

Every wound of the birth canal is a potential portal of entry for infection, a source of additional loss of blood, and a factor predisposing to shock. This triad of trauma, hemorrhage, and shock provides an ideal basis for puerperal infection.

Minimization of trauma involves the avoidance of unnecessary operations, the utmost gentleness in indicated procedures, the immediate repair of all wounds, the prevention of hemorrhage during the third stage, and prompt replacement of blood, when indicated.

During the Puerperium. The birth canal represents a wound for many days after delivery, but it is well protected against extraneous bacterial invasion by the closed vulva, provided fingers are not introduced. The fingers may be those of the patient herself, who should be warned accordingly. They may also be those of a nurse, who, in separating the labia during perineal cleansing, permits contaminated water to enter the vagina. The aim of routine perineal care in the puerperium is not antisepsis but comfort and cleanliness. Elaborate methods are therefore unnecessary and potentially harmful. The perineal pads must be sterile and should be changed frequently, at least every four hours during the first week and every eight hours thereafter. Bedpans should be cleansed and sterilized after each use. The patient should be encouraged to use the toilet or bidet as soon as early ambulation permits.

Although it is an obviously good precaution to separate patients with puerperal infection from other puerperal women, strict isolation is no longer considered mandatory.

TREATMENT

Antimicrobial Drugs. Effective antimicrobial drugs have revolutionized the treatment and the prognosis of puerperal infection. Although these agents are effective in most cases, they have not eliminated the necessity for older measures in the treatment of puerperal infection. Supportive therapy still plays an important role, particularly in the milder cases. Most slight elevations of temperature in the puerperium respond within a few days to simple measures; hence the indiscriminate administration of antibiotics in such cases serves only to augment the growing number of resistant organisms.

If antimicrobial therapy is to be used, the following program should be followed: (1) Uterine cultures should be made for isolation and identification of the pathogen. In the presence of chills or other evidence of a severe infection, a blood culture should also be obtained. (2) Since different species of organisms, and even strains within the species, show wide variations in sensitivity to the various antimicrobial agents, sensitivity tests should be done to ascertain what drug or drugs will be most efficacious against the particular organism involved. (3) The choice of the drug or drugs to be used should be based largely on the sensitivity tests, although other factors must sometimes be considered, such as the toxicity of some of these agents. (4) Until the laboratory reports are received, treatment should be instituted with broad-spectrum antibiotics. Penicillin and streptomycin or tetracycline have proved to be effective in many instances of puerperal infection. In our experience, penicillin G administered parenterally in daily doses of 10 million units or more combined with tetracycline in a dose of 1 to not more than 2 grams per day intravenously usually will effectively control infections caused by coliform organisms, anaerobic streptococci, enterococci, bacteroides, and sensitive staphylococci. If the puerperal infection is not controlled by such therapy, kanamycin, 1 gram per day, given in divided doses intramuscularly every six hours, may be substituted for the tetracycline. As with most antibiotics except penicillin, in case of renal impairment the amount administered after the initial dose should be sharply curtailed. Gentamicin given intramuscularly every eight hours to provide a total daily dose of 3 mg per kg is proving to be quite effective against a number of gram-negative and gram-positive bacteria resistant to other antibiotics. Gentamicin appears to be an even more effective drug than kanamycin. To avoid toxicity the same precautions must be applied as for kanamycin. Chloramphenicol is a potent broad-spectrum antibiotic that has been well demonstrated clinically to be quite effective even in severe cases of puerperal infection. Unfortunately bone marrow toxicity with fatal aplastic anemia has followed its use often enough for physicians to be reluctant to prescribe it and patients reluctant to receive it.

Although rather specific recommendations regarding antibacterial therapy can be made at this time, it is readily apparent that over the course of years both the pathogenic bacteria and their sensitivities to antibiotics tend to undergo change. Fortunately, the rate at which new potent antibiotics have been developed has, for the most part, thus far prevented this pattern of change from exerting a devastating effect on the successful treatment of puerperal infections. Physicians caring for such cases, however, must continue to look for and identify changes in bacterial flora and in bacterial sensitivity, and make appropriate changes in therapy.

Lesions of the Perineum, Vulva, and Vagina.   These infected, external wounds should be treated, like other infected surgical wounds, by establishing drainage. All stitches must be removed and the wound laid open. Reluctance in this regard may lead not only to infection of the paracervical and paravaginal connective tissue, but to a worse ultimate anatomic result. Local external antisepsis is indicated, but vaginal douches are obviously contraindicated. Relief of pain is afforded by warm compresses, hot sitz baths, or exposure of the perineum to a heat lamp for periods of half an hour two or three times a day. It is sometimes advisable to supplement these therapeutic measures with an appropriate antimicrobial drug, especially during the acute phase of the infection.

Endometritis.   Mild cases, with temperature under 101°F, pulse under 100, and no chills, are best handled by simple measures. In this group it is unnecessary to discontinue breast-feeding. In more severe cases, isolation is desirable to protect other patients and afford the mother greater rest. Fowler's position facilitates lochial drainage, ergonovine maleate four times daily for two days promotes uterine tone, and forced fluids provide additional support. In severe cases, breast-feeding is discontinued, not only because it exhausts the mother but also because it is usually futile in the presence of high fever. In addition to the routine measures, antimicrobial drugs are indicated.

Pelvic Cellulitis and Thrombophlebitis.   In addition to the usual supportive measures, including blood transfusions for overt anemia, antimicrobial drugs should be used. The physician should remain alert to signs of beginning suppuration, as suggested by spontaneous, severe pain, continuous elevation of temperature, and high leukocytosis. The diagnosis of an abscess, however, rests upon detection of fluctuation. The mass is often so tender that analgesia may be required to perform an adequate examination.

In the majority of cases, abscesses of this type are best opened through an incision just above and parallel to Poupart's ligament (Fig. 4), but occasionally a bulging, fluctuant mass in the posterior cul-de-sac is best opened through posterior colpotomy (Fig. 5). Colpotomy should be performed in the midline to avoid injury to a ureter or a large blood vessel. After the pus has been reached

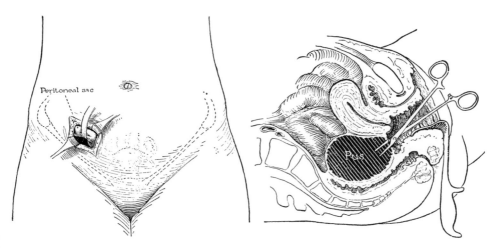

Fig. 4. Technic for opening localized collections of pus pointing above the inguinal ligament. (After Cullen. Surg Gynec Obstet 35:134, 1917.)

Fig. 5. Technic for opening collection of localized pus in the cul-de-sac of Douglas (posterior colpotomy).

by cautious blunt dissection, drainage is established and maintained by cigarette drains. Even if the main collection is not reached, a drain should be left in contact with the mass, which, as a rule, will spontaneously undergo necrosis and rupture subsequently in response to pressure. Pelvic thrombophlebitis usually accompanies parametritis and pelvic cellulitis. Treatment is customarily directed at parametritis or pelvic cellulitis rather than at pelvic thrombophlebitis alone. Anticoagulant drugs, which are successfully used in femoral thromboembolic disease (Ch. 35, p. 1001), are of less value in these cases, for the primary lesion is extravascular infection rather than thrombosis. Such treatment has been tried, however, particularly in cases of recurring septic pulmonary emboli. Rarely, ligation of the inferior vena cava and ovarian veins appears advisable to forestall extensive showering of septic emboli to the lungs.

Generalized Peritonitis.   The phases of treatment are specific, supportive, and symptomatic.

1. Specific.   The antimicrobial agent or agents most effective against the offending organism should be given parenterally in appropriate doses. As large a dose of penicillin as 30 million units per day may be beneficial. Gastrointestinal suction is a valuable aid in diminishing or perhaps preventing distention. Correction of hypokalemia is essential for proper intestinal function, but drugs used to stimulate peristalsis are of little value once distention has occurred; in fact, they may be dangerous.

2. Supportive.   Disturbances in fluid and electrolyte balance should be corrected. Fluids should be given intravenously. The volume is determined by the sum of the patient's urinary output, losses into the gastrointestinal tract, and an estimate of insensible loss and sweat. In general, oliguria can develop as the consequence of intense sequestration of extracellular fluid, as in the case of generalized peritonitis. Much less often, the oliguria is the result of bacterial shock with hypotension and inadequate renal perfusion pressure. With sequestration of fluid resulting from peritonitis, large volumes of electrolyte-containing solutions, such as lactated Ringer's, are essential to restore the functional extracellular fluid compartment. Only then is urine flow reestablished. Therapy to combat bacterial shock has been described in Chapter 20 (p. 521). Blood transfusions may be beneficial if the patient is anemic.

3. Symptomatic.   An analgesic agent may be used to relieve discomfort; a sedative, such as a barbiturate, is valuable in allaying restlessness and apprehension. Analgesia and sedation, however, should not be used to the point of obscuring or confusing the clinical picture. Oral feeding is withheld throughout the course of treatment until flatus is expelled and the bowel sounds return.

Procedures to Avoid.   Although countless local therapeutic measures have been recommended—such as intrauterine douches, swabbing of the endometrium with antiseptic solutions, continuous irrigation of the uterine cavity, instillations of glycerin, drainage with rubber tubes, and curettage—they have all been abandoned, since experience has shown them to be dangerous as well as futile. In the main, they tend to disseminate rather than halt the infection; nor does surgery merit a place in the treatment of puerperal infection, save for the incision and drainage of abscesses. Hysterectomy and laparotomy with drainage of the abdomen are to be avoided in the presence of generalized peritonitis.

The outcome of cases of puerperal infection is vastly different now from what it was a few decades ago. Today, not only are cases rarer but they are generally milder; therapy, furthermore, is more efficient and more specific. With the exception of cases of abortion, we have lost no patients from puerperal infection at Kings County Hospital in over 60,000 deliveries. There are many reasons for this decline in addition to the use of antibiotics. Certain of the pathogens are less virulent; prolonged labors and traumatic deliveries have all but disappeared; supportive measures—for example fluid therapy and intestinal decompression—are far more effective; and finally, most patients are in the hospital for delivery, with the result that there is no delay in the initiation of treatment. In cases of abortion in which trauma is superimposed and in which treatment is not rapidly initiated, the results are vastly different, as stressed in Chapter 20.

The prognosis for any case of puerperal infection depends primarily on the site and the extent of the infection. When confined to the perineum and the endometrium, infections respond quite promptly to proper supportive and antibiotic treatment. Even when the endometritis is caused by *Clostridium perfringens* (*welchii*), vigorous antibiotic treatment may yield good results.

When the infection extends to the parametrium, the response to treatment may not be so prompt, particularly in the event of the common complication, pelvic thrombophlebitis. Although most of these patients are eventually cured, the illness is likely to be prolonged.

Peritonitis is serious, but unless there has been undetected perforation of a hollow viscus, the eventual prognosis is good if treatment is prompt and vigorous. The same prognosis applies to septicemia accompanying puerperal infection. Most often tubal patency is maintained, and subsequent fertility is not impaired by the puerperal infection.

REFERENCES

Adams, J. Q., and Morton, R. F.   Puerperal tetanus. Amer J Obstet Gynec 69:169, 1955.

Bickerstaff, H. J.   The relationship between late prenatal hemoglobin levels and febrile puerperal morbidity. Amer J Obstet Gynec 43:997, 1942.

Burtenshaw.   The fever of the puerperium. New York and Philadelphia Med J, June and July, 1904.

Calman, R. M., and Gibson, J.. Bacteriology of the puerperal uterus. J Obstet Gynaec Brit Emp 61:623, 1954.

Douglas, R. G., and Stromme, W. B.   Operative Obstetrics, 2nd ed. New York, Appleton-Century-Crofts, 1965.

Eisenmann, G. E.   Die Wundfieber und die Kindbettfieber, Erlangen, 1837.

Galen.   Ars Medicinalis.

Gordon, A.   A Treatise on Epidemic Puerperal Fever of Aberdeen. London, C. G. and J. Robinson, 1795.

Guilbeau, J. A., and Schaub, I. G.   Uterine culture technic: simple method for avoiding contamination by cervical and vaginal flora. Amer J Obstet Gynec 58:407, 1949.

Halban, J., and Köhler, R.   Die pathologische Anatomie des Puerperalprozesses. Wien and Leipzig, 1919.

Hamilton, A.   Treatise on Midwifery, London, 1781.

Hill, A. M.   Why be morbid? Paths of progress in control of obstetric infection, 1931–1960. Med J Aust 1:101, 1964.

Hippocrates.   Liber prior De Muliebrum Morbis.

Holmes, O. W.   Puerperal Fever as a Private Pestilence. Boston, Ticknor & Fields, 1855.

Jewett, J. F., Reid, D. E., Safon, L. E., and Easterday, C. L.   Childbed fever—a continuing entity. JAMA 206:344, 1968.

Leake, J.   Practical Observations on the Child-bed Fever; also on the Nature and Treatment of Uterine Haemorrhages, Convulsions, and Such Other Acute Diseases, As Are Most Fatal to Women During the State of Pregnancy. London, J. Walter, 1772.

Lister, J.   On the antiseptic principle in the practice of surgery. Brit Med J 2:246, 1867.

Masterson, J. G., Nelson, J. H., and Valenti, C.   Acute monilial infection as a cause of death. Amer J Obstet Gynec 84:1799, 1962.

McCabe, W. R., and Abrams, A. A.   An outbreak of streptococcal puerperal sepsis. New Eng J Med 272:615, 1965.

Nuckols, H. H., and Hertig, A. T.   Pneumococcus infection of the genital tract in women, especially during pregnancy and the puerperium. Amer J Obstet Gynec 35:782, 1938.

Pearson, H. E., and Anderson, G. V.   Bacteroides infections and pregnancy. Obstet Gynec 35:31, 1970.

Peckham, C. H.   A brief history of puerperal infection. Bull Int Hist Med 3:187, 1935.

Puzos, N.   Premier mémoire sur les depôts laiteux, in Traités des accouchement, 1686, p. 341.

Sadusk, J. F., and Manahan, C. P.   Observations on the occurrence of *Clostridium welchii* in the vagina of pregnant women. Amer J Obstet Gynec 41:856, 1941.

Semmelweis, I. P.   Die Aetiologie, der Begriff u. die Prophylaxis des Kindbettfiebers, Pest, Wien und Leipzig, 1861.

Slotnick, I. J., Hildebrandt, R. J., and Prystowsky, H.   Microbiology of the female genital tract. IV. Cervical and vaginal flora during pregnancy. Obstet Gynec 21:312, 1963.

——— Stelluto, M., and Prystowsky, H.   Microbiology of the female tract. III. Comparative investigation of the cervical flora of parturients receiving either rectal or vaginal examinations. Amer J Obstet Gynec 85:519, 1963.

Strother.   Critical Essay on Fevers, London, 1716.

Watson, B. P.   An outbreak of puerperal sepsis in New York City. Amer J Obstet Gynec 16:157, 1928.

Weinstein, L.   The bacterial flora of the human vagina. Yale J Biol Med 10:247:1938.

White, C.   Treatise on the management of pregnant and lying-in women and the means of curing but more especially of preventing the principal disorders to which they are liable. London. E. C. Dilly, 1773.

Wierdsma, J. G., and Clayton, E. M.   The effects of certain antibiotics on the normal postpartum intrauterine bacteriologic flora. Amer J Obstet Gynec 88:541, 1964.

Willis, T.   Diatribae duae medico-philosophicae . . . de febribus . . . Londini, T. Roycroft, 1659.

35

DISORDERS OF THE PUERPERIUM OTHER THAN PUERPERAL INFECTION

DISORDERS OF THE BREAST

Engorgement of the Breasts.   For the first 24 or 48 hours after the development of the lacteal secretion it is not unusual for the breasts to become distended, firm, and nodular. This condition, commonly known as "caked breast," often causes considerable pain but is usually unaccompanied by an elevation of temperature. The disorder represents an exaggeration of the normal venous and lymphatic engorgement of the breasts, which is a regular precursor of lactation. It is not the result of overdistention of the lacteal system with milk.

Treatment consists of supporting and compressing the breasts with a binder or brassiere, applying an ice bag, and if necessary administering orally 60 mg of codeine sulfate or another analgesic. Pumping of the breast or manual expression of the milk may be necessary at first, but in a few days the condition is usually alleviated and the infant is able to nurse normally.

Suppression of Lactation.   When for a variety of reasons the infant is not to be breast-fed, suppression of lactation becomes important. Furthermore, since the majority of American women now prefer bottle feeding, it is not surprising that a great many methods have been suggested to relieve the discomfort and shorten the process of "drying up the milk." Perhaps the simplest method consists in support with a comfortably tight binder, ice bags, and mild analgesics for pain. Usually, all signs and symptoms will disappear in about a day if the breasts are not stimulated by pumping. Hormones, particularly natural estrogens or stilbestrol, either alone or combined with testosterone, have been widely used for this purpose. Womack and associates have investigated a number of currently employed hormonal preparations in a large series of puerperal women and concluded that satisfactory suppression of lactation can thus be achieved in the vast majority of cases. Their best results were obtained with a single intramuscular injection of 4 ml of long-acting steroid esters in the form of estradiol valerate and testosterone enanthate (Deladumone) at the time of delivery. In 900 patients so treated, only 45, or 5 per cent, had poor results. Although Womack and his group did not report delayed engorgement, pain, and increased lochia in their patients, general experience has been different. For example, Markin and Wolst in a controlled study found these complications in 20 to 40 per cent of their patients, although they too found the long-acting steroids to cause the least trouble in this regard. Tindall and Turnbull both have recently shown that administration of estrogen to suppress lactation was associated with an increase in thromboembolism in puerperal women.

Inflammation of the Breasts: Mastitis.   Parenchymatous inflammation of the mammary glands is a rare complication of pregnancy but is occasionally observed during the puerperium and lactation.

The symptoms of suppurative mastitis seldom appear before the end of the first week of the puerperium and, as a rule, not until the third or fourth week. Marked engorgement usually precedes the inflammation, the first sign of which is chills or actual rigor, which is soon followed by a considerable rise in temperature and an increase in pulse rate. The breast becomes hard and reddened, and the patient complains of pain. In some cases the constitutional symptoms attending a mammary abscess are severe, and very rarely, if neglected, may be fatal. Local manifestations may be so slight as to escape observation, however, Such cases are usually mistaken for puerperal infection. In still another group of patients the infection pursues a subacute or almost chronic course. The breast is somewhat harder than usual and more or less painful, but constitutional symptoms are either lacking or very slight. In such circumstances the first indication of the true diagnosis is often afforded by the detection of fluctuation.

Etiology.   By far, the most common offending organism is *Staphylococcus aureus* (coagulase-positive). The development of antibiotic-resistant staphylococci in hospitals has been accompanied by an increase in the frequency and severity of breast abscesses. The immediate source of the staphylococci causing mastitis is nearly always the nursing infant's nose and throat. At the time of nursing the organism enters the breast through the nipple at the site of a fissure or abrasion, which may be quite small. Whether the bacteria commonly cause mastitis simply by entering the lactiferous ducts of the breast with completely intact integument is not clear. Wysham and associates have shown that staphylococci in the throats of babies pass through the holes in rubber nipples to contaminate the contents of the bottle. Moreover, in cases of true mastitis the offending organism can be nearly always cultured from breast milk.

Suppurative mastitis among nursing mothers has at times reached epidemic levels. Such outbreaks most often coincide with the appearance of a new strain of antibiotic-resistant staphylococcus or the reappearance of one previously identified. Typically the infant becomes infected in the nursery as he comes in contact with nursery personnel who carry the organism. The attendants' hands are the major source of contamination of the newborn. Especially in a crowded, understaffed nursery it is a simple matter for the personnel inadvertently to transfer staphylococci from one colonized newborn to another. The colonization of staphylococci in the infant may be totally asymptomatic or may locally involve the umbilicus or the skin, but occasionally the organisms may cause a life-threatening, systemic infection.

Prevention.   Safeguards to prevent colonization of the newborn with virulent strains of staphylococci necessitate exclusion from the care of the infant and mother, of all personnel with a known or suspected staphylococcal lesion. Also, as a matter of daily routine, close inspection should be made of every infant, with prompt isolation of any who appear to be developing an infection of the cord or of the skin. The use of soap or detergent containing hexachlorophene to bathe the infants and for hand-scrubbing by personnel may be of value (Plueckhahn and Banks). However, it has been our experience that its use to bathe the infants increases the likelihood of infection with *E. coli.* All personnel should be checked periodically with appropriate cultures and phage typing of swabbings from the posterior nares to identify carriers of more virulent strains of staphylococci.

At the time of an epidemic the phenomenon of bacterial interference has been used successfully in our nursery as well as others to prevent colonization of the newborn with highly virulent strains of *Staphylococcus aureus* (Light and associates; Horne and colleagues). As each newborn arrives at the nursery the nares and umbilicus are directly inoculated with a strain of *Staphylococcus aureus* known to be nonvirulent. This procedure blocks subsequent colonization by virulent strains.

Treatment. Mastitis can be prevented in great part by suitable prophylactic measures that consist mainly in preventing the development of fissured nipples or treating them properly after they have appeared. The routine care of the lactating breasts should include the use of mild soap and water to cleanse the nipples before and after each nursing; the purpose is to remove encrusted flakes of inspissated milk, which may irritate the nipple. If cracks or fissures develop, the affected nipple is covered with tincture of benzoin or one of the commercial preparations available for this purpose (see Ch. 12, p. 341). If the cracks bleed or the nipples become too tender to allow the infant to nurse directly, a nipple shield is used or the breast pump is employed. Fissured nipples usually respond to this treatment; seldom is it necessary to discontinue breast-feeding for this reason.

The advent of antimicrobial drugs has markedly improved the prognosis in acute puerperal mastitis. Provided appropriate antibiotic therapy is started before suppuration begins, the infection can usually be aborted within 48 hours. Before initiating any antibiotic therapy, milk should be expressed from the affected breast onto a swab and promptly cultured. By so doing the offending organism can be identified and its bacterial sensitivity ascertained. At the same time the results of such cultures also provide information that is mandatory for a successful program of surveillance of nosocomial infections. The initial choice of antibiotic will undoubtedly be influenced to a considerable degree by the current experiences with staphylococcal infections at the institution in which the patient is receiving care. If at the time most staphylococcal infections are caused by organisms sensitive to penicillin, treatment with penicillin G is recommended. If the infection is caused by resistant, penicillinase-producing staphylococci, or if resistant organisms are suspected while awaiting the results of culture, a penicillinase-resistant compound should be used. It is important that treatment not be discontinued too soon. Even though clinical response may be prompt and striking, treatment should be continued for at least ten days.

Nursing should be discontinued when a diagnosis of suppurative mastitis is made, for it may be quite painful and the milk is infected; moreover, the infant often harbors the organisms and can therefore cause reinfection. Since the infant almost always is colonized by the offending organism, he should be observed very closely for signs of infection. Once established, staphylococcal infections tend to spread and recur among the family for protracted periods of time.

In the case of formation of frank abscesses, drainage in addition to antibiotic therapy is essential. The incisions should be made radially, extending from near the areolar margin toward the periphery of the gland, to avoid injury to the lactiferous ducts. In early cases a single incision over the most dependent portion of the area of fluctuation is usually sufficient, but multiple abscesses require several incisions. The operation should be done under general anesthesia, and a finger should be inserted to break up the walls of the locules. The resulting cavity is loosely packed with gauze, which should be replaced at the end of 24 hours by a smaller pack. If the pus has been thoroughly evacuated, the cavity of the abscess is obliterated and a complete cure is sometimes effected with great rapidity.

Galactocele.   Very exceptionally, as the result of the clogging of a duct by inspissated secretion, milk may accumulate in one or more lobes of the breast. The amount is ordinarily limited, but an excess may form a fluctuant mass that may give rise to pressure symptoms. Often the application of a binder will cause it to disappear.

Supernumerary Breasts.   One in every few hundred women has one or more accessory breasts (*polymastia*). The supernumerary breasts are sometimes so small as to be mistaken for pigmented moles. They rarely attain considerable size. They often have distinct nipples and are commonly situated in pairs on either side of the midline of the thoracic or abdominal walls, usually below the main breasts; less frequently they are found in the axillae, and occasionally on other portions of the body such as the shoulder, flank, or groin, and, in rare instances, the thigh. The number of supernumerary breasts varies greatly. When arranged symmetrically two or four are most common, although ten have been described.

The condition is usually regarded as atavistic, though it is not associated with an increased tendency toward multiple pregnancy. Polymastia has no obstetric significance, although occasionally the enlargement of supernumerary breasts in the axillae may result in considerable discomfort. Frequently a tongue of mammary tissue extends out into the axilla from the outer margin of a normal breast, whereas an isolated fragment is sometimes found in the same location. Such structures undergo hypertrophy during pregnancy. When lactation is established, they may become swollen and painful. Ordinarily, if disregarded, they soon undergo regression and give no further trouble.

Abnormalities of the Nipples.   The typical nipple is cylindric, projecting well beyond the general surface of the breast; its exterior is slightly nodular but not fissured. Variations, however, are not uncommon, some sufficiently pronounced to interfere seriously with suckling.

In some women the lactiferous ducts open directly into a depression at the center of the areola. In marked cases of depressed nipple, nursing is out of the question. When the depression is not very deep the breast may occasionally be made available by use of a breast pump.

More frequently, the nipple, although not depressed, is so greatly inverted that it cannot be used for nursing. In such a case daily attempts should be made during the last few months of pregnancy to draw the nipple out using traction with the fingers. Since the maneuver is rarely successful, however, if the nipples cannot be made available by the temporary use of an electric pump, suckling must be discontinued.

Nipples that are normal in shape and size may become fissured and therefore particularly susceptible to injury from the child's mouth during suckling. In such cases the fissures almost inevitably render nursing painful, sometimes with a deleterious influence upon the secretory function. Moreover, such lesions provide a convenient portal of entry for pyogenic bacteria. For these reasons every effort should be made to heal such fissures, particularly by protecting them from further injury with a nipple shield and topical medication. If such measures are of no avail, the child should not be permitted to nurse on the affected side. Instead the breast should be emptied regularly with a suitable pump until the lesions are completely healed.

Abnormalities of Secretion. There are marked individual variations in the amount of milk secreted, many of which are dependent not upon the general health and appearance of the woman but upon the development of the glandular portions of the breasts. A woman with large, well-formed breasts may produce only a small quantity of milk, whereas another with small, flat breasts may produce an abundant supply. Stout women with pendulous breasts are more likely to have a deficient secretion, for the bulk of the organ consists of fatty tissue, whereas the glandular elements are poorly developed. Deficient secretion is frequently noted in very obese young women, whose breasts may be poorly developed, and in elderly primiparas, in whom there may be early signs of atrophy.

Very rarely there is complete lack of mammary secretion (*agalactia*). As a rule, it is possible to express a small amount from the nipple on the third or fourth day of the puerperium. Relative deficiency is frequent, however, a large number of women secreting an amount of milk insufficient for the nutrition of the child. The variations in the quantity of milk, the various factors concerned in its production, and the endocrine control of mammary growth and lactation are discussed further in Chapter 8.

Occasionally the mammary secretion is excessive (*polygalactia*). Constant leakage of milk is called *galactorrhea*. In the Chiari-Frommel syndrome intractable galactorrhea may continue for years after birth of the child. As originally described the syndrome was accompanied by amenorrhea and related to a recent pregnancy. More recently a similar syndrome characterized by amenorrhea and galactorrhea but related to primary pituitary dysfunction rather than childbirth has been described by Ahumada and by Argonz and Del Castillo. In both the puerperal and nongestational forms of the disease there is a deficiency of FSH and low estrogen production. Prolactin continues to be secreted but the surge in luteinizing hormone appropriate for ovulation does not occur. Clomiphene (Clomid) has been used with some success to treat the Chiari-Frommel syndrome. Surprisingly, pregnancy has occurred in women with the nonpuerperal form of the disease (Maas).

DISEASES AND ABNORMALITIES OF THE UTERUS

Subinvolution. Subinvolution is an arrest or retardation of involution, the process by which the puerperal uterus is normally restored to its original proportions.

Involution is the result of autolysis, leading to atrophy of the myometrial fibers. Subinvolution may result from numerous factors that interfere with complete contraction of the myometrium. Among the more important causes are retention of placental fragments, endometritis, myomas, and pelvic infection. Since most cases of subinvolution result from local causes, they are usually amenable to early diagnosis and treatment.

Subinvolution is accompanied by prolongation of the period of lochial discharge and sometimes by profuse hemorrhage. It may be followed by prolonged leukorrhea and irregular or excessive uterine bleeding.

The diagnosis is established by bimanual examination. The uterus is larger and softer than normal for the particular period of the puerperium. Ergonovine maleate (Ergotrate) or methyl ergonovine maleate (Methergine), 0.2 mg every 3 to 4 hours for 24 to 48 hours, often leads to improvement. Retention of fragments of secundines is, of course, best treated by prompt curettage. Metritis may be best managed by antibiotic therapy.

Postpartum Cervical Erosions.   Cervical erosions are a complication of the late postpartum period. Weiner and Nelson report an incidence of 10 per cent. Shallow cauterization can be used to remove exuberant granulations without causing stenosis of the endocervix.

Relaxation of the Vaginal Outlet and Prolapse of the Uterus.   The frequent lacerations of the perineum during delivery, if not properly repaired, are commonly followed by relaxation of the vaginal outlet. Even when external lacerations are not visible, furthermore, overstretching or submucosal tears may lead to marked relaxation. The changes in the pelvic supports during parturition predispose, moreover, to prolapse of the uterus and to urinary stress incontinence. These conditions may escape detection unless an examination is made at the end of the puerperium and unless the patients are subjected to long-term follow-up.

In general, operative correction should be postponed till the end of the childbearing period, unless, of course, serious disability, notably urinary stress incontinence, demands intervention.

HEMORRHAGES DURING THE PUERPERIUM

If there is no serious loss of blood during the first hour or hour and a half after delivery, it may ordinarily be assumed that the danger of postpartum hemorrhage is past. Occasionally, however, in the latter part of the first week, and more often still later in the puerperium, uterine hemorrhages are encountered. They are most often the result of abnormal involution of the placental site (Gainey, Nicolay, and Lapi), but they may be caused also by retention of a portion of the placenta. Usually, the retained piece of placenta undergoes necrosis with deposition of fibrin, eventually forming a so-called placental polyp. By interfering with involution of the placental site the polyp may cause hemorrhage. A succinct survey of this complication has been made by Kurtz and Comando.

In a study of late postpartum hemorrhage by Wolfe and Pedowitz, the incidence of the complication was found to be once in about 1,000 cases. Most commonly, abnormal vaginal bleeding appeared between the sixth and tenth postpartum days.

Whether the hemorrhage is caused by subinvolution of the placental site or a retained placental fragment, curettage is usually necessary. This operation should, of course, be preceded by replacement of blood, when indicated. Curettage is usually curative, but the microscopic examination of the curettings fails to reveal large placental fragments in more than half of the cases, showing only the involuting placental site with large, partially organized veins with thrombosis and inflammatory cells (Lester and colleagues; Dewhurst). It has been our experience that occasionally severe hemorrhage may occur during the course of curetting the somewhat necrotic placental implantation site, especially in women of higher parity. Blood transfusion and even hysterectomy may be necessary.

Puerperal Hematomas. Blood may escape into the connective tissue beneath the skin covering the external genitalia or beneath the vaginal mucosa to form vulvar and vaginal hematomas, respectively, about once in every 500 to 1,000 deliveries. The condition usually follows injury to a blood vessel without laceration of the superficial tissues, and may occur with spontaneous, as well as operative, delivery. Occasionally the hemorrhage is delayed, probably as a result of sloughing of a vessel that had become necrotic from prolonged pressure. A hematoma may occasionally form during pregnancy and grow sufficiently large to obstruct delivery. Very exceptionally, if medical aid is not available, fatal hemorrhage may follow rupture of the hematoma at delivery.

Less frequently, the torn vessel lies above the pelvic fascia. In that event the hematoma develops above it. In its early stages it forms a rounded swelling that projects into the upper portion of the vaginal canal and may almost occlude its lumen. If the bleeding continues, it dissects retroperitoneally and thus may form a tumor palpable above Poupart's ligament, or it may dissect upward, eventually reaching the lower margin of the diaphragm.

Large vulvar hematomas (Fig. 1), particularly those that develop rapidly, may cause excruciating pain, often the first symptom that is noticed. Hematomas of moderate size may be absorbed spontaneously. The tissues overlying the hematoma may give way as a result of necrosis caused by pressure, and profuse hemorrhage may follow. In other cases, the contents of the hematoma may be discharged in the form of large clots.

In the subperitoneal variety the extravasation of blood beneath the peritoneum may be massive and occasionally fatal. Death may also follow secondary

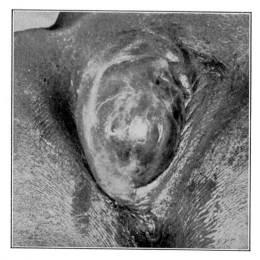

Fig. 1. Vulvar hematoma bulging into the right vaginal wall.

intraperitoneal rupture. Occasionally rupture into the vagina leads to infection of the hematoma and potentially fatal sepsis.

A vulvar hematoma is readily diagnosed by severe perineal pain and the sudden appearance of a tense, fluctuant, and sensitive tumor of varying size covered by discolored skin. When the mass develops in the vagina it may temporarily escape detection, but symptoms of pressure and inability to void should soon lead to a vaginal examination, which reveals a round, fluctuant tumor encroaching on the lumen. When the hematoma extends upward between the folds of the broad ligament it may escape detection unless a portion of the tumor can be felt on abdominal palpation or unlesss symptoms of anemia or infection appear.

The prognosis is usually favorable, though bleeding into very large hematomas has led to death.

Treatment. Small vulvar hematomas may be treated expectantly. If, however, the pain is severe, or if they enlarge, as they often do, the best treatment is incision and evacuation of the blood with ligation of the bleeding points. The cavity can then be obliterated with mattress sutures. Vaginal tamponade for about 24 hours may be helpful. Blood loss nearly always is considerably more than the clinical estimate. Shock and severe anemia should be prevented by adequate blood replacement. Broad-spectrum antibiotics are of value.

The subperitoneal and supravaginal varieties are more difficult to treat. They can be evacuated by incision of the perineum, but unless there is complete hemostasis, which is difficult to achieve by this route, laparotomy is advisable. A resume of this complication is presented by Pedowitz, Pozner, and Adler.

Diseases of the Urinary Tract

Evacuation of the uterus is associated with varying degrees of stretching and trauma of the base of the bladder. Cystoscopic examination after delivery shows not only edema and hyperemia but frequently submucous extravasations of blood. The edema of the trigone is occasionally sufficiently marked to cause obstruction of the urethra and acute retention. In addition, the puerperal bladder has an increased capacity and is not so sensitive to intravesical fluid tension as in the nonpregnant state. As a result, overdistention and incomplete emptying with residual urine are common. The effect of anesthesia, especially spinal, caudal, and epidural, and the temporarily disturbed neural control of the bladder are undoubtedly contributory factors.

Residual urine and bacteriuria introduced by catheterization in a traumatized bladder present the optimal conditions for the development of cystitis. The initial symptoms include dysuria, frequency, and urgency. In case of an atonic, overdistended bladder the patient voids only small volumes, even though a great deal more urine remains in the bladder. Signs and symptoms of infection subsequently will vary, depending upon whether the infection is localized to the bladder or ascends to involve the upper urinary tract.

After obtaining urine for culture, treatment should consist of appropriate antibiotic or chemotherapeutic agents, as discussed in Chapter 27 (p. 755). In case of overdistention of the bladder it is usually best to leave an indwelling catheter in place for 24 hours to empty the bladder completely and prevent prompt recurrence, as well as to allow recovery of normal bladder tone and sensation.

Incontinence of Urine. In multiparas, during the early part of the puerperium, coughing, sneezing, and other factors leading to a sudden increase in intraabdominal pressure often produce an involuntary discharge of a small quantity of urine. The condition usually disappears spontaneously but sometimes necessitates operative intervention at a later date.

More marked incontinence at this time is usually caused by a fistula at the bladder neck, the result of trauma from an operative delivery. These vesicovaginal fistulas may not become evident for five to ten days after delivery because of the slow necrosis of devitalized tissue. In this event scrupulous attention to cleanliness may be followed by spontaneous healing if the fistula is very small; most large or persistent openings, however, require subsequent surgical repair. The incidence of obstetric vesicovaginal fistulas has declined markedly over the past few decades, largely as a result of two changes in obstetric policy: (1) elimination of difficult, traumatic operative vaginal deliveries and (2) avoidance of prolonged labor and its consequence, ischemic necrosis of the bladder.

DISORDERS OF THE NERVOUS SYSTEM

Obstetric Paralysis. Pressure on branches of the sacral plexus during labor is demonstrated by complaints of intense neuralgia or cramplike pains extending down one or both legs as soon as the head begins to descend into the pelvis. As a rule the compression is rarely severe enough to give rise to grave lesions. In some instances, however, the pain continues after delivery and is accompanied by paralysis of the muscles supplied by the external popliteal nerve (the flexors of the ankles and the extensors of the toes). Occasionally the gluteal muscles are affected to a lesser extent. In modern obstetrics, paralysis of this kind is rare. Footdrop resulting from improper positioning of patients in stirrups or leg holders is more common and should be prevented.

Separation of the symphysis pubis or one of the sacroiliac synchondroses during labor may be followed by pain and marked interference with locomotion. In addition, the puerperal woman may occasionally suffer paralysis of central origin, usually resulting from cerebral vascular disease or preeclampsia-eclampsia.

Puerperal Psychoses. These conditions are discussed in Chapter 27.

THROMBOEMBOLIC DISEASE

Thrombophlebitis. Although it is common practice to divide thromboembolic disease into two categories—phlebothrombosis, denoting spontaneous intravascular clotting with a minimal inflammatory reaction, and thrombophlebitis, in which the thrombosis is accompanied or preceded by a severe and often symptomatic inflammation of the venous wall—it is obvious that all thromboses must cause some venous inflammation and vice versa. Often, therefore, a precise differential diagnosis is difficult, although in typical cases these two conditions are well defined.

Incidence. Although thromboembolic disease may occur during pregnancy, most cases are puerperal. The disease is more frequently associated with operative than with spontaneous deliveries. As traumatic obstetric operations have become less common, the incidence of thromboembolism has declined. It may also accompany pelvic thrombophlebitis in association with puerperal infection. Since the condition is associated also with venous stasis, early ambulation has contributed to its decreasing incidence (Ullery). Thromboembolism still, however, occurs in 1 in 270 puerperal women, according to Parker and associates, and 1.2 per cent according to Hiilesmaa. In contrast, thromboembolic disease occurs in between 0.018 and 0.3 per cent of antepartum women, and its incidence has shown little change during this century (Villasanta; Stamm). There is no clear explanation for this difference in incidence of embolic phenomena. During the prenatal period when several of the clotting factors are elevated and fibrinolytic activity is decreased, a high incidence of thromboembolic disease might be expected if these factors were the sole etiologic determinants. Obviously trauma and slowing of circulation in previously dilated veins must play a role.

Diagnosis. The veins of the lower extremities are most often involved, although thromboembolic disease of the pelvic veins is not rare. Thrombosis of uterine and pelvic veins is commonly associated with puerperal infection (Ch. 34, p. 989). Although phlebothrombosis may remain unsuspected, more often there are pain, edema, and elevation of temperature of the involved extremity. There may in addition be slight systemic elevation of temperature. Pressure over the deep veins of the leg and dorsiflexion of the foot cause pain in the calf (Homans' sign). Because the clot is loosely attached, it has a tendency to break off and cause pulmonary embolism, sometimes the first indication of phlebothrombosis.

Thrombophlebitis, sometimes called phlegmasia alba dolens, or milk-leg, is abrupt in onset with a chill, high fever, and severe pain and edema of the affected leg. Reflex arterial spasm sometimes produces the bluish white, tensely swollen extremity. There may be pain and tenderness along the entire course of the vessels of the leg. Pulmonary embolus in the primarily inflammatory variety of thromboembolic disease is less common because of the intense fixation of the thrombus.

Treatment. Thrombophlebitis limited strictly to the superficial veins of the saphenous system is treated with rest, elastic support, and analgesics. Some workers recommend intravenous dextran solution in these cases.

More aggressive therapy is indicated in cases of deep venous thrombosis, however. Anticoagulants and bed rest are usually effective in controlling the disease and in preventing pulmonary embolism. Heparin and Coumadin are usually used as anticoagulants in cases of deep venous thrombosis. Heparin is given intravenously in doses of 5,000 to 10,000 units every 4 to 6 hours; the amount injected should be sufficient to establish a whole blood clotting time that is two to three times the control value just before the next dose. If the heparin results in worrisome bleeding or if a surgical procedure is necessary while the heparin effect persists, protamine sulfate can be used to neutralize its anticoagulant action.

Coumadin interferes with the synthesis of clotting factors that are vitamin K–dependent (factors II, VII, IX, and X). Whereas the anticoagulant effect of heparin is maximal immediately after intravenous injection and decreases rapidly over the course of a few hours, the effect of Coumadin is negligible during the first 24 hours, the maximal effect being reached between 36 and 72 hours. Therefore, heparin is most often used initially, especially in cases of thrombophlebitis with obvious or suspected pulmonary embolism. It is discontinued a few days later when Coumadin therapy has become effective. To reduce the prothrombic activity to about 20 per cent of normal (approximately double the normal Quick one-stage prothrombin time) an initial dose of 40 to 50 mg of Coumadin is given, followed by a smaller daily dose of about 10 mg, but the exact dose must be ascertained individually to maintain this level of prothrombic activity.

The effect of Coumadin may be reversed by the intravenous administration of 50 to 150 mg of vitamin K_1 (phytonadione, Aquamephyton, Konakion) injected at a rate of not more than 10 mg per minute. The activities of the vitamin K–dependent clotting factors usually increase to safe levels within four to eight hours after vitamin K_1 injection. If a surgical procedure must be performed without delay, transfusions of blood or plasma can be used to correct them more promptly.

Therapy with Coumadin and related compounds may be hazardous prenatally, since they cross the placenta and may cause serious bleeding in the fetus. Therefore, heparin is the preferred anticoagulant during pregnancy (Mueller and Lebherz). Depot heparin can be used for long-term therapy to reduce the frequency of injections.

If pulmonary embolism develops while the patient is being treated with anticoagulants, ligation of the inferior vena cava just below the level of the renal veins and of the left ovarian vein is indicated. Recently, rather than ligating the vena cava some individuals have advocated partially occluding the vessel to such a degree that most emboli will not pass although blood can still flow. The advantages of these "straining" technics are not yet clearly established. In septic cases complicated by showering of septic emboli into the venous circulation, ligation of the inferior vena cava and ovarian veins may be lifesaving.

Ovarian vein thrombosis accompanied by localized pain, tenderness, fever, and variable degrees of leukocytosis is a relatively rare complication of the puerperium. Lotze and associates suggest ligation of both ovarian veins. Whether surgical intervention is desirable is debatable, however; O'Lane and Lebherz and also Montalto and associates recommend anticoagulant and antibiotic therapy without operation. Brown and Munsick have recently reviewed the clinical features of cases reported by others as well as 16 of their own. They endorse early diagnosis without laparotomy and recommend treatment with broad spectrum antibiotics plus effective doses of heparin. They find the prognosis for future pregnancies to be good. We have employed surgical interruption only in the rare case in which there was an obvious showering of septic emboli.

Pulmonary Embolism. The greatest danger from venous thrombosis is pulmonary embolism. The fatality rate among patients who have suffered pulmonary embolism is really not known, since many cases undoubtedly go undiagnosed. On the contrary, the diagnosis is occasionally made in instances in which another disease was the cause of findings suggestive, at least, of pulmonary embolism.

The reported incidence of pulmonary embolism varies widely from 1 in 2,700 deliveries (Stamm) to less than 1 in 7,000 deliveries (Mengert).

Chest pain, even if transient, accompanied by shortness of breath, air hunger, tachypnea, or just apprehension strongly suggests pulmonary embolism during the puerperium. Physical examination of the chest may or may not yield other findings such as an accentuated pulmonic valve second sound, rales, or friction rub. Right axis deviation may or may not be evident in the electrocardiogram. To date, our experiences with pulmonary angiography and with pulmonary scanning using isotopically labeled albumin macroaggregates have been rather disappointing. For the most part distinctly positive results have been limited to cases in which pulmonary embolism was obvious clinically. Immediate pulmonary artery embolectomy in case of a large embolus could prove lifesaving. In our limited experience it has not been successfully employed. The potential for this procedure will be more evident in the future.

The obstetrician must be ever alert to the possibility of pulmonary embolism, especially during the puerperium. Not infrequently at the time of embolism the source of the thrombus is not yet obvious. In general, whenever there is reasonable suspicion of pulmonary embolus, it is much safer to initiate an effective program of anticoagulation as outlined in this chapter rather than risk a second embolus, which may prove fatal. Dalen and Dexter have provided a succinct account of diagnosis and treatment of this complication of the puerperium, including a tabulation of emergency tests for pulmonary embolism (Table 1).

Table 1. **Emergency Diagnostic Tests for Pulmonary Embolism**

Test	Findings Suggestive of Pulmonary Embolism	Aids to Differential Diagnosis	Therapeutic Implication if Pulmonary Embolism is Present
ECG	Right axis shift (S1Q3T3) and right ventricular strain	To rule out acute myocardial infarction	Detection and treatment of arrhythmias
Chest roentgenogram	Enlargement of main pulmonary artery and right ventricle, infiltrate, pleural effusion, elevated diaphragm, or asymmetry of vasculature	To rule out pneumonia and congestive heart failure (may be secondary to pulmonary embolism)	Presence of acute right ventricular enlargement indicates life-threatening embolism
Arterial blood gases	Low pO_2 and pCO_2 are nearly constant findings in acute embolism	Normal pO_2 nearly excludes acute pulmonary embolism	Guide to oxygen therapy and guide to prognosis
Central venous pressure (CVP)	Elevated (if right ventricular failure is present)	If hypotension is present, low CVP nearly excludes pulmonary embolism as cause of hypotension	Central venous catheter provides route for administration of drugs or fluids and ready access to blood samples
Lung scan	Areas of oligemia (areas of the lung with a decreased concentration of radioactivity)	"Positive" scan can be caused by pneumonia, atelectasis, or other pulmonary lesions	Extent of avascular areas serves as a guide to severity of pulmonary embolism
Pulmonary angiography	Filling defects due to presence of emboli, cutoffs of pulmonary arteries, areas of decreased perfusion	Normal angiogram excludes large pulmonary embolus	Most accurate guide to extent of embolism

° pO_2 indicates arterial oxygen tension.
From Dalen and Dexter. JAMA 207:150, 1969.

References

Ahumada, J. C., and Del Castillo, E. B. (Amenorrhea and galactorrhea). Bol Soc Obst Ginec (Buenos Aires) 11:64, 1932.

Argonz, J., and Del Castillo, E. B. A syndrome characterized by estrogenic insufficiency, galactorrhea and decreased urinary gonadotropin. J Clin Endocr 13:79, 1953.

References

Brown, T. K., and Munsick, R. A.   Puerperal ovarian vein thrombophlebitis: A syndrome. Amer J Obstet Gynec 109:263, 1971.

Dalen, J. E., and Dexter, L.   Pulmonary embolism. JAMA 207:1505, 1969.

Dewhurst, C. J.   Secondary post-partum haemorrhage. J Obstet Gynaec Brit Comm 73:53, 1966.

Dippel, A. L., and Johnston, R. A.   Suppurative mastitis as a complication of pregnancy and the puerperium. Amer J Obstet Gynec 29:258, 1935.

Gainey, H. L., Nicolay, K. S., and Lapi, A   Noninvolution of the placental site: clinical and pathological studies. Amer J Obstet Gynec 69:558, 1955.

Hiilesmaa, V.   Occurrence and anticoagulant treatment of thromboembolism in gravidas, parturients and gynecologic patients: Study of 678 cases treated in women's clinic of the University of Helsinki in 1953–57. Acta Obstet Gynec Scand 39, Suppl 2, 1960.

Horne, J., Kay, J. L., Eichenwald, H. F., Jones, L., and James, N. K.   The use of bacterial interference to abort an outbreak of staphylococcal disease in a large newborn nursery population. Submitted for publication.

Hunt, A. B.   Postpartum amenorrhea. Obstet Gynec 1:522, 1953.

Knight, I. C. S., and Nolan, B.   Breast abscess. Brit Med J 1:1224, 1959.

Kurtz, G. R., and Comando, E. N.   Three cases of late puerperal hemorrhage caused by placental polyps. Amer J Obstet Gynec 66:663, 1953.

Lester, W. M., Bartholomew, R. A., Colvin, E. D., Grimes, W. H., Fish, J. S., and Galloway, W. H.   The role of retained placental fragments in immediate and delayed postpartum hemorrhage. Amer J Obstet Gynec 72:1214, 1956.

Light, I. J., Walton, R. L., Sutherland, J. M., Shinefield, H. R., and Brackvogel, V.   Use of bacterial interference to control a staphylococcal nursery outbreak. Amer J Dis Child 113:291, 1967.

Lotze, E. C., Kaufman, R. H., and Kaplan, A. L.   Postpartum ovarian vein thrombophlebitis. A review. Obstet Gynec Survey 21:853, 1966.

Maas, J. M.   Amenorrhea-galactorrhea syndrome. Before, during, and after pregnancy. Fertil Steril 18:857, 1967.

Markin, K. E., and Wolst, M. D.   A comparative controlled study of hormones used in the prevention of pospartum breast engorgement and lactation. Amer J Obstet Gynec 80:128, 1960.

Mengert, W. F.   Venous ligation in obstetrics. Amer J Obstet Gynec 50:467, 1945.

Montalto, N. J., Bloch, E., Malfetano, J. H., and Janelli, D. E.   Postpartum thrombophlebitis of the ovarian vein. Obstet Gynec 34:867, 1969.

Mueller, M. J., and Lebherz, T. B.   Antepartum thrombophlebitis. Obstet Gynec 34:874, 1969,

O'Lane, J. M., and Lebherz, T. B.   Puerperal ovarian thrombophlebitis. Obstet Gynec 26:676, 1965.

Parker, R. T., Anlyan, W. G., Mairs, D. A., and Carter, B.   Thromboembolic complications of pregnancy. Southern Med J 50:1228, 1957.

Pedowitz, P., Pozner, S., and Adler, N. H.   Puerperal hematomas: Analysis of 112 cases with a review of the literature. Amer J Obstet Gynec 81:350, 1961 (66 references cited).

Plueckhahn, V. D., and Banks, J.   Breast abscess and staphylococcal disease in a maternity hospital. Brit Med J 2:414, 1964.

Schwarz, R., and Trommer, R.   (Thromboembolic diseases at University of Leipzig Women's Clinic during 1937–56). Gynaecologia (Basel) 150:229, 1960.

Sherman, A. J.   Puerperal breast abscess. Report of an outbreak at Philadelphia General Hospital. Obstet Gynec 7:268, 1956.

Smith, C. O., and Varga, A.   Puerperal breast abscess. Amer J Obstet Gynec 74:1330, 1957.

Soltau, D. H. K., and Hatcher, G. W.   Some observations on the aetiology of breast abscess in the puerperium. Brit Med J 1:1603, 1960.

Stamm, H.   Obstetrical and gynecological mortality due to embolism in Central Europe and Scandinavia. Geburtsh Frauenheilk 20:675, 1960.

———   (Thromboembolic complications of pregnancy). Gynaecologia 164:137, 1967.

Tindall, V. R.   Factors influencing puerperal thromboembolism. J Obstet Gynaec Brit Comm 75:1324, 1968.

Turnbull, A. C.   Puerperal thromboembolism and the suppression of lactation. J Obstet Gynaec Brit Comm 75:1321, 1968.

Ullery, J. C. Thromboembolic disease complicating pregnancy in the puerperium. Amer J Obstet Gynec 68:1243, 1954.

Villasanta, U. Thromboembolic disease in pregnancy. Amer J Obstet Gynec 93:142, 1965 (109 references cited).

Weiner, A. E., and Nelson, H. B. The care of the postpartum cervix. Amer J Obstet Gynec 62:1106, 1951.

Wolfe, S. A., and Pedowitz, P. Late postpartum hemorrhage. Amer J Obstet Gynec 53:84, 1947.

Womack, W. S., Smith, S. W., Allen, G. M., Baker, R. L., Christensen, O., Gallaher, J. P., Hanson, I. R., Smith, W. B., and Gomez, A. A comparison of hormone therapies for suppression of lactation. Southern Med J 55:816, 1962.

Wysham, D. H., Mulhern, M. E., Navarre, G. C., LaVeck, G. D., Kennan, A. L., and Giedt, W. R. Staphylococcal infections in an obstetric unit. II. Epidemiological studies of puerperal mastitis. New Eng J Med 257:304, 1957.

36

INJURIES SUSTAINED BY THE FETUS IN PREGNANCY AND LABOR

Perinatal Mortality in General

This and the following chapter are devoted to injuries and diseases that affect the fetus and newborn and, as stated in Chapter 1, claim the lives of about 113,000 infants each year in the United States. These perinatal deaths comprise *fetal deaths* and *neonatal deaths*.

Fetal Mortality. "Fetal mortality" is death of infants before delivery in pregnancies of 20 or more weeks gestation. If an infant dies even immediately after birth, not a fetal death but a neonatal death results. The fact needs emphasis because the term "fetal mortality" is sometimes used incorrectly to include both fetal and neonatal mortality. Since a fetus of 20 weeks' gestational age weighs nearly 500 g, it is permissible to define fetal mortality also as deaths before or during labor of infants weighing 500 g or more. Because it is sometimes impossible to ascertain the exact duration of pregnancy, the definition based on weight is often preferred for statistical purposes.

Fetal mortality makes up about one half of all perinatal mortality. For example, the number of fetal deaths in 1967 was approximately 55,000 and the number of neonatal deaths about 58,000.

Fetal Death Before the Onset of Labor. Hypoxia is the major direct cause of fetal death prior to the onset of labor, but the precise mechanism responsible for the hypoxia is unknown in about half the cases, as shown by Goldstein and associates at the Boston Lying-In Hospital in their study of 492 such deaths (Table 1). In a study of fetal deaths before labor, Tricomi and Kohl found that if labor were allowed to begin spontaneously, 75 per cent of patients would be delivered by the end of the second week after fetal death, and 93 per cent would be delivered by the end of the third week. These data are quite similar to those from Boston Lying-In Hospital.

When a dead fetus has been retained for five or more weeks, the likelihood of potentially dangerous hypofibrinogenemia developing before spontaneous labor and delivery is about one in four, according to Pritchard. The hypofibrino-

Table 1. The Major Cause of Fetal Death Before Labor

	Number	Per Cent
Unexplained	258	53
Erythroblastosis	66	13
Congenital abnormalities	43	9
Cord complications	40	8
Diabetes	32	6
Toxemia	16	3
Abruptio placentae	16	3
External version	8	2
Other	13	3

genemia is the consequence, primarily intravascular coagulation caused by thromboplastic material from the degenerating placenta and probably from the necrotic fetus diffusing into the maternal circulation. The changes in the maternal coagulation mechanism are similar to those of placental abruption but most often occur over the course of weeks rather than within a few hours. Spontaneous correction of the defects in coagulation before delivery occurs only very infrequently.

Fibrinogen replacement is indicated if the patient either is in the process of delivering the necrotic products of conception or has recently done so and is bleeding excessively, there is no other demonstrable cause to account for the bleeding, and the clot observation test reveals a very small clot. The usual dose of fibrinogen is 4 g. If, on the other hand, hypofibrinogenemia is detected at a time when the patient is not in labor and is not actively bleeding, heparin intravenously may be of considerable value to block the consumptive coagulopathy, thereby allowing the deficiencies of fibrinogen and other coagulation factors to be corrected before delivery. Three cases have been described in detail by Jiminez and Pritchard in which heparin given for two to three days by continuous intravenous infusion successfully corrected the coagulation defects, after which delivery was accomplished without incident.

In general the management of patients with fetal death who failed to go into labor spontaneously has changed during the past decade from watchful waiting to active intervention. Although most of these patients will eventually go into labor spontaneously, the psychologic stress imposed upon the mother carrying a dead fetus, the dangers of blood clotting defects, and the advent of sure and safe methods of induction of labor have increased the desirability of early delivery. Because methods of early diagnosis of fetal death still lack certainty (Ch. 9, p. 288), and since 75 per cent of patients will deliver within two weeks, it is our practice

Table 2. Method of Labor and Delivery

Method	Per Cent
Spontaneous labor	58.9
Induction	
Amniotomy only	13.1
Oxytocin only	10.6
Amniotomy and oxytocin	8.6
Intraamniotic hypertonic saline	4.1
Hysterotomy	2.8
Hysterectomy	1.9

Courtesy of Goplerud, C. P., and White, C. A. Postgrad Med 43:167, 1968.

to delay induction of labor for at least that period of time. Suitable methods include amniotomy, the intravenous administration of increasing concentrations of oxytocin, and intraamniotic injection of hypertonic saline, as indicated in Table 2.

Neonatal Mortality.   More infants die during the first three days of life than during the remainder of the first year. The common causes of death in the first two weeks of life, as listed in Table 3 from Potter, show the predominant role of

Table 3. **Causes of Mortality During the Perinatal Period, Chicago Lying-In Hospital (17,000 Deliveries)**

Cause of Death	Weight (Grams)			
	400–1,000	1,001–2,500	2,500+	Total
Hypoxia	16	55	46	117
Malformations	10	39	21	70
Hyaline membrane	4	40	12	56
Erythroblastosis	9	19	16	44
Infection	4	8	9	21
No demonstrable cause	109	55	30	194

Modified from Potter, E. L. Pathology of the Fetus and Infant, 2nd ed. Chicago, Year Book Medical Publishers, Inc., 1961.

prematurity in neonatal mortality. Of the 194 deaths, 164, or 84.5 per cent, occurred in infants weighing 2,500 g or less. The commonest cause of death in this series was "hyaline membrane," which, although occasionally seen in mature infants, is characteristically a disease of premature babies. In the group including the smallest infants, 400 to 1,000 g in weight, there were no physical abnormalities in three quarters of the cases, indicating that gross prematurity itself was the direct cause of death. Aside from hyaline membrane disease and prematurity, the most common causes of neonatal death are malformations, brain damage from intrauterine hypoxia, cerebral hemorrhage from trauma, and infections.

In addition to injuries or diseases that may kill the infant, there are sublethal injuries to the fetus during pregnancy and labor that may cause mental retardation of the child, cerebral palsy, and other neurologic defects. If many babies actually die from hypoxia or trauma during birth, it seems likely that many others escape death but suffer permanent effects of cerebral injury. The late effects of birth injuries, both hypoxic and traumatic, are among the most important problems that require urgent and intensive study in modern obstetrics.

FACTORS AFFECTING THE CENTRAL NERVOUS SYSTEM

Fetal Distress.   There is no consensus regarding the precise definition of fetal distress. In referring to this syndrome, most obstetricians think in terms of labor, but efforts have recently been made to ascertain the status of the fetus before labor. Disturbances of fetal function might well be considered part of the syndrome of fetal distress. In the case of a diabetic mother with severe acidosis, for example, the fetus might be moribund. Research along these lines has been directed largely toward placental function, both endocrine and circulatory. Current research has also attempted to assess fetal and placental growth and maturation. Although methods have been developed that may generally differentiate seriously ill from normal fetuses, they are not yet sufficiently precise to be completely dependable in individual cases (Ch. 6, p. 181).

During labor, slowing of the fetal heart rate and, in vertex presentations, the passage of meconium are generally considered signs of fetal distress. There is still a difference of opinion as to whether the diagnosis of fetal distress is justified on the basis of just one criterion, such as fetal bradycardia alone. Irregularity of the fetal heartbeat and abnormally vigorous fetal movements are also sometimes included in the syndrome of fetal distress. More recently, small amounts of meconium discovered by amnioscopy or amniocentesis, as well as abnormalities in the pH of fetal scalp blood, have been employed as additional indications of fetal distress. Most observers agree that any single sign of fetal distress presages about a doubling of the stillbirth rate, whereas the combination of two, such as bradycardia and the passage of meconium, is associated with a fetal loss rate of between 20 and 30 per cent. For example, Cox as well as Fenton and Steer found an incidence of fetal distress in their respective series of about 10 per cent and a perinatal loss of about 5 per cent. In Cox's study, tachycardia alone was associated with a mortality of 3 per cent, bradycardia with 5.4 per cent, and the passage of meconium with 3.5 per cent. A combination of any two was associated with a mortality of 35 per cent.

Amnioscopy was reintroduced by Saling in 1962 to detect meconium in the amniotic fluid. With this technic, a small cone-shaped endoscope is passed through the somewhat dilated cervix and placed against the membranes. Although the procedure is painless and lacking in serious complications, it has not gained widespread popularity in this country. Bailey, who used the amnioscope first in 1948 and was so dissatisfied with the instrument that he did not publish his findings, states that meconium in the amniotic fluid is not always revealed by the amnioscope. Furthermore, although Kornacki and colleagues found meconium by means of this instrument in about 12 per cent of their patients with other signs of fetal distress, fewer than half of these women delivered asphyxiated infants.

Regrettably, extreme changes in pH do not always indicate fetal asphyxia. There still remain 8 per cent of babies in whom the pH before birth is higher than 7.25 and 20 per cent in whom the pH is lower than 7.15 who are vigorous at the time of delivery (Beard and Morris). Claims that the sampling of fetal scalp blood will save infants' lives and reduce the incidence of cesarean section have not been subjected to rigid statistical scrutiny and remain largely speculative. A prognostic error greater than 25 per cent places the method in the same class of accuracy as the more commonly used methods of detecting fetal distress.

Because of accessibility, efforts have been made to monitor the fetal heart throughout labor by means of the electrocardiograph. Recent years have brought marked refinements in the available instruments. It is still not clear, however, whether the improvements in instrumentation have resulted in increased fetal salvage. Two types of slowing of the fetal heart rate have been described by Hon and by Caldeyro-Barcia and his group. Both are approximately synchronous with the acme of uterine contractions, but as shown in Figure 1, the first type follows more directly than the second and is a transitory dip in rate, not very often to as low as 80 beats per minute, lasting less than 30 seconds. This first type of dip is the result of increased vagal tone induced by pressure on the fetal skull. It can be eliminated by the administration of atropine to the mother or directly into

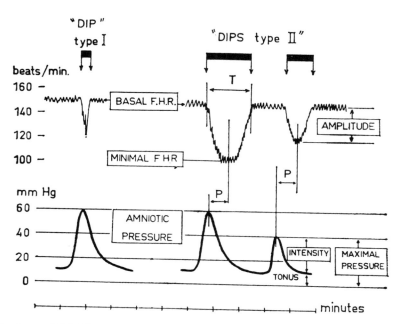

Fig. 1. Tracings of fetal heart rate and intraamniotic fluid pressure showing the difference in amplitude and timing between type I and type II "dips." (From Mendez-Bauer et al. Amer J Obstet Gynec 85:1033, 1963.)

the fetal scalp. The second type of dip is much more serious; the slowing is more profound and it often continues after cessation of the uterine contraction. Caldeyro-Barcia has shown that the second type of slowing is related to an increased perinatal loss. In some instances, fetal distress is associated with abnormal fetal electrocardiograms, a finding that is neither constant nor of clear significance.

Fetal distress is more prevalent in the conditions in Table 4, although it is often of unknown cause.

Table 4. **Conditions Associated with an Increased Prevalence of Fetal Distress**

Source	Cause
Infant	Prematurity
	Congenital malformations
Mother	Toxemia
	Diabetes
	Infection
	Dysfunctional labor
	Hypotension
Placenta	Placenta previa
	Abruptio placentae
Umbilical cord	Prolapse of the cord

The data on perinatal loss give a good indication of the gravity of the fetal distress syndrome. They do not, however, indicate the sequelae in infants who survive. Very few precise data are available. There is, however, a correlation between fetal distress and low Apgar scores at birth. Berendes has suggested, furthermore, that low scores are related to neurologic defects later in life. The seriousness of one or two episodes of fetal distress during labor is unknown. Many obstetricians have attended fearfully the birth of an infant whose heart rate has been slow and who has been passing meconium only to be astonished by its vigorous cry immediately after birth.

Treatment.   Little can be done to relieve many cases of fetal distress except delivery. It is obvious, however, that immediate search for the cause should be undertaken. In dysfunctional labor, oxytocin should be discontinued. Maternal hypotension caused by the supine position can sometimes be relieved by change in position or by antihypotensive agents if caused by conduction anesthesia. When it is the consequence of hypovolemia, vigorous fluid replacement, including whole blood, is mandatory.

The mother whose infant is showing fetal distress without obvious cause should have a thorough vaginal examination to ascertain whether the cord has prolapsed. In the absence of any obvious correctable abnormality the administration of oxygen to the mother may be of some transient value, but the only effective therapy is immediate delivery. In some cases cesarean section is required. In 2,547 primary cesarean sections recorded in the Obstetrical Statistical Cooperative series, fetal distress was an indication in 8.7 per cent.

Prolapse of the Umbilical Cord.   It is customary to speak of *prolapse* of the cord when the membranes are ruptured and the umbilical cord lies ahead of the presenting part in the vagina. If the cord lies alongside the presenting part and is palpable only by passing the examining finger into the cervical canal, it is often spoken of as an *occult prolapse* of the cord. If, however, the umbilical cord lies ahead of the presenting part but still within the intact membranes, it is termed a *cord* or *funic presentation.*

Etiology.   In general any factor that interferes with the accurate adaptation of the presenting part to the superior strait predisposes to prolapse of the cord. The accident, therefore, occurs most commonly in shoulder and foot presentations, less often with frank breeches, and with moderate frequency in multiple pregnancy.

It is rarely observed in cephalic presentations, however, unless there is interference with accommodation as a result of contracted pelvis (Fig. 2) or excessive development of the fetus.

Prematurity is associated with increased incidence of prolapsed cord, presumably because the small fetus is poorly applied to the pelvic inlet. Hydramnios and artificial rupture of the membranes seem to be of minor etiologic significance. The complication is more common in multigravidas than in primigravidas.

Incidence.   In a thorough study of prolapse of the cord at the Royal Maternity Hospital in Belfast, Myles cites the reported world incidence as varying between 0.3 and 0.6 per cent of deliveries. In a total of 255,759 reported deliveries collected from the literature there were 1,294 cases of prolapsed cord, an incidence of 0.50 per cent. In a current study of 83,624 deliveries at one hospital, the Kings County Medical Center in Brooklyn, Savage and co-workers report an incidence of 0.62 per cent. A difference in incidence of prolapsed cord in comparable groups of black and white patients has not been found consistently in reports in the literature.

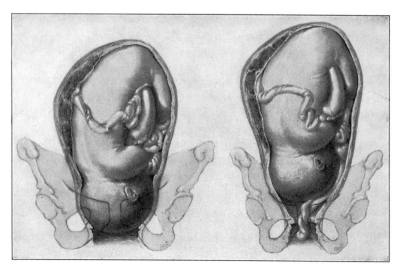

Fig. 2. Left, an engaged head, by filling the pelvic cavity, prevents prolapse of the cord. Right, an unengaged head, as in a case of contracted pelvis shown here, tends to favor prolapse of the cord after rupture of the membranes.

Diagnosis. The possibility of prolapsed cord should be considered whenever the membranes rupture with the presenting part still unengaged. If there is slowing of the fetal heart at that time or shortly thereafter, especially if the slowing continues beyond the uterine contraction, as shown in Figure 3, a careful vaginal examination should be performed to rule out the accident.

Presentation of the funis is diagnosed whenever a soft, pulsating, cordlike body can be felt through the cervix. Often, however, its recognition is possible only when the cord is in direct contact with the presenting part.

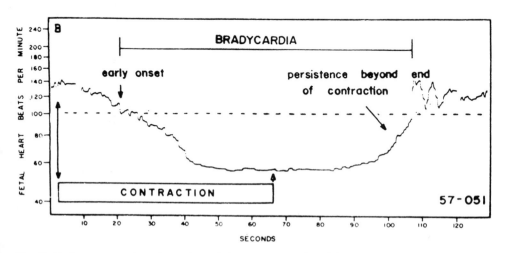

Fig. 3. Early onset and prolongation of fetal bradycardia with prolapsed cord. (From Hon. Amer J Obstet Gynec 77:1084, 1959.)

Prolapse of the cord is readily recognizable, since on vaginal examination the fingers come directly in contact with a loop, which occasionally may protrude from the vulva and make the diagnosis immediately evident. Even when the cord remains within the vagina, mistakes are hardly possible provided the fetus is alive, since distinct pulsations are felt.

Treatment. The treatment in any case depends mainly upon the extent to which the cervix is dilated and to a lesser extent upon the presentation of the fetus. In all instances, the head of the bed or table should be lowered or the patient placed in knee-chest position to relieve or minimize the pressure of the presenting part upon the cord and the danger of impaired umbilical circulation. In addition, the fetal head may be pushed upward by pressure from a finger in the rectum or a gloved hand in the vagina. With funic presentations there is danger to the fetus even though the membranes are intact. The treatment for a reasonably mature child is delivery by cesarean section.

In the absence of serious disproportion, if the cord prolapses under the observation of the obstetrician after the cervix has become fully dilated, the life of the child can usually be saved. No attempt at reposition should be made, but delivery should be effected at once. In cephalic and shoulder presentations, internal nodulic version may find one of its rare places in modern obstetrics, but forceps are indicated when the head is already deep down in the pelvis. In frank breech presentations, a foot, or preferably both feet, should be brought down and extraction promptly completed. Excessive haste in delivery must be avoided, since it is often attended by irreparable harm to the child and injury to the mother.

If the cervix is incompletely dilated, the chances of a favorable outcome for the child are greatly diminished unless prompt and decisive action is instituted. All available data indicate that if the fetus is mature and if the diagnosis is made promptly, cesarean section will yield excellent results. Such a course seems justified not only on the basis of the relative safety of section but because of the very poor results of attempts to reposit the cord and the danger to the mother of delivery through an incompletely dilated cervix. In Savage's large series from one hospital, cesarean section was employed in 28.5 per cent.

Upon diagnosis the mother should be placed in the knee-chest or deep Trendelenburg position and a hand covered by a sterile glove placed in the vagina to keep the head out of the pelvis. General anesthesia will prevent uterine contractions while preparations are made for cesarean section.

If the pulsations in the cord have slowed or ceased, no attempt at reposition should be made, inasmuch as the fetus has already died or will die before delivery can be effected. If, however, the cervix is fully dilated, there is little to be lost by immediate delivery. Occasionally a child that appears lost may be rescued. If, however, cesarean section is contemplated, immediate preparations for operation should be made. Before proceeding with the cesarean section, the operator should make certain that the fetal heart is still beating, since it is unjustifiable to subject the mother to an added risk without expectation of delivering a living child. Savage's current study concludes that the fetal salvage in face of prolapse of the umbilical cord can be improved by earlier detection of the accident by frequent vaginal examinations in high-risk situations and by greater use of cesarean section.

Prognosis. According to Savage and co-authors, the gross perinatal mortality associated with prolapse of the cord is 26.2 per cent. This figure is influenced by a very high rate of prematurity (45.5 per cent) and the large number of patients whose infants are dead on admittance (17.6 per cent). The perinatal mortality corrected to exclude fetuses dead on admittance and premature fetuses is 16.7 per cent. When cesarean section is employed under optimal conditions, the perinatal mortality for infants over 1,000 g may be reduced to 7.4 per cent.

Asphyxia of the Newborn. The three causes of intrauterine injury of the central nervous system—narcosis, hypoxia, and brain hemorrhage—produce a similar clinical picture, formerly known as *asphyxia neonatorum* and characterized by apnea as its prime objective manifestation. The course and prognosis of this syndrome vary with the degree of hypoxia, with the extent and location of hemorrhage, and, most important, with the degree of asphyxia. Asphyxia, as defined by the World Health Organization, "describes the condition of the infant's arterial blood and connotes hypoxia plus hypercapnea and acidosis." This acidotic asphyxial state is more injurious and more difficult to correct than hypoxia alone, as shown by the studies of James and others of Apgar's group.

Whereas the normal oxygen saturation of the arterial blood of the fetus at birth is approximately 60 per cent, in the severer degrees of asphyxia neonatorum the blood oxygen is reduced to one fifth or even one tenth that value. The blood of these infants, furthermore, has a high concentration of lactic acid and a very low pH. The alkali deficit caused by fixation of base by lactic acid and the primary excess of carbon dioxide resulting from inadequate diffusion from the fetus combine to raise markedly the partial pressure of carbon dioxide.

Narcosis of the respiratory center rarely causes asphyxia, provided that the infant is mature and that prompt, effective artificial respiration is given. Spontaneous respiration within a minute is the rule, and the outlook is excellent. If the infant has been profoundly narcotized, there will be areas of sclerosis and petechiae throughout the central nervous system. These lesions are probably caused by hypoxia rather than direct action of analgesic, narcotic, or anesthetic drugs.

Practically, therefore, it is impossible in any given case to be certain that narcosis is the only factor operative. The old term "asphyxia neonatorum" was therefore sometimes used to include cases of apnea at birth even though true asphyxia may have been absent. These infants are now classified as depressed. If they have been subjected to intrauterine narcosis, artificial respiration may be less effective in aerating the lungs. Consequently, varying degrees of hypoxia or asphyxia may result.

In addition to apnea, babies suffering from asphyxia often exhibit other evidence of injury in the color of their skin, their muscle tonus, and their heart rate. The Apgar score (p. 479) thus logically provides a better assessment of the newborn infant than any single observation, such as the breathing or crying time. In milder cases the infants are bluish, but when shock is superimposed they become white. In the presence of any significant degree of hypoxia, the muscle tone is weak, and in severe cases the infants are completely limp. A very slow heart beat is a characteristic finding, the rate often dropping below 50 per minute. The bradycardia responds dramatically to oxygen even in cases in which the ultimate termination is unfavorable. Since hypoxia may cause the rectal sphincter to relax, these infants are frequently covered with meconium.

Although minor degrees of oxygen deprivation increase the rate of respiration, profound levels of hypoxia invariably produce the opposite effect, namely, absence of respiration. A grave case of asphyxia at birth, with the low heart rate, the cold, white body covered with meconium, and the limp extremities, duplicates the reaction of any organism to hypoxia. In experimental animals, as well as in man, continued hypoxia produces a constant, well-defined sequence of phenomena that may readily be reproduced in the laboratory.

The sequence of events in experimental hypoxia is as follows: The reaction to mild hypoxemia includes increased respiration and accelerated heart rate. These are presumably compensatory mechanisms, the first designed to bring more oxygen to the blood and the second to deliver more oxygen to the tissues. With increasing hypoxemia these compensatory mechanisms ultimately fail to supply oxygen in amounts sufficient for cellular metabolism. Consciousness is lost and respirations stop. After respiratory failure there is an interval of three to five minutes during which the heart continues to beat, but there is a marked slowing of the rate. Electrocardiographic studies at this stage show suppression of the pacemaking function of the sinoatrial node and the assumption of that function by the atrioventricular node with its characteristic slow and regular rate. There is regularly partial or complete heart block with decrease in conduction in the internodal region to the point of suppression. Since this slowing of the heart in hypoxemia does not occur in animals in which the vagi are cut, it is apparently caused by vagotonia, which suppresses the sinoatrial rhythm. After respirations cease, or sometimes a little earlier, the blood pressure slowly declines through 40 to 60 seconds. It then may show a slight increase, but finally falls rapidly over two to three minutes, then more slowly for one or two minutes until a systolic pressure of 15 to 20 mm Hg is reached. Concomitant with the drop in blood pressure are blanching and cooling of the skin, as in shock. There is then skeletal muscular paralysis, producing flaccid extremities and relaxation of the sphincter ani. A few whiffs of oxygen or air, administered by artificial respiration, restore the animal at once to normal, provided they are given within three or four minutes after the oxygen crisis. To summarize the picture of experimental hypoxia immediately after crisis, there occur in rapid succession loss of consciousness, cessation of respiration, marked slowing of the heart, fall in blood pressure with the white, cold skin of shock, and skeletal muscular collapse causing general flaccidity of the extremities together with relaxation of the sphincter ani. Few clinical conditions can be simulated so completely as can asphyxia neonatorum by experimental hypoxemia.

Gruenwald has outlined the pathologic changes in hypoxic infants. Many of these features are lesions of shock. In combination, hypoxia and shock produce a variety of lesions in the viscera. Severe venous congestion and perhaps parenchymal damage to various organs increase the susceptibility of hypoxic infants to mechanical trauma. Gruenwald, Benitez, and others have shown fatty metamorphosis of the liver to be a prominent and frequent finding in hypoxic fetuses.

Treatment. In the presence of hypoxia, apnea is resistant to all types of treatment other than correction of the hypoxia itself. In other words, the only way in which respiration can be initiated when suppressed by hypoxia is by the administration of oxygen or air. Insufflation with oxygen, therefore, transcends all else in the treatment of apnea at birth. Attempts to stimulate respiration by adding carbon dioxide to the oxygen not only are futile but may even be dangerous, since these babies already suffer from hypercapnia.

Remote Sequelae. The residual effects of cerebral hypoxia are varied. In many instances there are no clearly defined episodes of apnea found in the infant ultimately destined to show crippling residual brain damage. Symptoms present at birth are often forgotten by the time trouble arises months later. There is great variation in the late effects of cerebral damage. There may be only a delay in normal behavior in some infants, whereas others manifest convulsions, mental deficiency, spastic paralysis, choreoathetosis, ataxia, disorders of speech, sensory disturbances, or combinations thereof. Courville states that behavioral disorders, isolated deficits in intellect and speech, and convulsive states heretofore considered idiopathic are probably the residual effects of overlooked hypoxia at birth.

An etiologic relation between hypoxia, both intrauterine and intrapartum, and a host of neurologic defects is commonly postulated. The evidence to support this concept is inconsistent, however. For example, Niswander and colleagues have followed children born of mothers with placenta previa, placental abruption, and prolapsed cord; although there was an increase in the incidence of low Apgar scores at birth, none of three complications appears to produce an increase in neurologic damage in term infants. In some circumstances the premature infant appeared at greater risk, but even considering the known effects of low birth weight, the relation of hypoxia to neurologic sequelae is inconstant. The data relating obstetric complications to mental retardation are less precise. It is probable that extremely low birth weights are positively correlated with lower intelligence quotients, but the relative role of hypoxia is uncertain (Drillien; also Ch. 37, p. 1033). Two recent studies bear on this subject. Drage and co-workers find a positive correlation between low Apgar scores and both fine and gross motor deficiencies. Less positive, but highly suggestive, are the findings of Neligan and Russell. These investigators showed a relation between breech delivery and low intelligence quotient. Presumably, infants presenting in this manner may be more hypoxic than those presenting by vertex.

Lilienfeld and Parkhurst; Levin, Brightman, and Burtt; and data from our own clinic emphasize antecedent obstetric complications in cases of cerebral palsy. From the data available on the incidence of cerebral palsy, any obstetric service with 3,000 deliveries annually should expect 12 to 15 of the babies born each year to develop this condition. In different terms, for every 5 perinatal deaths, 1 surviving infant will subsequently develop cerebral palsy.

The most thoroughly documented cause of cerebral palsy is prematurity, especially extreme prematurity, as demonstrated convincingly by Eastman and associates. In a retrospective analysis of the obstetric background, a large number of children afflicted with cerebral palsy were compared with a similar number of normal children. The incidence of premature birth of 30 per cent in the group with cerebral palsy, in contrast to only 8 per cent in the control series, is in keeping with previous reports. The new finding relates to extreme prematurity. Whereas in the control series of 750 cases only 3 children had weighed less than 1,500 g at birth, not less than 62 of the 750 palsied children had had a birth weight of less than 1,500 g. The mechanism by which extreme prematurity causes cerebral palsy is not known, but various evidence suggests that certain factors in the neonatal period may be responsible, particularly the respiratory distress syndrome and dehydration with resultant hypernatremia.

In mature infants, hyperbilirubinemia unassociated with isoimmunization is a less common cause of cerebral palsy; in grossly premature infants, the high levels of bilirubin in the tissues may be etiologically related to defective hearing and other neurologic deficits.

This study has also demonstrated rather conclusively that in present-day obstetrics the role played by traumatic delivery in the etiology of cerebral palsy is small. With exchange blood transfusions, moreover, the number of cases resulting from kernicterus associated with erythroblastosis has diminished dramatically. Hypoxia, as the result of abruptio placentae or prolapse of the cord, undoubtedly causes a substantial number of cases, but the number is far smaller than that caused by prematurity.

Cerebral Hemorrhage.   The head of the fetus may undergo molding during its passage through the birth canal. The skull bones, the dura mater, and the brain itself permit considerable alteration in the dimensions of the fetal head without untoward results, perhaps in part by changes in the distribution of the cerebrospinal fluid. The shape of the head is altered, with lengthening of the occipitofrontal and sagittal diameters of the skull (Fig. 4). As a result, stretching and even lacerations of the tentorium cerebelli and less often of the falx cerebri may

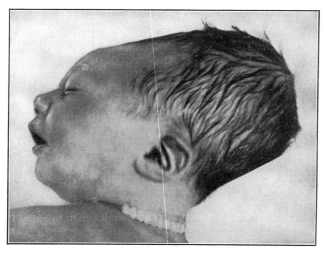

Fig. 4. Molding of head, newborn child.

occur. There may be edema and hyperemia in various parts of the brain, with the development of fetal distress during labor or hypoxia after delivery.

Intracranial hemorrhages were formerly encountered in 40 to 80 per cent of newborn infants upon whom an autopsy was performed, but in recent years most obstetric clinics have shown a substantial reduction in the incidence of traumatic brain hemorrhage. Former studies showing that one third to one half of all deaths within the first two weeks of life resulted from cerebral birth injuries are no longer valid. On the contrary, Potter and others state that the most significant decrease in mortality has been achieved in the group resulting from trauma. There is rather general agreement that refinements in the mechanical aspects of obstetrics, the choice of cesarean section in place of difficult vaginal deliveries, and the elimination of difficult forceps and of version and extraction have contributed to the downward trend.

Potter defines "birth injury" as any condition that affects the fetus adversely during labor or delivery. She distinguishes between "birth injury" resulting from primary oxygen deficiencies and that resulting from mechanical injury. In accordance with that concept, intracranial hemorrhage can be divided into cases initiated by hypoxia (ventricular and subarachnoid hemorrhages, subependymal hemorrhages, and isolated hemorrhages in the pia mater) and those produced by mechanical trauma associated with subdural hematomas or dural tears. The common types and locations of intracranial hemorrhages have been classified by Haller, Nesbitt, and Anderson, as illustrated in Figure 5.

In a study of 1,043 perinatal deaths (infants and fetuses weighing 1,000 g and over), Haller and associates attributed 94 deaths to intracranial hemorrhage.

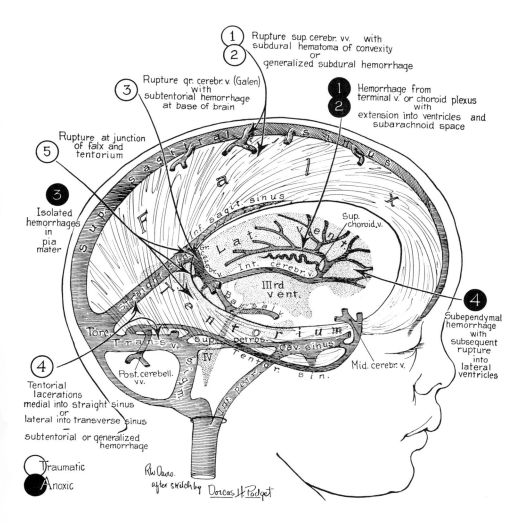

Fig. 5. The common types and locations of intracranial hemorrhage. (From Haller Nesbitt, and Anderson. Obstet Gynec Survey 11:179, 1956.)

The total number of deaths from brain hemorrhage was divided almost equally between premature infants (44 cases) and term infants (50 cases). Hypoxic brain hemorrhage was the principal type among premature infants (29 of 44 deaths), whereas trauma played the major etiologic role in term infants dying of intracranial hemorrhage (41 of 50 cases). Difficult midforceps delivery played an important role in the production of traumatic brain hemorrhage (19.6 per cent), but was a factor in only 2.6 per cent of the cases of hypoxic brain hemorrhage. Difficult deliveries were common in both groups, however. Even when evidence of mechanical trauma is lacking, extensive hemorrhage producing death often results from the hypoxia produced by the procedure itself. The fetus is rendered particularly susceptible to trauma when the cerebral vessels are congested and damaged by hypoxia.

The signs and symptoms are variable, including drowsiness, apathy, feeble cry, pallor, failure to nurse, dyspnea, cyanosis, vomiting, and convulsions. Ate-lectasis, asphyxia neonatorum, and forceps abrasions on the face may be asso-ciated findings. To rule out diaphragmatic hernia, congenital heart disease, atelectasis, and pneumonia, roentgenologic examination of the chest is useful.

Treatment consists of sedation to control convulsions, supportive measures, and oxygen for the dyspnea and cyanosis. If the anterior fontanel is bulging, a lumbar puncture is indicated to relieve pressure. The intramuscular administra-tion of vitamin K is indicated, because in many of these infants slow oozing of blood from the ruptured vessel continues for several days. Optimal coagulability of the blood is therefore essential if the process is to be checked.

The prevention of cerebral hemorrhage is of the utmost importance. Reduc-tion in the incidence of midforceps deliveries as well as the elimination of all difficult forceps operations, the use of cesarean section when there is definite cephalopelvic disproportion, the correct management of breech delivery, and the virtual elimination of internal version and extraction should contribute signif-icantly toward reduction in the incidence of all birth injuries, especially intra-cranial hemorrhage. The surviving infants may subsequently develop motor dis-turbances, including cerebral palsy, and about 10 per cent have residual mental deficiency. Certain cases of idiopathic epilepsy also are probably caused by intra-cranial injury sustained at birth.

PERIPHERAL INJURIES

Cephalhematoma.   Subperiosteal hemorrhages are most commonly found over one or both parietal bones, and they gradually increase in size during the first week of life. The lesion is differentiated from caput succedaneum by its periosteal limitations, with definite palpable edges (Fig. 6). Furthermore, it may not appear for hours or days after delivery, often growing larger and disappearing after weeks or months, whereas caput succedaneum is present at birth, grows smaller, and disappears usually within a few hours. A cephalhematoma is caused by injury to the periosteum of the skull during labor or delivery. Ingram and Hamilton have reported an incidence of cephalhematomas in their clinic of 1.66 per cent. Churchill and colleagues, from a review of the sparse literature on the subject, indicate that cephalhematomas occur about once in 50 deliveries. Although ex-pectant treatment is the rule in these cases, increasing size of the hematoma and other evidence of massive hemorrhage are indications for additional investigation. X-ray films may show a fracture of the skull, or more commonly, as indicated by Kozinn and associates, the infant may have defective blood clotting. A cephal-hematoma should not be aspirated because of the danger of infection.

Spinal Injury.   Overstretching of the spinal cord and associated hemorrhage may follow excessive traction during a breech delivery, and actual fracture or dis-location of the vertebrae may occur. Complete data on such lesions are lacking, since even the most careful autopsy does not always include examination of the spinal column, but fracture of the cervical vertebrae is not rare (Fig. 7).

Obstetric Paralyses.   As a result of a difficult labor, and in exceptional cases after an easy one, the child is sometimes born with a paralyzed arm. Commonly known as *Duchenne's* or *Erb's paralysis*, this condition involves paralysis of the deltoid, infraspinatus, and flexor muscles of the forearm, causing the entire arm

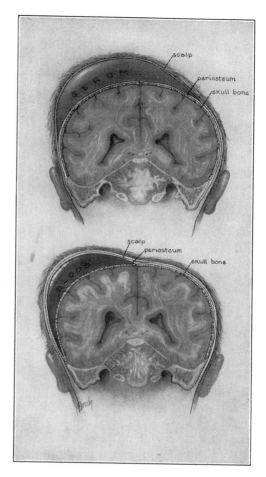

Fig. 6. Diagrammatic sketch to illustrate difference between caput succedaneum (above) and cephalhematoma (below). In a caput succedaneum the effusion overlies the periosteum and consists of serum; in a cephalhematoma it lies under the periosteum and consists of blood.

to fall close to the side of the body and rotate inward, with the forearm extended upon the arm. The function of the fingers is usually retained.

The lesion results from stretching or tearing of the upper roots of the brachial plexus, which is readily subjected to extreme tension as a result of pulling obliquely upon the head, thus sharply flexing it toward one of the shoulders. As traction in this direction is frequently employed to effect delivery of the shoulders in normal vertex presentations, Duchenne's paralysis may result without traumatic delivery. In extracting the shoulders, therefore, care should be taken not to bring about excessive lateral flexion of the neck. In breech extractions, moreover, particular attention should be devoted to preventing the extension of the arms over the head. Extended arms not only materially complicate delivery but increase the risk of paralysis.

The prognosis is usually fair, many of the children recovering. Occasionally, however, a case may resist all treatment, and the arm may remain permanently paralyzed, especially when mobility of the fingers has been lost. All of the infants personally observed by us have recovered, but in some, prolonged treatment was necessary. The child afflicted with this form of paralysis should be promptly placed under treatment by a competent specialist.

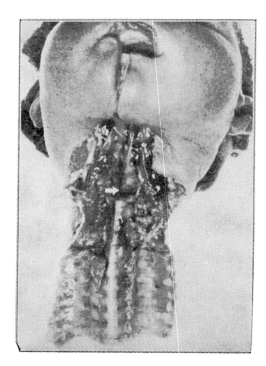

Fig. 7. Fracture of cervical vertebra following breech extraction.

Occasionally the child may be born with *facial paralysis,* a condition that may develop also shortly after birth (Fig. 8). It usually occurs in cases in which the head has been seized obliquely with forceps. It is caused by pressure exerted by the posterior blade of the forceps on the stylomastoid foramen, through which the facial nerve emerges. Not every case of facial paralysis following delivery by forceps should be attributed to the operation, however, since the condition is occasionally encountered after spontaneous delivery. Spontaneous recovery in a few days is the rule.

Skeletal Fractures.   Fractures of the clavicle and the humerus are found with about the same frequency. Difficulty encountered in the delivery of the shoulders in vertex presentations and extended arms in breech are the main factors in the production of such fractures. They are often of the greenstick type, although complete fracture with overriding of the bones is occasionally seen. Palpation of the clavicles and long bones should be performed on all newborn infants when a fracture is suspected, and any crepitation or unusual irregularity should be investigated by roentgenography.

Treatment of the clavicular fracture is simple, consisting of abduction of the arm, with outward and backward rotation. The position can be maintained by fastening the garment of the forearm to the bassinette above the child's head. The fractured humerus is maintained in a hand-on-hip position with a triangular splint, which keeps the arm in adduction. Application of a Velpeau bandage aids in further immobilization. Orthopedic consultation is desirable.

A fractured femur is relatively uncommon and is usually associated with breech delivery. It may be treated satisfactorily by extension of the leg and flexion of the thigh on the abdomen, maintaining the position by traction in an

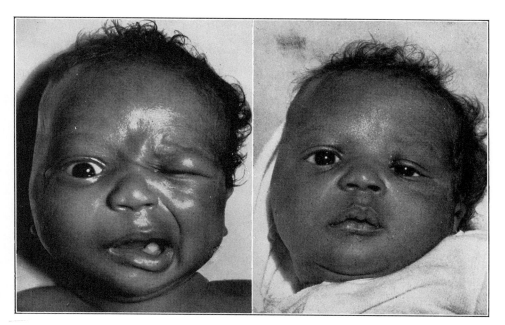

Fig. 8. Left, paralysis of left side of face 15 minutes after forceps delivery. Right, same infant 24 hours later. Recovery was complete in another 24 hours. (J.H.H. 296226.)

upward direction, as provided by a Bradford frame. Adhesive tape is used to attach the pulley and weight mechanism to the skin of the legs and thighs. Unilateral fractures are treated as though they were bilateral, that is, with traction applied to both legs.

Muscular Injuries. Injury to the sternocleidomastoid muscle may occur, particularly during breech delivery. There may be a tear of the muscle or possibly of the fascial sheath, leading to a hematoma and gradual cicatricial contraction. As the neck lengthens in the process of normal growth, the child's head is gradually turned to one side, since the damaged muscle is less elastic and does not elongate at the same rate as its normal counterpart on the opposite side, thus producing the deformity of *torticollis*. Roemer reports that 27 of 44 infants showing this deformity in his series had been delivered by breech or podalic version. He postulates that lateral hyperextension sufficient to rupture the sternocleidomastoid may occur as the aftercoming head passes over the sacral promontory. Thus, this condition is a birth injury and therefore must be considered possibly preventable.

References

Apgar, V., Holaday, D. A., James, L. S., Weisbrot, I. M., and Berrien, C. Evaluation of the newborn infant—second report. JAMA 168:1985, 1958.

Bailey, N. Amnioscopy. S Afr J Obstet Gynaec 5:12, 1967.

Beard, R. W., and Morris, E. D. Fetal distress—some biochemical considerations, in Kellar, R. J., (ed.), Modern Trends in Obstetrics. London, Butterworth, 1969, Vol. 4, Ch. 10, p. 273.

Benitez, R. E. Degenerative changes in liver associated with aspiration of vernix and hyaline membrane formation in lungs in intra-uterine anoxia. Arch Path 54:378, 1952.

Berendes, H. W. Proceedings of the International Congress on the Scientific Study of Mental Retardation, Copenhagen, Denmark, 1964.

Caldeyro-Barcia, R. (ed.). Transactions of the Symposium on the Effects of Labor on the Fetus and the Newborn, WHO, Geneva, 1965.

Churchill, J. A., Stevenson, L., and Habhab, G. Cephalohematoma and natal brain injury. Obstet Gynec 27:580, 1966.

Courville, C. B. Case studies in cerebral anoxia. Bull Los Angeles Neurol Soc 20:1:69, 1955.

Cox, L. W. Fetal distress. Aust New Zeal J Obstet Gynaec 1:99, 1961.

Drage, J. S., Berendes, H. W., and Fisher, P. D. Apgar scores and four-year psychological examination performance. Pan American Health Organization, Scientific Publication 185: 222, 1969.

Drillin, C. M. The Growth and Development of the Prematurely Born Infant. Baltimore, The Williams & Wilkins Co., 1969, p. 214.

Eastman, N. J. Fetal blood studies. Bull Hopkins Hosp 47:221, 1930; 48:261, 1931; 50:39, 1932.

——— Apnea neonatorum. Amer J Obstet Gynec 40:647, 1940.

——— Kohl, S. G., Maisel, J., and Kavaler, F. The obstetrical background of 753 cases of cerebral palsy. Obstet Gynec Survey 17:459, 1962.

Fenton, A. E., and Steer, C. M. Fetal distress. Amer J Obstet Gynec 83:355, 1962.

Goldstein, D. P., Johnson, J. P., and Reid, D. E. Management of intrauterine fetal death. Obstet Gynec 21:523, 1963.

Goplerud, C. P., and White, C. A. Delivering the dead fetus. Postgrad Med 43:167, 1968.

Gruenwald, P. Asphyxia, trauma and shock at birth. Arch Pediat 67:103, 1950.

Haller, E. S., Nesbitt, R. E. L., and Anderson, G. W. Clinical and pathologic concepts of gross intracranial hemorrhage in perinatal mortality. Obstet Gynec Survey 11:179, 1956.

Hon, E. H. Observations on "pathologic" fetal bradycardia. Amer J Obstet Gynec 77:1084, 1959.

Ingram, M. D., and Hamilton, W. M. Cephalohematoma in the newborn. Radiology 55:503, 1950.

James, L. S., Weisbrot, I. M., Prince, C. E., Holaday, D. A., and Apgar, V. The acid-base status of human infants in relation to asphyxia and the onset of respiration. J Pediat 52: 379, 1958.

Jimenez, J. M., and Pritchard, J. A. Pathogenesis and treatment of coagulation defects resulting from fetal death. Obstet Gynec 32:449, 1968.

Kornacki, Z., Biczysko, R., and Jakubowski, A. Amnioscopy as a routine obstetric examination in the later stages of pregnancy and at the beginning of labor. Amer J Obstet Gynec 101:539, 1968.

Kozinn, P. J., Ritz, N. D., Moss, A. H., and Kaufman, A. Massive hemorrhage—scalps of newborn infants. Amer J Dis Child 108:413, 1964.

Levin, M. L., Brightman, I. J., and Burtt, E. J. The problem of cerebral palsy. New York J Med 49:2793, 1949.

Lilienfeld, A. M., and Parkhurst, E. A study of the association of factors of pregnancy and parturition with the development of cerebral palsy. A preliminary report. Amer J Hyg 53:262, 1951.

Méndez-Bauer, C., Poseiro, J. J., Arellano-Hernandez, G., Zambrana, M. A., and Caldeyro-Barcia, R. Effects of atropine on the heart rate of the human fetus during labor. Amer J Obstet Gynec 85:1033, 1963.

Myles, T. J. M. Prolapse of the umbilical cord. J Obstet Gynaec Brit Emp 66:301, 1959.

Neligan, G., and Russell, J. K. Physical trauma as an etiological agent in mental retardation. Conference of National Institute of Neurological Diseases and Blindness. Lincoln, Nebraska, October, 1968.

Niswander, K. R., Friedman, E. A., Hoover, D. B., Pietrowski, H., and Westphal, M. C. Fetal morbidity following potentially anoxigenic obstetric conditions. Parts I, II, III. Amer J Obstet Gynec 95:838, 846, 853, 1966.

Potter, E. L. Pathology of the Fetus and Infant, 2nd ed. Chicago, Year Book Publishers, 1961.

Pritchard, J. A. Fetal death in utero. Obstet Gynec 14:573, 1959.

————and Ratnoff, O. D.   Studies of fibrinogen and other hemostatic factors in women with intrauterine death and delayed delivery. Surg Gynec Obstet 101:467, 1955.

Roemer, F. J.   Relation of torticollis to breech delivery. Amer J Obstet Gynec 68:1146, 1954.

Saling, E.   (Amnioscopy, a new method for diagnosis of conditions hazardous to the fetus when membranes are intact.) Geburtsh Frauenheilk 22:830, 1962.

Savage, E. W., Kohl, S. G., and Wynn, R. M.   Prolapse of the umbilical cord. Obstet Gynec 36:502, 1970.

Tricomi, V., and Kohl, S. G.   Fetal death in utero. Amer J Obstet Gynec 74:1092, 1957.

37

DISEASES OF THE NEWBORN

Definitions.   A premature infant is born so early in gestation that his organs have not reached adequate development; his chance of survival, therefore, is poorer than that of a term infant. Various criteria have been suggested for categorizing an infant as premature, such as gestational age (calculated from the mother's last menstrual period), length, weight, and various combinations of these factors. Since menstrual histories are often unreliable, estimations of gestational age on that basis may be erroneous. The length of the infant, furthermore, is not an entirely dependable criterion because of inaccuracies in measurement. The weight of a premature baby, therefore, is usually taken as the main index of gestational age, at least for purposes of classification. There has been general agreement that 2,500 g marks the lower limit of maturity. The value of 2,500 g, arrived at arbitrarily, was accepted by most professional organizations and by the World Health Organization as the dividing point between "mature" and "premature." Although there is no sharp change in survival at 2,500 g, choice of this end point was based on the ability of infants weighing more than 2,500 g to cope with extrauterine conditions about as well as do larger infants, as shown by many statistical studies. Infants weighing less than 2,500 g are less likely to survive, their handicap increasing progressively as the birth weight falls farther below 2,500 g. Closer scrutiny of this criterion, however, reveals that weight is at best an inaccurate index of the state of functional maturity. Some infants born at or near term weigh less than 2,500 g. Their low birth weight reflects intrauterine maldevelopment or retarded growth rather than prematurity, with its implication of functional immaturity. Conversely, infants with much edema, for example, or those born of diabetic mothers may weigh more than 2,500 g, although they are premature according to gestational age. Furthermore, although the arbitrary figure may be valid for the white race, it is hardly applicable to black infants, who, on the average, are slightly more than 100 g lighter; moreover, in parts of Asia such as India and China, this criterion of weight is totally inapplicable. The effects of race and other factors on the prevalence of "prematurity" are outlined in a review by Eastman.

The lower limits of prematurity—that is, the borderline between prematurity and abortion—are less well defined. Since an abortus is defined as a nonviable conceptus, the borderline between an abortus and a premature infant may be considered the weight below which survival is impossible.

This lower limit might logically be set at 400 g, because no fetus weighing less at birth has ever been known to survive. One fetus weighing 397 g on the second day of life, but doubtless slightly more than 400 g at birth, has survived, however, as reported by Monro. As shown in Figure 1, a fetus weighing approximately 400 g has a gestational age of about 20 weeks. Convenience is another reason for adopting this figure, since nearly all state departments of vital statistics require the reporting of all births in which the period of gestation is in excess of 20 weeks. Twenty weeks, of course, marks the midpoint of the normal duration of human pregnancy, counting from the last menstrual period. A premature infant might therefore be defined as weighing between 400 and 2,500 g at birth. The round figure of 500 g, however, has certain advantages as the definition of the limit between abortion and prematurity and is so employed elsewhere in this text.

Although infants weighing less than 800 g have been known to survive, such occurrences are rare. Even among those weighing between 800 and 1,000 g the

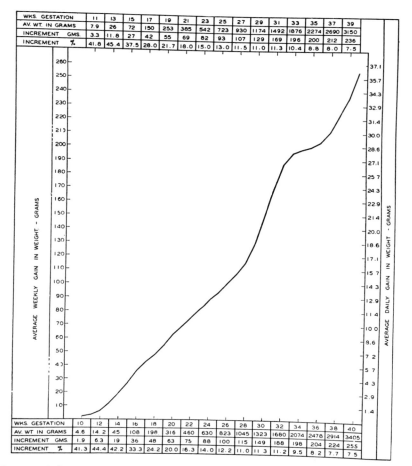

Fig. 1. Average daily and weekly fetal gain in weight, with average weight of fetuses plotted against their menstrual age. (From figures in Table 1. Streeter. Contrib Embryol, Vol. XI, Publ. No. 274, 1920.)

probability of survival is greatly reduced. Since formerly there was only a small
chance for survival of an infant markedly under 1,000 g, it might have been reasoned that all such fetuses should be classified as abortuses. Until recently that
view was widely held. It was customary to classify an infant as premature when
it weighed between 1,000 and 2,500 g at birth and to consider fetuses of less than
1,000 g as abortuses. Figure 1 shows that a fetus weighing 1,000 g has a gestational age of approximately 28 weeks. Since 28 weeks has long been cited in statutes as the lower limit of "viability," the figure of 1,000 g is consistent with a time-
honored concept. When an "abortus," as thus defined, survives, however, the
inconsistency of this definition becomes evident.

Although the problem of defining "prematurity" might seem to be of academic
interest only, its ramifications are surprisingly wide, since it enters into the definitions of abruptio placentae, therapeutic abortion, perinatal mortality, and other
important obstetric terms. Furthermore, the prognosis for the infant, both immediate and remote, depends on whether the low birth weight stems from true
prematurity, nutritional growth retardation, or congenital malformations. Few
data are available that record these factors. Ideally, a biologic marker of maturity
such as the activity of a specific enzyme would be of great value. This problem
is presently receiving much attention, but it has proved extremely difficult to
arrive at a universally satisfactory definition. Meanwhile, to obviate some of the
difficulties, it is becoming practical and customary to classify fetuses under 1,000
g in two categories: abortuses and "immature infants." Consistent with the convention of using weight groups of 500 g, an immature infant is defined as weighing between 500 and 999 g. The following definitions thus emerge:

1. *Abortuses.* Fetuses of birth weight under 500 g. No chance of survival.
2. *Immature Infants.* Fetuses of birth weight from 500 to 999 g. Poor chance
   of survival.
3. *Premature Infants.* Fetuses of birth weight from 1,000 to 2,499 g. Chances
   of survival range from poor to good according to weight.
4. *Mature Infants.* Fetuses of 2,500 g or more. Optimal chances of survival.

In 1935 the American Academy of Pediatrics recommended that an immature infant (premature) be classified as weighing 2,500 g or less at birth. This designation
was adopted by the National Vital Statistics Division of the U.S. Department of Health,
Education, and Welfare, and still appears in the World Health Organization's Manual
of International Statistical Classification of Diseases, Injuries, and Causes of Death.
In the strict sense of the definition, a mature infant weighs 2,501 g or more. The 1 g
is not statistically meaningful and is not consistent with customary groupings of data
or general computer programs that ordinarily break classification groups of 100 at 0
and 99. Furthermore, most obstetrical computer programs are now written in the customary statistical manner. Recent Committees on Terminology of the American College of Obstetricians and Gynecologists, and the International Federation of Gynecology and Obstetrics, have recommended that the customary statistical conventions be
followed and that premature and term infants be defined as 1,000 to 2,499 g, and
2,500 g or more, respectively. Throughout this text, as well as most other American
texts, this custom has been followed.

General Considerations.   It is common knowledge that prematurity is the
principal cause of death in the neonatal period, accounting for about one half of
all fatalities occurring at that time. Improved pediatric care and public health
programs have made significant gains, but the salvage, particularly among the

smaller infants, is still discouragingly low. There are two main ways of attacking this problem. First, mortality rates could be lowered substantially by wider dissemination of knowledge, together with better distribution of personnel, more precise diagnosis of the cause of low birth weight, and more intensive care of the newborn. At the Kings County Hospital the advent of a full-time neonatologist assigned to our service lowered our neonatal mortality by 15 per cent. Second is the prevention of premature birth, the obstetrician's greatest challenge.

Etiology.   Among a total of 28,493 deliveries at the Johns Hopkins Hospital during a period of about 20 years, 3,331 low-birth-weight infants (1,000 to 2,499 g) were born, an incidence of 12 per cent. Of these infants, about 12 per cent were associated with multiple pregnancies, in which the onset of labor was spontaneous. In 14 per cent of the total number of infants in this group, premature delivery of singletons was effected artificially because of maternal disease, chiefly toxemia, placenta previa, and abruptio placentae. In the remaining deliveries, almost two thirds of the low-birth-weight group, the precipitating cause was unknown.

The etiologic factors associated with infants of low birth weight in the Hopkins series are as follows: multiple gestation, 11.9 per cent; maternal disease necessitating operative termination of pregnancy, 14.3 per cent; maternal disease with spontaneous onset of labor, 10.3 per cent; and congenital abnormalities, 1.6 per cent. In other words, in the whole series of 3,331 small infants, a definite cause for the termination of pregnancy was demonstrable in only 1,269, or 38.1 per cent.

Other similar studies also indicate that the cause of more than half of all the births of infants of low birth weight is unexplained, although many investigators are convinced that these labors are more common in the lower economic groups. Even more controversial are the contention of Räihä that prematurity is related to maternal cardiac size and that of Kass that asymptomatic bacteriuria plays a role. Obviously these studies based solely on infant weight as a criterion of prematurity confuse the issue by grouping the gestationally premature infants with those who are nutritionally deprived or congenitally malformed.

Intrauterine Diagnosis of Maturity.   Although the intrauterine assessment of fetal maturity has received current attention, the diagnostic procedures lack precision. White and colleagues have examined the bilirubin and creatinine concentrations as well as the cytologic characteristics of the amniotic fluid. Although creatinine levels of at least 1.5 mg per cent and on optical density due to bilirubin of less than 0.010 at 450 mμ are usual after the thirty-fourth or thirty-fifth week of gestation, there is sufficient variation to cast doubt on the value of any single test. Henneman and associates along with many other investigators have made very similar observations. Similarly, although there are usually clumps of orange-colored cells after staining the amniotic fluid with Nile blue sulfate after the thirty-seventh week of gestation, Anderson and Griffiths have found some amniotic fluids with none of these cells at term. By using all three tests and applying a scoring technic, Thiede has suggested a more accurate evaluation of maturity.

Sonographic mensuration of the fetal head has also been used by Hellman and colleagues and Thompson and Makowski to ascertain fetal maturity. This method too appears promising.

Clinical Diagnosis of Maturity.   Usher and colleagues have pointed out that certain external physical features differentiate during the last month of pregnancy and are unaffected by growth retardation. The clinical signs that have proved to be most valuable are creases on the sole of the foot, size of breast nodule, texture of the hair, cartilaginous development of the earlobe, and in the male, testicular descent and scrotal creases (Table 1). Infants of 36 weeks and

Table 1. **Clinical Criteria for Gestational Age Assessment**

	To 36 Weeks	*Gestational Age 37–38 Weeks*	*39 Weeks or More*
Sole creases	Anterior transverse crease only	Occasional creases anterior two thirds	Sole covered with creases
Breast nodule diameter	2 mm	4 mm	7 mm
Scalp hair	Fine and fuzzy	Fine and fuzzy	Coarse and silky
Earlobe	Pliable, no cartilage	Some cartilage	Stiffened by thick cartilage
Testes and scrotum	Testes in lower canal	Intermediate	Testes pendulous
	Scrotum small		Scrotum full
	Few rugae		Extensive rugae

less have feet with smooth soles, small or absent breast nodules, fuzzy hair, pliable earlobes lacking cartilaginous support, and only partially descended testes with an empty scrotum. After 38 weeks the soles are well creased, the breasts are usually large, the hair is straight and silky, the earlobes are stiffened by cartilaginous support, and the testes are fully descended into a large scrotum. Intermediate conditions are found at 37 to 38 weeks' gestation.

Before 36 weeks' gestation, neurologic and electroencephalographic findings have proved useful in estimating true gestational age. The Moro, grasp, and rooting reflexes, as well as pupillary contraction, glabellar tap, automatic walk, and cry have proved most useful diagnostically. At Kings County Hospital a simple composite gestational age sheet is included on the chart of each newborn infant (Table 2).

Infants Small for Gestational Age.   Certain infants weighing less than 2,500 g, which have previously been erroneously classified as premature, suffer instead from intrauterine growth retardation. Their low birth weights may result from either sudden interruption of a normally developing gestation or long-term deprivation of nutrients. A practical classification of newborn infants based upon gestational age and birth weight has been proposed by Battaglia and Lubchenco. Figure 2 identifies infants who deviate from the normal pattern of intrauterine growth.

The "small-for-gestational-age infant" can be subclassified into three categories:

A. Intrauterine undernutrition
B. Congenital malformation
C. Intrauterine infection

Intrauterine malnutrition includes the postterm infant who commonly has a small, infarcted placenta; he is easily recognized by his alert facies, emaciation, and peeling skin (p. 590). In the preterm infant suffering from intrauterine undernutrition caused by inadequate uterine blood flow or by placental insufficiency, growth in head circumference and length are unaffected whereas weight is diminished. Morbidity is related to long-term fetal undernourishment, as well as

Table 2. Downstate University–Kings County Hospital Assessment of Gestational Age

Feature		Week Usually Present	24	25	26	27	28	29	30	31	32	33	34	35	36	37	38	39	40	41	42	43
Sole creases	Anterior transverse	36 or less													Transverse							
	Anterior 2/3	37–38														Ant. 2/3						
	Sole covered	39 or more																Covered				
Breast nodule	2 mm	36 or less													2 mm							
	4 mm	37–38														4 mm						
	7 mm	39 or more																7 mm				
Scalp hair	Fine-fuzzy	38 or less														Fuzzy						
	Coarse-silky	39 or more																Silky				
Ear lobe	Without cartilage	36													None							
	Some cartilage	37–38														Some						
	Thick cartilage	39 or more																Thick				
Genitalia	Testes in canal	36													Canal							
	Testes in scrotum	38															Scrotum					
	Rugae few	36														Few						
	Rugae extensive	39																Extensive				
Posture	Lateral	24		Lateral																		
	Supine	28						Supine														
	Froglike	34												Froglike								
	Full flexion	38															Total flexion					
Popliteal angle	180°	24		180°																		
	120°	34												120°								
	90°	38															90°					
Moro		24–32		Present											Complete							
Grasp		24–28		Feeble								Solid				"Pick Up"						
Rooting		24–28		Minimal						Good												
Suck		28–34						Present						Strong								
Pupillary contraction		32										Present										
Glabellar tap		30–32								Present												
Automatic walk		34												Minimal								
Crossed extension		24–28						Slight								Withdrawal						
Cry		24–28		Feeble					High pitch			Good										

Neurologic examination must be done after the first 24 hours of life.

Summary

I. True Premature: Gestational Age _____ wk

II. Low-Birth-Weight Infant: Gestational Age _____ wk

III. Mature Newborn: Gestational Age _____ wk

1031

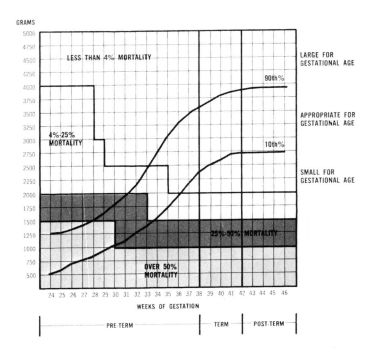

Fig. 2. Mortality and size for gestational age. (From Battaglia, F. C., and Lubchenco, L. O. J Pediat 71:161, 1967.)

hypoglycemia in the neonatal period. The brain of these infants grows to nearly normal size, whereas the growth of the liver is markedly stunted. The ability of the liver to supply glucose to the brain is therefore compromised, and the blood glucose is sharply lowered. Compensatory mechanisms seem to be impaired (Cornblath). Maternal conditions associated with a decreased rate of fetal weight gain after the thirty-fifth week include hypertensive cardiovascular diseases, preeclampsia-eclampsia, and multiple pregnancies. In addition, low birth weight may result from residing at high altitude or from cigarette smoking.

Some congenital and genetic malformations are associated with infants that are small for their gestational ages, including those with 16-18 and 13-15 trisomy. Twenty per cent of mongoloid babies are small at birth; the head size is reduced although the length is normal.

Low birth weight is associated also with Turner's, DeLange's, Silver's, and Seckle's syndromes and with osteogenesis imperfecta. Intrauterine infections such as rubella, cytomegalic inclusion body disease, toxoplasmosis, and listeriosis are also related to growth retardation, according to Lubchenco and colleagues.

Infants that are small for gestational age do not form an etiologically homogeneous group. Their prognosis depends upon the cause of the growth retardation. In general, these infants appear more mature than their weights would indicate, at least with respect to their temperature responses. Hyperbilirubinemia in these infants seems to follow a milder course. They rarely attain normal growth, however. This lasting effect of intrauterine growth retardation is well exemplified in the case of twins, one of which is small and the other of normal size. These twins maintain this differential in size throughout life (Faulkner).

Prognosis.   If standard medical and nursing care is available, the prognosis for a premature infant depends almost entirely on its gestational age, which is related, of course, to its weight at birth.

About 80 per cent of the neonatal deaths in premature infants occur within the first 24 hours. If a premature infant survives this period, the likelihood of his ultimate survival is greatly increased. Since well over 90 per cent of neonatal deaths in premature infants take place in the first week of life, the prognosis for an infant surviving this period is immeasurably improved. The liveborn survival rates for both white and black patients at the Kings County Hospital are shown in Figure 3, which illustrates graphically the effect of weight upon the infant's

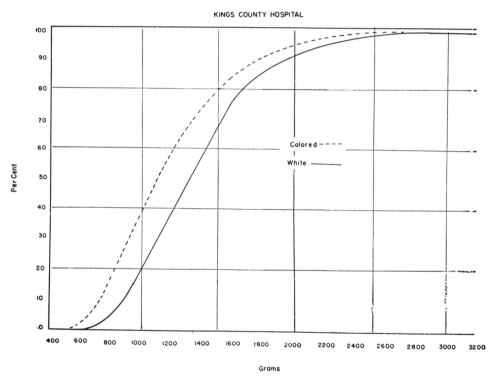

Fig. 3. Liveborn infant survival rate for both white and black patients at the Kings County Hospital.

prognosis. This effect must be carefully considered when early delivery for maternal disease, as in preeclampsia or hypertension, is contemplated.

Respiratory Distress Syndrome.   The cause of the respiratory distress syndrome remains obscure, but it appears to involve to a considerable degree the inability of the negative pressure from inspiration to overcome the surface tension of the collapsed alveoli. The ability of the fetal lung to secrete significant amounts of surface tension reducing phospholipids, collectively termed *surfactant*, is ordinarily acquired relatively late in pregnancy. It has been demonstrated recently that pulmonary maturation and surfactant activity can be induced in utero by administering cortisol to the premature sheep fetus and probably other species as well (Brumley and de Lemos and co-workers). It is also of considerable interest that if the amount of cortisol infused exceeds a critical level, labor is induced. Strang and colleagues reported that elective cesarean section itself does not increase the risk of "hyaline membrane disease." Usher and his associates at the Royal Victoria Hospital showed, however, that cesarean section did predispose to the respiratory distress syndrome in infants of less than 270 days' gestation. A history of maternal diabetes or bleeding also predisposes the infant to hyaline membrane disease (Cohen). James indicates that hypoxia is a definite contributing factor and Keuth reports a higher incidence of respiratory distress in twins. Moss, Duffie, and Fagan, as well as others, suggest that early clamping of the cord plays a role in its causation; the relation is difficult to prove, however, and at least one group of investigators (Taylor, Bright, and Birchard) concluded that "placental transfusion did not benefit premature infants." A condition resembling hyaline membrane disease has been produced experimentally in animals by a variety of insults, such as injection of vernix into the trachea, x-irradiation of the lungs, carbon dioxide poisoning, vagotomy, and injection of toxins that produce capillary damage.

Clinically the infants exhibit an increased respiratory rate accompanied by severe retraction. The upper portion of the chest appears overinflated. Expiration is often accompanied by a whimper or grunt. A tendency toward a fixed heart rate of 110 to 120 beats per minute has been noted. Poor peripheral circulation and systemic hypotension are evident. Hypoxia and hypothermia are usually found along with a combined metabolic and respiratory acidosis. The single most useful diagnostic aid is a chest roentgenogram, which reveals a diffuse, reticulo-granular infiltrate throughout the lung fields with an air-filled tracheobronchial tree. Deaths from "hyaline membrane disease" almost always occur before 72 hours of age. An incubator kept at 95°F or more is required occasionally to raise body temperature to normal levels. Metabolic acidosis should be corrected, and assisted ventilation may be beneficial when infants appear to be tiring.

The death rate for seriously affected premature infants is nearly 30 per cent, but it is somewhat less than 4 per cent for term infants. There is an inverse pro-portion between the length of life and the extent of membrane found. Latham, Nesbitt, and Anderson correlated the clinical and pathologic findings in 124 infants dying with associated pulmonary hyalinelike membranes. They empha-size that the severe grades were associated with 70 per cent or more of pulmonary atelectasis. These cases, representing 30 per cent of their total group, comprised those in which the condition was considered the primary cause of death. The remaining cases were milder and usually associated with other major extrapul-monary lesions to which death could be attributed.

Graven and Misenhimer have reported that the risk of recurrence of the respiratory distress syndrome in a subsequent low-birth-weight infant is nearly 90 per cent. This risk is reduced to 5 per cent if a normal low-birth-weight-infant intervenes.

The concentration of oxygen administered to these infants depends on the degree of hypoxia and acidosis. The ambient oxygen and the pH must be care-fully monitored. Humidity also is important in the management of these infants, and antibiotics should be administered as protection against pneumonitis. For details of this problem the monograph by Avery should be consulted.

Retrolental Fibroplasia. Terry described retrolental fibroplasia as a disease of very premature infants, in which an opaque tissue forms behind the lens of the eye during the first few months after birth. Before the etiologic role of oxygen was understood the highest incidence of the disease was in infants weighing between 1,000 and 1,500 g. Retrolental fibroplasia developed in about 10 to 15 per cent of infants weighing less than 1,360 g (3 pounds) at birth and in about 1 per cent of infants weighing between 1,360 and 2,000 g. The prognosis was grave, most of the affected infants developing partial or total blindness.

The earliest changes are retinal edema and proliferation of the capillary-forming mesenchymal cells in the nerve fiber layer. Capillary buds and whorl-like proliferations break through the intimal limiting membrane and grow along the inner side of the retina, forming a preretinal capillary plexus. Retinal hemorrhages and gliosis characterize secondary stages of the disease.

Retrolental fibroplasia is almost always caused by exposure of premature infants to high concentrations of ambient oxygen (above 40 per cent) over periods longer than a day or two. The disease is thus almost wholly preventable, although, rarely, highly susceptible infants have been reported to develop the disease after breathing normal air (Silverman). It was therefore highly desirable that the following policies with respect to administration of oxygen be adopted by all hospitals caring for newborn infants, as recommended by the Committee on Maternal and Child Welfare of the Medical and Chirurgical Faculty of Maryland:

1. All babies under 1,500 g shall continue to receive routine oxygen in their incubators, for 24 hours, the concentration of which shall be kept between 30 per cent and 40 per cent as checked by measurement with an oxygen analyzer every 8 hours. These infants shall be removed as soon thereafter as qualified nursing and medical estimates of the infant's status permit.

2. Oxygen shall be prescribed for individual infants by the physician on the basis of clinical symptoms, particularly cyanosis.

3. In no circumstances shall oxygen be administered continuously in concentrations exceeding 40 per cent.

4. The actual concentration of oxygen during administration shall be checked by measurement with an oxygen analyzer at least every 8 hours.

5. The continuous administration of oxygen for periods in excess of three days should be prescribed only in case of real need. The indications for continued oxygen therapy should be reevaluated by the physician daily. When oxygen is administered for periods longer than three days, extreme caution should be exercised to measure the oxygen concentration to see that it does not exceed 40 per cent.

Klaus and Meyer indicate that there is no contraindication to the use of 100 per cent oxygen during resuscitation. In these instances the actual pO_2 is low, and high concentrations of oxygen for short periods of time can only be helpful and do not cause retrolental fibroplasia.

In infants with chronic hypoxia, it may be necessary to administer high concentrations of oxygen for several days in order to maintain life. In these circumstances the infant's arterial pO_2 must be monitored with extreme caution. Although there are differences of opinion, the arterial pO_2 should probably be kept below 100 mm Hg.

HYPERBILIRUBINEMIA OF THE NEWBORN

Hyperbilirubinemia of the newborn is a serious and often life-threatening derangement that may precipitate neonatal death. In other cases it predisposes to kernicterus, an encephalopathy caused by unconjugated bilirubin concentrated within the brain substance. The obstetrician, fortunately, now can prevent or greatly modify the clinical course of the disease.

"Hemolytic disease of the newborn" caused by Rh incompatibility well exemplifies the problem of hyperbilirubinemia. With the advent of specific measures to prevent Rh sensitization, the incidence of this form of hemolytic disease should decrease. Hyperbilirubinemia in its less severe manifestation, nevertheless, remains a threat to the life and neurologic status of the newborn. ABO incompatibility, prematurity, sepsis, and many drugs are all etiologically related to hyperbilirubinemia. In addition, even mild hyperbilirubinemia may predispose to kernicterus when it is associated with asphyxia, hypothermia, acidosis, hypercapnia or hypoglycemia. Some infants affected with erythroblastosis fetalis are severely edematous and stillborn, whereas others in the early neonatal period exhibit a clinical picture of varying severity, characterized by jaundice, anemia, and cardiac, hepatic, and splenic enlargement. This immunologic disease is nearly always dependent upon differences between the blood groups of mother and fetus.

The discovery of immunologic basis of hemolytic disease is an impressive scientific achievement. In its hydropic form the disease was probably known to Hippocrates but was firmly established clinically and pathologically by Ballantyne in 1892. Rautmann was the first to use the term "erythroblastosis," and Diamond, Blackfan, and Baty showed that the three forms—hydrops, icterus gravis, and anemia of the newborn —were all manifestations of the same disease.

Before the discovery in 1939–1940 of the Rh factor and its relation to the disease, considerable evidence suggested that erythroblastosis was caused by immunization of the mother by a genetically inherited antigen in the fetus. In 1938 Hellman and Hertig reemphasized the rarity of erythroblastosis among firstborn infants and demonstrated clearly the peculiar familial occurrence of the disease. In 1938 Darrow reported that the illness was caused by a maternally formed antibody against a component of fetal blood. Subsequent research has shown that this effect is brought about by the passage of minute quantities of Rh-positive fetal red blood cells through the placenta of an Rh-negative mother.

In 1940, while engaged in research on red cell antigens, Landsteiner and Wiener announced the discovery of the Rh antigen, so called because it was found originally on the red cell of the rhesus monkey. This event had been, to a certain extent, foreshadowed by a report of Levine and Stetson in 1939, which described an atypical agglutinin in the blood of a woman who had just given birth to a stillborn, macerated fetus and subsequently experienced a severe reaction when given a transfusion of apparently compatible blood. This reaction was classified as an intragroup hemolytic transfusion reaction, since both donor and recipient were of the same major (ABO) blood group. It was postulated by the observers that maternal immunization was the result of stimulation by some fetal antigen inherited from the father but absent in the mother. This phenomenon is known as isoimmunization, since the antigen originated from an individual of the same species as the patient. The antibody was found to react best at 37°C (warm agglutinin), producing agglutination of 80 per cent of a series of bloods with which it was tested. It appeared to be independent of the properties of M, N, and P. No name was given to the antigen or its antibody at that time.

Since 1937 Landsteiner and Wiener had been studying a property of the red blood cell of the rhesus monkey that was apparently related to, but not identical with, human blood group antigen M. These investigators studied the reactions of human erythrocytes to a rabbit antirhesus immune serum. In 1940 they reported that the erythrocytes of 85 per cent of a group of Caucasians reacted positively with this antirhesus serum and therefore contained the antigen, whereas 15 per cent did not. The antigen of human erythrocytes thus discovered was termed *Rh* to indicate its relation to a similar property of the rhesus erythrocytes. Those that reacted were designated *Rh-positive* and those that did not, *Rh-negative*. This antigen was subsequently shown to be only one member of the group now known as the *Rh system*.

In 1940–1941 Wiener and Peters, as well as Levine and associates, not only explained a whole group of transfusion reactions on the basis of Rh isoimmunization but also defined the Rh factor's relation to erythroblastosis fetalis. Levine's theory proposed that the disease was the result of the intrauterine activity of anti-Rh agglutinins produced by the mother in response to antigenic stimulation by the Rh-positive fetal erythrocytes.

Blood Group Factors. Originally the Rh concept was extremely simple, defined by one antiserum and two blood group factors, Rh (Rh-positive) and Rh (Rh-negative). In the past two decades, however, the Rh factors have become increasingly complex, and a host of other factors have been discovered. Although some of them are immunologically and genetically important, many are so rare as to be of little clinical significance in the genesis of erythroblastosis. Their most outstanding common characteristic is their antigenicity when introduced into the circulation of a person lacking the peculiar factor. Such a person will then create antibodies to that specific factor that might be harmful in case of a transfusion or pregnancy. The vast majority of human beings have at least one such factor inherited from their father and lacking in their mother. In these cases the mother could be sensitized if enough red cells in the fetus reach her circulation. In these terms, hemolytic disease is a possibility in nearly every pregnancy. That the disease occurs in only about 1 per cent of pregnancies is a result of several circumstances, among which are the varying rates of occurrence and antigenicity of the factors, the failure of sufficient transplacental crossing, the variability of host response to the antigen, and the presence or absence of the factors in tissues other than the blood.

The number and interrelations of red cell factors are becoming highly complex. They belong to at least nine genetically independent "systems" or "families," as shown in Table 3. Some are quite common; others are rare. The frequency of occurrence plays a large role in determining whether a given factor will be of clinical importance. If a factor is exceedingly common, sensitization is necessarily relatively uncommon. Conversely, if a factor is rare, the chance of exposure and sensitization will be infrequent. If the prevalence is 50 per cent, one quarter of the transfusions will consist of positive blood given to negative recipients unless the recipients are typed before transfusion for the specific effect. For detailed information about the genetics of the Rh system see the 13th edition of this textbook.

Rh Antibodies. The detection of antibodies as indicative of isoimmunization to a red cell antigen is the first important step in the clinical management of a specific pregnancy. Sensitization by pregnancy or transfusion induces a variety of antibody responses in the host. At first Rh antibodies were detected by the incubation of known Rh-positive cells in saline to which a suspected serum was added. Such agglutinins, known as saline antibodies, were soon found to be rather rare and unimportant in the causation and detection of erythroblastosis. Methods that involve suspending red cells in solutions of albumin, dextran, polyvinyl pyrrolidone (PVP), acacia, and a number of other substances have improved the detection of even the most elusive antibodies. In addition, pretreatment of the red cells with various enzymes, such as trypsin, has increased the sensitivity of these

Table 3. **Blood Group Antigens***

Family		*Name†*		
ABO	A 0.45	B 0.14	H 0.52	
	D (Rh₀) 0.85	Term "Rh," otherwise unqualified, usually refers to this antigen		
Rh	C (rh′) 0.70	c (hr′) 0.80	Cʷ (rh ʷ) 0.01	Cˣ (rare)
	E (rh″) 0.30	e (hr″) 0.98	Eʷ (rare)	
	f (rh) 0.64	G (rhᵍ) 0.86	V (rare)	
MNS	M 0.79	N 0.71	S 0.55	s 0.89
	Miᵃ (rare)	Vw (rare)	He (rare)	Hu (rare)
Kell	K 0.10	k 0.998	Kpᵃ 0.02	Kpᵇ 0.9999
Duffy	Fyᵃ 0.66	Fyᵇ 0.83		
Kidd	Jkᵃ 0.77	Jkᵇ 0.73		
P	P₁ 0.79	P₂ 0.21		
Lewis	Leᵃ 0.20	Leᵇ 0.71		
Lutheran	Luᵃ 0.08	Luᵇ 0.998		
Unclassified	Levay (rare)	Gr (rare)	Ven (rare)	Ca (rare)
	Beᵃ (rare)	Wrᵃ (rare)	Diᵃ (rare)	Byᵃ (rare)
	Rm (rare)	Vel (extremely common)		Ytᵃ 0.997
	Chrᵃ (rare)	I (extremely common)		

* *Antigens in Rh family generally designated by two names; those in parentheses are preferred by Wiener.*
† *Figures after names refer to approximate frequency of antigens in Caucasian population of United States.*
From Allen and Diamond, Erythroblastosis Fetalis, Including Exchange Transfusion Technique. Boston, Little, Brown & Co., 1957.

tests. Most important in this area is the *Coombs test*, which utilizes the serum of rabbits immunized to human gamma globulin. In the detection of hemolytic disease in a newborn, the baby's Rh-positive red cells from the cord blood, although coated with Rh antibodies from the mother, may not in themselves agglutinate. Inasmuch as these maternal antibodies are globulins, the addition of rabbit immune antiglobulin causes agglutination (direct Coombs positive). The test may also be used to measure the titer of maternal antibody by mixing her serum with Rh-positive cells and testing with antiglobulin (indirect Coombs test).

Titration of antibodies is a simple matter of serial dilution of the serum to find the end point of agglutination: a titer of 1:64 indicates that dilution of the serum to 64 volumes is the last tube (highest dilution) in which agglutination of a 2 or 3 per cent suspension of red cells occurs.

In general terms, a higher titer is more dangerous; furthermore, the intensity of the hemolytic disease is likely to be greater when the titer is rising than when it is stationary or falling. Allen and co-workers have shown that the chances for survival are excellent if the mother has a titer of 1:64 or less, whereas if it is higher, the probability is reduced to about 60 per cent.

A previously immunized mother may have a rise in titer, known as an *anamnestic reaction*, during a subsequent pregnancy, even with an Rh-negative fetus. Conversely, in the face of severe fetal disease maternal titers may not increase appreciably but may appear to drop. If titers are considered in relation to such factors as history and zygosity of the parents, however, they become increasingly meaningful in prognosis of the infant.

The Rh antigens are inherited independently of all other blood group antigens. There is apparently no difference in the distribution of the various Rh antigens with regard to sex; there are, however, important racial differences. The

Chinese and other Asiatic peoples thus far studied are almost all Rh-positive (99 per cent). Among American Negroes there is a lesser incidence of Rh negatives (7 to 8 per cent) than among white Americans (13 per cent). Of all the racial groups studied thus far, the Basques show the highest incidence of Rh-negativity (33.6 per cent).

Prevention. The ideal approach to hemolytic disease of the newborn is prevention. Fortunately, isoimmunization rarely is a problem in the first pregnancy unless the patient has received the antigen in a transfusion. Fortunately also, most hemolytic disease is caused by the antigen Rho(D), which induces antibody formation in the mother after delivery. Freda and his colleagues used these several coincidental facts to prevent maternal sensitization by giving 300 to 400μg of human anti-D gamma globulin intramuscularly to the mother within 72 hours after delivery. This procedure has proved highly successful even with doses as low as 250 μg of anti-D immunoglobulin (DeWit and colleagues). Rhogam is currently recommended for previously unsensitized women who have been delivered of D-positive infants or those who have aborted infants of an unidentified Rh type or who have had an ectopic pregnancy.

Clinical Management of Rh-Negative Pregnant Women. Hemolytic disease of the newborn now should be a problem almost totally limited to Rh-negative women who were sensitized before anti-Rho globulin was available and to the 2 or 3 per cent of Rh-negative women who become sensitized without apparent cause. Approximately 13 per cent of all marriages among whites in this country take place between an Rh-negative woman and an Rh-positive man. The potential for isoimmunization, therefore, exists in a considerable proportion of pregnant women. As a result, analysis of the Rh type of every pregnant woman and of her serum for abnormal blood group antibodies has become routine in prenatal care. History of previous blood transfusions must also be ascertained and recorded.

If blood typing indicates that a patient is Rh-negative, it becomes essential to type the father of the fetus. Should he be Rh-negative also, there will be no danger of hemolytic disease on this basis, since all offspring of such a union will be Rh-negative.

If, however, the father is Rh-positive, an effort should be made in several ways to ascertain his genotype. If the husband's parents are living they should be typed; if one of them is found to be Rh-negative, the male in question must be heterozygous positive. The other living children of the couple may also be Rh-typed. The detection of an Rh-negative child likewise implies that the husband is heterozygous positive. If all children are Rh-positive, no certain conclusions can be drawn about the husband's genotype. Were anti-d (Hr$_0$) serum available, the DD-(R$_0$R$_0$) genotype could be distinguished from the Dd (R$_0$r). A somewhat indirect approach is possible, however, through the use of the more readily available anti-c(hr') serum, which permits division of the relatively common phenotype CDe (Rh$_1$) into two groups. Negative reactors are probably homozygous positive, whereas those that react positively are probably heterozygous. There is, however, a certain margin of unavoidable error in the serologic detection of genotypes. For example, no antiserum could distinguish between such genotypes of CDE/cde (R^{z}r) and CdE/cDe (r^{y}R$_0$).

Although antibody titers give a good indication of the outcome of series of cases, their prognostic value for the individual is uncertain. In a series of investigations beginning in 1950, Bevis showed that certain characteristics of the amniotic fluid were of diagnostic and prognostic value in hemolytic disease of the newborn. In particular, the nonhematin iron, the oxyhemoglobin, and especially the bilirubin concentration in the fluid correlate positively with the severity of the infant's involvement. Both Walker and Liley pursued these studies by serial examination of amniotic fluid obtained by amniocentesis during pregnancy. Amniotic fluid has a relatively linear absorption curve when plotted on semilogarithmic paper (Figs. 4 and 5). The absorption curve will be curvilinear (exponential) when an arithmetic tracing is made, and the deviations of the optical density at the 450 mμ peak will be slightly smaller, with peaks at 415 and 450 mμ. The 415 mμ peak probably reflects oxyhemoglobin. The 450 mμ peak produced by bilirubin and its height in fresh amniotic fluid correlates well with the severity of fetal hemolytic disease.

Various interpretations are given to the different values of OD 450. Freda, on the one hand, believes that his values indicate the status of the fetus at the time of the amniocentesis. On the other hand, the zoned graphic method of Liley at-

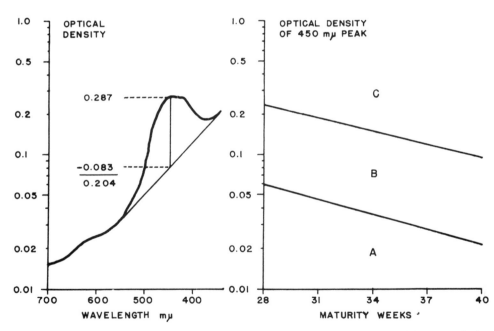

Fig. 4. Spectral absorption curve of amniotic fluid in hemolytic disease. The optical density is plotted on semilog paper and the 450 mμ peak is measured on a line drawn from the peak to an intersection with a tangent connecting the beginning and ending curves of the rise. (From Liley. In Greenhill, ed. Yearbook of Obstetrics and Gynecology, 1964–1965 Series, p. 256. Courtesy of Year Book Medical Publishers.)

Fig. 5. Clinical significance of the height of the peak of pigment in the amniotic fluid at different maturities. Zone A, mild or no hemolytic disease. Zone B, moderate. Zone C, severe. (From Liley. Amniocentesis and amniography in hemolytic disease. Year Book of Obstetrics and Gynecology, 1964–1965 Series. Chicago, Year Book Medical Publishers, 1964, p. 256.)

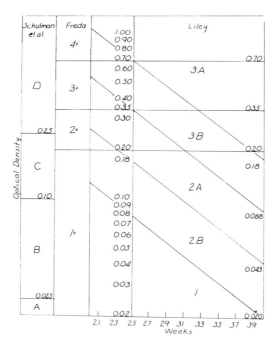

Fig. 6. Composite graph showing critical zones according to Liley, Freda, and Schulman and colleagues. (From Halitsky, V., Krumholz, B. A., Schwalb, E., and Gromisch, D. S. Obstet Gynec Survey 23:308, 1968.)

tempts to predict the severity of the hemolytic disease if delivery should occur within one week of the measurement. The various methods of interpretation are illustrated in Figure 6 and are briefly described as follows.

According to Freda:
1.   *OD 450, 0–0.21.* Similar to a normal tracing. May change and therefore amniocentesis should be repeated at two-week intervals.
2.   *OD 450, 0.2–0.34.* Without a history of previous severe hemolytic disease, delivery before 37 weeks is not indicated. Weekly tracings to be performed until thirty-seventh to thirty-eighth week. With significant history of hemolytic disease, perform exchange transfusion before 37 weeks.
3.   *OD 450, 0.35–0.7.* Fetus is in some degree of circulatory failure. There will be inevitable progression to a next stage (4) and fetal death. Deliver if beyond 32 weeks. Exchange transfusion may be attempted before 32 weeks but may prove fatal.
4.   *OD 450, 0.7 or higher.* Fetal death within one week. Outlook poor but infant may survive if sufficiently mature.

According to Liley:
Zone I at 28 to 31 weeks. The fetus will be unaffected or will have mild hemolytic disease. Repeat tap in two or three weeks.
Zone II. The prognosis is less accurate here and may require repeated taps to indicate a trend. In Zone IIB the infant's expected hemoglobin at birth will be between 11.0 and 13.9 g, whereas in Zone II the infant's anticipated hemoglobin will range from 8.0 to 10.9 g. Trends and time of gestation will obviously indicate the necessity for early delivery or intrauterine transfusions.

Zone III. A severely affected infant or fetal death within one week to ten days may be expected. The treatment (early delivery or intrauterine transfusion) will depend on the stage of gestation.

According to Schulman (linear tracing):
Group A.   OD 450, 0–0.025. Delivery at time anticipated.
Group B.   OD 450, 0.025–0.10. Amniecentesis to be repeated within two weeks. Delivery should be accomplished between 37 and 40 weeks.
Group C.   OD 450, 0.10–0.25. Repeat amniocentesis weekly. Delivery at 34 to 36 weeks.
Group D.   OD 450, 0.25 or greater. Immediate delivery or intrauterine transfusions.

Amniocentesis can be done on an outpatient basis. If sonographic apparatus is available, it may be used to ascertain the location of the placenta. After the patient empties her bladder she is placed in the supine position. The abdominal skin is cleansed with an antiseptic solution and draped with sterile towels. The puncture is made with a 3½-inch, 20- or 21-gauge needle through an anesthetized area of the skin. An area distant from the fetus at about the level of the umbilicus is usually chosen. From 5 to 15 ml of amniotic fluid are withdrawn, centrifuged at 2,000 rpm for 30 minutes, and passed through a Whatman No. 42 filter paper. Exposure of the fluid to light should be as brief as possible. If performed with care, amniocentesis rarely proves hazardous.

Schindler and associates have indicated that the concentrations of estriol in the amniotic fluid may have a predictive value. Estriol levels below 60 μg/L are found with severely affected infants.

Intrauterine Fetal Transfusions.   The refinement in prognostic precision furnished by the analysis of amniotic fluid led Liley to try intrauterine transfusion of blood into the fetal abdomen. The procedure should be limited to cases in which, between the twenty-sixth and thirtieth weeks, the spectrophotometric tracings and history forecast certain death of the fetus by the thirty-second week. Based on the sparse data available, the salvage rate in "salvageable" fetuses is about 50 per cent. "Salvageable" fetuses are those without hydrops. As shown by Liley, this technic is of no value in the presence of hydrops, because the injected blood does not seem to be absorbed from the peritoneal cavity, probably because of lymphatic obstruction. Bowman and colleagues report 218 transfusions carried out on 100 fetuses. In the last 61 cases the survival rate was 62 per cent. Eleven centers forming a cooperative study group reported, at a Ross Conference on Pediatric Research, the results of 238 fetuses receiving 399 intrauterine transfusions. The series included 132 intrauterine deaths; 26 were attributed to some complications of the procedure. Data on the success of intrauterine transfusions are not meaningful because of lack of unanimity regarding indications for initiating the transfusions. The mortality is obviously high and the subsequent infant morbidity unknown. Gregg and Hutchinson, who were able to test 15 of these infants ranging from nine months to three years of age, state: "It appears that intrauterine transfusion, judiciously administered before serious intrauterine damage occurs, is not intrinsically harmful to the neonate." Our experience has been similar to that of Gregg and Hutchinson. In carefully selected, otherwise hopeless cases, it seems to merit consideration.

Our recommended technic is similar to that described by Liley. Some time after the twenty-sixth week when evidence of severe disease has become manifest, the position of the fetus is ascertained roentgenologically in relation to opaque markers placed on the mother's abdomen as close to the fetal abdomen as possible. More precise localization of the fetal abdomen may be obtained by injecting 10 to 15 ml of Renografin into the amniotic cavity 10 to 12 hours before the proposed transfusion. This contrast medium is swallowed with amniotic fluid. It passes into the fetal intestine and is clearly visible in a roentgenogram or by fluoroscopy with an image intensifier. After approximate localization of the fetal abdomen, the mother's abdomen is cleansed and draped. With attention to asepsis, a small area of the mother's abdomen is anesthetized with 1 per cent lidocaine, and a 16-gauge Tuohy needle is passed through the maternal abdomen into the amniotic sac. A sterile syringe containing physiologic saline is then attached to the needle, which is pressed against the fetal abdomen and passed gently through it. This procedure is carried out under roentgenographic or fluoroscopic visualization with an image intensifer. Passage through the abdominal wall can be tested by injections of small amounts of saline. Once the needle has traversed the fetal abdominal wall, resistance to the injection disappears. A polyethylene catheter is then passed through the needle, with the catheter directed downward. The needle is then removed, and to make certain of the proper placement of the catheter, a small amount of water-soluble contrast medium (Renografin) is injected into the fetal abdomen and a roentgenogram is obtained. Dispersion in the fetal peritoneal cavity produces a typical picture of crescents of contrast medium surrounding loops of bowel (Fig. 7). Transfusion is accomplished with fresh group O, Rh-negative packed red cells crossmatched against the mother's blood. Transfusion may be repeated at biweekly intervals.

The reader is referred to the recent review of amniotic fluid analysis and intrauterine transfusion by Halitsky and associates.

Delivery Before Term. In many circumstances delivery before term is advantageous. Obviously when intrauterine transfusions have been performed, delivery is desirable at the earliest date compatible with sufficient maturity to yield a reasonable chance of survival. The exact timing of delivery in these cases depends on both clinical judgment and the results of the various laboratory tests. Delivery before the thirty-second week is contraindicated by the extreme prematurity. In many cases delivery can be carried out at about the thirty-fourth week.

When intrauterine transfusion has not been performed, delivery may be considered for several of the following reasons: (1) previous history of an infant with unmistakable evidence of erythroblastosis; (2) a high titer of antibodies during a considerable portion of the present pregnancy; (3) reasonable evidence of homozygosity of the husband; (4) progressive and sharp rise in antibody titer during the last trimester of pregnancy; and (5) evidence of fetal disease from analysis of the amniotic fluid. The efficacy of early induction of labor is attested by Sundal, who has reduced the stillbirth and neonatal death rates markedly by the procedure, and by Lind and colleagues, who report an 82 per cent survival rate for infants of isoimmunized mothers delivered before the thirty-eighth week of gestation.

The choice of the method of delivery (induction of labor or cesarean section) must depend upon the clinical judgment of the obstetrician. Cesarean section

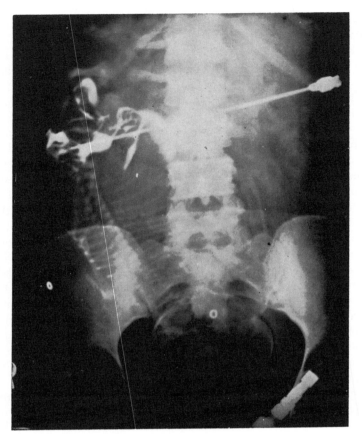

Fig. 7. Roentgenogram illustrating injection of contrast medium into the peritoneal cavity of a fetus. (Courtesy of Drs. R. A. H. Kinch and T. O. Ramsay.)

may be necessitated by a cervix unfavorable for induction three or four weeks before term. Whenever a decision is reached to terminate pregnancy before term, adequate facilities for care of premature infants should be available, as well as the necessary equipment for carrying out an exchange transfusion. The pediatrician should be advised of the situation well in advance of delivery, so that blood and equipment can be immediately available in the delivery room. If the infant appears jaundiced at time of delivery, he is most probably severely compromised and will require immediate exchange transfusion.

Pathologic Changes in Hemolytic Disease of the Fetus and Newborn.   Maternal isoimmunization results in the varied clinical and pathologic manifestations of the syndrome of hemolytic disease of the fetus and newborn.

Maternal antibodies gain access to the fetal circulation. In Rh-positive infants such antibodies are both adsorbed upon the Rh-negative erythrocytes and exist in a free form in the infant's serum. The adsorbed antibodies act as hemolysins, leading to an accelerated rate of destruction of the red blood cells. The earlier this process begins in utero and the greater its intensity, the more severe will be the effect upon the fetus; the variability of the syndrome is thus explained in part. Careful and widespread prenatal study of the maternal serum led not only to the recognition of intermediate forms of the disease but also to the detection of many cases that because of their relative mildness would probably have been overlooked in the past.

Maternal antibodies, detectable at birth, gradually disappear from the fetal circulation over a period of four to eight weeks. Their rate of disappearance is influenced to some extent by the treatment employed in the management of the infant. Detection of adsorbed antibodies is best accomplished by the direct Coombs test. If cells coated with antibody are typed with an anti-Rh saline agglutinin serum, they may be reported incorrectly as Rh-negative because of the blocking effect produced by the adsorbed antibody. Red cells reported to be Rh-negative cells from a potentially erythroblastotic infant must always be checked by the Coombs test.

The pathologic changes in the organs of the fetus and newborn vary with the severity of the process. The severely affected fetus or infant may show considerable subcutaneous edema as well as effusion into the serous cavities (hydrops fetalis). Sometimes the edema of the scalp is so severe that the diagnosis can be made simply by roentgenography (Fig. 8). In these cases the placenta too is markedly edematous and boggy, with large, prominent cotyledons and edematous villi (Fig. 9). Excessive and prolonged hemolysis results in marked erythroid hyperplasia of the bone marrow as well as large areas of extramedullary hematopoiesis, particularly in the spleen and liver. Histologic examination of the liver may reveal, in addition, fatty degenerative parenchymal changes as well as deposition of hemosiderin and engorgement of the hepatic canaliculi with bile. There may be cardiac enlargement and pulmonary hemorrhages. Important lesions may occur in the brain, collectively known as kernicterus and characterized by yellowish pigmentation of the basal nuclei and, to a lesser extent, other portions of the brain. Certain infants that survive the neonatal period may later exhibit serious neurologic defects resulting from neuronal degeneration in the areas mentioned, with subsequent gliosis. Affected infants may be hypoglycemic.

Fetuses with hydrops fetalis may die in utero; death is believed to result from profound anemia and circulatory failure. The liveborn hydropic infant appears pale, edematous, and limp at birth, often requiring resuscitation. The spleen and liver are enlarged, and there may be widespread ecchymoses or scattered petechiae. Dyspnea and circulatory collapse are common. Death may occur within a few hours, again largely as the result of severe anemia and circulatory collapse.

Less severely affected infants may appear well at birth only to become jaundiced within a few hours. Hepatomegaly and splenomegaly are usually found. Hematologic and immunologic tests are extremely important in diagnosis and prognosis. Increasing jaundice may be associated with lethargy, stiffness of the extremities, retraction of the head, squinting, a high-pitched cry, poor feeding, and convulsions. These signs are indicative of kernicterus. In such cases death usually occurs within the first week of life. Surviving infants are physically helpless, unable to support their heads or to sit. Ability to walk is delayed or never acquired. In less severe forms there may be varying degrees of motor incoordination, whereas some infants demonstrate residual nerve deafness as the only manifestation of neurologic injury.

Some infants affected by erythroblastosis fetalis exhibit none of the signs or symptoms listed in the preceding text; they can be detected only by immunologic studies. Some go through a completely uneventful neonatal period,

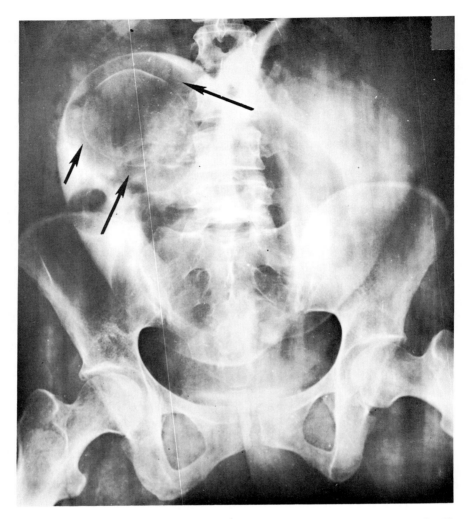

Fig. 8. Amniogram of a fetus with hydrops fetalis showing severe edema of the scalp. (Courtesy of Dr. John T. Queenan.)

whereas others develop a slowly progressive anemia that may be quite marked at two to four weeks of age.

The hematologic and biochemical changes in hemolytic disease caused by Rh isoimmunization must be viewed against the background of normal values for the first day of life. Mollison has provided pertinent data: in 134 normal infants the cord hemoglobin ranged from 13.6 to 19.6 g per cent with a mean of 16.6 g per cent. Samples of venous blood obtained during the first day of life showed a range of hemoglobin values from 14.5 to 22.5 g per cent, with a mean of 18.5 g per cent. Capillary blood hemoglobin during this period was approximately 0.5 g higher. Whereas the normal infant during the first two days of life may have from 200 to 2,000 nucleated red blood cells per cubic millimeter, the infant with erythroblastosis usually has from 10,000 to 100,000 nucleated erythro-

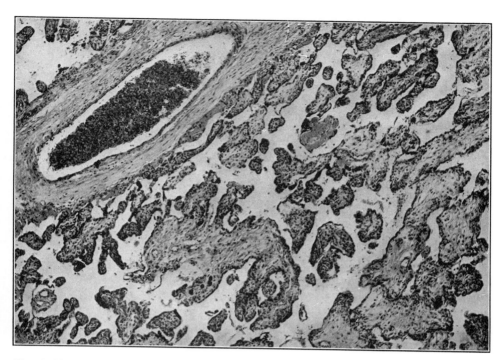

Fig. 9. Photomicrograph of a hydropic placenta. Note the large edematous villi and the fetal vessels containing immature erythrocytes.

cytes per cubic millimeter, in addition to a high percentage of reticulocytes. In the normal infant at birth, serum indirect bilirubin seldom exceeds 3 mg per 100 ml. A peak of 5 to 6 mg per cent may be seen by the third day of life. Deviations from these norms provide an index of the severity of the hemolysis and a basis for management of the patient.

The significance of hyperbilirubinemia is its association with kernicterus. This complication occurs with greater frequency in premature infants. The yellow staining of the basal ganglia is indicative of profound degeneration in these areas. If the infants survive, they show spasticity and muscular incoordination. There is a positive correlation between kernicterus and bilirubin levels above 18 to 20 mg per 100 ml. In a group of 30 infants studied by Crawford, Cutbush, and Mollison, in which the highest serum level of bilirubin remained below 18 mg per 100 ml, no cases of kernicterus occurred; in contrast, among 11 infants in which the concentration of bilirubin exceeded 18 mg, 5 died of kernicterus and 2 others survived with signs of motor damage. Allen and Diamond, among others, have shown that the early and repeated use of exchange transfusion has significantly reduced the incidence of kernicterus. Factors other than the serum bilirubin concentration contribute to the development of kernicterus. For example, sulfonamides and salicylates such as aspirin may increase the incidence of kernicterus because they compete with bilirubin for protein-binding sites and conjugation with glucuronic acid. Caffeine sodium benzoate uncouples bilirubin from albumin; and excessive doses of vitamin K analogues, as well as novobiocin, may be associated with hyperbilirubinemia.

The effect of bilirubin may be exaggerated if hypoxia or acidosis is superimposed. Quite recently Levi and co-workers have described 2 hepatic intracellular proteins, called by them Y and Z, that specifically bind organic anions including unconjugated bilirubin. The intracellular concentration of Y is low in the liver of the fetus and newborn monkey but increases rapidly to adult levels during the first 10 days of life. Quite likely these observations are pertinent to the problem of impaired conjugation and excretion of bilirubin in instances of jaundice due to hemolytic disease as well as physiologic jaundice of the newborn.

Both hypothermia and hypoglycemia predispose the infant to kernicterus by raising the level of nonesterified fatty acids, which also compete with bilirubin for the binding sites of albumin. Sepsis also contributes to kernicterus, although the mechanism of action is not clear.

The low albumin levels that accompany hypoproteinemia militate against the binding of bilirubin and increase the danger of kernicterus. Premature infants suffer from hypoproteinemia because of biochemical immaturity of their liver. As a result, they often manifest more prolonged and more intense jaundice than do term infants.

A small number of nursing mothers excrete in their milk an unusual isomer, pregnane-3(alpha),20(beta)-diol, that inhibits glucuronyl transferase (Arias and colleagues). Their infants manifest prolonged jaundice from the fourth week of life until breast-feeding ceases. Rarely significant hyperbilirubinemia may result from the ingestion by the fetus of a large volume of maternal blood. Egan and associates have reported this to occur associated with partial placental abruption and we have observed this phenomenon.

The infant with hemolytic disease who survives the neonatal period without evidence of involvement of the central nervous system has in the main no serious residual disease, with the possible exception of a hearing defect. There is no significant deficit in intellectual achievement in the infants that escape other neurologic lesions.

The pathologic changes in the placenta in hemolytic disease have been thoroughly studied by Hellman and Hertig. These lesions vary with the severity of the process and are grossly recognizable only in fetal hydrops, in which the placenta is pale and grossly increased in size, sometimes attaining double or triple the normal weight. The villi are correspondingly enlarged, showing marked edema, prominence of the Langhans layer and Hofbauer cells, foci of erythropoiesis, and immature endothelial cells of the fetal blood vessels. Such changes are compensatory in part for the low oxygen-conveying capacity of fetal blood.

Toxicity and Disposal of Bilirubin.   Day, and also Waters and Bowen, found that bilirubin inhibits the uptake of oxygen by rat brain tissue in vitro. The effect is more marked in preparations of brains from newborn animals than in those from adults. As a result of the associated effect of loss of respiratory cofactors, DPN and cytochrome C, metabolism is both depressed and less efficient. These effects appear at concentrations of bilirubin of about 20 mg per 100 ml, coinciding with the critical levels for the development of kernicterus in the human infant.

Free (unconjugated, indirect) bilirubin cannot be excreted in the urine or to any extent in the bile. Normally the liver conjugates bilirubin with glucuronic acid. The glucuronide is water-soluble and is normally excreted into the bile by the liver predominantly and by the kidney. Glucuronic acid is made available for this reaction by transfer from uridine diphosphoglucuronic acid (UDPGA), catalyzed by the enzyme glucuronyl transferase. Since many other biologic substances also are conjugated with glucuronic acid, such as steroids, phenolic compounds, carboxylic acids, and sulfonamides, they may compete with bilirubin for conjugation and lead to higher levels of unconjugated, toxic bilirubin.

Several studies, notably those of Dutton, of Lathe and Walker, and of Brown and Zuelzer, have shown that the fetal livers of several mammals are deficient not only in the enzyme but in uridine diphosphoglucuronic acid as well. Since during most of pregnancy the conjugating activity of the fetal liver is negligible, the fetus depends to a great extent on placental transfer for disposal of its bilirubin.

Treatment of Hemolytic Disease. In most instances of erythroblastosis fetalis resulting from Rh isoimmunization, the birth of a potentially affected child can be anticipated by knowledge gained from the prenatal studies already described. These infants are best delivered in a hospital equipped to carry out prompt hematologic, biochemical, and immunologic studies and exchange transfusions. Some infants have undoubtedly suffered during a long trip to such a center after jaundice and anemia had already appeared.

Labor and delivery of isoimmunized mothers should be conducted with minimal trauma to the infant. It is perhaps wise to employ conduction analgesia and anesthesia or at least to minimize the use of narcotizing drugs. Caffeine sodium benzoate is without merit for resuscitation and may augment hyperbilirubinemia.

Prompt clamping of the cord in all such affected infants is important, since the additional load of erythrocytes from the placenta poses a greater problem for the immature hepatic conjugating systems.

The umbilical cord should be left about four inches long to facilitate possible future exchange transfusions. At the same time samples of anticoagulated and clotted blood should be obtained. The anticoagulated blood is used for hemoglobin and hematocrit measurements, reticulocyte count, white blood cell count, and blood smear. Clotted blood is used for blood types, Coombs test, and measurement of serum bilirubin. All cells types as Rh-negative must be checked by the Coombs test, in view of the possibility of a falsely negative result in the case of Rh-positive cells heavily coated with incomplete antibodies.

Exchange transfusion is often the most effective method of treatment of the infant with hemolytic disease. In reaching a decision to use exchange transfusion, certain aspects of the maternal obstetric history are important. If there is a history of previous stillbirths resulting from isoimmunization or of severely affected liveborn infants, and the newborn infant has a positive Coombs test, some authorities believe that exchange transfusion is indicated despite the initially adequate level of hemoglobin. Premature infants with Coombs-positive red cells should have exchange transfusion because of the high incidence of kernicterus in that group. For the term infant that is Rh-positive and Coombs-positive but is not hydropic, the laboratory data should be evaluated before arriving at a decision. Crawford, Cutbush, and Mollison found the cord hemoglobin to be the best single index of the severity of the disease. The infant with a cord hemoglobin of 17 g per 100 ml or higher should be followed during the first 24 hours with serial observations of the levels of hemoglobin and bilirubin. The vast majority of these infants will require no treatment. With hemoglobin levels of 14 to 17 g per 100 ml the serum bilirubin may be used as an adjunct in arriving at a decision. If the bilirubin in this group exceeds 3 mg per 100 ml during the first 24 hours, exchange transfusions will probably be needed. Infants with a cord hemoglobin concentration of less than 14 g should receive exchange transfusion.

Considerable stress has been placed upon the serum bilirubin concentration in prognosis. There is general agreement that if jaundice appears early and increases rapidly, exchange transfusion is imperative. The hemoglobin concentration and the bilirubin concentration in the cord blood are negatively correlated; the more anemic the infant, the more likely it is to have a high bilirubin. Should the hemoglobin level remain satisfactory but the serum bilirubin rise beyond 14 mg per 100 ml in the first 24 hours, exchange transfusion is often indicated. Diamond has recommended a second, third, or even fourth exchange transfusion if the serum bilirubin level remains above 20 mg per cent. Elevation of the reticulocyte count and an increased number of nucleated red cells provide supporting evidence of active hemolysis and may also be considered in evaluating the necessity for exchange transfusion. Blood to be used for exchange transfusion preferably should be as fresh as possible, certainly less than one week old. Group O, Rh-negative blood is employed. The blood should always be crossmatched against the mother's serum.

The method of choice for exchange transfusion is the umbilical vein technic of Diamond. The infant is placed under a radiant heater and his temperature is carefully maintained. In the crib the extremities are immobilized. The periumbilical area is cleansed in the manner usual for surgical procedures and is draped. The umbilical cord is divided completely with a pair of scissors 1 cm from the skin. A tie is placed on the proximal stump of the cord. The umbilical vein, recognized as the largest vessel in the cord, is picked up with a mosquito clamp, and plastic tubing approximately 1 mm in diameter is passed into it. The plastic tubing should have been previously attached by a special Tuohy adapter to two stopcocks in series, which in turn are connected to the bottle of blood and to an empty bottle, which is to receive the "waste blood." The catheter is introduced as far as a large hepatic vein or the inferior vena cava (usually 6 or 7 cm), as a rule. If obstruction is encountered after the tip of the catheter has been introduced, the stump of the umbilical cord should be pulled downward toward the pubes. If the infant's venous pressure is high, blood may well up through the catheter. As a rule it is necessary to exert gentle suction with the syringe to obtain blood. The failure of blood to appear may be caused by a clot in the vessel. In such a case, withdrawal of the cannula with constant gentle suction will clear the vessel; clots should not be pushed into the circulation. The initial sample of blood removed should be placed in appropriate containers for study in the laboratory. Samples may also be obtained midway through the procedure and at its termination.

An assistant keeps accurate records of the amounts of blood introduced and withdrawn. Gastric contents are sometimes aspirated before starting, to avoid the possibility of aspiration pneumonia. A pacifier is useful to prevent the infant from crying during the procedure. After transfusion of every 100 ml sample of blood, 1 ml of 10 per cent calcium gluconate solution is given intravenously to prevent hypocalcemia. During the next seven days the infant should be given antibiotics. After the procedure, glucose feedings may be resumed.

Exchange transfusion is not an innocuous procedure. Boggs and Westphal have defined the mortality from exchange transfusion as the number of infants dying during or within six hours of the procedure. If moribund, hydropic, and kernicteric infants are excluded, the mortality rate should be less than 1 per cent.

Several experimental studies have demonstrated that phenobarbital and other barbiturates enhance the conjugation and excretion of bilirubin by accelerating the induction of the glucuronyl transferase system. McMullin and associates have recently reported that the administration of phenobarbital to infants with Rh hemolytic disease decreased the need for exchange transfusion. While their results appear quite promising, the advantages from decreased need for exchange transfusions have to be weighed carefully against the possible harmful effects of the phenobarbital. Further well-controlled studies are needed before this mode of therapy is generally used.

Sensitization to Other Blood Group Factors. The "major" blood groups factors A and B are other important causes of hemolytic disease. For example, group O women may from early life have anti-A and anti-B agglutinins, which may be augmented by pregnancy, particularly if the fetus is a secretor. About 20 per cent of all babies have a "major" maternal blood group incompatibility, but only 5 per cent of them (1 per cent of all babies) show signs of hemolytic disease; moreover, when they do, the disease is usually much milder than that concerned with the Rh factor. Although the reason is not entirely clear, it may relate to the fact that the A and B factors are not confined to red cells but are found in all tissues; the antibodies are therefore widely absorbed and are not so free to attack the red cells alone, as in the Rh system.

Criteria for diagnosis include the following: (1) mother usually group O, with anti-A and anti-B in her serum, while the fetus is A, B, or AB; (2) onset of jaundice within the first 24 hours; (3) varying degrees of anemia, reticulocytosis, and erythroblastosis (increased hypotonic saline fragility of the red cells is also found as a rule); (4) careful exclusion of other blood group sensitization.

Unlike the result in Rh hemolytic disease, the Coombs test in ABO incompatibility is usually negative or weakly positive. Hemolysis has been definitely proved by cell survival studies. Transfused group A cells are more rapidly destroyed in the circulation of an infant with a hemolytic disease than are simultaneously administered group O cells.

The principles of management of Rh disease may be applied to ABO hemolytic disease, particularly with reference to the behavior of hemoglobin and bilirubin. For simple transfusion or exchange transfusion, group O blood is used. Lucey and others advocate exposing the infant with hyperbilirubinemia to ultraviolet light in an attempt to degrade and detoxify bilirubin.

Since there is no adequate method of antenatal diagnosis, careful observation is essential in the neonatal period if cases are to be detected. Although the infants with ABO hemolytic disease are less severely affected than those with Rh hemolytic disease, they are equally incompetent in dealing with excess bilirubin and its toxic effects on the central nervous system. Zuelzer and Kaplan have reported an incidence of 15 per cent of neurologic damage in a group of infants with ABO hemolytic disease. Unlike Rh-hemolytic disease, ABO disease frequently occurs in infants of primigravidas and may or may not recur in subsequent pregnancies. Most of the cases occur in group O mothers with A or B babies, although other combinations of heterospecificity may occur.

Rh incompatibility and ABO heterospecificity account for approximately 98 per cent of all cases of hemolytic disease. A few instances of hemolytic disease resulting from rare blood factors have been reported, but the detection of such cases requires extensive serologic study.

HEMORRHAGIC DISEASE OF THE NEWBORN

Hemorrhagic disease of the newborn is a syndrome characterized by spontaneous internal or external bleeding accompanied by hypoprothrombinemia and very low levels of other vitamin K dependent coagulation factors. Bleeding may begin any time after birth but is often delayed for a day or two. The infants may be at term and healthy in appearance, although a greater incidence of the disease has been noted in premature infants. The bleeding and clotting times are usually within the elevated physiologic range for newborn infants, although both occasionally may be markedly increased. The red cell count, hemoglobin, and white count are within the normal range for the newborn infant unless continued hemorrhage has produced anemia. The platelets may be slightly decreased and the prothrombin is markedly reduced, even below the low values normally seen at birth. Icterus neonatorum is not more frequent. The placenta is usually of average weight and shows no distinctive lesion. In the differential diagnosis, hemophilia, congenital syphilis, sepsis of the newborn, thrombocytopenic purpura, erythroblastosis, and traumatic intracranial hemorrhage must be considered.

In the treatment of hemorrhagic disease of the newborn, the intramuscular injection of 1 mg of vitamin K_1 (phytonadione) has proved the most efficacious therapy. Not only does vitamin K_1 given parenterally to the infant raise the plasma prothrombin rapidly, but as shown by Hellman, Moore, and Shettles, the administration of vitamin K to the mother in pregnancy or labor also prevents serious hypoprothrombinemia.

Upon these facts all observers agree, but whether the prophylactic administration of vitamin K to mothers in pregnancy or labor will improve fetal mortality through reducing the incidence of certain types of cerebral hemorrhage is a moot question. In our opinion it virtually eliminates hemorrhagic disease of the newborn. The extent to which this prophylactic practice improves fetal mortality naturally depends upon the frequency in any given locality of hemorrhagic disease in newborn infants.

Serious reduction of vitamin K dependent clotting factors during the first week after birth in infants of women with epilepsy treated with anticonvulsant drugs has been described by Mountain and associates. They recommend giving vitamin K to the epileptic mother during labor. In our experience the administration of 1 mg of phytonadione to the infant immediately upon admittance to the nursery has proved effective in preventing bleeding from hypoprothrombinemia and related coagulation defects.

The toxic effects of menadione and its derivatives in causing hyperbilirubinemia resulted from unnecessarily large doses, particularly to premature infants. Allison's original report, and the deluge of subsequent publications relating the administration of vitamin K to the development of hyperbilirubinemia and kernicterus, without exception dealt with excessive doses of the drug. In short, there is no convincing evidence that the small but effective dose of 1 to 2 mg of vitamin K_1 (phytonadione) to the infant or 2.5 to 5 mg given to the mother in labor is associated with significant hyperbilirubinemia or its sequelae. The recommendation of the prophylactic administration of vitamin K to either the mother during labor or the infant immediately after birth remains valid today. The subject has been discussed in detail by Wynn.

INFECTIONS OF THE NEWBORN

Fetal Syphilis.   In the past, syphilis was one of the most important infections of the fetus. It formerly accounted for nearly one third of all fetal deaths. Indeed, delivery of a macerated fetus was considered diagnostic of syphilis. Today syphilis plays a much smaller but persistent role in the causation of fetal death. There is, nevertheless, a need for specific criteria that support the diagnosis of fetal syphilis, particularly since the absolute criterion of spirochetes in the fetal tissues or placenta has been largely eliminated by the widespread use of penicillin in the general population, as well as by the great expansion of venereal disease clinics and rapid treatment centers.

Syphilitic lesions in the internal organs comprise essentially interstitial changes in the lungs (pneumonia alba of Virchow), liver (hypertrophic cirrhosis), spleen, and pancreas, and osteochondritis in the long bones (Fig. 10). These

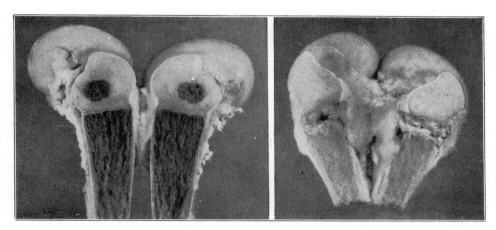

Fig. 10. Left, normal fetal epiphysis. Right, syphilitic fetal epiphysis. (Courtesy of Dr. J. Furth.)

lesions are most readily recognizable at the lower end of the femur and at the lower ends of the tibia and radius, and may be detected radiologically (Fig. 11).

Under the influence of syphilitic infection the placenta becomes larger and paler and often dull and greasy. Microscopically, the villi appear to have lost their characteristic arborescent appearance and to have become thicker and more club-shaped. There is a marked decrease in the number of blood vessels, which in advanced cases almost entirely disappear as a result of endarteritis and proliferation of the stromal cells (Fig. 12). Spirochetes are sparsely scattered through the placenta even when they are present in large numbers in the fetal organs. They can frequently be demonstrated, however, by examination under the dark-field microscope of scrapings from the intima of the vessels of the fresh cord.

Syphilis is discussed further in Ch. 27, p. 800.

Nonsyphilitic Infections.   Nonsyphilitic infections of the newborn are still an important cause of morbidity in term infants and of morbidity and mortality in premature infants. Infection exerts its greatest effect in causing death in term infants during the first 28 days of life. In that group, infection is the cause of

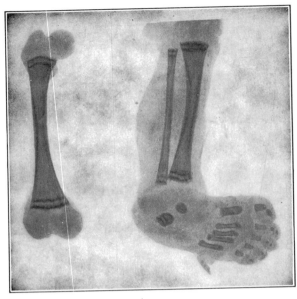

Fig. 11. Roentgenogram of leg bones of syphilitic fetus.

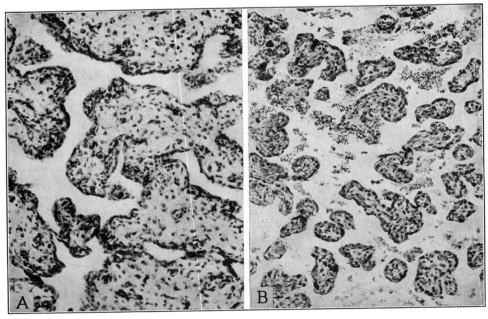

Fig. 12. Photomicrographs of placentas at term. A, syphilitic, showing large, club-shaped villi with increased amount of fibrous tissue in stroma. B, normal placenta.

roughly one quarter of the deaths. Pneumonia is fairly common; septicemia, omphalitis, and other infections are less frequent causes of death. Pneumonia that occurs within the first few days of life usually results from intrauterine infection, and is a frequent finding in term infants dying in the neonatal period. Long labors, prolonged rupture of the membranes, and intrapartum fevers are often associated with contamination of the amniotic fluid with bacteria. Usually ascending from the vagina, bacteria gain access to the fetal respiratory passages and gastrointestinal tract or to the liver through the umbilical cord. There is an increase in the incidence of pneumonia in the infants of mothers whose membranes are ruptured three or more days before delivery, despite the liberal administration of antibiotics to the mother. Tetanus neonatorum, though still common in underdeveloped countries, is a rarity in the United States.

Epidemic Diarrhea of the Newborn.   Outbreaks of epidemic diarrhea of the newborn may occur at any time, and many have been reported. Certain cities have enacted rigid sanitary codes for the conduct of maternity hospitals with the aim of preventing this disease; the sanitary code of the Department of Health of the City of New York is such an example. No code alone can fully prevent outbreaks of this dreadful disease. Its very contagiousness, well described by Stulberg and associates, makes control inordinately difficult. Although it is unlikely that a single pathogen is responsible for all epidemics, certain pathogenic strains of *E. coli* (0-26, 0-55, 0-86, 0-111, 0-125, and 0-126) have been isolated in many outbreaks. The possibility that a virus may be involved has not been entirely ruled out, but it is probable that many of the epidemics are caused by these pathogenic colon bacilli and that the organism is brought into the nursery either by infected personnel, with or without symptomatic disease, or by an already infected infant.

The clinical symptoms are diarrhea with loose, watery, greenish stools, lethargy, dehydration, unstable temperature, and anorexia. Loss of weight is always great. The mortality varies, at times ranging as high as 6 per cent in term infants and 35 per cent in prematures. To stem the tide, no more infants should be admitted to the nursery; those affected should be isolated, and after the unit is evacuated, rigid cleansing of all equipment and of the nursery itself should be carried out. A stool culture should be obtained from all exposed infants to identify carriers and potentially ill babies.

Prophylactic measures against outbreaks of epidemic diarrhea consist in rigid adherence to sanitary codes and technic, adequate space between the bassinets, and small unit nurseries. Strict hand-washing technic for all personnel must be enforced before the handling of each newborn. Recently built nurseries are equipped with ultraviolet light for serilization of entering air and higher pressure of air in the unit than outside, leading to outward flow. As a further precaution, they have small, four- to six-bed units with individually assigned personnel. In a study of early hospital discharge, Hellman, Kohl, and Palmer pointed out that these epidemics are minimized or practically eliminated if the patients and their babies remain in the hospital 48 hours or less.

The treatment of epidemic diarrhea includes antibiotics, maintenance of fluid and electrolyte balance, correction of acidosis, and prevention of dehydration. The infant is given parenteral fluids when oral feedings are not tolerated and when it is desirable to rest the gastrointestinal tract. Sodium bicarbonate is employed to combat acidosis. In addition, transfusions of whole blood may be necessary. As the infant improves, he should receive small quantities of 5 per cent glucose in a solution containing electrolytes, starting with 5 ml and increasing by 5 ml at alternate feedings, with sterile distilled water every two hours until the total fluid requirements are tolerated by mouth. Skimmed milk preparations of hydrolyzed casein are then gradually substituted. Subsequently the interval between feedings is gradually decreased until the infant receives six feedings a day.

Staphylococcal Infection of the Newborn. The resistance of the staphylococcus to antibiotics often poses a very serious hazard to the newborn infant. When staphylococcal infection of the newborn is confined solely to the skin, it is frequently called *impetigo neonatorum*. The number of cases in any nursery is related to the physical facilities and the technic of handling the babies. Overcrowding, inadequate numbers of nurses, and carelessness in technic lead to an increase in such infections. The lesions may appear as early as the second or third day of life or as late as the second week. They are characterized by vesicles that contain turbid fluid; when the vesicles break there is usually a round, moist, denuded area. Localized treatment with gentian violet or even with antibiotic ointments has been generally discontinued; the treatment of choice is now parenteral antibiotics. As a rule the skin clears very quickly, but the newborn infant, especially the premature, is susceptible to generalized systemic infection that may be fulminating and fatal if the organism is inappropriately treated or if it proves to be resistant to antibiotics.

Herpes Simplex. Disseminated herpes simplex is an uncommon but frequently fatal disease of the newborn (Ch. 27, p. 812). Disseminated infection of a neonate may be related to maternal herpetic vulvovaginitis during pregnancy (Nahmias and co-workers). Originally it was thought that the infant was inoculated with the virus during passage through the birth canal. Recent reports, however, have raised the possibility of transplacental passage in some cases. Both term and premature infants are affected. At four to seven days of age, listlessness, irritability, and lethargy occur. Instability of temperature and involvement of the respiratory and central nervous system ensue. Physical findings include hepatosplenomegaly, vesicular lesions of the skin, tongue, mucous membranes, and conjunctivae, and respiratory and neurologic abnormalities. Hemostatic defects frequently lead to multiple areas of hemorrhage. Neurologic deficiencies among the survivors are frequent. The presenting symptoms in the mother are frequently vaginal pain and dysuria, with a sudden onset of vaginal discharge. Single or multiple vesicles followed by shallow ulcers appear on the cervix or vulva. The virus can be cultured from these lesions. Cytologic smears show enlarged nuclei with inclusions characteristic of herpes simplex virus. Elective cesarean section without labor may be justified to prevent fetal contamination (Nahmias). When premature rupture of the membranes occurs, termination of pregnancy by the abdominal route without delay should be considered. An infant born to a mother with a primary herpetic infection should be isolated. Maternal contact while the mother is still shedding the virus should be avoided. Large (10 to 12 ml) doses of gamma globulin may be administered to the infant, although the clinical effectiveness is still speculative. The use of idoxuridine is under consideration.

Spontaneous Pneumothorax. Spontaneous pneumothorax is always a possibility when a newborn infant shows persistent dyspnea and cyanosis. The diagnosis is made in most cases by the fluoroscope or roentgenogram, since the physical findings may be vague and misleading. Frequently, pneumothorax produces no symptoms in the newborn and thus escapes diagnosis unless the chest is x-rayed. The cause is often obscure, for it may develop in infants that breathe spontaneously at birth and require no artificial respiration. It appears to be more common in males than in females. The prognosis of pneumothorax is believed to be somewhat better when it occurs in the neonatal period than when it develops later on, but it is always grave, with a fatal outcome in about half the cases. Although withdrawal of the air with a needle and syringe is often successful, the relief may be only temporary, and chest tube attached to underwater drainage may be required. Treatment is designed to prevent mediastinal shift and to promote expansion of the collapsed lung.

POSTMATURITY

Any fetus born two weeks or more after the calculated date of confinement is often considered postmature. Although such a definition would include at least 12 per cent of all pregnancies, many of them are not prolonged pregnancies but results of errors in the date of the last menstrual period. A more logical estimate of the prevalence of postmaturity is about 4 per cent of all pregnancies. The effects of prolonged pregnancy on the fetus are quite variable. In some instances the fetus continues to grow at a significant rate, as reflected in a high birth weight, and does not appear to suffer any serious harm in this circumstance. In other instances the fetus fails to grow as the pregnancy continues; at times he is starved in utero to the extent that loss of soft tissue and low birth weight is obvious at the time of birth.

The typical postmature infant has an absence of lanugo hair, long nails, abundance of scalp hair, pale skin with desquamated epithelium, diminished vernix, and apparently increased alertness. The amniotic fluid may be scant and meconium-stained.

In the United States, pregnancies extending beyond the expected date have created less concern than abroad. Many clinicians deny that postmaturity predisposes to infants of excessive size or dystocia. In England, however, the policy of elective induction of labor has evolved in many clinics, based principally on the assumption of a progressive diminution in oxygen content and saturation in the cord blood as pregnancy advances beyond term. This belief has gained support through the studies of Walker. Some statistical studies corroborated the experimental work and showed a significant progressive rise in rates of stillbirth as pregnancy advances beyond term. Several investigators in England and many in the United States, however, have cast serious doubt on these clinical findings. Even if postmaturity possibly imposes a slightly increased risk of fetal death, it is probable that this hazard is less than that associated with the induction of labor in the presence of an unripe cervix. We believe, therefore, that postmaturity is not an indication for the induction of labor unless the cervix is favorable. There are several exceptions to this complacent attitude. Pregnancies that go more than three weeks past term have an increased stillbirth rate, especially if there is associated placental dysfunction. Placental dysfunction may be assessed by studies of urinary estriol, amniotic fluid, fetal scalp blood, and ultrasonic estimation of placental volume (Hellman and colleagues). These infants have been classified into three groups by Clifford:

1. Infants with the usual signs of postmaturity
2. Infants with the usual signs of postmaturity and meconium staining
3. Infants with signs of group 1 and 2 with bright yellow staining of the skin, nails, and umbilical cord.

Infants in the first group have no increase in mortality, although a few have respiratory distress. Infants in group 2 have a 35 per cent mortality, resulting principally from the respiratory distress and cerebral hypoxia. Few infants in group 3 are born alive. Those that are suffer from respiratory distress and aspiration pneumonia. The mortality rate is about 15 per cent.

All postmature infants may have high hematocrits, dehydration, and hypoglycemia. Elderly primigravidas, especially those over 40, should not be allowed to go more than a week beyond term. In these patients, however, cesarean section rather than induction of labor is often the procedure of choice. For an extensive discussion of this subject, the papers by Beischer and colleagues should be consulted.

REFERENCES

Allen, F. H. Induction of labor in the management of erythroblastosis fetalis. Quart Rev Pediat 12:1, 1957.
——— and Diamond, L. R. Erythroblastosis Fetalis, Including Exchange Transfusion Technic. Boston, Little, Brown & Co., 1958.
——— Diamond, L. K., and Jones, A. R. Erythroblastosis fetalis. IX. The problems of stillbirth. New Eng J Med 251:453, 1954.
Allison, A. C. Danger of vitamin K to newborn (Letters to the Editor). Lancet 1:669, 1955.
Anderson, A. B. M., and Griffiths, A. D. Estimation of duration of gestation by amniotic fluid cytology. J Obstet Gynaec Brit Comm 75:300, 1968.
Arias, I. M., Gartner, L. M., Seifter, S., and Furman, M. Prolonged neonatal unconjugated hyperbilirubinemia associated with breast feeding and steroid, pregnane-3(alpha),20 (beta)-diol in maternal milk that inhibits glucuronide formation in vitro. J Clin Invest 43: 2037, 1964.
Avery, M. E. The Lung and Its Disorders in the Newborn Infant. Philadelphia, W. B. Saunders, 1968.
Ballantyne, J. W. The diseases and deformities of the foetus. Edinburgh, Oliver & Boyd, 1892–1895.
Battaglia, F. C., and Lubchenco, L. O. A practical classification of newborn infants by weight and gestational age. J Pediat 71:159, 1967.
Beischer, N. A., Evans, J. H., and Townsend, L. Studies in prolonged pregnancy. I. The incidence of prolonged pregnancy. Amer J Obstet Gynec 103:476, 1969.
——— Brown, J. B., Smith, M. A., and Townsend, L. Studies in prolonged pregnancy. II. Clinical results and urinary estriol excretion in prolonged pregnancy. Amer J Obstet Gynec 103:483, 1969.
——— Brown, J. B., and Townsend, L. Studies in prolonged pregnancy. III. Amniocentesis in prolonged pregnancy. Amer J Obstet Gynec 103:496, 1969.
Bevis, D. C. A. Composition of liquor amnii in haemolytic disease of newborn. Lancet 2:443, 1950.
Boggs, T. R., and Westphal, M. C. Mortality of exchange transfusion. Pediatrics 26:745, 1960.
Bowman, J. M., Friesen, R. F., Bowman, W. D., McInnis, A. C., Barnes, P. H., and Grewar,

D. Fetal transfusion in severe Rh isoimmunization. Indications, efficiency and results based on 218 transfusions carried out on 100 fetuses. JAMA 207:1101, 1969.

Brown, A. K., and Zuelzer, W. W. Studies on the neonatal development of the glucuronide conjugating system. J Clin Invest 37:332, 1958.

Brumley, G. W. Personal communication.

Chen, H., Lin, C., and Lien, I. Vascular permeability in experimental kernicterus. An electron-microscopic study of the blood-brain barrier. Amer J Path 51:69, 1967.

Clifford, S. H. Postmaturity—with placental dysfunction; clinical syndrome and pathologic findings. J Pediat 44:1, 1954.

Cohen, M. M., Weintraub, D. H., and Lilienfeld, A. M. The relationship of pulmonary hyaline membrane to certain factors in pregnancy and delivery. Pediatrics 26:42, 1960.

Conway, D. J. Prematurity. J Obstet Gynaec Brit Emp 58:236, 1951.

Cornblath, M. Neonatal hypoglycemia: A summons to action, in Wynn, R. M. (ed.), Fetal Homeostasis, IV. New York, Appleton-Century-Crofts, 1969, p. 122.

Crawford, H., Cutbush, M., and Mollison, P. L. Hemolytic disease of the newborn due to anti-A. Blood 8:620, 1953.

Darrow, R. R. Icterus gravis (erythroblastosis) neonatorum. Examination of etiologic considerations. Arch Path 25:378, 1938.

Day, R. L. Inhibition of brain respiration in vitro by bilirubin. Reversal of inhibition by various means. Proc Soc Exp Biol Med 85:261, 1954.

de Lemos, R. A., Shermata, D. W., Knelson, J. H., Kotas, R. V., and Avery, M. E. Acceleration of appearance of pulmonary surfactant in the fetal lamb by administration of corticosteroids. Amer Rev Resp Dis 102:459, 1970.

DeWit, C. D., Borst-Eilers, E., Van deWeerdt, CHM v.d., and Kloosterman, G. J. Prevention of rhesus immunization. A controlled trial with a comparatively low dose of anti-D immunoglobulin. Brit Med J 4:477, 1968.

Diamond, L. K. Replacement transfusion as a treatment for erythroblastosis fetalis (technic of exchange transfusion via umbilical vein). Pediatrics 2:520, 1948.

———— Blackfan, K. D., and Baty, J. M. Erythroblastosis fetalis and its association with universal edema of the fetus, icterus gravis neonatorum and anemia of the newborn. J Pediat 1:269, 1932.

Drillien, C. M. The growth and development of the prematurely born infant. Baltimore, The Williams & Wilkins Co., 1964.

Driscoll, S. G., Benirschke, K., and Curtis, G. W. Neonatal deaths among infants of diabetic mothers. Amer J Dis Child 100:818, 1960.

———— and Smith, C. A. Neonatal pulmonary disorders. Pediat Clin N Amer 9:325, 1962.

Dutton, G. J. Glucuronide synthesis in foetal liver and other tissues. Biochem J 71:141, 1959.

Eastman, N. J. The great deterrent; prematurity. Bull Sloane Hosp Wom 10:181, 1964.

Faulker, F. A pair of monozygotic twins. in Faulkner, F., (ed.). Human Development. Philadelphia, W. B. Saunders, 1966.

Fisher, R. A. Cited by Race, R. R. An "incomplete" antibody in human serum. Nature 153: 771, 1944.

———— The rhesus factor. Amer Sci 35:95, 1947.

Freda, V. J. The Rh problem in obstetrics and a new concept of its management using amniocentesis and spectrophotometric scanning of amniotic fluid. Amer J Obstet Gynec 92:341, 1965.

———— Gorman, J. G., Pollack, W., Robertson, J. G., Jennings, E. R., and Sullivan, J. F. Prevention of Rh isoimmunization. JAMA 199:390, 1967.

Gitlin, D., and Craig, J. M. Nature of hyaline membrane in asphyxia of the newborn. Pediatrics 17:64, 1956.

Glass, B. The relation of Rh incompatibility to abortion. Amer J Obstet Gynec 57:323, 1949.

Goodlin, R. C. Erythroblastosis fetalis. Obstetrical management. Calif Med 96:312, 1962.

Gray, C. H., and Nicholson, D. C. Pathways of bile pigment metabolism. Ann NY Acad Sci 111:281, 1963.

Graven, S. N., and Misenhimer, H. R. Respiratory distress syndrome and the high risk mother. Amer J Dis Child 109:489, 1965.

Gregg, G. S., and Hutchinson, D. L. Developmental characteristics of infants surviving fetal transfusion. JAMA 209:1059, 1969.

Halitsky, V., Krumholz, B. A., Schwalb, E., and Gromisch, D. S.   The current role of intrauterine fetal transfusion in the management of erythroblastosis fetalis. A review of indications and methods. Obstet Gynec Survey 23:301, 1968 (103 references cited).

Hellman, L. M., and Hertig, A. T.   Erythroblastosis. Amer J Obstet Gynec 36:137, 1938.

—— and Hertig, A. T.   Pathological changes in the placenta associated with erythroblastosis of the fetus. Amer J Path 14:111, 1938.

—— Kobayashi, M., Tolles, W. E., and Cromb, E.   Ultrasonic studies on the volumetric growth of the human placenta. Amer J Obstet Gynec 108:740, 1970.

—— Kohl, S. G., and Palmer, J.   Early hospital discharge in obstetrics. Lancet 1:227, 1962.

—— Moore, W. T., and Shettles, L. B.   Factors influencing plasma prothrombin in the newborn infant. Bull Hopkins Hosp 66:379, 1940.

Henneman, C. E., Anderson, G. V., TeJavej, J. A., Gross, H. A., and Heiman, M. L.   Fetal maturation and amniotic fluid. Amer J Obstet Gynec 108:302, 1970.

Huntington, R. W., and Jarzynka, J. J.   Sudden unexpected death in infancy with special reference to so-called crib deaths. Amer J Clin Path 38:637, 1962.

James, L. S.   Physiology of respiration in newborn infants and in the respiratory distress syndrome. Pediatrics 24:1069, 1959.

Kass, E. H.   Pyelonephritis and bacteriuria. Ann Intern Med 56:46, 1962.

Keuth, U.   Das Membransyndrom der Früh-und Neugeborenen. Berlin, Springer-Verlag, 1965.

Klaus, M., and Meyer, B. P.   Oxygen therapy for the newborn. Pediat Clin N Amer 13:731, 1966.

Landsteiner, K., and Wiener, A. S.   An agglutinable factor in human blood recognized by immune sera for rhesus blood. Proc Soc Exp Biol Med 43:223, 1940.

—— and Wiener, A. S.   Studies on an agglutinogen (Rh) in human blood reacting with anti-rhesus sera and human isoantibodies. J Exp Med 74:309, 1941.

Latham, E. F., Nesbitt, R. E. L., and Anderson, G. W.   A clinical and pathological study of the newborn lung with hyalinelike membranes. Bull Hopkins Hosp 96:173, 1955.

Lathe, G. H., and Walker, M.   The synthesis of bilirubin glucuronide in animal and human liver. Biochem J 70:705, 1958.

Levi, A. J., Gatmaitan, Z., and Arias, I. M.   Deficiency of hepatic anion binding and jaundice in newborn monkeys. New Eng J Med 283:1136, 1970.

Levine, P.   Iso-immunization in pregnancy and the pathogenesis or erythroblastosis fetalis, in H. T. Karsner and S. B. Hooker, 1941 Yearbook of Pathology and Immunology. Chicago, Year Book Publishers, 1941, p. 505. (First report in literature on Hr.)

—— Burnham, L., Katzin, E. M., and Vogel, P.   The role of isoimmunization in the pathogenesis of erythroblastosis fetalis. Amer J Obstet Gynec 42:925, 1941.

—— and Katzin, E. M.   Isoimmunization in pregnancy and the varieties of isoagglutinins observed. Proc Soc Exp Biol Med 45:343, 1940.

—— and Stetson, R. E.   An unusual case of intragroup agglutination. JAMA 113:126, 1939.

—— and Waller, R. K.   Erythroblastosis fetalis in the first born. Blood 1:143, 1946.

—— Wigod, M., Backer, A. M., and Ponder, R.   The Kell-Cellano (K-k) genetic system of human blood factors. Blood 4:869, 1949.

—— and Wong, H.   The incidence of the Rh factor and erythroblastosis fetalis in Chinese. Amer J Obstet Gynec 45:832, 1943.

Liley, A. W.   Liquor amnii analysis in the management of the pregnancy complicated by rhesus sensitization. Amer J Obstet Gynec 82:1359, 1961.

—— Intrauterine transfusion of foetus in haemolytic disease. Brit Med J 2:1107, 1963.

—— Amniocentesis and amniography in hemolytic disease, in J. P. Greenhill (ed.), Yearbook of Obstetrics & Gynecology, 1964–1965 series. Chicago, Year Book Publishers, 1964, p. 256.

—— The technique of foetal transfusion in the treatment of severe haemolytic disease. Aust New Zeal J Obstet Gynaec 4:145, 1964.

Lind, T., Anderson, K. J., and Tacchi, D.   Early induction of labour in cases of rhesus isoimmunization. Lancet 1:585, 1969.

Lubchenco, L. O., Hausman, C., and Bäckström, L.   Factors influencing fetal growth, in

Jonxis, J. H. P., Visser, H. K. A., and Troelstra, J. H. (eds.), Aspects of Praematurity and Dysmaturity. Springfield, Ill., Charles C Thomas, 1968, p. 149.

———— Delivoria-Popadopoulos, M., and Searls, D. Long-term follow-up studies of prematurely born infants. II. Influence of birth weight and gestational age on sequelae. J Ped Clin Amer 17:125, 1970.

Lucey, J., Ferreiro, M., and Hewett, J. Prevention of hyperbilirubinemia of prematurity by phototherapy. Pediatrics 41:1047, 1968.

McElin, T. W., Buckingham, J. C., and Danforth, D. N. The outcome and treatment of Rh-sensitized pregnancies. Amer J Obstet Gynec 84:467, 1962.

McMullin, G. P., Hayes, M. F., and Arora, S. C. Phenobarbitone in rhesus haemolytic disease. Lancet 2:949, 1970.

Miller, H. C. Respiratory distress syndrome of the newborn infant. I. Diagnosis and incidence. II. Clinical study of pathogenesis. J Pediat 61:2,9, 1962.

Mollison, P. L. Blood Transfusion in Clinical Medicine. Springfield, Ill., Charles C Thomas, 1951.

Monro, J. S. Premature infant weighing less than one pound at birth who survived and developed normally. Canad Med Ass J 40:69, 1939.

Moss, A. J., Duffie, E. R., and Fagan, L. M. Respiratory distress syndrome in the newborn. Study on the association of cord clamping and the pathogenesis of distress. JAMA 184:48, 1963.

Mountain, K., Hirsh, J., and Gallus, A. S. Neonatal coagulation defect and maternal anticonvulsant treatment. Lancet 1:265, 1970.

Nahmias, A. J., Josey, W. E., and Naib, Z. M. Neonatal herpes simplex infection. Role of genital infection in mother as a source of virus in the newborn. JAMA 199:164, 1967.

Nesbitt, R. E. L. Prolongation of pregnancy: a review. Obstet Gynec Survey 10:311, 1955.

———— and Anderson, G. W. The pathologic aspects of fetal death in utero, in Engle, E. T. (ed.), Pregnancy Wastage. Springfield, Ill., Charles C Thomas, 1953.

Potter, E. L. Reproductive histories of the mothers of 322 infants with erythroblastosis. Pediatrics 2:369, 1948.

Räihä, C. E., Lind, J., Johanson, C. E., Kihlberg, J., and Vara, P. Relationship of premature birth to heart volume and hemoglobin per cent concentration in pregnant women: preliminary report. Ann Paediat Fenn 2:69, 1956.

Rautmann, H. (On blood formation in classes of general fetal edema). Beitr Path Anat 54:332, 1912.

Report of the 53rd Ross Conference on Pediatric Research. Intrauterine transfusion and erythroblastosis fetalis, in Lucey, J. F., and Butterfield, T. J. (eds.). Columbus, Ross Laboratories, 1966.

Schenker, S. Disposition of bilirubin in the fetus and the newborn. Ann NY Acad Sci 111:303, 1963.

Schindler, A. E., Ratanasopa, B., Lee, T. Y., and Herrmann, W. L. Estriol and Rh isoimmunization: a new approach to the management of severely affected pregnancies. Obstet Gynec 29:625, 1967.

Schulman, H., Mann, L., and Hayashi, T. T. The Rh sensitized pregnant woman. JAMA 196:177, 1966.

Silverman, W. A. Dunham's Premature Infants. New York, Hoeber Medical Division, Harper and Row, 1964, p. 265.

Strang, L. B., Anderson, G. S., and Platt, J. W. Neonatal death and elective cesarean section. Lancet 272:954, 1957.

Stulberg, C. S., Zuelzer, W. W., Nolke, A. C., and Thompson, A. L. *Esch. coli* 0127B8. A pathogenic strain causing infantile diarrhea. I. Epidemiology and bacteriology of a prolonged outbreak in a premature nursery. Amer J Dis Child 90:125, 1955.

Sundal, A. Erythroblastosis foetalis. A survey of 491 consecutive cases of Rh-immunization in pregnancy. Part I. Stillbirths due to erythroblastosis foetalis. Acta Paediat 51:Suppl. 135, 203, 1962.

———— Erythroblastosis foetalis. A survey of 491 consecutive cases of Rh-immunization in pregnancy. Part II. Liveborn affected by erythroblastosis foetalis. Acta Paediat 52:65, 1963.

Taylor, P. M., Bright, N. H., and Birchard, E. L.   Effect of early versus delayed clamping of the umbilical cord on the clinical condition of the newborn infant. Amer J Obstet Gynec 86:893, 1963.

Terry, T. L.   Extreme prematurity and fibroblastic overgrowth of persistent vascular sheath behind each crystalline lens. Preliminary report. Amer J Ophthal 25:203, 1942.

Thiede, H. A.   Discussion of White, C. A., Doorenbus, D. E., and Bradbury, J. T.   The role of chemical and cytologic analysis of amniotic fluid in determination of fetal maturity. Amer J Obstet Gynec 104:668, 1969.

Thompson, H. E., and Makowski, E. L.   Estimation of birth weight and gestational age. Obstet Gynec 37:44, 1971.

Tovey, G. H., and Valaes, T.   Prevention of stillbirth in Rh haemolytic disease. Lancet 2:521, 1959.

Usher, R., McLean, F., and Maughan, G. B.   Respiratory distress syndrome in infants delivered by cesarean section. Amer J Obstet Gynec 88:806, 1964.

——— McLean, F., and Scott, K. E.   Judgment of fetal age. II. Clinical significance of gestational age and an objective method for its assessment. Pediat Clin N Amer 13:835, 1966.

Walker, A. H. C.   Liquor amnii studies in the prediction of haemolytic disease of the newborn. Brit Med J 2:376, 1957.

Walker, J.   Foetal anoxia. J Obstet Gynaec Brit Emp 61:162, 1954.

Walker, W., Fairweather, D. V. I., and Jones, P.   Examination of liquor amnii as a method of predicting severity of haemolytic disease of the newborn. Brit Med J 2:141, 1964.

Waters, W. J., and Bowen, W. R.   Bilirubin encephalopathy: studies related to cellular respiration. Amer J Dis Child 90:603, 1955.

White, C. A., Doorenbos, D. E., and Bradbury, J. T.   The role of chemical and cytologic analysis of amniotic fluid in determination of fetal maturity. Amer J Obstet Gynec 104:664, 1969.

Wiener, A. S.   Blood Groups and Transfusions, 3rd ed. Springfield, Ill. Charles C Thomas, 1943.

——— and Peters, H. R.   Hemolytic reactions following transfusions of blood of the homologous group, with three cases in which the same agglutinogen was responsible. Ann Intern Med 13:2306, 1940.

World Health Organization.   Manual of International Statistical Classification of Disease, Injuries and Causes of Death. Geneva, 1957.

Wynn, R. M.   The obstetric significance of factors affecting the metabolism of bilirubin, with particular reference to the role of vitamin K. Obstet Gynec Survey 18:333, 1963 (109 references cited).

Zuelzer, W. W., and Kaplan, E.   ABO heterospecific pregnancy and hemolytic disease: A study of normal and pathologic variants. Amer J Dis Child 88:158, 179, 307, 319, 1954.

38

MALFORMATIONS OF THE FETUS

Incidence. Malformations of the fetus range from trivial defects, such as tiny supernumerary digits, to grave deformities incompatible with life, such as anencephalus. Malformations incompatible with life, resulting in stillbirth, form a fairly discrete group, occurring once in about 200 viable births. In an additional 0.5 per cent of viable births, there are deformities of sufficient gravity to cause the death of the infant in the first year of life, usually during the neonatal period (Table 1).

Table 1. Congenital Malformations
(Hartford, Connecticut, 1957–1959)

	Number	*Incidence*
1. Incompatible with life	124	0.5
2. Of clinical significance	260	1.1
3. Inconsequential	212	0.9
Subtotal #1 and #2	384	1.6
Total	596	2.5

From Kohl. Community Obstetrical Study, Hartford, Conn., 1960.

Accordingly, about 1 per cent of all fetuses alive at the twenty-eighth week of pregnancy die from congenital malformations before their first birthday (Record and McKeown). Deaths in this category are an important cause of stillbirth and neonatal mortality, accounting for about 15 per cent of all perinatal fatalities. Most of these lethal malformations involve the central nervous system in the form of anencephalus or hydrocephalus, with or without spina bifida.

Malformations compatible with survival beyond one year (with or without surgical correction) are a less discrete group, ranging widely from the inconsequential to the serious. If, however, deformities of clinical significance only are considered, their incidence is probably between 1 and 2 per cent, depending on the extent to which the minor defects are included. "Deformities of clinical significance" are malformations that require special surgical, medical, or pediatric management. Malformations in this category include such conditions as congenital heart disease, harelip, cleft palate, mongolism, pyloric stenosis, tracheo-esophageal fistula, imperforate anus, hypospadias, clubfoot, and certain other bony deformities. If this group of conditions is added to the lethal deformities discussed in the previous paragraph, the total incidence of malformations of clinical significance rises to the order of 2 or 3 per cent. McIntosh and associates make the pertinent observation that less than half of the malformations diagnosed in a group of children followed from birth to 1 year of age were discovered at birth.

The incidence of five relatively common malformations in various regions of the world is shown in Table 2, as summarized by Boon. Similar variations in the

Table 2. The Incidence per 1,000 Births of Five Relatively Common Congenital Malformations in Various Regions of the World

Author	Place	Spina Bifida	Hydro-cephalus	Anencephaly	Cleft Lip	Mongolism
McIntosh (1954)	New York	1.57	0.87	1.40	0.87	1.92
Coffey & Jessop (1959)	Dublin	4.20	3.50	5.10	0.88	0.64
Pleydell (1957)	Northamp-tonshire	1.86	0.45	0.87	1.57	1.63
Edwards (1958)	Scotland	1.70	1.90	2.80	—	—
Pitt (1961)	Melbourne	1.08	0.54	0.58	1.25	0.98
Neel (1958)	Japan	0.20	0.19	0.63	2.68	—
Wong (1964)	Singapore	0.17	0.12	0.21	1.36	0.88

From Boon. Bull Kandung Kerbau Hosp 3:1, 1964.

incidence of major malformations appear in the worldwide prospective survey carried out under the supervision of WHO (Carter) and in an examination of the world literature (Kennedy). These deformities are obvious at birth and, with the possible exception of certain cases of mongolism, can hardly be missed; hence, the geographic and racial differences shown cannot be questioned. Why the frequency of spina bifida, hydrocephalus, and anencephalus is 5 to 20 times greater in Dublin than in Japan or Singapore, for instance, awaits explanation.

The incidence of congenital malformations may be affected by maternal age, parity, race, and the sex of the infant. The effects wrought by these factors, however, are not uniform but are more or less specific for particular deformities. In other words, these factors appear to favor the development of certain malformations, whereas in the case of other deformities they may exert no influence at all. The most striking effect of age on the frequency of congenital deformities is seen in mongolism, which is much more common in mothers over 35. With other malformations the relation between age and incidence is less pronounced, but hydrocephalus is definitely more frequent in older mothers. In general, malformations of the central nervous system are somewhat more common at the very beginning of the reproductive period (under 15) and during its last decade (over 35). Because of the high correlation between age and parity, it is difficult to analyze the effects of either alone, but there is evidence that, irrespective of age, first births and those after the sixth are more likely to be associated with anencephalus and spina bifida. Except for supernumerary digits, malformations are more common in whites than in the blacks. For example, as reported by the National Office of Vital Statistics, the neonatal mortality rate from malformations in whites (4.7 per 1,000 births) is almost twice that in nonwhites (2.7). Murphy found the death rate from malformations to be 5.7 and 3.2 per 1,000 live births for whites and blacks, respectively. Supernumerary digits, however, are seen much more frequently in black than in white infants, indeed almost 10 times more often, according to the data of Shapiro and associates. The data from the Kings County

Hospital bear out this differential. Although the total rate of malformations for both groups is 2.5 per cent (Table 3), there is a predominance of inconsequential

Table 3. Congenital Malformations
(Kings County Hospital, 1956–1958)

	White		Nonwhite	
	Number	Per Cent	Number	Per Cent
1. Incompatible with life	29	0.6	76	0.5
2. Of clinical significance	68	1.5	140	1.0
3. Inconsequential	18	0.4	145	1.0
Subtotal #1 and #2	97	2.1	216	1.5
Total	115	2.5	361	2.5

From Hellman. First International Conference on Congenital Malformations, National Foundation, London, 1960.

malformations in the Negro, with an increase of those of clinical significance in the white race.

The occasional relation between fetal sex and malformations is exemplified by anencephalus, in which about 70 per cent of viable fetuses so affected are female.

If a mother has already given birth to a malformed child, there is an increased likelihood that she will have malformed infants in subsequent pregnancies, because malformations tend to repeat and, moreover, tend to repeat in kind. Following spina bifida, as stated by MacMahon, Pugh, and Ingalls, the risk of spina bifida in subsequent siblings is about 12 times greater than in the general population and the risk of anencephalus or hydrocephalus about 6 times greater. Following anencephalus, the risk of anencephalus, hydrocephalus, and spina bifida in subsequent siblings is about 6 times that in the general population. Hydrocephalus as a single malformation seems to be different etiologically. Following malformations of the central nervous system in general, the likelihood of another such deformity in subsequent siblings is about 1 in 20. Following anencephalus and spina bifida it appears to be somewhat higher. These forecasts seem to apply to malformations of other systems also. For example, for cleft lip, with or without cleft palate, the risk of repetition is between 3.4 and 5.7 per cent, according to Fraser.

Finally, since congenital malformations are often multiple, the presence of one deformity should always lead to suspicion of others. For instance, spina bifida is frequently accompanied by talipes, presumably because of a disturbance of the nerve tracts supplying the lower extremities. Another common combination is hydrocephalus and spina bifida. This association is of considerable clinical importance, since the discovery of a spina bifida in the course of a breech delivery should always suggest the possibility of hydrocephalus. A single umbilical artery occurred in 0.94 per cent of 12,078 infants surveyed by Ainsworth and Davies. In 33.6 per cent there were accompanying major malformations.

Etiology. "A minority of congenital malformations have a major environmental cause. A minority of congenital malformations have a major genetic cause. Most malformations probably result from complicated interactions between genetic predispositions and subtle factors in the intrauterine environment" (Fraser, 1959). This succinct statement is a lucid summary of the relative roles of environment and heredity in the causation of congenital malformations in the light of modern thought.

Environmental Defects.   Perhaps the most familiar example of a major environmental cause of human malformation is maternal rubella during early pregnancy. It produces congenital cataracts, cardiac defects, anomalies of the middle ear, microcephalus, and mental retardation (p. 811). Eichenwald believes that viral infections cause only a small proportion of congenital malformations and that in most instances the cause is unknown. Radiation damage to the fetus might also be cited, as exemplified in Plummer's study of the population exposed at Hiroshima. He showed that defects of the fetal central nervous system may be produced by atomic irradiation. In support of this hypothesis Le Vann has shown an increase in the rate of congenital abnormalities in the province of Alberta corresponding to the increase in the fallout of radioactive dust containing cesium-137, cerium-144, and strontium-90. The role of maternal intoxication with carbon monoxide in the causation of fetal hydrocephalus and microcephalus is another example of pure environmental effect (Muller and Graham).

In experimental animals, chiefly rodents, fetal malformations have been produced by withdrawing various vitamins from the maternal diet (Warkany and Nelson), by injecting certain chemicals at particular stages in pregnancy, by the administration of cortisone, by irradiation, and by numerous other means. Although in many respects the results of these investigations may not be applicable to man, such research has brought out certain principles underlying induced malformations that bear on the etiology of many human deformities. They are outlined by Wilson as follows:

1. The susceptibility of an embryo to a teratogen depends upon the developmental stage at which the agent is applied. The real determinant is the degree of differentiation within a susceptible tissue. Generally, all organs and systems seem to have a susceptible period early in the differentiation of their primordia. Ingalls has prepared a calendar of "anomaly potential," showing the stage specificity and potential malformations according to week of gestation. Susceptibility to teratogenic agents in general decreases as organ formation advances and usually becomes negligible after organogenesis is substantially completed.

2. Each teratogenic agent acts on a particular aspect of cellular metabolism. Different teratogenic agents therefore tend to produce different effects, although acting at the same period of embryonic development and on the same system. The same agent, moreover, may produce different effects when acting at different stages of embryonic development.

3. The genotype influences to a degree the animal's reaction to a teratogenic agent. In most malformations, therefore, both a genetic predisposition and a teratogenic agent are required to produce an anomaly.

4. An agent capable of causing malformations also causes an increase in embryonic mortality. This concept provides one explanation for early abortions.

5. A teratogenic agent need not be deleterious to the maternal organism. Subclinical cases of rubella, for instance, may cause congenital malformations (p. 809).

The influence of purely genetic factors in the causation of congenital malformations is demonstrable in experimental animals and human beings. In certain strains of mice, for instance, about 15 per cent of newborn young have cleft palate, but none have microphthalmia; in another strain, however, about 8 per cent of the young have microphthalmia, but none have cleft palate (Fraser, 1959). These two examples indicate that the genes predispose one variety of embryo to cleft palate and the other to microphthalmia. In human beings, the high frequency of supernumerary digits in Negroes, not only in this country but throughout the world, requires a genetic explanation.

The vast majority of congenital malformations, however, appear to have a dual etiology, environmental *and* genetic. In human beings, the factors involved may be so subtle and complex as to preclude unequivocal demonstration, but it is possible in rodents to show this synergistic action. For example, when a certain strain of pregnant mice is treated with cortisone, cleft palate occurs in 100 per cent of the offspring, whereas following the same treatment in another strain, only 17 per cent of the young are so affected (Fraser, 1955).

Among the few drugs known to be definitely teratogenic in the human being are certain antifolic acid compounds and thalidomide. In addition some progestational compounds masculinize the human fetus. There are strong but by no means conclusive suggestions that lysergic acid diethylamide (LSD) is teratogenic in man. This subject has been reviewed by Smart and Bateman. A great many other drugs are suspect, either because they are teratogenic in animals or because there are clinical impressions of prevalence of congenital malformations associated with their use. Evidence from experimental animals can be misleading in support and elucidation of an etiologic relation between drugs and human congenital malformations. For example, on one hand, it has been difficult to find an animal that demonstrates the teratogenic effect of thalidomide. On the other hand, some antihistaminic drugs are teratogenic in rodents but not in man (Yerushalmy and Milkovich). Although proof of these suspicions is virtually nonexistent and will be difficult to obtain, pregnant women should restrict the intake of all but essential drugs, especially during the early months of gestation.

Chromosomal Anomalies.   Chromosomal anomalies associated with the conditions listed in Table 4 reflect either an absence of chromosomal material, as in Turner's syndrome, or an excess, as in the other diseases listed.

Whether the involved chromosome is an autosome or a sex chromosome, the pathogenetic mechanism seems to be the same. During meiotic division in the gonad a chromosome may "drop out" of the dividing cell (anaphase lagging) and thus be lost. Fertilization of such a gamete results in a zygote with one chromosome too few. In trisomies, one of the explanations of a chromosomal gain is nondisjunction, or failure of the gamete to split equally at meiotic division. If the cell with the extra chromosome is fertilized, the zygote becomes trisomic. These errors of meiotic division produce individuals whose cells are all chromosomally equal but abnormal. If, however, nondisjunction occurs during mitosis after fertilization, the result is an individual with cells of two or more different chromosomal constitutions, or a chromosomal mosaic.

The obstetrician may suspect many of these aberrations at birth of the infant. In addition to a careful physical examination, the observation of a single umbilical artery or particular palmar dermatoglyphic patterns may suggest further investigations. A single umbilical artery, for example, has been found in 10 to 50 per cent of infants with trisomy E (Smith).

Ascertaining "nuclear sex" from buccal smears and karyotypes from peripheral blood, skin, and bone marrow cultures may provide a definite diagnosis.

In mosaicism, appraisal is more difficult, since the major phenotypic defects

Table 4. Major Findings in Established Chromosomal Anomalies in Man
Frequency per 1,000*

Syndrome	Chromosomal Complement	Sex Chromatin	Newborn Babies	Institution Populations	Signs Recognizable at Birth	Mean Parental Age† Maternal	Paternal
Turner	45/XO	Neg.‡	0.4		Lymphangiectatic edema of hands and feet Webbed neck	27.5	30.3
Klinefelter	47/XXY	Pos.	2.0	10–30	None	33.6	37.7
Triple X	47/XXX	Double	0.6	4–7	None	32.5	35.8
YY	47/XYY	Neg.	1.4–4§	10–30**	None		
Down's trisomy, 21	47	Depends on sex. Ordinarily not abnormal	1.6	100	Mongoloid facies Simian line	36.7	
Translocation	46		Rare		Same		
Trisomy, 13–15	47		Rare		Cleft palate Harelip Eye defects Polydactyly		
Trisomy, 16–18	47		Rare		Finger flexion Low set ears Digital arches	32.8	35.2
Cat cry	46 (Deletion B 5)		Rare		Cat cry Moon face		

* Data from Maclean and associates. Lancet 1:286, 1964.
† Data from Hamerton, J. L. (ed.). Chromosomes in Medicine. London, W. J. Heinemann Medical Books Ltd., and from Rohde, R. A., Hodgeman, J. E., Cleland, R. S. Pediatrics 33:258, 1964.
‡ May be positive with iso-X complement.
§ Ratcliffe and associates. Lancet 1:121, 1970; Sergovich and associates. New Eng J Med 280:851, 1969.
** Court Brown, W. M. J Med Genet 5:341, 1968. Refers to penal institutions.

may be much less obvious, and karyotypes may be misleading unless many cells are examined.

The changes that are detectable with the technics presently available represent gross genetic damage to the cell. Even with the loss of the smallest possible chromosomal fragment, a very large number of genes is probably involved. Before more precise diagnoses can be made, new technics to demonstrate subtler chromosomal anomalies must be developed. For general reviews of human chromosomal anomalies see the book by Hamerton.

Inborn Errors of Metabolism. There are several rare but heritable inborn errors of metabolism, most of which result from the absence of crucial enzymes, with resulting incomplete metabolism of proteins, sugars, or fats. In some cases, there are consequent high levels of toxic metabolites in the blood, causing mental retardation and other defects. These metabolic errors are true congenital defects, which may be inherited as autosomal recessives.

Phenylketonuria is a defect in the conversion of phenylalanine to tyrosine. Nationally, it is reported to occur about once in 10,000 births. Because the associated mental retardation can often be prevented by proper diet, early diagnosis is important and in many cases can be made by the second or third day of life.

Galactosemia is an inborn error of sugar metabolism, also resulting in mental retardation and other defects.

Current annotated bibliographies of these two congenital defects have been prepared by the Children's Bureau. Widespread screening of the newborn is currently employed only for phenylketonuria. In some states, for example New York, this test is mandatory. It is likely that screening for a host of other heritable diseases will be practicable in the near future (Hsia).

Phocomelia. Phocomelia is a congenital malformation characterized by severe deformities of the long bones. Either the radius is absent or both radius and ulna are defective; in extreme cases the radius, ulna, and humerus are lacking and the hand buds arise from the shoulders. The legs may be affected in the same manner. In extremely severe cases both arms and legs are missing (Fig. 1). The mental development of the vast majority of the children is normal, and about two thirds of them survive (Taussig).

In 1961–1962 an outbreak of phocomelia occurred in West Germany and conclusive evidence indicated that it was attributable to the widespread use by pregnant women of a sedative and tranquilizing drug, thalidomide. In a large proportion of the cases the drug was administered early in pregnancy for the treatment of nausea and vomiting. The fetus was most vulnerable to the teratogenic action when the drug was ingested by the mother between the thirtieth and fiftieth day of pregnancy. It has been estimated that the thalidomide tragedy involved at least 5,000 infants and possibly many more.

The most important practical lesson to be drawn from the experience with thalidomide is that no drug should be administered to pregnant women unless it is urgently indicated. This injunction applies particularly to drugs administered during the first half of pregnancy for nausea and insomnia. Since we do not know which drugs are teratogenic to the highly vulnerable fetus in its early stages of development, it is best to abstain from the use of any drugs during the first half of pregnancy unless a specific agent is indispensable to maternal health.

Anencephalus. Anencephalus is a malformation characterized by complete or partial absence of the brain and the overlying skull. In most such cases there is

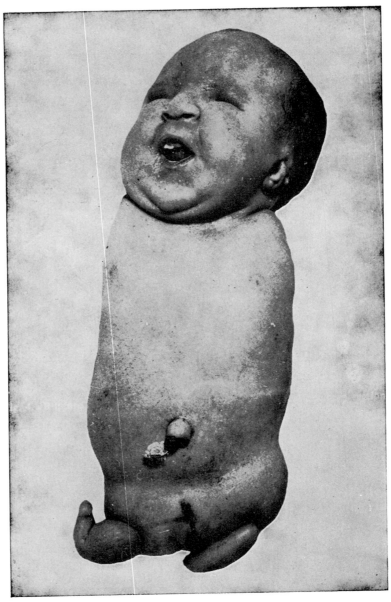

Fig. 1. Phocomelia due to thalidomide. (Courtesy of Prof. Scott Russell, Sheffield, England.)

no brain tissue except a small mass composed of a few glial cells distributed between the larger vessels. The pituitary gland also is either absent or very hypoplastic. The absence of the cranial vault renders the face very prominent and somewhat extended; the eyes often protrude markedly from their sockets, and the tongue hangs from the mouth. About 70 per cent of anencephalic fetuses are females.

In addition to the virtual absence of brain tissue in anencephalic fetuses there is extreme diminution in the size of the adrenal glands, the combined weight of which may be well under 1 g, in contrast to the usual weight of 5 g of the adrenals in normal term infants. The small size of the gland reflects the absence of the fetal, or provisional, cortex. Although it is commonly conjectured that the adrenal hypoplasia is secondary to the absence of the pituitary gland, some authorities believe that the factor producing the anencephalus also produces the adrenal defect.

Nothing definite is known about the cause of anencephalus, but it again appears that both genetic and environmental factors are involved. A genetic factor is strongly suggested, of course, by the frequency with which this malformation recurs in subsequent pregnancies. Yen and MacMahon point out, however, that the relatively small increase (4.5 per cent) in sibship risk over the rate in the general population furnishes a strong argument against a single major-gene hypothesis. A polygenic predisposition is possible, but the very rare occurrence of concordance in twins is difficult to reconcile with any genic hypothesis. Extreme examples of recurrence in siblings have been reported, in which women have produced four successive anencephalic infants (Horne). The reported geographic differences in the incidence of anencephalus, however, have led to the belief that different environmental conditions in these several areas, notably poor living conditions and inadequate diets, predispose to the anomaly. Anderson, Baird, and Thomson, in Scotland, believe that as social status falls there is a steady increase in the incidence of anencephalus. They do not conclude, however, that environmental influences are necessarily major causes of malformations of the central nervous system, but suggest that they probably act by bringing out latent tendencies.

Clinical Aspects. Inability to palpate a fetal head abdominally and increased fetal movement on rectal examination suggest anencephalus (Figs. 2 and 3), but radiologic confirmation is necessary for definitive diagnosis. Since accompanying hydramnios occurs in about 90 per cent of cases, it too suggests anencephalus or, perhaps, another malformation. Anencephalus is the most common cause of gross hydramnios, which may occasionally be sufficiently massive to require paracentesis (p. 599). Because of the diminutive size and abnormal shape of the fetal head, malpresentations, especially breech and face, are frequent.

Dystocia is uncommon, but the very small head is a poor dilator, which occasionally passes through the cervix before complete dilatation. Shoulder dystocia may thus result.

The most frequent practical question posed by pregnancies complicated by anencephalus is whether to initiate labor as soon as the diagnosis is confirmed. Awaiting spontaneous labor is generally the most judicious plan, but oxytocin by intravenous drip in a dose two or three times that ordinarily used for uterine dysfunction sometimes initiates labor. The uterus containing an anencephalic fetus, however, is refractory to oxytocic administration in about 40 per cent of patients. The slow removal of a large portion of the amniotic fluid in addition to the administration of oxytocin almost always accomplishes delivery.

Especially in the absence of hydramnios, the duration of anencephalic pregnancies may be remarkably long, exceeding that reported in any other form of gestation with a living fetus. In the well-authenticated case of Higgins, for ex-

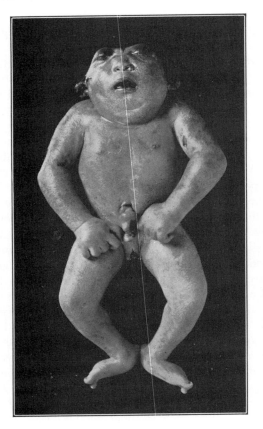

Fig. 2. Anencephalus.

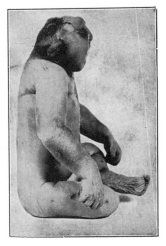

Fig. 3. Anencephalic monster. Note protruding eyes and relatively long arms, which usually accompany this deformity.

ample, the duration of pregnancy was one year and twenty-four days after the last menstrual period, with fetal movements present until the moment of delivery. Several such cases have been reported, but they defy explanation. Comerford cites placental abruption, amniotic fluid embolism, and shoulder dystocia as possible obstetric complications.

Hydrocephalus. Because of the clinical importance of hydrocephalus as a cause of dystocia and rupture of the uterus, this malformation is discussed on page 885 together with other fetal causes of dystocia.

Spina Bifida. This condition consists of a hiatus, usually in the lumbosacral vertebrae, through which a meningeal sac may protrude, forming a *meningocele;* if the sac contains the spinal cord as well, the anomaly is called a *meningomyelocele.* In the presence of complete rachischisis the spinal cord is represented by a ribbon of spongy, red tissue lying in a deep groove. In these circumstances the infant dies soon after birth. In other instances, the defect may be very slight, as in *spina bifida occulta.* Immediate treatment consists in prevention of trauma and infection. Care is required to keep the surface of the protrusion clean. It should be covered with a large pad of absorbent cotton and protected from ulceration with a ring cushion. Neurosurgical consultation should be obtained. Associated malformations, particularly hydrocephalus (Fig. 4), anencephalus, and clubfoot, are common.

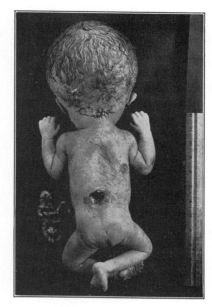

Fig. 4. Hydrocephalus with spina bifida.

Iniencephalus.   Iniencephalus is a rare malformation characterized by pronounced retroflexion of the head, defective occipital bones, and cerebral and spinal meningoceles.

Down's Syndrome (Mongolism).   This congenital malformation presents a striking clinical picture often recognizable at birth. The facies of the infants are mongoloid, with narrow, slanting, closely set palpebral fissures. The tongue is thick and fissured, and the palatal arch often high. Fingers are stubby and the hands present clear-cut dermatoglyphic patterns, particularly a simian line (Fig. 5). Mental retardation is almost always present. Currently, these children may live to a nearly normal age.

Most cases of Down's syndrome result from an extra chromosome, trisomy 21 (Lejeune; Jacobs), which has a prevalence in the general population of about 1 in 700. There is a marked variation in the occurrence of Down's syndrome with maternal age, as shown by Collmann and Stoller in a study of 1,134 mongoloid infants among 780,168 births in Victoria, Australia (Fig. 6). In contrast to the modal maternal age for all births of 25–29 years, that for mongoloid births lies in the 35–39 lustrum. One quarter of all these children were born to mothers over 40 years of age. Whereas in mothers up to the age of 30 the risk of a mongoloid birth is less than 1 in 1,000, this risk increases to 1 in 100 at age 40, and to 1 in 45 when the maternal age is 45 or above.

There is a bimodality in the curves shown in Figure 6 that is not statistically significant, but similar shapes characterize the curves presented by both Øster and Penrose. Consequently, Penrose suggests two disparate distributions of etiologically distinct groups, one of younger and one of older mothers. This suggestion is consistent with the now recognized dual chromosomal abnormality in Down's syndrome: the more common, trisomy 21; and the less common, a translocation defect that occurs in only 8.9 per cent of mothers less than 30 years of age and in 2.1 per cent of those older (Lilienfeld and Beneṣch). Translocation is

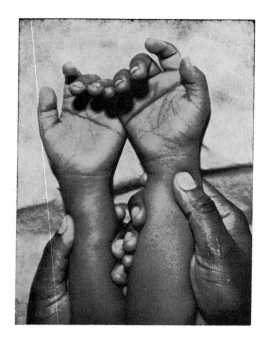

Fig. 5. Hands of an infant with Down's syndrome. The simian lines on the palms are striking.

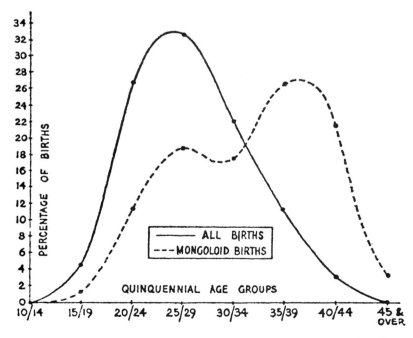

Fig. 6. Maternal age distributions for all births and mongoloid births in Victoria, Australia, 1942–1957. (Collman and Stoller. Amer J Public Health 52:813, 1962.)

the transfer of a segment of one chromosome to a different site on the same chromosome or to a different chromosome. In mongolism, such translocations are recognized by study of the karyotype. The important translocations in mongolism are 13–15/21, 21/21, and 21/22. A female carrier with a 13–15/21 translocation has a 20 per cent chance of producing a mongoloid infant. If either parent is a 21/21 carrier, 100 per cent of the children will be affected; but if any normal children have been produced or if one of the carrier's parents has the same balanced translocation, the carrier almost certainly has a 21/22 defect. The rate of recurrence of this specific type of translocation is reported to be low. A 21/21 translocation cannot be distinguished from 21/22 except by the birth of a normal child, which rules out the 21/21 translocation. The obvious importance of this rare defect lies in the differential probability of recurrence of mongolism in these families. Lilienfeld and Benesch have recently written a monograph on the epidemiology of mongolism, including an extensive reference list.

Congenital Heart Disease. Because of the irregularity with which cases of congenital heart disease are reported, the frequency of this malformation cannot be stated precisely, but it is not uncommon. The cardiac malformations include such conditions as patent ductus arteriosus (often asymptomatic), coarction of the aorta, septal defects, pulmonary stenosis, and tetralogy of Fallot. They often occur as part of a syndrome, such as Down's, Marfan's, Ellis–van Creveld's, and other chromosomal disorders. Infants with severe congenital heart disease may look and react quite normally at birth, only to deteriorate later. Therefore one should consider the possibility of a cardiovascular defect in the mature infant who appears normal at birth and then develops tachypnea, cyanosis, marked tachycardia, and hepatomegaly in the early hours or days after birth. Arrhythmias are rare in the newborn. These changes are often difficult to distinguish clinically from those of so-called idiopathic respiratory distress syndrome.

Renal Agenesis. The incidence of complete absence of the kidney is about 1 in 4,000 births (Potter). The malformation occurs more frequently in male infants and is characteristically accompanied by oligohydramnios. The infant has prominent epicanthic folds, a flattened nose, and large low-set ears. The skin is loose and the hands often seem large. A cardiac malformation is common. One third of the infants are stillborn; the longest reported survival is 48 hours. Pulmonary hypoplasia is found in practically all infants.

Clubfeet (Talipes Equinovarus). The extremities are involved in a large number of congenital defects, most of which are rare. Clubfeet, however, are common, occurring about once in 1,000 births. Since the borderline between the normal and the pathologic is not sharp in this malformation, early orthopedic consultation is essential.

Congenital Dislocation of the Hip. This fairly common malformation is six times more frequent in girls than in boys (Record and McKeown) and more common in breech than in vertex deliveries. It shows geographic variations, having been noted with unusual frequency in northern Italy, for example. It is almost never seen in the Negro. The cause is defective formation of the acetabulum, particularly its upper lip. As a result the head of the femur may migrate upward and backward. In most cases, the displacement probably does not begin until after birth, developing gradually during the early weeks or months of life. From an obstetric point of view, this fact is worthy of note because it is sometimes alleged that these malformations were overlooked in the neonatal period. Carter, reviewing the genetic aspects of the disease, found concordance in 40 per cent of monozygous twins with congenital dislocation of the hip but in only 3 per cent of dizygous twins. One per cent of subsequent male siblings and 5 per cent of later female siblings were affected.

Polydactylism.   Supernumerary digits are occasionally seen, especially in Negro newborns. They usually consist of a small amount of skin and cartilage attached by a fine pedicle to the base of the fourth finger or toe. Simple ligation of the stalk with a silk thread is generally sufficient treatment. If the base is broad and the digit is well developed, however, surgical removal may be required.

Harelip and Cleft Palate.   A cleft in the lip, either unilateral or bilateral, may or may not be associated with a cleft in the alveolar arch or a cleft in the palate. It is one of the most frequent congenital deformities, with an incidence of approximately 1.3 per 1,000 births. Because of difficulties in feeding, it is advisable to operate upon a harelip as soon as the weight of the infant permits. Cleft palate may present even greater difficulties in feeding, requiring use of a prosthesis until the age of 2 or 2½ years. A common error is to confuse simple cleft palate and harelip with the more serious 13–15 trisomy.

Meningocele.   Meningocele is a herniation of the meninges in the suture lines, usually in the occipital region (Fig. 7), and less commonly lower in the spinal

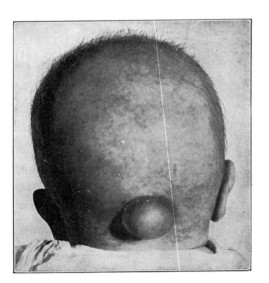

Fig. 7. Meningocele in infant four months of age. (Courtesy of Dr. S. Z. Levine.)

column. It may be associated with spina bifida. If part of the brain protrudes into the sac, an *encephalocele* results. Attempts at closure often result in hydrocephalus. Early closure of these defects, nevertheless, leads to a decreased incidence of infection and superior neurologic results.

Hernia: Umbilical and Inguinal.   Umbilical hernias are common, especially in blacks. They are rarely serious, and strangulation of the bowel is almost unknown. Most small umbilical hernias disappear spontaneously within a few months, whereas the larger varieties are generally treated successfully by simple mechanical measures, such as strapping the surrounding skin with a band of adhesive tape.

Similarly inguinal hernias are rarely serious, often correcting themselves spontane-ously during the first year of life. Incarceration of the bowel is uncommon, and strangulation is even rarer in term infants. In small premature infants, however, these inguinal hernias frequently undergo incarceration. Inguinal herniorrhaphy should be performed before these infants leave the hospital.

Undescended Testicles.   Occasionally the testes do not descend in the first month of life. Treatment is usually expectant until just before puberty, when surgical correction may be necessary. Indications for the use of gonadotropins in this condition may be found in textbooks of pediatrics or clinical endocrinology. Inguinal hernia is often associated.

Imperforate Anus.   In this abnormality, because of atresia of the anus, the rectum ends in a blind pouch. Examination of the newborn in the delivery room usually reveals the condition. More commonly perhaps, it is discovered on the first attempt to record the infant's rectal temperature. Surgical intervention is, of course, imperative.

Harlequin Fetus.   Infants with this rare anomaly, the exact cause of which is unknown, have a pronounced ichthyosis at birth, characterized by thick, horny, armorlike plates, which cover the entire skin and lead to fetal or early neonatal death. MacLaverty and Kidney report two cases in which the fetal thyroid was exceptionally small and the thymus enlarged. The mother of these two infants was thought to show marked evidence of hypothyroidism. Reference has been made to this association previously in the literature.

INTRAUTERINE DIAGNOSIS

Only a small percentage of congenital malformations are diagnosed before birth. Some major defects can be demonstrated by roentgenographic or sonographic technics (Figs. 8 and 9).

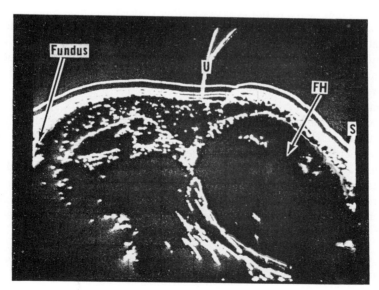

Fig. 8. Sonogram of a hydrocephalic fetus (36 weeks). A huge head is seen occupying one half of the uterine cavity. FH, fetal head; S, symphysis pubis; U, umbilicus.

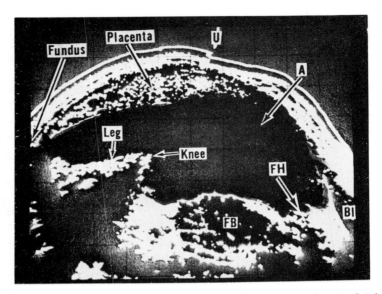

Fig. 9. Sonogram of an anencephalic fetus (33 weeks). There is no discrete fetal head demonstrable. There is moderate hydramnios as shown by large amniotic cavity. A, amniotic cavity; Bl, bladder; FB, fetal body; FH, fetal head area; U, umbilicus.

At about the same time in different parts of the world Serr and associates, Fuchs and Riis, Makowski and co-workers, and Shettles noted that the sex of the fetus often could be ascertained by examining the nuclear chromatin (Barr body) of the fetal cells obtained by amniocentesis. Thus it was theoretically possible to detect sex-linked heritable conditions. More recently it has been shown that in cell culture the Y chromosome fluoresces when treated with atabrine and examined microscopically with ultraviolet light. Determination of sex by either of these methods is in error about 15 per cent of the time (Miller).

Various hereditable diseases in which there are cellular enzyme deficiencies can be diagnosed if enough of the fetal cells in aspirated amniotic fluid will replicate in culture. These diseases include Lesch-Nyhan syndrome, type II glycogenosis, lysosomal acid phosphatase deficiency, and Tay-Sachs disease (Schneck and co-workers).

Valenti and associates and others have diagnosed Down's syndrome in utero in cells cultured from amniotic fluid. Miller suggests karyotyping of cells cultured from amniotic fluid from those pregnant women who are over 40 or who previously had a child with Down's syndrome.

If removal of a significant volume of amniotic fluid early in the second trimester of pregnancy continues to prove to be quite safe, intrauterine diagnosis will play an important role in providing rational grounds for therapeutic abortion. Milunsky and associates have quite recently reviewed the subject of prenatal genetic diagnosis.

Genetic Counseling

Genetic counseling supplies information to families with genetic problems, helping them to make intelligent decisions regarding future childbearing. A malformed child often precipitates the request for such guidance, although other problems leading to consultation include inheritable diseases in the family and consanguineous marriages. Human genetic counseling is by no means an exact science, but it becomes increasingly complex with the accumulation of additional information (Fraser). Amateurish advice, particularly of the unjustifiably optimistic variety, may produce tragic results.

Forecasting the probability of an inherited disorder is an important step, but it requires a precise medical history and construction of a family tree. Statistics alone, however, do not suffice, for the total impact of a heritable defect on the family, including emotional, social, and religious aspects, must be considered. The likelihood of recurrence must be presented to the patient positively. For example, if the chance of recurrence is 5 per cent, the probability for a normal child is 95 per cent. Finally, all such advice should be permissive, for the family must make the decision.

Diagnosis and History.   Accurate diagnosis is required to distinguish similar effects resulting from abnormalities of different genes or from nongenetic causes. Hydrocephalus, microcephalus, microphthalmus, cataract, cleft lip, cleft palate, clubfoot, and polydactylism may result from different genetic mechanisms or from nongenetic prenatal disturbances. A detailed medical pedigree carried through several generations and collateral lines is a prerequisite to sound genetic advice. In addition to the entire history of the mother's pregnancy, the medical histories of the maternal and paternal relatives should be explored, and the information concerning their general health and their ages and causes of death should be recorded. Consanguinity of husband and wife, often deliberately hidden, must be investigated.

Upon completion of the detailed history, it is often possible to decide whether the disease follows an easily recognized pattern of inheritance or represents an isolated congenital defect.

Dominant Inheritance.   A mutant gene producing its effect when present on one or both chromosomes of a given pair is referred to as a dominant gene. A recessive gene produces its effect only when present on both chromosomes. A dominantly inherited disease caused by a single dominant gene is transmitted from one generation to the next in a direct line so that each affected individual has an affected parent and there are no skipped generations. There is a 50 per cent chance that the children of an affected parent married to an unaffected mate will inherit the condition. These affected children will in turn transmit the defect to half of their offspring.

A dominant trait may be sex-linked (located on the X chromosome) or autosomal (located on any one of the other 22 pairs of autosomes in the genome). If the trait is dominant and sex-linked, one half of the daughters of an affected father whose wife is normal will inherit the gene, and none of the sons will be affected. If, however, the mother is heterozygous and affected and the father normal, she will transmit the condition to half of her daughters and half of her sons; but if the mother is homozygous and affected, she will transmit the condition to all of her children.

Nongenetic factors may mimic inherited determinants in the production of disease, but these phenocopies can often be detected by adequate history, appropriate clinical examination, and studies in the laboratory. Familial recurrence is unlikely with phenocopies. Affected individuals are nearly always males in

X-linked inheritance, for the female must have mutations in both her X chromosomes in order to manifest the disease. Red-green color blindness and hemophilia are well-known examples of sex-linked recessive inheritance.

Penetrance.   A dominant gene with phenotypic expression in all individuals who carry the gene is said to be 100 per cent penetrant. If not expressed in some individuals even though they have the gene, the gene is not completely penetrant. The degree of penetrance may be quantitatively expressed as the percentage ratio of carriers who show the trait to the total number of individuals who have the gene. A gene that is 80 per cent penetrant is expressed in only 80 per cent of the people who have that gene. The term "penetrance" is applicable not only to heterozygous dominant genes but also to homozygous genes, whether dominant or recessive.

The same gene may express itself in a variety of ways in different people. This characteristic is known as the *expressivity* of the condition. The expressivity of a gene varies from complete manifestation of the condition to complete absence.

Recessive Inheritance.   A child with an inherited disease that requires for its clinical expression the contribution of a duplicate mutant gene from each of its parents is affected by a recessively inherited disease. The parents in these circumstances may be either heterozygous carriers of the mutant gene or homozygous and therefore affected.

If the recessively inherited disease is autosomal, either sex may be similarly affected, and the parents and more remote ancestors are usually unaffected. Frequently in this type of inheritance the parents are related to each other and presumably have brought together in their affected offspring genes received from a common ancestor. The probability of a subsequent child's being affected in such a family is one in four. The likelihood that a normal sibling of an affected child is a carrier of the defect is two chances out of three. The carrier child will not produce affected children, however, except by mating with another carrier or an affected individual. If a recessive gene is rare, there is, of course, only a remote chance that unrelated carriers will marry.

Muller estimated that each normal individual in the general population is heterozygous for at least eight mutant genes, each of which in the homozygous condition would produce a genetic disease. In the normal population, therefore, there is about 1 to 1.5 per cent probability of homozygosity and, therefore, of genetic defects among the children of normal unrelated parents.

In sex-linked recessive inheritance, the affected individuals are nearly always males. The mothers of the affected males are the carriers, and, as with all sex-linked inheritance, male-to-male transmission does not occur. Positive information in this type of inheritance comes from the maternal side of the family pedigree, whereas the paternal history is of little consequence.

Multifactorial or Polygenic Inheritance.   The largest source of genetic variability comes from the combined actions of a number of genes, each with a very small individual effect. The great range of effects so produced is thought to be responsible for the continuous variation seen in the vast majority of differences among normal human beings, as expressed in stature, intelligence, blood pressure, and quite likely in the susceptibility to a number of common diseases (Roberts and Fraser).

Many of the more common congenital malformations have a genetic factor in their causation. The increased incidence in relatives, compared with the incidence in the general population, is difficult to explain in terms of any known environmental factors and is much below that found in single-gene transmission. Carter has suggested that common congenital malformations with an incidence at birth of at least 1 in 1,000, such as cleft lip, pyloric stenosis, talipes equinovarus, congenital dislocations of the hip, spina bifida, anencephalus, and congenital heart defects, are polygenically inherited. In addition, the family patterns of some common diseases of adult life, such as the major psychoses, early-appearing ischemic heart disease, rheumatoid arthritis, ankylosing spondylitis, and diabetes mellitus, appear to be consistent with a multiple genic origin and with varying degrees of environmental modification.

Empiric Risks.   In the majority of cases, a simple pattern of inheritance cannot be demonstrated. In such patients, prognosis is derived from data on empiric risk, based on the pooled experience of many investigators. Such pooled data may be inapplicable to the individual case and occasionally misleading because they include "high-risk" and "low-risk" families. The average so obtained may thus either overestimate or underestimate the true risk. In many instances, however, such average data represent the only estimates available. As a rule of thumb, the risk of a significant malformation in any pregnancy is approximately 1-1.5 per cent. The risk of a second malformed child is about 5 per cent, increasing with subsequent malformed children. Examples of some empiric risks are:

Anencephalus, spina bifida, or both: 5 per cent.

Hydrocephalus: Likelihood of sibling's being affected much less than in anencephalus, but exact statistics are scarce.

Harelip with or without *cleft palate:* 5 per cent. If two children or one child and a parent are affected: 10 to 15 per cent.

Congenital heart disease: 2 per cent.

Clubfoot: (a) When the parents are normal and unrelated and have a child with clubfoot (without spina bifida or dislocated hips), the risk is about 3 per cent that any other child of theirs will be similarly affected. (b) When the parents are normal but *related* and have a child with clubfoot (without spina bifida or dislocated hips), the risk is between 3 and 25 per cent that any other child of theirs will be similarly affected (Fraser, 1958).

Consanguinity.   The risk of recurrence of affected offspring is obviously greater for related than nonrelated parents, and the closer the relationship, the greater is the risk. Even for closely related couples, however, such as first cousins, the chance of having a significantly abnormal child, although twice that expected for children of nonrelatives, is estimated by Motulsky and Hecht not to exceed 2 per cent. Reed has reported a risk of malformation of about 10 per cent in a child resulting from a brother-sister union. Stevenson and colleagues indicate, from the 1958 WHO survey, that malformations of the neural tube occur in 1.42 per cent of the offspring of first-cousin marriages, 0.8 per cent of those from more remote cousin marriages, and 0.5 per cent of the children from marriages of nonrelatives. These data suggest a relation between consanguinity and central nervous system malformations, but they are not conclusive. Because the likelihood of a normal child's resulting from a cousin marriage is greater than that of an affected child, there is no compelling genetic reason to discourage cousin marriage unless there is familial evidence of recessive disease.

In addition to supplying positive information, genetic counseling helps to dispel many misapprehensions and ill-founded rumors concerning congenital malformations. It also helps relieve the feeling of guilt after the birth of a defective child.

Advances in cytogenetics and in the detection of heterozygosity have rendered estimates of the true risk of inheritable defects more accurate. There is every indication of continued progress in the field of genetic counseling.

REFERENCES

Ainsworth, P., and Davies, P. A.   The single umbilical artery: a five-year survey. Develop Med Child Neurol 11:297, 1969.

Anderson, W. J. R., Baird, D., and Thomson, A. M.   Epidemiology of stillbirths and infant deaths due to congenital malformations. Lancet 1:1304, 1958.

Boon, W. H.   Congenital malformations in Singapore. Bull Kandung Kerbau Hospital 3:1, 1964.

Carter, C. O.   Genetic factors in congenital dislocation of the hip. Proc Roy Soc Med 56:803, 1963.

———— Congenital malformations. WHO Chron 21:287, 1967.

———— Genetics of common disorders. Brit Med Bull 25:52, 1969.

Coffey, V. P., and Jessop, W. J.   Rubella and the incidence of congenital abnormalities. Irish J Med Sci 397:1, 1959.

Collmann, R. D., and Stoller, A.   A survey of mongoloid births in Victoria 1942–1957, Australia. Amer J Public Health 52:813, 1962.

Comerford, J.   Pregnancy with anencephaly. Lancet 1:679, 1965.

Edwards, J. H.   Congenital malformations of the central nervous system in Scotland. Brit J Prev Soc Med 12:115, 1958.

Eichenwald, H. F., in Woodside, G. L., and Mitchell, S. C. (eds.), Viral Etiology of Congenital Malformations (189 references). The National Heart Institute of Child Health and Human Development, N.I.H., U.S. Govt Printing Office, Washington, D. C. 1967.

Fraser, F. C.   Thoughts on the etiology of clefts of the palate and lip. Acta Genet (Basel) 5:358, 1955.

———— Causes of congenital malformations in human beings. J Chronic Dis 10:97, 1959.

———— Genetic counselling. Hospital Practice, p. 49, Jan. 1971.

Fuchs, F., and Riis, P.   Antenatal sex determination. Nature 177:330, 1956.

Galactosemia, a selected bibliography compiled by D. O'Brien. U.S. Dept. of Health, Education, and Welfare, Welfare Administration, Children's Bureau, Washington, D.C., 1963.

Hamerton, J. L.   Cytogenetics of mongolism, in Hamerton, J. L. (ed.), Chromosomes in Medicine, London, W. Heinemann Medical Books, Ltd., 1962, p. 137.

———— Chromosomes in Medicine. London, W. Heinemann Medical Books, Ltd., 2nd ed. 1968.

Hellman, L. M.   First International Conference on Congenital Malformations. London, National Foundation, 1960.

Higgins, L. G.   Prolonged pregnancy. Lancet 2:1154, 1954.

Horne, H. W.   Anencephaly in four consecutive pregnancies. Fertil Steril 9:67, 1958.

Hsia, D. Y.   The screening of hereditary metabolic defects among newborn infants. Canad Med Ass J 95:247, 1966.

Ingalls, T. H.   Calendar of anomaly potential, in Mechanisms of Congenital Malformation. The Second Scientific Conference, Association for the Aid of Crippled Children, 1955, p. 16.

Jacobs, P. A., Court Brown, W. M., Baikie, A. G., and Strong, J. A.   The somatic chromosomes in mongolism. Lancet 1:710, 1959.

Kennedy, W. P.   Epidemiologic aspects of the problem of congenital malformations. Birth Defects original article Series 3:No. 2, 1967 (217 references cited).

Kohl, S. G.   Community Obstetrical Study. Hartford, Connecticut, 1960.

Lejeune, O. J., Gauthier, M., and Turpin, R.   (Human chromosomes in tissue culture). C R Acad Sci 248:602, 1959.

Le Vann, L. J.   Congenital abnormalities in children born in Alberta during 1962. A further communication. Alberta Med Bull 1965.

Lilienfeld, A. M., and Benesch, C. H.   Epidemiology of Mongolism. Baltimore, The Johns Hopkins Press 1969 (515 references cited).

MacLaverty, M., and Kidney, W.   The harlequin foetus. J Irish Med Ass 31:295, 1952.

MacLean, N., Harnden, D. G., Court Brown, W. M., Bond, J., and Mantle, D. J.   Sex-chromosome abnormalities in newborn babies. Lancet 1:286, 1964.

———— Mitchell, J. M., Harnden, D. G., Williams, J., Jacobs, P., Buckton, K. A., Baikie, A. G., Court Brown, W. M., McBride, J. A., Strong, J. A., Close, H. G., and Jones, D. C.   A survey of sex-chromosome abnormalities among 4,514 mental defectives. Lancet 1:293, 1962.

MacMahon, B., Pugh, T. F., and Ingalls, T. H.   Anencephalus, spina bifida, and hydrocephalus; incidence related to sex, race, season of birth and incidence in siblings. Brit J Prev Soc Med 7:211, 1953.

Makowski, E. L., Prene, K. A., and Kaiser, I. H.   Detection of sex of fetuses by the incidence of sex chromatin body in nuclei of cells in amniotic fluid. Science 123:542, 1956.

McIntosh, R., Merritt, K. K., Richards, M. R., Samuels, M. H., and Bellows, M. T.   The incidence of congenital malformations: a study of 5,964 pregnancies. Pediatrics 14:505, 1954.

Miller, O. J.   Personal communication.

Milunsky, A., Littlefield, J. W., Kanfer, J. N., Kolodny, F. H., Shih, V. E., and Atkins, L.   Prenatal genetic diagnosis. New Eng J Med 283: No. 25, p. 1370, 283: No. 26, p. 1441, 283: No. 27, p. 1498 (3 parts), 1970. (250 refs. cited.)

Motulsky, A., and Hecht, F.   Genetic prognosis and counseling. Amer J Obstet Gynec 90:1227, 1964.

Muller, G. L., and Graham, S.   Intrauterine death of the fetus due to accidental carbon monoxide poisoning. New Eng J Med 252:1075, 1955.

Muller, H. J.   Our load of mutations. Amer J Hum Genet 2:111, 1950.

Murphy, D. P.   Maternal age at conception of the congenitally malformed child; study based on 607 cases. Amer J Dis Child 51:1007, 1936.

———— Intervals between pregnancies of mothers giving birth to congenitally malformed children. A study of 531 families. Surg Gynec Obstet 63:593, 1936.

———— Congenital Malformations, 2nd ed. Philadelphia, J. B. Lippincott Co., 1947.

National Office of Vital Statistics.   Relation of weight at birth to cause of death and age at death in neonatal period: United States early 1950, Vol. 36, No. 6, February 23, 1956.

Neel, J. V.   A study of major congenital defects in Japanese infants. Amer J Hum Genet 10:398, 1958.

Øster, J.   The causes of mongolism. Danish Med Bull 3:158, 1956.

Penrose, L. S.   Mongolian idiocy (mongolism) and maternal age. Ann NY Acad Sci 57:494, 1954.

———— Genetics of anencephaly. J Ment Defic Res 1:4, 1957.

Pitt, D. B.   Study of congenital malformations, II.   Aust New Zeal J Obstet Gynaec 2:82, 1962.

Pleydell, M. J.   Mongolism and other congenital abnormalities; an epidemiological study in Northamptonshire. Lancet 1:1314, 1957.

Plummer, G. W.   Anomalies occurring in children exposed in utero to the atomic bomb. Pediatrics 10:687, 1952.

Potter, E. L.   Bilateral absence of ureters and kidneys. A report of 50 cases. Obstet Gynec 25:3, 1965.

Record, R. G., and McKeown, T.   Congenital malformations of the central nervous system. I. A survey of 930 cases. Brit J Soc Med 3:183, 1949.

Reed, S. C.   Counseling in Medical Genetics, 2nd ed. Philadelphia, W. B. Saunders Co., 1963.

Roberts, J. A., and Fraser, F.   An Introduction to Medical Genetics. New York, Oxford University Press, 1967.

Rohde, R. A., Hodgman, J. E., and Cleland, R. S.   Multiple congenital anomalies in the E_1-trisomy (group 16-18) syndrome. Pediatrics 33:258, 1964.

Schneck, L., Friedland, J., Valenti, C., Adachi, M., Amsterdam, D., and Volk, B. W.   Prenatal diagnosis of Tay Sachs disease. Lancet 1:582, 1970.

Serr, D. M., Fechs, L., and Denon, N.   The diagnosis of sex before birth using cells from the amniotic fluid. Bull Res Council Israel, 5B2:137, 1955.

Shapiro, R. N., Eddy, W., Fitzgibbon, J., and O'Brien, G. The incidence of congenital anomalies discovered in the neonatal period. Amer J Surg 96:396, 1958.

Shettles, L. B. Nuclear morphology of cells in human amniotic fluid in relation to sex of infant. Amer J Obstet Gynec 71:834, 1956.

Smart, R. G., and Bateman, K. The chromosomal and teratogenic effects of lysergic acid diethylamide. A review of the current literature. Canad Med Ass J 99:805, 1968 (20 references cited).

Smith, D. W. Autosomal abnormalities. Amer J Obstet Gynec 90:1055, 1964 (118 references cited).

Stern, C. Human Genetics. San Francisco, W. H. Freeman & Co., 1968, p. 297.

Stevenson, A. C., Johnston, H. A., Stewart, M. I. P., and Golding, D. R. Congenital malformations. A report of a study of series of consecutive births in 24 centres. Bull WHO 34:Suppl. 9, 88, 1966.

Taussig, H. B. A study of the German outbreak of phocomelia. JAMA 180:1106, 1962.

Valenti, C., Schutta, E. J., and Kehaty, T. Prenatal diagnosis of Down's syndrome. Lancet 2:220, 1968.

Warkany, J., and Nelson, R. C. Appearance of skeletal abnormalities in offspring of rats reared on a deficient diet. Science 92:383, 1940.

——— Weinstein, E. D., Soukup, S. W., Rubinstein, J. H., and Curless, M. C. Chromosome analyses in a children's hospital. Selection of patients and results of studies. Pediatrics 33:454, 1964 (129 references).

Wilson, J. G. Experimental studies on congenital malformations. J Chron Dis 10:111, 1959.

Wong, N. B., and Chua, T. S. The D (13-15) trisomy syndrome. J Singapore Paed Soc 6:19, 1964.

Yen, S., and MacMahon, B. Genetics of anencephaly and spina bifida. Lancet 2:623, 1968.

Yerushalmy, J., and Milkovich, L. Evaluation of the teratogenic effect of meclizine in man. Amer J Obstet Gynec 93:553, 1965.

39

THERAPEUTIC ABORTION, INDUCTION OF LABOR, STERILIZATION, AND CONTRACEPTION

THERAPEUTIC ABORTION

Definitions. Therapeutic abortion is the termination of pregnancy before the period of fetal viability for the purpose of saving the life of the mother or safeguarding her health. Because concepts are changing rapidly, the definition of therapeutic abortion lacks precision. The word "health" in particular is variously interpreted. In its broadest sense, as defined by the World Health Organization, it applies not only to physical health but also to mental health and social well-being. Therapeutic abortion, unlike any other surgical operation, is governed by statute or common law in all states, but the wording of the regulations differs widely. In the strictest sense the law in most states does not permit the procedure for reasons such as illegitimacy, poverty, or rape, or on the basis that the infant is likely to be gravely malformed. Despite its apparent simplicity the law remains vague because the definitions of "life," "save," and "preserve" are subject to widely varying interpretation. For example, one English high court has acquitted a physician for performing therapeutic abortion in a case of rape of a young girl (*Rex* v. *Bourne.* For details see Harper). Abortions are commonly performed in cases of rubella, as a result of which the child may be malformed. In a time of rapidly changing laws, concepts, and mores, therapeutic abortion cannot be defined nor can the listing of its indications carry any degree of accuracy or permanence.

Legal Status. Contrary to popular belief today's stringent abortion laws are of fairly recent origin. Before quickening (the term applied to the first definite perception of fetal movement, which occurs between the sixteenth and twentieth weeks of gestation), abortion was either lawful or widely tolerated in both the United States and Great Britain until 1803. In that year, as part of a general overhaul of British criminal law, a basic criminal abortion law was enacted that made abortion before quickening illegal. The Catholic Church's traditional condemnation of abortion did not receive the ultimate sanction of universal law (excommunication) until 1869 (see Pilpel and Norwick).

The British law of 1803 became the model for similar laws in the United States, but it was not until 1821 that Connecticut enacted the nation's first abortion law. Throughout the nation abortion became illegal except to save the life of the mother. In a few states, the word "health" was added. Until very recently therapeutic abortion in most states was legally permissible only if it was necessary to save the *life* of the mother. Two states extended the exception to "to prevent serious or permanent bodily injury"; and in another two, the exception read "to preserve the life or health of the woman." If the "health of the woman" be construed to include her mental health, still in only two states was therapeutic abortion legally permissible on psychiatric indications or to prevent the birth of a malformed child (as in rubella), which might affect the mother's mental health. Since therapeutic abortion to save the *life* of the woman is rarely necessary, it follows that the great majority of such operations performed in this country went and still go beyond the letter of the law. Nevertheless, experience has shown that if a reputable physician, with the written approval of two other reputable physicians, carries out the operation openly in an accredited hospital, the propriety of the operation is rarely questioned by officers of the law. (For details of the legal status of therapeutic abortion in the United States, consult Harper). Many hospitals have set up abortion committees to decide the permissibility of abortion. Because the intent of these committees is to protect the reputation of the hospital, they have, in general, tended to be restrictive.

There is a growing body of both professional and lay opinion in favor of liberalization of the abortion laws. In 1943, the prestigious New York Academy of Medicine was among the first medical organizations to recognize the need for reform. Since that time the Academy has issued three statements on the subject; the last in 1969 favors repeal of existing abortion laws.

In 1959, the American Law Institute suggested a Model Penal Code governing abortion. This code would authorize therapeutic abortion when a licensed physician believes there is substantial risk that continuance of the pregnancy would gravely impair the physical or mental health of the mother, or that the child would be born with grave physical or mental defects, or that the pregnancy resulted from rape by force, or incest. Two physicians must certify in writing their belief in the justifying circumstance.

In 1967 the House of Delegates of the American Medical Association went on record as supporting reform of the abortion laws conforming to the general guidelines set forth in the Model Penal Code. In 1965 the American College of Obstetricians and Gynecologists recommended, in addition to the provision of the Model Penal Code, that social and total economic environment, actual or reasonably foreseeable, be considered as having a bearing on the health of the mother.

Between 1967 and 1969 eleven states amended their abortion laws by extending the indications for therapeutic termination of pregnancy. The new abortion act in Great Britain (1967) is among the most permissive of all recently enacted statutes. It contains two significant clauses in respect to the ascertainment of health of the mother:

1. "Account be taken of the pregnant woman's actual or reasonably foreseeable environment.
2. "Account be taken not only of the effect of pregnancy on the mother but on any existing children of her family."

If liberally construed, the current British abortion law is tantamount to virtually unrestricted abortion.

The report of Governor Rockefeller's special commission to review the New York State Abortion Law was published in March, 1968. The recommendations follow the Model Penal Code, but add two additional indications for abortion as follows:

1. "The pregnancy commenced while the female was unmarried and under 16 years of age, and is still unmarried.
2. "When the female already has four living children."

The principal arguments in favor of a more permissive abortion statute have been summarized by the Governor's special commission as follows:

1. "The deaths, sterility and harmed physical and mental health, resulting from the large number of illegal abortions each year could largely be prevented if such abortions were performed by competent physicians in proper hospital surroundings, within the framework of reasonable legislation.
2. "The wide disparity between the statutory law and actual practice encourages disrespect for the law and places upon the conscientious physician an intolerable conflict between his medical duty to his patients and his duty as a citizen to uphold the law.
3. "The present law places an unfair discrimination on the poor. Persons with money may obtain safe abortions either by traveling to other jurisdictions, by going to high-priced, competent though illegal abortionists, or by obtaining legal abortion here based on 'sophisticated' psychiatric indications."

The divergence between the literal interpretation of the law and current medical practice has led today's physician into an area of grave legal risk. There are indications that the courts may take action when reputable medical practice in accredited hospitals does not conform to strict interpretation of rigid abortion laws.

In 1969 there were two court decisions of major importance in this field. On September 5 the California Supreme Court in the case of *People* v. *Belous* declared the pre-1967 California abortion law unconstitutional on the following grounds:

1. The phrase "necessary to preserve life" is unconstitutionally vague;
2. "The fundamental rights of the woman to choose whether to bear children" is a right of privacy which the statute unconstitutionally abridges;
3. The statute violates the Fourteenth Amendment because of the "delegation of decision making power to a directly involved individual" (i.e., the doctor might be penalized for approving a request for abortion but not for denying a request).

In November, 1969, a decision in the United States District Court for the District of Columbia declared unconstitutional that part of the statute outlawing abortions other than those done "for the preservation of the mother's life or health." The reasoning was similar to, and in part relied upon, that in the *Belous* decision.

The New York law was recently challenged in the Federal Court for the Southern District of New York. The complaint in this case alleged that the abortion law is unconstitutional on grounds similar to those cited in the California case.

Minority reports accompanying many of these reports and resolutions are best summarized by the conclusion to The Minority Report of the Governor's Commission Appointed to Review New York State's Abortion Law, as follows: "Because we consider the proposals of the majority of our Committee to be violative of the fundamental rights of the human child *in utero* and detrimental to our traditional and still viable ideals of the sanctity of human life and the integrity of the family unit, we dissent."

The reform of abortion laws along the guidelines drawn by the American Law Institute has not worked well. Although the number of abortions has increased markedly, the poor still find it difficult to obtain abortions even in situations of obvious merit. Illegal abortions have probably not decreased. The laws are vague and in many instances capriciously interpreted (Monroe; Russell and Jackson; Droegemueller and co-workers; and Overstreet).

Although some states, notably Hawaii, Alaska, Washington, and New York have repealed their abortion laws, in most instances the solution to this complex problem may stem not from legislative reform of existing statutes but from action of the courts on the constitutionality of abortion laws. (For full discussion of the constitutional questions, see Lucas.)

Indications.   The indications for therapeutic abortion are discussed with the diseases that most commonly lead to the operation. A well-documented indication is heart disease in the wake of previous decompensation (p. 783). Another commonly accepted indication is advanced hypertensive vascular disease (p. 738). Still another is carcinoma of the cervix (p. 641).

Currently the two most frequently encountered indications for therapeutic abortion are psychiatric disease and potential abnormalities of the fetus. Among 4,675 therapeutic abortions performed in New York City between 1951 and 1962, inclusive, the major indication for the operation was a mental disorder (Gold and co-workers). Many, however, believe that interruption of pregnancy on psychiatric grounds is often a double-edged sword, which may aggravate rather than ameliorate psychotic tendencies. In the opinion of both Pearce and Martin, when the operation is carried out on mentally unstable women, 25 to 59 per cent are left with remorse and guilt. Even in the case of abortion for nonpsychiatric indications, Gebhard and associates found evidence of prolonged psychiatric trauma in 9 per cent of a sample of American women in whom the operation had been performed therapeutically or criminally. McCoy found that 27 percent of 62 women questioned at least one year after therapeutic abortion expressed varying degrees of regret. Seventy-three per cent of his patients were satisfied, and those for whom pregnancy was socially untenable rarely regretted the operation. Niswander and Patterson found that a similar percentage of their patients regretted the operation. Sim, an English psychiatrist, makes the sweeping statement: "There are no psychiatric grounds for termination of pregnancy." There is little information about the psychologic impact on the patient of refusal of her request for abortion. These women rarely commit suicide even though they may threaten to do so; however, among 249 Swedish women who were denied abortion, Hook found only 23 per cent who had accepted the situation and made a satisfactory adjustment.

Potential abnormality of the fetus as an indication for therapeutic abortion comes up most frequently in connection with maternal rubella. We believe that the operation is justified in selected cases (p. 808). As intrauterine diagnostic technics improve, the problem of serious fetal malformation will present more frequently. Valenti and colleagues have reported a therapeutic abortion performed on the basis of a firm diagnosis of Down's syndrome. Recently Schneck and colleagues have made an intrauterine diagnosis of Tay Sachs enzymatic disease. Other enzymatic disorders can be diagnosed with reasonable accuracy (Ch. 38, p. 1078).

It is impossible to predict what the future acceptable indications for therapeutic abortion will be. It is certain, however, that public opinion will not tolerate much longer the disregard of patients with unwanted pregnancies complicated by serious social problems. The new abortion policy of the American College of Obstetricians and Gynecologists succinctly states the matter as follows:

Therapeutic abortion may be performed for the following established medical indications:
1. When continuation of the pregnancy may threaten the life of the woman or seriously impair her health. In determining whether or not there is such risk to health, account may be taken of the patient's total environment, actual or reasonably foreseeable.

2. When pregnancy has resulted from rape or incest: In this case the same medical criteria should be employed in the evaluation of the patient.
3. When continuation of the pregnancy is likely to result in the birth of a child with grave physical deformities or mental retardation.

Incidence. Tietze and Lewit estimate that about 8,000 therapeutic abortions per year were performed in hospitals in the United States from 1963 to 1965 (see also Rosen). This ratio of about 2 abortions per 1,000 live births contrasts with 79 per 1,000 live births in Sweden. In Hungary the number of abortions exceeds the number of live births. As the result of a sharp and continuing decline in traditional medical indications (heart disease, hypertension, pulmonary tuberculosis, and hyperemesis, for example), the number of operations performed on these grounds has fallen dramatically over the past two decades, with the result that interruption of pregnancy on physical indications is becoming rare.

Technic. Vaginal therapeutic abortion may be performed by the traditional dilatation and curettage or by the more recently introduced suction technic. The likelihood of uterine perforation, cervical laceration, hemorrhage, incomplete removal of the placenta, and infection increases sharply after the twelfth week, and perhaps somewhat earlier in primigravidas; for this reason neither dilatation and curettage nor suction curettage should be performed when the duration of pregnancy has exceeded that limit. If interruption of more advanced pregnancy is urgent, abdominal hysterotomy, hysterectomy, or intraamniotic injection of hypertonic saline are preferable.

There are other circumstances in which abdominal hysterotomy or hysterectomy is preferable to the vaginal operation. If, for example, sterilization is to be included in the procedure, combining hysterotomy with tubal ligation in a single operation or performing a hysterectomy is sometimes preferable to the two separate procedures. If the therapeutic abortion is done for medical or serious psychiatric indications, it is often carried out abdominally, because many of these indications for the operation are sound reasons for sterilization also. Still another advantage of abdominal hysterotomy is the greater likelihood of complete evacuation of the uterine contents, particularly if care is exercised in incising the uterine wall, so that the gestational sac may be delivered intact.

Light inhalation anesthesia with or without a muscle relaxant is usually satisfactory for the vaginal operation. The cervix is more easily dilatable if 1 per cent procaine or xylocaine is injected bilaterally into the paracervical tissues. Warming of the dilators is also helpful. To lessen the likelihood of uterine perforation an infusion of 10 units of oxytocin in 500 ml of saline or Ringer's lactate solution is sometimes given slowly during the operation. After the usual preparations for a vaginal operation, the cervix is grasped with a tenaculum and the depth of the uterine cavity is measured by a sound. Care is taken that no instrument be introduced into the uterus beyond that depth. The cervix is very gradually dilated with a series of Hegar dilators (Fig. 1). As shown in Figure 2, the fourth and fifth fingers of the hand introducing the Hegar dilators should rest on the patient's buttock as a further safeguard against uterine perforation. It is our opinion that a sharp curette is more efficacious and that its dangers are not greater than those of the dull instrument in the usual therapeutic abortion. Perforations of the uterus rarely occur on the downstroke of the curette but may occur when any instrument is introduced into the uterus; since the knife edge of a sharp curette is directed downward, it can have no bearing on this hazard. Any curette, however, is a

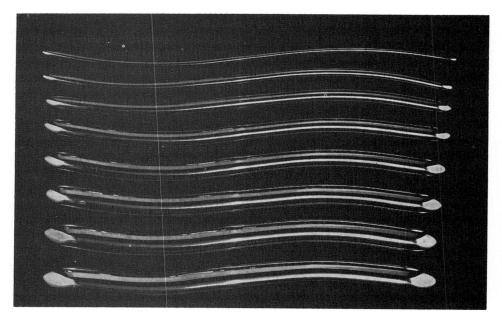

Fig. 1. Hegar graduated dilators.

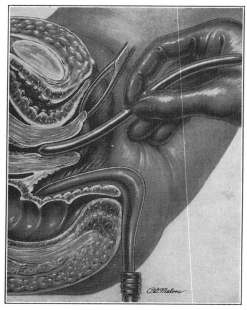

Fig. 2. Dilatation of cervix with Hegar dilator. Note that the fourth and fifth fingers rest against the buttock. This maneuver is a most important safety measure because, if the cervix relaxes abruptly, these fingers prevent a sudden and uncontrolled thrust of the dilator, a common cause of perforation of the uterus.

dangerous instrument if injudicious force is applied to it. As shown in Figure 3 the necessary manipulations should be carried out with the thumb and forefingers only.

Suction curettage, introduced by Wu and Wu in China in 1958, has furnished

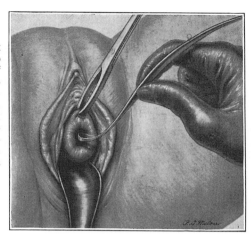

Fig. 3. Introduction of the curette. Note that the instrument is held merely with the thumb and forefinger; in the upward movement of the curette only the strength of these two fingers should be used. Moreover, just as soon as the curette has entered the cervical canal, the fourth and last fingers rest on the buttock as further protection against uterine perforation. Still another safeguard is the administration of 5 units of oxytocin 15 minutes before the operation and again as the patient is being draped.

a quick, nearly painless and almost completely safe method of performing therapeutic abortions before the twelfth week of gestation. This technic is now the method of choice in the U.S.S.R. (Reid) and in other countries of eastern Europe. It is receiving increasing attention in Great Britain (Kerslake and Casey) and in the United States. The suction curettes are hollow tubes of different diameters, with a moderate-sized opening at or near the tip. A glass trap is interposed between the curette and a vacuum pump. Under paracervical block or light general anesthesia the cervix is dilated sufficiently to allow passage of the curette. Oxytocin is usually administered, and suction up to 760 mm Hg is obtained by covering the bypass at the base of the curette with the thumb. The curette is swept gently around the interior of the uterus until no further products of conception can be seen entering the trap. The entire procedure takes from two to three minutes. It is too soon to predict whether current enthusiasm for this method will be sustained. Perforation of the uterus is not unknown, however.

After the fourteenth week of pregnancy, when the fundus can be palpated through the abdominal wall, abortion may be brought about by the intraamniotic injection of hypertonic saline or 50 per cent glucose solution. The exact mechanism of action is still uncertain. Klopper has shown a rapid fall in estriol excretion after the injection of hypertonic saline. Pregnanediol remains at the same level, however, until the abortion is terminated. Such technics are not new, Boero having produced abortion with an intraamniotic injection of dilute formalin as early as 1935. In 1958, Brosset passed a needle through the abdominal wall into the uterine cavity, withdrew 50 ml of amniotic fluid, and injected an equivalent amount of 50 per cent dextrose in water. In his series, the interval between injection and abortion averaged 38 hours. Since then, articles by numerous authors (Jaffin and associates; Wood and colleagues; Weingold and co-workers; and Gochberg and Reid) have attested the efficacy of this method, using 50 to 200 ml of either 50 per cent dextrose or the even more effective 20 per cent saline. These technics may obviate the necessity for hysterotomy in therapeutic abortion. Although they are far safer than the original technic utilizing formalin, there is danger of infection, especially when dextrose solution is employed. Peel has reported a death from this procedure, caused by the staphylococcus, and Briggs and MacDonald and colleagues have reported deaths caused by *Clostridium perfringens.*

Inadvertent introduction of hypertonic saline into the maternal circulation carries the likelihood of serious central nervous system and cardiopulmonary reactions. Cameron and Dayan have reported two new deaths as well as five others collected from the literature. All the patients had a high concentration of sodium in the blood and damage to the brain. Six patients showed extreme dehydration. Another reported complication following hypertonic saline is defective hemostasis caused by hypofibrinogenemia and related coagulation defects (Goldstein and also Quilligan). Between 1946 and 1950, more than 70 papers on this technic were published. There were 18 deaths between 1949 and 1952 alone (Wagatsuma). The method is no longer used in Japan. In contrast, both Goodlin and Schiffer report good results in moderately large series. Eastman comments on these studies as follows: "The intraamniotic injection of hypertonic saline for the induction of labor, if without substantial hazard, fills a real need in obstetrics; but only time will tell whether precautionary measures against hypernatremia will prevent such catastrophes as here reported."

In 22,179 cases, both gynecologic and obstetric, in which dilatation and curettage were performed for various reasons in two Baltimore hospitals, perforation of the uterus was recognized in 47, or once in about 500 operations, as reported by Radman and Korman. This figure agrees fairly well with that of Kushner and Dill, who report one known perforation in 700 operations. Although it is customary to regard the curette as the main offending instrument, Kushner and Dill point out that in their series of 21 perforations the curette caused less than one third. In the remainder a sponge stick, a sound, or dilators (both Hegar and Goodell) were the perforating instruments in about equal numbers.

The management of perforation of the uterus depends on the clinical events following the accident, particularly with regard to the extent of damage to other pelvic or abdominal viscera. Constant close observation of the patient for signs of peritoneal irritation or abdominal hemorrhage is therefore required. In the Baltimore series cited, abdominal exploration was deemed advisable in about one half the cases. In other series the comparable fraction has been somewhat smaller, averaging perhaps one third or less. In doubtful cases of perforation expectant treatment is the best course.

The morbidity and mortality rates from therapeutic abortion can be documented only from countries with permissive laws. In 23,666 therapeutic abortions performed in Denmark, the mortality rate was 0.7 per 1,000 operations, and serious but nonfatal sequelae ensued in 3.2 per cent (Berthelsen and Østergaard). These sequelae included 82 cases of perforation of the uterus and 122 cases of salpingitis, peritonitis, and septicemia. In addition, 113 cases of nonfatal but serious complications followed 5,320 abdominal hysterotomies, or 2.1 per cent.

The mortality rates appear to be correlated closely with the ease of obtaining abortion and the period in pregnancy when the operation is performed. Thus there is a mortality rate of about 4 per 100,000 abortions in the countries of eastern Europe and Japan, where abortion is not permitted after the third month of pregnancy and is entirely permissive. In contrast, the mortality rate is nearly 70 per 100,000 abortions in Denmark, where abortion may be performed later in pregnancy and is relatively more frequently done for serious medical disease.

Rupture of Membranes.   At or very close to term, it is usually possible to induce labor successfully by simple rupture of the membranes, provided the cervix is favorable. For a cervix to be favorable for induction, or "ripe," it is essential that it be anterior soft, more than half effaced, and sufficiently dilated to admit the index finger with ease. If any of these three conditions is unmet, it is prudent to abandon attempts to initiate labor immediately. In those circumstances any attempted induction is more likely to be unsuccessful; furthermore, if labor does ensue, it is likely to be desultory and prolonged.

Artificial rupture of the membranes is an extremely simple procedure, which does not require anesthesia. It entails merely the introduction of a sterile-gloved finger through the cervix, stripping the membranes from the uterus for a distance of about 5 cm, and rupturing the amniotic sac with a suitable instrument. The fetal head should be held up slightly with the finger to allow amniotic fluid to escape. If the cervix meets all of the above criteria, labor usually begins within an hour or two after this procedure.

If the cervix is not favorable, as is usually the case two weeks or more before term, and if there is a good indication for delivery such as preeclampsia, an attempt is occasionally justified to "ripen" the unfavorable cervix. The conversion may be effected by an intravenous infusion of oxytocin or by stripping the membranes. The most effective method is a combination of intravenous oxytocin and rupture of the membranes, but it commits the obstetrician to delivery of the infant within about 24 hours even if labor is not effected.

Intravenous Drip Oxytocin.   The administration of oxytocin by the intravenous drip technic, as described on page 845, is carried out for 8 or 10 hours with meticulous control of the dose and careful auscultation of the fetal heart tones. When induction of labor is indicated by maternal disease, delivery must be accomplished reasonably quickly in one of several ways. Intravenous oxytocin may be given for several hours or the membranes may be ruptured. Labor is most likely to ensue if intravenous oxytocin is administered at the time of rupture of the membranes. If these attempts fail and if the original indication was valid, delivery should be accomplished by cesarean section. In any induction the safeguards enumerated on page 845, with respect to parity and other factors, must be observed if risks are to be minimized.

Stripping of the Membranes.   Digital stripping of the membranes in the region of the cervix sometimes suffices to initiate labor at term, and earlier in pregnancy it often effects appreciable softening and effacement of the cervix. The method is, of course, not feasible if the cervix is so tightly closed as to prohibit the introduction of a finger. That stripping of the membranes has an effect on the initiation of uterine contractions has been demonstrated in a controlled study by Swann, who found that the method was successful in a high percentage of patients at term but of little value when the presenting part was high.

Intraamniotic Injections.   Provided the fetus is dead, transabdominal injections of hypertonic solutions into the amniotic cavity are a relatively safe and efficient means of inducing labor in the latter half of pregnancy. After the bladder has been emptied and local anesthesia administered, a size 16 needle with a 50 ml syringe attached is introduced into the uterus in the midline about 5 cm below the umbilicus. Up to 200 ml of amniotic fluid are withdrawn and the same volume of 20 per cent saline is carefully injected.

Prostaglandins. These 20-carbon fatty acids are ubiquitous hormone-like substances that have a variety of biologic effects. The term prostaglandins was introduced by Van Euler in 1935. The oxytocic effect of human semen, however, was noted by Kurzrok and Lieb five years earlier. Bergstrom synthesized the pure compounds in 1957. Experiences are rapidly accumulating with the use of prostaglandins E_1 and F_2, for the induction of labor and abortion (Karim and colleagues). The drugs are not yet released for general use in this country but they hold great promise. (For a brief review of the clinical use of these compounds see Brit Med J 4:253, 1970). The subject is more extensively reviewed by Speroff and Ramwell.

Indications. The most common indication for the induction of labor is preeclampsia, as discussed on page 689. Whether to induce labor in preeclampsia depends on the condition of the cervix and the intensity of the disease. If the patient is far from term, with a long, firm, and closed cervix, it is usually wiser to persist in medical therapy than to risk the dangers of induction with such a cervix, provided the preeclampsia is mild. If the preeclampsia is severe and resistant to treatment, however, and a course of oxytocin stimulation proves ineffective, cesarean section is the best treatment.

The *elective induction of labor* (with no medical indication) may be justifiable occasionally, as in a multipara who has a history of rapid labors and lives far from the hospital. In the long run, however, the conveniences of elective induction are somewhat offset by the hazards, primarily prematurity, prolonged latent period with intrapartum infection, and prolapse of the umbilical cord.

Prolonged latent periods and prolapse of the cord rarely occur if the patient is within a week or ten days of term, with a favorable cervix and the fetal head engaged. The incidence of prematurity, moreover, can be reduced by sonographic measurements of the fetal skull before attempted induction. In 6,860 elective inductions of labor reported by Keettel, Randall, and Donnelly, the incidence of prematurity was 3.1 per cent, with a 9.9 per cent perinatal mortality rate in these premature infants. Latent periods over 24 hours occurred in 5 per cent of the cases. The overall perinatal mortality rate was 1.4 per cent; in the opinion of these authors, 39 of the 92 total perinatal deaths in the series, or 0.6 per cent of the babies delivered, were directly related to the elective induction. In a more recent study of 2,862 elective inductions (Niswander and Patterson), 0.7 per cent of perinatal deaths were related to the induction.

STERILIZATION

Many conditions that justify therapeutic abortion make permanent prevention of pregnancy also desirable, especially heart disease, chronic hypertension, and chronic renal disease. Other circumstances frequently warranting sterilization are a history of two or more previous cesarean sections and, less frequently, various psychiatric disorders. If a complication of pregnancy such as placenta previa requires cesarean section in a multipara, it is our practice to offer sterilization at the time of the operation.

In a strict sense multiparity *alone* cannot be regarded as an indisputable medical indication for sterilization, but it will often reinforce other indications, especially chronic hypertensive vascular disease or advanced varicosities. Moreover, multiparity is now widely regarded as a justifiable indication for sterilization in the presence of a variety of social and economic factors.

Many American couples now complete their desired families at an early age. Since the long-term use of contraception is uncertain and perhaps undesirable, many more women are now requesting sterilization after they have had their desired number of children. In short, the proportion of sterilizations performed primarily for social reasons is increasing quite rapidly. For example at Parkland Memorial Hospital the majority of women with 3 or more children request and receive tubal sterilization early in the puerperium.

Prevalence.   The prevalence of sterilization in the United States is unknown. There has been, however, a marked increase in both male and female sterilizing operations. Ryder and Westoff in their recent publication estimate that 13 per cent of white married couples between the ages of 20 and 39 have had a sterilizing operation. In contrast, Phillips presented data from a western suburban population as follows: tubal ligations, 6.4 per cent; remedial operations, 4.8 per cent; vasectomies, 14.4 per cent. The total for all sterilizations was approximately 26 per cent. Phillips' study not only indicates the increasing frequency of sterilization, but also the greater use of vasectomy. Despite these data, tubal sterilization is still about twice as prevalent as vasectomy for the entire United States.

Time of the Operation.   The operation can be done at any time, but the first two days of the puerperium are particularly convenient. Because the fundus is at a high level in the abdomen, the operation is technically simple and hospitalization is not prolonged.

Types of Operation.   The Irving procedure is probably the most dependable technic of tubal sterilization. It is illustrated in Figure 4 and described in the accompanying legend.

The simplest method of performing abdominal tubal sterilization is the Pomeroy technic, as illustrated in Figure 5. It is important that plain catgut be used to ligate the knuckle of tube, since the rationale of the procedure is based on absorption of the ligature and subsequent separation of the severed tubal ends, which become sealed over by fibrosis. The Madlener operation for tubal sterilization may appear similar to the Pomeroy but is quite different in principle and efficacy. The technic of the Madlener procedure differs in three important respects from that of the Pomeroy operation.

1. In the Madlener operation, the tube is crushed with a clamp at the site of the intended ligation; in the Pomeroy technic it is not crushed.
2. In the Madlener procedure, silk or other nonabsorbable suture is used; in the Pomeroy method, an absorbable suture is employed.
3. In the Madlener technic, the knuckle of tube is not cut; in the Pomeroy operation, which is correctly termed a tubal resection, the knuckle of tube is excised.

The objective of the Madlener operation is to produce occlusion of the tube by crushing and the use of a silk suture; the aim of the Pomeroy technic is separation of the tubal ends and their occlusion by fibrosis. The Pomeroy method is much more dependable than the Madlener.

Trends in family planning and population control require the development

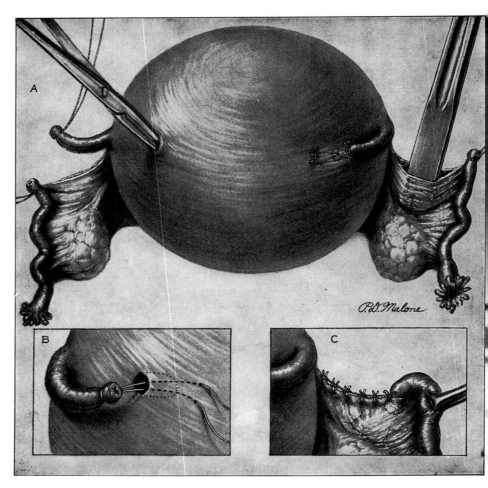

Fig. 4. Modified Irving sterilization. A, fallopian tubes have been cut and are being buried in musculature of posterior uterine wall. B, method of burying proximal tubal end. C, broad ligament is closed and distal end of tube buried. (From Te Linde. Operative Gynecology, 2nd ed. Courtesy of J. B.Lippincott Co.)

of methods for sterilization that not only are simple, safe and effective, but also do not necessitate extended hospitalization. Laparoscopy with fiber optic illumination permits surgical sterilization by electrocauterization of the isthmic tubal segments and division of the coagulated areas with biopsy forceps. The procedure is done under endotracheal anesthesia after pneumoperitoneum is produced with carbon dioxide. The patients may be discharged from the hospital as early as the first postpartum day and may resume normal activity without additional delay. The method is not applicable during the puerperium, nor are sufficient data available to assess the failure or morbidity rates.

The place of cesarean-hysterectomy as a sterilizing procedure is discussed on page 1176. Hysterectomy for sterilization in the absence of uterine disease appears difficult to justify statistically.

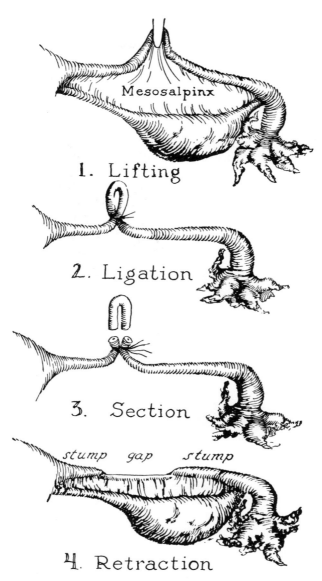

1. Lifting

2. Ligation

3. Section

4. Retraction

Fig. 5. Pomeroy tubal sterilization. The use of plain catgut for the ligation is mandatory in order to permit the subsequent retraction of the stumps as shown in stage 4. (From Dickinson. Techniques of Conception Control. The Williams & Wilkins Co.)

Efficacy. In a review of the literature covering 35,000 tubal sterilizations, Thomas found that the rate of failure to prevent subsequent pregnancies was 0.5 per cent. Based on ten major studies from three continents, Tietze found 34 failures in 20,000 sterilizations. Garb's extensive review of this problem quotes similar figures for the incidence of failure of Pomeroy operation, namely, 0.4 per cent in 5,447 cases. In 1,830 Pomeroy sterilizations analyzed by Prystowsky and Eastman,

456 were performed in association with cesarean section and the remainder were carried out in the early puerperium after vaginal delivery. In the former group, the failure rate was 1:57, whereas in the latter it was only 1:340. Similar figures have been reported by Lee, Randall, and Keettel, using the Madlener technic. Husbands, Pritchard, and Pritchard have been unable to substantiate this increased rate of failure of the operations associated with cesarean section. One curious aspect of failures of tubal sterilization is the occasional long interval that may intervene between the operation and conception. In one of our cases, for example, the interval was seven and a half years; in another, over four years; and in three others, more than three years. Most patients with failed tubal sterilization return pregnant within 18 months.

Hazards.   The two main hazards are the rare occurrence of pulmonary embolism and subsequent tubal pregnancy. In the series of 1,830 tubal sterilizations reported by Prystowsky and Eastman, four tubal gestations occurred, of which one proved fatal (Fig. 6). There have been no fatalities in 714 tubal ligations at

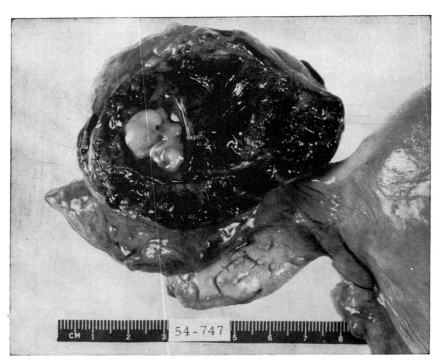

Fig. 6. Autopsy specimen of ruptured tubal pregnancy following Pomeroy sterilization. Sudden, massive abdominal hemorrhage, occurring seven and a half years after the Pomeroy operation, caused death before patient could be transported to hospital.

the Kings County Hospital. Haynes and Wolfe in a current paper indicate that about 10 per cent of patients with tubal ligations eventually develop unrelated gynecologic complaints, which combined with the previous tubal sterilization led to a decision to perform a hysterectomy (p. 1176). Tubal sterilization carries certain risks, which must be carefully balanced before undertaking the operation. Moreover, as pointed out by Barnes and Zuspan, as well as McCoy, a few women regret the operation; most often they were women with small families who underwent tubal sterilization because of their own illness. Thompson and Baird reported that 87 per cent of 162 women studied were satisfied with their sterilizations. Very rarely do women request to have their fallopian tubes reunited. Restitution of tubal continuity is technically feasible, with a rate of success no more than 50 per cent.

CONTRACEPTION

The term "contraception," as generally used, refers to the *temporary* prevention of pregnancy by various methods, in contradistinction to the *permanent* prevention of pregnancy effected by surgical sterilization. The obstetrician's attention will be focused on this problem most intimately at the time of the postpartum visit, when the majority of women inquire about family planning. Advice is also often requested during the premarital examination or at one of the prenatal visits. Obstetricians will vary in their attitudes toward contraception, but they cannot avoid their responsibility, since the health of the mother and her family are dependent in part on the spacing and limitation of her children. The modern obstetrician should, moreover, bear in mind his specialty's role in population control whenever he is consulted by a patient in the childbearing years. From a global viewpoint, concern over population growth and its bearing on public health as well as on economic development has stimulated widespread interest in family limitation as a major public health and demographic problem. Accordingly, the American Public Health Association has endorsed a statement that cites the threat to health, nutrition, and standards of living of unrestricted population growth. It concludes as follows:

The American Public Health Association believes therefore that:
Public health organizations at all levels of government should give increasing attention to the impact of population change on health. . . .
Public and private programs concerned with population growth and family size should be integral parts of the health program, and should include medical advice and services which are acceptable to the individuals concerned.
Full freedom should be extended to all population groups for the selection and use of such methods for the limitation of family size as are consistent with the religion and mores of the individuals concerned.

The American Medical Association and the American College of Obstetricians and Gynecologists, as well as numerous other national and international organizations, have issued similar statements endorsing control of fertility. The burgeoning of the population has finally become evident to governments throughout the world. The leaders of thirty nations representing nearly half of the world's population issued the following statement: "We believe that the population problem must be recognized as a principal element in long-range national planning if governments are to achieve their economic goals and fulfill the aspirations of their people" (United Nations).

President Nixon in a historic message to Congress on population (July 18, 1969) declared: "One of the most serious challenges to human destiny in the last third of this century will be the growth of population. Whether man's response to that challenge will be a cause for pride or for despair in the year 2000 will depend very much on what we do today."

The challenge is largely to the obstetricians, for it is to them that women turn for advice and help in their reproductive years. Contraception is vital to the health of these women and their children. It is a requisite of good obstetric care.

Relative Effectiveness. Effectiveness of contraceptive methods may be classified as *theoretical effectiveness* and *use effectiveness*. Theoretical effectiveness refers to the antifertility action of a contraceptive method under ideal conditions, used without omissions or errors of any kind. Use effectiveness refers to protection achieved by a method under realistic conditions of life. The use effectiveness therefore varies not only with the motivation of the individual but also with the cultural characteristics of the couple and their socioeconomic status.

Since theoretical effectiveness is not susceptible to direct measurements because of the absence of ideal conditions, it can only be inferred from the performance of the most successful groups of users. These observations can be supplemented by *a priori* anatomic and physiologic considerations and by data from laboratory animals (Johnson and Masters).

Use effectiveness usually is quantitatively evaluated in terms of failure rates per 100 woman-years of exposure according to the following formula:

$$\text{Pregnancy rate} = \frac{\text{Number of pregnancies} \times 1,200}{\text{Patients observed} \times \text{Months of exposure}}$$

For example, if 100 couples have used a method for an average of 2 years and if 20 pregnancies have occurred despite its use, the equation reads:

$$\text{Pregnancy rate} = \frac{20 \times 1,200}{100 \times 24} = \frac{24,000}{2,400} = 10$$

The cumulative failure rates according to the life table method furnish more informative data that may be used to compare different methods used for varying periods (Potter).

All failure rates must be interpreted with caution, since their levels reflect not only the behavior of particular populations, but also the decisions of the investigators with regard to inclusion or exclusion of periods of "non-use" or irregular use of the prescribed contraceptive and of pregnancies occurring during these periods. A compilation of failure rates from several or many sources may be more confusing than informative (Tietze).

METHODS

According to Segal and Tietze, virtually all of the temporary contraceptive practices used in the world today can be classified under the nine headings listed in Table 1.

The modern methods of contraception came into extensive use during the second half of this century. Their effectiveness in preventing pregnancy is vastly superior to the folk or traditional methods. More important is their temporal dissociation from the sexual act. Despite the accompanying adverse reactions, the obvious advantages led to widespread use among the poor as well as the socially

Table 1

Folk Methods
  1. Coitus interruptus
  2. Postcoital douche
  3. Prolonged lactation

Traditional Methods
  4. Condom
  5. Vaginal diaphragm
  6. Spermicides
  7. Rhythm, or safe period

Modern Methods
  8. Oral contraceptives
  9. Intrauterine devices

and economically privileged. According to reports from the Food and Drug Administration, in 1969 between one and two million women in the United States were using the intrauterine devices and more than eight million were taking the oral contraceptives.

Coitus Interruptus.   Withdrawal of the penis before ejaculation may be the oldest contraceptive procedure known to man. It makes great demands on the self-control of the male, and although widely practiced in parts of Europe, it does not appear to be popular in the United States. Studies by Westoff and colleagues show that coitus interruptus may have a failure rate only slightly higher than those of the mechanical methods of contraception.

Postcoital Douche and Prolonged Lactation.   These methods of contraception are largely ineffective. Prolonged breast-feeding is not practiced commonly in the Western Hemisphere; moreover, the length of time that lactation inhibits ovulation is highly variable.

The Condom.   Before the introduction of the oral contraceptives, the condom was a widely used method of birth control in the United States and throughout the world. As pointed out by Tietze, the rate of change to other methods tends to be lower for the condom than for other contraceptive technics. As used by married couples studied in a variety of situations, the condom offers greater protection against unwanted pregnancy than do most other barrier contraceptive methods. When the condom is of high quality and is used with regularity, pregnancy rates as low as 7 per 100 women per year have been reported (Tietze). This rate is slightly higher than the theoretical effectiveness of the diaphragm, but somewhat lower than that of withdrawal and substantially lower than that of douches alone. Most failures with this method have been attributed to irregular use, tearing of the sheath, or escape of semen.

The Diaphragm.   The diaphragm is a dome-shaped rubber cup, usually from 5.5 to 10 cm in diameter, which before intercourse is inserted digitally into the vagina and over the cervix and removed subsequently. A spermicidal jelly or cream is usually applied to the rim of the diaphragm to afford more effective sealing.

The diaphragm was formerly regarded as the "standard" and most dependable method. When used *properly* and *consistently* the diaphragm offers excellent protection against unwanted pregnancies. In these circumstances Sage and associates report a failure rate of 2 to 3 pregnancies per 100 women per year. For this reason, it has been the method of choice by strongly motivated, intelligent women who demand the utmost in protection. In view of the important role played by motivation in clinical efficacy, the excellent results reported with the diaphragm may be largely the result of regular and meticulous usage, rather than of any intrinsic superiority of this technic over other procedures, for in general clinic practice the pregnancy rate is about 10 per 100 women per year (Tietze and Lewit). The chief objection to the diaphragm is the vaginal manipulation necessary to insert it properly and to remove it several hours after intercourse, procedures that are repugnant to many women. Furthermore, privacy, which is not always available, especially to the poor, is required for insertion.

Fitting the diaphragm is of paramount importance. Before the pelvic examination and after the history is taken, pelvic anatomy should be explained to the patient. Charts and models are helpful. The patient should be taught to examine herself and should be made aware of the feel of the pubic bone and the cervix. The physician then selects a diaphragm ring from a fitting set usually ranging in size from 55 to 95 mm. The selection is made on the basis of the depth of the vagina; 75 and 80 mm fitting rings are usually tried first, since they are the most frequently used sizes. The rim of the diaphragm may cover a coiled, flat, or arc spring. The arc spring diaphragm is popular since it is easier to insert and generally provides a better fit. If this type of diaphragm is uncomfortable or fits poorly, the other forms should be tried until a comfortable fit is obtained. The testing ring is inserted into the vagina by the physician. The ring of proper size will fit snugly along the anterior wall of the vagina between the posterior fornix and the pubic arch without undue pressure.

The Safe Period, or Rhythm.   The rationale of the safe period, or rhythm method, is as follows. (1) Ovulation *usually* occurs at *approximately* the same date in any given menstrual cycle. (2) The ovum is capable of being fertilized for a period of about only 48 hours after ovulation. (3) Spermatozoa also are short-lived and are incapable of fertilizing an ovum for more than 48 hours after ejaculation. Theoretically, therefore, if the date of ovulation could be ascertained with precision *beforehand*, abstinence from sexual intercourse on that day and for the two days before and after would forestall conception.

Ovulation, of course, does not occur with any such clocklike precision (p. 63). Hence, when the rhythm method is used, only an approximate ovulation date can be estimated in advance. Abstinence must therefore be practiced for several days before and after that date to allow for errors in its estimation. The precision with which the date can be calculated is the decisive factor in the dependability of this method. Calculation of the expected date of ovulation is usually the responsibility of the physician for the first few months during which the method is used and at intervals of approximately six months thereafter.

Before the probable date of ovulation can be calculated, the record of at least three previous dates of menstruation is required. Women whose menstrual cycles vary in length by 8 days or more and those with cycles of 25 days or fewer are advised not to rely on this method. Women are advised to postpone use of the rhythm method after delivery and during lactation until they have had at least three successive menstrual cycles of similar length. The method of calculating the fertile period has been described by Fleck, Snedeker, and Rock as follows:

The sixteenth to twelfth days inclusive before the next expected menstruation constitute for us the period during which ovulation may occur. An admittedly generous allowance of three days before and after this period is added for the viability of spermatozoa and susceptibility of ova, respectively. The theory may be expressed thus: The fertile period extends from and including the nineteenth day before the *earliest* likely menstruation up to and including the ninth day before the *latest* likely menstruation. In each case the apprehended dates of menstruation are derived from the patient's record of previous catamenial dates.

The accuracy of the estimated day of ovluation can be increased if the woman will take her oral temperature each day during three cycles, record the figures, and submit them to her physician for analysis.

The advantages of this method are as follows: no mechanical devices or spermicidal chemicals are required; no local manipulations are necessary; and it is approved in principle by all religious faiths. The objections are the period of abstinence required, the somewhat complicated calculations entailed, and its lack of suitability for a considerable number of months after childbirth as well as in women with irregular or short cycles. As for efficacy, Tietze, Poliakoff, and Rock reported a conception rate of 14.4 in a series of very carefully supervised women. The rate is probably lower if intercourse is interdicted until two days after apparent ovulation, gauged by the oral temperature. The same authors conclude from their extensive experience that

. . . the rhythm method offers a satisfactory degree of protection against unwanted pregnancy to rigorously selected and carefully instructed wives who, with their husbands, are intelligent and strongly motivated. For others, and for those to whom pregnancy would be dangerous, the effectiveness of the method in preventing conception is not considered adequate.

Westoff and Ryder indicated that there has been a decline in the use of rhythm among Catholics to only about one third of those practicing contraception.
Spermicides. Jellies and creams are inserted into the vagina by means of a nozzle, which can be attached to a tube of some spermicidal jelly or cream. Suppositories are simply inserted with the finger and allowed to melt for a period of 5 to 10 minutes. Various chemicals have been employed in these preparations; phenylmercuric acetate is one of the more common, especially in suppositories.

Foam tablets are inserted into the vagina before coitus and pushed up with a finger as high as possible. Upon contact with moisture of the vagina, the tablet crumbles and dissolves. Carbon dioxide is released to produce a dense foam, which is believed to serve as a mechanical barrier as well as a means to distribute the spermicidal agent in the foam tablet. A wait of several minutes is required for the disintegration of the tablet. Certain aerosol foams, which are easy to apply, obviate the waiting period.

Reported pregnancy rates with spermicides range from 8 to 37, depending on the population for which they are prescribed. Used alone they are less effective than when employed with a diaphragm. All spermicides require a high degree of motivation. The jellies and creams are messy and they may furnish too much lubrication; foam may be irritating to the male. Spermicides are of minor contraceptive importance in the United States.
Intrauterine Devices. In 1928 Gräfenberg of Berlin reported on his experience with an intrauterine ring. After a brief period, gynecologists, the majority of whom had never had any experience with it, almost universally condemned this method of contraception.

The development of modern intrauterine devices awaited the availability of new chemically inert stainless steel and plastics that would assume their original shape after having been narrowed in order to pass through the cervical canal. In 1962 the Population Council inaugurated an intensive research program that included laboratory investigations as well as clinical and field trials. The largest body of clinical data was assembled under the Cooperative Statistical Program directed by Tietze. Nine reports have been issued involving experience with 31,767 women and covering 546,787 woman-months of use (Tietze and Lewit). These studies represent the first attempt to evaluate a method of fertility control from the time of its inception. In 1965 sufficient data had been accumulated for the Food and Drug Administration to issue a report on the intrauterine devices.

The mode of action of the devices is not known. They probably do not cause abortion of the implanted egg, but interfere with implantation.

These devices have singular advantages: they are very cheap, they require only one period of motivation for use (the time of insertion); removal also requires motivation. Most important, the pregnancy rates are of the order of 1.5 to 3 per 100 woman-years of use.

The most common adverse effects include pelvic inflammation, spotting, and cramps. The spotting and cramps tend to disappear after several months of use. In 5 to 6 per cent of women, however, they are severe enough to require removal of the device. Pelvic inflammation, diagnosed by parametrial tenderness and thickening, occurs in 2 to 3 per cent of patients. The incidence is higher in the first month after insertion than in later months. Spontaneous expulsion occurs in 1.5 to 18 per cent of patients, depending on the size and shape of the device.

Perforation of the uterus occurs about once in 2,500 insertions according to Tietze and his group. Scott reported fatalities from peritonitis following uterine perforation. Rarely the uterus is perforated with a closed ring, which can cause death if a loop of bowel passes through the device and becomes strangulated. The death rate is estimated by the Food and Drug Administration to be about 2 per 100,000.

The number of insertions of intrauterine devices in the United States is not known. It has been estimated to be between 1 and 2 million. Discontinuance of use depends on the severity of the adverse reactions and, to some extent, on the experience of the physician and his rapport with the patient. Tietze and Lewit estimate that 70 to 80 per cent of users will still be retaining the devices at the end of one year and that the rate of continuance at two years will be between 60 and 70 per cent. Lower continuance rates at two years have been reported by Mauldin and associates.

Insertion of the Intrauterine Device. A carefully obtained history and satisfactory pelvic examination are necessary before insertion to ascertain the most suitable intrauterine device and to prevent its use when it is not indicated. The usual contraindications are:

1. Suspected pregnancy.
2. Acute or subacute pelvic infection, including infected abortion or postpartum endometritis within the preceding three months
3. Myomas distorting the uterine cavity
4. Recent abnormal uterine bleeding, undiagnosed gynecologic disease, or suspicion of uterine cancer
5. Extreme flexion of the corpus or fixation of the uterus in marked malposition

Optimal time of insertion is during the menstrual period, two or more cycles after a pregnancy has ended. The uterus should be fully involuted. Insertion of an intra-uterine device into the uterus of a woman who is lactating is more dangerous and must be performed with great care.

At present the Lippes loop is the most widely used device. It is shaped like a double S and is made of barium-impregnated polyethylene. The second most widely employed device is the Ota ring, which has been in continuous use since the early 1930's. Many other devices are available or being tested throughout the world. Among the plastic devices are the Saf-T-Coil, the Ancor, and the Antecon. Three stainless steel devices are in use: the Majzlin spring, the M device, and the Hall-Stone ring. Each has useful properties, but to date no single device has been developed that is suitable for all women (Fig. 7). Recently, however, the T device, with a copper coil on the stem, has shown great promise.

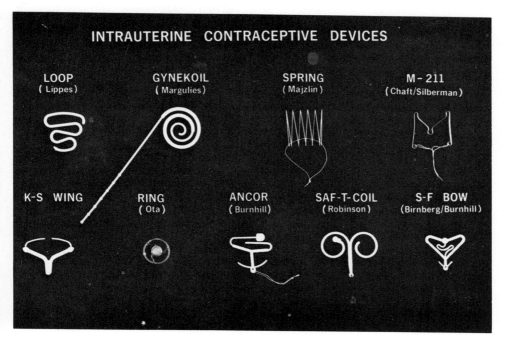

Fig. 7. Various intrauterine contraceptive devices.

Sterile precautions should be followed in loading and inserting an intrauterine device. Sterile gloves should be worn for loading the devices when the commercially packaged products are not sterile and when it is not possible to load the device without contaminating the sterile uterine end of the introducer. When such packages are not available, the introducer and device should be soaked in a solution of 1:750 aqueous benzalkonium chloride for 24 hours before the insertion.

To load the loop, the large end (the end opposite the suture) is placed into the end of the inserter, which is capped with a flanged indicator. Figure 8 shows the loop and the inserter. The loading is continued until the loop is entirely within the inserter. The plunger is then inserted, pushing the large end of the loop to the front end of the inserter. Whenever possible the loading of a plastic device should take place immediately before insertion. If the inserter remains loaded for more than five minutes, the plastic may not return to its original shape.

The following instructions for insertion should be followed:

1. The loaded inserter, sterile sound, and sterile tenaculum (or Allis, White, or Teale clamp) are placed on a sterile surface adjacent to the patient.

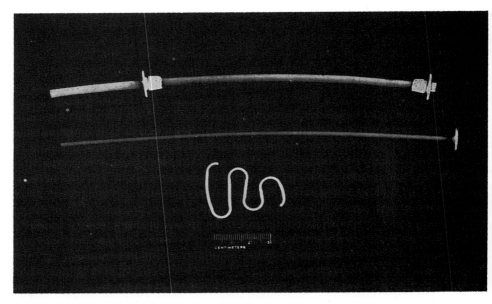

Fig. 8. Lippes loop D and inserter. (From Southam. Clin Obstet Gynec 7:814, 1964.)

2. A careful bimanual examination, noting especially the position, size, and shape of the uterus, is performed and, if appropriate, smears for cervical cytology are obtained.
3. The cervix is then grasped with a tenaculum, and gentle traction is applied to reduce the angle between the uterine corpus and the cervix.
4. The uterus is then sounded to rule out cervical stenosis and marked deformities of flexion and to be certain that the cavity is at least two and one half inches in depth. If the cavity is smaller, the rate of expulsion is higher.
5. The position of the intrauterine device within the inserter must be visually checked prior to insertion. The loaded inserter is then slowly and gently inserted into the cervical canal until the flange, or depth stop, reaches the external os. Care must be taken to place the device in the same plane as the widest diameter of the endometrial cavity.
6. Slowly and gently push on the plunger until it is fully within the inserter. Stop the insertion if any resistance is encountered and resound the uterus.
7. Withdraw the plunger completely to avoid pulling on or bending the tail; then remove the inserter.
8. Pass a sound or a small dilator into the cervical canal to be certain that the device is entirely within the endometrial cavity. The terminal portion of the device is frequently left in the upper cervical canal, especially in the presence of cervical hypertrophy, thereby increasing side effects and expulsions.

After inserting the device, the physician should instruct the patient as follows:

1. Call immediately if the device is expelled or if any part of the device is felt to protrude through the cervix.
2. Use mild analgesics if cramping takes place and if needed during the menses. Patient should be informed that these cramps will become gradually milder during successive menses.
3. Spotting or heavier menses may occur during the first few months after a device is inserted.

4. Report any increase in body temperature, any purulent vaginal discharge, or any unpleasant odors emanating from the vagina.
5. Return after two menstrual periods. At this time, and annually thereafter, the position of the device should be checked.

Despite the many advantages of the intrauterine devices, they have not been so popular in the United States as the oral contraceptives. As mentioned, the Food and Drug Administration estimates that between 1 and 2 million devices have been inserted in this country.

Oral Contraceptives.   The oral contraceptives in current use consist of estrogens and progestins. They comprise synthetic or semisynthetic compounds that in general are more potent than the naturally occurring hormones. In dosages currently used these compounds suppress ovulation. As the dosage decreases, however, ovulation may occur in a few women, but pregnancy is still prevented. The mechanism of this additional antifertility effect is currently under investigation.

The oral contraceptives are prescribed in either *combined* or *sequential* methods. In the combined regimen, the simplest dosage schedule is to take a tablet containing both a synthetic progestin and an estrogen daily, from the fifth to the twenty-fourth or twenty-fifth day of the cycle. In the sequential regimen, 15 or 16 tablets containing estrogen only are followed by 5 tablets containing both progestin and estrogen. In both regimens, suspension of the medication ordinarily results in withdrawal bleeding after two to three days. The drugs may be resumed on the fifth day of the new cycle. An alternative procedure is the use of the combination pills for three weeks and the substitution of an inert tablet for the fourth week. This regimen has the advantage that the patient takes a pill every day.

The theoretical effectiveness of the combined hormonal contraceptives leads to a pregnancy rate of approximately 0.1 per hundred women per year. The theoretical effectiveness of the sequential oral contraceptives is somewhat lower, as indicated by a pregnancy rate of 0.5 per hundred women per year. The usually quoted pregnancy rates reflecting use effectiveness average 0.7 per hundred women per year for the combined regimen and 1.4 per hundred women per year for the sequential regimen.

According to the Food and Drug Administration, effectiveness judged by the total number of pregnancies is significantly greater with the oral contraceptives, combined or sequential, than with the intrauterine devices or any of the traditional methods. The pregnancy rates among users of diaphragms with contraceptive jellies or creams appear to be 10 to 30 times higher than those among users of oral contraceptives; those among users of intrauterine devices are 2 to 4 times higher. The only important reason for failure is the omission of one or more tablets during the cycle of medication.

According to Tietze, the minor adverse reactions associated with the hormonal contraceptives are related to estrogen and are similar to the symptomatic complaints associated with early pregnancy. They include nausea, vomiting, breast engorgement, and breakthrough bleeding during medication. Other minor complaints comprise weight gain, headache, dizziness, and occasionally chloasma. In general these symptoms disappear or decrease after a few months of use. Some users, however, find them so objectionable that they discontinue the hormonal contraceptives.

A wide range of more serious adverse reactions has been noted. An etiologic relation between these findings and the hormonal contraceptives has been extremely difficult to prove because the effects under consideration occur naturally in women who are not taking the oral contraceptives, albeit at a low rate. Statistical resolution of this epidemiologic problem has proved formidable, not only because of the small numerators (occurrence of the adverse effect) and large denominators (users) but also because the data on the natural incidences of the disorders in question are not available. Therefore, in most instances it is impossible to ascertain whether the adverse reaction under observation represents an effect of the medication or is merely a chance occurrence. Available data have failed to confirm or refute a statistically valid etiologic relation between the oral contraceptives and most of the adverse experiences reported in the literature.

Thromboembolic disease represents an exception to this generalization. An etiologic relation between oral contraceptives and an increase in thromboembolic disorders has been disclosed by several groups of investigators using retrospective methods of inquiry and studies on mortality trends.

In 1967 the Royal College of General Practitioners in Great Britain undertook interviews of young women with vascular disease. By comparing patients with superficial thrombophlebitis with a suitably matched series of controls, it was shown that the risk of thrombophlebitis was tripled in women using oral contraceptives.

In a second study, Vessey and Doll investigated young women admitted to several hospitals in the northwest of London with a diagnosis of idiopathic thrombophlebitis. These patients also were matched with suitable controls. A third study, conducted by Inman and Vessey, involved all the deaths that occurred in England, Wales, and Northern Ireland during 1966 in women between the ages of 20 and 40 whose death certificates referred to thrombosis or embolism of the pulmonary, cerebral, or coronary vessels.

According to these British investigators, in the absence of other predisposing causes the risk of developing deep vein thrombosis, pulmonary embolism, or cerebral thrombosis is increased about eight times by the use of oral contraceptives. The risk of developing coronary thrombosis is apparently unchanged. The likelihood of hospitalization from thromboembolic disease in users of oral contraceptives is about 1 in 2,000 as compared with 1 in 20,000 among nonusers. Since that time Vessey and Doll have expanded their retrospective study, including a larger group of patients with matched controls. The results of this study confirm the findings of the previous investigation.

Another retrospective study of cases of thromboembolism with an equal number of matched controls was conducted by Sartwell and colleagues in the United States. This study necessitated a search for cases in five large cities. The subjects were women of reproductive age who were discharged alive over a recent three-year period from 43 teaching hospitals. Additional requirements for inclusion in the study were the absence of a history of any acute or chronic condition that might predispose to thromboembolism, absence of history of a prior attack of the disease, reasonable certainty of diagnosis, and presumption of fertility. The controls were women admitted to the same hospital in the same six-month period. These controls were matched by race, age, marital status, parity, residence, and financial status. The controls were in good health prior to hospitalization with no evidence of sterility. The cases and controls were interviewed in their homes after discharge from the hospital. Topics other than the use of oral contraceptives were included in the questionnaires.

Most of the acceptable cases had thrombophlebitis, pulmonary embolism, or both; a few had cerebral or retinovascular disease. The risk of thromboembolism to a woman using hormonal contraceptives was estimated by indirect methods to be 4.4 times that of the nonuser. The excess risk did not persist after cessation of use, nor did prolonged continuation of use enhance the risk. No striking differences among contraceptive products were found except for an excess use of sequential compounds among the cases as compared with the controls.

These studies establish an etiologic relation between thromboembolic disorders and the use of oral contraceptives. Quantitatively they suggest that the mortality from thromboembolic disorders attributable to oral contraceptives is about 3 per 100,000 women per year, adding slightly less then 3 per cent to the total age-specific mortality in users of these drugs.

The cause of thromboembolic disease associated with the oral contraceptives is not clearly understood. Thromboembolism is increased during pregnancy and is presumably related to the changes in blood flow and blood volume and changes in coagulability of the blood associated with the increased secretion of estrogen. Strangely, however, the disease is much more frequent in the puerperium, when the levels of estrogen are relatively low (p. 1002), than during pregnancy. In the Second Report on the Oral Contraceptives by the Advisory Committee on Obstetrics and Gynecology of the Food and Drug Administration, Dugdale and Masi conclude that pregnant women appear in danger of abnormal blood clotting in that some coagulation rates as well as amounts of procoagulant and coagulant are increased at the same time that fibrinolysis is depressed. Dugdale and Masi add that platelets are little affected by pregnancy, whereas the steroid contraceptives increase the number of platelets and possibly their tendency to clump. The answer may well lie not in increased coagulability of the blood, but in changes in the endothelium of the blood vessel walls or in blood flow.

Inman and Vessey believe there is a positive correlation between the amount of estrogen in the oral contraceptives and the occurrence of thromboembolic disease.

Much indirect evidence suggests that estrogens may be carcinogenic in man. These data are derived from experiments on laboratory animals in which long-term administration of estrogen resulted in cancer in five species. The exception is the subhuman primate. Although all physical and chemical agents that are carcinogenic in man produce malignant tumors in experimental animals also, evidence of the carcinogenicity of estrogen in other species cannot be transposed directly to man. Suspicion lingers, however, that the results in laboratory animals may be pertinent to man. Many difficulties arise in the epidemiologic elucidation of this suspected relation. The principal obstacle is the long latent period between administration of a known carcinogen and the development of cancer in man. Thus far, no properly devised prospective or retrospective studies have provided an adequate solution to this problem.

Estrogens may produce a variety of epithelial changes of uncertain prognostic significance in the human cervix. In 1969 Melamed and co-workers conducted a survey of women attending the clinics of Planned Parenthood of New York City. This study revealed a higher prevalence of epithelial abnormalities, diagnosed as carcinoma in situ, among women using oral contraceptives, compared with those using the diaphragm. Because of epidemiologic considerations, the Advisory Committee on Obstetrics and Gynecology of the Food and Drug Administration did not believe that this study proved or disproved an etiologic relation between the oral contraceptives and the cervical changes described.

Estrogen causes epithelial changes in the human breast, but its carcinogenic effect there has never been proved. Even in women with frank mammary carcinoma, estrogen produces variable changes in the clinical course of the disease. For example, ovariectomy leads to regression of metastatic carcinoma in 30 to 50 per cent of premenopausal women. Exogenous estrogens cause either regression or stimulation of similar tumors in menstruating women, but induce regression in approximately half of postmenopausal women. The reasons for these paradoxical effects of estrogen on breast cancer are not clear.

Currently available data on death rates from genital and mammary cancer in women in the United States do not clarify the problem of the association of steroids and carcinoma. The long latent period of the known carcinogens (10 years) and the length of time between diagnosis and death eliminate vital statistics as a possible source of information about this association until perhaps the mid-1970's or later.

The massive campaign of prophylaxis launched against cervical cancer in the United States has accomplished a steady decline in deaths from the disease. It is good practice to repeat cervical smears annually in women taking oral contraceptives. Although these practices have contributed to the decline of the disease, they have clouded the question of the relation of effective oral contraceptives and cervical cancer. It is obvious, however, that oral contraceptives should never be administered to women without continuing surveillance.

The hormonal contraceptives produce numerous effects on many organs, for example, the liver, the thyroid, and the adrenal. They also affect some of the body's homeostatic mechanisms. They alter metabolism of sodium and water and occasionally induce hypertension, presumably by altering plasma renin, renin substrate, and aldosterone excretion (Laragh and co-workers). Recently they have been shown to produce changes in the endothelium of blood vessels.

The contraceptive steroids are known to increase the concentration of triglycerides and phospholipids, particularly lecithin. Wynn and colleagues, as well as Spellacy, have noted elevations of mean plasma insulin levels and impairment of the glucose tolerance test during use of oral contraceptives. These changes do not occur in all women, and they apparently revert to normal after discontinuance of the oral contraceptives.

Although these metabolic changes are widespread and fundamental, there is little evidence that any of these drug-induced metabolic alterations are serious hazards to health. Further information is available in the Food and Drug Administration's Second Report on the Oral Contraceptives and in the comprehensive review by Salhanick and colleagues.

The oral contraceptives have proved highly acceptable in the United States, and the number of women using these compounds has increased rapidly. These compounds are most popular among younger women with better than average education. They have also proved highly acceptable to less well educated and to socioeconomically deprived clinic patients. It appears that the continuation rate is about 73 per cent after 12 months and 62 per cent after 24 months (Westoff and Ryder).

Each of the many methods of contraception has its advantages and disadvantages. No single method is best or suitable for all patients. The proper prescription of a contraceptive method requires thorough discussion between the patient and her physician. It demands, in addition, extensive knowledge on the part of the physician. Because the data concerning modern methods of contraception are accumulating at a remarkable rate, it also requires that the physician take steps to remain informed. The patient must be aware of the risks, real or suspected, of the hormonal contraceptives.

No challenge is of greater importance to the specialty of obstetrics and gynecology than is the control of fertility. No field offers a broader and more fascinating opportunity for basic and clinical research.

REFERENCES

American College of Obstetricians and Gynecologists, Statement on Therapeutic Abortion, Approved by the Executive Board, The American College of Obstetricians and Gynecologists, Chicago, Ill., May 8, 1968.

American Law Institute. Model Penal Code, Section 230.3, Proposed Official Draft, 1962.

American Medical Association, House of Delegates, Resolution on Therapeutic Abortion, adopted June 1967. JAMA 201:544, 1967.

American Public Health Association. Governing council policy statement on the population problem. Amer J Public Health 49:1703, 1959.

American Public Health Association Resolution on Therapeutic Abortion. Amer J Public Health 59:153, 1969.

Barnes, A. C., and Zuspan, F. P. Patient reaction to puerperal surgical sterilization. Amer J Obstet Gynec 75:65, 1958.

Bergström, S., and Sjövall, J. The isolation of prostaglandin. Acta Chem Scan 11:1086, 1957.

Berthelsen, H. G., and Østergaard, E. Techniques and complications in therapeutic abortion. Danish Med Bull 6:105, 1959.

Boero, E. A. (Interruption of incompatible pregnancy before viability; a new concept and method). Gynec Obstet (Paris) 32:502, 1935.

Briggs, D. W. Induction of labour with hypertonic glucose. Brit Med J 1:701, 1964.

British Abortion Act, 1967, Chapter 87 (English Statutes).

Brosset, A. The induction of therapeutic abortion by means of a hypertonic glucose solution injected into the amniotic sac. Acta Obstet Gynec Scand 37:519, 1958.

Calderone, M. S. Manual of Contraceptive Practice, 2nd ed. Baltimore, The Williams & Wilkins Co., 1969.

Cameron, J. M., and Dayan, A. D. Association of brain damage with therapeutic abortion induced by amniotic fluid replacement: report of two cases. Brit Med J 1:1010, 1966.

Droegemueller, W., Taylor, E. S., and Drose, V. E. First year of experience in Colorado with the new abortion law. Amer J Obstet Gynec 103:694, 1969.

Dugdale, M., and Masi, A. T. Effects of the oral contraceptives on blood clotting, in Food and Drug Administration Advisory Committee on Obstetrics and Gynecology, Second Report on the Oral Contraceptives. Superintendent of Documents, U.S. Government Printing Office, 1969, p. 43.

Eastman, N. J. Editorial: Intra-uterine saline. Obstet Gynec Survey 21:739, 1966.

Fleck, S., Snedeker, E. F., and Rock, J. Contraceptive safe period: clinical study. New Eng J Med 223:1005, 1940.

Food and Drug Administration Advisory Committee on Obstetrics and Gynecology. Report on the Oral Contraceptives. Superintendent of Documents, U.S. Government Printing Office, 1966.

Food and Drug Administration Advisory Committee on Obstetrics and Gynecology. Report on Intrauterine Contraceptive Devices. U.S. Government Printing Office, 1968.

Food and Drug Administration Advisory Committee on Obstetrics and Gynecology. Second Report on the Oral Contraceptives. Superintendent of Documents, U.S. Government Printing Office, 1969.

Garb, A. E. A review of tubal sterilization failures. Obstet Gynec Survey 12:291, 1957.

Gebhard, P. H., Pomeroy, W. B., Martin, C. E., and Christenson, C. V. Pregnancy, Birth and Abortion. London, Heinemann, 1959.

Gochberg, S. H., and Reid, D. E. Intra-amniotic injection of hypertonic saline for termination of pregnancy. Obstet Gynec 27:648, 1966.

Gold, E. M., Erhardt, C. L., Jacobziner, H., and Nelson, F. G. Therapeutic abortions in New York City: a twenty-year review. Amer J Public Health 55:964, 1965.

Goldstein, P. J. Amniotic fluid embolism complicating intrauterine saline abortion. Amer J Obstet Gynec 101:858, 1968.

Goodlin, R. C.   Intra-amniotic saline. Obstet Gynec 34:897, 1969.

Gräfenberg, E.   Silk as a contraceptive, in Bendix, K. (ed.), Geburten-Regelung: Vorträge und Verhandlungen des Ärztekursus. Berlin, Selbstverlag, Dec. 28–30, 1928, pp. 50–64.

Harper, F.   Abortion laws in the United States, Appendix A, in Calderone, M. S. (ed.), Abortion in the United States. New York, Paul B. Hoeber, Inc., 1958.

Haynes, D. N., and Wolfe, W. M.   Tubal sterilization in an indigent population: report of fourteen years' experience. Amer J Obstet Gynec (in press, 1970).

Hook, K.   Refused abortion. A follow-up study of 249 women whose applications were refused by the National Board of Health in Sweden. Acta Psychiat Scand 39(Suppl. 168):1, 1963.

Husbands, M. E., Jr., Pritchard, J. A., and Pritchard, S. A.   Failure of tubal sterilization accompanying cesarean section. Amer J Obstet Gynec 107:966, 1970.

Inman and Vessey, M. P.   Investigation of deaths from pulmonary, coronary, and cerebral thrombosis and embolism in women of child-bearing age. Brit Med J 2:193, 1968.

Irving, F. C.   A new method of insuring sterility following cesarean section. Amer J Obstet Gynec 8:335, 1924.

Jaffin, H., Kerenyi, T., and Wood, E. C.   Termination of missed abortion by the induction of labor in mid-trimester pregnancy. Amer J Obstet Gynec 84:602, 1962.

Johnson, V. E., and Masters, W. H.   Intravaginal contraceptive study: Phase II: physiology. Western J Surg 71:144, 1963.

Karim, S. M. M., Hillier, K., Trussell, R. R., Patel, R. C., and Tamusange, S.   J Obstet Gynaec Brit Comm 77:200, 1970.

Keettel, W. C., Randall, J. H., and Donnelly, M. M.   The hazards of elective induction of labor. Amer J Obstet Gynec 75:496, 1958.

Kerslake, D., and Casey, D.   Abortion induced by means of the uterine aspirator. Obstet Gynec 30:35, 1967 (52 references cited).

Klopper, A.   The assessment of feto-placental function by hormone assay. Amer J Obstet Gynec 107:807, 1970.

Kurzrok, R., and Lieb, D. C.   Biochemical studies of human semen: action of semen on human uterus. Proc Soc Exp Bio Med 28:268, 1930.

Kushner, D. H., and Dill, L. V.   A ten-year survey of dilatation and curettage complicated by uterine perforation. Med Ann DC 32:130, 1963.

Laragh, J. H., Newton, M. A., Sealey, J. E., and Ledinghaur, J. G. G.   Oral contraceptives and high blood pressure: changes in renin, renin substrate and aldosterone excretion, in Salhanick, J. A., Kipnis, D., and Vande Wiele, R. (eds.), Metabolic Effects of Gonadal Hormones and Contraceptive Steroids. New York, Plenum Press, 1969.

Lee, J. G., Randall, J. H., and Keettel, W. C.   Tubal sterilization; a review of 1,169 cases. Amer J Obstet Gynec 62:568, 1951.

Lucas, R.   Federal constitutional limitations on the enforcement and administration of state abortion statutes. North Carolina Law Review 46:730, 1968.

MacDonald, D., O'Driscoll, M. K., and Geoghegan, F. J.   Intra-amniotic dextrose—a maternal death. J Obstet Gynaec Brit Comm 72:452, 1965.

Martin, M. E.   Puerperal mental illness: Follow-up study of 75 cases. Brit Med J 2:773, 1958.

Mauldin, W. P., Nortman, D., and Stephan, F. F.   Retention of IUD's: an international comparison. Studies in Family Planning 18:1, 1967.

McCoy, D. R.   The emotional reaction of women to therapeutic abortion and sterilization. J Obstet Gynaec Brit Comm 75:1054, 1968.

Melamed, M. R., Koss, L. G., Flehinger, B. J., Kelisky, R. P., and Dubrow, H.   Prevalence rates of uterine cervical carcinoma in situ for women using the diaphragm or contraceptive oral steroids. Brit Med J 3:195, 1969.

Monroe, K.   How California's abortion law isn't working. (New York Times Magazine, December 29, 1968). ASA Reprints (from the Association for the Study of Abortion, Inc.), New York, 1969.

Niswander, K. R., and Patterson, R. J.   Hazards of elective induction of labor. Obstet Gynec 22:228, 1963.

————— and Patterson, R. J.   Psychologic reaction to therapeutic abortion. I. Subjective patient response. Obstet Gynec 29:702, 1967.

Overstreet, E. W.   Experience with the new California law, in Hall, R. E. (ed.), Abortion in a Changing World. New York, Columbia University Press, 1970.

Pearce, J. D. W. The psychiatric indications for the termination of pregnancy. Proc Roy Soc Med 50:321, 1957.

Pearl, R. Contraception and fertility in 2000 women. Human Biology 4:363, 1932.

Peel, J. Introducing labour by intra-amniotic injection. Letter to the editor. Brit Med J 2:1397, 1962.

Phillips, N. The prevalence of surgical sterilization in a suburban population. Demography, May, 1971.

Pilpel, H. F., and Norwick, K. P. When should abortion be legal? Public Affairs Pamphlet #429, Public Affairs Committee, 1969, New York.

Potter, R. G. Application of life table techniques to measurement of contraceptive effectiveness. Demography 3:297, 1966.

Prystowsky, H., and Eastman, N. J. Puerperal tubal sterilization; report of 1,830 cases. JAMA 158:463, 1955.

Quilligan, E. J. Personal communication.

Radman, H. M., and Korman, W. Uterine perforation during dilatation and curettage. Obstet Gynec 21:210, 1963.

Reid, S. Obstetrics and gynaecology in U.S.S.R. Aust New Zeal J Obstet Gynec 6:112, 1966.

Report by the Records Unit and Research Advisory Service. Oral contraception and thromboembolic disease. Roy Coll Gen Pract 13:267, 1967.

Report of the Governor's Commission Appointed to Review New York State's Abortion Law, Hon. Charles W. Froessel, Chairman, State of New York, 1968.

Resolution 69-96, Criteria for Revision of Abortion Laws Introduced by the Medical Society of the County of New York. New York J Med, June 1, 1969, p. 1660.

Rosen, H. Abortion in America: Medical, Psychiatric, Legal, Anthropological and Religious Considerations (formerly Therapeutic Abortion). New York, Beacon Press, 1967.

Russell, K. P., and Jackson, E. W. Therapeutic abortions in California. First Year's Experience. Amer J Obstet Gynec 105:757, 1969.

Ryder, N. B., and Westoff, C. F. Reproduction in the United States, 1965. Princeton, New Jersey, Princeton University Press, 1971.

Sagi, P. C., Potter, R. G., and Westoff, C. F. Contraceptive effectiveness as a function of desired family size. Population Studies 15:291, 1962.

Salhanick, H. A., Kipnis, D., and Vande Wiele, R. Metabolic Effects of Gonadal Hormones and Contraceptive Steroids. New York, Plenum Press, 1969.

Sartwell, P. E., Masi, A. T., Arthes, F. G., Greene, G. R., and Smith, H. E. Thromboembolism and oral contraceptives: An epidemiologic case-control study. J Epidemiol 90:365, 1969.

Schiffer, M. A. Induction of labor by intra-amniotic instillation of hypertonic solution for therapeutic abortion or intrauterine death. Obstet Gynec 33:729, 1969.

Scott, R. B. Critical illness and deaths associated with intrauterine devices. Obstet Gynec 31:322, 1968.

Segal, S. J., and Tietze, C. Contraceptive Technology: Current and Prospective Methods. Reports on Population/Family Planning. Population Council and the International Institute for the Study of Human Reproduction. Columbia University, October 1969 (142 references cited).

Siegler, A. M., and Berenyi, K. J. Laparoscopy in gynecology. Obstet Gynec 34:572, 1969.

Sim, M. Abortion and the psychiatrist. Brit Med J 2:145, 1963.

Southam, A. L. Intrauterine devices. Clin Obstet Gynec 7:814, 1964.

Spellacy, W. N. A review of carbohydrate metabolism and the oral contraceptives. Amer J Obstet Gynec 104:448, 1969.

Speroff, L., and Ramwell, P. W. Prostaglandins in reproductive physiology. Amer J Obstet Gynec 107:1111, 1970 (80 refs. cited).

State Laws:
  Ark.: Arkansas Statutes Annotated, Section 41-301, 1970 Supplement.
  Calif.: California Penal Code, Section 274, 1969 Supplement, and California Health and Safety Code, Section 25950-54, 1970 Supplement.
  Colo.: Colorado Revised Statutes Annotated, Section 40-2-50, 1970 Supplement.
  Del.: Delaware Code Annotated, title II, Section 301, 1970 Supplement.
  Ga.: Georgia Code Annotated, Section 26-1101 to 1103, 1970 Supplement.
  Hawaii: Hawaii Revised Laws, Section 309-3, 1970 Supplement.

Kans.: Kansas General Statutes Annotated, Section 21-3407, 1970 Supplement.

Md.: Maryland Annotated Code, Article 27, Section 3, 1970 Supplement.

N.C.: North Carolina General Statutes, Section 14-44, 1970 Supplement.

N.M.: New Mexico Statutes Annotated, Section 40 A-5-1, 1970 Supplement.

N.Y.: New York Revised Penal Law, Section 125.05, 1970 Supplement.

Ore.: Oregon Revised Statutes, Section 163.060, 1970 Supplement.

S.C. South Carolina Code Annotated, Section 16-82, 1970 Supplement.

Va.: Virginia Code Annotated, Section 5923, 1970 Supplement.

Steptoe, P. C.   Laparoscopy in Gynecology. Edinburgh, E. & S. Livingstone, Ltd., 1967.

Swann, R. O.   Induction of labor by stripping membranes. Obstet Gynec 11:74, 1958.

Thomas, W. L.   Prevenception: Panhysterectomy versus tubectomy. Southern Med J 46:787, 1953.

Thompson, B., and Baird, D.   Follow-up of 186 sterilised women. Lancet 1:1023, 1968.

Tietze, C.   The condom as a contraceptive. Publ. No. 5, National Committee on Maternal Health, Inc., New York, 1960.

———   Statistical assessment of adverse experiences associated with the use of oral contraceptives. Clin Obstet Gynec 11:698, 1968.

———   Contraception: relative effectiveness, in Calderone, M. S. (ed.), Manual of Contraceptive Practice, 2nd ed. New York, The Williams & Wilkins Co., 1969.

———   Effectiveness of contraceptive methods. 15th Nobel Symposium on Control of Human Fertility, Stockholm, Sweden, May 27–29, 1970.

———   and Lewit, S.   Comparison of three contraceptive methods: diaphragm with jelly or cream, vaginal foam, and jelly/cream alone. J Sex Research 3:295, 1967.

———   and Lewit, S.   Abortion. Sci Amer 220:21, 1969.

———   and Lewit, S.   I.U.D.: Ninth Progress Report, Cooperative Statistical Program for the Evaluation of Intrauterine Devices. Studies in Family Planning 55:1, 1970.

———   Poliakoff, S. R., and Rock, J.   The clinical effectiveness of the rhythm method of contraception. Fertil Steril 2:444, 1951.

United Nations, World Leaders Declaration on Population, Human Rights Day, New York, December 1967.

Valenti, C., Schutta, E. J., and Stambler, J.   Octoploid endoreduplication. Mammal Chrom Newsletter 9:235, 1968.

Vessey, M. P., and Doll, R.   Investigation of the relation between the use of oral contraceptives and thromboembolic disease. Brit Med J 2:199, 1968.

———   and Doll, R.   Investigation of relation between use of oral contraceptives and thromboembolic disease. A further report. Brit Med J 2:651, 1969.

Von Euler, U.S.   A depressor substance in the vesicular gland. J Physiol (London) 84:21, 1935.

Wagatsuma, T.   Intra-amniotic injection of saline for therapeutic abortion. Amer J Obstet Gynec 93:743, 1965.

Weingold, A. B., Seigal, S., and Stone, M. L.   Intra-amniotic hypertonic solutions for the induction of labor. Obstet Gynec 26:622, 1965.

Westoff, C. F., Potter, R. G., Sagi, P. C., and Mishler, E. G.   Family Growth in Metropolitan America. Princeton, Princeton University Press, 1961.

———   and Ryder, N. B.   United States: methods of fertility control, 1955, 1960, and 1965. Studies in Family Planning 17:1, 1967.

———   and Ryder, N. B.   Duration of use of oral contraception in the United States 1960–1965. Public Health Rep 83:277, 1968.

Wood, C., Booth, R. T., and Pinkerton, J. H. M.   Induction of labour by intra-amniotic injection of hypertonic glucose solution. Brit Med J 2:706, 1962.

Wu, Y. T., and Wu, H. C.   Suction and artificial abortion: 300 cases. Chinese J Obstet Gynec 6:447, 1958.

Wynn, V., and Doar, J. W. H.   Some effects of oral contraceptives on carbohydrate metabolism. Lancet 2:761, 1969.

———   Doar, J. W. H., and Mills, G. L.   Effect of oral contraceptives on serum-lipid and lipoprotein levels. Lancet 2:720, 1966.

Zipper, J. A., and Tatum, H. J.   Metallic copper as an intrauterine contraceptive adjunct to the T device. Amer J Obstet Gynec 105:1274, 1969.

40

FORCEPS

The obstetric forceps is an instrument designed for the extraction of the fetus. It consists of two crossing branches designated right and left according to the side of the maternal pelvis into which they are inserted. They are introduced separately into the vagina and articulated after being placed in position. Each branch is made up of four portions: the *blade, handle, shank,* and *lock.*

The instruments vary considerably in size and shape. The blades have two *curves,* the *cephalic* and the *pelvic;* the former conforms with the shape of the fetal head and the latter with that of the birth canal. The blades are more or less elliptical, tapering toward the shank, and usually *fenestrated* to permit a firm hold upon the head. Certain authorities consider *solid* blades less traumatic to the infant.

The cephalic curve (Fig. 1) should be large enough to grasp the child's head firmly without compression, but not so large that the instrument slips. The greatest distance between the two blades should not exceed 7.5 cm when they are articulated. The pelvic curve (Fig. 2) corresponds more or less to the axis of the birth canal, but varies considerably among different instruments. With the forceps on a plane surface, the tips of the blades should be about 8.8 cm higher than the handles. The blades are connected to the handles by the shanks, which give the requisite length to the instrument.

The two blades articulate at the lock, which varies among different instruments. The English type (Fig. 3) consists of a socket upon each branch, into which fits the shank of the other half of the instrument. That arrangement allows simple but not firm articulation. In the French lock (Fig. 4) a pivot is screwed into the shank of the left branch, which fits into an opening on the right; the screw is then tightened after articulation. The German lock is a combination of the two, the shank of the left branch bearing a pivot with a broad, flat head, while the right is provided with a notch that corresponds to the pivot. When the instrument is properly articulated, the handles are approximated and the forceps may be conveniently grasped by one hand.

History. Crude forceps are an ancient invention, several varieties having been described by Albucasis, who died in 1112. Since their inner surfaces were provided with teeth to penetrate the head, however, it appears that they were intended for use only on dead fetuses.

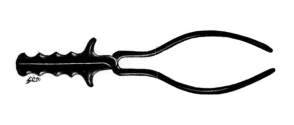

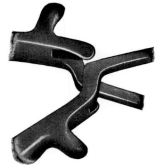

Fig. 1. Simpson's forceps, cephalic curve.   Fig. 3. English lock.

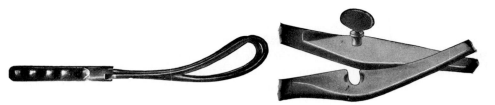

Fig. 2. Simpson's forceps, pelvic curve.   Fig. 4. French lock.

The true obstetric forceps was devised in the latter part of the sixteenth or the beginning of the seventeenth century by a member of the Chamberlen family. The invention was not made public at the time, but was preserved as a family secret through four generations, not becoming generally known until the early part of the eighteenth century. Previously, version had been the only method that permitted the operative delivery of an unmutilated child. When that operation was impossible, imperative delivery was accomplished with hooks and crochets, which usually led to the destruction of the child. Thus, before the invention of forceps, the use of instruments was synonymous with the death of the child, and frequently of the mother as well.

William Chamberlen, the founder of the family, was a French physician who fled from France as a Huguenot refugee and landed at Southampton in 1569. He died in 1596, leaving a large family. Two of his sons, both of whom were named Peter, and designated the elder and younger, respectively, studied medicine and settled in London. They soon became successful practitioners, devoting a large part of their attention to midwifery, in which they became very proficient. They attempted to control the instruction of midwives and, to justify their pretensions, claimed that they could successfully deliver patients when all others failed.

The younger Peter died in 1626 and the elder in 1631. The elder left no male children, but the younger was survived by several sons, one of whom, born in 1601, was likewise named Peter. To distinguish him from his father and uncle, he is usually spoken of as Dr. Peter, since the other two did not possess that title. He was well educated, having studied at Cambridge, Heidelberg, and Padua, and on his return to London was elected a Fellow of the Royal College of Physicians. He was most successful in the practice of his profession and counted among his clients many of the royal family and nobility. Like his father and uncle, he attempted to monopolize control of the midwives, but his pretensions were set aside by the authorities. These attempts gave rise to much discussion, and many pamphlets were written about the mortality of women in labor attended by men. He answered them in a pamphlet entitled "A Voice in Ramah, or the Cry of Women and Children as Echoed Forth in the Compassions of Peter Chamberlen." He was a man of considerable ability, combining some of the virtues of a religious enthusiast with many of the devious qualities of a quack. He died at Woodham Mortimer Hall, Moldon, Essex, in 1683, the place remaining in the possession of his family until well into the succeeding century. He was formerly considered the inventor of the forceps, a fact now known to be incorrect.

Chamberlen left a very large family, and three of his sons, Hugh, Paul, and John, became physicians who devoted special attention to the practice of midwifery. Of them, Hugh (1630–?), was the most important and influential. Like his father, he was a man of considerable ability who took a practical interest in politics. Since some of his views were out of favor, he was forced to leave England for Paris, where in 1673 he attempted to sell the family's secret to Mauriceau for 10,000 livres, claiming that with forceps he could deliver in a very few minutes the most difficult case. Mauriceau placed at his disposal a rachitic dwarf whom he had been unable to deliver, and Chamberlen, after several futile hours of strenuous effort, was obliged to acknowledge his inability to do so. Notwithstanding his failure, he maintained friendly relations with Mauriceau, whose book he translated into English. In his preface he refers to the forceps in the following words: "My father, brothers, and myself (though none else in Europe as I know) have by God's blessings and our own industry attained to and long practiced a way to deliver women in this case without prejudice to them or their infants."

Some years later he went to Holland and sold his secret to Roger Roonhuysen. Shortly afterward the Medico-Pharmaceutical College of Amsterdam was given the sole privilege of licensing physicians to practice in Holland, to each of whom, under the pledge of secrecy, was sold Chamberlen's invention for a large sum. The practice continued for a number of years until Vischer and Van der Poll purchased and made public the secret, whereupon it was discovered that the device consisted of only one blade of the forceps. Whether that was all Chamberlen sold to Roonhuysen, or whether the Medico-Pharmaceutical College had swindled the purchasers, is not known.

Hugh Chamberlen left a considerable family, and one of his sons, Hugh (1664–1728), practiced medicine. He was a highly educated, respected, and philanthropic physician, who numbered among his clients members of the best families in England. He was an intimate friend of the Duke of Buckingham, who had a statue erected in his honor in Westminster Abbey. During the later years of his life he allowed the family secret to leak out, and the instrument soon came into general use.

For more than one hundred years Dr. Peter Chamberlen was considered the inventor of the forceps, but in 1813 Mrs. Kemball, the mother of Mrs. Codd, who was the occupant of Woodham Mortimer Hall at the time, found in the garret a trunk containing numerous letters and instruments, among them four pairs of forceps together with several levers and fillets. As the drawings indicate (Fig. 5), the forceps were

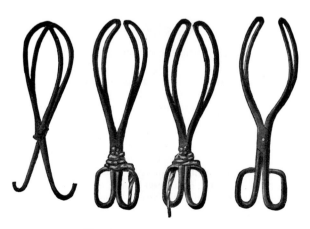

Fig. 5. Chamberlen's forceps.

in different stages of development, one pair hardly applicable to the living woman, although the others were useful instruments. Aveling, who carefully investigated the matter, believes that the three pairs of available forceps were used respectively by the three Peters, and that in all probability the first was devised by the elder Peter, son of the original William. The forceps came into general use in England during the lifetime of Hugh Chamberlen, the younger. The instrument was employed by Drinkwater, who died in 1728, and was well known to Chapman and Giffard.

In 1723, Palfyn, a physician of Ghent, exhibited before the Paris Academy of Medicine a forceps he designated *mains de fer*. It was crudely shaped and impossible to articulate (Fig. 6). In the discussion following its presentation, De la Motte stated that it would be impossible to apply it to the living woman, and added that if by chance anyone should happen to invent an instrument that could be so used, and kept it secret for his own profit, he deserved to be exposed upon a barren rock and have his vitals plucked out by vultures. He had little knowledge that at the time he spoke such an instrument had been in the possession of the Chamberlen family for nearly one hundred years.

The Chamberlen forceps, a short, straight instrument with only a cephalic curve, is perpetuated in the short forceps of today (Fig. 5). It was used, with but little modification, until the middle of the eighteenth century, when Levret, in 1747, and Smellie, in 1751 (Figs. 7 and 8), independently added the pelvic curve and increased the length of the instrument. Levret's forceps was longer, with a more decided pelvic curve than that of Smellie. From these two instruments the long forceps of the present day are descended.

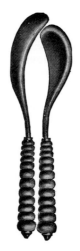   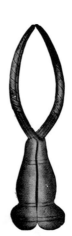   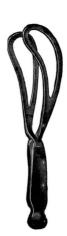

Fig. 6. Palfyn's forceps.   Fig. 7. Smellie's short forceps.   Fig. 8. Smellie's short forceps.

As soon as forceps became public property they were subjected to various modifications. As early as 1798, Mulder's atlas included illustrations of nearly 100 varieties. The modifications attempted in improving the instrument are pictured in Witkowski's *Obstetrical Arsenal*, illustrating several hundred forceps but representing only a small fraction of those devised. The monograph of Das contains excellent historical sketches of the development of the instrument. It is remarkable, however, that little advance was made over the instruments of Levret and Smellie until Tarnier, in 1877, clearly enunciated the principle of axis traction. These forceps were designed to cope with high stations of the fetal head and contracted pelves. Such problems today, however, are generally solved by other means. Episiotomy, furthermore, has eliminated many of the difficulties stemming from the pelvic curve, and severe traction at the fenestra, as in the axis-traction forceps, is therefore unnecessary and probably undesirable (Rhodes).

Except for two specialized forceps, those of Barton and Kielland, very little that is both new and useful in modern obstetrics has been added to the development of the instrument in over 200 years (Figs. 42 and 33).

Definitions and Classification.   Forceps operations on a fetus presenting by the vertex are classified as follows, according to the level and position of the head at the time the blades are applied:

Low forceps operations are those in which the instrument is applied after the fetal head has reached the perineal floor with the sagittal suture in the anteropos-terior diameter of the outlet (Figs. 9 and 10).

Midforceps operations are those in which forceps are applied before the criteria for low forceps are met but after engagement has taken place. Clinical evidence of engagement is usually afforded by the descent of the lowermost part of the skull to or below the level of the ischial spines, since the distance between the

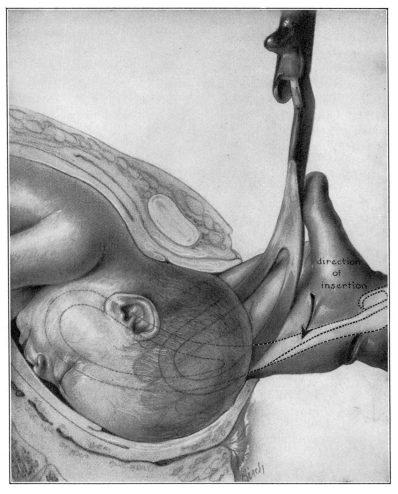

direction
of
insertion

Fig. 9. Low forceps. The **left** blade is being introduced into the **left** side of the pelvis by the **left** hand of the operator. The fingers of the right hand are being used to protect the maternal soft parts, while the thumb helps guide the instrument into place.

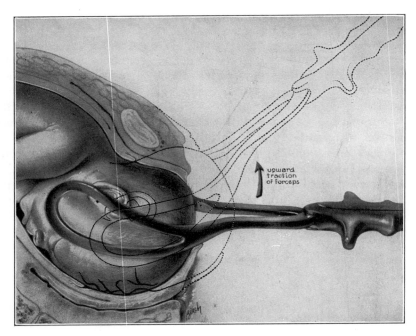

Fig. 10. Direction of traction in low forceps: outward and upward. (See also Figs. 14 through 22.)

ischial spines and the plane of the inlet is greater than the distance between the biparietal diameter and the leading point of the fetal head (Ch. 10, p. 302). Occasionally, however, after vigorous labor the combination of a great degree of molding of the fetal head and extensive formation of caput will create the erroneous impression that the head is engaged, since the occiput is thought to be at the level of the ischial spines.

High forceps operations are those in which forceps are applied before engagement has taken place. No variety of high forceps has any place in modern obstetrics except in the rarest circumstances.

On the basis of this classification, 63,238 deliveries were reviewed from 22 hospitals in the Obstetrical Statistical Cooperative. The overall incidence of forceps operations was 32.8 per cent, with low forceps elective, 23.9 per cent; low forceps, indicated, 3.9 per cent; midforceps, elective, 2.4 per cent; and midforceps, indicated, 2.0 per cent. High forceps represented 0.008 per cent; vacuum extractor, elective, 0.2 per cent; and vacuum extractor, indicated, 0.2 per cent.

Undoubtedly the incidence of forceps operations in any given institution depends upon the attitude of its staff and perhaps also upon the obstetric population, as indicated in Table 1.

Our definition of midforceps avowedly includes many levels of the fetal head and, therefore, a wide range of difficulty. Dennen has subdivided midforceps operations as follows:

A midforceps delivery is one performed when the leading bony portion of the head is at or just below the plane of the ischial spines, with the biparietal diameter below the superior strait. The head nearly fills the hollow of the sacrum.

Table 1. Percentage Distribution of Forceps Operations
1965–1966

	Kings County Hospital	Royal Victoria Hospital	Long Island Jewish Hospital
Deliveries	12,002	6,337	4,768
Elective	17.3	16.1	10.9
Indicated	5.5	19.7	5.6
Total forceps (per cent)	22.8	35.9	16.8

A low-midforceps delivery is one performed when the biparietal diameter is at or below the plane of the ischial spines, with the leading part within a finger's breadth of the perineum between contractions. The head completely fills the hollow of the sacrum.

With great experience or roentgenographic aid shortly before the operation, these two types of midforceps operations may usually be differentiated. Molding of the fetal head and asynclitism, however, may distort the findings. We therefore present the simpler classification as perhaps most dependable for general clinical use, as well as for statistical analysis of forceps deliveries.

Choice of Forceps. Any properly shaped instrument will give satisfactory results, provided it is used intelligently. For general purposes, however, the ordinary Simpson forceps is probably the most useful.

When the progress of labor ceases with the fetal head in the transverse position, well down in the pelvis with the leading point below the spines, the situation is referred to as *deep transverse arrest*. If the diameters of the pelvis are normal, such arrest is often overcome with oxytocin stimulation, with resulting descent to the perineum and anterior rotation there. If, however, there are indications for delivery, as in instances of fetal distress, the Kielland forceps with its sliding lock (p. 1131) or the Barton forceps with its hinged anterior blade (p. 1135) may have definite advantages.

Functions of the Forceps. The forceps may be used as a tractor or rotator, or both. Its most important function is *traction*, although particularly in transverse and posterior positions of the occiput it is often successfully employed for rotation.

Forces Exerted by the Forceps. Obstetricians have long been interested in the forces exerted by the forceps blades on the fetal skull and maternal tissues. If excessive, these forces can damage both mother and baby. From experiments done on women in labor many years ago, Joulin estimated that a pull in excess of 60 kg might damage the fetal skull. These crude studies furnish only a gross approximation, for the force produced by the forceps on the fetal skull is a complex function of pull and compression by the forceps and friction produced by the maternal tissue. Kelly and Sines have used multiple strain gauges built into the blades and shank of a Simpson forceps to assess the magnitude of the various forces. They state that the first pull of an elective low forceps procedure exerts 24.8 pounds of traction and 15.1 pounds of compression. The field of forceps mechanics is worthy of further study.

Indications for the Use of Forceps. The termination of labor by forceps, provided it can be accomplished without great danger, is indicated in any condition threatening the life of the mother *or* child that is likely to be relieved by delivery. Such maternal indications include eclampsia, heart disease, acute pulmonary edema, hemorrhage from premature separation of the placenta, intrapartum infection, or exhaustion. Fetal indications include prolapse of the umbilical cord, premature separation of the placenta, pressure exerted upon the head from prolonged perineal arrest, and especially changes in cardiac rhythm and the escape of meconium in vertex presentations. A fetal heart rate below 100 per minute that persists between contractions indicates fetal distress and possible death unless delivery is promptly effected. In vertex presentations the discharge of amniotic fluid tinged with meconium likewise usually indicates fetal distress. In breech presentations, however, the escape of meconium may result merely from pressure exerted upon the fetal abdomen.

One of the most frequent indications for forceps is uterine dysfunction when oxytocin is ineffective with the head well down in the pelvis. In nulliparas, furthermore, the marked resistance of the perineum and the vaginal outlet may sometimes present a serious obstacle to the passage of the child, even when the expulsive forces are normal. In such cases an episiotomy is of great value.

Elective Low Forceps.   Prolonged pressure of the fetal head against a rigid perineum sometimes results in injury to the brain. To prevent cerebral injury and to spare the mother the strain of the last few minutes of the second stage, DeLee recommended the "prophylactic forceps operation," more commonly called "elective low forceps" on the grounds that the obstetrician elects to interfere knowing that it is not absolutely necessary, for spontaneous delivery may normally be expected within approximately 15 minutes. The vast majority of forceps operations performed in this country today are elective low forceps. One reason is that all methods of analgesia interfere to a certain extent with the mother's voluntary expulsive efforts, in which circumstances low forceps delivery becomes the most reasonable procedure.

The fact that these methods for relief of pain frequently necessitate forceps delivery is not an indictment of the procedures, provided the obstetrician adheres strictly to the definition of low forceps. The fetal head must be on the perineal floor with the sagittal suture anteroposterior. In these circumstances, forceps delivery preceded by episiotomy is a very simple and safe operation requiring only gentle traction. By allowing the patient ample time, the criteria for low forceps can usually be met despite the influence of analgesia. If, however, the head does not descend and rotate, any forceps operation performed thereon is not a low forceps but an indicated or elective midforceps. Although midforceps operations, especially those in which anterior rotation is the only criterion of low forceps not met, may occasionally be easy in expert hands, in general, the head is higher before rotation and more traction is usually required. For maximal safety of both mother and infant, therefore, forceps should not be used *electively* until the criteria of a low forceps operation, as here defined, are fulfilled.

Prerequisites for Application of Forceps.   1. *The head must be engaged, preferably deeply engaged.* Application of the blades before engagement, that is, high forceps, is an extremely difficult operation, often entailing brutal trauma to the maternal tissues and death of a large proportion of the babies. Many years ago when cesarean section was also a highly dangerous operation, high forceps had a certain place in operative obstetrics; it is rarely employed today, however, and is mentioned here only to condemn it. Even after engagement occurs, the higher the station of the fetal head, the more difficult and traumatic the forceps delivery becomes. Whenever the blades are applied before the head has reached the perineal floor, moreover, it is common to find the head decidedly higher than rectal or vaginal examination had indicated, because of extensive caput succedaneum and partial deflection.

These difficulties of midforceps operation obtain even in the presence of a valid maternal indication for forceps delivery. For instance, it is generally agreed that patients with heart disease and preeclampsia should be spared the bearing-down efforts of the second stage if at all feasible; such efforts, however, may be much less harmful than a difficult midforceps. Forceps should, therefore, not be used until the station of the head promises an easy operative procedure. The same generalization applies to forceps for fetal distress when the skull is not close to the perineal floor. Granted that the fetal heart rate in such a case may suggest that the infant is hypoxic, it may still be judicious to allow more time for the head to descend rather than to superimpose the trauma of a difficult midforceps operation on an already distressed infant. In these circumstances more infants have been killed than saved by operations for fetal distress. In brief, except for cases in which the fetal head has become arrested in the midpelvis because of maternal exhaustion or intractable inertia (in which case the obstetrician has little choice), it is best to defer the application of the blades until a low forceps operation is possible, even in the presence of maternal disease or fetal distress. If delivery is mandatory, cesarean section is preferable to a difficult and damaging forceps operation.

2. The fetus must present either *by the vertex or by the face with the chin anterior.* The use of forceps is not applicable, of course, to transverse lies, nor is it intended for the breech.

3. The *position of the head must be known* so that rotation, if necessary, can be effected in the proper direction.

4. The *cervix must be completely dilated* before the application of forceps. Even a small rim of cervix may offer great resistance when traction is applied, causing extensive cervical lacerations that may also involve the lower uterine segment. If prompt delivery becomes imperative before complete dilatation of the cervix, cesarean section is generally preferable. In exceptional circumstances, Dührssen's incision may be performed (p. 1142).

5. The *membranes must be ruptured* to permit a firm grasp of the head by the blades of the forceps.

6. There should be *no disproportion* between the size of the head and that of the midpelvis or the outlet. Since forceps should not be employed until after the head has passed through the inlet, contraction at the superior strait as a contraindication to forceps is not pertinent to present-day practices.

Preparations for Operations.   When anesthesia is complete, the patient's buttocks should be brought to the edge of the table, and her legs held in position by an appropriate leg holder or by stirrups. The patient is then prepared for operation, as previously described. Catheterization of the bladder is necessary only if a midforceps delivery is planned.

Application of Forceps.   Forceps are so constructed that their cephalic curve is closely adapted to the sides of the fetal head, the biparietal diameter corresponding to the greatest distance between the blades. Consequently, the head is perfectly grasped only when the long axis of the blades corresponds to the occipitomental diameter, with the fenestrae including the parietal bosses and the tips of the blades lying over the cheeks, while the concave margins of the blades

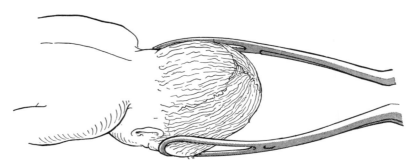

Fig. 11. INCORRECT application of forceps over brow and mastoid region.

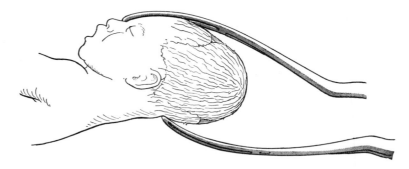

Fig. 12. INCORRECT application of forceps, one blade over occiput and the other over the brow. Note that the forceps cannot be locked.

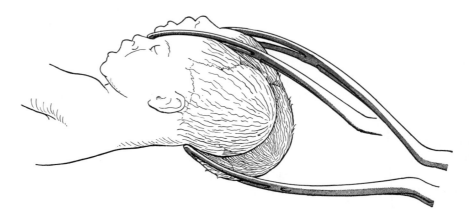

Fig. 13. Forceps applied INCORRECTLY as in Figure 12. Note extension of head and tendency of blades to slip off with traction.

are directed toward either the occiput or the face. Thus applied, the forceps should not slip, and traction may most advantageously be applied. When forceps are applied obliquely, however, with one blade over the brow and the other over the opposite mastoid region, the grasp is less secure, and the head is exposed to injurious pressure. If one blade is applied over the face and the other over the occiput, the instrument cannot be locked, whereas if the blade over the face is moved down to permit articulation, the grasp becomes insecure and each traction tends to increase extension of the head (Figs. 11, 12, and 13).

For these reasons, the forceps should be applied directly to the sides of the head along the *occipitomental diameter,* in what is termed the cephalic, biparietal, or bimalar application. In contradistinction, the term *pelvic application* is employed when the left blade is applied to the left and the right blade to the right side of the mother's pelvis, regardless of the position of the fetal head. It follows that the head is grasped satisfactorily only when the sagittal suture happens to be directed anteroposteriorly. Pelvic applications may be injurious to the infant and are not advocated in this country.

Precise knowledge of the exact position of the fetal head is essential to a proper cephalic application. With the head low down, diagnosis of position is made on examination of the sagittal suture and the fontanels, but when it is at a higher station, an absolute diagnosis can be made by locating the posterior ear.

Low Forceps (Figs. 14–23). With the head at the low station required in the definition of low forceps, the obstacle to delivery is usually insufficient expulsive forces or abnormally great resistance of the perineum. In such circumstances the sagittal suture occupies the anteroposterior diameter of the pelvic outlet, with the small fontanel directed toward either the symphysis pubis or the concavity of the sacrum. In either event the forceps, if applied to the sides of the pelvis, grasps the head ideally. The left blade is introduced into the left and the right blade into the right side of the pelvis, as follows: Two fingers of the right hand are introduced past the left and posterior portion of the vulva into the vagina past the landing point of the fetal head. The handle of the left branch is then grasped between the thumb and two fingers of the left hand, as in holding a pen,

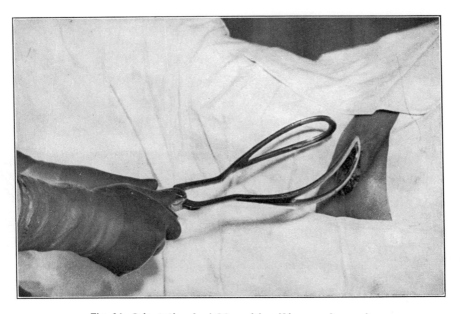

Fig. 14. Orientation for LOA position (Simpson forceps).

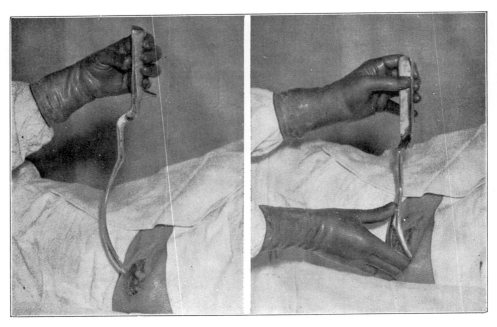

Fig. 15. The left handle held in the left hand. Fig. 16. Introduction of left blade into left
Simpson forceps.   side of pelvis.

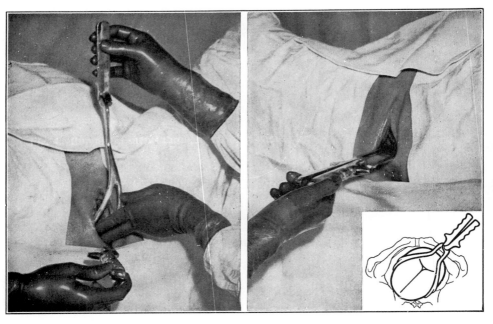

Fig. 17. Left blade in place; introduction of   Fig. 18. Forceps has been locked.
right blade by right hand.

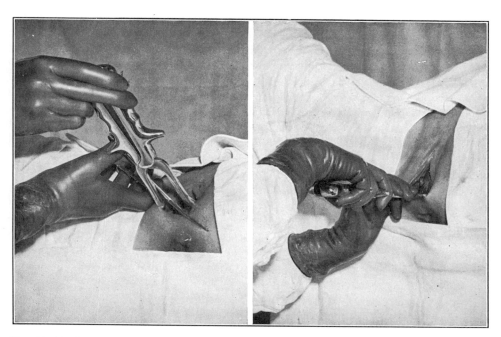

Fig. 19. Median or mediolateral episiotomy may be performed at this point. Left mediolateral episiotomy shown here.

Fig. 20. Horizontal traction; operator seated.

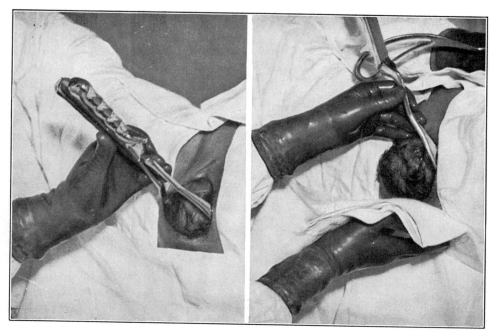

Fig. 21. Upward traction.

Fig. 22. Disarticulation of branches of forceps. Beginning modified Ritgen maneuver.

and the tip of the blade is gently passed into the vagina along the palmar surface of the fingers of the right hand, which serve as a guide. The branch is held at first almost vertically, but as the blade adapts itself to the head, the forceps is depressed, eventually to a horizontal position. The guiding fingers are then withdrawn, and the handle is left unsupported or held by an assistant. Similarly, two fingers of the left hand are then introduced into the right and posterior portion of the birth canal to serve as a guide for the right blade, which is held in the right hand and introduced into the vagina. These guiding fingers are then withdrawn and the branches are articulated. They may usually be locked without difficulty; otherwise, first one and then the other blade should be gently moved until the handles are repositioned to effect easy articulation. Episiotomy is performed either just before application of the blades or more often when traction on the head begins to distend the perineum.

Examination then reveals whether the blades have been correctly applied. If cervical tissue has been grasped, the forceps should be loosened and the incompletely retracted cervix pushed up over the head. When it is certain that the blades are satisfactorily placed, the handles are held with one hand, and gentle, intermittent, horizontal traction is exerted until the perineum begins to bulge. As soon as the vulva is distended by the occiput, the handles are gradually elevated, eventually pointing almost directly upward as the parietal bones emerge. During upward traction, the four fingers should grasp the upper surface of the handles and shanks, while the thumb exerts the necessary force upon their lower surface, as shown in Figure 21.

During birth of the head, spontaneous delivery should be simulated as closely as possible, employing minimal force. Traction should therefore be intermittent, and the head should be allowed to recede in the intervals, as in spontaneous labor. Except when urgently indicated, as in fetal distress, delivery should be sufficiently slow, deliberate, and gentle to allow for gradual stretching of the pelvic tissues.

After the vulva is well distended by the head, and the brow can be felt through the perineum, the delivery may be completed in several ways. We frequently keep the forceps in place, in the belief that greatest control over the advance of the head is thus maintained. The thickness of the blades may at times add to the distention of the vulva, however, thus increasing the likelihood of laceration. In such cases, we remove the forceps and complete the delivery by the modified Ritgen maneuver (p. 412), slowly expressing the head by using upward pressure upon the chin through the posterior portion of the perineum, covering the anus with a towel to minimize contamination from the bowel. Occasionally when the forceps is removed prematurely, the modified Ritgen maneuver proves a tedious and inelegant procedure.

When the occiput is directly posterior, horizontal traction should be applied until the forehead or root of the nose engages under the symphysis. The handles should then be slowly elevated until the occiput gradually emerges over the anterior margin of the perineum. Then by imparting a downward motion to the instrument, the forehead, nose, and chin successively emerge from the vulva. The extraction is more difficult than when the occiput is anterior, and because of greater distention of the vulva, perineal tears are more common (Fig. 23).

Midforceps Operations. When the head lies above the perineum, the sagittal suture usually occupies an oblique or transverse diameter of the pelvis. In such cases the forceps should always be applied to the sides of the head. The applica-

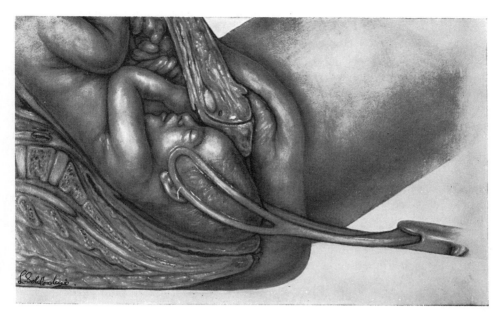

Fig. 23. Low forceps. Occiput directly posterior; horizontal traction.

tion is best accomplished by introducing two or more fingers into the vagina to a sufficient depth to feel the posterior ear, over which, whether right or left, the first blade should be applied.

In left occipitoanterior positions the entire right hand, introduced into the left posterior segment of the pelvis, should locate the posterior ear and at the same time serve as a guide for introduction of the left branch of the forceps, which is held in the left hand and applied over the posterior ear. The guiding hand is then withdrawn, and the handle is held by an assistant or left unsupported, the blade usually retaining its position without difficulty. Two fingers of the left hand are then introduced into the right posterior portion of the pelvis, but no attempt is yet made to reach the anterior ear, which lies near the right iliopectineal eminence. The right branch of the forceps, held in the right hand, is then introduced along the left hand as a guide. It must then be applied over the anterior ear of the child by gently sweeping it anteriorly until it lies directly opposite the blade that was introduced first. Of the two branches, now articulated, one occupies the posterior and the other the anterior extremity of the left oblique diameter.

In right positions, the blades are introduced similarly but in opposite directions, for in those cases the right is the posterior ear, over which the first blade must accordingly be placed. After the blades have been applied to the sides of the head, the left handle and shank lie above the right. Consequently, the forceps does not immediately articulate; locking of the branches is easily effected, however, by rotating the left around the right to bring the lock into proper position.

If the occiput is in a *transverse position*, the forceps is introduced similarly, with the first blade applied over the posterior ear, and the second rotated anteriorly to a position opposite the first. In this case one blade lies in front of the sacrum and the other behind the symphysis. The conventional Simpson or the special Kielland or Barton forceps may be used. Regardless of the original position of the head, delivery is effected by exerting traction downward until the occiput appears at the vulva; the rest of the operation is completed as described. When the occiput is obliquely anterior, it gradually rotates spontaneously to the symphysis pubis as traction is exerted; but when it is directed transversely, in order to bring it anteriorly a *rotary motion* of the forceps is sometimes required. The direction of rotation, of course, varies with the position of the occiput. Rotation from the left side toward the midline is required when the occiput is directed toward the left, and in the reverse direction when it is directed toward the right side of the pelvis. In certain circumstances, particularly when the Barton forceps is used in transverse positions in anteroposteriorly flattened pelves, rotation should not be attempted until the fetal head has reached or approached the pelvic floor. Premature attempts at anterior rotation under such conditions may result in injury to the fetus and maternal soft parts.

In exerting traction before the head appears at the vulva, one or both hands may be employed according to the force required. With the Simpson forceps, one hand grasps the handles of the instrument while the fingers of the other are hooked over the transverse projection at their upper ends. To avoid excessive force the operator should sit with his arms flexed and elbows held closely against the thorax, since the effect of the body weight must not be applied.

Application of Forceps in Obliquely Posterior Positions. Prompt delivery may become necessary when the small fontanel is directed toward one of the sacroiliac synchondroses—namely, in ROP and LOP positions. When interference is required in either of these cases, the head is often found imperfectly flexed. In many cases, when the hand is introduced to locate the posterior ear, the occiput rotates spontaneously to a transverse position. Delivery by forceps is then accomplished, as described. If, however, rotation does not occur, the head should be grasped with four fingers over the posterior ear and the thumb over the anterior. An attempt should then be made to rotate the occiput to a transverse position. Rotation can usually be accomplished with ease, occasionally even to an anterior position. The forceps is then applied as previously described. In other cases, after manual rotation has been effected, the head slips back into its original position before the forceps can be applied.

If manual rotation cannot be accomplished promptly and easily, application of the blades to the head in posterior position and delivery as such is the safest procedure in the hands of the average operator, as emphasized by Douglass and Kaltreider. In many of these cases the cause of the persistent occiput posterior position and of the difficulty in accomplishing rotation is an anthropoid pelvis, the architecture of which plainly predisposes to posterior delivery and opposes rotation. Somewhat more traction is often required for delivery of an occiput posterior as such, and a liberal episiotomy is advisable. Except in the hands of experts with extensive experience in manual rotation or the Scanzoni maneuver, however, it probably produces less maternal and fetal injury than does difficult rotation of the head.

Scanzoni Maneuver (Figs. 24–32). The occiput may be rotated 45 degrees to the posterior position or 135 degrees to the anterior (Fig. 24). Unfortunately, in rotating the occiput forward with forceps, the pelvic curvature, originally

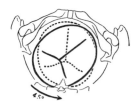 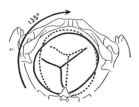

Fig. 24. Diagrams showing rotation of obliquely posterior occiput to sacrum (left) and symphysis pubis (right).

directed upward, at the completion of rotation is inverted and directed posteriorly. Attempted delivery with the instrument in that position is likely to cause serious injury to the maternal soft parts. To avoid the trauma, it is essential to remove and reapply the instrument as described in the following text.

The *double application for forceps*, which was first described by Smellie and rediscovered by Scanzoni nearly a century later, has given satisfactory results in some hands, but it is rarely necessary and is generally employed in only a small percentage of all obliquely posterior occipital positions. Since the right posterior variety is much more frequent, the steps of the operation in that case are here detailed.

In the first application the blades are applied to the sides of the head with the pelvic curve toward the face of the child, whereas in the second manipulation it is directed toward the occiput. For the first application (Figs. 25 and 26) the right hand is passed into the left posterior segment of the pelvis, and the posterior (right) ear is located. The left blade is applied over it and held in position by an assistant, while the operator's left hand is passed into the right side of the vagina to control the introduction of the right blade, which is then rotated anteriorly until it lies opposite the blade first introduced. The forceps is then locked, the blades occupying the left and the sagittal suture the right oblique diameter of the pelvis. The forceps is then rotated 45 degrees, bringing the occiput to the transverse or an obliquely anterior position. Both blades are then removed and reapplied in the usual manner, whereupon with the next rotation the occiput is brought directly under the pubic arch (Figs. 28, 30, and 32).

Some difficulty may arise in proper articulation, since the handle of the left branch lying above the right cannot be locked, but this can be readily overcome by rotating the left around the right branch to bring the lock into proper position. In left positions the blades are applied similarly, but in the reverse direction.

To avoid confusing the left with the right branch of the forceps, the beginner, after having made an accurate diagnosis of the position of the head, should articulate the forceps and hold the blades in front of the vulva of the patient, in the position in which they are to be applied (Fig. 14). He should remember that the *left* blade of the forceps always goes to the *left* side of the mother and is introduced by the *left* hand of the operator.

Kielland in 1916 described a forceps with narrow, somewhat bayonet-shaped blades that he claimed could readily be applied to the sides of the head and surpassed all other models as a *rotator*. He held that his forceps were particularly useful when the station of the fetal head was high and when the sagittal suture

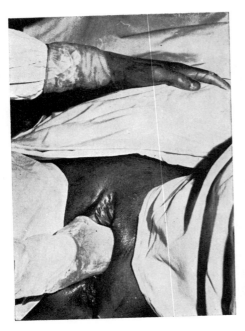

Fig. 25. Vaginal examination and location of posterior ear.

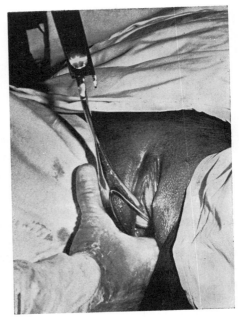

Fig. 26. Introduction of posterior blade.

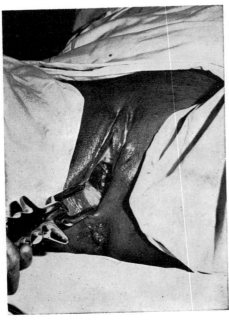

Fig. 27. Forceps locked in first application; ROP.

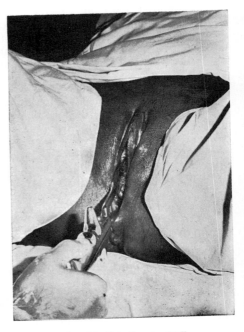

Fig. 28. Rotation to ROT.

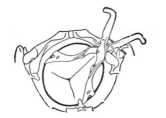 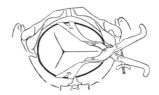

Fig. 29. Rotation from ROP to transverse as shown in Figures 27 and 28.

was directed transversely. These forceps have also been advocated as of particular value in the delivery of posterior positions. The Kielland forceps have almost no pelvic curve, but they have a sliding lock and are very light. On each handle is a small knob that indicates the direction of rotation. There are two methods of applying the anterior blade. In one, the anterior blade is introduced first with its cephalic curve directed forward and, after it has entered sufficiently far into the uterine cavity, is turned through 180 degrees to adapt the cephalic curvature to the head. This rotation of the anterior blade must take place in the direction of the side on which the concave margin of the blade points, as indicated by the small knob on the blade. The shank now rests on the perineum. The second blade is introduced posteriorly. When the blades are locked, traction may be exerted downward in the direction in which the handles point. The head may be gently rotated to an anterior position. Rotation and traction are not performed at the same time. In all cases of transverse arrest, rotation should be performed at the station at which it may most easily be accomplished. It may be performed above or below, but rarely at, the point of arrest (Figs. 33–41).

Keilland advises a "gliding method" of application for the anterior blade when the uterus is tightly contracted about the head and the lower uterine segment is stretched and thin. In such cases, when the pelvis is slightly contracted, it is dangerous to introduce the anterior blade with its cephalic curvature directed upward to be followed by rotation of the blade. In the wandering or gliding method the anterior blade is introduced at the side of the pelvis over the brow or face of the child. It is made to glide over the child's face to an anterior position, the handle of the blade held close to the opposite buttock throughout the maneuver. The posterior blade is introduced in the manner described.

In our experience the Kielland forceps is of particular value in transverse arrest of the head unless there is anteroposterior flattening of the pelvis, since the anterior blade may be applied without excessive difficulty. We prefer the gliding method of application to the classical introduction of the anterior blade with the cephalic curvature directed forward, because the risk of injury to the uterus or bladder is lower in the former method.

Figure 42 illustrates the forceps described by Barton, Caldwell, and Studdiford and recommended by Decker, Dickson, and Heaton, as well as others. It differs from the usual types in that the anterior blade is hinged where it joins the shank. It appears to be particularly useful when the sagittal suture occupies the transverse diameter of a platypelloid pelvis with a straight sacrum. For such

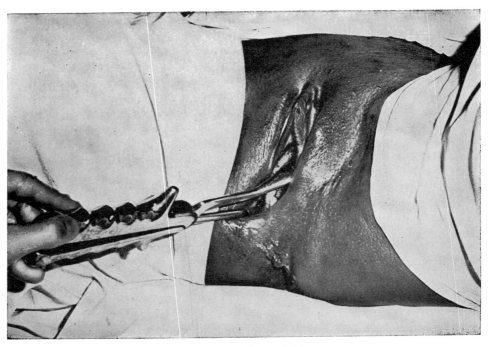

Fig. 30. Rotation to ROA.

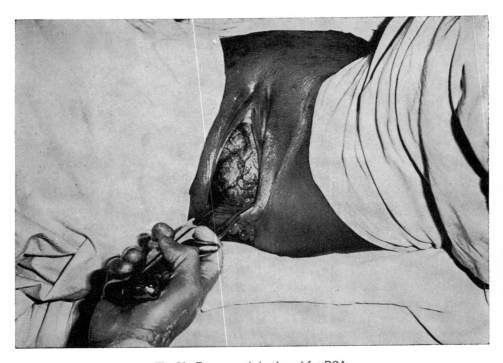

Fig. 31. Forceps reintroduced for ROA.

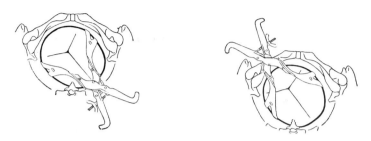

Fig. 32. Left, forceps after rotation to ROA (Fig. 30) with pelvic curve of forceps directed downward. Right, the forceps reapplied for ROA (Fig. 31) with pelvic curve upward and properly directed.

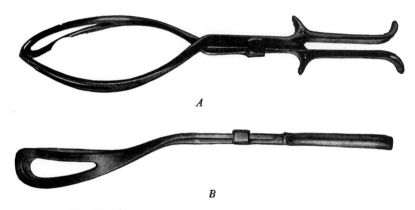

A

B

Fig. 33. Kielland's forceps. A, front view; B, side view.

cases it is used with satisfactory results in several clinics in this country. The usual method of employing the Barton forceps involves wandering the hinged blade over the occiput or, less frequently, over the face. The posterior blade is then inserted directly into the hollow of the sacrum and the two branches of the forceps are articulated, adjusting the application, when necessary, by means of the sliding lock. Traction is applied in the transverse diameter of the pelvis, with rotation effected at or near the pelvic floor. Traction and rotation should not be performed simultaneously.

Application of Forceps in Face Presentations. In face presentations the application of forceps is occasionally necessary but is usually successful only in the transverse and anterior varieties. The blades are applied to the sides of the head along the occipitomental diameter, with the pelvic curve directed toward the neck. Downward traction is exerted until the chin appears under the symphysis. Then by an upward movement the face is slowly extracted, the nose, eyes, brow, and occiput appearing in succession over the anterior margin of the perineum (Fig. 43).

Forceps should not be applied when the chin is directed toward the hollow of the sacrum, since delivery cannot be effected in that position.

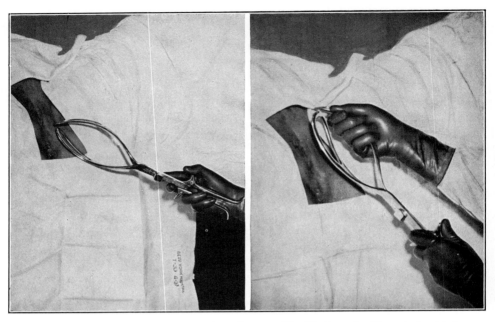

Fig. 34. Orientation for transverse (ROT) posi-   Fig. 35. Grasping the anterior blade.
tion. Kielland forceps.

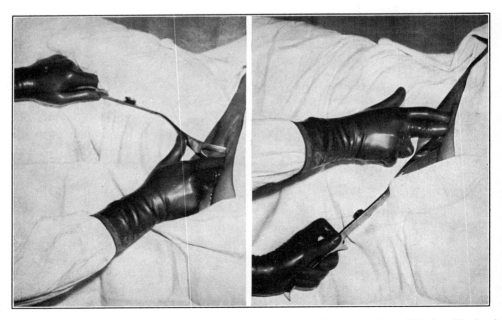

Fig. 36. Introduction and anterior wandering   Fig. 37. Further wandering of blade with shank
of blade.   of forceps against buttock.

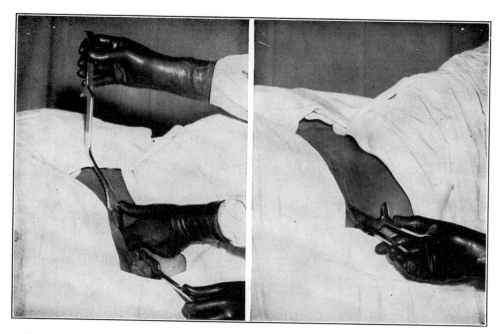

Fig. 38. Introduction of posterior blade.

Fig. 39. Forceps is locked. Note overlapping of handles possible with sliding lock.

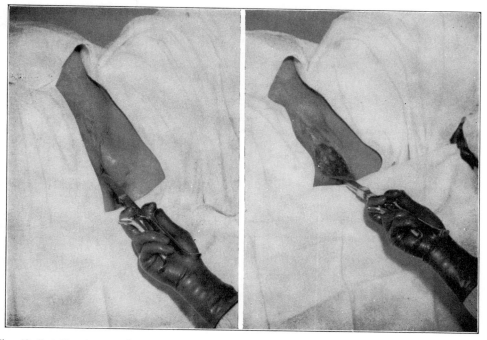

Fig. 40. Rotation to anterior position followed by downward traction.

Fig. 41. Further downward traction. Occiput emerging at introitus.

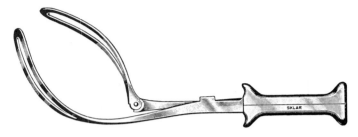

Fig. 42. Barton's forceps. (Courtesy of J. Sklar Mfg. Co.)

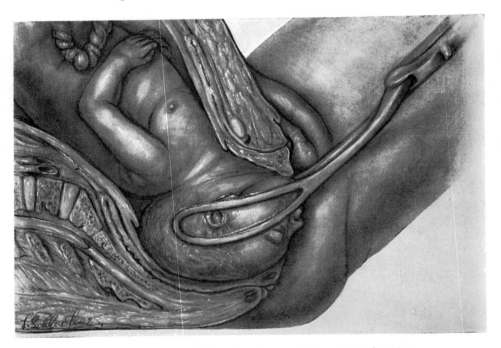

Fig. 43. Forceps applied to face along occipitomental diameter.

Prognosis.   The perinatal mortality associated with forceps deliveries depends on the condition of the fetus at the time the operation is undertaken, as well as the station of the head. It should be practically zero when the head is on or very close to the perineum. The application of forceps at higher stations, however, is attended by perinatal loss or damage in direct proportion to the height of the skull above the perineal floor. In such cases the head may be subjected to injurious pressure that may lead to intracranial hemorrhage. Fortunately, the difficult forceps delivery has been largely supplanted by cesarean section or oxytocic stimulation.

TRIAL FORCEPS; FAILED FORCEPS

In "trial forceps" the operator attempts midforceps delivery with the full knowledge that a certain degree of disproportion at the midpelvis may make the procedure incompatible with safety for the child. After a good application has been achieved, several firm, downward pulls on the instrument are made. If no descent occurs, the procedure is abandoned and cesarean section is performed (Douglass and Kaltreider).

The term "failed forceps" is applied to a case in which a frank attempt has been made to deliver with forceps but without success. The three fundamental factors responsible for such failures are disproportion, incomplete cervical dilatation, and malposition of the fetal head, usually an unrecognized occiput posterior position. Most but not all such cases stem from inexperience and gross ignorance of obstetric fundamentals. In most areas of the United States these cases are becoming much less frequent. If an attempt to apply the forceps is unsuccessful for technical reasons, the procedure may also be classed as a failed forceps.

Since incomplete dilatation of the cervix is the cause of many cases of failed forceps, additional time in labor will frequently solve the problem. Similarly, if the head does not rotate in occiput posterior positions the case should be managed according to the principles set forth on page 853. In the presence of disproportion, cesarean section may be the only recourse with a living fetus, or craniotomy after fetal death. Since many of these women are infected, dehydrated, and exhausted, antibiotics, general supportive treatment, and rest are often indicated. The prognosis for the infant is usually poor because of the trauma it has received. The outlook for the mother, however, is usually better, although it varies with the extent of trauma and infection. In a study based on the annual reports of nine hospitals in England, Law found that the maternal mortality rate in "failed forceps" was 2.0 per cent and the perinatal loss was 36.2 per cent.

THE VACUUM EXTRACTOR

There have been numerous attempts in the past to apply suction to the fetal scalp as a means of traction in place of forceps. The advantages of such a procedure over the forceps include the avoidance of a space-occupying instrument and potentially less damage to the infant. All previously described instruments were unsuccessful until Malmström applied a new principle—namely, suction and traction on a metal cup so designed that the suction creates an artificial caput within the cup that holds firmly and allows adequate traction (Fig. 44). The instrument is simple and easy to use. In spite of the early enthusiasm for the instrument in this country (Tricomi, Amorosi, and Gottschalk), the vacuum extractor is not used extensively here, partly because of numerous reports of fetal damage—such as lacerations of the scalp, cephalhematomas, and intracranial hemorrhage—and loss of infants. In contradistinction to the American hesitancy about the instrument, there has been an enthusiastic reception in many other parts of the world. Typical examples of such acceptance are indicated by the reports of Lillie in Ireland; Lasbrey, Orchard, and Crichton in South Africa; Chalmers in Great Britain; Hammerstein and Gromoltke in Germany; and Filimonov in the Soviet Union. The subject has been reviewed by Sjöstedt, who compared the results of use of the vacuum extractor with those of the forceps in two separate series of deliveries in his hospital in Helsinki. He found, in contrast to experience in the United States, that vacuum extraction was superior to forceps delivery with respect to perinatal mortality and morbidity of infants and mothers. The divergence of opinion is perplexing, but according to Donald, who has had good results with

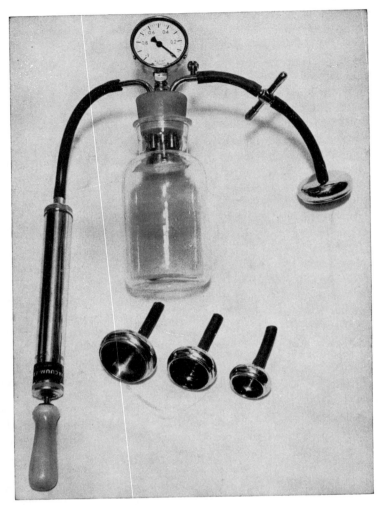

Fig. 44. Malmström vacuum extractor with metal cups, vacuum pump, and pressure gauge.

the vacuum extractor in his clinic, the instrument is safer than a trial of forceps in midpelvic and deep transverse arrest and is often successful. Although we agree with that concept, in our experience the vacuum extractor provides no advantage over forceps when the head is sufficiently deep in the pelvis to permit a low forceps delivery.

We believe, furthermore, that use of the vacuum extractor should be restricted to cases in which the cervix is fully dilated.

CRANIOTOMY

The term *craniotomy*, as used in obstetrics, means any operation that effects a decrease in the size of the fetal head for the purpose of facilitating its delivery.

It comprises puncture of the fetal skull and evacuation of its contents. After the skull collapses, the infant is extracted with suitable instruments that grasp the collapsed cranium. Widespread prenatal care, more astute management of pelvic contraction, antibiotics, and improvements in cesarean section have rendered craniotomy an exceedingly rare operation in modern obstetrics.

Except in the presence of hydrocephalus, craniotomy should not be performed on a living child. As indicated on page 889, moreover, cases of hydrocephalus are normally managed better by needle puncture and drainage than by craniotomy.

In the presence of a dead fetus, craniotomy is indicated whenever delivery of the intact head by other means threatens to be difficult. The operation is absolutely contraindicated in the extremely rare instances in which the obstetric conjugate is less than 5.5 cm.

The patient should be placed in the lithotomy position and prepared as for other obstetric operations. Craniotomy usually includes the perforation of the head and evacuation of its contents (Fig. 45) and the delivery of the mutilated

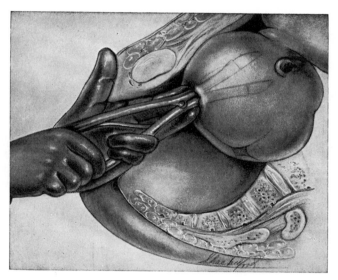

Fig. 45. Craniotomy. Perforation of head. (From Titus. Management of Obstetric Difficulties, 2nd ed., St. Louis, C. V. Mosby Co., 1949.)

child. Of the numerous instruments devised for perforating the head, the most suitable is *Smellie's scissors* (Fig. 46). If the head is engaged and firmly fixed, perforation is accomplished with little difficulty. With two fingers the large or small fontanel, whichever is more convenient, is located and the perforator is plunged through it. The opening is then enlarged and the instrument is briskly moved about within the skull to disintegrate the brain. As a result of the pressure to which the skull is subjected in these circumstances, the cranial contents flow out spontaneously without the need to flush them out. After the brain has been evacuated, the collapsed head may be expelled by spontaneous or oxytocin-stimulated uterine contractions.

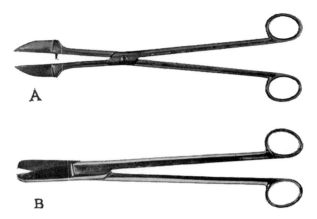

A

B

Fig. 46. A, Smellie scissors for perforation of skull. B, Dubois scissors for incision of scalp.

In modern obstetrics, there is rarely an indication for this operation, but in face of uterine inertia in a patient with a contracted pelvis and a dead fetus, the mother may thereby be spared a cesarean section.

OPERATIONS PREPARATORY TO FORCEPS

Dührssen's Incisions, or Hysterostomatomy.   When immediate delivery is desirable before the cervix is fully dilated, multiple radial incisions may be made in the cervix and repaired with sutures after the completion of labor. They are usually called Dührssen's incisions, after the German obstetrician who first described them in 1890. The operation is sometimes referred to as *hysterostomatomy*. The technic of the operation is simple: three incisions, corresponding approximately to the hours 2, 6, and 10 on the face of a clock, are made as shown in Figures 47, 48, and 49, extending to the junction of the cervix with the vagina. Delivery is then effected by forceps or breech extraction, depending on the presentation. The

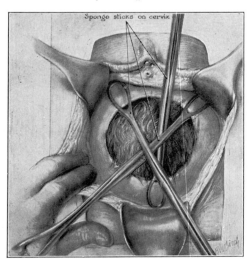

Fig. 47. Dührssen's incisions. Sponge forceps are applied to the cervix at 2, 6, and 10 o'clock, the sites where incisions are to be made. Once the first incision has been made, the remaining rim of cervix tends to retract and becomes more difficult to reach unless it has been grasped previously and held by a clamp as here shown. Although the two extra forceps may interfere somewhat at the time of the first incision, their use is justified in making the operation more thorough.

operation should never be done unless the cervix is fully effaced and more than 5 cm dilated, lest profuse or even fatal hemorrhage result. The procedure is, of course, contraindicated in placenta previa.

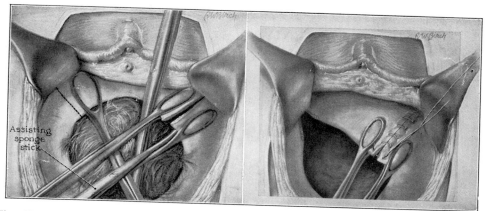

Fig. 48. Dührssen's incisions. The first incision has been made.

Fig. 49. Dührssen's incisions. Repair of incision with interrupted sutures of chromic catgut.

Many modern obstetricians consider the operation obsolete. It is included here only because of the rare possibility of its use in fetal distress when the cervix is almost fully dilated or when prolapse of the umbilical cord occurs in a similar situation.

Although the incisions themselves are simple to perform, the procedure involves major potential hazards, and cesarean section is often preferable. For instance, in cases of uterine dysfunction in which the cervix is not yet fully dilated, the head is usually well above the pelvic floor, and a difficult midforceps operation with its attendant trauma to mother and child is often required. In such circumstances severe maternal hemorrhage is common. The incisions heal satisfactorily in only about half the cases, moreover. Poor anatomic results, such as deep scars and adhesions between the cervix and the vaginal mucosa are often found.

There is no such procedure as "manual dilatation of the cervix." What actually occurs when it is attempted is manual laceration of the cervix. The operation has no place in modern obstetrics.

Symphysiotomy and Pubiotomy. *Symphysiotomy* is the division of the pubic symphysis with a wire saw or knife to effect an increase in the capacity of a contracted pelvis sufficient to permit the passage of a living child. In *pubiotomy*, the pubis is severed a few centimeters lateral to the symphysis. Because of interference with subsequent locomotion, bladder injuries, and hemorrhage, and because of the greater safety of modern cesarean section, these two operations have been abandoned in the United States. They are still performed in Africa, among other places, where it is almost impossible to follow a patient in a subsequent pregnancy. Since, in these circumstances, a woman delivered by cesarean section for a mildly contracted pelvis might well die with a ruptured uterus in her next pregnancy, symphysiotomy is indicated in such a case in an attempt to produce sufficient enlargement of the pelvis to allow subsequent vaginal delivery (Rendle-Short).

References

Aveling, J. H.   The Chamberlens and the Midwifery Forceps. London, J. & H. Churchill, 1882.

Barton, L. G., Caldwell, W. E., and Studdiford, W. E.   A new obstetrical forceps. Amer J Obstet Gynec 15:16, 1928.

Chalmers, J. A.   Five years' experience with the vacuum extractor. Brit Med J 1:1216, 1964.

Das, K.   The Obstetric Forceps, Its History and Evolution. Calcutta, Art Press, 1929, p. 913.

Decker, W. H., Dickson, W. A., and Heaton, C. E.   An analysis of five hundred and forty-seven midforceps operations. Amer J Obstet Gynec 65:294, 1953.

DeLee, J. B.   The prophylactic forceps operation. Amer J Obstet Gynec 1:34, 1920.

Dennen, E. H.   Forceps Deliveries, 2nd ed. Philadelphia, F. A. Davis Co., 1964.

Donald, I.   Practical Obstetric Problems, 4th ed. Philadelphia, J. B. Lipincott, 1969.

Douglass, L. H., and Kaltreider, D. F.   Trial forceps. Amer J Obstet Gynec 65:889, 1953.

Dührssen, A. (On the value of deep cervical incisions and episiotomy in obstetrics). Arch Gynaek 37:27, 1890.

Filimonov, N. N.   (Experience in the use of the vacuum extractor). Akush Ginek (Moskva) 37:16, 1961.

Hammerstein, J., and Gromoltke, R.   The value of Malmström's vacuum extractor in operative obstetrics. J Int Coll Surg 37:458, 1962.

Hunt, A. B., and McGee, W. B.   Dührssen's incision. An analysis of 592 cases. Amer J Obstet Gynec 31:598, 1936.

Joulin, M.   (Study on the use of force in obstetrics). Arch Gén de Méd, 6th Series 9:149, 1867.

Kelly, J. V., and Sines, G.   An assessment of the compression and traction forces of obstetrical forceps. Amer J Obstet Gynec 96:521, 1966.

Kielland, C.   (On the application of forceps to the unrotated head, with description of a new model of forceps). Mschr Geburtsh Gynäk 43:48, 1916.

Lasbrey, A. H., Orchard, C. D., and Crichton, D.   Study of the relative merit and scope of the vacuum extractor as opposed to forceps delivery: preliminary report. S Afr J Obstet Gynaec 2:1, 1964.

Law, R. G.   "Failed forceps": a review of 37 cases. Brit Med J 2:955, 1953.

Lillie, E. W.   The use of the vacuum extractor in labour. Irish J Med Sci 7:309, 1962.

Malmström, T.   The vacuum extractor, an obstetrical instrument. Acta Obstet Gynec Scand Suppl 4:33, 1954.

Rendle-Short, C. W.   Causes of maternal death among Africans in Kampala, Uganda. J Obstet Gynaec Brit Comm 68:44, 1961.

Rhodes, P.   A critical appraisal of the obstetric forceps. J Obstet Gynaec Brit Emp 65:353, 1958.

Scanzoni, F. W.   Lehrbuch der Geburtshülfe, 2nd ed. Wien, L. W. Seidel, 1853, pp. 838–840.

Sjöstedt, J. E.   The vacuum extractor and forceps in obstetrics. A clinical study. Acta Obstet Gynec Scand 48:(Suppl. 10):1, 1967 (360 references).

Smellie, W.   A Treatise on the Theory and Practice of Midwifery. London, D. Wilson & T. Durham, 1752.

Tricomi, V., Amorosi, L., and Gottschalk, W.   Preliminary report of the use of Malmström's vacuum extractor. Amer J Obstet Gynec 81:681, 1961.

41

BREECH EXTRACTION AND VERSION

There are three types of breech deliveries:

1. In spontaneous breech delivery the entire infant is expelled by natural forces without any traction or manipulation other than support of the infant. This form of delivery of mature infants is uncommon.

2. In partial breech extraction the infant is delivered spontaneously as far as the umbilicus, but the remainder of the body is extracted.

3. In total breech extraction the entire body of the infant is extracted by the obstetrician.

Since the technic of breech extraction differs in complete and incomplete breeches, on the one hand, and frank breeches, on the other, it is necessary to consider the conditions separately. In all cases, the prerequisites for successful extraction are complete dilatation of the cervix and absence of mechanical obstacles. Although extraction through an imperfectly dilated cervix is sometimes possible, it is usually accompanied by deep cervical tears with resulting hemorrhage and the likelihood of considerable trauma to the infant. Dilatation of the cervix of sufficient degree for passage of the breech, furthermore, does not necessarily imply that the cervix is sufficiently dilated to allow the head to pass through without laceration of the cervix or further stretching. The difficulty is compounded by the additional resistance that generally causes extension of the head. The arms at the same time are extended over the head, complicating and delaying delivery to the extent that the child is almost invariably lost.

Indications for Extraction. In all breech presentations, preparations should be made for extraction as soon as the feet or buttocks appear at the vulva. Extraction is indicated when progress in delivery ceases or when fetal distress ensues. The passage of meconium is of much less significance in breech presentation, since it may result simply from abdominal compression of the infant. Regularity and rate of the fetal heart, however, are of singular importance and must be followed meticulously. Both gross irregularity and slowing to below 100 beats per minute are indications for extraction.

EXTRACTION OF COMPLETE OR INCOMPLETE BREECH

The patient should be placed in lithotomy position on the delivery table. Complete anesthesia is desirable, even when the body of the child has already been born and only the head remains to be extracted. As a rule, extraction is a much simpler operation when the breech has been born spontaneously (partial breech extraction) than when the feet are still high, requiring total breech extraction. During total extraction the entire hand should be introduced into the vagina and both feet of the fetus seized; the ankles should be grasped with the second finger lying between them. The feet are then brought down into the vagina, and traction applied until they appear at the vulva. If difficulty is experienced in seizing both feet, however, one foot should be brought into the vagina first, and the hand immediately reintroduced in order to grasp and extract the other.

As soon as the feet have been drawn through the vulva, they should be wrapped in a sterile towel to obtain a firmer grasp, for the vernix caseosa renders them slippery and difficult to hold. Downward traction is then continued (Fig. 1);

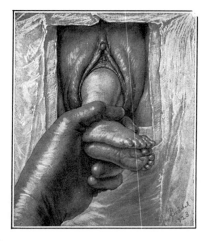

Fig. 1. Breech extraction. Traction upon the feet.

as the legs emerge, successively higher portions are grasped, first the calves and later the thighs. When the breech appears at the vulva, upward traction is applied until the hips are delivered. The thumbs are then placed over the sacrum and the fingers over the hips, and downward traction is continued until the costal margins, and later the scapulae, become visible (Figs. 2, 3, and 4). As the buttocks emerge, the back of the child faces more or less upward, but as further traction is exerted it tends to turn spontaneously toward the side of the mother to which it was originally directed. If turning does not occur, however, slight rotation should be added to the traction, with the object of bringing the bisacromial diameter of the child into the anteroposterior diameter of the outlet.

The cardinal point in successful extraction is steady downward traction until at least the lower halves of the scapulae are outside the vulva, with no attempt at delivery of the shoulders and arms until one of the axillae becomes visible. Failure to follow this rule will frequently make an otherwise simple procedure

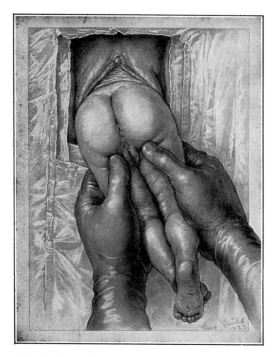

Fig. 2. Breech extraction. Traction upon the thighs. Sterile towel not illustrated.

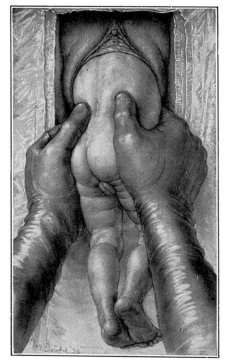

Fig. 3. Breech extraction. Extraction of body with operator's thumbs over sacrum.

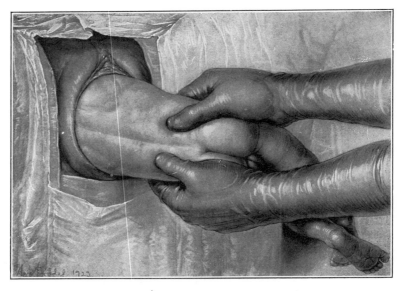

Fig. 4. Breech extraction. Scapulae visible.

difficult. The appearance of one of the axillae indicates that the time has arrived for delivery of the shoulders. Provided the arms are maintained in flexion, it makes little difference which shoulder is delivered first. Occasionally, while plans are made to deliver one shoulder the other is born spontaneously.

There are two methods of delivery of the shoulders:

1. With the scapulae visible (Fig. 4), the trunk is rotated in such a way that the anterior shoulder and arm appear at the vulva and can easily be released and delivered first. Figure 4 shows the operator rotating the trunk of the infant counterclockwise to deliver the right shoulder and arm. The body of the child is then rotated in the reverse direction to deliver the other shoulder and arm.

2. If the method of trunk rotation is unsuccessful, the posterior shoulder must be delivered first. The feet are grasped in one hand and drawn upward over the groin of the mother toward which the ventral surface of the child is directed; in that way leverage is exerted upon the posterior shoulder, which slips out over the perineal margin, usually followed by the arm and hand (Fig. 5). Then by depressing the body of the child the anterior shoulder emerges beneath the pubic arch, the arm and hand usually following spontaneously (Fig. 6). Thereafter, the back tends to rotate spontaneously in the direction of the mother's symphysis; if upward rotation fails to occur, it is effected by manual rotation of the body. Delivery of the head may then be accomplished.

Unfortunately, however, the process is not always so simple, and it is sometimes necessary first to free and deliver the arms. These maneuvers are much less frequently required today, presumably because of adherence to the principle of continuing traction without attention to the shoulders until an axilla becomes visible. Attempts to free the arms immediately after the costal margins emerge should be avoided.

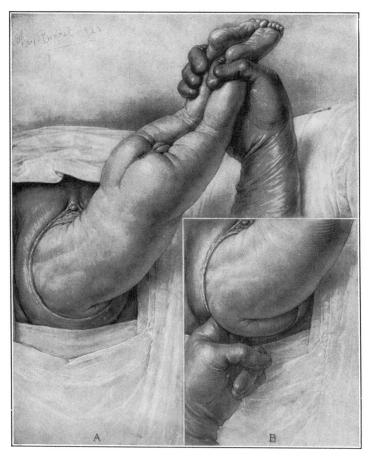

Fig. 5. Breech extraction. A, upward traction to effect delivery of posterior shoulder. B, freeing posterior arm.

Since there is more space available in the posterior and lateral segments of the normal pelvis than elsewhere, the posterior arm should be freed first. Since the corresponding axilla is already visible, upward traction upon the feet is continued, and two fingers of the other hand are passed along the humerus until the elbow is reached (Fig. 5). The fingers are now used to splint the arm, which is swept downward and delivered through the vulva. To deliver the anterior arm, depression of the body of the infant is sometimes all that is required to allow it to slip out spontaneously. In other cases it can be wiped down over the thorax using two fingers as a splint. Occasionally, however, the body must be seized with the thumbs over the scapulae and rotated to bring the undelivered shoulder near the closest sacrosciatic notch. The legs are then carried upward to bring the ventral surface of the child to the opposite groin of the mother; thereafter the arm can be delivered as described previously.

If the arms have become extended over the head, their delivery, although more difficult, can usually be accomplished by the maneuvers just described. In so doing, particular care must be taken to carry the fingers up to the elbow and

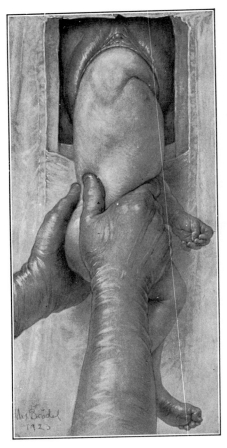

Fig. 6. Breech extraction. Delivery of anterior shoulder by downward traction.

to use them as a splint, for if they are merely hooked over the arm, the humerus or clavicle is exposed to great danger of fracture. Very exceptionally, the arm is found around the back of the neck (nuchal arm), and its delivery becomes still more difficult. If it cannot be freed in the manner described, its extraction may be facilitated by rotating the child through half a circle in such a direction that the friction exerted by the birth canal will serve to draw the elbow toward the face. Should rotation of the infant fail to free the nuchal arms, it may be necessary to push the child upward in an attempt to relase them. If the rotation is still unsuccessful, the arm is often forcibly extracted by hooking a finger over it. In that event, fracture of the humerus or clavicle is very common. Fortunately, good union almost always follows appropriate treatment.

After the shoulders have been born, the head usually occupies an oblique diameter of the pelvis with the chin directed posteriorly, and it may be extracted by *Mauriceau's maneuver* (Figs. 7 and 8). In that procedure, the index finger of one hand is introduced into the mouth of the child and applied over the maxilla, while the body rests upon the palm of the hand and the forearm, which is straddled by the legs. Two fingers of the other hand are then hooked over the neck and, grasping the shoulders, apply downward traction until the suboccipital region appears under the symphysis. The body of the child is now elevated toward

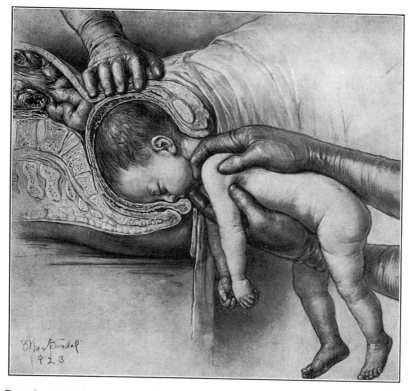

Fig. 7. Breech extraction. Suprapubic pressure and horizontal traction have caused the head to enter the pelvis. Mauriceau's maneuver.

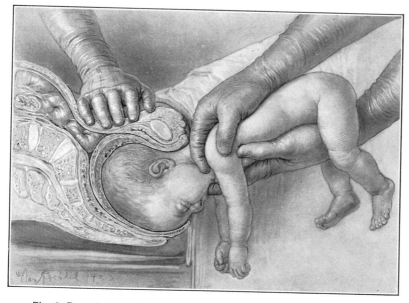

Fig. 8. Breech extraction. Mauriceau's maneuver; upward traction.

the mother's abdomen, and the mouth, nose, brow, and eventually the occiput emerge successively over the perineum. Traction should be exerted only by the fingers over the shoulders and not by the finger in the mouth, which may slip from the maxilla and rest upon the mandible and base of the tongue, creating a source of potential serious injury to the child.

This maneuver was first practiced by Mauriceau in the eighteenth century but for some reason fell into disfavor. Nearly a hundred years later Smellie described a similar procedure but rarely made use of it, since he preferred forceps. In the meantime, other devices were used until Veit in 1807 redirected attention to the superiority of Mauriceau's method of extraction. In Germany, therefore, the procedure is frequently named after Veit. The most accurate designation, however, is the Mauriceau-Smellie-Veit maneuver.

In the vast majority of cases the back of the child eventually rotates toward the front, regardless of its original position, but when rotation fails to occur spontaneously, the movement may be initiated by using stronger traction upon the leg. If even then the back remains posterior after birth of the shoulders, extraction must be begun with the occiput posterior. As a rule, rotation can still be effected by means of the finger in the mouth, and the head then extracted by Mauriceau's maneuver. When rotation is not possible, however, delivery of the head in its abnormal position must be attempted by the modified *Prague maneuver*, so called because it was strongly recommended by Kiwisch of that city. The Prague maneuver, as employed today with the fetal back down, is actually the reverse of the original procedure in which the fetal back was directed upward. In the procedure two fingers of one hand grasp the shoulders from below, while the other hand draws the feet up over the abdomen of the mother. The Prague maneuver, as well as most breech extractions, is more easily performed after an adequate episiotomy, to be described.

In an effort to simulate the forces of nature, Bracht described a maneuver whereby the breech is allowed to deliver spontaneously to the umbilicus. The baby's body is then held, not pressed, against the mother's symphysis. The force applied in this procedure should be equivalent to that of gravity. The mere maintenance of this position, added to the effects of uterine contractions and moderate suprapubic pressure by an assistant, often suffices to complete the delivery spontaneously. The *Bracht maneuver* has been popular in Europe but has not gained wide acceptance in this country. The procedure has been thoroughly reviewed by Plentl and Stone.

Episiotomy.   The episiotomy is an important adjunct to any type of breech delivery. Performed properly and at the appropriate time it can facilitate what otherwise might be a difficult and traumatic procedure. In contrast to the timing of episiotomy in delivery of a vertex, the operation should be performed in breech extraction only when the buttocks distend the vulva. A mediolateral episiotomy is usually preferred with a term-sized infant because it furnishes greater room and is less likely to extend into the rectum. With small infants a median episiotomy will provide ample space.

EXTRACTION IN FRANK BREECH PRESENTATIONS

When indications for delivery of a frank breech arise, the extraction becomes somewhat more difficult. In such cases, it is advisable to try to decompose the

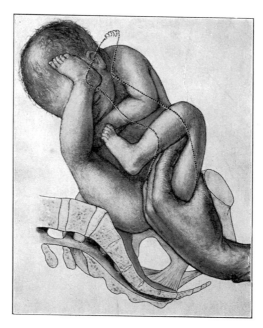

Fig. 9. Pinard's maneuver for bringing down a foot in frank breech presentation.

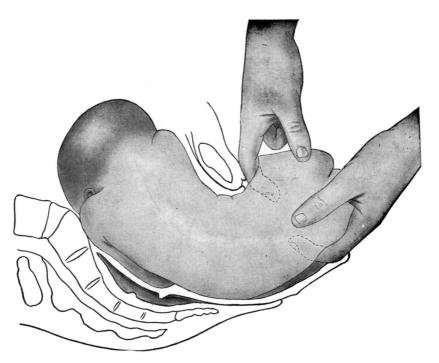

Fig. 10. Extraction of frank breech; fingers in groins.

wedge and bring down one or, preferably, both feet. The procedure is often readily accomplished in the presence of recently ruptured membranes but becomes extremely difficult if considerable time elapses after the escape of the amniotic fluid and if the uterus is tightly contracted over the fetus.

In many cases the *Pinard maneuver* aids materially in bringing down the feet. In that procedure two fingers are carried up along one extremity to the knee to push it away from the midline. Spontaneous flexion usually follows, and the foot of the child is felt to impinge upon the back of the hand. It may then be readily grasped and brought down (Fig. 9). As soon as the buttocks are born, first one leg and then the other are drawn out and extraction accomplished as described (Fig. 10).

FORCEPS TO THE AFTERCOMING HEAD

Piper forceps (Figs. 11 to 16) should be applied when the Mauriceau maneuver cannot be easily accomplished, as in the case of a small baby; or they may advantageously be applied electively instead of the Mauriceau procedure. The

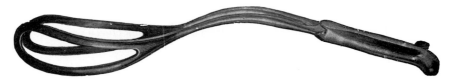

Fig. 11. Piper's forceps.

blades should not be applied to the aftercoming head until it has been brought into the pelvis by gentle traction and is engaged. As shown in Figure 17, suspension of the body of the infant in a towel, as recommended by Savage, keeps the arms out of the way and prevents excessive abduction of the trunk.

Entrapment of the Aftercoming Head. Occasionally with small premature infants the incompletely dilated cervix will not allow delivery of the aftercoming head. Prompt action is necessary if the infant is to be delivered alive. With gentle traction on the infant's body the cervix can be manually slipped over the occiput. If this maneuver is not readily successful, Dührssen's incisions should be made in the cervix at 10 and 2 o'clock. This is one of the few indications for this procedure in modern obstetrics.

ANESTHESIA FOR BREECH DELIVERY

It is wise to allow the breech to deliver spontaneously to the umbilicus. Extraction is then easily accomplished with a pudendal block, which may be administered at the onset of delivery. If, for any reason, general anesthesia is desired, it can be quickly induced with thiopental and maintained with nitrous oxide or cyclopropane.

Anesthesia for decomposition and extraction must provide sufficient relaxation to allow intrauterine manipulation. Although successful extraction has been ac-

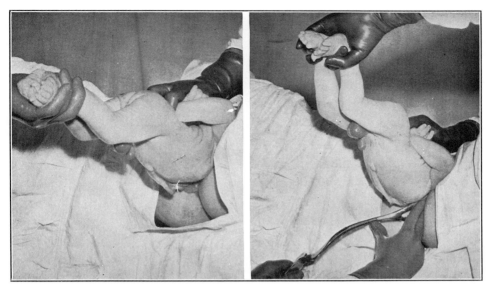

Fig. 12. Position of infant with head in pelvis prior to application of Piper's forceps.

Fig. 13. Introduction of left blade to left side of pelvis. Note upward direction of forceps.

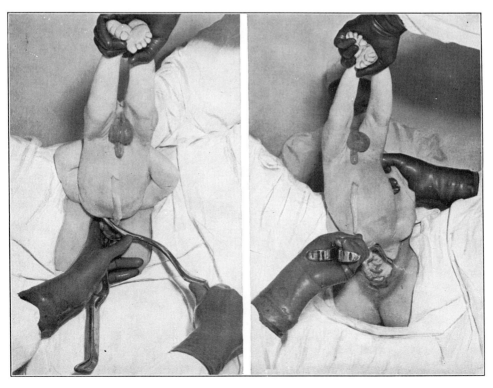

Fig. 14. Introduction of right blade, completing application.

Fig. 15. Forceps locked and traction applied; chin, mouth, and nose emerging over perineum.

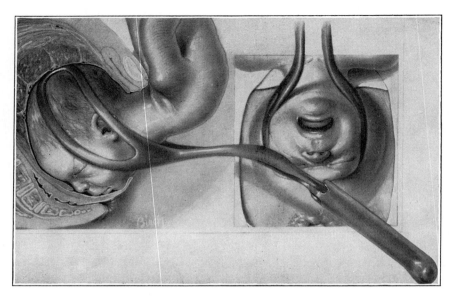

Fig. 16. Piper's forceps on the aftercoming head.

complished under caudal or spinal anesthesia, the increased uterine tone may render the operation difficult. In most instances, cyclopropane gives adequate uterine relaxation; if not, ether or halothane can be used.

PROGNOSIS

In all forms of breech extraction the prognosis for the mother is good, although it is more serious in frank breech than in the other varieties. Increased manipulation of the frank breech may predispose to infection, and the attempt to reach the posterior groin often causes deep and sometimes complete perineal tears before the buttocks have reached the perineum. In extraction by the feet, however, the likelihood of perineal tears is not greater than in cephalic presentations. Moderate degrees of disproportion between the size of the head and the pelvis scarcely influence the maternal prognosis, since the pressure of the head upon the soft parts lasts but seconds or minutes, rather than hours as in cephalic presentations.

For the fetus, however, the outlook is not so favorable and it becomes more serious the higher the presenting part is situated at the beginning of the operation. In addition to the increased risk of tentorial tears and intracerebral hemorrhage, which are inherent in breech presentations, the perinatal mortality is augmented by the greater probability of trauma during extraction. In incomplete breech presentations, moreover, prolapse of the umbilical cord is much more common than in vertex presentations and aggravates further the prognosis for the infant.

Fractures of the humerus and clavicle cannot always be avoided when freeing the arms, and fracture of the femur may occur in difficult frank breech extractions. Hematomas of the sternocleidomastoid muscles occasionally develop after

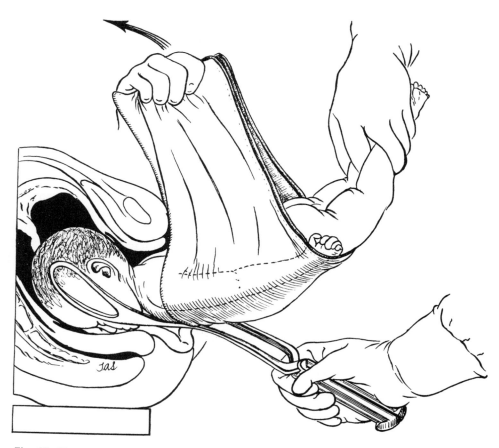

Fig. 17. Management of fetal arms in breech extraction. (From Savage. Obstet Gynec 3:55, 1954.)

the operation, though they usually disappear spontaneously. More serious results, however, may follow separation of the epiphyses of the scapula, humerus, or femur. Exceptionally, paralysis of the arm follows pressure upon the brachial plexus by the fingers in exerting traction, but more frequently it is caused by overstretching the neck while freeing the arms. When the child is forcibly extracted through a contracted pelvis, spoon-shaped depressions or actual fractures of the skull, generally fatal, may result. Occasionally even the neck may be broken when great force is employed. In general, the prognosis for the child in simple extractions is good, whereas in complicated operations it is dubious.

VERSION

Version, or turning, is an operation in which the presentation of the fetus is artificially altered, either substituting one pole of a longitudinal presentation for the other, or converting an oblique or transverse lie into a longitudinal presentation.

According to whether the head or breech is made the presenting part, the operation is designated cephalic or podalic version, respectively. It is also named according to the method by which it is accomplished. Thus in *external version* the manipulations are performed exclusively through the abdominal wall; in *internal version* the entire hand is introduced into the uterine cavity; and in *combined version* one hand manipulates the fetus through the abdominal wall while two or more fingers of the other hand are introduced through the cervix.

EXTERNAL CEPHALIC VERSION

The object of the operation is to substitute a vertex for a less favorable presentation.

Indications. If a breech or shoulder presentation is diagnosed in the last weeks of pregnancy, its conversion into a vertex may be attempted by external maneuvers, provided there is no marked disproportion between the size of the fetus and the pelvis. Cephalic version is thought by many to be indicated because of the increased perinatal mortality attending breech delivery. If the fetus lies transversely, a change of presentation is usually the only alternative to cesarean section.

External cephalic version may be attempted only under the following conditions: (1) the presenting part must not be engaged; (2) the abdominal wall must be sufficiently thin to permit accurate palpation; (3) the abdominal and uterine walls must not be highly irritable; (4) the uterus must contain a sufficient quantity of amniotic fluid to permit the easy movement of the fetus. Anesthesia should never be used, lest undue force be applied.

In the early stages of labor, before the membranes have ruptured, the same indications apply. They may then be extended to oblique presentations as well, though these unstable lies usually convert spontaneously to longitudinal lies as labor progresses. External cephalic version can rarely be effected, however, after the cervix has become fully dilated or the membranes have ruptured.

Method. Cephalic version in modern obstetrics is performed solely by *external manipulations* (Fig. 18). In the recommended technic the patient's abdomen is bared, and the presentation and position of the fetus are carefully ascertained. Each hand then grasps one of the fetal poles. The pole that is to be converted into the presenting part is then gently stroked toward the pelvic inlet while the other is moved in the opposite direction. After version has been completed, the fetus will tend to return to its original position unless engagement occurs. During labor, however, the head may be pressed down into the pelvic inlet and held firmly in position until it becomes fixed under the influence of the uterine contractions.

INTERNAL PODALIC VERSION

Internal podalic version is turning of the fetus by seizing one or both feet and drawing them through the cervix. The operation is followed by breech extraction.

Indications. The very few indications for internal podalic version include occasional examples of the following situations:

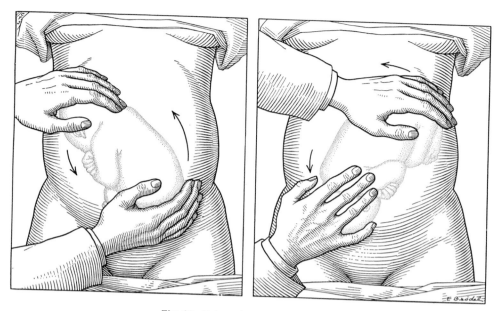

Fig. 18. External cephalic version.

1. Transverse lie with the cervix fully dilated and the membranes intact.
2. Prolapse of the umbilical cord with the cervix fully dilated, vertex unengaged, and membranes very recently ruptured.
3. Second twin.

The only favorable time for performing internal podalic version is just after the cervix has become fully dilated but before the membranes have ruptured. At that time the amniotic fluid is still in utero and the fetus is readily movable. It should never be attempted when the cervix is imperfectly dilated. Occasionally the patient is not seen until some time after rupture of the membranes, when conditions usually make the operation extremely difficult or even impossible. For example, the uterus may be so tightly applied to the body of the fetus as to render the introduction of a hand extremely difficult. In other cases, the lower uterine segment may be so thin that the operation becomes extremely dangerous, probably leading to rupture of the uterus.

Technic. For internal podalic version the patient should be placed in lithotomy position and the usual preoperative preparations carried out. An intravenous infusion system for administering oxytocics continuously after delivery and for administering fluids, including whole blood, in case of hemorrhage caused by uterine atony or rupture should be started. Version should never be attempted without an accurate diagnosis of presentation and position of the fetus (Fig. 19) or with a contracted pelvis. Version is greatly facilitated by the use of long rubber gloves reaching to the elbow and by preliminary wide episiotomy. It is most easily accomplished while the membranes are intact, and it becomes increasingly difficult after their rupture. The anesthetic of choice is ether or halothane, since uterine relaxation is of paramount importance for satisfactory performance of internal podalic version. Although succinylcholine and curarelike drugs produce

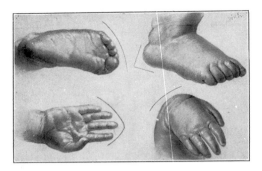

Fig. 19. Internal podalic version. Differentiation of a foot from a hand, parts that feel very much the same in the uterus unless the foot is identified by its heel. A hand presents nothing that resembles a **heel,** a fact that serves to distinguish the two. To attempt to differentiate fingers from toes is less practical. At classical cesarean section, moreover, recognizing a heel avoids pulling out a hand.

relaxation of the abdominal wall and to a lesser degree the pelvic floor, they have no effect on the myometrium.

The operative technics vary somewhat in cephalic and transverse presentations. In the first instance the well-lubricated, sterile-gloved hand and arm must be introduced considerably farther into the vagina and uterus. The choice of the hand to be employed depends upon the location of the fetal small parts. If, for example, the back is directed to the mother's left, the feet can be most conveniently seized with the left hand.

If the membranes are still intact, the hand is passed through the cervix and carried up into the uterine cavity to the feet. The membranes are then ruptured, and, if possible, both feet are seized and downward traction is applied (Figs. 20 and 21). Ordinarily the fetus turns without difficulty, and the feet are readily

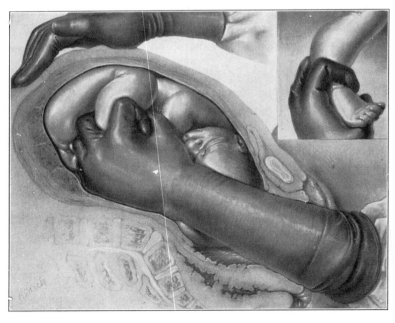

Fig. 20. Internal podalic version. Grasping both feet makes the turning much easier. Note use of long version gloves.

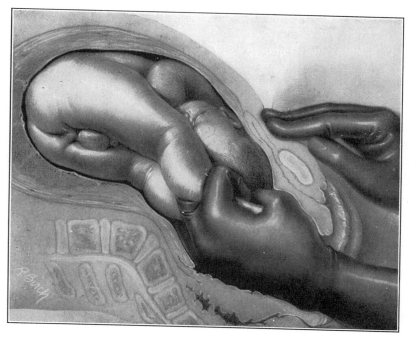

Fig. 21. Internal podalic version. Upward pressure on head is applied as downward traction is exerted on feet.

brought down into the vagina and thence through the outlet. When the knees emerge, version has been effected, and delivery is completed by extraction.

Again it is emphasized that (1) if the amniotic fluid has drained away and the uterus is tightly applied over the fetus, version is difficult or impossible, and (2) any attempts after the lower uterine segment has become markedly stretched may result in rupture of the uterus.

In shoulder presentations, it is preferable to bring down both feet, but one foot will suffice. When only one extremity is brought down, however, the choice of the foot is very important. When the back is directed anteriorly, the lower foot should be seized, for by so doing the fetal back is kept toward the symphysis, whereas if the upper foot is seized, the back may turn in the opposite direction. When the back is directed posteriorly, however, the upper foot is the extremity of choice, since traction upon it will cause the back to rotate to the front. If, however, the lower foot is seized, although anterior rotation will usually occur, the upper buttock is likely to impinge upon the anterior portion of the pelvic brim, and great force may be required to dislodge it. Version and extraction should always be followed by internal exploration of the uterus to make certain that rupture has not occurred.

Prognosis.   For the mother the prognosis after podalic version is good in properly selected cases, provided the patient is in good condition and the operator is skilled. In the case of a tetanically contracted uterus or an over-stretched lower segment, however, forcible attempts at version may lead to uterine rupture and death. In general, the most common cause of traumatic rupture of the uterus is version and extraction.

The prognosis for the singleton fetus is uncertain, depending upon the indication and the difficulty of extraction. In version and extraction for delivery of the second twin, the prognosis for the infant is excellent. In singletons, however, if the operation is undertaken through an imperfectly dilated cervix and the fetal head is arrested by the external os, the time required for extraction is usually so great that death from hypoxia is inevitable. With marked pelvic contraction, moreover, the fetal mortality is very high. In many such cases forcible traction may eventually lead to delivery, but usually not until prolonged compression of the cord has caused pronounced hypoxia and fetal death. Injuries to the head resulting from pressure are additional causes of perinatal death during delivery or shortly thereafter.

REFERENCES

Bracht, E.   (Manual aid in breech presentation). Z Geburtsh Gynaek 112:271, 1936.
Kiwisch, F. H.   Beiträge zur Geburtskunde. Würzburg, I. Abth., 69, 1846.
Mauriceau, F.   (The method of delivering the woman when the infant presents one or two feet first). Traité des Maladies des Femmes Grosses, 6me éd., 1721, pp. 280–285.
Pinard, A.   (On version by external maneuvers). Traité du Palper Abdominal, Paris, 1889.
Plentl, A. A., and Stone, R. E.   Bracht maneuver. Obstet Gynec Survey 8:313, 1953.
Savage, J. E.   Management of the fetal arms in breech extraction. Obstet Gynec 3:55, 1954.
Smellie, W.   Smellie's Treatise on the Theory and Practice of Midwifery, Vol. 1, A. H. McClintock (ed.). London, The New Sydenham Society, 1876, pp. 305–307.
Veit, G.   (On version by external manipulation). Hamburgisches Magazin für die Geburtshülfe, 1807.

42

CESAREAN SECTION

Cesarean section may be defined as delivery of the infant through incisions in the abdominal and uterine walls. Incision of the uterus (hysterotomy) is the essence of the operation; therefore it does not include removal of the fetus from the abdominal cavity in cases of rupture of the uterus or abdominal pregnancy. The origin of the term is obscure.

Three principal explanations have been suggested:

1. According to legend, Julius Caesar was born in this manner, with the result that the procedure became known as the "Caesarean operation." Several circumstances weaken this explanation, however. First, the mother of Julius Caesar lived for many years after his birth. Even as late as the seventeenth century, the operation was almost invariably fatal, according to the most dependable writers of that period. It is thus improbable that Caesar's mother could have survived the procedure in 100 B.C. Second, the operation, whether performed on the living or dead, is not mentioned by any medical writer before the Middle Ages. Historical details of the origin of the family name "Caesar" are found in Pickrell's monograph.

2. It has been widely believed that the name of the operation is derived from a Roman law, supposedly created by Numa Pompilius (eighth century, B.C.), ordering that the procedure be performed upon women dying in the last few weeks of pregnancy in the hope of saving the child. This explanation then holds that this *lex regia*, as it was called at first, became the *lex caesarea* under the emperors, and the operation itself became known as the *caesarean* operation. The German term "Kaiserschnitt" reflects this derivation.

Numa Pompilius, however, was said to be the successor to Romulus, the mythical "first king" of Rome. Any writings later attributed to Numa Pompilius are dismissed by modern historians as sheer forgeries. If, moreover, this operation had actually been a legal requirement in antiquity, it would certainly have been mentioned by medical writers of the period; but, it was not.

3. The word "caesarean," as applied to the operation, was derived sometime in the Middle Ages from the Latin verb *caedere*, "to cut." An obvious cognate is the word "caesura," a "cutting," or pause, in a line of verse. This explanation of the term "caesarean" seems most logical, but exactly when it was first applied to the operation is uncertain. Since "section" is derived from the Latin verb "seco," which also means "cut," the term "caesarean section" seems tautological.

It is customary in the United States to replace the "ae" ligature in the first syllable of "caesarean" with the letter "e"; in Great Britain, however, the "ae" is still retained.

History. From the time of Virgil's Aeneas to Shakespeare's Macduff, poets have repeatedly referred to persons "untimely ripped" from their mother's womb. Ancient historians such as Pliny, moreover, say that Scipio Africanus (the conqueror of Hannibal), Martius, and Julius Caesar were all born thus. In regard to Julius Caesar, Pliny adds that it was from this circumstance that the surname arose by which the Roman emperors were known. Birth in this extraordinary manner, as described in ancient mythology and legend, was believed to confer supernatural powers and elevate the heroes so born above ordinary mortals.

In evaluating these references to abdominal delivery in antiquity, it is pertinent that no such operation is even mentioned by Hippocrates, Galen, Celsus, Paulus, Soranus, or any other medical writer of the period. If cesarean section were actually employed at that time, it is particularly surprising that Soranus, whose extensive work written in the second century A.D. covers all aspects of obstetrics, does not refer to it. In Genesis (II:21) it is written: "And the Lord God caused a deep sleep to fall upon Adam, and he slept: and he took one of his ribs, and closed up the flesh instead thereof." Are we to conclude from this statement that general anesthesia and thoracic surgery were known in pre-Mosaic times? It would probably be just as logical to draw comparable conclusions about the beginnings of cesarean section from the myths and fantasies that have come down to us.

Several references to abdominal delivery appear in the Talmud, compiled between the second and sixth centuries A.D., but whether they had any background in terms of clinical usage is conjectural. There can be no doubt, however, that cesarean section on the dead was first practiced soon after the Christian Church gained dominance, as a measure directed at baptism of the child. Faith in the validity of some of these early reports is rudely shaken, however, when they glibly state that a living, robust child was obtained 8 to 24 *hours* after the death of the mother.

Some of the early reports of cesarean section on the living excite similar skepticism. The case often cited as representing the first cesarean section performed on a living woman is that attributed to a German gelder named Jacob Nufer, who is said to have carried out the operation on his wife in the year 1500. Not only did his wife survive (a miracle in itself) but she lived to give birth to two subsequent children after normal labors, in a period when suturing of the uterine wound during cesarean section was unknown. The case was not reported until almost a hundred years later (1591), by an author who based his description on hearsay handed down through three generations.

Cesarean section on the living was first recommended, and the current name of the operation used, in the celebrated work of François Rousset entitled "Traité Nouveau de l'Hystérotomotokie ou l'Enfantement Césarien," published in 1581. Rousset had never performed or witnessed the operation, his information having been based chiefly on letters from friends. He reported 14 successful cesarean sections, a fact in itself difficult to accept. When it is further stated that 6 of the 14 operations were performed on the same woman, the credulity of the most gullible is exhausted.

The apocryphal nature of most early reports on cesarean section has been stressed because many of them have been accepted without question. Authoritative statements by dependable obstetricians about early use of the operation, however, did not appear in the literature until the mid-seventeenth century, as for instance in the classic work of the great French obstetrician François Mauriceau, first published in 1668. These statements show without doubt that the operation was employed on the living in rare and desperate cases during the latter half of the sixteenth century, and that it was usually fatal. Details of the history of cesarean section are to be found in Fasbender's classic text.

The appalling maternal mortality of cesarean section continued until the beginning of the twentieth century. In Great Britain and Ireland, the maternal death rate from the operation had mounted in 1865 to 85 per cent. In Paris during the 90 years ending in 1876, not a single successful cesarean section had been performed. Harris noted that as late as 1887 cesarean section was actually more successful when performed by the patient herself, or when the abdomen was ripped open by the horn of a bull. He collected 9 such cases with 5 recoveries from the literature, and contrasted them with 12 cesarean sections performed in New York City during the same period, with only 1 recovery.

The turning point in the evolution of cesarean section came in 1882 when Max

Sänger, then a 28-year-old assistant of Credé in the University Clinic at Leipzig, introduced suturing of the uterine wall. The long neglect of so simple an expedient as uterine suture was not the result of oversight, but stemmed from a deeply rooted belief that sutures in the uterus were superfluous as well as harmful. In meeting these objections Sänger, who had himself used sutures in only one case, documented their value, not from the sophisticated medical centers of Europe, but from frontier America. There, in outposts from Ohio to Louisiana, 17 cesarean sections had been reported in which silver wire sutures had been used, with the survival of 8 mothers, an extraordinary record in those days. In a table included in his monograph, Sänger gives full credit to these frontier surgeons for providing the supporting data for his hypothesis. The problem of hemorrhage was the first and most serious problem to be solved. Details are found in Eastman's review.

Although the introduction of uterine sutures reduced the mortality of the operation from hemorrhage, generalized peritonitis remained the dominant cause of death; hence, various types of operations were devised to meet this scourge. The earliest was the Porro procedure, in use before Sänger's time, which combined subtotal cesarean hysterectomy with marsupialization of the cervical stump. The first extraperitoneal operation was described by Frank in 1907 and with various modifications, as introduced by Latzko, Sellheim, and Waters, was employed until recent years. The next phase in development of the modern technic of cesarean section was concerned with simpler operations designed to reduce infection.

In 1912 Krönig contended that the main advantage of the extraperitoneal technic consisted not so much in avoiding the peritoneal cavity entirely as in opening the uterus through its thin lower segment and then covering the incision with peritoneum. To accomplish this end he cut through the vesical reflection of the peritoneum from one round ligament to the other and separated it and the bladder from the lower uterine segment and cervix. The lower portion of the uterus was then opened through a vertical median incision and the child extracted by forceps. The uterine incision was then closed and buried under the vesical peritoneum. With minor modifications this low segment technic was introduced into the United States by Beck and popularized by DeLee and others. A particularly important modification was recommended by Kerr in 1926, who preferred a transverse rather than a longitudinal uterine incision. The Kerr technic is the most commonly employed type of cesarean section today.

The two main hazards of cesarean section have long been *infection* and *hemorrhage;* accordingly, the history of cesarean section over the past 75 years is largely an account of the conquest of these two threats. Improvements in operative and aseptic technic have done much to forestall infection, while the introduction of antibiotics has made death from peritonitis and other postoperative infections a rarity. Blood banks and transfusions have, during the same period, virtually eliminated death from hemorrhage. As a result of these advances, cesarean section, once the deadliest of operations, is now one of the safest.

Indications   The indications for cesarean section have been discussed in connection with the various conditions that sometimes require the operation. In about one half of the cesarean sections performed in this country today, the main and often the only indication is a previous cesarean section scar. These operations are usually called "repeat sections" and are justified on the basis that the scar may possibly rupture, especially during labor (Ch. 32, p. 937). The other half of all cesarean sections, "primary sections," are performed for a variety of reasons as shown in Figure 1, which is based on 9,680 primary cesarean sections performed in 10 clinics in the Obstetrical Statistical Cooperative.

The most frequent indication for primary cesarean section is dystocia. A major component of dystocia is "fetopelvic disproportion," often called "cephalopelvic disproportion." These two terms are widely employed to designate a large group of cases in which dystocia is the result of some kind of *spatial* inadequacy.

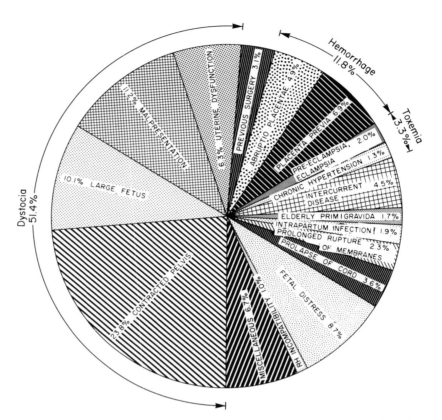

Fig. 1. Indications for primary cesarean section in 2,547 operations. (From the Obstetrical Statistical Cooperative, 1965 through 1968.)

The clearest examples are pelvic contraction, a tumor blocking the birth canal, or a huge child. Not infrequently, a combination of factors may place a case in this category. For example, two or more of the following may be associated: a moderately large child, a minor aberration in pelvic size or architecture, faulty flexion of the head causing a larger diameter to present, and uterine dysfunction.

Occasionally a cesarean section may be required because of several indications, no single one of which in the particular instance would justify the operation. For example, a preeclamptic patient with moderate pelvic contraction and an unengaged head may have uterine dysfunction. In the presence of several "partial indications" the hazards of vaginal delivery may be additive, and when taken together these "fractions" of an indication may sometimes make a whole. Nicety of judgment is required, however, and sweeping statements are therefore improper. In the preparation of Figure 1, cases with multiple indications were carefully scrutinized and only the main indication used.

Another, possibly more informative, method of analyzing statistics on cesarean section is ascertaining in what proportion of cases of a given condition abdominal delivery was performed. To this end the percentage of patients delivered by cesarean section for a number of complications is shown in Table 1.

Primary cesarean section is occasionally indicated in multiparas. For example,

Table 1. Incidence of Cesarean Section by Specific Complication
(Obstetrical Statistical Cooperative, 1965–1968)

Indication	No. of Cases	No. of C.S.	Per Cent of C.S.
Placenta previa	289	194	67.1
Abruptio placentae	908	141	15.5
Preeclampsia and eclampsia	2,326	52	2.2
Diabetes	578	110	19.0
Prolapse of cord	793	95	12.0
Term breech	1,459	142	9.7

rather than to allow vaginal delivery in all instances of nonrepetitive indications, of the abdominal deliveries reported by Klein, Robbins, and Gabaeff, about 15 per cent were primary sections in multiparas. The indication was hemorrhage in the majority of cases, and cephalopelvic disproportion in about one fourth. In a more recent study, Van Praagh and Tovell report that 1 out of every 6 primary cesarean sections performed at the Women's Hospital in New York were in multiparas. Diabetes and previous pelvic operations also contributed to the indications in this group of patients.

Incidence.   In a former medical era the excellence of an obstetric service was judged by the paucity of cesarean sections performed. In the past decade, however, there has been a considerable shift in viewpoint regarding the validity of this criterion. Not only has cesarean section become progressively safer for the mother, but the focus of obstetric thinking has been directed increasingly toward perinatal survival and the prevention of trauma to the child during birth. The idea that cesarean section converts a healthy gravida into an obstetric cripple, furthermore, is now viewed by many obstetricians with increasing skepticism. Not only may a cesarean delivery be followed by a series of vaginal deliveries, but according to Piver and Johnston, repeated abdominal deliveries entailing four, five, and even six such operations are not uncommon. Although cesarean section remains more hazardous than normal vaginal delivery, there are many series of 1,000 consecutive cesarean sections without a single maternal death. The hazards of abdominal delivery, both immediate and remote, have been so reduced that the shift in viewpoint is both understandable and commendable.

Although it is still more common in this country to repeat cesarean sections many foreign reports deny the necessity for this practice. O'Driscoll, for example, prefers vaginal delivery, whenever possible, after low segment but not classical cesarean sections. McGarry makes the point even more strongly by suggesting that only 12 per cent of patients delivered abdominally need subsequent cesarean sections. He even permits the use of oxytocin to stimulate a uterus with a scar. Schilling reports a fourfold increase in vaginal delivery after cesarean section between the years 1946 and 1964. He even mentions vaginal delivery after section for disproportion. In evaluating the occasional successful result in an inherently risky situation, however, the obstetrician must distinguish luck from sound judgment and must understand that similar management in similar circumstances may lead to tragedy on a subsequent occasion. The recent report of Stephens and Brown indicates that the maternal and perinatal mortalities from uterine rupture are 4 per cent and 75 per cent, respectively.

The incidence of the operation in the United States is given by Chase as between 4.2 and 5.7 per cent. Comparable figures for England and Wales and for the Netherlands are 2.7 per cent and 1.25 per cent, respectively. However, the incidence varies rather markedly among clinics according to the types of patients and the policy of the staff, particularly in regard to repeating cesarean sections. An idea of modern incidence rates can be obtained from Table 2, which contains

Table 2. Incidence of Cesarean Section

Source	Year	Deliveries	Per Cent Cesarean Section
Obstetrical Statistical Cooperative	1965–68	63,238	7.0
Kings County	1967	4,971	6.8
Royal Victoria	1966	3,230	6.7
Hartford, Connecticut	1964	5,287	9.7
Long Island College Hospital	1968	2,186	7.7
University of Maryland	1967	2,185	9.1
San Francisco General	1967	1,095	5.0
University of Oklahoma	1967	1,098	6.0
University of Utah	1967	822	4.0

data not only from the Obstetrical Statistical Cooperative and the city of Hartford, Connecticut, but also from some of the leading teaching hospitals in the United States.

A study of Table 2 shows that the incidence of cesarean section in these institutions hovers around the 6 to 7 per cent mark, a figure that has gradually risen over the past few decades. With the increase in cesarean section rate has come a progressive decrease in the perinatal mortality rate in most clinics. The same decrease has been reported from European clinics (Raics). Although the increment in abdominal deliveries is not the only explanation for this fall, it must play a significant role.

Timing of Repeat Cesarean Section. The question of a previous cesarean section as an indication for abdominal delivery has been discussed in Chapter 32 (p. 939). Once a decision has been made in the course of pregnancy to repeat a cesarean section, however, the timing of the operation is of the greatest importance to prevent the delivery of a premature infant. The threat is so serious and errors in estimating the maturity of the fetus so common that many clinics follow a policy of awaiting the onset of labor before repeating the cesarean section. In many cases this program may be best, but it has the disadvantages of any emergency operation, including lack of preparation of the patient, possible lack of anesthesia personnel, and in some hospitals, difficulty in obtaining an operating room at once. It therefore seems better to set a definite date and perform the operation as an elective procedure but only *if the maturity of the fetus can be estimated with confidence.* We have recently evaluated the degree of accuracy achieved through clinical estimation of the weight of the fetus prior to cesarean section. Fifty per cent of the time the examiners' estimates based on history, inspection, and palpation were quite acceptable, being within 10 per cent of the actual birth weight. Nonetheless, the discrepancy on occasion was quite marked. In general, when the infant weighed less than 5 pounds the estimate was too high. Conversely, when the infant weighed more than 7 pounds, the estimate frequently was too low. Niswander and associates have evaluated the use of external uterine measurements to estimate birth weight. Neither of 2 methods yielded more accurate estimates than did simple abdominal palpation. For confidence about the maturity of the baby, the following three findings should be in agreement: (1) the expected date of confinement, based on the last menstrual period as stated with apparent accuracy by the patient; (2) an estimated fetal weight of 3,000 g or more, as estimated by experienced examiners; (3) *definite auscultation of the fetal heart by a competent examiner at or before the twentieth week of pregnancy,* and quickening at 16 to 18 weeks calculated from the last menstrual period as stated by the patient. If these findings are not in agreement, the patient should be allowed to go into labor before the cesarean section is repeated. The date set for repeating the section should not be more than 10 days before the calculated date of confinement unless some other complication forces the issue.

Additional help may be provided by the laboratory in assessing fetal maturity. Analysis of the amniotic fluid of a mature fetus will often provide the following data: a concentration of *creatinine* of at least 2 mg per cent, negligible *bilirubin*, and *orange-staining epithelial cells* after treatment with Nile blue sulfate. Sonography can provide a reasonable estimate of fetal maturity by measurements of the fetal skull and volume of the placenta (Hellman and associates). For a further discussion of fetal maturity see Chapter 37 (p. 1029).

Contraindications. In modern obstetric practice there are virtually no contraindications to cesarean section, provided the proper operation is selected. Cesarean section is less frequently indicated, however, if the infant is dead or too small for survival. Exceptions to this generalization include pelvic contraction of such a degree that vaginal delivery by any means is impossible; placental abruption with the cervix firm, long, and undilated; most cases of placenta previa; and most cases of neglected transverse lie. Debate still centers about the validity of fetal indications alone, which formerly were not considered adequate grounds for cesarean section. In current practice, however, there is an increasing tendency to resort to abdominal delivery in the face of fetal distress manifested by a slow or irregular fetal heart rate and the passage of meconium, as discussed on page 1009.

Lower Segment Cesarean Section. In general, the lower uterine segment cesarean section utilizing the transverse uterine incision is the operation of choice for the following reasons: (1) it reduces the danger of postoperative infection; (2) it reduces the danger of intestinal obstruction; (3) it places the uterine incision in the area of least uterine activity; (4) it is associated with loss of less blood and is easier to repair than the classical incision; and (5) the probability of rupture of the scar in any subsequent pregnancy is lower than after classical section.

Operative Technic. After the bladder is emptied through an indwelling catheter, the patient is placed supine or in slight Trendelenburg position. An abdominal incision 12 to 15 cm long should be made, extending from above the symphysis to just below the umbilicus. The margins of the abdominal incision are then drawn apart by suitable retractors and the lowermost portion of the uterus exposed. The loose peritoneum is grasped with dissecting forceps just below its firm attachment to the anterior wall of the uterus and is incised transversely for almost the entire distance between the round ligaments (Fig. 2). Then, the peritoneum and upper posterior surface of the bladder are bluntly separated

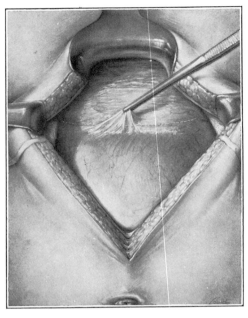

Fig. 2. Low segment cesarean section (the umbilicus below, the symphysis pubis above). The transverse incision in the peritoneum is made about 1 inch below the point where the peritoneum is firmly attached to the uterus. Incision of the peritoneum, as indicated by the dotted line, creates an upper and a lower flap of peritoneum.

from the uterine wall (Figs. 3 and 4). In this way two flaps are formed, a short upper flap of uterine peritoneum, and a somewhat longer lower flap, which consists of peritoneum and the posterior surface of the bladder.

The uterine incision may be made either transversely (Fig. 5) or longitudinally (Fig. 6). The former incision is often called the "Kerr technic" and the latter the "Krönig technic." In either case care must be exerted to penetrate completely the uterine wall but not cut the fetus. Once the initial incision is made with

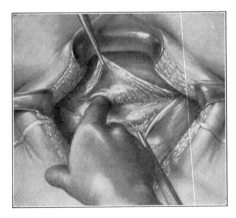

Fig. 3. Low segment cesarean section (symphysis pubis above). Dissection of peritoneum and bladder off uterus to expose lower uterine segment.

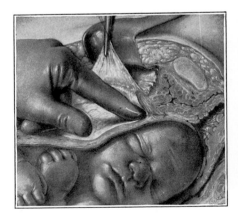

Fig. 4. Low segment cesarean section. Cross section showing dissection of bladder off uterus to expose lower uterine segment.

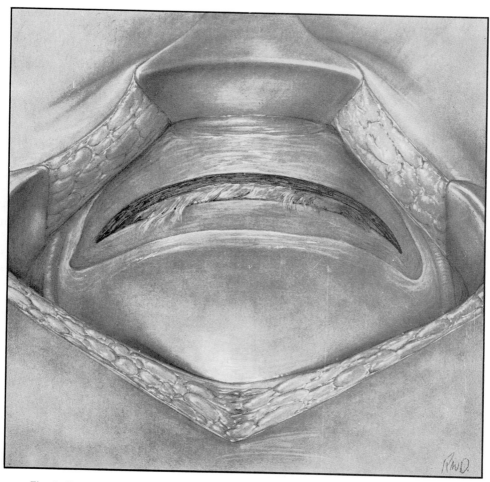

Fig. 5. Transverse uterine incision in low segment cesarean section (Kerr technic).

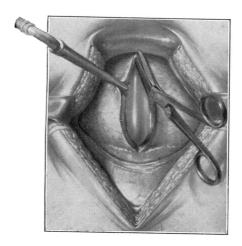

Fig. 6. Low segment cesarean section; vertical incision. The bladder is protected by the retractor, which at the same time helps expose the lower uterine segment while the incision is made.

a scalpel, it is usually completed with bandage scissors, or in case of the transverse incision sometimes bluntly with the fingers.

In most cases the transverse incision is probably preferable because much less undermining of the bladder is required, delivery of the fetal head is easier, and the entire incision is more likely to remain in the lower segment. The transverse incision should be semilunar with the concavity upward, and care should be taken to direct its terminal ends upward and to keep an inch away from the uterine arteries. These two admonitions should forestall extension of the incision into the uterine arteries, the chief hazard of the transverse incision. Should the transverse incision extend to sever the uterine artery, however, the vessel usually can be promptly ligated and bleeding thus controlled without resorting to hysterectomy.

Delivery of the fetal head from the lower segment incision may pose considerable problems for the beginner, but with a little experience it becomes simple. It may frequently be facilitated by drawing the head up from the pelvis before making an incision in the lower uterine segment. If the vertical incision is used, a hand should be inserted between the pubis and the head, and the face rotated anteriorly. The hand is then removed, and in most instances with this incision, the head is delivered by forceps. This technic is illustrated in Figures 7 and 8. If the transverse incision is used, delivery of the fetal head presents little or no problem. A hand is inserted between the head and the symphysis, and the face is rotated slightly posteriorly. Simple upward traction serves to deliver the

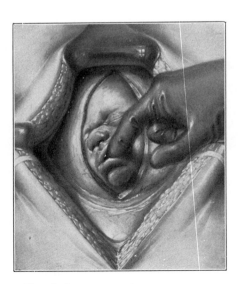

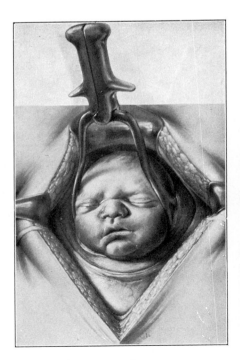

Fig. 7. Low segment cesarean section. A finger in the baby's mouth rotates the face anteriorly, and the chin is delivered over the upper edge of the incision.

Fig. 8. Low segment cesarean section. Delivery of infant's head **slowly** with forceps.

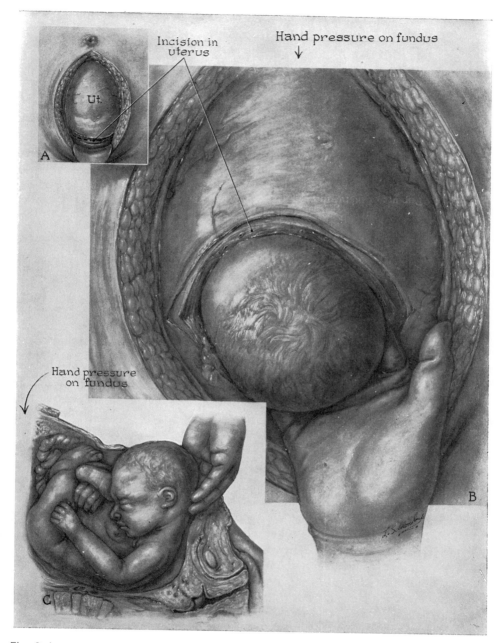

A

Incision in uterus

Hand pressure on fundus

Ut.

Hand pressure on fundus

B

C

Fig. 9. Low segment cesarean section; transverse incision. The head is easily delivered manually.

head by extension (Fig. 9). There are, of course, numerous other satisfactory methods of delivery of the head. If the head is quite deep in the birth canal it may be advantageous to have an attendant wearing a sterile glove dislodge it upward through the vagina.

Repair of both incisions in the lower segment is similar. After delivery of the

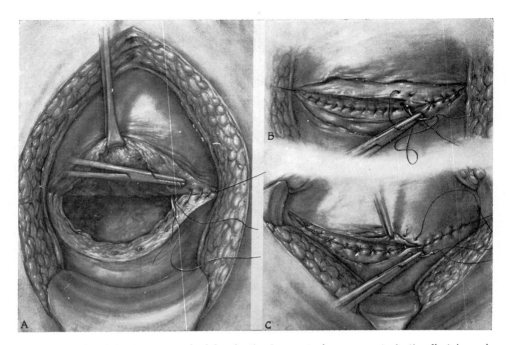

Fig. 10. Repair of the transverse incision in the lower uterine segment. A, the first layer is a continuous suture including the endometrium. Some authorities believe that this suture should exclude the endometrium, but in our experience better approximation is attained by the method illustrated. B, the second layer consists of interrupted figure-of-eight sutures including the myometrium and serosa. C, a continuous suture repairs the divided flap of vesicouterine peritoneum.

placenta the edges of the incised myometrium are grasped, and ovum forceps, T-clamps, or instruments such as those shown in Figure 10A are applied. They should hold the tissue firmly without injury. Repair is begun at one end of the incision, using a continuous closure. In some clinics both layers are closed with continuous sutures. The usual material employed for suture is #0 or #1 chromic catgut. Many obstetricians prefer to place this suture in the uterine muscle without incorporating the decidua. It is questionable, however, whether this detail of technic is of great importance in eventual healing of the scar. A second layer of suture includes more superficial layers of the myometrium (Fig. 10B). Once the lower segment has been repaired the bladder flap is brought up and sewed to the upper layer of visceral peritoneum with a continuous suture, usually # 00 chromic catgut (Fig. 10C).

Hysterographic studies by Poidevin and, more recently, by Waniorek suggest that continuous sutures, excessive numbers of sutures, and inclusion of decidua are detrimental to healing of the scar. Schiøler and co-workers in an extensive study concluded that hysterography two and five months postpartum was not helpful in predicting the ultimate integrity of the uterine scar.

Except in special circumstances, lower segment cesarean section should be the standard procedure. This technic is in fact neither more difficult nor time-consuming than the classical operation. With minimal experience it can be performed with just as much facility and speed as the classical operation. Indeed, suturing of the classical incision is more difficult and time-consuming than repair of the lower segment incision.

Classical Cesarean Section. Although classical cesarean section has been largely and correctly superseded by the lower segment procedure, it is valuable in special circumstances: (1) When *dense adhesions* from previous cesarean sections make access to the lower segment difficult or render the bladder tightly adherent to the uterus, stubborn insistence on performing a lower segment operation may produce extensive hemorrhage and injury to the bladder. (2) When the fetus is in *transverse lie,* unless it is small, its extraction through a transverse lower segment incision may prove very difficult, sometimes causing an upward or downward extension of the incision and resulting in a jagged T-shaped wound. (3) In certain cases of anterior placenta previa, the classical incision may be preferable (Ch. 23, p. 621).

Operative Technic. A midline abdominal incision 12 to 15 cm long is made. If markedly rotated, the uterus should be repositioned to permit vertical incision approximately in the midline. It is desirable to avoid spillage of amniotic fluid and blood into the peritoneal cavity, thereby increasing the likelihood of a smoother convalescence. Packing around the uterine incision and aspiration of amniotic fluid through a small hole in the membranes aid in keeping the field dry. The anterior surface of the uterus is then opened longitudinally in the midline, with the lower end of the incision terminating just above the reflection of the

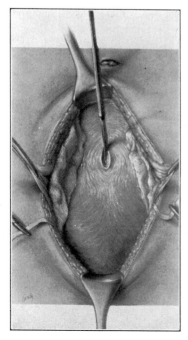

Fig. 11. Classical cesarean section (the umbilicus above, the symphysis pubis below). Beginning incision in uterus with scalpel.

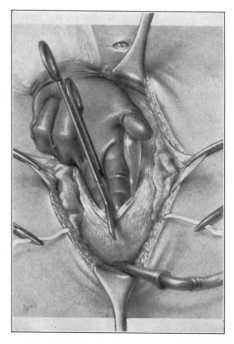

Fig. 12. Classical cesarean section. Uterine incision extended with bandage scissors.

vesicouterine peritoneal flap (Fig. 11). The incision is then enlarged to a length of about 10 cm (Fig. 12). The membranes are ruptured and the obstetrician's hand is inserted through the uterine incision to grasp one or both feet of the baby and effect extraction (Fig. 13). Two clamps are applied to the cord, which is cut between them. The child is then handed to an assistant. If the placenta lies under the incision, it should be displaced to one side if possible or at least rapidly transected to minimize fetal hemorrhage. Shortly after delivery of the child, the uterus usually contracts and maternal hemorrhage is greatly decreased. To ensure rapid contraction of the uterus, 0.2 mg of ergonovine should be administered intramuscularly or, preferably, 10 units of oxytocin should be given by intravenous infusion just as the child is delivered.

After extracting the infant, if excessive bleeding occurs or if disease of the pelvic organs is suspected, the uterus may be exposed by lifting it through the abdominal incision for inspection. The adnexa may be examined at the same time. If portions of the placenta and membranes are still attached to the uterus, they should be removed promptly and completely (Fig. 14). Even when the operation is performed before the onset of labor, it is usually unnecessary to dilate the cervix, since it is sufficiently patulous to permit free drainage.

The uterine wound is then closed in such a manner that the cut edges are evenly and completely coapted and hemorrhage is adequately controlled. One satisfactory method employs a layer of continuous chromic catgut (#0 or #1) to approximate the inner halves of the cut edges, followed by a continuous chromic catgut suture for the outer half, and finally a continuous suture for the peritoneum and the immediately subjacent superficial myometrium (Fig. 15). Blood should be removed from the pelvis and gutters, and the abdominal wound should be closed in separate layers.

Cesarean Hysterectomy.   The greatest usefulness of cesarean section followed by hysterectomy is in certain cases of myomas and in multiparas with gross infections, as in a neglected transverse lie. Stevenson and co-workers recently reported that 45 of the 85 maternal deaths from puerperal sepsis in their series were in women who underwent cesarean section. These figures support the practice of removal of infected uteri, as in cases in which cesarean section is performed after prolonged rupture of the membranes. As stated on page 630, a Couvelaire uterus in itself is a very rare indication. Of the 23,490 transabdominal deliveries in the series of the Obstetrical Statistical Cooperative, 2.5 per cent were cesarean hysterectomies; the figure varies considerably from clinic to clinic, however, according to the extent to which the procedure is used for sterilization.

Two advantages of cesarean hysterectomy over tubal sterilization operations are often mentioned. First, hysterectomy is 100 per cent effective, whereas tubal sterilization sometimes fails to prevent pregnancy. Second, total hysterectomy prevents later uterine disease, especially cancer. The first alleged advantage is weakened if the Irving technic for tubal sterilization is employed, since the rate of failure of that procedure approaches zero. In considering the question of cancer, it is necessary to know how many deaths from uterine cancer can be prevented if 100 total cesarean hysterectomies are performed in women around 30 years of age. On the average, there will be only one or two deaths from uterine cancer over the course of the following 50 years. This estimate is based on the following assumptions: 2 to 4 per cent of women 30 years of age will develop uterine cancer in the future, a 50 per cent cure rate, and the unduly pessimistic assumption that this

Fig. 13. Classical cesarean section. Delivery of the infant after version. The calf of the infant's leg may be grasped with a towel rather than with the gloved hand as shown, in order to secure better traction.

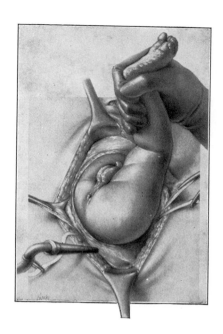

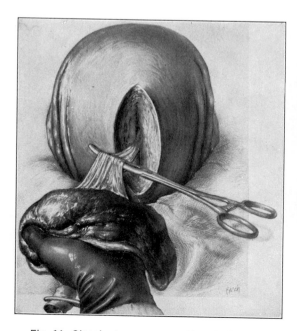

Fig. 14. Classical cesarean section. Delivery of placenta and membranes. The membranes must be carefully and completely removed.

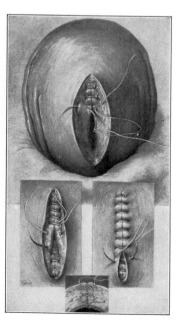

Fig. 15. Classical cesarean section. Three-layer closure.

figure will not be improved in the next few decades. To compare this expectancy of death from uterine carcinoma with the operative mortality of cesarean hysterectomy, however, is meaningless, since fatalities from hysterectomy are immediate whereas most of the deaths from cancer will not occur until the hypothetical 30-year-old woman is between 45 and 70 years of age. It therefore does not seem justified, as a rule, to impose on the 98 or 99 women in 100 who desire to be sterilized this unnecessarily extensive operation in order to prevent perhaps one or two deaths from uterine cancer many years later. The main support for this viewpoint is the operative mortality of cesarean section–total hysterectomy, which, except in the hands of expert gynecologic surgeons, approaches or even exceeds the estimated mortality of future uterine cancer in these women. In a 1964 review of total cesarean hysterectomies performed at the Sloane Hospital for Women, O'Leary and Steer point out that the operation is followed by a higher morbidity rate than that of cesarean section with tubal sterilization. They indi-

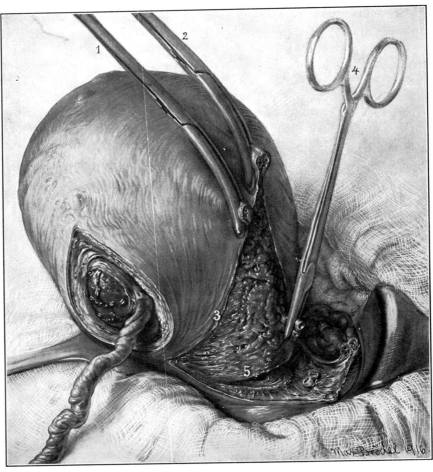

Fig. 16. Supravaginal hysterectomy following cesarean section. Placenta in utero. 1, clamp applied to round ligament; 2, clamp applied to severed fallopian tube and broad ligament; 3, anterior peritoneal flap; 4, clamp applied to uterine artery; 5, transverse incision through cervix.

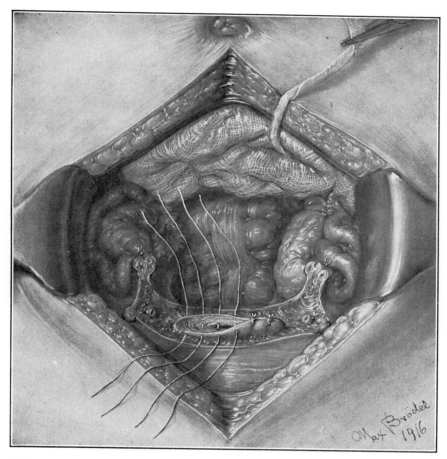

Fig. 17. Cesarean section followed by supravaginal hysterectomy. Note the tubes and ovaries in situ, the method of suturing the cervical stump, and the defects in the broad ligaments, which are later closed with continuous sutures.

cated, furthermore, that in some cases difficulty in identification of the limits of the cervix led to incomplete removal of the cervix. That consequence, of course, invalidates the argument that the operation always provides prophylaxis against the subsequent development of cervical carcinoma.

Blood loss typically is greater with cesarean section followed by total hysterectomy than with cesarean section and tubal sterilization. Pritchard and associates, for example, identified a mean blood loss of nearly 1½ liters with cesarean section accompanied by elective total hysterectomy, or a half liter more than with cesarean section alone. As a consequence the majority of patients who undergo hysterectomy are transfused. Brenner and associates, for example, note that two-thirds of their patients who at the time of cesarean section underwent hysterectomy just for sterilization received one or more blood transfusions.

Many recent reports, such as those of Webb and Gibbs, however, provide clinical support for the practice of more widespread cesarean hysterectomy in preference to tubal sterilization at the time of cesarean section. In a recent study of 800 tubal sterilizations, Haynes and Wolfe reported that 50 of their 800 patients followed for more than three and a half years after the tubal sterilization developed gynecologic disease that resulted in hysterectomy. The incidence of cervical carcinoma was high in this group, which included 9 preinvasive and 6 invasive cancers.

When the uterus is diseased with myomas or a defective scar for example, cesarean hysterectomy may often be the procedure of choice. How often to perform elective cesarean hysterectomy solely as a means of sterilization, however, remains debatable.

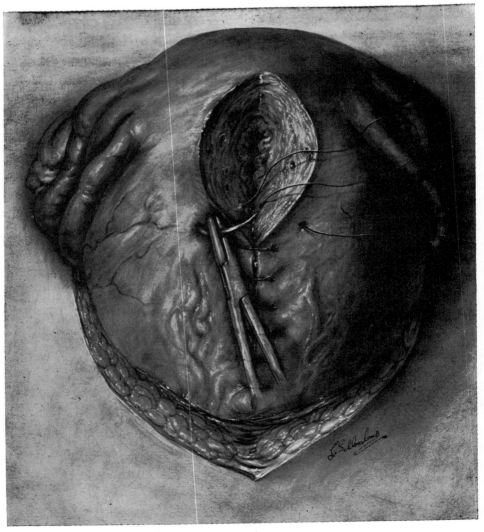

Fig. 18. Closure of uterine incision of classical cesarean section with a single layer of interrupted sutures prior to total abdominal hysterectomy.

Technic of Cesarean Hysterectomy. After delivery of the infant by classical or low segment cesarean section, supravaginal or total hysterectomy, usually with retention of the adnexa, can be carried out according to standard operative technics (Figs. 16 and 17). Although the vessels in the gravid uterus are larger than those in the nonpregnant organ, hysterectomy is usually facilitated by the ease of development of tissue planes. The incision in the uterus is repaired with a continuous or a few interrupted sutures to prevent excessive bleeding (Fig. 18). The uterus is then elevated out of the abdominal cavity and the round ligaments

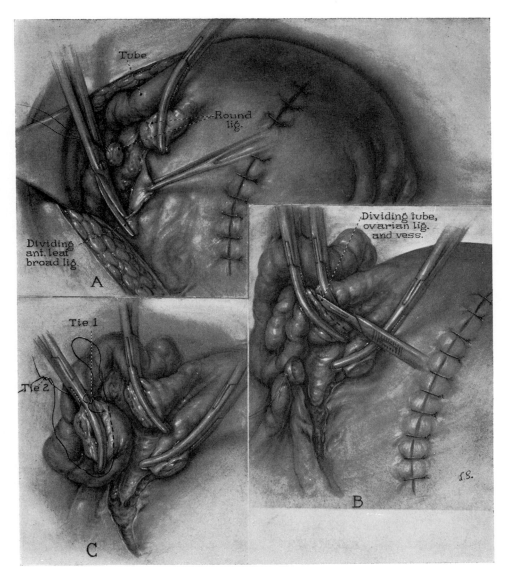

Fig. 19. Total abdominal hysterectomy. A, division of round ligament. B, beginning division of the anterior leaf of the broad ligament. C, ligation of severed fallopian tube and utero-ovarian vessels.

on either side are divided between clamp and ligature (Fig. 19). An incision is made into the anterior leaf of the broad ligament on either side and carried across the midline above the bladder, forming a flap of vesicouterine peritoneum (Fig. 20). The fallopian tubes, uteroovarian ligaments, and ovarian vessels are then doubly clamped, severed, and doubly ligated. The posterior leaf of the broad ligament is next divided (Fig. 21). The bladder and attached peritoneal flap are then dissected off the lower uterine segment and retracted out of the operative field. The uterine arteries on either side are then skeletonized, doubly clamped

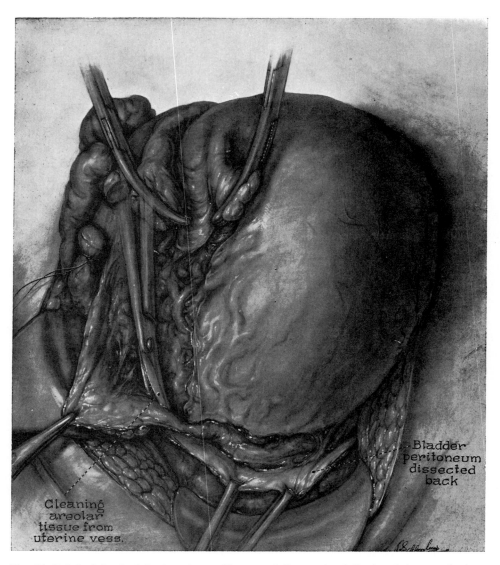

Fig. 20. Total abdominal hysterectomy. The round ligaments, fallopian tubes, and utero-ovarian vessels and ligaments have been divided. The anterior leaf of the broad ligament and the bladder flap have been cut and the bladder reflected downward. The uterine vessels may be skeletonized under direct vision.

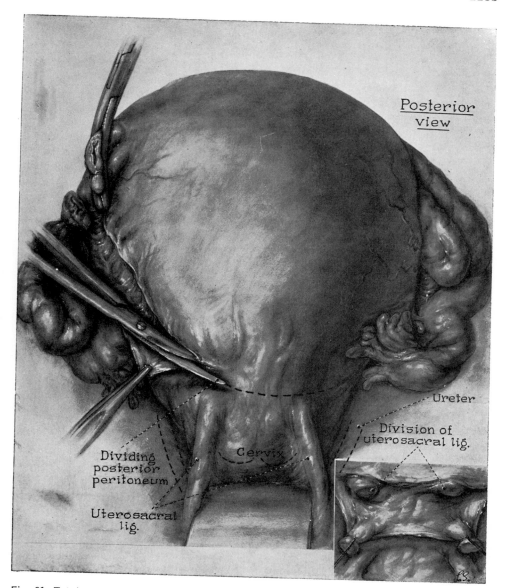

Fig. 21. Total abdominal hysterectomy. Division of the posterior leaf of the broad ligament and division and ligation of the uterosacral ligaments. The ureters are in close approximation to the uterosacral ligaments.

and divided, and doubly ligated immediately adjacent to the uterus. At this point care is necessary to avoid injury to the ureters, which pass beneath the uterine arteries (Fig. 22). To perform a subtotal hysterectomy, it is necessary only to amputate the corpus at this level (Fig. 16). The cervical stump is usually closed with interrupted catgut sutures and covered with peritoneum. Reperitonization is performed as for total hysterectomy.

To perform a total hysterectomy, it is advisable to incise the pubocervical

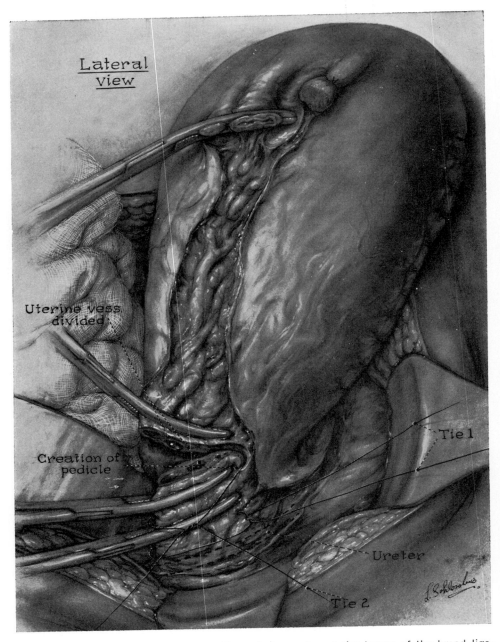

Fig. 22. Total abdominal hysterectomy. The anterior and posterior leaves of the broad ligament have been divided, and the uterine vessels have been doubly clamped and severed. The position of the ureter in relation to the clamps is shown.

fascia immediately after ligation of the uterine arteries (Fig. 23). This layer of connective tissue is better defined anteriorly than on the posterior aspect of the cervix. The anterior incision in the pubocervical fascia is carried around the cer-

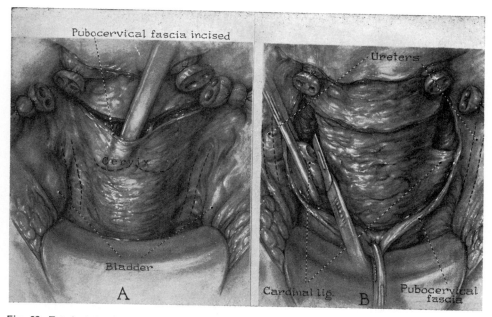

Fig. 23. Total abdominal hysterectomy. A, division of paracervical tissue through transverse incision and dissection off the cervix. B, division of the cardinal ligaments. The technic of dividing these ligaments within the paracervical cuff obviates the danger of damage to the ureters, which are indicated by the dotted lines.

vix, and a cuff of pubocervical fascia is developed. The peritoneum covering the posterior aspect of the cervix is then reflected downward. At this point it is ordinarily advantageous to divide the uterosacral ligaments between clamps and ligatures. The parametrial connective tissue on either side is then grasped with Kocher, Phaneuf, or Heaney clamps and is divided and ligated. If the cervix is long, several more parametrial bites are usually necessary. In performing total hysterectomy after cesarean section when the cervix is partially or wholly effaced, there may be difficulty in identifying the lower limits of the cervix. A finger inserted through the uterine incision into the vagina may aid in locating the cervico-vaginal junction and removing the entire cervix. Occasionally even this technic will not identify the junction of the cervix and the vagina, especially if there has been complete cervical effacement. In this situation the cervix can be opened anteriorly by incising downward from the lower pole of the uterine incision. In this way the upper limit of the vagina can be visualized and the cervix completely excised. Usually, however, there is little difficulty in identifying the lower limits of the cervix after the pubocervical fascia has been developed. The vagina can then be cut across (Fig. 24).

The vaginal vault is closed with interrupted catgut sutures, as shown in Figure 25, with special care to provide adequate hemostasis at the angles. The innermost stumps of the cardinal ligaments are then sutured to the angles of the vault, and the severed ends of uterosacral ligaments are incorporated into the vaginal cuff by means of a continuous suture of catgut. Defects in the pelvic peritoneum are repaired, and the bladder flap is sutured to the posterior peritoneum behind the vaginal vault (Fig. 26). The abdomen is then closed in layers.

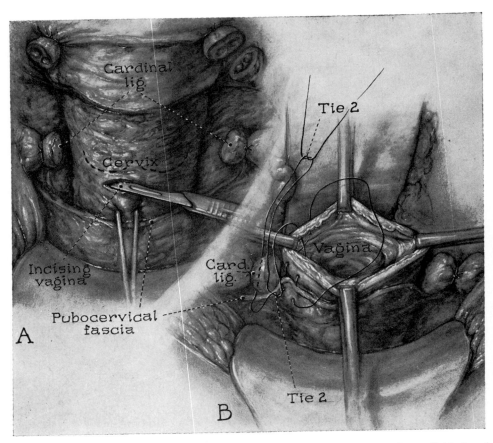

Fig. 24. Total abdominal hysterectomy. After the cardinal ligaments have been divided and ligated, the vagina is cut across at the level of the external cervical os, which may sometimes be difficult to identify, particularly if the cervix is widely dilated. If the vagina is transected below the junction of the cardinal ligaments, however, the entire cervix is usually thus removed. The vagina and endopelvic fascia are closed with interrupted figure-of-eight sutures; the stumps of the cardinal and uterosacral ligaments are included in these sutures; and the stitches at the vaginal angles, the frequent site of postoperative hemorrhage, are carefully placed.

Although total hysterectomy is far more commonly employed than the subtotal operation, certain unusual circumstances render the incomplete operation the more logical and safer procedure. If the patient's condition is precarious, it may be necessary to terminate the procedure after amputation of the corpus. In the vast majority of cases, however, total operation is relatively safe to employ, and is the procedure of choice.

Extraperitoneal Cesarean Section. Before the advent of efficacious antimicrobial drugs, this operation afforded a means of reducing the likelihood of peritonitis in infected cases. With the availability of such agents and the proven efficacy of the technically easier low segment operations, the extraperitoneal procedures are now obsolescent.

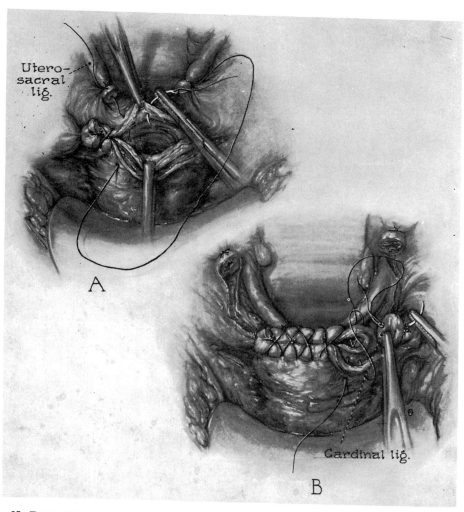

Fig. 25. Total abdominal hysterectomy. Repair of vaginal cuff. Both the cardinal and utero-sacral ligaments are sutured to the cuff. The endopelvic fascia and vaginal cuff are then closed.

Prognosis. The maternal mortality of cesarean section in competent hands is 0.2 per cent or less. Many clinics cite series of more than a thousand cases without a maternal death. Davis, for example, reports a mortality of only 0.1 per cent in 1,962 cesarean sections at the Chicago Lying-In Hospital, the 2 deaths resulting from pulmonary emboli. In 3,285 elective repeated cesarean sections in the large Obstetricial Statistical Cooperative series, comprising patients not in labor and without complications of pregnancy, there was not a single maternal death. Among 242 cesarean deaths reported by Gordon, 48 were anesthetic fatalities. Anesthesia may in fact be a greater hazard today than the operation itself.

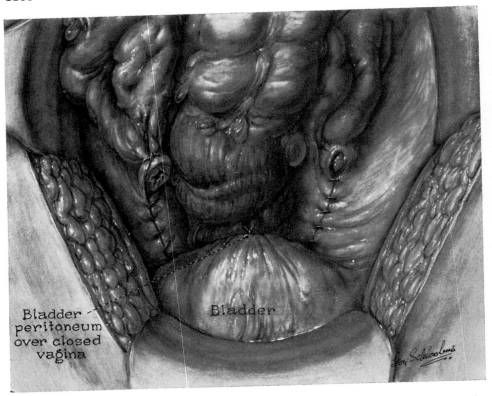

Bladder peritoneum over closed vagina

Bladder

Fig. 26. Total abdominal hysterectomy. The pelvic peritoneum is sutured together over the vaginal cuff. Sutures bury the ovarian vessels retroperitoneally.

The gross perinatal mortality from cesarean section may range as high as 12 per cent. Pedowitz, Schwartz, and Goldberg point out, however, that this statistic is biased because it combines the perinatal loss in both indicated and elective operations. The indicated cesarean sections include those in which there is an obstetric complication that is often deleterious to the fetus and, furthermore, may force the delivery of a premature infant. In the indicated group the perinatal mortality is necessarily high, whereas in the elective group the perinatal wastage should be much closer to the basic loss in vaginal delivery. Hall, Kohl, and Schecter have indicated, however, the inherent error of performing elective cesarean section so early that prematurity becomes a factor. In their series of 3,285 cesarean sections electively repeated, the total perinatal mortality was 0.91 per cent, and that for term infants was 0.85 per cent.

Postmortem Cesarean Section. As reviewed by DeKruif, Rockwood, and Baker in 1957, there had been 113 successful postmortem cesarean sections reported in the world's literature during the past 250 years. Cloud added 10 additional cases. Only a very small fraction of those performed have been recorded. Although the outlook for the infant is notoriously poor, the 4 infants followed by Weil and Graber and by Cloud appear to be normal. Successful cases have been recorded in which the operation was performed as long as 20 minutes after maternal death, but the usual interval has been 2 to 10 minutes.

REFERENCES

Beck, A. C.   Observations on a series of cases of cesarean section done at the Long Island College Hospital during the past six years. Amer J Obstet Gynec 79:197, 1919.

Brenner, P., Sall, S., Sonnenbick, B.   Evaluation of cesarean section hysterectomy as a sterilization procedure. Amer J Obstet Gynec 108:355, 1970.

Chase, H. C.   Perinatal and infant mortality in the United States and six west European countries. Amer J Public Health 57:1735, 1967.

Cloud, I. G.   Cesarean section on the dead and moribund. Obstet Gynec 16:27, 1960.

Cosmi, E. V., and Marx, G. F.   Acid-base status of the fetus and clinical condition of the newborn following cesarean section. Amer J Obstet Gynec 102:378, 1968.

Davis, M. E.   Complete cesarean hysterectomy: a logical advance in modern obstetric surgery. Amer J Obstet Gynec 62:838, 1951.

DeKruif, H., Rockwood, P. M., and Baker, N. H.   Postmortem cesarean section with survival of infant. JAMA 163:938, 1957.

DeLee, J. B., and Cornell, E. L.   Low cervical cesarean section (laparototrachelotomy). JAMA 79:109, 1922.

Döderlein, A.   Transperitonealer Cervikaler Kaiserschnitt, in Döderlein and Krönig (eds), Operative Gynäkologie, 1912, p. 879.

Eastman, N. J.   The role of Frontier America in the development of cesarean section. Amer J Obstet Gynec 24:919, 1932.

Fasbender, H.   Geschichte der Geburtshülfe, Jena, 1906, pp. 979–1010.

Frank, F.   (Suprasymphysial delivery and its relation to other operations in the presence of contracted pelvis). Arch Gynaek 81:46, 1907.

Gordon, C. A.   Cesarean section death. Amer J Obstet Gynec 63:284, 1952.

Hall, J. E., Kohl, S. G., and Schecter, H. R.   Current aspects of cesarean section and perinatal mortality. Amer J Obstet Gynec 75:387, 1958.

Harris, R. P.   Lessons from a study of the caesarean operation in the City and State of New York. Amer J Obstet 12:82, 1879.

Haynes, D. M., and Wolfe, W. M.   Tubal sterilization in an indigent population: report of fourteen years' experience. Amer J Obstet Gynec 106:1044, 1970.

Hellman, L. M., Kobayashi, M., Fillisti, L., and Lavenhar, M.   Sources of error in sonographic fetal mensuration and estimation of growth. Amer J Obstet Gynec 99:662, 1967.

———— Kobayashi, M., Tolles, W. E., and Cromb, E.   Ultrasonic studies on the zolumetric growth of the human placenta. Amer J Obstet Gynec 108:740, 1970.

Kerr, J. M. M.   The technic of cesarean section with special reference to the lower uterine segment incision. Amer J Obstet Gynec 12:729, 1926.

Klein, M. D., Robbins, R., and Gabaeff, L.   Primary cesarean section in the multipara. Amer J Obstet Gynec 87:242, 1963.

Krönig, B.   Transperitonealer Cervikaler Kaiserschnitt, in Döderlein and Krönig (eds.), Operative Gynäkologie, 1912, p. 879.

McGarry, J. A.   The management of patients previously delivered by caesarean section. J Obstet Gynaec Brit Comm 76:137, 1969.

McNally, H. B., and Fitzpatrick, V.   Patients with four or more cesarean sections. JAMA 160:1005, 1956.

———— and Fitzpatrick, V.   Patients with four or more cesarean sections: second series. Southern Med J 54:360, 1961.

Niswander, K. R., Capraro, V. J., and Van Coevering, R. J.   Estimation of birthweight by quantified external uterine measurements. Obstet Gynec 36:294, 1970.

O'Driscoll, K. Catastrophes in labour: rupture of the uterus. Proc Roy Soc Med 59:65, 1966.

O'Leary, J. A., and Steer, C. M.   A 10-year review of cesarean hysterectomy. Amer J Obstet Gynec 90:227, 1964.

Pedowitz, P., Schwartz, R. M., and Goldberg, M.   Perinatal mortality in primary cesarean section. Obstet Gynec 14:764, 1959.

Pickrell, K.   An inquiry into the history of cesarean section. Bull Soc Med Hist, Chicago, 4:414, 1935.

Piver, M. A., and Johnston, R. A.   The safety of multiple cesarean sections. Obstet Gynec 34:690, 1969.

Pliny the Elder.   Natural History, Book VII, Chapter IX. Cambridge, Mass., Harvard University Press. Translated by H. Rackham, 1942.

Poidevin, L. O. S.   Cesarean Section Scars. Springfield, Ill., Charles C Thomas, 1965.

Porro, E.   Della amputazione utero-ovarica. Milan, 1876.

Pritchard, J. A., Baldwin, R. M., Dickey, J. C., and Wiggins, K. M.   II. Red blood cell loss and changes in apparent blood volume during and following vaginal delivery, cesarean section, and cesarean section plus total hysterectomy. Amer J Obstet Gynec 84:1271, 1962.

Raics, J.   (The influence of the changes in indications for cesarean section on perinatal mortality). Zbl Gynaek 89:91, 1967.

Rousset, F.   Traité Nouveau de l'Hystérotomotokie ou l'Enfantement Césarien. Paris, Denys duVal, 1581.

Sänger, M.   Der Kaiserschnitt bei Uterusfibromen. Leipzig, 1882.

Schilling, H.   (Vaginal delivery after cesarean section). Zbl Gynaek 88:245, 1966.

Schiøler, H., Eiken, M., Øvlisen, B., and Trolle, D.   Hysterographic changes following transverse lower segment cesarean section. Acta Radiol (Diagn) (Stockholm) 6:145, 1967.

Schwartz, R. M., Pedowitz, P., and Goldberg, M.   Perinatal mortality in repeat cesarean section. Obstet Gynec 14:773, 1959.

Sellheim, H.   (The extraperitoneal uterine incision). Zbl Gynaek 32:133, 1908.

Stephens, S. R., and Brown, W. E.   Rupture of the gravid uterus. Southern Med J 60:359, 1967.

Stevenson, C. S., Behney, C. A., and Miller, N. F.   Maternal death from puerperal sepsis following cesarean section. A 16-year study in Michigan. Obstet Gynec 29:181, 1967.

Van Praagh, I. G., and Tovell, H. M. M.   Primary cesarean section in the multipara. Obstet Gynec 32:813, 1968.

Waniorek, A.   Hysterography after cesarean section for evaluation of suturing technic. Obstet Gynec 29:192, 1967.

Waters, E. G.   Supravesical extraperitoneal cesarean section. Presentation of a new technique. Amer J Obstet Gynec 39:423, 1940.

Webb, C. F., and Gibbs, J. V.   Preplanned total cesarean hysterectomies. Amer J Obstet Gynec 101:23, 1968.

Weil, A. M., and Graber, V. R.   The management of the near-term pregnant patient who dies undelivered. Amer J Obstet Gynec 73:754, 1957.

INDEX

(Italicized numbers refer to illustrations)

Aardvark placentation, 190
Abdomen
  abortion and surgery of, 500
  auscultation, 277-78
    fetal heart and, 395
    presentation of fetus and, 330-31
    twin diagnosis and, 668
  binder, 474
  delivery through, 1163 ff. *See also* Cesarean
    section.
  changes of wall, 245-46
  diastasis of rectus muscles, 246, 468, 652-53
  engagement detected through, 303
  enlargement, 280-81
    dystocia and, 890
  first stage of labor and, 402
  linea nigra, 269
  local infiltration anesthesia, 458
  localization of fetus, 1043
  pain
    decompression in labor, 458-59
    tubal pregnancy and, 545-46, 548-49
  palpation. *See also* Palpation.
    abdominal pregnancy and, 555
    lower uterine segment, 354
    presentation of fetus and, 326 ff., 374,
      382, 383
    twin diagnosis and, 668
  pendulous, 650
    face presentation and, 865
  pregnancy of, 554 ff.
    cesarean section, 1163
    diagnosis, 555-56
    frequency, 554-55
    intraperitoneal rupture of tubal pregnancy
      and, 543
    missed labor and, 851
    palpation, 555
    prognosis, 558
    at term, *556*
    treatment, 556-58
  prenatal care, 341
  pressure, eclampsia and, 717
  puerperium and, 468
  shape, uterine contraction and, *357*
  striae gravidarum, 246, 286

Abdomen (*cont.*)
  umbilical hernia, 652
Ablatio placentae, 623. *See also* Abruptio
    placentae.
ABO incompatibility, 513, 518, 1036 ff., 1051
Abortifacients, vaginal atresia and, 922
Abortion, 493 ff.
  abnormal development and, 496 ff.
  abruptio placentae and, 623
  blood group incompatibility, 513, 518
  blood mole, 502
  cervix, incompetence of, 512-13, 515, 516-18
  chronic diseases, 500, 521
  classification, pathologic, 504
  coagulation and, 506, 509, 522, 524
  complete, 494
  consequences and complications, 520 ff.
  consumptive coagulopathy and, 506, 509,
      522, 524
  criminal, 494, 519
    Clostridium perfringens and, 975
    complications, 520 ff.
    perforation of uterus, 949
  cytogenetic studies, 498
  definitions, 493-94, 509-10, 1085
  dissolution of fetus, 503
  eclampsia and, 718
  endocrine defects, 500
  germ plasm defects, 497-98, 510-11, 514
  habitual, 509 ff.
    clinical investigation, 513 ff.
    definition, 509-10
    etiology, 510 ff.
    prediction of, 510
    prognosis, 518-19
  hemorrhage, 501, 504 ff., 521
  hormonal abnormalities, 511, 514
  hypertension, 513, 736, 738
  illegal. *See* Abortion, criminal.
  imminent, 508
  incomplete, 505-6
    definition, 494
    treatment, 508-9
  induced, 493, 519. *See also* Abortion, thera-
    peutic.
    definition, 494

Abortion (*cont.*)
  inevitable, 505, 508
  infections, 499-500, 520-21
  laparotomy, 500
  maceration of fetus, 503
  malaria and, 814
  maternal disease, 499-501, 511-13
  McDonald operation, *515*
  missed, 506
    treatment, 509
  mummification, 503
  myoma and, 926
  nutritional factors, 511-12, 514
  ovarian tumors, 509
  oxytocin, 509
  pain, 507-8
  perforation of uterus, 526, 949
  perinatal mortality, 13
  placenta and, 499, 586
  renal failure, acute, 524-26
  repeated, 509 ff. *See also* Abortion, habitual.
  reproductive organs, abnormalities of, 500-1
  rubella and, 811, 1088
  septic, 520-21
  sex differences, 498-99
  Shirodkar operation, *516 ff.*
  shock, 505
    bacterial endotoxic, 521 ff.
  spontaneous, 494 ff.
    clinical aspects, 504-6
    definition, 493
    etiology, 496 ff.
    incidence, 494-96
    pathology, 501 ff.
    placenta membranacea and, 586
    treatment, 506 ff.
  syphilis, 513
  teratogens, 123, 499, 1066
  therapeutic, 1085 ff.
    definition, 493, 1085
    glomerulonephritis and, 759
    heart disease and, 782-83, 785
    hypertension and, 738
    incidence, 1089
    indications, 1088-89
    induction, 951, 1091-92
    legal status, 1085 ff.
    morbidity and mortality, 1092
    nervous system and, 819-20
    psychiatric disorders, 1088
    retinitis gestationis and, 824
    rubella and, 811
    sex differences, 498
    technic, 1089 ff.
  threatened, 504-5
    treatment, 506-8
  thyroid dysfunction, 511, 514
  toxic compounds for production of, 524
  trauma, psychic and physical, 501, 513
  tubal pregnancy, 541-42
    intrauterine vs., 548
    signs and symptoms, 545 ff.
  tuberous mole, 503
  uterine anomalies, 512-13, 516, 649
  vaginal bleeding, 504

Abortus, defined, 1026-27
Abruptio placentae, 623 ff.
  anemia and, 769
  anesthesia, 458
  apoplexy, uteroplacental, 630-31
  clinical diagnosis, 627-29
  complications, 629 ff.
  consumptive coagulopathy, 629-30
  Couvelaire uterus, 630-31
  etiology, 625-27
  fibrinolysis, 630
  frequency, 624-25
  hypertension, 624
  nomenclature, 623-24
  pathology, 627
  recurrence, 626
  prognosis, 634-35
  renal disease, 631-32, 760
  shock, 628, 629
  stillbirths, eclampsia and, 724
  toxic and nontoxic, 635
  treatment, 633-34
  urine, 633, 635
  vascular changes, 626
Abscesses
  abdominal pregnancy, 555
  Bartholin's glands, 640
  breast, 995-96
  pelvic, 989
    abortion and, 521
Acanthopelyx, 916
Acardius, 664, 884, 885
Acetonuria, diabetes and, 794
Acid-base balance, 252
Acidosis
  anesthesia and, 432
  asphyxia of newborn, 1015
  bilirubin and, 1048
  diabetic, 791
  eclampsia and, 716
Acini, breast, 468-69
Acormus, 885
Acromion presentation, 321-22, 872. *See also* Shoulder presentation.
Actinomycin D, choriocarcinoma and, 583
Addison's disease, 180, 797
  pernicious anemia, 769-70
Adenomyosis, 654
Adipocere, 555
Admittance procedures, 401-2, 697-99
Adolescents, 396-97
Adenitis, inguinal, 803
Adrenal glands, 268-69
  bilateral excision, 797
  dysfunction, 797
  eclampsia and, 710
  endotoxic shock and, 524
  estrogens and, 178, 179-80
  fetal, 178, 222, 223
Adrenocorticosteroids, placenta and, 185-86. *See also* Steroids; specific hormones.
Adrenocorticotropic hormone, fetal, 222
Aerobacter, puerperium and, 974
Afterpains, 471-72, 474
Agalactia, 997

Age
  fetal, 199, 236, 496, 1026, 1030 ff.
  maternal
    chromosomal anomalies and, 1068
    hydatidiform mole and, 569
    labor and, 396-97
    mongolism and, *1074*
    mortality and, 5, *6*
    placenta previa and, 611, 612
    precocious and late pregnancy, 238
    twinning and, 658
    uterine rupture and, 943
  menarche onset, *104*
  neonatal, mortality and, *10*
  placental, 148-49, 154, 591
Agglutinins, 1037
Air-rebound technic .in anesthesia, *454, 455, 456*
Airway conductance, 260
Albumin, 262
  bilirubin and, 1048
  -globulin ratio, 716
  mature fetal, 218
Alcock's canal, 437
Alcohol, 342
  intravenous, premature labor arrest and, 530
Aldosterone, 268, 269, 797
  eclampsia and, 714-15
  fetal, 223
  placenta and, 185
Alimentary tract diseases, 806 ff. *See also* specific structures.
Alkaline phosphatase
  heat-stable, 149
  leukocyte, 256
  serum, liver and, 262
Alkaline-resistant hemoglobin, 216
Alkaloids, eclampsia and, 731
Alkalosis, respiratory, 252
Alkylating agents, 111
Allantois, 137, 139-40, 171
  comparative anatomy, 186-87
Aluminum hydroxide, 345
Ambulation, 474, 697
Amebiasis, 814-15
Amenorrhea
  lactation and, 475
  missed abortion and, 506
  tubal pregnancy and, 546
American Board of Obstetrics and Gynecology, mortality and, 8
American College of Obstetricians and Gynecologists
  abortion and, 1088-89
  contraception and, 1099
American Committe on Maternal Welfare, hypertension classification of, 685, 686, 687, 734
American Law Institute, abortion laws and, 1086
American Medical Association,
  abortion laws and, 1086
  contraception and, 1099
American Public Health Association, contraception and, 1099

Amnesia, labor and, 432-34
Amino acids from oxytocin peptide, *418*
Aminocaproic acid therapy, 630
Aminopeptidase, 262
Amniocentesis, 227
  dangers, hydramnios and, 603
  hyperbilirubinemia and, 1042
  malformations of fetus, 1078
  meconium detection, 1010
Amniography, hydrops fetalis and, *1046*
Amnion, 170-71, 226
  blood vessels and nerves, 170
  caruncles, 171, 604
  chorion fusion with, 147
  cuboidal cells, 170
  cysts, 604
  development, 133-34, 135, 139
  disorders, 599 ff.
  hydrostatic action, 361
  inflammation, 604
  injections for abortion, 1093-94
  nodosum, 604
  separation of placenta and, *370, 371*
  squamous metaplasia, 604
  thickness, 170
  twins and, 622
  vacuoles, 171
Amniotic fluid, 226 ff.
  abruptio placentae and, 630
  breech presentation and, 324, 326
  cervical dilatation and, 361
  composition, 227
  death of fetus and, 288
  disorders, 599 ff.
  embolism, 630, 849, 950 ff.
  estriol, 1042
  excessive, 599 ff. *See also* Hydramnios.
  kidneys of fetus and, 218
  labor and, 361, 391, 849
  monitoring, 228-29
  osmolality, *227*, 228
  pelvic contraction and, 900
  pH, 405
  precipitate labor and, 849
  prematurity and, 1029
  pressure, 601, *1011*
  Rh negative women and, 1040-42
  sodium chloride, 406
  somatomammotropin (chorionic), 176
  swallowing, *219*, 220
  urine in, 228
  volume, 227
  water content, 248
Amobarbital, eclampsia and, 730
Ampicillin, 755
Amylophagia, 345-46
Analgesia, 430 ff.
  amnesia, 432-34
  ataractic drugs, 433
  caudal, 446, 449-50
  chloroform, 436
  diagram of methods, *438*
  fetal homeostasis, distress and oxygenation, 432
  forceps and, 1122

Analgesia (*cont.*)
  hypnosis, 459
  local infiltration, 437
  multiparas, 431
  nalorphine (Nalline), 433-34
  narcotic, 432
  newborn respiratory depression, 432
  nitrous oxide, 434
  optimal time, 431
  oxygen dissociation curves, 432
  paracervical, *445*
  premature labor, 530
  primigravidas, 431
  program, 431, 432
  psychologic methods, 459
  scopolamine, 432
  sensory pathways involved, 437 ff.
  uterine contraction impairment, 449
Anamnestic reaction, 1038
Anaphylactoid shock, amniotic fluid embolism
      and, 951
Anatomy of female reproductive organs, 19 ff.
  external, 19 ff.
  internal, 30 ff.
Ancor, 1105
Androgens, 82, 178
Android pelvis, 316
Androstenedione, 82, 178
Anectine, 457
Anemia, 761 ff.
  abortion and premature labor, 500
  acquired, 763 ff.
  acute loss of blood, 766
  aplastic, 770-71
  definition, 761-62
  drug-induced, 770
  etiology, 762-63
  frequency, 762
  genetic counseling, 776
  hemoglobin and, 761-62, 774-75
  hemolytic, 770 ff.
    renal failure and, 760-61
  hereditary, 771 ff.
  hydatidiform mole, 569
  hypoplastic, 770-71
  inflammation, 767
  iron-deficiency, 763 ff.
  megaloblastic, 767 ff.
    malaria, 814
  multiple pregnancy, 674
  pernicious (Addisonian), 769-70
  physiologic, 763
  puerperal infection and, 976, 985, 986
  refractory, 767
  renal failure and, 760-61
  sickle-cell, 772 ff.
  thalassemia, 771-72, 775
  tubal pregnancy, 547
Anencephaly, 1069 ff.
  adrenocorticotropic hormone and, 222
  breech presentation, 325
  cause, 1071
  clinical aspects, 1071-72
  digestive system, 220
  duration of pregnancy, 237
  estrogens and, 178, 179

Anencephaly (*cont.*)
  face presentation, 865
  hydramnios and, 599-600, 603
  incidence, 1064, 1065
  labor onset and, 351
  risk of, 1081
Anesthesia, 430 ff.
  abdominal decompression, 458-59
  abdominal wall infiltration, 458
  abortion and, 508, 1089
  aspiration of gastric contents, 430-31, 434
  breech delivery, 1154, 1156, 1159
  caudal, 352, 446 ff.
    doses, 448
    maternal mortality, 449
  cesarean section, 452 ff.
  chloroform, 436
  cyclopropane, 434, 435, 457, 458
  diabetes and, 796
  eclampsia, 732, 733
  endotracheal intubation, 434, 436
  epidural, 352, 448, 450, 453 ff.
  ether, 435
  fetal homeostasis, 432
  food withholding and, 407
  gas, 434-35
  general, 434
  halothane (Fluothane), 435-36
  headache and, 451
  heart disease and, 780
  hypotension, 449, 450, 452, 457
  inhalation, 434 ff., 457-58
  intravenous, 436-37
  local infiltration, 437-39, 448
  lumbar epidural block, 450, 453 ff.
    doses, 448
  multiple pregnancy, 677
  neurologic damage, 451
  nitrous oxide, 434, 436, 457, 458
  occipitoposterior position, 854
  oxygen dissociation curves, 432
  paracervical block, 442 ff.
  parasacral and paravertebral block, 442
  peridural, air-rebound technic and, 455, *456*
  placental barrier, 434
  pneumonia and, 786
  pudendal nerve, 437
    transperineal block, 439-40
    transvaginal block, 440-42
  regional, 437 ff.
  saddle block, 451
  shock, postural, 452
  spinal, 450 ff.
    cesarean section, 452-53
    vaginal delivery, 352, 450-51
  subarachnoid block, 450 ff., 457
  succinylcholine, 436, 457, 458
  thiopental sodium, 436-37
  trichlorethylene (Trilene), 436
  d-tubocurarine (curare), 457
  uterosacral block, 442 ff.
  volatile, 435-36
Angiogenesis, 144
Angiography
  placental localization, 617
  pulmonary embolism, 1004

Angioma, 269
  placental, 584
Angiotensin, 269
Anovulation, 99, 661
Antacids, 345
Antecon, 1105
Antecubital venous pressure, 258, 259
Anteflexion of uterus, 649-50
Antepartum
  eclampsia, 704
  hemorrhage, 609 ff., 678
  thromboembolic disease, 1002
Anthropoid
  multiple pregnancy, 656
  pelvis, 316
Antibiotics
  discharge from hospital and, 476
  gonorrhea and, 802
  mortality, perinatal, 398
  ophthalmia neonatorum and, 487
  puerperal infection and, 987-88
  staphylococci and, 1056
  syphilis and, 800-1
  tuberculosis and, 787-88
  urinary tract infections and, 755-56
Antibodies
  fetal, 224
  Rh, 1037 ff.
  rubella, 809
  saline, 1037
Anticoagulants
  cardiac valvar prosthesis and, 783
  thromboembolic disease and, 1002-3
Anticonvulsants, 819
  eclampsia and, 728 ff.
Antidiuresis, oxytocin and, 418
Antidiuretic hormone
  fetal, 222
  renal function and, 263
Antigens
  Australia, 804
  epidemic-hepatitis, 804
  fetal, 168-69, 224
  Rh, 1038-39
  transplantation, 169, 170
Antihistamines, 1067
Antihypertensives, 728 ff., 739
Antimicrobials. *See* Antibiotics.
Antisepsis in second stage of labor, 407, 410
Anuria
  abortion, 522
  abruptio placentae, 633
  renal necrosis, 760
Anus
  imperforate, 1077
  sphincter laceration, *427*
Aorta
  coarctation, 784
  compression by uterus, 259
Aortic valve prosthesis, 783-84
Apgar scoring system, 479-80, 1015, 1017
  fetal distress syndrome and, 1012
  paracervical block anesthesia and, 444
Aplastic anemia, 770-71
Apnea, newborn, 478, 481, 484, 1015, 1016
  analgesia, 433

Apoplexy, uteroplacental, 630-31, 635
Appendicitis, 806-7
  tubal pregnancy and, 548
Appetite
  pica, 345-46
  puerperal, 474
Apresoline, 731
Aramine, abortion and, 524
Arcuate arteries, 37
Arias-Stella phenomenon, 540, 576
Arm
  delivery, breech extraction and, 1149-59
  prolapse, 879
Arteries
  arcuate, 37
  basal, 37
  blood gases, pulmonary embolism and, 1004
  brachial, 258
  cervicovaginal, 40
  coiled, 37, 93, 241
  endometrial, 37
  hypogastric, 947-49
  ovarian, 41
  pressure, 258, 259, 703. *See also* Blood
    pressure.
  spiral, 163, 167, 241-42
  umbilical, 172
    single, 598-99, 1065, 1067
  uterine, 37, 40-41, 259
    cesarean section hysterectomy and, 1182,
      1184
    rupture and, 947
  uteroplacental, 163, 167
Arteriograms
  hydatidiform mole, 569
  placenta previa, *619*
Arterioles
  abruptio placentae and, 626
  eclampsia and, 711-12
  retinal, 691, 712
  spiral, 626
Arteriovenous shunt, placental, 259
Arthritis, rheumatoid, 815-16
Ascites
  dystocia and, 890
  hydramnios vs., 601
Ascorbic acid
  placental transfer of, 210
  pregnancy requirements, *337*
Asepsis in labor, 407, 410
Asian influenza, 813
Asphyxia, 1015-17
Aspiration
  Bartholin's duct cysts, 640
  gastric contents, 430-31, 434, 786
  meconium, 479
  mucus, in newborn, 479
  pharyngeal, *482*
  pneumonitis, 786
Asthma, 787
Asynclitism, 376, 899
Ataractic drugs, 433
Atresia
  esophageal, 228
  urethral, 228
  vulvar and vaginal, 921

Attitude of fetus, 320
Auscultation, 277-78. *See also* Abdomen, auscultation.
Australia antigen, 804
Autoimmune disease, placental barrier and, 168
Automobile accidents, birth canal injuries and, 949-50
Autonomic nervous system, labor pains and, 437
Autosomes, 110, 125
    abortion and, 498
    dominant inheritance and, 1079
    recessive inheritance and, 1080
Azathioprine, 761
Azotemia, 759

Backache, 344
    abortion and, 504
Bacteremia
    abortion and, 521 ff.
    puerperal infection and, 982
Bacteria, 813-14. *See also* Infections.
    cholera, 814
    endocarditis, 785-86
    erysipelas, 814
    mastitis, 994-95
    newborn infection, 1053 ff.
    puerperal infection, 973-75
    scarlet fever, 813-14
    septic abortion, 521
    shock, 755, 990
        renal necrosis and, 760
    typhoid fever, 814
Bacteriuria, 749 ff.
    asymptomatic, 750 ff.
        sickle-cell trait and, 775
    diagnosis, 750
    perinatal mortality, 751-53
    prematurity and, 529-30, 751
Bacteroides, puerperal infection and, 974
Ballottement, 281
Bandl's ring, 355, 850
Barbiturates, 432-33
    eclampsia and, 730
    placental crossing, 437
Barr body, 124, 229. *See also* Sex chromatin.
    fetal malformations and, 1078
Bartholin's glands, 22
    cysts, 640
    inflammation, 640
Barton forceps, 1130, 1135, *1138*
Basal metabolic rate, 267
Basal plate of placenta, 144, 152, 154
Bathing, 340
Battledore placenta, 594
Bearing-down efforts, 407
Bicarbonate, pH of infant blood and, 483
Bilirubin
    fetal, 221, 229
    hepatosis and, 805
    newborn, 415, 488
        hemolytic disease, 1036 ff.
        toxicity and disposal, 1048-49
    prematurity and, 1029

Bilirubin (*cont.*)
    serum, *488*, 1047, 1050
Binder, abdominal, 474
Bioassays for diagnosis of pregnancy, 284
Biochemistry in eclampsia, 713 ff.
Biopsy
    cervical, 642, 644
    hepatic, 706
    renal, *709*, 760
Biparietal diameter, 206
Birth canal, 362. *See also* Cervix; Uterus; Vagina; Vulva.
    injuries, 932 ff.
Birth certificate, 13-14, *15*
Birth injury. *See also* Newborn.
    definition, 1018
Birth rate, 3-4
    definition, 2
    projections, 4
Bisischial diameter, 304
Bitemporal diameter, 206
Bladder, urinary, 266
    bacterial infection, 749-50
    calculi, 757
    distention, dystocia and, *922*
    fetal, enlargement of fetal body and, *891*
    full, labor and, 407
    herniation, 641, 930
    inflammation, 749
        puerperal, 1000
    tumors, dystocia and, 930
    uterine retrodisplacement, 650
Blastocyst, 123, 125, 128, 129, 144-45, 200
    implantation, 130, 132
    sex chromatin, 230
Blastomere, 125, *126*
Bleeding. *See* Hemorrhage.
Blindness
    eclampsia and, 705
    retrolental fibroplasia and, 1035
Blood, 761 ff. *See also* Plasma; Serum.
    anemia, 761 ff. *See also* Anemia.
    bacteria, 521 ff., 982
    bicarbonate, eclampsia and, 715
    bilirubin, 805, 1050
    coagulation, 256. *See also* Coagulation.
        puerperal, 473
    culture, puerperal infection and, 986
    cutaneous flow, 260
    electrolytes, 252
    factors, 256, 1037
        abruptio placentae and, 630
        hyperbilirubinemia and, 1037, 1051
        thromboembolism and, 1002
    fetal, 215 ff.
        volume, 215-16
    gases. *See also* Carbon dioxide; Oxygen.
        pulmonary embolism and, 1004
    Hodgkin's disease, 777
    hormonal levels in menstruation, *83*
    incompatibility
        abortion and, 513, 518
        eclampsia and, 717
    insulin levels, *250*
    leukemia, 777
    lipid levels, *251*

Blood (*cont.*)
  loss. *See* Hemorrhage.
  mole, 502
  pH, 252
    fetal, 1010
    newborn, 483
  polycythemia, 776
  pressure, 258, 259
    anesthesia and, 451
    fetal, 208
    hypertensive, 687, 689, 690, 725, 738
      eclampsia, 687, 703, 725
      preeclampsia, 689, 690
    intervillous space, 208
    labor, 393
    tubal pregnancy, 547
  progesterone, 79
  protein, eclampsia and, 715-16
  puerperal, 473
  sedimentation rate, 256
  thrombocytopenic purpura, 776-77
  transfusions. *See* Transfusions, blood.
  urinary. *See* Urine, blood.
  vessels. *See also* Arteries; Capillaries; Veins.
    size increase, 239
  volume,
    fetal, 215-16
    iron metabolism and, 252 ff., 764, 766
    maternal, 778-79
Bloody show, 387-88
Body stalk, 135, 171
  variations of insertion of cord, 595
Bonadoxin, 344
Bone
  estrogen effects, 78
  marrow, erythroid hyperplasia and, 253
  pain, sickle-cell anemia and, 773
  phocomelia, 1069
  syphilis and, 1053, *1054*
Bonine, 344
Bowel habits, 340-41
  newborn, 487-88
  puerperal care, 475
Brachial plexus
  paralysis, 1021
  stretching in delivery, 413
Bracht maneuver, 1152
Bradycardia, fetal, 395, 402, 442 ff., 1010
  anesthesia and, 442 ff.
  prolapsed cord and, *1013*
Brain
  anencephalic, 1069 ff. *See also* Anencephaly.
  eclampsia and, 708, 710
  fetal, compression, 1010
  hemorrhage, 1018-20
  hypoxia and, 1016
  meningocele, 1072, 1076
  pelvic contraction and, 901
Braxton Hicks contractions, 241, 281, 359
  placenta previa and, 620
Breast(s), 468 ff., 993 ff.
  abscesses, 995-96
  agalactia, 997
  caked, 993
  carcinoma, 823-24, 1109-10
  changes in pregnancy, 246, *247*

Breast(s) (*cont.*)
  Chiari-Frommel syndrome, 997
  colostrum, 246, 469-70
  diagnosis of pregnancy and, 286
  engorgement, 471, 993
  estrogen effects, 78
  feeding, 470-71
    duration, 489
    frequency, 489
    mastitis and, 995
  galactocele, 996
  galactorrhea, 997
  hormones and, 470
  inflammation, 994-96
  lactation, 419, *469*, 997. *See also* Lactation.
  nodule, 1030, 1031
  nonlactating, *247*
  oral contraceptives and, 1109-10
  oxytocin and, 419
  polygalactia, 997
  prenatal care, 341
  progesterone effects, 81-82
  puerperal care, 468 ff.
  pumping, 993, 997
  supernumerary, 996
Breech presentation, 321, 324, 855 ff., 1145 ff.
  anesthesia, 1154-56, 1159
  cesarean section, 862-63
  complete, 855-56, 1146 ff.
  contracted pelves, 897, 899, 906
  decomposition, 862
  decompression, 890
  diagnosis, 855-56
  etiology, 856 ff.
  extraction, 1145 ff. *See also* Extraction, breech.
  footling, 321, 856, *858*, 862
  forceps to aftercoming head, 1154
  frank, 321, *856*, 862, 1152-54
  habitual, 859
  hydrocephalus and, 885, 886, 890
  hyperextension of fetal head, 863
  incidence, 855
  incomplete, *856*, 1146 ff.
  management, 862-63, 1145 ff.
  mechanism, 859-60
  paralysis and, 1021
  placenta previa, 614
  premature rupture of membranes and, 863
  prognosis, 860-61, 1156-57
  prophylaxis, 861-62
  twins, 674
  uterine dysfunction, 863
  vaginal examination, 329-30
  vasa previa, *596*
  version, 1157 ff.
    external cephalic, 861, 1158
    internal podalic, 1158 ff.
  vertex vs., 860
  weight of fetus, 324
British abortion law, 1086
Broad ligament, 38, *39*
  cesarean section and, 1182, *1183*
  enlargement of uterus and, 241
  pregnancy, 544
  puerperal infection, 981

Broad ligament (*cont.*)
  trophoblast in blood, *169*
  tubal pregnancy rupture into, 543-44
Brow presentation, 321, 870-72
  incidence, etiology, diagnosis, 870
  mechanism and treatment, 871-72
Brucella abortus, 500
Butanol-extractable iodine, 267, 798
  abortion and, 511

Calcification, placental, 594
Calcium, 252
  dietary, 338
  fetal, 225, 338
  parathyroids and, 268
Calculi, urinary, 757
Caldwell-Moloy method, 310-11, 313
Candida albicans, 347
Canon law, abortion and, 1085
Capillaries
  glomerular endotheliosis, 692, 707
  permeability, 249
Caput succedaneum, 384, *385*, 871, 1020
Carbocaine, 442
Carbohydrate metabolism, 225, 250-51
Carbonic acid, eclampsia and, 715
Carbonic anhydrase, 132
Carbon dioxide
  accumulation in newborn, 477-78
  placental transfer, 209-10
  progesterone and, 260
Carbon monoxide, fetal malformations and,
      1066
Carcinoma
  breast, 823-24, 1109-10
  cervical, 641 ff., 1110
    in situ, 643-45
  chorionic, 478 ff. *See also* Choriocarcinoma.
  hydatidiform mole and, 564 ff.
  oral contraceptives and, 1109-10
  ovarian, 929
  rectal and colonic, 808
Cardiac disease. *See also* Heart.
  embarrassment, 781
  output
    fetal, 209, 214
    maternal, 258, 778
    postural hypotension and, 452
    puerperal, 471
    supine position and, 259
  sounds, 257-58
Cardinal ligament, 39, 40
Cardiomegaly, 257
Cardiovascular system, 257 ff. *See also* Arter-
      ies; Capillaries; Circulation; Heart;
      Veins.
  circulation, 258-60
  fetal and newborn, *212-13*
  heart, 257-58
Carnegie classification, 504
Carneous mole, 502
Carnivore placentation, 190
Caruncles, amniotic, 171, 604
Casserian fontanel, 204

Casts, hemoglobin, eclampsia and, 708
Catecholamines, fetal, 223
Catheterization
  anesthesia and, 443 ff.
  urethral, bacterial infection and, 750
Cat cry syndrome, 1068
Caudal analgesia and anesthesia, 352, 446 ff.
Caul, 362
Cellulitis, pelvic, 980-81, 983-84, 989
Cephalhematoma, 1020
Cephalic presentation, 321, 324-26. *See also*
      Brow, Face, Occiput presentations.
  predominance, 324-26
Cephalic version, external, 1158
Cephalometry, 903-4, *905*
Cephalopelvic disproportion, 1165
  uterine rupture and, 943
Cerebral palsy
  asphyxia and, 1017
  precipitate labor and, 849
Cerebrospinal fluid accumulation, 885 ff. *See*
      also Hydrocephaly.
Cerebrum
  hemorrhage, 1018-20
    in eclampsia, 708, 710
  mortality
    maternal, 819-20
    perinatal, 861, 1019
  hypoxia, 1016-17
  injury, fetal, 901, 1009
Ceruloplasmin, 252
Cervicovaginal artery, 40
Cervix, 639 ff.
  abdominal pregnancy and, 555
  abortion and
    anomalies, 501
    decidual bleeding, 505
    dilatation, 512-13, *1090*
    Hegar dilators and, *1090*
    incompetent, 512-13, 516-18
    inevitable, 505
    polyp, bleeding and, 507
  anatomy, 31 ff.
  annular detachment, 934-35
  anomalies, 501, 646
  biopsy, 642, 644
  carcinoma, 641 ff., 1110
    in situ, 643-45
  cesarean section hysterectomy and, 1185
  changes in pregnancy, 242-44
  circular detachment, 934-35
  conglutination, 923
  connective tissue, 244
  cyclic changes of glands, 99
  diagnosis of pregnancy and, 281
  dilatation, 351, 357, 361, 403
    abortion and, 512-13, 1089, *1090*
    forceps and, 1123
    Hegar dilator, *1090*
    manual, 1143
    pelvic contraction and, 899-900
    perforation of uterus, 526
    resistance, 358
    uterine dysfunction and, 836, *837*
  double, 646

Cervix (*cont.*)
Dührssen's incisions, 1142-43
dystocia and, 923-24, 934-35
edema, 652, 934
effacement, 358-59, 403
complete, *362*
epithelial cells, 35-36, 1109
erosions, 243-44, 998
eversion, 243
examination, 403 ff.
external os, 32
Ferguson reflex, 352
glands, 33, 99, 243
hydrostatic action of membranes, *360*
hypertrophy, 652
incompetent, 512-13, 516-18
inflammation, 476
injuries, 934-35
pelvic cellulitis, 980-81
postpartum
erosions, 998
hemorrhage, 957, 958-59, 961-62
symptoms, diagnosis, treatment, 935
mucosa, anatomy, 33, 35
mucus, 67, 99, 346
beading, 101, 243
ferning, 67, 100, 102
ovulation and, 67
Spinnbarkeit, 67, 99
necrosis, 843
oral contraceptives and, 1109, 1110
papilloma, 641
placenta previa and, 614, 618
preeclampsia and, 700
in pregnancy and nonpregnancy, *243*
pregnancy of, 561
prolapse, 651
puerperal changes, 468
infection, 977, 982, 988-89
progesterone effects, 81
reserve cells, 36
rigidity, 842, 923-24
rupture of membranes, 406, 1093
septate, 646
stenosis, cicatricial, 923
Cesarean section, 1163 ff.
abdominal pregnancy subsequent to, 554
abruptio placentae and, 634
atresia of vagina and, 921
blood loss, 255
breech presentation and, 862-63
classical, 937-39, 1175-76
contraindications, 1169
Couvelaire uterus at, *628*
definition, 1163
Dührssen's incisions, 1143
eclampsia and, 726, 733
enlargement of fetus and, 891
ether and, 435
extraperitoneal, 1186
fetal distress and, 1012
hemorrhage as indication, 1167
history, 1163-65
hysterectomy, 878, 1176 ff.
technic, 1181 ff.

Cesarean section (*cont.*)
incidence, 1167-68
incisions, 1143, 1169 ff.
indications, 1165-67
lower segment, 937-39, 1169 ff.
technic, 1169 ff.
mortality, 435, 902, 939, 1187-88
myoma and, 927
pelvic contraction and, 902
placenta previa and, 620-21
postmortem, 1188
preeclampsia and, 700
premature rupture of membranes and, 398
primary, indications for, 1165, *1166*
prognosis, 1187-88
repeat
incidence, 1167
indications, 1165
timing of, 1168-69
scar rupture, 947 ff.
classical vs. lower segment, 937-39
dehiscence, 937 ff.
healing, 939
perinatal mortality, 939
subsequent delivery and, 939 ff.
shoulder presentation, 878
twins and, 677
umbilical cord prolapse and, 1014
uterine anomalies and, 648
Chadwick's sign, 245
Chamberlen forceps, 1116-17
Chancroid, 803
"Change of life," 104. *See also* Menopause.
Chemotherapy. *See also* Antibiotics.
choriocarcinoma and, 583-84
hydatidiform mole and, 573, 574
tuberculosis and, 787-88
Chest
pain, pulmonary embolism and, 1003
x-ray, prenatal, 334
Chiari-Frommel syndrome, 997
Chiasmata in meiosis, 110
Childbed fever, 971. *See also* Puerperal infection.
Children's Bureau, maternal mortality decline and, 9
Chills, postpartum, 471
Chimerism
placental barrier and, 168
twins and, 666
Chloasma, 269
Chloramphenicol, puerperal infection and, 988
Chlorides
eclampsia and, 714
fetal, 225
Chloroform, 436
Chloroprocaine, 448
Chlorothiazide, preeclampsia and, 695
Chlorpromazine, 120, 732
Cholecystitis, 805-6
Cholelithiasis, 805-6
Cholera, 814
Cholestasis, 805
Cholesterol
progesterone and, 185

Cholesterol (*cont.*)
  serum, *251*
Cholinesterase, 262
Chondrodystrophia, 890, 917, 918
Chorea, 820
Chorioadenoma destruens, 564. *See also* Invasive mole.
Chorioamnionitis, 604
Chorioangioma, 584
Choriocarcinoma, 578 ff.
  clinical history, 581-82
  definition, 564
  diagnosis, 583
  etiology, 578
  frequency, 578
  gonadotropin and, 159, 175
  hydatidiform transformation to, 572, 573
  pathology, 578 ff.
  perforation of uterus, 582
  transplanted, 580
  treatment, 583-84
  trophoblast similarity to, 143
Chorion, *144*
  abortus classification and, 504
  amnion fusion with, 147
  carcinoma, 578 ff. *See also* Choriocarcinoma.
  comparative anatomy, 187
  cysts, 584
  development, 135
  frondosum, 145, *150*
  gonadotropin, 173-75. *See also* Gonadotropin, chorionic.
  laeve, 146, *150*
    separation of placenta and, *370, 371*
  plate, 144
  somatomammotropin, 175-77. *See also* Somatomammotropin, chorionic.
  twins and, 662
  vesicle, 135, *146*
    hydatidiform mole and, 564 ff.
    spontaneous abortion and, 496-97
  villus, transfer, 208
Chromatin, sex, 124. *See also* Barr body; Sex chromatin.
Chromosomes
  abortion and, 498
  dominant inheritance, 1079
  Down's syndrome and, 1073
  fetal malformations and, 1067-69, 1078
  hydatidiform mole and, 567
  mosaicism, 124-25
  nondisjunction, 124, 125
  number, 108
  sex, 110-11
    abnormal differentiation, 123-25
    normal cell, *112*
    ratios, 229
  translocation, 1073, 1075
Circulation, 159 ff.
  fetal, 159 ff., 162, 207-8, 211 ff.
    Rh antibodies and, 1044
  maternal, 162 ff., 207, 242, 258-60
    eclampsia and, 712
    in labor, 393-94
    saline, hypertonic, introduction into, 1092
    time, 258

Circumcision, 490
  thrombocytopenic purpura and, 776
Circumference of fetal head, 206
Circumvallate placenta, 586 ff.
Cirrhosis, 806
Clavicle, fracture of, 1022
  breech extraction and, 1150, 1156
Clay, ingestion of, 345-46
Cleft lip and palate, 1076
  incidence, 1064, 1065
  risk of, 1081
Climacteric. *See* Menopause.
Clinistix, 789
Clitoris, 21-22
Clomiphene (Clomid), 997
Clostridium
  perfringens
    abortion and, 521
    anemia and, 770
    enlargement of fetus and, 891
    puerperal infection and, 974-75, 991
    renal necrosis and, 760
  tetani, 975
Clot observation test, 633
Clothing, 340
Clotting factors, 256. *See also* Coagulation.
Clubfeet, 1075
  risk of, 1081
Coagulation
  abortion and, 522
    missed, 506, 509
  abruptio placentae and, 629-30, 633
  amniotic fluid embolism and, 951, 952
  eclampsia and, 711, 718
  factors, 217, 256
  fetal, 217
  fetal death and, 1007-8
  maternal, 256
  oral contraceptives and, 1109
  puerperal, 473
    thromboembolism and, 1002-3
  tubal pregnancy and, 549
Coagulopathy, consumptive, renal failure and, 761
Coccidioidomycosis, 815
Coccyx, 290, 299
Coiled arteries, 37, 93, 241
Coitus
  interruptus, 1101
  ovulation and, 65
  pregnancy and, 341
  puerperal infection and, 987
  superfecundation and superfetation, 667
  vaginal bleeding and threatened abortion, 507
Colcher-Sussman pelvimetry method, 310
Cold, common, 813
Coliform organisms, 974
Colitis, ulcerative, 808
Collagen diseases, 815-17
Collision in multiple pregnancy, 677
Colonic carcinoma, 808
Colostomy, 803, 808
Colostrum, 246, 469-70
  corpuscles, 470
Colporrhexis, 932, 933

Colpotomy
 pelvic cellulitis and, 989
 tubal pregnancy and, 549
Coma, eclampsia and, 702-3, 730
Committee on Maternal Nutrition, 336, 337, 338
Compound presentation, 879-80
Conception age of fetus, 199
Condom, 1101
Conduplicato corpore, 875
Condylomas, 640-41, 921
Cone biopsy of cervix, 642, 644
Confinement, calculated date of, 236
Connective tissue
 cervical, 244
 ovarian, 50
 pelvic, puerperal infection and, 982
 uterine, 32, 36-37, 39
Consanguinity
 choriocarcinoma and, 578
 fetal malformations and, 1081-82
Constipation, 341
 puerperal, 475
Constriction ring, 679
Contraception, 1099 ff.
 coitus interruptus, 1101
 condom, 1101
 diaphragm, 1101-2
 douche and prolonged lactation, 1101
 effectiveness, 1100
 intrauterine devices, 1103 ff.
  ectopic pregnancy and, 535
 methods, 1100 ff.
 oral, 1107 ff.
  adrenals and, 268
  chloasma and, 269
  sickle-cell anemia and, 774
 rhythm, or safe period, 1102-3
 rubella and, 810
 spermicides, 1103
Contractions
 pelvic. See Pelvis, contractions.
 uterine, 281, 351 ff., 835 ff. See also Uterus, contractions.
Conversion operation, face presentation and, 869-70
Convulsions
 eclamptic, 700, 702, 704, 727 ff.
 magnesium sulfate and, 728-30
 preeclampsia and, 696
Coombs test, 1038, 1045, 1049, 1051
Copper
 fetal, 225
 maternal, 252
Cord, umbilical. See Umbilical cord.
Cornual resection, 551
Coronal sutures, 204
Corona radiata, 115
Coronary thrombosis, 785-86
Cor pulmonale, 785, 952
Corpus
 albicans, 71-72
 luteum, 67 ff.
  ablation, 71
  atretic, 72
  hypophysectomy and, 85

Corpus (cont.)
 luteum (cont.)
  K cells, 69, 70
  luteinizing hormone and, 85
  of menstruation, 70
  of pregnancy, 69, 70-71, 244
  progesterone secretion and, 78
  regressive changes, 69-70
  ultrastructure, 70
 uteri, 31, 36-38
Corticosteroids. See also Steroids.
 placenta and, 185-86
Corticotropin, 173
 fetal, 222
 premature labor and, 351
Cortisol
 circulating, 268
 placenta and, 185-86
 premature labor and, 351
Cortisone
 glucose tolerance test, 790
Cotyledon, placental, 147, 148, 167
Coumadin, thromboembolic disease and, 1002-3
Countercurrent flow, 167
Cousins, marriage of, 1081
Couvelaire uterus, 630-31
 at cesarean section, 628
Coxalgic pelvis (coxitis), 914-16
Coxarthrolisthetic pelvis, 916
Coxsackie virus disease, 812
Cramps
 abortion and, 504
 second stage of labor, 411
Craniopagus, 668, 882
Craniotomy, 1140-42
Cranium. See also Head, fetal; Occiput.
 stresses in labor, 386
Creatinine, 263
 prematurity and, 1029
Credé's maneuver, 966
Cretin dwarf, 918
Criminal abortion, 494, 519, 520 ff. See also Abortion, criminal.
Crista dividens, 211
Crohn's disease, 808
Crowning, 390, 411
Cry, newborn, 1031
Cul-de-sac of Douglas, 24, 30
 abscess, 989
Culdocentesis, tubal pregnancy diagnosis and, 549
Cullen's sign, 547
Culture, puerperium and, 986, 995
Cumulus oophorus, 59, 115
Curare, 457
Curettage
 abortion and, 508-9, 1089 ff.
  perforation of uterus, 526
 choriocarcinoma diagnosis, 583
 hydatidiform mole and, 572
 puerperal hemorrhage and, 998-99
 technic, 1089
Cushing's syndrome, 797
Cutaneous blood flow, 260
Cyanosis, pneumothorax and, 1056-57

Cyclopropane, 435, 457, 458
Cyst(s)
  amniotic, 604
  Bartholin's glands, 640
  chorionic, 584
  kidney, 890
  ovarian
    abortion and, 507
    hydramnios vs., 601
    lutein, 567-68
      choriocarcinoma and, 580
      incidence, 567-68
    tubal pregnancy vs., 548
  placental, 584-85
  umbilical cord, 598
  vaginal, 641
Cystine aminopeptidase, 262
Cystitis, 749
  puerperal, 1000
Cystocele, 641, 930
Cytogenetic studies
  abortion and, 498-99
  hydatidiform mole and, 567
Cytomegalovirus, 811-12
Cytotrophoblast, 133, 144, 155
  circulation and, 167
  thymidine, 155

Decidua, *144*, 149 ff.
  abruptio placentae and, 626-27
  aging, 154
  basalis, 145, 150, 151
    abortion and, 505
    hematoma, 592
  capsularis, 145, *146*, 150
    placenta membranacea and, 586
    tubal pregnancy and, 539, 541
  hemorrhage, 501, 627
  histochemistry and ultrastructure, 154
  histology, 152-53
  implantation and, 130
  involution of uterus and, 466
  parietalis (vera), *146*, 150, *151*, 152, 369
  placenta previa and, 612
  placental separation and, 368-70, 626-27
  zones, 151
Decomposition, anesthesia for breech delivery
    and, 1154
Decompression, abdominal, anesthesia and,
    458-59
Dehydrocorticosterone, placenta and, 185
Dehydroisoandrosterone, 82, 178-80
  fetal adrenal production, 223
Deladumone, 993
DeLee-Hillis stethoscope, 394
Delirium tremens, newborn, 342
Delivery. *See also* Labor.
  principal movements, *381*
Demerol, 732
Dental treatment, 342
Deoxyribonucleic acid
  double helix, *112*
  gametogenesis and, 111

Deoxyribonucleic acid (*cont.*)
  syncytial, 155
Dermatoglyphics, 485
Dermatologic diseases. *See* Skin.
Descent, 377
Desmosomes, syncytial, 156
Destructive mole, 575
Dextran, anemia and, 765, 774
Dextrose
  eclampsia and, 730
  preeclampsia and, 698
Diabetes
  insipidus, 796-97
    lactation and, 470
  mellitus, 250, 788 ff.
    clinically evident, 794-96
    delivery and, 795-96
    diagnosis, 789
    eclampsia and, 718
    effects of pregnancy on, 791-93
    effects on pregnancy of, 790-91
    fetal size and, 226, 791, 792, 881
    glucose
      plasma, 789
      tolerance test, 789-90
      urinary, 264
    heredity and, 789
    hydramnios and, 601
    incidence, 789
    infertility and, 788
    management, 794
    maternal mortality, 791, 793
    perinatal loss, 791-92
    preclinical (chemical), 794
    prognosis, 793
Diad, 110
Diagnosis of pregnancy, 277 ff. *See also* Preg-
    nancy, diagnosis.
Diagonal conjugate, 299 ff., 306, 405, 894
Diameters of fetal head, 204-6
Diaphragm
  air under, perforation of uterus and, 526,
    528
  contraceptive, 1101-2
  elevation in pregnancy, 260
  hiatal hernia, 824
  pelvic, 364
  urogenital, 367
Diarrhea, epidemic, of newborn, 1055-56
Diastasis of recti, 468, 652-53
Diastolic blood pressure, 686, 687. *See also*
    Blood pressure.
Diazepam, 433
Dibucaine, 450, 451
Dicephalic monsters, 882
Dictyotene stage, 113, 125
Diet, 335 ff. *See also* Nutrition.
  recommended daily allowances, 337
Diethazine, 732
Diffusion, placental, 208-10
Digestive system. *See also* specific structures.
  fetal, 220-21
  maternal, 260-61
    labor and, 394

Digitalis, heart disease and, 781
  eclampsia, 732
Dilatation and curettage. *See also* Cervix, dilatation; Curettage.
  abortion and, 1089 ff.
Dimenhydrinate, 344
Dionne quintuplets, 656, 661
Diparcol, 732
Diphtheroids, 975
Diplotene stage, 110
Diprosopus dipagus, 882
Discharge from hospital, 475-76
Discus proligerus, 59, 115
Diuresis. *See also* Antidiuretic hormone; Diabetes insipidus.
  oxytocin and, 418
  preeclampsia and, 695, 698
  puerperal, 472
Diverticula, fallopian tube, 47
Dizygotic twins, 657, 658
Donovania granulomatis, 803
Doppler principle, 278, 288, 394
Doptone, 394
Dorsoanterior and dorsoposterior shoulder, 872
Douches, 341, 1101
Down's syndrome, 125, 1068, 1073-75
  incidence, 1064
  intrauterine diagnosis, 1078
DPN-diaphorase, 149
Drainage
  breast abscesses, 995-96
  puerperal infection, 988
Dramamine, 344
Draping, 409
Drugs. *See also* Antibiotics; Chemotherapy.
  fetal malformations and, 1067
  prenatal use, 342-43
Duchenne's paralysis, 1020
Duct(s)
  Bartholin's, 22, *23,* 640
  Gartner's, 38
  lactiferous, 469
  mesonephric (wolffian), 51
  müllerian, 51, 641
    fusion, 645
  paraurethral, 22
  Skene's, 22, *23*
Ductus
  arteriosus, 211, 214, 219, 784
  venosus, 173, 211, 214
Dührssen's incisions, 1142-43, 1154
Duration of pregnancy, 236-38, 1057-58
Dwarf pelvis, 917-18
Dye excretion tests, 263
Dysentery, 814
Dysfibrinogenemia, 630
Dyspnea
  heart disease and, 778, 780
  pneumothorax and, 1056-57
Dystocia, 835 ff. *See also* Labor.
  amniotic fluid embolism, 950 ff.
  breech presentations, 855 ff.
  brow presentation, 870-72

Dystocia (*cont.*)
  causes, 835
  cervical abnormalities, 923-24, 934-35
  cesarean section, 937 ff., 1165
  compound presentations, 879-80
  developmental abnormalities, 880 ff.
  echinococcal cysts, 930
  enterocele, 930
  excessive-sized child, 880-81, 890-91
  expulsive forces, 835 ff.
  face presentations, 863 ff.
  fetal malformations, 882 ff.
  generative tract abnormalities, 921 ff., 949-50
  hemorrhage, postpartum, 956 ff.
  hydrocephalus, 885 ff.
  injuries to birth canal, 932 ff.
  mortality, perinatal, *840,* 843, 848
  occiput posterior positions, 853-55
  pelvic contractions, 894 ff.
    atypical deformities, 916-17
    combinations, 910
    dwarf, 917-18
    femurs and, 913 ff.
    inlet, 894 ff.
    midpelvic, 906-8
    outlet, 908-10
    rare types, 910 ff.
  position or presentation abnormalities, 853 ff.
  precipitate labor, 849
  retention of placenta, 962-64
  shoulder, 881-82
    presentation, 872 ff.
  spleen and, 930
  third stage of labor abnormalities, 956 ff.
  tumors, 924 ff.
  twins, conjoined, 668
  uterine dysfunctions, 836 ff., 924
    accidental injury, 949-50
    instrumental perforation, 949
    inversion, 965 ff.
    rupture, 936 ff.
      cesarean scar, 937 ff.
  vaginal abnormalities, 921-23, 932-33
  vulvar abnormalities, 921, 932-33

Ear
  bilirubin and, 1048
  fetal, 223
  otosclerosis, 824
Earlobe, 1030, 1031
Echinococcal cysts, 930
Eclampsia, 700 ff.
  anatomy, 705 ff.
  anesthesia, 732, 733
  barbiturates, 730
  biochemistry, 149, 713 ff.
  blindness, 705
  blood pressure, 703
  brain lesions, 708, 710
  cause, 716 ff.

Eclampsia (*cont.*)
  cesarean section and, 726, 733
  chronic hypertension and, 725-26
  classification, 686-87
  clinical course, 702 ff.
  coagulation and, 718
  coma, 702-3, 730
  convulsions, 700, 702, 704, 727 ff.
  dextrose and, 730
  diagnosis, 722 ff.
  diet and, 720-21
  digitalis and, 732
  drugs, 728 ff.
  Eden's criteria, 722-23
  familial tendency, 701
  heart and, 710, 712
  hemoconcentration, 715
  hemolysis, 770
  hepatic lesions, 705-7
  hormones and, 719-20
  hydatidiform mole and, 569, 701
  incidence, 689, 700-2
  intercurrent, 704
  kidney and, 707-8, 716-17, 760
  lumbar puncture, 732
  magnesium sulfate, 728-30
  mortality, maternal, 722, 725, 727
  multiparas, and 718
  nulliparas and, 721
  paraldehyde and, 730
  parity and, 718, 722
  perinatal loss, 722
  physiology, 711-13
  placental changes, 710-11
  primigravidas and, 721
  prognosis, 723-25
  proteinuria, 703
  socioeconomic factors, 721
  subsequent pregnancies, 723, 724
  treatment. 726 ff.
  twins and, 670, 672
  venesection, 732
Economic factors. *See* Socioeconomic factors.
Ectoderm, 136, 139
Ectopic pelvic kidney, 929
Ectopic pregnancy, 535 ff.
  abdominal, 554 ff. *See also* Abdomen, pregnancy of.
  anatomic considerations, 538 ff.
  cervical, 561
  chronic ruptured, 547-48
  combined and multiple, 553
  diagnosis, 548-50, 555
  etiology, 535 ff.
  incidence, 535, 554
  infection, 537
  interstitial, 551-52
  ovarian, 559-61
  prognosis, 550-51, 558
  terminology, 535
  treatment, 551, 556-58
  tubal, 535 ff. *See also* Tubal pregnancy.
  tubouterine, tuboabdominal, and tuboovarian, 544-45
Ectropion, congenital, 35

Edema
  cervical, 652, 934
  dependent, 248
  eclamptic, 704, 712
  face presentation and, 866, *867*
  glomerulonephritis, 757-58
  heart disease, 778
  hemolytic disease, 1045
  hypertensive, 686, 691, 695, 704
  pulmonary, 704, 710, 712
  renal failure and, *525*
  retinal, 691
  umbilical cord, 598
Eden's criteria, 722-23
Effacement, cervical, 358-59, *362*, 403
Electrical stimulation for labor, 352
Electrocardiography, 258
  fetal, 278
    in labor, 395
  pulmonary embolism and, 1004
Electrolytes, 252
  epidemic diarrhea and, 1055-56
Electroshock therapy, 823
Elderly primigravida labor, 397
Elephantiasis congenita cystica, 890
Embolism
  amniotic fluid, 630, 849, 950 ff.
  oral contraceptives and, 1108-9
  puerperal, 978, 1001 ff.
  pulmonary, 1003-4
    contraceptives and, 1108
    diagnostic tests, 1004
    postpueral, 1103
    sterilization and, 1098
  septic, 1003
Embryo, 50 ff., 125
  abortion and, 499
    classification, 504
  beginning of period, 200
  comparative embryology, 138-40
  disc, 133, 200
  early human, *200, 201*
  genital abnormalities and, 645-47
  germ layers, 136
  gonads and metanephros, *52-53*
  hemoglobin, 216
  measurements, 200
  nutrition and, 224
  ovary development, 50 ff.
  rubella and incidence of affection, *811*
  somites, development of, 136-37
  uterus, development of, 45
Emesis, 343-44, 569, 806. *See also* Vomiting.
Emotional factors, 270
  abortion and, 501, 513
  labor and, 400-1
  nausea and vomiting, 343
  pain and, 459
Employment, 340
Encephalocele, 1076
Endarteritis, abortion and, 499
Endocarditis, bacterial, 785-86
Endocervical glands, cyclic changes, 99
Endocervicitis, 641
Endocervix, ectopic pregnancy and, 561

Endocrine function, 266 ff., 788 ff. *See also* specific glands and hormones.
  abortion and, 500, 511, 514
  adrenal dysfunction, 797
  diabetes insipidus and, 796-97
  diabetes mellitus and, 788 ff.
  diagnostic tests for pregnancy, 283
  fallopian tube effects, 120
  fetal, 221-23, 351
  obesity and, 799-800
  parathyroid disease, 799
  pheochromocytoma, 797
  thyroid disease, 797-99
Endoderm, 136, 139
Endometriosis, 654
  tubal pregnancy and, 537
Endometritis, 977-78, 980, 982-83, 989
Endometrium, 30, 90 ff.
  anatomy, 36-37
  cycle, 90 ff.
    anovulatory, 99
    dating, 99
    menstrual phase, 93-94
    ovarian cycle correlated with, 97
    ovulatory, 90-99
    premenstrual phase, 92-93
    proliferative phase, 90-91
    secretory phase, 91-92, 96
    ultrastructure, 94 ff.
  ectopic pregnancy and, 548
  involution of uterus and, 466
  lymphatics, 43
  necrosis, 982
  postovulatory, 95-97, 99
  preovulatory, 94
  progesterone effects, 80
  tubal transport of ovum and, 120
  ultrastructure, 94 ff.
  vasculature, 37
  zones, 91-92
Endopelvic fascia, 28
Endoplasmic reticulum, syncytial, 156-57
Endosalpingitis, tubal pregnancy and, 536-37
Endotheliosis, glomerular capillary, 692, 707
Endotoxins, placental, 717
Endotracheal intubation
  general anesthesia, 434
  newborn, 482-83
  thiopental sodium, 436
Engagement, 302-4
  breech presentation, 859
  forceps and, 1119-20, 1122
  station of head, 404
  vertex presentation, 302, 375-77
Entamoeba histolytica, 814
Enteritis, regional, 808
Enterocele, 652
  dystocia and, 930
Enterococcus, 974
Environment, fetal malformations and, 1066-67
Enzymes
  amniotic fluid, 229
  bilirubin and, 1048, 1049
  liver, 221

EPH-Gestosis, 686
Epidural anesthesia, 352, 450
  doses, 448
  intermittent, 453 ff.
Epilepsy, 819
  hemorrhagic disease of newborn and, 1052
  intracranial injury and, 1020
Epinephrine, infant heart rate and, 483
Epiphysis, syphilis and, *1053*
Episiotomy, *389*, 423 ff.
  blood loss, 957
  breech delivery, 1152
  forceps and, 1122, *1127*
  infection, 977
  median vs. mediolateral, 425-26
  occiput posterior position, 854
  pain, 428
  purpose, 424
  technic, 427-28
  timing of, 424-25, 427
Epithelium, cervical, 35-36
  oral contraceptives and, 1109
Epoophoron, 38, 54
Epulis, *261*, 808
Erb's paralysis, 1020
Ergastoplasm, syncytial, 156
Ergonovine, 419-21
  postpartum hemorrhage and, 960
Ergot, history of, 420
Ergotrate, 418, 419
Erysipelas, 814
Erythema, palmar, 269
Erythroblastosis, 1045, 1049
  estriol and, 183
  gonadotropin and, 175
  hydramnios and, 601
  placental barrier and, 168
  placental size and, 585
  thalassemia and, 772
  treatment, 1049
Erythrocytes
  anemia and, 762 ff.
  fetal, 215 ff.
  hemolytic disease and, 1046
  life-span, 215
  loss in delivery, 255
  sedimentation rate, 762-63
  volume of circulating, 253
Erythroid hyperplasia, 253
Erythromycin, gonorrhea and, 802
Erythropoiesis, 764, 767 ff., 771
Erythropoietin, 215, 253
Escherichia coli
  abortion and, 521
  diarrhea and, 1055
  mastitis and, 995
  puerperal infection and, 974
  pyelonephritis and, 749
Escutcheon, 19
Esophagus
  atresia, 228, 599
  reflux of gastric contents, 261, 345
Estradiol, 72, *73*, 74
  diabetes and, 795
  lactation and, 993

Estradiol (*cont.*)
  luteinizing hormone and, 84
  placental, 177, 179
  plasma levels, 177
  production, 76
Estriol, 72, 73, 74
  abortion and, 511
  amniotic fluid, 1042
  fetal endocrines and, 223
  nonpregnant, 178
  placental conversion, 179
  Rh-negative women and, 1042
  urinary, interpretation of, 183
    diabetes and, 795-96
    placental function and, 181 ff.
Estrogens, 72 ff., 177 ff.
  actions, 76-78
  adrenals and, 268
  alkaline phosphatase and, 262
  in biologic fluids, 76
  biosynthetic pathways, 74-75, 178
  carbohydrate metabolism and, 251
  chemistry, 73-74
  eclampsia and, 720
  lactation and, 993
  mammary growth and, 470
  melanocyte-stimulating hormone and, 269
  oral contraceptives and, 1107, 1109
  placenta and, 177 ff.
  plasma levels, 177
  precursors, 178-80
  secretion, 75
  site of origin, 177
  sources, 74
  sulfobromphthalein and, 262
  terminology, 72-73
  thyroid function and, 267, 268
  transferrin levels and, 255
  tubal function and, 120
  uterine wall hypertrophy and, 239
Estrone, 72, 73, 74, 178, 179
Ether, 435
  breech presentation and, 1159
Eutheria, placentation in, 186
Exercise, 340
Exocelomic membrane, 133, 172
Expressivity, genetic, 1080
Expulsion of fetus, 382
Extension, 379 ff., 390
External cephalic version, 1158
External generative organs, anatomy of, 19 ff.
External rotation, 382, 391, 412, 860
External version, breech presentation and,
    861-62
Extraction, breech, 1145 ff.
  anesthesia, 1154-56
  complete or incomplete, 1146 ff.
  forceps to aftercoming head, 1154
  frank, 1152-54
  indications, 1145
  prognosis, 1156-57
Extremities
  lameness, 914-16
  presentation, 870. See also Breech presenta-
    tion.

Extremities (*cont.*)
  varicosities, 344-45
Eye
  fetal, 223
  newborn, 486-87
  retinitis gestationis, 824
  retrolental fibroplasia, 1035

Face
  maternal, 269
    in eclamptic convulsions, 702
  paralysis, newborn, 1022, *1023*
  presentation, 321, *325*, 863 ff.
    contracted pelves and, 897, 906
    diagnosis, 864-65
    etiology, 865
    forceps use, 1135
    incidence, 863
    mechanism, 865-66
    palpation, 864
    prognosis, 866 ff., 869, 870
    treatment, 869-70
    vaginal examination, 329-30
Factors, clotting
  fetal, 217
  maternal, 256
Fallopian tubes, *30*, 45 ff.
  ampulla, 45, 47
  anatomy, 45 ff.
  blood supply, *42*
  changes in pregnancy, 245
  ciliated cells, 47, 48
  cyclic changes, 102
  diverticula, 47
  estrogen effects, 77
  hormonal effects, 77, 81, 120
  inflammation, 535. See also Salpingitis.
    tubal pregnancy and, 536-37
  infundibulum, 45
  interstitial portion, 45
  isthmus, 45, 47
  ligation, 1089. See Sterilization.
  mucosa, 47
  musculature, 45, 47
  pregnancy in, 535 ff. See also Tubal preg-
    nancy.
  progesterone effects, 81
  removal, 551
  secretory cells, 47, 48
  sphincter, 119
  sterilization, 1089, 1176, 1180. See also
    Sterilization.
  transport of ovum, 119-20
Falx cerebri, 1018
Fascia, 28
  pelvic, 28, 363
  perineal, 28, 367-68
  vagina, 28, 367
Fatigue, 286, 346
Fat metabolism, 251-52
  fetal, 225
Fatty acids
  fetal, 225
  induction of labor and, 1094
  insulin and, 250-51

Index

Fatty acids (*cont.*)
  serum levels, *251*
  somatomammotropin and, 176
Febrility. *See also* Fever.
Feet. *See also* Breech presentation.
  differentiation from hand, 1160
  internal podalic version and, 1158 ff.
Femoral vein
  pressure, 258, *259*
  thrombophlebitis, 978
Femurs
  forces exerted by, 913 ff.
  fracture, fetal, 1022
  lameness and, 914-16
Ferguson reflex, 352
Ferning of cervical mucus, 67, 100, 102
Ferrous compounds, 765
Fertility
  control of, 1111. *See also* Contraception.
  puerperal infection and, 991
  rate, 2, 3-4
  of twins, 668
Fertilization, 122 ff.
  abnormal sexual differentiation and, 123-25
  aging of gametes and, 125
  in vitro, 122
  ovum changes, 123
  preimplantation stages, *127*
  superfecundation and superfetation, 667
  zona pellucida and, 123
Fetopelvic disproportion, 1165
Fetus, 125, 199 ff.
  abdomen, localization of, 1043
  abdominal pregnancy, 544-55. *See also* Abdomen, pregnancy of.
  adrenals, 179-80
  age determination, 199, 236
  albumin, 218
  alcoholism and, 342
  amniotic fluid and, 226 ff. *See also* Amniotic fluid.
  anesthesia and, 430, 432, 442 ff.
  antigens, 168-69
  ascorbic acid transfer, 210
  attitude, 320
  axis pressure, 357
  barbiturates and, 437
  bilirubin, 221, 229
  blood, 215 ff., 229
    ingestion, 1048
    pH, 1010
    pressure, 208
  bradycardia, 442 ff., 1010, *1013*
  calcium content, 338
  cardiac output, 209, 214
  circulation, 162, 207-8, 211 ff., 1044
  coagulation factors, 217
  compressus, 503
  cotyledon, 147
  dead. *See also* Mortality, perinatal.
    craniotomy, 1140-42
    dissolution, 503
    identification of, 288-89
    probability, *494*
    rate of, definitions, 2

Fetus (*cont.*)
  dead (*cont.*)
    villous degenerative disease, 592
  diabetes and size of, 226, 791, 792, 881
  digestive system, 220-21
  distress, 1009 ff.
  drugs affecting, 343
  dystocia and, 835 ff., 853 ff. *See also* Dystocia; Labor.
  electrocardiography, 278, 395
  endocrines, 221-23, 351
    estriol and, 181 ff.
    estrogens and, 178, 179-80
    labor onset and, 351
  erythrocytes, 215 ff.
  gas in, 289
  goiter, 787, 798
  growth, 202-4, 224, 226
  head, 204-6. *See also* Head, fetal; Occiput.
    fontanels, 204, *205*, 330
    measurements, 204-6
    sutures, 204, 206
  heart, 211. *See also* Heart, fetal.
  height increase, 202-3
  hemoglobin, 215, 216
  hemolytic disease, 1044 ff.
  hemorrhage, 206, 1018-20
  hepatitis and, transmission to, 804
  histidine transfer, 210
  hypoxia, 209-10, 352, 402, 783, 1016-17
    mortality, 1007
  immunology, 168, 218, 223-24
  infections, 211, 224
  injuries, 1007 ff.
    asphyxia, 1015-17
    cephalhematoma, 1020
    cerebral hemorrhage, 1018-20
    fractures, 1022-23
    mortality in general, 1007-9. *See also* Mortality, perinatal.
    muscular injuries, 1023
    nervous system, central, 1009 ff.
    paralyses, 1020-22
    peripheral, 1020 ff.
    spinal, 1020, *1021*
    umbilical cord prolapse, 1012 ff.
  insulin, 221
  iron, 210, 254, 764
  kidneys, enlargement of body and, 890
  lie of, 320-21
  liver, 221, 890-91
  living, identification of, 288
  lunar months, 202
  lungs, 211, 214, 218-20
    expansion, 477-79
  maceration, 503
  magnesium, 729
  malformations, 1063 ff.
    anemia and, 769
    anencephaly 220, 228, 1069 ff., 1081. *See also* Anencephaly.
    anus, imperforate, 1077
    chromosomes and, 1067-69, 1078 ff.
    clubfeet, 1075, 1081
    consanguinity, 1081-82

Fetus (*cont.*)

  malformations (*cont.*)

    diagnosis, 1077-78, 1079

    Down's syndrome, 125, 1064, 1068, 1073-75

    dystocia and, 882 ff.

    environmental defects and, 1066-67

    etiology, 1065-66

    genetic counseling and, 1078 ff.

    harelip and cleft palate, 1076, 1081

    harlequin, 1077

    heart disease, 1075, 1081. *See also* Heart, fetal.

    hernia, umbilical and inguinal, 1076-77

    hip dislocation, 1075-76

    hydramnios and, 599, 601

    hydrocephalus, 885 ff., 1072, 1081

    incidence, 1063-65

    iniencephalus, 1073

    influenza and, 813

    meningocele, 1076

    metabolism and, inborn errors of, 1069

    phocomelia, 1069

    polydactylism, 1076

    protozoal infections and, 814

    renal agenesis, 1075

    respiratory system, 211, 214, 218-20

    rubella and, 810-11

    spina bifida, 1072, 1081

    testes, undescended, 1077

  meconium, 221

  minerals, 225

  monitoring, 228-29

  mortality. *See* Mortality, perinatal.

  movements, 202, 278

  multiple, 656 ff. *See also* Multiple pregnancy.

    gonadotropin and, 175

  mummification, 503

  nervous system, 223

  nutrition, 224-26

  ossification, beginning of, 202

  outlining of, 281, 283

  oxygen

    analgesia and anesthesia and, 432

    and carbon dioxide transfer, 209-10

    dissociation curve, 216, *217*

    IQ and, 458-59

  pancreas, 221-22

  papyraceus, 503, *666*

  pelvis, 297, 298

  physiology, 211 ff.

  placental transfer, 206 ff.

  polyuria, 228

  preeclampsia and function of, 699

  presentation and position, 320 ff. *See also* Presentation and position; and specific presentations.

    dystocia and, 853 ff.

  protein, 249

  respiration, intrauterine, 478-79

  rotation. *See* Rotation.

  sacs. *See also* Amnion; Chorion.

    cervical pregnancy and, *560*

    ovarian pregnancy and, 559

Fetus (*cont.*)

  sacs (*cont.*)

    tubal pregnancy and, 540

  sensory organs, 223

  sex, 229-30

    prediction of, 230

  size, 202-4, 224, 397

    abortion and, 493

    breech delivery and, 324

    diabetes and, 226, 791, 792, 881

    dystocia and, 890-91

    excessive, 880-81, 890-91

    pelvic contraction and, 897

  socioeconomic factors and, 204

  sounds, 278

  spinal curvature, 289

  swallowing, *219*, 220, 228

  syphilis, 224, 800, 1053

  at term, 203

  thorax compression in delivery, 477-78

  transfusion, intrauterine, 216

  umbilical cord

    loops around neck, 596-97

    prolapse. *See* Umbilical cord, prolapse.

    velamentous insertion, 595, 597

  urinary system, 218, 228

  vaccinia, 813

  villous degenerative changes, 592

  viral disease and, 808, 810-11, 812

  water content, 248

  weight, 202-4, 225, 226. *See also* Fetus, size.

  x-ray pelvimetry dosage, 317

Fever. *See also* Temperature.

  abortion and, 520

  genital infection and, 982

  milk, 470, 471

  puerperal, 971

  rheumatic, 817

  scarlet, 813-14

  tubal pregnancy and, 547

  typhoid, 814

Fibrin

  abruptio placentae and, 630

  eclampsia and, 711

Fibrinogen, 217, 256

  abortion and, 524

  abruptio placentae and, 629-30, 633-34

  eclampsia and, 719

  fetal death and, 1007-8

Fibrinogenopenia

  abruptio placentae and, 629-30, 635

  amniotic fluid embolism and, 951

  retention of dead fetus and, 1007-8

Fibrinoid, placental, 154, 591

  immunology and, 169-70

Fibrinolysin, 256

Fibroplasia, retrolental, 1035

FIGLU, 769

Fimbria ovarica, 45

Finger edema, hypertension and, 695

Fingernails, eclampsia and, 711

Fingerprinting, 485

First stage of labor, 358 ff. *See also* Labor, first stage.

Fistulas
  pelvic inlet contraction and, 900
  rectovaginal, 425, 900
  vesicocervical, 900, 950
  vesicovaginal, 900, 950, 1001
Fixation of fetal head, 304
Flagyl, 347
Flexion, 377
Fluid balance
  bacterial endotoxic shock and, 522, 523
  epidemic diarrhea and, 1055
Fluoride, supplemental, 339
Fluothane, 435-36
Foam tablets, 1103
Folic acid, 339, 765 ff.
  abortion and, 512
  abruptio placentae and, 627
  anemia and, 765, 767-69, 774
  choriocarcinoma, 583
  epilepsy and, 819
  fetal malformation and, 339
Follicles, ovarian
  atretic, 72
  development, 113-15
  graafian, 59 ff., 64
  of Montgomery, 246
  nabothian, 33, 246
  primordial, 51, *54*, 55, 58, 59
Follicle-stimulating hormone, 78, 82, 83-84
Follow-up examination, 476
Fontanels, fetal, 204, *205*, 330
  flexion and, *378*
  occipitotransverse position, 375
Food and Nutrition Board, 336, 337, 338
Foot
  club, 1075, 1081
  differentiation from hand, *1160*
Footling presentation, 321, 856, 862
  double, *858*
Footprinting, 485
Foramen ovale, 211, 214
Forceps, 1115 ff.
  application, 1123 ff.
  Barton, 1130, 1135, *1138*
  blades, 1115
  breech presentation and aftercoming
    head, 1154
  Chamberlen, 1116-17
  choice of, 1121
  curves, 1115
  definitions and classification, 1119-21
  Dührssen's incisions, 1142-43, 1154
  English lock, *1116*
  face presentations, 1135
  failed, 1138-39
  forces exerted, 1121
  French lock, *1116*
  functions, 1121
  high, 1120
  history of, 1115 ff.
  incidence of use, 1120
  incorrect applications, *1124*
  indications for use, 1121-22
  Kielland, 855, 1130, 1131, 1133, *1135, 1136*

Forceps (*cont.*)
  low, 1119, 1122, 1125 ff.
  midforceps, 1119, 1120, 1123, 1128-30
    cerebral hemorrhage and, 1019
    occiput posterior position and, 855
    pelvic contraction and, 907
  obliquely posterior positions, 1130
  occiput posterior positions, 853, 855
  operation prepatory to use, 1142-43
  Palfyn's, *1118*
  pelvic application, 1125
  Piper, 1154, *1155, 1156*
  preparations for operations, 1123
  prerequisites for application, 1122-23
  prognosis, 1138
  pubiotomy, 1143
  Scanzoni maneuver, 1130 ff.
  Simpson, *1116, 1125*, 1130
  Smellie's, *1118*
  symphysiotomy, 1143
  trial, 1138-39
  Willett's, 620
Foreign body in peritoneal cavity, abortion
    and, 526, *527*
Formiminoglutamic acid, 769
Fornices, vaginal, 26
Fourchet, 21
Fractures, 1022-23
  breech extraction and, 1150, 1156
  clavicular, 1022
  femoral, 1022
  humerus, 1022
  pelvic, 917
  skull, 901
  vertebral, 1020, *1022*
Frankenhäuser's ganglion, 43, 239, 437
Fraternal twins, 657, 658
Freemartin, 668
Frenulum of clitoris, 21
Frontal sutures, 204
Functional residual capacity, 260
Fungal infections, 815
Funis. *See* Umbilical cord.
Furadantin, 756
Furosemide, 766, 781

Galactocele, 996
Galactorrhea, 997
Galactosemia, 1069
Gallbladder, 262
  inflammation and stones, 805-6
Gametes. *See also* Ovum; Spermatozoon.
  aging of, 125
Gametogenesis, 108 ff.
  biochemistry, 111
  meiosis, 108 ff.
  mitosis, 109
  oogenesis, 111 ff.
  spermatogenesis, 116
  spermiogenesis, 116 ff.
Gamma globulin
  Rh antibodies and, 1039
  rubella and, 809

Gangrene, 982, 985
Gartner's duct, 38, 641
Gas
    anesthetics, 434-35
    fetal, 289
    gangrene, 985
Gastric contents, aspiration of, anesthesia and, 430-31, 434
Gastric emptying, 261
Gastrointestinal tract, 806 ff. *See also* specific structures.
    fetal, 220-21
    labor and, 394
    maternal physiology, 260-61
General anesthesia, 434
Genetics
    abortion and, 498-99, 510
    anemia and, 771 ff., 776
    anencephaly and, 1071
    counseling, 1078 ff.
    dominant genes, 1079
    expressivity, 1080
    fetal malformations and, 1065
    hypertension and, 735
    Marfan's syndrome and, 817
    penetrance, 1080
    polygenic inheritance, 1080-81
    recessive genes, 1080
Genital ridge, 51
Genitourinary tract, 19 ff., 639 ff. *See also* Urinary system.
    abnormalities, 500-1, 639 ff.
        dystocia and, 921 ff.
    accidental injury, 949-50
    anatomy, 19 ff.
    infection
        herpesvirus, 812
        puerperal, 971 ff., 977, 982, 988-89
        temperature rise and, 471
        venereal, 800 ff.
    nerve supply, 22
    perforation following necrosis, 950
    prematurity and, 1031
Gentamicin, 756, 988
Gentian violet, 347
Geophagia, 345-46
Germ cells, 108. *See also* Ovum; Spermatozoon.
    maturation, 113
    migration, 111
    primordial ovarian, 50-51
Germ layers of embryo, 136
Germ plasm defects, abortion and, 497-98, 510-11, 514
German measles, 808 ff.
Germinal epithelium, ovarian, 50
Gestational age, 199, 236, 496, 1026, 1030 ff.
Gestosis, 686
Gibbus, 910 ff.
Gingivitis, 808
Glabellar tap, 1031
Glandulae vestibulares majores and minores, 22
Globin fetal, 216

Globulin
    -albumin ratio, eclampsia and, 716
    liver and, 262
    rubella and, 809
Glomeruli
    capillary endotheliosis, 692, 707
    filtration rate, 263, 715
Glomerulonephritis
    acute, 708, 757-58
    chronic, 758-59
    hypertension and, 734
    poststreptococcal, 758
Gloving, surgical, 410-11
Gluconeogenesis, somatomammotropin and, 176
Glucose
    fetal, 225-26
    metabolism, 250-51
    somatomammotropin and, 176
    tolerance test, 251, 789-90
Glucose-6-phosphate dehydrogenase
    anemia and, 770
    placental, 149
    urinary tract infection and, 756
Glucosuria, 251, 264, 789, 794
Glucuronyl transferase, bilirubin and, 1048, 1049
Glycerophosphatase, 149
Glycogen, fetal, 221, 225
Glycosuria, 789
Goiter, 267, 787, 798
Golgi bodies, 94, 156
Gonadotropin, 82 ff.
    chorionic, 173-75
        abdominal pregnancy and, 558
        abortion and, 508, 511
        assaying, 174
        chemical structure, 174
        choriocarcinoma diagnosis, 583
        diagnosis of pregnancy, 283-84
        eclampsia and, 720
        fetal death and, 288
        hydatidiform mole and, 173, 343, 568, 571, 573-74
        molecular weight, 174
        nausea and vomiting and, 343
        origin of, controversy over, 159
    multiple pregnancy and, 661
    pituitary
        diagnosis of pregnancy, 283
        fetal, 222
        lactation and, 475
        ovarian and endometrial cycles, 98
Gonads
    embryonic, 52-53
    x-ray pelvimetry and, 317
Gonorrhea, 801-3, 975, 985
    asymptomatic, 801
    Bartholin's glands and, 640
    eye care of infant and, 486-87
    incidence, 801
    salpingitis, 535, 985
    treatment, 802

Gower hemoglobin, 216
Graafian follicle, 59 ff., 64
    maturation, 115
Graft-vs.-host reaction, placental barrier and, 168
Granuloma
    anemia and, 767
    inguinale, 803
Granulosa cells, 59, 60, 64, 67, 70, 72, 74
Grasp, newborn, 1031
Graves' disease, 799
Gravida, definition of, 332
Grosser classification, 187, 190
Growth hormone, 176, 222. *See also* Somato-mammotropin.
Gums, 261
    epulis, *261*, 808
    inflammation, 808
Gunshot wounds, 950
Gynecoid pelvis, 315-16

Habitual abortion, 509 ff. *See also* Abortion, habitual.
Habitus of fetus, 320
Hall-Stone ring, 1105
Halothane, 435-36, 1159
Hand
    differentiation from foot, *1160*
    presentation, 879
    scrubbing, mastitis and, 995
Harelip and cleft palate, 1076
    incidence, 1064, 1065
    risk of, 1081
Harlequin fetus, 1077
Hartman's sign, 504-5
Head, fetal, 204-6. See also Occiput.
    birth of, 388 *ff.*
    cerebral injury, 901, 1009
    craniotomy, 1140-42
    cesarean section and, 1172
    crowning, 390, 411
    descent, 377
    engagement, 302-4, 375-77. *See also* Engagement.
    extension, 379 ff., 390
    external rotation, 382, 391
    face presentation, 863 ff.
    flexion, 377
    fontanels, 204, *205*, 330, 375, 378
    hyperextension, 863
    internal rotation, 377-79
    method of controlling, *411*
    measurements, 204-6, 903
    molding, 384, *385*. *See also* Molding.
    onset of labor and, 374
    restitution, 382, 391
    shape changes, 384-86
    station, 403
    sutures, 204, 206, 330, 375
Headache, 346
    preeclampsia, 691
    spinal anesthesia, 451
Hearing defects, bilirubin and, 1048

Heart
    fetal, 211
        bradycardia, 395, 402, 442 ff., 1010
        congenital disease, 1075, 1081
        detectable signs, 277-78
        forceps and, 1123
        hypoxia, 783
        labor and, 394-96, 402
        maternal disease and, 783
        monitoring, 394-95
        output, 209, 214
        sounds and rate, 277-78, 330-31, 402
        twins, 664
        vertex presentation, 375, 383
    maternal disease, 777 ff.
        abortion and, 785
        bacterial endocarditis, 785-86
        classification, 779
        diagnosis, 778
        displacement, 257
        dyspnea, 778, 780
        eclampsia, 710, 712. *See also* Eclampsia.
        failure, 780 ff.
        functional capacity, 779
        hypertension, 685 ff. *See also* Hypertension.
        hypertrophy, 257
        kyphoscoliosis, 912
        multiple pregnancy and, 674
        output, 258, 259, 452, 471, 778
        physiology, 257-58
        postpartum, 785
        prognosis, 778-79
        rheumatic fever, 817
        treatment, 779 ff.
        work in pregnancy, 258
    newborn, resuscitation and, 483-84
Heartburn, 261, 345
Hegar dilators, 1089, *1090*
Hegar's sign, 281, *282*
Hemagglutination inhibition, 283, 284
    rubella and, 809, 810
Hemangioma, placental, 584
Hematocele, tubal pregnancy and, 541, 547
Hematocrit, 253
    abruptio placentae and, 633
Hematologic disorders, 252 ff., 776-77
Hematoma
    abruptio placentae and, 627, 631
    broad ligament, 544
    decidual, 592, 627
    myometrial, 631
    placental, 368, 372, 590, 592
    puerperal, 999-1000
    retroplacental, 417, 627, 628
    sternocleidomastoid muscle, 1156-57
    subdural, 1018
    tuberous subchorial, 503
    umbilical cord, 598
    uterine rupture and, 947
    vulvar, 999-1000
Hematopoiesis, 215, 583, 1045
Hematosalpinx, 541
Hematuria. *See also* Urine, blood.
    urinary tract infection and, 749, 757, 758

Hemiacardius, 885
Hemoconcentration, eclampsia and, 715
Hemoglobin
  A, 216, 771
  anemia, 761 ff., 771
  Bart's, 772
  C diseases, 774-75
  concentration, 253, 761-62
  D, 775
  eclampsia, 708
  fetal, 215, 216
  Gower, 216
  hemolytic disease, 1046
  iron, 253
  S (sickle cell), 772 ff.
  umbilical cord, 1049
Hemoglobinopathies. *See also* Anemia.
  genetic counseling and, 776
Hemolytic disease, 770, 1036 ff.
  bilirubin, 1050
  newborn, 1036 ff.
  perinatal mortality, 1042
  renal failure, 760
  streptococcal infection, 813
  transfusion, 1050
  treatment, 1049-51
Hemoperitoneum, tubal pregnancy and, 549
Hemophilus ducreyi, 803
Hemoptysis, 780
Hemorrhage
  abdominal pregnancy, 556-57
  abortion, 501, 504 ff., 521, 541
  abruptio placentae, 623 ff.
  anemia from, 766
  antepartum, 624, 678-79
    perinatal loss, 609
  brain, 708, 710, 819-20, 861, 1018-20
  carcinoma of cervix, 642
  cervical tears, 935, 961-62
  cesarean section, 255, 1167, 1179
  concealed, 624, *625,* 627, 632
  fetal, 206
  hemorrhoidal, 345
  hepatic, 705-7
  hydatidiform mole, 569, 572, 574
  hypotonic uterus, 421
  menstrual, 93
  mortality, 7, 819-20, 1019
  newborn, 1052
  peptic ulcer, 807
  placental separation, 416-17, 505
  placenta previa, 609, 613, 618
  postpartum, 417, 473, 956 ff.
    causes, 957-58
    cervical lacerations, 935, 961-62
    clinical picture, 958
    definition, 956
    diagnosis, 958-59
    halothane and, 436
    management, 959-61
    mortality, 956
    multiple pregnancy, 679
    prognosis, 959
    retained placental fragments, 962
    twins, 678

Hemorrhage (*cont.*)
  puerperal, 998-1000
    infection and, 976
    late, 466
  retroperitoneal, 933
  retroplacental, 417, 627, 628
  show, 387-88
  subdural, 386
  subperiosteal, 1020
  tubal pregnancy, 541, 546
  twins and, 678-79
  unavoidable, 610, 623
  vaginal, 255
    diagnosis of pregnancy, 285
    threatened abortion, 506-7
  vulvar, 639
Hemorrhoids, 345
Hemovillous degeneration, 590
Heparin
  abortion and, 524
  abruptio placentae and, 634
  amniotic fluid embolism and, 951
  fetal mortality and, 1008
  heart surgery and, 783
  sickle-cell anemia and, 773-74
  thromboembolic disease and, 1002
Hepatic disease. *See* Liver.
Hepatitis, viral, 803-4
  abruptio placentae transfusion and, 634
  fibrinogen therapy and, 633
Hepatosis, obstetric, 805
Hereditary disorders. *See* Genetics.
Hernia
  diaphragmatic, 824
  inguinal, 1077
  umbilical, 1076
    maternal, 652
Herpes
  gestationis, 817-18
  hominis infections, 812
  simplex, 1056
Hertig-Rock ova, 129, 130
Heterozygosity, 1079, 1080
Heuser's membrane, 133
Hiatal hernia, 824
High-risk infants, 484-85
Hip
  breech presentation and, 859
  congenital dislocation, 1075-76
Histidine transfer, 210
History taking, 333
Hoboken, folds of, 173
Hodges' pelvimetry method, 310-11
Hodgkin's disease, 777
Hofbauer cells, 148, 157
Holocardius, 885
Homans' sign, 1002
Homografts, 169
Homozygosity, 1079, 1080
"Horizons," 200
Hormones. *See also* Endocrine function; and
    specific hormones.
  abortion and, 500, 511, 514
  cervical mucus ferning and, 102
  eclampsia and, 711, 719-20
  fetal, 222

Hormones (*cont.*)
  lactation and, 993
  menstrual cycle and, *98*
  oral contraceptives and, 1107, 1110
  placental, 173 ff.
  pressor, 711
  tests for pregnancy, 283
Hospitalization
  admittance procedures, 401-2, 697-99
  diabetes and, 795
  discharge, 475-76
  eclampsia and, 727
  heart disease and, 782
  preeclampsia and, 697-99
Humerus, fracture of, 1022
  breech extraction and, 1150, 1156
Humpback, 910 ff.
Huntington's chorea, 820
Hyaline membrane disease
  neonatal mortality, 1009
  prematurity and, 1034
Hydatidiform mole, 564 ff.
  abortion and, 496, 502
  age and, 569
  anemia and, 569
  blood volume and, 252
  clinical history, 569
  definition, 564
  diagnosis, 569-71
  eclampsia and, 701
  follow-up procedures, 573-75
  gonadotropin and, 175, 343, 568, 571, 573-74
  hemorrhage and, 569, 572, 574
  histology, 567
  incidence, 568-69
  invasive, 575 ff.
  nausea and vomiting, 343
  partial, 565
  pathology, 564 ff.
  prognosis, 571-72
  sonography, 567
  subsequent pregnancies and, 573
  transition theory, 567
  treatment, 572-73
  ultrastructural features, 567
Hydralazine, 731
Hydramnios, 228, 599 ff.
  anencephaly and, 1071
  diagnosis, 601
  etiology, 600
  incidence, 599-600
  pressure, 601, 603
  prognosis, 601-2
  symptoms, 601
  treatment, 602-3
  twins and, 665, 670
Hydrocephaly, 885 ff., 1072
  breech presentation, 325
  craniotomy, 1141
  diagnosis, 886-87
  incidence, 1064, 1065
  prognosis, 888-89
  risk of, 1081
  sonogram, *1077*

Hydrocephaly (*cont.*)
  treatment, 889-90
Hydrochloric acid, 261
Hydrocortisone, placenta and, 186
Hydrops fetalis, 1045
  amniogram, *1046*
  hydatidiform mole and, 567
  intrauterine transfusions, 1042
Hydrorrhea gravidarum, 653
Hydrostatic pressure, intracapillary, 249
Hydroxyzine, 433
Hymen, 23-24
  puerperium and, 468
Hyperbaric oxygen, 210
Hyperbilirubinemia, 415, 488, 1036 ff., 1052
  hepatosis and, 805
  prematurity and, 1032
Hyperemesis gravidarum, 343-44, 569, 806
Hyperestrogenemia, 251
Hyperextension of head, 863
Hyperglycemia
  fetal size and, 226
  newborn, 792
Hyperinsulinism, diabetes and, 794
Hyperparathyroidism, 268, 799
Hyperplasminemia, 630
Hyperprogesteronemia, 251
Hyperreflexia, eclampsia and, 702
Hypertension, 685 ff.
  abortion, 513
  abruptio placentae, 624, 626, 635
  blood pressure, 738
  chronic, 687-88, 733 ff.
    heredity and, 735
    management, 738-39
    prognosis, 736-38
    superimposed preeclampsia, 688, 735-36, 739
  classification, 685 ff.
  concealed hemorrhage and, 624
  diuretics, 695
  eclampsia, 686-87, 700 ff., 725. *See also* Eclampsia.
  edema, 686, 691, 695, 704
  essential, 687, 734
  fixed, 738
  glomerulonephritis and, 757-58
  incidence, 689
  kidney function, 737
  lupus erythematosus and, 815
  mortality, 689, 736, 737
  preeclampsia, 686 ff., 725. *See also* Preeclampsia.
  proteinuria, 686, 687, 691
  pulmonary, 784
  recurrence, 723, 724
  retinal changes, 735
  somatomammotropin, 176-77
  transient, 688-89
  twins and, 670
Hyperthyroidism, 267, 268, 798
Hypertonic uterine dysfunction, 842, 848-49
Hyperventilation, 260
Hypervolemia, 252
  twins and, 664
Hypnosis, 459

Hypofibrinogenemia
abruptio placentae and, 629-30, 635
fetal death and, 1007
Hypogastric artery legation, uterine rupture and, 947-49
Hypogastric plexus, 352
Hypoglycemia, 791, 794
kernicterus and, 1048
postmaturity and, 1031
prematurity and, 1032
tolbutamide effect, 251
Hypokalemia, pica and, 346
Hypoparathyroidism, 799
Hypophysial-portal system, 83, 86
Hypophysis
excision, 266-67
corpus luteum and, 85
puerperium and, 470
Hypoplastic anemia, 770-71
Hypoplastic dwarf pelvis, 917, 918
Hypoproteinemia, bilirubin and, 1048
Hypoprothrombinemia, newborn, 1052
Hypotension, anesthesia and, 449, 450, 452, 457
Hypothalamus, 85-86
Hypothyroidism, 799
eclampsia and, 719-20
Hypotonic uterine dysfunction, 841 ff.
Hypovolemia
iron-deficiency anemia and, 766
tubal pregnancy and, 546
Hypoxia
bilirubin and, 1048
eclampsia and, 711
experimental, 1016
fetal, 209-10, 352
cerebral, 1016-17
heart disease and, 783
mortality, 1007
nitrous oxide and, 434
respiratory distress syndrome, 1034
retrolental fibroplasia, 1035
Hysterectomy
cesarean, 878, 1176 ff.
hydatidiform mole and, 573, 577
mortality, 1178
myoma and, 926, 927
postpartum hemorrhage, 961
subtotal, 1186
supravaginal, 1178, 1179
total abdominal, 1181 ff.
Hysterography, 647, 941, 942
Hysterostomatomy, 1142-43
Hysterotomy, 1163
abortion, 1089
hydatidiform mole, 572

Ice, ingestion of, and iron deficiency, 346
Icterus gravidarum, 805
Icterus neonatorum, 488-89
Identa-bands, 485
Identical twins, 657 ff.
Identification of infant, 485
Ilioinguinal nerve, 439
Imaginary pregnancy, 287

Immature infant, definition of, 1028
Immunization, 342
Rh antibody and, 1038
rubella, 342, 809-10
smallpox, 342
Immunoglobulins, 218, 224, 809
Immunology
eclampsia, 717
fetal, 223-24
hemolytic disease, 1036 ff.
placental, 168-70
tests for pregnancy, 283-84
Impetigo neonatorum, 1056
Implantation, 130-32. See also Ovum, implantation.
Incision, cesarean section, 1169 ff.
classical, 1175
Kerr, 1170, 1171
Krönig, 1170
transverse, 1172
vertical, 1171
Incision, Dührssen's, 1142-43, 1154
Inertia, uterine, 836 ff.
Infant. See Newborn.
Infarcts, placental, 590-92, 710, 717
Infection
abortion, 499-500, 520-21
amniotic, 900
anemia, 766-67
cesarean section, 1176
dystocia, 843
genitourinary, 471, 748 ff., 800 ff., 971 ff.
gonorrheal, 801-3. See also Gonorrhea.
newborn, 1053 ff.
placental, 593, 622
puerperal, 971 ff. See also Puerperium, infection.
mortality, 7
rupture of membranes, 530
syphilitic, 800-801. See also Syphilis.
tubal pregnancy, 535, 536-37
umbilical cord, 486, 597
urinary tract, 748 ff.
eclampsia and, 717
management, 755-57
puerperal, 468
uterus. See Uterus, infection.
Infertility
diabetes, 788
thyroid disease, 799
Influenza, 342, 812-13
Infundibulopelvic ligament, 38, 49
Inguinal adenitis, 803
Inguinal hernia, 1077
Inhalation anesthesia, 434 ff., 457-58
Inheritance. See Genetics.
Iniencephalus, 1073
Inlet. See Pelvis.
Innominate bones, 290, 295, 297
Instruction to patients, 335
Insulin
diabetes mellitus and, 788, 791, 796
fetal, 221
metabolism, 250-51
plasma levels, 250
resistance, 791

Insulin (*cont.*)
 shock, 791
 somatomammotropin and (chorionic), 266
Intelligence quotient, 458-59, 792
Intercourse. *See* Coitus.
Internal generative organs, anatomy of, 30 ff.
Internal podalic version, 1158 ff.
Intersex, human, 124
Interspinous diameters, 295
Interstitial cell-stimulating hormone, 82, 84
Interstitial pregnancy, 551-52
Intertuberous diameter, 304
Intervillous space, 200
 blood flow, 162, 166-68, 208, 242
 formation, 144
 infarcts, 590
 placental transfer, 207-8
Intestinal displacement, 241
Intestinal obstruction, 807-8
Intraabdominal pressure, 357-58
Intraamniotic injections, labor induction and,
  1093-94
Intracapillary hydrostatic pressure, 249
Intracranial hemorrhage, 1018. *See also* Cerebrum, hemorrhage.
Intraepithelial carcinoma, 643-45
Intraligamentous pregnancy, 544
Intrapartum. *See also* Labor.
 eclampsia, 701
 infection, 900
Intrauterine. *See also* Uterus.
 devices, 120, 1103 ff.
  ectopic pregnancy and, 535
  insertion of, 1104 ff.
 diagnosis of fetal malformations, 1077-78
 parabiosis, 664
 pressure during contraction, 352
 transfusions, blood, 1042-43
Intravascular coagulation. *See also* Coagulation, consumptive coagulopathy.
 abruptio placentae and, 630
 amniotic fluid embolism and, 951, 952
 dead fetus and, 1007-8
 eclampsia and, 719
Intravenous anesthesia, 436-37
Intubation, endotracheal, 434, 436, 482-83
Invasive mole, 575 ff.
 definition, 564
 hydatidiform mole transformation into, 572
 terminology, 575
Inversion of uterus, 416, 965 ff.
Involution
 placental site, 466-67
 uterine, 465-66, 470
Iodine
 abortion and, 411
 asthma and, 787
 butanol-extractable, 267, 411, 798
 placental transport, 222, 616
 protein-bound, 267, 411, 798
 thyroid disease, 798
  fetal, 798
  maternal, 798
Iron, 252 ff.
 absorption, 254
 -deficiency anemia, 763 ff.

Iron (*cont.*)
 -dextran, 765
 dietary requirements, 254, 338
 ferrous compound content, 765
 fetal, 225
 menstrual loss, 105
 metabolism, blood volume and, 252 ff.
 multiple pregnancy and, 674
 newborn, 415
 pica and, 346
 placental transfer, 210
 storage, 255, 762, 763-64
 therapy, 338, 764-65, 774
 total body, 253
Irradiation. *See also* Radiography.
 therapy of cervical carcinoma, 643
Irving sterilization, *1096*, 1176
Ischemia
 heart disease, 784-85
 kidney, 760
 necrosis of villi, 590
 uterine eclampsia, 718-19
Ischiopagus twins, 882
Ischiorectal fossa, 367
Ischium, 292, 295, 314, 379
Isoimmunization, 169, 1046, 1049
Isoproterenol, abortion and, 524
Isotopes, placental localization and, 616-17
Isoxsuprine hydrochloride, 530

Jaundice
 maternal, 805
 newborn, 488-89
Jellies and creams, vaginal, 1103
Joints, 269, 295-97

K cell, 69, 70
Kanamycin
 puerperal infection and, 988
 urinary tract infection and, 756, 802
Karyotype, abortion and, *498*
Kernicterus, 1036, 1045, 1047-48
 sulfonamides and, 755
Kerr technic, 1170, *1171*
Ketoacidosis, maternal, 337
Ketonemia and ketonuria, 251
Kidney, 263-64
 agenesis, 647, 1075
 anemia and, 767
 biopsy, 760
 calculi, 757
 dilatation, infection and, 750
 eclampsia and, 707-8, 714 ff.
 failure
  abortion and, 524-26
  abruptio placentae and, 631-32
  hypotension and, 632
  postpartum, 760-61
 fetal, 218
  enlargement of body and, 890
 function tests, 263
 glomerulonephritis, 708, 734, 757-59
 hypertension and, 737
 necrosis, 708, 760
 nephrosis, 759

Kidney (*cont.*)
  pelvic ectopic, 929
  polycystic disease, 759
  preeclampsia and, 692
  pyelonephritis, 749 ff., 986. *See also* Pyelo-
      nephritis.
  removal, pregnancy after, 759-60
  transplantation, pregnancy after, 761
  tuberculosis, 757
Kielland forceps, 1130, 1131, 1133, 1135 ff.
Klebsiella, 974
Klinefelter's syndrome, 124, 1068
Kreiselman resuscitator, 479, *480*
Krönig, cesarean section technic, 1170
K-value, 790
Kyphorachitic and kyphoscoliorachitic pelvis,
    913
Kyphoscoliosis, 910 ff.
  heart disease and, 785

Labia majora, anatomy of, 19-20
Labia minora, anatomy of, 20-21
Labor
  abdominal examination, 402
  admittance procedures, 401
  age of mother, 396-97
  amnesia, 432-34
  amniotic fluid, 361
  anesthesia and analgesia, 430 ff. *See also*
      Analgesia; Anesthesia.
  artificial termination, 371-72
  blood volume, 255
  cardiac output, 258
  cardinal movements, 375 ff.
  cervical dilatation, 351. *See also* Cervix,
      dilatation.
  circulation, 393-94
  clinical course, 387 ff.
  delivery procedures, 411 ff.
  descent, 377
  duration, 391, 396
    breech presentation, 860
    occiput posterior position, 853
    twins, 675
    uterine dysfunction, 840
  dystocia, 835 ff. *See also* Dystocia.
  eclampsia and, 704
  elderly primigravida, 397
  electrical stimulation, 352
  emotional aspects, 400-401
  engagement, 375-77. *See also* Engagement.
  episiotomy and repair, 423 ff.
  ergonovine, 419-20, 421
  false, 387
    diagnosis, 402
    twins and, 675
  first stage, 358 ff., 388
    management, 402 ff.
    prolongation, 840
  flexion, 377
  forceps, 1115 ff. *See also* Forceps.
  forces, 349 ff.
    cause of onset, 349-51

Labor (*cont.*)
  forces (*cont.*)
    characteristics, 351 ff.
    intraabdominal pressure, 357-58
    ligamentous action, 357
    lower uterine segment, 353-54, 355
    resistance, 358
    shape of uterus changes, 357
    stages, 351
    upper uterine segment, 355
  "fourth stage," 427
  gastrointestinal tract, 394
  heart disease, 780-81
  heart rate, fetal, 394-96
  induction of, 398, 1093-94
    abruptio placentae, 634
    anenencephaly, 1071
    diabetes, 796
    eclampsia, 732-33
    indications, 1094
    intraamniotic injections, 1093-94
    oxytocin, 398, 796, 1093. *See also* Oxy-
        tocin.
    postmaturity, 1057
    preeclampsia, 700
    prostaglandins, 1094
    rupture of membranes, 1093
    stripping of membranes, 1093
    twins, 674-75
  injuries to fetus, 1007 ff.
  interval between births and, 397
  kyphosis and, 912
  lacerations of birth canal, 421-23
  lameness and, 358, 915
  leukocyte count, 255, 394
  lightening, 387
  mechanism, 375 ff.
  methylergonovine, 419-20, 421
  missed, 851, 875
  natural childbirth, 400-401, 459
  normal, 400 ff.
  onset, fetal head position and, 374
  pain, 352, 388, 400
    diagnosis, 402
    relief, 430 ff., 459. *See also* Analgesia;
        Anesthesia.
  palpation of lower uterine segment, 329
  parity and, 396
  pelvic contractions, 897 ff. *See also* Pelvis,
      contractions.
  perineum, 368
    lacerations, 421-23
    preparation, 401-2
  placental separation, 368 ff., 415-16
  precipitate, 849
  premature, 526 ff. *See also* Prematurity.
    anemia and, 500
    bacteriuria and, 751
    etiology, 499-501
    hormones, 350-51
    incidence, 526, 529
    placental abnormalities, 499
    viruses and, 812

Labor (*cont.*)
presentations, 320 ff., 853 ff. *See also* specific presentations.
principal movements, *381*
progesterone deprivation, 349-50
prognosis, 305, 396-98
prolonged, 362, 835 ff. *See also* Dystocia.
proteinuria, 264, 394
puerperal infection, 976, 987
rectal examination, 402 ff.
rupture of membranes, spontaneous, 388, 397-98
detection of, 405-7
scrubbing and gloving, 410-11
second stage, 361-62, 388 ff.
extension, 840
intraabdominal pressure, 358
management, 407 ff.
vaginal and pelvic floor changes, 362 ff.
sedation, 432-34
show, 387-88
sickle-cell disease, 773
size of baby, 397
test of, 906
third stage, 368 ff., 391-93, 415 ff., 956 ff.
atony of uterus, 473
drugs, 418 ff.
hemorrhage, 956 ff.
intraabdominal pressure, 358
physiology, 368 ff.
placental retention, 962-64
placental separation and expulsion, 368 ff., 415-16
uterine inversion, 965 ff.
trial, 904, 906
twins, 674-75
tying the cord, 414-15
vaginal examination, 402 ff.
vaginal lacerations, 421-23, 425, 957, 958-59
vertex presentations, 374 ff.
vulvar preparation, 401-2
work involved, 358
Laboratory tests, 334. *See also* specific tests.
Lacerations, degrees of, 421-22, 425
Lactation
amenorrhea and, 475
breast during, *469*
contraception and, 1101
diet and, 337
drug secretion, 470-71
hormones and, 993
menstruation return and, 475
oxytocin and, 419
puerperium and, 468-70
suppression of, 993-94
Lactiferous ducts, 469
Lactobacillus, 245
Lactogen, human placental, 176, 575
Lacunae, trophoblastic, 135
Lambdoid sutures, 204
Lameness, 914-16
Langhans cells, 145, 149, 156, 159
choriocarcinoma, 579

Langhans cells (*cont.*)
transfer, 208
Laparoscopy
sterilization and, 1096
tubal pregnancy and, 549
Laparotomy
abdominal pregnancy, 557
abortion, 500
instrumental perforation of uterus, 949
tubal pregnancy, 550
Largactil, 732
Laryngoscopy for newborn, 483
Lash and Lash operation, 518
Lasix, 766, 781
Latex inhibition and agglutination tests, 283, 284
LATS, 222, 799
LE factor, 815
Leg(s)
cramps, 411
fractures, 1022-23
holders, 407, *408*
lameness, 914-16
milk, 1002
phocomelia, 1069
syphilis and, *1054*
varicosities, 344-45
Legal factors. *See* Medicolegal problems.
Lens, fibroplasia of, 1035
Leopold maneuvers, 326, *327-28*, 374-75
Leptotene stage of meiosis, 109
Leucine aminopeptidase, 262
Leukemia, 777
Leukocytes, 255-56
hypersegmentation of neutrophiles, 767
tubal pregnancy, 547
Leukocytosis
endometritis, 983
labor and, 394
puerperal, 473
thrombophlebitis, 984
Leukopenia, 767
Leukorrhea, 346-47, 641
Levator ani, 28, 30, 363, 364
injuries, 932
tetanic contraction, 923
Lidocaine, 442, 451
doses, 448
Life tables
contraception and, 1100
perinatal mortality, 496
Ligaments, 38-40
action in labor, 357
broad, 38, *39. See also* Broad ligament.
cardinal, 39, 40
infundibulopelvic, 38
ovarian, 49
round, 40, 357
suspensory, 49
umbilical, 215
uterosacral, 40
Ligamentum
arteriosum, 215
flavum, anesthesia and, 455

Ligamentum (*cont.*)
  teres, 215
  venosum, 215
Lightening, 387
Linea nigra, 269
Linea terminalis, 291
Lipid metabolism, 251-52
Lipolysis
  fetal, 225
  somatomammotropin (chorionic) and, 176
Lippes loop, 1105, *1106*
Liquor folliculi, 60, 61
Listeria monocytogenes, abortion and, 500
Lithiasis, 757
Lithopedion
  abdominal pregnancy, 555
  tubal pregnancy, 543
Litzmann pelvis, 913
Liver, 261-62, 803 ff.
  atrophy, acute yellow, 804-5
  blood flow, 262
  cholelithiasis and cholecystitis, 805-6
  cirrhosis, 806
  eclampsia and, 705, *706*, 707
  fatty metamorphosis, *805*
  fetal, 221
    body enlargement, 890-91
  hemolytic disease, 1045
  hepatitis, 634, 803-4
  hepatosis, obstetric, 805
  physiology, 261-62
  umbilical vein and, 211
Local anesthesia, 437-39, 448
Lochia, 472
  endometritis, 983
Lockwood v. *Lockwood,* 237
Long-acting thyroid stimulator, 222, 799
Longitudinal lie of fetus, 320
Lordosis, 269, 910, 911
LSD, fetal malformations and, 1067
Lumbar epidural block, 448, 450, 453 ff.
Lumbar puncture, 732
Lumbar sympathectomy, 352
Lunar months, 202
Lungs. *See also* Respiratory system.
  compliance, 260
  initial expansion, 477-79
  resection, 787
  scan, pulmonary embolism and, 1004
Lupus erythematosus, 708, 815
Lutein cells, 60, 70, 72
  ovulation and, 67
Lutein cysts, 567-68, 580
Luteinizing hormone, 84, 86
  diagnosis of pregnancy, 283, 284
  estradiol and, 84
  progesterone and, 84
Luteinizing releasing factor, 86
Luteolytic factors, 85
Luteoma of pregnancy, 244
Luteotropic hormones, 84-85
Luxation of femurs, 915
Lymphatics
  endometrial, 43
  puerperal infection, 978, 980
  uterine, size increase, 239

Lymphopathia venereum, 803
Lysergic acid diethylamide, 1067
Lysol, 524

M device, 1105
Madlener operation, 1095, 1098
Magnaflux MD 500, 394
Magnesium, 252
  antacids, 345
  fetal, 225
  sulfate
    in eclampsia, 728-30
    in preeclampsia, 698
Majzlin spring, 1105
Malaria, 814
Mälmstrom vacuum extractor, *1140*
Malnutrition, prematurity and, 1030
Mammary gland. *See also* Breast(s).
  hormones and, 470
Mannitol, 633
  preeclampsia and, 698
Manometer, venous pressure and, *523*
Marfan's syndrome, 817
Marginal sinus rupture, 624
Marginate placenta, 587
Marriage rate, definition, 2
Mastectomy, 823
Mastitis, 994-96
Maternal mortality. *See* Mortality, maternal.
Maternal physiology, 236 ff.
  abdominal wall, 245-46
  adrenal glands, 268-69
  bladder, 266
  blood volume, 252 ff.
  breasts, 246, *247*
  cardiovascular system, 257 ff.
  circulation, 258-60. *See also* Circulation,
      maternal.
  coagulation, 256
  diet, 225
  emotional changes, 270
  endocrine glands, 266 ff.
  gallbladder, 262
  gastrointestinal tract, 260-61
  heart, 257-58
  hematologic changes, 252 ff.
  kidney, 263-64
  leukocytes, 255-56
  liver, 261-62
  metabolic changes, 248 ff.
    acid-base balance, 252
    carbohydrate and insulin, 250-51
    fat, 251-52
    iron, 252 ff.
    minerals, 252
    protein, 249
    water, 248-49
    weight gain, 248. *See also* Weight.
  musculoskeletal system, 269
  ovaries and oviducts, 244-45
  parathyroids, 268
  pituitary, 266-67
  respiratory tract, 260
  skin, 269
  thyroid, 267-68

Maternal physiology (*cont.*)
  ureters, 264-66
  urinary system, 262 ff.
  uterus, 238 ff.
    blood flow, 242
    cervical changes, 242-44
    contractility, 241
    musculature, 239-40
    size and shape changes, 240-41
    spiral artery changes, 241-42
  vagina and perineum, 245
Mauriceau's maneuver, 1150, *1151*, 1152
McDonald operation, *515*, 517
Measles
  German (rubella), 342, 808 ff., 1088
  rubeola, 812
Meclizine, 344
Meconium, 221, 487-88
  amnioscopy and, 1010
  amniotic fluid embolism and, 951
  aspiration of, 479
Medications, prenatal, 342-43
Medicolegal problems
  abortion, 1085 ff.
  legitimacy, 237
  superfetation, 667
Megaloblastic anemia, 767 ff.
Meiosis, 108 ff.
  fetal malformations and, 1067
  nondisjunction, 124
Melanocyte-stimulating hormone, 269
Melanoma, 818
  malignant placental, 584
Membrana granulosa, 60, 61, 72
Membranes
  abnormalities, 564 ff.
  festooning, *370*
  multiple pregnancy, 661 ff., 674
  placental separation, 370
  rupture
    abruptio placentae, 634
    cervical dilatation, 361
    detection of, 405-7
    inevitable abortion, 505
    infection of newborn, 1055
    nitrazine test, 406
    placenta previa, 620
    premature, 389, 397-98, 530
      breech presentation, 863
    shoulder presentation, 877
    spontaneous, 388, 397-98
    uterine dysfunction, 844-45
  stripping, 361, 1093
Menadione, 1052
Menarche, 102
  age of, *104*, 238
Meningocele, 1072, 1076
Meningomyelocele, 1072
Menopause
  menstruation and, 102, 104
  spurious pregnancy, 287
  vagina, 24, 27
Menstruation, 93-94, 102 ff.
  beginning of, mean age of, 238
  blood loss, amount of, 105
  breast-feeding and, 475

Menstruation (*cont.*)
  cessation, diagnosis of pregnancy and, 285
  character and amount, 105-6
  clinical aspects, 102 ff.
  corpus luteum of, *68*, 69
  fetal age and, 199, 203, 236
  flow variability, 105
  histologic changes, *91*, 99, *100*
  hormonal relationships, 79, 80, *98*
  interval and duration, 104-5
  iron loss, 105
  irregularity of length, 104
  menopause, 102, 104
  ovulation, 65
  postpartum, 475
  prematurity, 1026
  progesterone and, 79, 80
  puberty and, 102
  safe period, 1102-3
  tubal pregnancy and, 546
  vaginal smears, *103*
  weight changes, 106
Meperidine, 433, 732
Mepivacaine, 442, *448*
Mercaptopurine, 583
Mesenchyme, body stalk, 135
Mesoderm, 136, 139
  amnion-chorion fusion, 147
Mesonephric ducts, 51
Mesonephric ridge, 113
Mesosalpinx, 38
Mesovarium, 49, 54
Metabolism, 248 ff. *See also* Maternal physiology, metabolic changes.
  inborn errors, 1069
  insulin, 250-51
  oral contraceptives and, 1110
  porphyria, 797
  progesterone and, 79
  somatomammotropin (chorionic) and, 176
Metanephros, *52-53*
Metaraminol, 524
Metastases
  choriocarcinoma, 580
  hydatidiform mole, 574
  placental tumors, 584
Metatherian placentation, 187
Methergine, 418, 419, 472
Methotrexate, 573, 583
Methylergonovine, 419-21, 472
Methylprednisolone, 786
Metritis dissecans, 982
Metronidazole, 347
Metycaine, 457
Microvilli, syncytial, 156
Midforceps, 1119, 1120, 1123, 1128-30
  cerebral hemorrhage and, 1019
  occiput posterior position and, 855
  pelvic contraction and, 907
Midpelvis, 295
  contractions, 906-8
  size estimation, 305
Midwifery, definition of, 2
Milk
  abnormalities of secretion, 997

Milk (*cont.*)
  bilirubin and, 1048
  drug secretion, 470-71
  "drying up," 993
  duration of feeding and, 489
  ejection, or "letting down," 470
  fever, 470, 471
  mammary development and, 470
  mastitis and, 995
  puerperal, 469
Milk-leg, 1002
Minerals, 252
  prenatal dietary, 338
Minute volume, 260
Miscarriage. *See* Abortion.
Mitochondria, 94, 156, *157*
Mitosis, 109, *110*
Mitral valvotomy, 783
Mittelschmerz, 66
Model Penal Code, 1086
Molding of fetal head, 384, *385*
  brow presentation, 871
  cerebral hemorrhage, 1018
  pelvic contraction, 901
Mole
  blood, 502
  carneous, 502
  destructive, 575
  hydatidiform, 564 ff. *See also* Hydatidiform
    mole.
  invasive, 564, 575 ff.
  penetrative, 575
  tuberous, 503
Monad, 110
Mongolism, 125, 1068, 1073-75
  incidence, 1064
  intrauterine diagnosis, 1078
Moniliasis, 347
Monsters, 882 ff. *See also* Fetus, malforma-
    tions.
Mons veneris, 19
Montgomery, follicles of, 246
Morning sickness, 286
Moro, 1031
Morphine, 433
  eclampsia and, 727
  heart disease and, 781
  preeclampsia and, 698
Mortality
  maternal, 4 ff.
    abdominal pregnancy, 558
    abortion, 520, 521, 525-26, 1029
    abruptio placentae, 634
    age and, 5, *6*
    appendicitis, 807
    breech presentation, 860
    brow presentation, 871
    carcinoma of cervix, 643
    caudal anesthesia, 449
    causes, common, 7-8
    cesarean section, 1187-88
    decline, 8-9
    definition, 3
    diabetes, 793
    eclampsia, 722, 725, 727

Mortality (*cont.*)
  maternal (*cont.*)
    geographic distribution, 6
    hemorrhage, 7, 819-20
    hepatitis, 804
    hydatidiform mole, 571
    hydrocephalus, 888
    hypertension, 736
    hysterectomy, 1178
    infection, 7
    influenza, 812
    intracranial hemorrhage, 819-20
    kidney, ectopic, 929
    multiple pregnancy, 681-82
    parity and, 5
    placenta previa, 623
    preeclampsia, 696
    racial differences, 4, 5, 6, *8*
    sickle-cell disease, 774
    toxemia, 7
    tubal pregnancy, 550
    U.S. vs. other nations, 9-10
    uterine rupture, 946
    weight, 336
  perinatal, 10 ff., 1007-9
    abdominal pregnancy, 554-55, 558
    abnormal development, 496 ff.
    abruptio placentae, 635
    age, gestational, *494*
    anesthesia, 435, 442
    antepartum hemorrhage, 609
    appendicitis, 807
    bacteriuria, 751-53
    brow presentation, 871
    causes, 11-12, 1008
    cerebral hemorrhage, 1019
    cesarean section, 435, 902, 939, 1188
    compound presentation, 880
    definition, 2
    diabetes, 791, 793
    dystocia, 840, 843
    eclampsia, 722, 724
    ether, 435
    face presentation, 869, 870
    forceps, 1138, 1139
    hyaline membrane disease, 1034
    hydramnios, 601
    hypotonic uterus, 848
    hypertension, 685, 689, 736, 737
    kidney, ectopic, 929
    latent period in labor, 398
    life tables, 496
    malformations, 1063
    multiple pregnancies, 681
    oxytocin, 848
    pelvic contraction, 902
    placenta previa, 623
    poliomyelitis, 813
    preeclampsia, 694, 696
    prematurity, 529, 1028, 1029, 1033, 1094
    racial differences, *12*
    shoulder presentation, 877
    sickle-cell disease, 772, 774
    social and economic factors, 12, 1029
    twins, 662, 680
    umbilical cord prolapse, 1014-15
    U.S. vs. other nations, 13

Mortality (*cont.*)
  perinatal (*cont.*)
    uterine rupture, 946
    weight, 336, 680
Morula, 128
Mosaicism, 124-25, 1067
Mucus
  aspiration in newborn, 479
  cervical, 67, 99. *See also* Cervix, mucus.
Müllerian ducts, 51, 641, 645
Müller's method of impression, 903
Multigravida, definition of, 332
Multipara
  abruptio placentae, 626
  afterpains, 474
  analgesia, 431
  cesarean section, 863, 1166
  definition, 333
  diagnosis of pregnancy, 287-88
  duration of labor, 396
  eclampsia, 700, 718
  face presentation, 865
  menstruation return, 475
  mortality
    maternal, 5
    perinatal, 10
  placenta previa, 611, 612, 622
  vaginal relaxation, 641
Multiple pregnancy, 553, 656 ff.
  anesthesia, 677
  cesarean section, 677
  clinical course, 670-71
  collision, 677
  conjoined twins, 667-68
  constriction ring, 679
  delivery, 675 ff.
  diagnosis, 668-70
  estriol excretion in urine, 183
  etiology, 657 ff.
  fertility of twins, 668
  frequency, 657
  gonadotropin, 175
  hemorrhage
    antepartum and intrapartum, 678-79
    postpartum, 679, 957
  infant, 679-81
  interval between infants, 676
  labor, 674-75
  management, 671 ff.
  monsters, 882
  mortality, 681-82
  myoma, 926
  placenta and membrane relations, 661 ff.
  presentation, 674
  superfecundation and superfectation, 667
  sex of children, 661
  tubal pregnancy and, 553
  velamentous insertion of cord, 594-95
Mummification, 503, 555
Mumps, 812
Murmurs, systolic, 258, 778
Musculcskeletal system, 269
Muscle
  dermatomyositis, 816
  eclamptic contractions, 702
  fallopian tube, 45, 47

Muscle (*cont.*)
  injuries, 1023
  pelvic, 363 ff.
  perineal, 30, 364
  relaxants, 457
  uterine, 37-38, 239-40. *See also* Myometrium.
  vaginal, 28
Myasthenia gravis, 820
Mycobacterium tuberculosis, 788
Mycostatin, 347
Myocardium
  eclampsia and, 710
  infarction, 785
Myoma, 924 ff.
  abortion and, 501, 512
  carneous degeneration, 925, 926
  diagnosis of pregnancy, 283
  interstitial, 926
  intramural, 925
  subserous, 926
Myomectomy, 926-27
  scar rupture, 940
Myometrium, 37-38
  cell size, 238-39
  circulation, 163
  hematoma, abruptio placentae and, 631
  invasive mole, 564, 575 ff.
  labor and, 352
  necrosis, 982
  onset of labor, 349
Myrtiform caruncles, 24, 468

Nabothian follicles, 33
Naegele pelvis, 913
Naegele's rule, 236, 237
Nail bed, eclampsia and, 711
Nalline (Nalorphine), 433-34
  resuscitation of newborn, 484
Narcotic analgesics, 432
Nasopharynx, puerperal infection and, 987
National Research Council, 336, 337, 338
Natural childbirth, 400-1, 459
Nausea, 286, 343-44
Neck
  maternal, 269
  umbilical cord coils, 413
Necrosis
  cervical, 843
  endometrial, 982
  genital tract perforation following, 950
  hepatic, 705-7
  renal, 760
  villous, 590
Neisseria gonorrhoeae, 801-3. *See also* Gonorrhea.
Neonatal mortality, 2, 10. *See also* Mortality, perinatal.
Neonate. *See* Newborn.
Nephrectomy, pregnancy after, 759-60
Nephritis, lupus, 815
Nephrons, fetal, 218
Nephrosclerosis, 760
Nephrotic syndrome, 759

Nervous system, 819-20
  anesthesia, 439-40, 446, 451
  consanguinity and, 1081
  epilepsy, 819
  external genitalia supply, 22
  fetal, 223, 1009 ff.
  Huntington's chorea, 820
  incidence of malformations, 1064
  intracranial hemorrhage, 819-20
  labor pain and, 437
  multiple sclerosis, 820
  myasthenia gravis, 820
  paraplegia, 820
  parasympathetic, 43, 437
  perineal block, 439-40
  puerperal disorders, 1001
  sacral anesthesia, 446
  Sydenham's chorea, 820
  sympathetic, 43, 352, 437
  uterine supply, 43-45, 239, 352
Nervus erigens, 352
Neural groove, 137
Neuraminidase, 170
Neurenteric canal, 137
Neurohormonal control of pituitary, 85-86
Neurohypophysis, puerperium and, 470
Neutrophils, anemia and, 767
Nevus, 269, 818
Newborn, 477 ff., 1026 ff.
  antibiotics, 487
  Apgar scoring, 444, 479-80, 1012, 1015,
      1017
  apnea, 433, 478, 481, 484, 1015, 1016
  asphyxia, 1015-17
  bilirubin, 415
  blood
    group factors, 1037 ff., 1051
    pH, 483
    Rh antibodies, 1037 ff.
  carbon dioxide accumulation, 477-78
  cerebral hemorrhage, 1018-20
  circumcision, 490
  delirium tremens, 342
  diabetes, maternal, 793
  diarrhea, 1055-56
  drugs affecting, 343, 1067
  endotracheal intubation, 482-83
  evaluation, 479-80
  eye care, 486-87
  feeding, 489
  fibrinogen, 217
  footprinting, 485
  growth retardation
    prematurity, 529
    twins, 680
  head measurements, 204-6
  heart disease and, maternal, 783
  heart rate, 483-84
  hemolytic disease, 1036 ff.
  hemorrhagic disease, 1052
  herpes simplex, 1056
  high-risk, 484-85
  hyaline membrane disease, 1009, 1034
  hyperbilirubinemia, 488, 1036 ff.
  hypercapnea, 477-78

Newborn (cont.)
  hypoxia, 1015, 1016
  icterus neonatorum, 488, 1036 ff.
  identification, 485
  infections, 1053 ff.
  injuries during pregnancy and labor, 1007 ff.
  IQ, 458-59, 792
  iron stores, 415
  ketoacidosis, 337
  largest on record, 880
  length, 1026
  magnesium sulfate and, 729
  malformations, 1063 ff. See also Fetus, mal-
      formations.
  mastitis, 994
  mortality, 10, 1009. See also Mortality, peri-
      natal.
    definition, 2
  mucus aspiration, 479
  multiple pregnancy, 679-81
  myasthenia gravis, 820
  oxygen, 478, 481, 1015, 1016
  paralysis, 1020-22
  pelvis, 297-99
  pneumonia, 1055
  pneumothorax, 1056-57
  postmature, 1057-58
  premature, 1026 ff. See also Labor, prema-
      ture; Prematurity.
    definition, 493
  respiration, initiation of, 477-79
  respiratory distress, 415, 432, 1033-35
  resuscitation, 480 ff.
  retrolental fibroplasia, 1035
  rooming-in, 489
  rubella and, 810-11
  skin care, 487
  small-sized, 1030 ff.
  staphylococcal infection, 1056
  stools, 487-88
  supravalvar syndrome, 339
  syphilis, 1053
  temperature, 478, 485
  tetany, 799
  transfusions, 1042-43
  umbilical cord, 485-86
  urine, 488
  weight, 203-4
    bacteriuria and, 753
    cesarean section and, 863, 1168-69
    diabetes and, 791, 792
    gain, 1027
    mortality and, 336, 398
    prematurity and, 1026 ff.
    smoking and, 342, 529
    twins, 679
Nipples
  abnormalities, 995, 996-97
  puerperal care, 475
  shield, 475, 997
Nitrazine test, 406
Nitrofurantoin, 755, 756
Nitrogen
  eclampsia and, 715
  fetal, 225

Nitrous oxide, 434, 457
    thiopental sodium and, 436
    twins and, 677
Nondisjunction, 124, 125
    abortion and, 499
Norethynodrel, 120
Nosocomial infections, 995
Notochord, 137
Novocaine, 451
Nulliparas
    cesarean section in breech presentation, 863
    diagnosis of pregnancy, 287
Nupercaine, 450, 451
Nutrition, 335 ff.
    abortion and, 511-12, 514
    eclampsia and, 720-21
    emotional changes, 270
    fetal, 224-26, 880
    preeclampsia, 697-98
    prematurity and, 529, 1030
    prenatal, 335
    puerperal, 474, 986
    recommended daily allowances, 337
Nymphae, 20-21
Nystatin, 347

Obesity, 799-800
    abortion and, 514
    diet and, 337
    excessive development of fetus, 880
Oblique lie, 872, 1157 ff.
Obstetric conjugate, 294, 299
Obstetrics
    aims, 2
    definition, 1
    etymology, 1
    future, 16-17
    related branches of medicine and other
        fields, 14, 16
    statistical definitions, 2-3
Occipital bone, 901
Occipitofrontal diameter, 206
Occipitomental diameter, 9, 206, 1125
Occiput, 322, 323
    anterior, 380, 382
        forceps, 1125 ff., 1129, 1135
        pelvic contractions and, 897
    posterior, 382-84
        forceps, 1128, 1130, 1132
        lacerations, 422
        pelvic contractions and, 897
        persistent, dystocia and, 853-55
        prognosis of labor, 397
    transverse, 374 ff.
        forceps, 1129-30
        pelvic contractions and, 897
Oligohydramnios, 228, 603-4
    renal agenesis, 1075
Oliguria
    abortion and, 522
    abruptio placentae, 633, 635
    hypertension, 687
    preeclampsia, 698
Omentum, ovum implantation on, 554
Omphalopagus twins, 667

Omphalopleure, 187
Oocytes
    graafian follicle, 62
    meiosis, 108-9
    migration, 113
    morphology, 55
    number at birth, 54
    primary, 51, 54, 113
    primordial follicle, 51, 55, 58, 59
    secondary, 115
Oogenesis, 55, 111
Oogonia, 51, 108
Oophorectomy, tubal pregnancy and, 551
Ophthalmia neonatorum, 487
Optical density 450, 1040-41
Orinase, 794
Osmotic pressure, colloidal, 249
Ossification, beginning of, 202
Osteomalacic pelvis, 913
Ota ring, 1105
Otosclerosis, 824
Outlet contractions, 908-10
Ovarian artery, 41
Ovarian veins, 245
    ligation, bladder infection and, 750
    puerperal infection and, 978
    thrombosis, 1003
Ovary, 50 ff., 244-45
    accessory, 59
    anatomy, 48 ff.
    blood supply, 42
    carcinoma, 929
    cysts, 928
        abortion and, 507
        hydramnios vs., 601
        lutein, 567-68
        tubal pregnancy vs., 548
    cycle, 58 ff.
        corpora albicantia, 71-72
        corpus luteum, 67 ff.
        development of follicle, 58-59
        endometrial cycle correlated with, 97
        hormonal plasma levels, 83
        mature follicle, 59 ff.
        ovulation, 64 ff.
        postovulatory phase, 95-97, 99
        preovulatory phase, 94
    decidualike reaction, 244
    development, 50 ff.
    fetal, 223
    hormones, 72 ff.
        androgens, 82
        estrogens, 72 ff. See also Estrogens.
        neurohormonal control, 85-86
        pituitary effects, 82 ff.
        progesterone, 78 ff. See also Progesterone.
        relaxin, 82
    hydatidiform mole and, 567
    ligaments, 49
    microscopic structure, 54
    pregnancy in, 122, 559-61
    removal, 551
    sclerocystic, 67
    tumors, 928-29
    x-ray pelvimetry dosage, 317
Oviducts. See Fallopian tubes.

Ovulation, 64 ff.
  age of fetus, 199
  agents to introduce, multiple pregnancy and,
      661
  ferning, 67, 100, 102
  gonadotropin and, 173-74
  hormonal plasma levels, *83*
  hypothalamus and, 85-86
  lactation and, 475
  Mittelschmerz, 66
  pregnancy and, 244
  pregnanediol in urine, 67
  progesterone and, 67, 81
  in rat, *65*
  rhythm method and, 1102-3
  signs and symptoms, 66-67
  temperature change, 66
  tests, 66-67
  time of, 64-66
Ovum, 58 ff., 200
  abortion and, 497-98, 510, 514
  aging, 125
  blastocyst, 125, 128, 129, 130. *See also*
      Blastocyst.
  blighted, 496, 498, 502
  cleavage, 125 ff.
  comparative embryology, 138-40
  cumulus oophorus, 59
  development, 111 ff., 132 ff.
  discus proligerus, 59
  dropsical, 502
  early human, 129-30, *145*
  fertilization, 122, 125 ff.
    changes preceding, 123
    ectopic pregnancy and, 538
  germ layers, 136
  implantation, 130-32
    cervical, *560, 561*
    ectopic pregnancy and, 535
    peritoneal, 554
    placenta previa and, 611-13
  intraperitoneal rupture, 542-43
  loss, 497
  maturation, 59 ff., 116
  migration, 120-21
  morphology, 62
  morula, 128
  neogenesis, 113
  previllous stage, *134*
  preimplantation stages, *127*
  somite formation, 136-37
  sonograms, *495*
  tubal transport, 119-20, 538
  tuberculosum, 503
  twinning and, 657. *See also* Twins.
  youngest human, *131*
  zona pellucida, 59, 64, 115, 123, 129
  zygote, 125
Oxygen
  administration to newborn, 481
  analgesia and anesthesia, 432, 435
  asphyxia of newborn, 1015, 1016
  brain damage and, 1016
  cyclopropane and, 435
  dissociation curves, 216, *217*, 432
  eclampsia, 732

Oxygen (*cont.*)
  heart disease and, 781
  hyperbaric, 210
  hypoxia, newborn, 478, 1016
  IQ and, 458-59
  nitrous oxide mixture with, 434
  placental transfer, 209-10
  respiratory distress syndrome, 1034
  retrolental fibroplasia and, 1035
  tension
    ductus arteriosus, 214
    pulmonary embolism, 1004
  uterine consumption, 242
Oxytocin, 350-52, 418 ff., 845 ff.
  abortion, 508, 509
  abruptio placentae, 629, 634
  antidiuresis, 418
  breech presentation, 863
  diabetes, 796
  hemorrhage, postpartum, 959, 960
  hydatidiform mole, 572
  intravenous drip, 845 ff., 1093
  involution of uterus, 472
  linguets, 846
  milk ejection, 419
  multiple pregnancy, 674-75, 676
  nasal spray, 846
  onset of labor, 350-52
  pelvic contraction, 906, 908
  precautions in use, 845, 848
  premature rupture of membranes, 398
  puerperal, 470
  test for abdominal pregnancy, 555
  third stage of labor, 418 ff.
  twins, 676
  uterine dysfunction, 845 ff.

Pacemakers, uterine, 352
Pachytene stage, 110
Pain
  abortion, vaginal bleeding and, 507-8
  bone, sickle-cell anemia and, 773
  chest, pulmonary embolism and, 1003
  episiotomy, 428
  false labor, 387
  forceps, 1122
  heart disease and, 780
  labor, 352, 388, 400, 430 ff.
  puerperal, 471-72
  relief, 430 ff. *See also* Analgesia; Anesthesia.
  symphysial, 824
  tubal pregnancy, 545-46, 548-49
  urinary calculi, 757
Palfyn's forceps, *1118*
Palmar erythema, 269
Palpation, 326 ff.
  abdominal pregnancy, 555
  breech presentation, 855, 857
  brow presentation, 870
  face presentation, 864
  lower uterine segment, 354
  placenta previa, 613-14
  position of fetus, 326 ff., 374, 382, 383
  pubic arch, kyphosis and, 912
  twin diagnosis, 668, *669*

Palsy, 849, 1017
Pancreas, fetal, 221-22
Pancreatitis, 807
Papanicolaou smear, 334, 642
Papilloma, cervical, 641
Parabiosis, intrauterine, 664
Paracentesis, hydramnios and, 603
Paracervical block, 442 ff.
Paraldehyde
    eclampsia and, 730
    preeclampsia and, 698
Paralysis
    maternal, 352, 358, 820
    newborn, 1001, 1020-22
Parametrium, 39
    inflammation, 980-81, 983-84, 989
        abortion and, 521
        prognosis, 991
Paraplegics, 352, 358, 820
Parasacral block, 442
Parasitic infections, 814-15
Parasympathetic nerves, 43, 437
Parathyroids, 268, 799
Paraurethral ducts, 22
Paravertebral block, 442
Parietal bone, pelvic contraction and, 901
Parity, 493
    abruptio placentae and, 626
    eclampsia and, 722
    maternal mortality and, 5
    oxytocin and, 846
    perinatal mortality and, 10
    placenta previa and, 612
    prognosis of labor and, 396
    shoulder presentation and, 872
    twinning and, 658
    uterine rupture and, 943
Paroophoron, 38-39
Parotitis, epidemic, 812
Parovarium, 38
Parthenogenesis, 122
Parturient, definition of, 333
Pelvimetry. See Pelvis, measurements.
Pelvis, 290 ff.
    abscess, 521, 989
    adult, 290 ff.
        sex differences, 297, 916, 950
    anatomy, 291 ff., 315
    android, 316
    anthropoid, 316
    assimilation, 913
    atypical deformities, 916-17
    axis, 296
    bisischial diameter, 304
    cellulitis, 980-81, 983-84, 989
    chondrodystrophic dwarf, 918
    conjugates
        diagonal, 299 ff., 306, 405, 894
        obstetric, 294, 299, 894, 903
    contractions, 894 ff.
        cesarean section and, 1166
        combinations, 910
        inlet, 895 ff.
            breech presentation, 906
            cervical dilatation, 899-900

Pelvis (cont.)
    contractions (cont.)
        inlet (cont.)
            child, effects on, 900
            course of labor, 899-901
            effect on pregnancy, 896 ff.
            etiology, 894-96
            face presentation, 865, 897, 906
            fistula production, 900
            head of fetus, 900 ff.
            incidence, 897
            infection, 900
            mechanism of labor, 897-99
            presentation and position of fetus, 896-
                97, 906
            prognosis, 901-3
            scalp and skull, 900-1
            size of fetus, 897, 903 ff.
            transverse, 302
            treatment, 906
            umbilical cord prolapse, 900
            uterine position, 896
            uterine rupture, 900
        midpelvic, 906-8
        outlet, 908-10
        rare, 910 ff.
    coxalgic, 914-16
    coxarthrolisthetic, 916
    cretin dwarf, 918
    diameters, 292 ff., 299 ff., 894, 902, 909
    diaphragm, 364
    dwarf, 917-18
    engagement, 302-4. See also Engagement.
    excessively large infant and, 881
    false, 291-92, 895
    fascia, 363
    femoral forces, 913 ff.
    floor, changes in labor, 362 ff.
    forceps application, 1125
    fractures, 917
    funnel, 911
    greatest dimensions, 294
    gynecoid, 315-16
    hypoplastic, 918
    inclination, 295
    inferior strait, 292
    inflammatory disease, 549, 653, 980 ff.
    inlet, 292, 293, 294
        anatomy, 313-14
        asynclitism and, 376
        contractions, 895 ff. See also Pelvis, con-
            tractions, inlet.
        round, 293
    intermediate types, 316
    interspinous diameter, 295
    intertuberous diameter, 304
    joints, 295
    kidney, ectopic, 929
    kyphotic, 910 ff.
    lameness and, 914-16
    linea terminalis, 291
    Litzmann, 913
    measurements, 292 ff., 299 ff.
        inlet, 894
        midpelvic, 295, 305, 907

Pelvis (*cont.*)
  measurements (*cont.*)
    outlet, 304-5
    shoulder presentation, 877
    uterine dysfunction, 844
    x-ray, 305 ff., 317
      hazards, 316-17
  midpelvis, 295, 305, 906-8
  muscles, 363 ff.
  Naegele, 913
  nana, 918
  newborn, 297
  obtecta, 910
  osteomalacic, 913
  outlet, 292, 294, 304-5, 908-10
  planes, 292 ff., 906-7
  platypelloid, 316
  posterior sagittal diameter, 295
  rachitic, 894-96, 913, 918
  Robert, 913
  sexual differences, 297, 916, 950
  shape, 313 ff.
  spinosa, 916, 950
  split, 913
  spondylolisthesis, 913, *914*
  superior strait, 292, 293
  thrombophlebitis, 978, 984, 989
  transformation of fetal into adult, 298-99
  tuberculosis, 788
  tumors, 916-17, 924 ff.
    benign ovarian, 928-29
    carcinoma of ovary, 929
    myomas, 924 ff.
    pregnancy complications, 653-54
Penetrance, genetic, 1080
Penetrative mole, 575
Penicillin. *See also* specific disease.
  gonorrhea, 487, 802
  mastitis, 995
  ophthalmia neonatorum, 487
  syphilis, 800
Penicillinase, mastitis and, 995
Penis, circumcision of, 490
Pentothal, 436-37, 453, 508
Pepsin, 261
Peptic ulcer, 807
Peptide, oxytocin, *418*
Periarteritis nodosa, *816-17*
Peridural anesthesia, *454, 455, 456*
Perinatal mortality, 10-11. *See also* Mortality,
      perinatal.
  definition, 2
Perineal body, 30
Perineotomy, 423
Perineum, *29*, 30, 245, 390
  anesthetic nerve block, 439-40
  care, 987
  episiotomy, 423 ff. *See also* Episiotomy.
  fascia, 367-68
  lacerations, 421-23, 425, 932-33
    face presentation, 868
  muscles, 364
  preparation for delivery, 401-2
  puerperal infection, 977, 982, 988-89
Periosteal hemorrhage, 1020

Peritoneal cavity
  foreign body, abortion and, 526, *527*
  pregnancy, 554 ff. *See also* Abdominal preg-
      nancy.
  tubal pregnancy rupture, 539, 542-43
  uterine rupture, 943
Peritoneum
  perforation in dystocia, 933
  puerperium and, 468
Peritonitis
  abortion and, 521, 526
  appendicitis and, 807
  generalized, 980, 990
  prognosis, 991
  puerperal, 978-80, 984-85, 990, 991
Perivitelline fluid, 127, 129
Pharynx, aspiration of, *482*
Phenergan, 433
Phenobarbital, 730
Phenolsulfonphthalein excretion, 263
Phenylketonuria, 1069
Pheochromocytoma, 797
Phlebothrombitosis, puerperal, 1001
Phlegmasia alba dolens, 1002
Phocomelia, 1069
Phosphatase
  leukocyte, 256
  liver, 262
  placental, 149
Phospholipids, 1033
Phosphorus, fetal, 225
Physical examination, 333-34. *See also* specific
      procedures.
Physiology, maternal, 236 ff. *See also* Maternal
      physiology.
Phytonadione, 819, 1052
Pica, 270, 345-46
Pigmentation, 819
  hyperbilirubinemia, 1036, *1040*
Pinard maneuver, *1135*, 1154
Pinocytosis, syncytial, 158
Piper forceps, 1154, *1155, 1156*
Piperocaine, 448, 457
Pitocin, 418. *See also* Oxytocin.
Pituitary gland, 266-67
  ACTH, fetal, 222
  eclampsia and, 720
  estrogen effects on, 78
  follicle-stimulating hormone, 78, 82, 83-84
  gonadotropic hormones, 82 ff., *98*, 222, 283,
      475
  lactation and, 475
  luteinizing hormone, 84, 86, 283, 284
  luteotropic hormones, 84-85
  neurohormonal control of, 85-86
  progesterone and, 82
  puerperium and, 470
  releasing factor, 85-86
  shock and, 419
  somatomammotropin, 222
  thyrotropin, 222
Pituitrin, 419. *See also* Oxytocin.
Placenta, 143 ff., 564 ff.
  abdominal pregnancy, 557-58

Placenta (*cont.*)
  abnormalities, 499, 564 ff.
  abortion, 499, 504
  abruptio, 623 ff. *See also* Abruptio placentae.
  accessory lobes, 586
  accreta, 612-13, 621, 963-64
  aging, 148-49, 154, 591
  amnion, 170-71. *See also* Amnion.
  anesthesia, 434
  angiogenesis, 144
  angioma, 584
  arteriovenous shunt, 259
  barrier, 157, 168, 187, 208
  battledore, 594
  bipartita, 586
  calcification, 594
  carnivore, 190
  chorioallantoic and chorioamnionic, 187
  chorionic villi. *See* Chorion; Villi.
  choriovitelline, 145, 187
  circulation, 159 ff., 207 ff., 242. *See also*
      Circulation, fetal and maternal.
    countercurrent flow, 167-68
    factors regulating, 167
    radiogram, *166*
    volume of blood, 215-16
  circumvallate, 586 ff.
  comparative anatomy, 186 ff.
  cotyledon, 147, 148, 167
  cysts, 584-85
  decidua, 149-51, 154
  definition, 143
  degenerative changes, 592
  development, 143 ff.
  diffusion, 208-10
  dimidiata, 586
  diminution of size of site, *369*
  duplex, 586
  eclampsia, 710-11, 717
  electron micrograph, *156*
  endotheliochorial, 187, 190
  endotoxins, 717
  enzymes, 149, 262
  epitheliochorial, 187, 190
  expression, 416
  expulsion, 371-72
  extrachorial, 587
  fenestrata, 586
  fetal surface, *163*
  fragments, postpartum hemorrhage and, 957,
      962
  Grosser classification, 187, 190
  hemangioma, 584
  hematoma, 590, 592
  hemochorial, 187, 190, 192
  hemodichorial, hemomonochorial, hemotrichorial, and hemotrophic, 190
  hemolytic disease, 1048
  histology, 149, 152-53, 154, 156-58
  histotrophic, 190
  hormones, 173 ff. *See also* specific hormones.
    adrenocorticosteroids, 185-86
    estriol excretion, 181 ff.
    estrogens, 177 ff.
    gonadotropin, 173-75

Placenta (*cont.*)
  hormones (*cont.*)
    localization, 158-59
    maternal crossing, 222
    progesterone, 184-85
    somatomammotropin, 175-77
  hydatidiform mole, 564 ff. *See also* Hydatidiform mole.
  hypertrophy of uterus and site of, 239
  immunology, 168-70
  increta, 963
  infarcts, 590-92, 710, 717
  infections, 211
  inflammation, 593
  intervillous space. *See* Intervillous space.
  involution, 466-67
  localization, 614
  manual removal, 417, 962-63
    multiple pregnancy, 679
    postpartum hemorrhage, 960
    puerperal infection, 976
  marginata, 587
  maternal surface, *162*
  membranacea, 586
  membrane (barrier), 158
  metastatic tumors, 584
  multiple, in single pregnancies, 586
  multiple pregnancy, 661 ff.
  percreta, 963
  polyp, 589-90
  postmaturity, 1058
  preeclampsia, 699
  previa, 589, 609 ff.
    accreta, 612-13, 621
    anesthesia, 458
    degrees of abnormality, 609-10
    diagnosis, 613 ff.
    etiology, 611-13
    frequency, 610-11
    hemorrhage, 609, 613, 618
    localization of placenta, 614
    low-lying, 609, 622
    marginal, 609
    partial, 609-10
    percreta, 964
    prevalence and perinatal loss, 609
    recurrence, 612
    signs and symptoms, 613
    total, 609-10, *616*
    treatment, 618 ff.
      cesarean section, 620-21
      delivery, 622-23
      expectant, 621-22
      prognosis, 623
      vaginal methods, 620
    twins and, 678
  protein, 249
  radiography, 615
  retention, 962-64, 976
  separation, 368 ff., 392, 393, 415-16
    abdominal pregnancy, 557-58
    incomplete abortion, 505
    involution of uterus, 465
    premature, 623 ff. *See also* Abruptio placentae.
    twins, 678

Placenta (*cont.*)
  septa, 147-48, 161
  septuplex, 586
  size, 148, 161, 585-86
  sonography, 615, *616*
  spuriae, 586
  succenturiata, 586
  syncytium, 154 ff.
  syndesmochorial, 187, 190
  syphilis, 585, 1053, 1054
  thrombi, 590
  transfer, 206 ff.
    ascorbic acid, 210
    barbiturates, 437
    chorionic villi, 208
    diffusion, 208-10
    histidine, 210
    intervillous space, 207-8
    iron, 210
    oxygen and carbon dioxide, 209-10
    selective, 210-11
  transfusion, 415
  triplex, 586
  trophoblast, 154 ff.
  tubal pregnancy, 539
  tuberculosis, 594
  tumors, 564 ff.
  ultrastructure, 154, 156-58
  umbilical cord, 171-73. *See also* Umbilical
    cord.
  vasochorial, 187, 190
  water content, 248
  weight, 148, 161, 600
"Placental sign" bleeding, 99
Placentitis, 593
Plasma
  bicarbonate, 252
  estrogens, 177
  fibrinogen, 633-34
  insulin, *250*
  iron-binding capacity, 255
  lipids, 251
  osmotic pressure, 249
  sugar, 789
  urea nitrogen, 756
  volume, 252, 546, 664, 715, 766
Plasminogen, maternal, 256
Platelets, eclampsia and, 719
Platypelloid pelvis, 316
Plural births, 656 ff. *See also* Multiple preg-
    nancy.
Pneumococcus, 975
Pneumonia, 786-87
  aspiration, 786-87
  influenza and, 813
  newborn, 1055
  varicella, 787
Pneumonitis
  aspiration, 434
  sickle-cell disease, 774
Pneumothorax, newborn, 1056-57
Podalic version, internal, 1158 ff.
Podophyllin, 641
Poisoning
  abortion and, 500
  eclampsia and, 722

Polar body, 115, 127, 129
Poliomyelitis, 342, 813
Polyarteritis nodosa, 816-17
Polycystic disease, 759
Polycythemia, 776
Polydactylism, 1076
Polygalactia, 997
Polyhydramnios, 599 ff.
Polymastia, 996
Polyploidy, hydatidiform mole and, 567
Polyps
  bleeding, abortion and, 505, 507
  placental, 589-90
Polyuria, fetal, 228
Polyzygotic births, 657
Pomeroy technic, 1095, *1097*
Pontocaine, 451, 453, 457
Popliteal angle, 1031
Porphyria, 797
Portio vaginalis, 32
Position of fetus, 320 ff., 853 ff. *See also* Pres-
    entation and position; and specific
    presentations.
Postmaturity, 880, 1057-58
Postpartum
  eclampsia, 701
  heart disease, 785
  hemorrhage, 417, 473, 956 ff. *See also* Hem-
    orrhage, postpartum.
  psychiatric problems, 822
  urologic investigations, 754
Poststreptococcal glomerulonephritis, 758
Postural hypotension, 452
Postural relaxation, 355
Posture
  kidney function and, 263
  prematurity and, 1031
Potassium
  fetal, 225
  pica and, 346
Pouch of Douglas, 24, 30
Precipitate labor, 849
Prednisone, 761
Preeclampsia, 689 ff.
  abruptio placentae, 626
  cause and pathologic anatomy, 692
  chronic hypertension, 688, 725-26, 735-36
  classification, 686-87, 688
  clinical course, 690-91
  diagnosis, 692-94
  diet, 697-98
  diuresis, 472-73
  familial tendency, 701
  forceps and, 1123
  glomerulonephritis, 758-59
  headache, 691
  histochemical changes, 149
  hormones and, 720
  hydatidiform mole and, 569, 701
  incidence, 689
  induction of labor, 1094
  kidney and, 714-15, 760
  mortality, 694, 696
  nail bed changes, 711
  physiologic changes, 713
  predisposition, 689-90, 694

Preeclampsia (*cont.*)
  prognosis, 694, 696
  retinal changes, 691-92
  treatment, 694 ff.
    ambulatory, 697
    hospital management, 697-99
    objectives, 696-97
    prophylaxis, 694-96
    termination of pregnancy, 699-700
  twins, 670, 672, 674
  weight gain, 690, 695
Pregnancy
  broad ligament, 544
  combined, 553
  confinement, calculated date of, 236
  diagnosis, 277 ff.
    differential, 286-87
    fetal life or death identification, 288
    first vs. subsequent, 287-88
    positive signs, 277-79
    presumptive evidence, 285-86
    probable evidence, 279 ff.
    spurious, 287
    tests, 283-85
  duration, 236-38, 1057-58
  ectopic, 535 ff. *See also* Abdomen, pregnancy of; Ectopic pregnancy; Tubal pregnancy.
  extramembranous, *653*
  initial reactions to, 820-21
  injuries to fetus, 1007 ff.
  interstitial, 551-52
  mask of, 269
  maternal physiology, 236 ff. *See also* Maternal physiology.
  multiple, 656 ff. *See also* Multiple pregnancy.
  ovarian, 122, 559-61
  precocious or late, 238
  prenatal care, 332 ff. *See also* Prenatal care.
  prolongation, 237, 880, 1057-58
  spurious, 287
  tubal, 535 ff. *See also* Tubal pregnancy.
  tubouterine, tuboabdominal, and tuboovarian, 544-45
  Weight gain. *See* Weight.
Pregnanediol, 78, 79
  ovulation and, 67
  placenta and, 184
  urinary excretion, 184
Pregnanolone, 79
Prematurity, 526 ff., 1026 ff.
  anesthesia, local, 442
  birth weight and mortality, 398
  breech presentation, 860
  cerebral palsy, 1017
  definitions, 1026-28
  diagnosis, 1029-30
  economic factors, 527
  etiology, 1029
  hydramnios, 600, 601
  incidence, 526, 529
  induction of labor, 1094
  jaundice, 488-89
  labor, 526 ff. *See also* Labor, premature.

Prematurity (*cont.*)
  mortality, 398, 442, 621-22, 681, 1028-29, 1033
  nutrition and, 529
  preeclampsia and, 698
  placenta previa, 621
  prognosis, 1033
  respiratory distress syndrome, 1033-35
  retrolental fibroplasia, 1035
  rupture of membranes, 389, 397-98, 530, 863
  small-sized infants, 1030 ff.
  twins, 672, 679
  umbilical cord prolapse, 1012
  uterine anomalies, 649
  viruses and, 812
Prenatal care, 332 ff.
  alcohol, 342
  backache, 340, 344
  bathing, 340
  bowel habits, 340-41
  breast and abdominal care, 341
  chest x-ray, 334
  clothing, 340
  coitus, 341
  common complaints, 343 ff.
  definitions of terms, 332-33
  douches, 341
  employment, 340
  exercise, 340
  fatigue and somnolence, 346
  general hygiene, 340 ff.
  headache, 346
  heartburn, 345
  hemorrhoids, 345
  history, 333
  immunization, 342
  instruction to patients, 335
  laboratory tests, 334
  leukorrhea, 346-47
  medications, 342-43
  minerals, 338-39
  nausea and vomiting, 343-44
  nutrition, 335 ff., 345-46
  physical examination, 333-34
  pica, 345-46
  protein, 338
  ptyalism, 346
  return visits, 334-35
  smoking, 341-42
  teeth, care of, 342
  travel, 340
  varicosities, 344-45
  vitamins, 339
Prepuce, 21
Presentation and position, 320 ff., 374 ff., 853 ff. *See also* specific presentations.
  acromion, 321-22, 872
  auscultation, 330-31
  breech, 855 ff.
  brow, 321, 870-72
  cephalic, 321, 324-26
  contracted pelves, 896-97
  diagnosis, 326 ff.
  face, 321, 324, 863 ff.

Presentation and position (*cont.*)
  foot, 321, 856, 862
  forceps, 1125 ff.
  frequency of various, 322-23
  myoma and, 926
  nomenclature, 321-22
  occiput, 322, 323, 374 ff., 853-55
  palpation, 326 ff.
  placenta previa, 613, 614
  shoulder, 872 ff.
  sonography, 331
  station, 403-4
  transverse, 374 ff. *See also* Shoulder presen-
      tation; Transverse lie.
  twins, 674
  vaginal examination, 329-30
  variety, 321-23
  vertex, 321, 324, 374, ff.
  x-ray, 331
Pressor agents, abortion and, 524
Pressor hormones, eclampsia and, 711
Pressure
  abdominal, eclampsia and, 717
  amniotic fluid, 601, *1011*
  arterial, 258, 259, 703. *See also* Blood pres-
      sure.
  blood. *See* Blood pressure.
  fetal axis, 357
  intraabdominal, 357-58
  intracapillary hydrostatic, 249
  uterine, 352, 356-57, 841
  venous, 258, *259*
    abruptio placentae, 633
    antecubital and femoral, 258
    bacterial endotoxic shock, 522-24
    pulmonary embolism, 1004
Preston-Jones v. *Preston-Jones*, 237
Primigravidas
  analgesia, 431
  definition, 332
  duration of labor, 396, 397
  eclampsia, 721
  elderly, 397
    postmaturity, 1058
    vulvar atresia, 921
  preeclampsia, 689
  placenta previa, 611, 612, 622
  shoulder presentations, 877
Primiparas
  afterpains, 474
  definition, 333
  menstruation return, 475
Primitive groove and streak, 136
Primordial follicles, 51, *54*, 55, 58, 59
Primordial germ cells, 50-51, 108, 116
Procaine, 458, 451
  doses, 448
Profibrinolysin, 256
Progesterone, 78 ff.
  adrenals and, 269
  in blood, 79
  breasts and, 81-82
  carbon dioxide and, 260
  cervical effects, 81
  chemistry, 79

Progesterone (*cont.*)
  cholesterol and, 185
  definition, 79
  diagnosis of pregnancy, 284
  digestion and, 261
  eclampsia and, 720
  effects, 80-82
  endometrial effects, 80
  fallopian tubes, 81
  fat metabolism and, 252
  ferning of cervical mucus, 102
  insulin and, 251
  labor onset, 349-50
  luteinizing hormone and, 84
  mammary growth and, 470
  melanocyte-stimulating hormone and, 269
  menstruation and, 79, 80
  metabolism and, 79
  ovulation and, 67, 81
  pituitary effects, 82
  placental, 184-85
  pregnancy maintenance, 80-81
  sources, 79
  synthetic, 82
  thermogenic effects, 82
  urinary, 79, 184, *185*
  uterine hypertrophy, 239
  uterine motility, 81
Progestin, diagnosis of pregnancy and, 284
Promethazine, 433
Propylthiouracil, 798
Prostaglandins, 1094
Protamine sulfate, 1002
Protein
  eclampsia and, 715-16
  metabolism, 249
  prenatal dietary, 338
  thyroxin-binding, 267, 268
Protein-bound iodine, 267, 268
  abortion and, 411
  thyroid disease and, 798
Proteinuria, 264
  eclampsia, 703
  hypertension, 686, 687, 691
  labor and, 394
Prothrombin time, 256
Prototherian placentation, 187
Protozoal infections, 211, 814-15
Pruritus, 819
Pseudocyesis, 287
Pseudopreeclampsia, 714
Psychiatric and psychologic aspects, 820 ff.
  abortion, 501, 513, 1088
  approach to patient, 400-401
  dystocia complications, 843
  eclampsia, 704
  electroshock therapy, 823
  initial reactions to pregnancy, 820-21
  nausea and vomiting, 344
  pain relief, 459
  postpartum problems, 822
  psychosomatic therapy, 822-23
  second and third trimester complications,
      821-22
  Sydenham's chorea, 820

Ptyalism, 346
Puberty
 estrogens and, 77
 menstruation and, 102
 precocious, 238
Pubiotomy, 1143
Pubis, 292 ff. *See also* Symphysis pubis.
Pudenda
 anatomy, 19 ff.
 episiotomy, 423 ff.
Pudendal nerve, 437
 local infiltration, *441*
 transperineal block, 439-40
 transvaginal block, 440-42
Puerperium, 465 ff., 993 ff.
 afterpains, 471-72, 474
 ambulation, 474
 anatomic changes, 465 ff.
 blood, 473
  volume, 255
 bowels, 475
 breasts and lactation, 468-70, 471, 475,
  993 ff.
 care of patient, 473 ff.
 cervical and vaginal changes, 468
 chills, 471
 clinical aspects, 471-73
 definition, 333
 diet, 474
 discharge from hospital, 475-76
 fever, 971
 follow-up examination, 476
 heart disease, 781
 hematoma, 999-1000
 hemorrhage, 998-1000
 infection, 971 ff.
  antimicrobial drugs, 987-88
  anemia and, 976, 985, 986
  bacteremia, 982
  bacteriology, 973-75
  bacteroides, 974
  cellulitis, 980-81, 983-84, 989
  Clostridium, 974-75, 991
  definition, 971
  diagnosis, 986-87
  diphtheroides, 975
  endometritis, 977-78, 980, 982-83, 989
  erysipelas, 814
  gangrene of uterus, 982
  genitalia, 977, 982, 988-89
  gonococcal, 975, 985
  history, 972-73
  incidence, 972
  metritis dessicans, 982
  modes of, 975-76
  parametritis, 980-81, 983-84, 989
  pathology, 976 ff.
  peritonitis, 978-80, 984-85, 990, 991
  penumococcal, 975
  predisposing causes, 976
  prevention, 986-87
  prognosis, 991
  pyelonephritis, 750
  pyemia, 978

Puerperium (*cont.*)
 infection (*cont.*)
  salpingitis, 985
  staphylococcal, 974
  streptococcal, 813, 814, 973-74, 980, 983
  thrombophlebitis, 978, 984, 989
  treatment, 987 ff.
 insulin requirements, 791
 lochia, 472
 menstruation return, 475
 milk, 469
 morbidity, 971
 nervous system disorders, 1001
 nursing, 470-71
 oxytocin and, 470
 peritoneal and abdominal wall changes, 468
 placental site involution, 466-67
 pulse, 471
 sepsis, 971
 septicemia, 971
 temperature, 471
 thromboembolic disease, 1001 ff.
 urinary tract changes, 468, 472 ff., 1000-1
 uterus, 997-98
  involution, 465-66, 470
  vessels, 467-68
 vulva, 474
 weight loss, 473
Pulmonary disease. *See also* Respiratory system.
 edema, 704, 710, 712
 embolism, 1003-4, 1098, 1108
 function, 260
 resection, 787
Pulse rate, 258
 puerperal, 471
 tubal pregnancy, 547
Punch biopsy of cervix, 642, 644
Pupillary contraction, newborn, 1031
Purpura, thrombocytopenic, 776-77
"Pyelitis of pregnancy," 748
Pyelography, *264, 265*
 bacterial infection, *751, 752, 754*
 genital malformations, 647
Pyelonephritis
 acute, 749-50
 bacteriuria, 753
 chronic, 755, 756
 prognosis, 756
 puerperal, 986
Pyemia, 978
Pyopagus twins, 667, 882

Quadruplets, *665, 672*
 frequency, 657
Quelicin, 457
Quickening, 202
 abortion and, 1085
 diagnosis of pregnancy, 286
Quintuplets, 656, 661

Rachitis pelvis, 913, 918

Racial differences
  anemia, 770, 772, 774
  appearance of newborn, 203
  duration of gestation, 237
  eclampsia, 721
  fetal malformations, 1064-65
  maternal mortality, 4, *5*, *6*, *8*
  multiple pregnancy, 657, 658
  neonatal mortality, *12*
  pelvic contractions, 894
  premature labor, 527
  Rh antibodies, 1038-39
  twin pregnancies, 679-80
Radioactivity, fetal malformations and, 1066
Radiography
  abdominal pregnancy, 556
  accumulated doses, 317
  calcification of placenta, *593*
  cesarean scar rupture, 941, *942*
  chest, prenatal, 334
  diagnosis of pregnancy, 279
  face presentation, 865
  hazards of pelvimetric, 316-17
  hydatidiform mole, 571
  hydrocephalus, 886, *887*
  multiple pregnancy, 670
  pelvimetry, 305 ff., 316-17
  placenta previa, 615
  presentation of fetus, 331, 865, *874*
  pulmonary embolism, 1004
  thoracopagus, *883*
  transverse lie, *874*
  uterine anomalies and dysfunction, 647, 844
Radioiodine
  fetal hazards, 222
  uptake, 267, 798
Radioisotopes, placental localization and, 615
Radiotherapy
  cervical carcinoma, 643
  Hodgkin's disease, 777
Rape, alleged, 24
Rat
  ovarian hyperemia test, 284
  ovulation, *65*
Receptive relaxation, 355
Receptors, uterine, for internal pressure, 356-57
Recessive inheritance, 1080
Rectocele, 641, 930
Rectouterine pouch, 24, 30, 989
Rectovaginal fistula
  episiotomy and, 425
  pelvic contraction and, 900
Rectovaginal septum, 24
Rectum
  anesthesia and, 439
  carcinoma, 808
  examination
    breech presentation, 855
    first stage of labor, 402-3, 404
    puerperal infection, 987
    vertex presentations, 375, 383
  sphincter episiotomy, 425
  stricture, lymphopathia venereum and, 803
Rectus muscles, diastasis of, 468, 652-53

Red blood cells. *See* Erythrocytes.
Regional anesthesia, 437 ff.
Regional enteritis, 808
Relaxin, 82
Releasing factors, 85-86
Renal disease. *See also* Kidney.
  failure, abortion and, 524-26
Renal plasma flow, 263
Renin, 268-69
  eclampsia and, 716
Renografin, 1043
Reproductive tract, 639 ff. *See also* Genito-urinary tract; and specific organs.
  abortion and, 500-501
Reserpine, oval transport and, 120
Reserve cells, cervical, 36
Residual capacity, functional, 260
Respiratory alkalosis, 252
Respiratory distress, newborn, 415, 432, 1033-35
Respiratory system, 260, 786 ff.
  amniotic fluid embolism, 952
  asthma, 787
  eclampsia and, 704, 710, 712
  edema, 704, 710, 712
  embolism, 787, 952, 1003-4, 1098, 1108
  fetal, 211, 214, 218-20
  narcosis, 1015
  pneumonia, 786-87, 813, 1055
  puerperal infection, 986
  pulmonary embolism and, 1003-4, 1098, 1108
  resection, 787
  sarcoidosis, 788
  thromboembolism and pulmary infarction, 787
  tuberculosis, 787-88
Restitution of fetal head, 382, 391
Resuscitation, newborn, 480 ff.
Retina
  eclampsia and, 705, 712
  preeclampsia and, 691-92, 712
  retrolental fibroplasia, 1035
Retinitis gestationis, 824
Retraction rings, 329, *353*, 355, 360, 849-51
Retrolental fibroplasia, 1035
Retroplacental hemorrhage, 417, 627, 628
Rh antibodies, 1037 ff. *See also* Blood factors; Hemolytic disease; Transfusions, blood.
Rho(D), 1039
Rheumatic fever, 817
Rheumatic heart disease, 777, 778
Rheumatoid arthritis, 815-16
Rhythm method, 1102-3
Ribonucleoprotein, placental, 149
Rickets, pelvic contractions and, 894-96, 913, 918
RISA, 616
Ritgen maneuver, 412, *1127*, 1128
Robert pelvis, 913
Rooming-in, 489
Rooting, newborn, 1031
Rotation
  breech extraction, 859, 1148 ff.

Rotation (*cont.*)
 brow presentation, 871
 external, 382, 391, 412, 860
 forceps, 1121, 1130 ff.
 internal, 377-79
  breech presentation, 859
  face presentation, 866, 869
  occipitoposterior position, 853-54
  vertex presentation, 377-79
Round ligaments, 40, 357
Rubella, 808 ff.
 abortion, 1088
 diagnosis, 809
 frequency of malformations, 810-11
 vaccines, 342, 809-10
Rubeola, 812

Sacculation of uterus, 648-49
Sacroiliac synchondrosis, 296
Sacrosciatic notch, 314
Sacrum, 291, 292, 295, 315
 caudal anesthesia and, 446, 448
 posterior position, *323*
Saddle block anesthesia, 451
Saf-T-Coil, 1105
Sagittal sutures and fontanel, 204, 330
Saline. *See also* Sodium.
 abortion and, 951, 1091-92
 antibodies, 1037
Salmonella typhosa, 975
Salpingectomy, 551
Salpingitis
 gonorrheal, 535, 801, 985
 puerperal, 985
 tubal pregnancy and, 536-37, 551
Saluretic drugs, preeclampsia and, 695
Sarcoidosis, 788
Scalp
 blood, fetal, pH and, 1010
 hair, 1030, 1031
 hemolytic disease and, 1045
 pelvic contraction and, 900-1
Scanzoni maneuver, 854-55, 1130 ff.
Scarlet fever, 813-14
Schultze's mechanism, 372
Scissors, Smellie's, 1141, *1142*
Sclerocystic ovary, 67
Scleroderma, 816
Sclerosis, multiple, 820
Scoliosis, 912-13
Scopolamine, 432
Scrubbing, surgical, 410-11
Second stage of labor, 361-62. *See also* Labor, second stage.
Secundines, retention of, 998
Sedation, 432-34
 preeclampsia, 698
 uterine dysfunction, 849
Sensory organs
 anesthesia and, 437 ff.
 fetal, 223
Septicemia
 abdominal pregnancy, 555
 abortion, 521
 prognosis, 991

Sepsis
 abortal, 521
 cesearean section, 1176
Serologic test for syphilis, 334, 800
Serum
 bilirubin, *488*, 1047, 1050
 fatty acids, *251*
 gonadotropin, 573-74
 hepatitis, 803
 iron, *253*
 lipids, *251*
 osmolality, 252
 proteins, eclampsia and, 715-16
Sex chromatin, 124, 1068
 abortion and, 498
 blastocyst, 230
 hydatidiform mole, 567
 masses, 124
 nuclear, 230
 sex ratios and, 229
Sex differences
 abortion, 498-99
 multiple pregnancies, 661
 pelvis, 297
Sex, fetal, 229-30
 prediction of, 230
Sex-linked traits, 1079
Sexual differentiation
 abnormal, 123-25
 estrogens and, 76-77
Sexual intercourse. *See also* Coitus.
 during pregnancy, 341
Sextuplets, 656
Sheehan's syndrome, 470, 959
Shirodkar-Barter operation, *516 ff.*
Shock
 abortion, 505, 521 ff.
 abruptio placentae, 628, 629
 amniotic fluid embolism, 951
 bacterial, 755, 990
  abortion, 521 ff.
  renal necrosis, 760
 pituitary extract and, 419
 therapy, 823
 tubal pregnancy, hypovolemic, 546
 uterine inversion, 965, 966
 uterine rupture, 946
Shoulder
 delivery, breech extraction, 1148
 descent of anterior, *413*
 dystocia, 881-82
 external rotation, 412
 presentation, 872 ff.
  Denman's mechanism, *876*
  diagnosis, 872-74
  Douglas' mechanism, *876*
  etiology, 872
  external cephalic version, 1158, 1161
  incidence, 872
  labor, course of, 874 ff.
  pelvic inlet contraction, 897
  prognosis, 877
  retraction ring of uterus, *850*
  treatment, 877-78
  twins, 674

Show, bloody, 387-88
Sialomucins, 170
Siamese twins, 659, 667
Sickle-cell anemia, 772 ff.
Silver nitrate, 487
Simian line, 1073
Simpson forceps, *1116, 1125,* 1130
Sims' classification of hypertension, 734
Sincipital presentation, 321
Sinus, marginal, rupture, 624
Skeletal system, 269
    estrogen effects, 78
Skene's ducts, 22, *23*
Skin, 269, 817-19
    care of newborn, 487
    dermatomyositis, 816
    herpes gestationis, 817-18
    melanoma, 819
    pigmentation, 819
        diagnosis of pregnancy, 286
    pruritus, 819
Skull
    pelvic contraction and, 900-1
    hematoma, 1020
Sleep, twilight, 433
Smallpox, 813
Smellie's forceps, *1118*
Smellie's scissors, *1142*
Smoking, 341-42
    prematurity and, 529
Snow's method, 312
Soap, 524
Socioeconomic factors
    eclampsia, 721
    ectopic pregnancy, 535
    fetal growth, 204
    oral contraceptives, 1110
    maternal mortality, 5
    perinatal mortality, 12, 1029
    pica, 345-46
    premature labor, 527
Sodium
    antacids, 345
    bicarbonate, pH of infant blood and, 483
    chloride, membrane rupture test, 406
    eclampsia, 714-15
    fetal, 225
    preeclampsia, 695, 697
    retention, 249
    space, puerperium and, 473
Sole creases, 1030, 1031
Solu-Cortef and Solu-Medrol, 524, 786
Somatomammotropin
    chorionic, 175-77, 266, 267
        chemical structure, 176
        fatty acids and, 226
        hydatidiform mole, 575
        insulin and, 251
        mammary growth, 470
        metabolic activity, 176
        placental function, 176
        time of detection, 176
    pituitary, 222, 266
Somites, formation of, 136-37
Somnolence, 346

Sonography
    cephalometry, 903-4
    diagnosis of pregnancy, 279
    fetal malformations, *1077-78*
    hydatidiform mole, 567, 571
    normality of conception products, 508
    ovum, *495*
    placenta previa, 615, *616*
    presentation, 331
    tubal pregnancy, 550
    twins, *659,* 668
Souffles, 278, 555
Spalding's sign, 289
Sparteine sulfate, 846-47
Spermatids, 116, 118
Spermatocytes, 108-9
Spermatogenesis, 116
Spermatogonia, 108, 116
Spermatozoa, 116 ff.
    abortion and, 510-11, 514
    acrosomic granule, 118
    aging, 125
    capicitation, 121-22
    count, 121
    development, *118*
    fertilization, 122
    flagellum, 118
    motility, 121
    transport, 121
Spermicides, 1103
Spermiogenesis, 116-18
Spherocytosis, 776
Spiders, vascular, 269
Spiegelberg criteria, *558, 559*
Spina bifida, 885, 1072
    incidence, 1064, 1065
    risk of, 1081
Spinal anesthesia, 450 ff.
Spinal cord injury, 1020
Spine, kyphosis of, 910 ff.
Spinnbarkeit, 67, 99
Spiral artery, 163, 167, 241-42
Spironolactone, 714
Splanchnopleure, 187
Spleen
    dystocia and, 930
    hemolytic disease and, 1045
    rupture of, 824
Spondylolisthetic pelvis, 913, *914*
Spontaneous abortion, 494 ff., 586
Spontaneous evolution of dead fetus, 875
Spotting, tubal pregnancy and, 545, 546
Spurious pregnancy, 287
Staphylococci
    mastitis, 994-95
    newborn infection, 1056
    puerperal infection, 974
Starch ingestion, 345-46
Starvation
    diabetes and, 794
    fat metabolism and, 251
Station of presenting part, 403-4
Statistics. *See also* Vital statistics.
    definitions, 203

Sterilility, salpingitis and, 985
Sterilization, 1094 ff., 1176, 1180
    abortion and, 1089
    asthma and, 787
    cesarean hysterectomy, 1176
    diabetes and, 796
    efficacy, 1097-98
    epilepsy and, 819
    hazards, 1098-99
    hypertension, 738
    prevalence, 1095
    time of operation, 1095
    types of operation, 1095-96
Sternocleidomastoid muscle, 1023, 1156-57
Steroids. *See also* specific hormones.
    asthma, 787
    bacterial endotoxic shock, 524
    fetal synthesis, 223
    lactation, 993
    oral contraceptives and, 1110
    placental, 185-86
Stereoscopic x-ray pelvimetry, 310-12
Stethoscope, DeLee-Hillis, 394
Stillbirths, 11-12
    anesthesia and, 442
    diabetes and, 792
    eclampsia and, 724
    fetal malformations and, 1063
    hypertension and, 736
    postmaturity and, 1057
    rate, 2, 10-12
Stirrups, leg, *408*, *409*
Stomach
    absorption, labor and, 394
    aspiration of contents, 430-31, 434, 786
    emptying, 261
    reflux of contents, 261, 345
Stools
    epidemic diarrhea, 1055
    newborn, 487-88
Straps for labor, 407
Streptococci
    abortion and, 521
    beta hemolytic, 974, 980, 983
    erysipelas, 814
    faecalis, 974
    kidney infection, 758
    lochia, 472
    puerperal infection, 813, 814, 973-74, 980, 983
    pyogenes, 813
Streptomycin, 756
Striae gravidarum, 246, 286
Subarachnoid block, 250 ff.
Subclavian vein, *523*
Subchorionic infarcts, 590
Subdural hemorrhage, 386
Suboccipitobregmatic diameter, 206
Subpubic arch, 315
Succinic dehydrogenase, 149
Succinylcholine, 436, 457, 458
Suck, newborn, 1031
Suction
    abortion, 508, 509, 1089, 1090-91
    fetal scalp, 1139-40

Sugar level, plasma, 789
Sulfobromophthalein, 262
Sulfonamide, 755
Superfecundation and superfetation, 667
Supernumerary digits, 1076
Supine position
    hypotensive syndrome, 452
    kidney studies, 263
    vascular compression, 259
Suppuration
    mastitis, 994
    pelvic cellulitis, 989
Supravalvar syndrome, 339
Surfactants, 1033-34
Suspensory ligament of ovary, 49
Sutures, fetal head, 204, 206, 330, 375
Suturing, cesarean section, 1174, 1176, *1180*,
        1185
Swallowing, fetal, *219*, *220*, 600
Sydenham's chorea, 820
Sympathectomy, lumbar, 352
Sympathetic nerves, 43
    labor pain and, 437
Symphysiotomy, 1143
Symphysis pubis, 292 ff.
    anatomy, 292 ff.
    extension, 379
    fracture, 917
    kyphosis, 912
    paralysis, 1001
    separation, 824-25
Synapsis in meiosis, 110
Synclitism, 376
Syncope, tubal pregnancy and, 546
Syncytiotrophoblast, 133, 135, 145, 155
    choriocarcinoma, *582*
    first trimester, *157*
    gonadotropin and, 159
    transfer, 208
Syncytium, 133, *144*, 145, 154 ff.
    choriocarcinoma, 579
    degeneration, infarcts and, 590
    differentiated form of trophoblast, 159
    desmosomes, 156
    DNA in, 155
    endoplasmic reticulum, 156, 157
    ergastoplasm, 156
    giant cells, 154
    hormones, 158-59
    knots, 148, 149
    microvilli, 156
    mitochondria, 156, *157*
    organelles, 156
    origin of, 154-55
    pinocytosis, 158
    thymidine and, 155
    ultrastructure, 156-58
Syntocinon, 418
Syphilis, 211, 800-1
    abortion and, 500, 513
    condyloma and, 640
    fetal, 224, 800, 1053
    placenta and, 585
    serologic test, 334, 800
    treatment, 800-1

Systemic vascular resistance, fetal, 214
Systolic pressure, 686, 688. *See also* Blood
    pressure.

Talipes equinovarus, 1075
Taste buds, fetal, 223
Teeth, care of, 342
Telangiectasis, 269
Telegony, 667
Temperature. *See also* Fever.
  abortion and, 520
  eclampsia and, 703
  genital infection and, 982
  newborn, 478, 485
  puerperal, 471, 971
  tubal pregnancy and, 547
  ovulation and, 66
  progesterone and, 82
Temporal sutures and fontanel, 204
Tentorium cerebelli, 1018
Teratogens, 123, 1066
  abortion and, 499
Testosterone, 82, 178
  lactation and, 993
Testes
  fetal, 223
  normal human, *117*
  newborn, 1030
  undescended, 1077
Tetany
  hyperparathyroidism and, 799
  levator ani, 923
Tetrabenazine, 120
Tetracaine, 451, 453, 457
Tetracycline
  gonorrhea, 802
  ophthalmia neonatorum, 487
  puerperal infection, 988
  urinary tract infection, 756
Tetrad, 110
Tetralogy of Fallot, 784
Thalassemia, 771-72
  sickle-cell disease, 775
Thalidomide, 1067, 1069, 1070
Theca
  cells, estrogen secretion and, 74
  folliculi, 60-61, 69
  lutein cells, 60, 70, 72
  lutein cysts, 568
Thiazide diuretics, 695
Thiopental sodium, 436-37, 453, 508
Third stage of labor, 368 ff. *See also* Labor,
    third stage.
Thoms' method, 309, *312*
Thoracic cage, expansion of, 260
Thoracopagus, 882, *883, 884*
Thorazine, 732
Thorotrast, 218, 219, 220
Threatened abortion, 504 ff.
Thrombocytopenia, 776-77
  anemia and, 770, 767

Thromboembolism
  fibrinolysis and, 256
  oral contraceptives and, 1108-9
  puerperal, 1001 ff.
Thrombophlebitis, 978, 984, 989
  endometritis and, 983
  oral contraceptives and, 1108
  pelvic, 981
  puerperal, 1001 ff.
Thromboplastin
  abruptio placentae and, 630
  eclampsia and, 719
  time, partial, 256
Thrombosis
  cerebral, eclampsia and, 708
  coronary, 784-85
  fibrinolysis and, 256
  hemorrhoidal, 345
  placental, 466, 590
Thymidine, 155
Thyroid, 267-68, 797 ff.
  abortion and, 511, 514
  basal metabolic rate and, 267
  disease, 797 ff.
  eclampsia and, 719
  estrogen and, 268
  fetal, 222
  releasing factor, 86
  -stimulating hormone, 173, 222, 267
Thyroidectomy, 798
Thyrotropin, 173, 222, 267
Thyroxin
  -binding proteins, 267, 268
  circulation, 267
  estrogen and, 267
  thyroid disease and, 798
Tidal volume, 260
Tocopherol, 512
Tokodynamometer, 355-56
Tolbutamide
  diabetes and, 794
  hypoglycemic effect, 251
  response test, 790
Torticollis, 1023
Toxemia. *See also* Eclampsia; Hypertension;
    Preeclampsia.
  definition, 685
  maternal mortality, 7
  recurrent, 688
Toxoplasma, abortion and, 500
Toxoplasmosis, 814
Trachea
  fluid, 220, 228
  intubation, 434, 436, 482-83
Traction
  breech presentation, 1146 ff.
  forceps, 1121
Tranquilizers, 433
Transcortin, 268
Transferrin, 255
Transfusions, blood
  abdominal pregnancy, 556-57
  abruptio placentae, 633
  anemia, 766, 772-73, 774

Transfusions, blood (*cont.*)
hemolytic disease, 1044, 1049, 1050
hydatidiform mole, 572
intrauterine, 216, 1042-43
placental, 415
tubal pregnancy, 551
uterine rupture, 948
Transperineal pudendal block, 439-40
Transplanted choriocarcinoma, 580
Transplantation antigens, 169, 170
Transvaginal pudendal block, 440-42
Transverse diameter of pelvis, 304
Transverse incision, 1172
Transverse lie, 320, 374 ff.
arrest, 383
contracted pelves, 897
forceps, 1129-30
internal podalic version, 1159
neglected, 875
shoulder presentation, 872. *See also* Shoulder presentation.
version, 1157 ff.
Trauma
abortion and, 501
abruptio placentae and, 625
rupture of uterus, 943 ff.
Travel, 340
Treponema, 211, 640, 800
Trichlorethylene, 436
Trichomonas vaginalis, 346-47
Triiodothyronine, 267, 268, 798
Trilene, 436
Trimesters, 199
Triple X syndrome, 1068
Triplets, 661, 662, 663, *665,* 676
frequency, 657
velamentous insertion of cord, 595
Triploidy, hydatidiform mole and, 567
Trisomies, 125, 1067, 1068, 1073
abortion and, 498
prematurity and, 1032
Trophoblast, 128, 132-34, *144,* 154 ff.
abdominal pregnancy, 561
blood, from broad ligament, *169*
cellular, 144, 148
cervical pregnancy, 561
choriocarcinoma and, 143, 578-79
eclampsia and coagulation, 719
enzymes, 149
fibrinoid degeneration, 591
giant cells, 153
hydatidiform mole, *566,* 567 ff.
invasive, 575 ff.
origin of, 154-55
ultrastructure, 156-58
Trophotropism, 663
Trunkless monster, 885
Tubal pregnancy, 535 ff.
abdominal pregnancy and, 554
abortion, 541-42, 548
amenorrhea, 546
anemia, 547
culdocentesis, 549
Cullen's sign, 547

Tubal pregnancy (*cont.*)
decidua, 539, 541
diagnosis, 545 ff.
endosalpingitis and, 536-37
etiology, 535 ff.
fetal sac structure, 540
hemorrhage, 541, 546
implantation of ovum, 538-39
incidence, 535
interstitial, 551-52
laparoscopy and laparotomy, 549-50
leukocyte count, 547
pain, 545-46, 548-49
pelvic mass, 546
placenta, 539
prognosis, 550-51
rupture
into broad ligament, 543-44
chronic, 547-48
clinical picture, 545
intraperitoneal, 539, 542-43
signs and symptoms, 545 ff.
sterilization and, 1098
subsequent pregnancies, 550-51
syncope and hypovolemic shock, 546
temperature, 547
termination of, 541 ff.
treatment, 551
uterine changes, 540-41, 546
vaginal signs, 546
Tuberculosis, 787-88
pelvic, 788
placental, 594
renal, 757
Tuboabdominal pregnancy, 544-45
Tubocurarine, 457
Tuboovarian pregnancy, 545
Tubouterine pregnancy, 544
Tubules, renal
eclampsia and, 708, 714-15
glucose reabsorption, 264
Tumors
dermatomyositis, 816
differential diagnosis of pregnancy, 286
liver, fetal enlargement and, 890-91
ovarian, 928-29
pelvic, 653-54, 916-17, 924 ff.
placental, 564 ff.
umbilical cord, 598
urinary bladder, 930
vaginal, 641, 923
Tuohy needle, 453, 455
Turner's syndrome, 124, 1068
Twilight sleep, 433
Twins, 657 ff.
ascertaining zygosity, 663
cesarean section, 677
collision, 677
conjoined, 667-68
craniopagus, 668
diagnosis, 668-70
differential size, 1032-33
dizygotic, 657, 658, 662, 664
eclampsia, 701

Twins (*cont.*)
etiology, 657 ff.
fertility of, 668
fraternal, 657, 658, 662, 664
frequency, 657
heart, 664
hemorrhage, 678-79
heredity, 658
hydramnios, 599-600
identical, 657, 658, 660, 662, 664
internal podalic version, 1159
kidney transplantation, 761
locking, 677, *678*
malformations, congenital, 680-81
monoamniotic, 597, 662
monozygotic, 600, 657, 658, 660, 662, 664
monsters, 882 ff.
mortality, 681-82
omphalopagus, 667
postpartum hemorrhage, 957
pyopagus, 667
Siamese, 659, 667
single-ovum, 600, 657, 658, 660, 662, 664
size and weight, 666
spontaneous delivery, 676
tubal pregnancy, 553
velamentous insertion of cord, 595
Typhoid fever, 814

Ulcer, peptic, 807
Ulcerative colitis, 808
Ultradop, 394
Ultrasonography. *See* Sonography.
Umbilical arteries, 172
single artery, 598-99, 1065, 1067
Umbilical cord, 171-73, 211, 485-86
abnormalities, 594 ff.
clamping, Rh isoimmunization and, 1049
coils around neck, 413
compression, hypoxia and, 210
cysts, 598
desiccation, *486*
development, 171-72
diameter and length, 173, 595-96
edema, 598
hematoma, 598
hemoglobin, 1049
infections, 486, 597
insertion variations, 594-95
knots, 596
ligaments, 215
loops, 596-97
newborn, 485-86
prolapse, 1012 ff.
breech presentation, 861, 862
compound presentation, 879
diagnosis, 1013-14
etiology, 1012
incidence, 1012
internal podalic version, 1159
multiple cord, 679
occult, 1012
pelvic contraction, 900
premature rupture of membranes, 398
prognosis, 1014-15

Umbilical cord (*cont.*)
prolapse (*cont.*)
treatment, 1014
separation, 486
souffle, 278
structure and function, 173
torsion, 597
tumors, 598
twin, 662, 668, 676
tying of, 414-15
varices, 597
velamentous insertion, 594-95, *611*, 679
Umbilical hernia, 595, 652, 1076
Umbilical vein, 172, 211
oxygen, 209, 210
transfusion, hemolytic disease and, 1050
United States
birth certificate, *15*
intrauterine devices, number of, 1104
maternal mortality, 9-10
neonatal mortality, 13
perinatal mortality, 10
Urea, 263, 737
Ureter, 264-66
calculi, 757
cesarean section and, 1183
dilatation, 264, 265
Urethra
anatomy, 22, *23*
atresia, 228
catheterization, bacterial infection and, 750
Urinary system, 262 ff., 748 ff., 757 ff. *See also* Genitourinary system.
anomalies, 647
antimicrobials, 755-56
bacteriuria, 750 ff.
bladder, 266. *See also* Bladder, urinary.
calculi, 757
cystitis, 749, 1000
dead space, 263
diagnosis of pregnancy, 286
eclampsia and, 717
embryologic development, 50 ff.
failure, postpartum, 760-61
fetal, 218
glomerulonephritis, 708, 734, 757-59
infections, 468, 748 ff., 800 ff.
kidney, 263-64. *See also* Kidney.
necrosis, 760
nephrectomy, pregnancy after, 759-60
nephrosis, 759
polycystic disease, 759
puerperium, 468, 1000-1
pyelonephritis, 749 ff., 986
temperature and, 471
transplantation of kidney, pregnancy after, 761
tuberculosis, 757
ureters, 264-65
venereal diseases, 800 ff.
Urination
diminished, 633, 635, 687, 698, 760
eclampsia, 722-23
frequent, diagnosis of pregnancy and, 286
oxytocin and, 418
polyuria, fetal, 228

Urination (*cont.*)
  puerperal, 474-75
Urine, 334
  abruptio placentae, 633
  bacteria, 750 ff., 775
    prematurity and, 529-30, 751
  blood
    renal necrosis, 760
    urinary tract infection, 749, 757, 758
    uterine rupture, 946
  concentration tests, 263
  diabetes, 789, 795-96
  dye excretion tests, 263
  estriol, 181 ff., 795-96
  estrogens, 76, 181 ff., 795-96
  fetal, 218
  formiminoglutamic acid, 769
  glucose, 251, 264, 789, 794
  gonadotropin, 174
  incontinence, 1001
  newborn, 488
  progesterone, 79, 184, *185*
  protein, 264
    eclampsia, 703
    labor and, 394
    preeclampsia, 686, 687, 691
  puerperal, 472-73
  retention, fetal, 890, *891*
  sodium, 714
Urogenital diaphragm, 367
Uterine arteries
  abruptio placentae and, 626
  cesarean section and, 1182, 1184
  uterine rupture and, 947
Uterine veins, 41-43
Uteroabdominal pregnancy, 943
Uteroplacental apoplexy, 630-31, 635
Uteroplacental arteries, 163, 167
Uterorenal reflex, 717
Uterosacral block, 442 ff.
Uterosacral ligaments, 40
Uterovaginal fascia, 28
Uterus, 238 ff.
  abortion and suboptimal environment of,
    499
  accidental injury, 949-50
  anatomy, 30 ff.
    defects, abortion and, 512, 516, 518
  anomalies, 645 ff.
  anteflexion, 649-50, 924
  atony
    postpartum hemorrhage and, 957, 958,
      962
    puerperal, 473
  Bandl's ring, 355, 850
  bicornuate, 646, *647*, 661
  blood supply, 37, 40 ff., 208, 242, 467-68,
    718
  breech presentation cause and, 325
  cervix, 31 ff. *See also* Cervix.
  compression
    bimanual, postpartum hemorrhage and,
      960, *961*
    of blood vessels, 259
  connective tissue, 32, 36-37, 39
  contractions, 241, 351 ff.

Uterus (*cont.*)
  contractions (*cont.*)
    Braxton Hicks, 241, 281, 359
    caudal analgesia, 449
    dysfunction, 836 ff.
    involuntary nature, 352
    pacemakers, 352
    pelvic inlet and, 896
    podalic version and, 1161
    pressure, 352, 841
    tokodynamometer, 355-56
  cornua, 31
  corpus, 31, 36-38
  Couvelaire, 630-31
    at cesarean section, *628*
  culture, puerperium and, 986
  curettage, 1089 ff. *See also* Curettage.
  cystic degeneration, 565
  development, embryologic, 45
  didelphys, *648*
  differential growth, 239
  displacement, 649 ff., 924
  double, 512, 516, 518, 646
  dysfunction (inertia), 836 ff.
    active phase, 836
    breech presentation, 863
    complications, 842-43
    deceleration phase, *838*
    etiology, 842
    forceps and, 1122
    latent phase, *838*
    oxytocin and, 845 ff.
    treatment, 843 ff.
    types of, 841-42
  endometrium, 36-37. *See also* Endometrium.
  enlargement, hydramnios and, 601
  ergot effects, 420
  estrogen effects, 77
  external os, 32
  first stage of labor changes, 358 ff.
  fundus, 31
  gangrene, 982
  glands, 36
  hemorrhage, 613, 957 ff.
  hydatidiform mole, 565 ff. *See also* Hydatidiform mole.
  hypertonic, 842, 848-49
  hypertrophy in pregnancy, 239
  hypotonic, 421, 841 ff.
  hysterectomy, 1176 ff. *See also* Hysterectomy.
  incarceration, 650
  incomplete fusion, 512
  inertia, 836 ff.
  infections, 211, 569
    puerperal, 971 ff. *See also* Puerperium, infection.
  instrumental perforation, 949
  intrauterine devices, 1103 ff.
  inversion, 416, 965 ff.
  involution, 465-66, 470, 997
  ischemia, eclampsia and, 718-19
  ligaments, 38-40
  lower segment
    cesarean section technic, 1169 ff.
    in contraction, 352-54, 355, 361

Uterus (*cont.*)
  lower segment (*cont.*)
    palpation in labor, 329
    relaxation, 355
    separation of placenta, 371
  lymphatics, 43
  motor pathways, 437
  multiple pregnancy, 676
  musculature, 37-38, 238-40, 355. *See also*
    Myometrium.
  myomas, 924 ff.
    abortion and, 501, 512
  myometrium, 37-38, 238-40, 355. *See also*
    Myometrium.
  myxomatous degeneration, 565
  nerve supply, 43-45, 239, 437
  oxygen consumption, 242
  oxytocin sensitivity, 350
  pacemakers, 352
  packing, 960
  parametrium, 39. *See also* Parametrium.
  perforation
    abortion and, 526, 527, 528, 1089, 1092
    choriocarcinoma and, 582
    instrumental, 949
    intrauterine contraceptive devices and,
      1103 ff.
  placenta and. *See also* Placenta.
    in situ, *160*
    retention, 392
  plastic repair, 648
  position, 40
  progesterone and motility of, 81
  prolapse, 651-52, 924, 998
    of completely inverted, 965, *966, 967*
  pudendal nerve, 437
  puerperal pain (afterpains), 471-72
  receptor measurement of pressures, 356-57
  removal, 1176 ff. *See also* Hysterectomy.
  retraction rings, 329, 353, *353*, 355, 360,
    849-51
  retrodisplacement (retroversion), 650, 924
  rigidity and tenderness, 627-28
  rotation, 241
  rudimentary horns, 648
  rupture, 936 ff.
    cesarean scar, 937 ff.
    classification, 937
    complete vs. incomplete, 944-46
    hydrocephalus and, 888
    incidence, 936
    lower segment, *847, 848,* 937-39, 944
    mortality, 939, 942, 946
    oxytocin and, *847, 848*
    pelvic inlet contraction, 900
    prolonged labor, 362
    shoulder presentation, 878
    spontaneous, of intact, 942-43
    traumatic, 943 ff.
  sacculation, 648-49, 924
  second stage of labor changes, 361-62
  septate, 646
  shape changes, 31, 240-41, 281, 357, 392,
    393
  size, 31, 238, 240-41, 281
  souffle, 278

Uterus (*cont.*)
  stretch theory, 351
  subinvolution, 997-98
  torsion, 652
  tubal pregnancy changes, 540-41, 546
  upper segment in contraction, 355
  vaginal outlet relaxation and, 998
  weight, 238

Vaccination, 342, 809-10
  poliomyelitis, 813
  rubella, 342, 809-10
  smallpox, 813
Vacuum extractor, 1139-40
  incidence, 1120
  midpelvic contraction, 908
Vagina, 23 ff., 639 ff.
  anatomy, 23 ff.
  annular strictures, 922
  atresia, 921
  bleeding. *See* Vagina, hemorrhage.
  cervical relation, 32
  Chadwick's sign, 245
  classification of anomalies, 646
  cyclic changes of epithelium, 102
  cysts, 28, 641
  discharge, prenatal, 346
  diseases, 639 ff.
  double, 646
  embryologic origin, 25
  epithelium, 102, 245
  estrogen effects, 77
  examination
    breech presentation, 855
    brow presentation, 870
    face presentation, 864-65
    first stage of labor, 402 ff.
    gonorrhea, 803
    occipitoposterior position, 375, 383
    placenta previa, 618-20
    presentation, 329-30
    puerperal infection, 987
    safety, 405
    shoulder presentation, 872
    twin diagnosis, 668
    umbilical cord prolapse, 1014
    uterine dysfunction, 843
  exfoliated cells, 124
  fascia, 28, 367
  fistulas, 425, 900, 950, 1001
  fornices, 26
  hemorrhage
    abortion and, 504, 506-7
    abruptio placentae, 627
    diagnosis of pregnancy, 285
    hydatidiform mole, 574
    placenta previa, 613, 614, 618-20
    postpartum, 957, 958-59
    tubal pregnancy and, 545, 546
  hydrorrhea gravidarum, 653
  hysterectomy and, 1185, *1187*
  infection, 346-47, 640, 977, 982, 988-89
  injuries, 932-33
  jellies and creams, 1103
  in labor, changes in, 362 ff.

Vagina (cont.)
  lacerations, 421-23, 425
    postpartum hemorrhage and, 957, 958-59
  lochia, 472
  longitudinal septum, 921
  menopause, 24, 27
  menstrual cycle smears, 103
  mucosal discoloration, 286
  muscles, 28
  myrtiform caruncles, 24
  packing, 619
  Papanicolaou smears, 642
  pH, 28, 245, 405
  placenta previa and, 619, 620
  prolapse of uterus, 651
  pudendal nerve block, 440-42
  puerperium, 468
    infections, 977, 982, 988-89
  rectouterine pouch, 24, 30, 989
  relaxation of outlet, 641, 998
  rugae, 27
  rupture, 932-33
  secretions, 28, 245, 405
  septa, 24, 922
  septate, 646, 648
  tenderness, tubal pregnancy and, 546
  transverse septum, 922
  tumors, 641, 923
  vascularity, 28, 245
Valium, 433
Valvotomy, mitral, 783
Varicella pneumonia, 787
Varices (varicosities), 344-45
  umbilical cord, 597
  vulvar, 639
Vasa previa, 595, 679
Vascular disorders. See also Arteries; Veins.
  spiders, 269
Vasodilation, abortion and, 524
Vasopressin, eclampsia and, 692, 711-12
Veins
  antecubital, 258
  arcuate, 43
  compression in supine position, 259
  femoral, 258
  ovarian, 43, 245, 627, 978, 1003
  pampiniform plexus, 43
  puerperal infection extension, 978
  thromboembolic disease, 1002
  umbilical, 172
    oxygen, 209, 210
    transfusion, hemolytic disease and, 1050
  uterine, 41-43
  varicose, 344-45
Velamentous insertion of cord, 594-95, 611,
    679
Vena cava
  abruptio placentae and, 627
  ligation, puerperal thromboembolism and,
    1003
  postural hypotension, 452
Venereal diseases, 800 ff. See also specific dis-
    eases.
  chanchroid, 803
  gonorrhea, 801-3
  granuloma inguinale, 803

Venereal diseases (cont.)
  lymphopathia venereum, 803
  syphilis, 800-1
Venesection, eclampsia and, 732
Venous pressure, 258, 259
  abruptio placentae, 633
  antecubital and femoral, 258
  bacterial endotoxic shock, 522-24
  pulmonary embolism, 1004
Veratrum, 351, 730-31
Vernix caseosa, 487
Version
  breech presentation, 861-62, 1157 ff.
    external, 861-62, 1158
    internal, 957, 1158 ff.
  face presentation, 869-70
  shoulder presentation, 877
  postpartum hemorrhage, 957
Vertebrae
  fractures, 1020, 1022
  kyphosis, 910 ff.
Vertex presentation, 374 ff. See also Occiput.
  attitude, 320
  breech vs., 1158
  cardinal movements of labor, 375 ff.
  descent, 377
  diagnosis, 374, 382, 383
  engagement, 375-77
  extension, 379 ff.
  expulsion, 382
  external rotation, 382, 1158
  flexion, 377
  head shape, 384-86
  hydrocephalus and, 887
  internal rotation, 377-79
  occipitoanterior, 380, 382
  occipitoposterior, 382-84
  occipitotransverse, 374 ff.
  pelvic inlet contraction, 897
  twins, 674
  vaginal examination, 329-30
Vesicocervical fistula, 900, 950
Vesicovaginal fistula, 900, 950, 1001
Vesicovaginal septum, 24
Vestibular bulbs, 22-23
Vestibule, 22
Villus (villi)
  abortion and, 496, 502
  anchoring, 147
  avascular, 592
  choriocarcinoma and, 575 ff.
  degenerative changes in vessels, 592
  development, 135, 144, 145
  eclampsia and, 711
  hydatidiform mole, 564 ff.
  hypertrophic lesions, 592
  infarcts, 590
  ischemic necrosis, 590
  oviduct wall, 538
  surface area, 208
  transfer, 208
Viral infections, 808 ff.
  cold, 813
  Coxsackie, 812
  cytomegalovirus, 811-12
  hepatitis, 634, 803-4

Viral infections (*cont.*)
　herpes, 812, 1056
　influenza, 342, 812-13
　mumps, 812
　placental, 211
　poliomyelitis, 813
　rubella, 342, 808 ff., 1088
　rubeola, 812
　smallpox, 813
Vision, 266
　eclampsia and, 705
　gonorrhea and, 486-87
　preeclampsia and, 691-92
Vistaril, 433
Vital statistics, 2 ff.
　birth rate, 2, 3-4
　　live, *3*
　　　by color, *8*
　　　projection, 4
　definitions, 2
　fertility rate, 2, 3-4
　fetal death, 2
　　rate, 2
　infant mortality, 2, *10*
　marriage rate, 2
　maternal death rate, 3, 4 ff.
　neonatal death rate, 2, 10
　　malformations and, 1064
　perinatal death rate, 2, 10-11
　precocious and late pregnancy, 238
　stillbirth, 2, 10-11
Vitamins
　B$_{12}$, anemia and, 769
　D, 339, 799
　deficiencies, abortion and, 512
　E, abortion and, 512
　K
　　epilepsy and, 819
　　hemorrhagic disease of newborn and,
　　　1052
　　prophylactic, for fetus, 217
　　thromboembolism and, 1003
　prenatal dietary, 339
Vitelline duct, 172
Volatile anesthetics, 435-36
Volvulus, 807-8
Vomiting, 343-44
　anesthesia and, 430-31, 434
　diagnosis of pregnancy, 286
　hydatidiform mole and, 569
　pernicious, 806
　treatment, 344
Voorhees bag, 620
Vulva, 19 ff., 639 ff.
　anatomy, 19 ff.
　atresia, 921
　discoloration, 286
　diseases, 639 ff.
　distention, face presentation and, *868*
　hematoma, 999-1000
　hemorrhage, 639
　injuries, 932-33
　preparation for delivery, 401-2

Vulva (*cont.*)
　puerperal care, 474
　　infection, 977, 982, 988-89
　varicosities, 345

Walcher position, 297
Water, 248-49
　eclampsia, 714
　fetal, 225
　hydramnios, 600
　intoxication, oxytocin and, 418
　metabolism, 248-49
　retention, 248-49
Weight
　abortion and, 514
　birth, 203-4
　　bacteriuria and, 753
　　cesarean section and, 863, 1168-69
　　diabetes and, 791, 792
　　mortality, fetal and, 336, 398
　　prematurity and, 1026 ff.
　　smoking and, 342, 529
　fetal, 202-4, 225, 226
　gain
　　metabolism and, 248
　　newborn, *1027*
　　preeclampsia and, 690, 695
　　prematurity and, 529
　　prenatal, 336
　initial newborn loss, 489
　menstrual cycle and, 106
　obesity. *See also* Obesity.
　puerperal loss, 473
　uterine, 238
Wharton's jelly, 173
White blood cells, 255-56, 547, 767
Willett's forceps, 620
Withdrawal bleeding, 284

X-linked inheritance, 1080
X-ray. *See* Radiography.
Xylocaine, 442, 451

Yellen clamp, 490
Yellow atrophy of liver, 804-5
Yolk sac, 145
　comparative anatomy, 187
　electron microscopic studies, 172
　formation of, 135
YY syndrome, 1068

Zinc, fetal, 225
Zona basalis, 91, 151, 152-53
Zona compacta, 151, 152
Zona functionalis, 92, 151
Zona pellucida, 59, 64, 115
　fertilization and, 123, 129
　preimplantation stages, *127*
Zona spongiosa, 92, 151, 152
Zygote, 125
　twins and, 663
Zygotene stage, 109